WITHDRAWN
WRIGHT STATE UNIVERSITY LIBRARIES

SUDDEN CARDIAC DEATH: PREVALENCE, MECHANISMS, AND APPROACHES TO DIAGNOSIS AND MANAGEMENT

SUDDEN CARDIAC DEATH: PREVALENCE, MECHANISMS, AND APPROACHES TO DIAGNOSIS AND MANAGEMENT

Masood Akhtar, M.D.
*Professor of Medicine
University of Wisconsin Medical School
Milwaukee Clinical Campus
Director for Arrhythmia Services
Sinai Samaritan Medical Center
Staff Electrophysiologist
St. Luke's Medical Center
Milwaukee, Wisconsin*

Robert J. Myerburg, M.D.
*Professor of Medicine and Physiology
Director, Division of Cardiology
University of Miami School of Medicine
Miami, Florida*

Jeremy N. Ruskin, M.D.
*Associate Professor of Medicine
Harvard Medical School
Director, Cardiac Arrhythmia Service
Massachusetts General Hospital
Boston, Massachusetts*

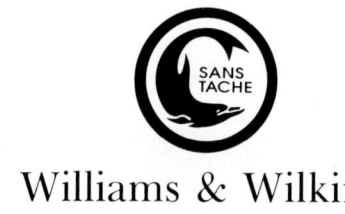

Williams & Wilkins
PHILADELPHIA • BALTIMORE • HONG KONG
LONDON • MUNICH • SYDNEY • TOKYO
A WAVERLY COMPANY
1994

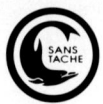

Executive Editor: R. Kenneth Bussy
Development Editor: Tanya L. Lazar
Production Coordinator: Peter J. Carley
Project Editor: Jessica Howie Martin

Copyright © 1994
Williams & Wilkins
200 Chester Field Parkway
Malvern, PA 19355 USA

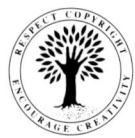

All rights reserved. This book is protected by copyright. No part of it may be reproduced in any form or by any means, including photocopying, or utilized by any information storage and retrieval system without written permission from the copyright owner.

Accurate indications, adverse reactions, and dosage schedules for drugs are provided in this book, but it is possible they may change. The reader is urged to review the package information data of the manufacturers of the medications mentioned.

Printed in the United States of America

94 95 96 97 98
1 2 3 4 5 6 7 8 9 10

Dedication

SUDDEN CARDIAC DEATH is dedicated to our patients and their families, and to:

Rashi, wife of Masood Akhtar, MD and his sons, Ayad and Shazad;

Wilhelmina, wife of Robert J. Myerburg, MD, his son, Michael and daughter, Laura;

and

Barbara, wife of Jeremy N. Ruskin, MD, and his sons, Jesse and Matthew.

Preface

Sudden cardiac death remains a problem of enormous dimensions, accounting for more than 300,000 deaths per year among adults in the United States. This figure represents approximately 50% of all cardiac deaths and 25% of *all* natural deaths. It is not a specific *cause* of death, but rather a specific *mechanism* of death, crossing all categories of cardiac disease, as well as resulting from cardiac manifestations of non-cardiac disorders. This fact has led to the evolution of a heterogeneous body of information on the topic, taken from the perspectives of different disciplines in medicine. Accordingly, access to this information is hampered by a diversity of sources. The purpose of this text is to bring together relevant information, derived from the key sources of data, about this multi-disciplinary problem.

In designing the content of this text, we began by identifying the disciplines that have large bodies of information, and then developed a format that would provide the reader with a natural evolution of concepts and thought processes relative to the problem. We were fortunate in being able to attract a large number of individuals who have made prominent contributions to their fields to participate in the preparations of this text.

The problem of sudden cardiac death is viewed from multiple perspectives. We begin with discussions of the epidemiology and pathology of the syndrome and then develop information on the pathophysiology of sudden cardiac death. To achieve this, both experimental and clinical discussions are included. Subsequently, specific causes and anatomic associations are described, followed by functional disorders and the mechanisms of potentially fatal arrhythmias. Both acute interventions and long-term therapy are discussed in considerable detail, highlighting the latest information available on advanced interventions, such as implantable defibrillators, arrhythmia, and surgical and ablative techniques.

A multidisciplinary approach is necessary to achieve a major impact on the problem of sudden cardiac death. Our hope is that this text may serve as a useful focal point of information covering the multiple factors. It is intended for both practicing clinicians and researchers.

Milwaukee, Wisconsin	Masood Akhtar, M.D.
Miami, Florida	Robert J. Myerburg, M.D.
Boston, Massachusetts	Jeremy N. Ruskin, M.D.

Contributors

Masood Akhtar, M.D.
Professor of Medicine
University of Wisconsin Medical School
Milwaukee Clinical Campus
Director for Arrhythmia Services
Sinai Samaritan Medical Center
Staff Electrophysiologist
St. Luke's Medical Center
Milwaukee, Wisconsin

Kelley P. Anderson, M.D.
Associate Professor of Medicine
Director, Cardiac Electrophysiology
  Laboratory
Cardiology Division
University of Utah Medical Center
Salt Lake City, Utah

Philippe Aouate, M.D.
Service de Rythmologie et de Stimulation
  Cardiaque
Hôpital Jean Rostand
Ivry, France

Kathi Axtell, R.N.
Electrophysiology Laboratory
University of Wisconsin Medical School
Milwaukee Clinical Campus
Sinai Samaritan Medical Center
Milwaukee, Wisconsin

David G. Benditt, M.D.
Professor of Medicine
Section of Cardiology
University of Minnesota Medical School
Twin Cities Campus
Minneapolis, Minnesota

Saroja Bharati, M.D.
Professor of Pathology
Rush-Presbyterian St. Lukes Medical Center
Rush Medical College
Chicago, Illinois;
Director, Congenital Heart and Conduction
  System Center
Heart Institute for Children
Christ Hospital and Medical Center
Oak Lawn, Illinois

J. Thomas Bigger Jr., M.D.
Division of Cardiology
Department of Medicine
Columbia University
New York, New York

Susan M. Blanchard, Ph.D.
Basic Arrhythmia Laboratory
Duke University Medical Center
Durham, North Carolina

Zalmen Blanck, M.D.
Assistant Professor
Electrophysiology Laboratory
University of Wisconsin Medical School
Milwaukee Clinical Campus
Sinai Samaritan Medical Center
Staff Electrophysiologist
St. Luke's Medical Center
Milwaukee, Wisconsin

Alfred E. Buxton, M.D.
Director, Clinical Electrophysiology
  Laboratory
Cardiovascular Section
Department of Medicine
Hospital of the University of Pennsylvania
Philadelphia, Pennsylvania

Agustin Castellanos, M.D.
Division of Cardiology
Department of Medicine
University of Miami School of Medicine
Miami, Florida

Peter B. Corr, Ph.D.
Professor of Medicine (Cardiology) and
  Molecular Biology and Pharmacology
Cardiovascular Division
Department of Internal Medicine
Washington University School of Medicine
St. Louis, Missouri

Michael J. Davies, M.D.
British Heart Foundation Professor of
  Cardiovascular Pathology
Department of Cardiological Sciences
St. George's Hospital Medical School
University of London
London, United Kingdom

Contributors

Susan W. Denfield, M.D.
The Lillie Frank Abercrombie Section of
  Cardiology
Department of Pediatrics
Baylor College of Medicine and Texas
  Children's Hospital
Houston, Texas

Sanjay S. Deshpande, M.D.
Assistant Professor
Electrophysiology Laboratory
University of Wisconsin Medical School
Milwaukee Clinical Campus
Sinai Samaritan Medical Center
Staff Electrophysiologist
St. Luke's Medical Center
Milwaukee, Wisconsin

Anwer A. Dhala, M.D.
Assistant Professor
Electrophysiology Laboratory
University of Wisconsin Medical School
Milwaukee Clinical Campus
Sinai Samaritan Medical Center
Staff Electrophysiologist
St. Luke's Medical Center
Milwaukee, Wisconsin

Linda W. Dickerson, Ph.D.
Department of Pharmacology
Georgetown University School of Medicine
Washington, D.C.

John P. DiMarco, M.D., Ph.D.
Director, Clinical Electrophysiology
  Laboratory
Associate Division Head
Division of Cardiology
Department of Medicine
University of Virginia Health Sciences Center
Charlottesville, Virginia

Arnold L. Fenrich, Jr., M.D.
Fellow in Pediatric Cardiology and
  Electrophysiology
The Lillie Frank Abercrombie Section of
  Cardiology
Department of Pediatrics
Baylor College of Medicine and Texas
  Children's Hospital
Houston, Texas

Guy Fontaine, M.D., Ph.D.
International Consultant
Director of Clinical Electrophysiology and
  Pacemaker Department
Hôpital Jean Rostand
Ivry, France

Fabrice Fontaliran
Service de Rythmologie et de Stimulation
  Cardiaque
Hôpital Jean Rostand
Ivry, France

Robert Frank, M.D.
Service de Rythmologie et de Stimulation
  Cardiaque
Hôpital Jean Rostand
Ivry, France

Curt D. Furberg, M.D., Ph.D.
Professor and Chairman
Department of Public Health Sciences
Bowman Gray School of Medicine
Winston-Salem, North Carolina

Hasan Garan, M.D.
Cardiac Arrhythmia Service
Massachusetts General Hospital and
Harvard Medical School
Boston, Massachusetts

Arthur Garson, Jr., M.D., M.P.H.
Professor and Chief, Pediatric Cardiology
Associate Vice Chancellor for Health Affairs
Duke University Medical Center
Durham, North Carolina

Bernard J. Gersh, M.D., Ch.B., D. Phil.
Professor of Medicine, Mayo Medical School
Consultant, Division of Cardiovascular
  Diseases and Internal Medicine
Mayo Clinic and Foundation
Rochester, Minnesota

Leonard S. Gettes, M.D.
Professor of Medicine
Division of Cardiology
University of North Carolina
Chapel Hill, North Carolina

J. Anthony Gomes, M.D.
Professor of Medicine
The Mount Sinai School of Medicine
Director Electrocardiography and
  Electrophysiology Section
Division of Cardiology
The Mount Sinai Medical Center
New York, New York

Ronnell Hansen, B.A.
Cardiac Arrhythmia Service
Department of Medicine (Cardiovascular Division)
University of Minnesota Medical School
Minneapolis, Minnesota

W. Clark Hargrove, M.D.
Department of Surgery
Division of Cardiothoracic Surgery
Presbyterian Medical Center
Philadelphia, Pennsylvania

Raymond E. Ideker, M.D., Ph.D.
Duke University Medical Center
Durham, North Carolina

John Ip, M.D.
Instructor of Medicine
The Mount Sinai School of Medicine
Attending in Electrophysiology
Electrocardiography and Electrophysiology Section
Division of Cardiology
The Mount Sinai Medical Center
New York, New York

Toru Iwa, M.D.
Service de Rythmologie et de Stimulation Cardiaque
Hôpital Jean Rostand
Ivry, France

Michiel J. Janse, M.D.
Department of Clinical and Experimental Cardiology
University of Amsterdam and the Interuniversity Cardiology Institute
Amsterdam, The Netherlands

Mohammad R. Jazayeri, M.D.
Associate Professor
Electrophysiology Laboratory
University of Wisconsin School of Medicine
Milwaukee Clinical Campus
Sinai Samaritan Medical Center
Staff Electrophysiologist
St. Luke's Medical Center
Milwaukee, Wisconsin

Eric E. Johnson, M.D.
Duke University Medical Center
Engineering Research Center for Emerging Cardiovascular Technologies and the Department of Biomedical Engineering of the School of Engineering
Duke University
Durham, North Carolina

Mark E. Josephson, M.D.
Director, Harvard-Thorndike Electrophysiology Institute and Arrhythmia Service
Department of Medicine
Beth Israel Hospital
Boston, Massachusetts

Katherine M. Kavanagh, M.D.
Department of Medicine
University of Alberta School of Medicine
Edmonton, Alberta
Canada

Stephen G. Keim, M.D.
Cardiac Electrophysiology
University of Pittsburgh Heart Institute
Pittsburgh, Pennsylvania

Kenneth M. Kessler, M.D.
Division of Cardiology
Department of Medicine
University of Miami School of Medicine
Miami Veterans Administration Medical Center
Miami, Florida

You-Ho Kim, M.D.
Cardiac Arrhythmia Service
Massachusetts General Hospital and Harvard Medical School
Boston, Massachusetts

Robert Kinn, M.D.
Cardiac Electrophysiology
University of Pittsburgh Heart Institute
Pittsburgh, Pennsylvania

George J. Klein, M.D., FRCP(C)
Distinguished Research Professor of the Heart and Stroke Foundation of Ontario
Department of Medicine
University of Western Ontario
Arrhythmia Service, Cardiac Investigation Unit
University Hospital
London, Ontario
Canada

Timothy K. Knilans, M.D.
Assistant Professor of Pediatrics and Medicine
University of Cincinnati College of Medicine
Cincinnati, Ohio

Maria Teresa La Rovere
Centro Medico di Montescano
Divisione di Cardiologia
Montescano (PV), Italy

Gilles Lascault, M.D.
Service de Rythmologie et de Stimulation
   Cardiaque
Hôpital Jean Rostand
Ivry, France

Ralph Lazzara, M.D.
Department of Medicine
Cardiovascular Section
University of Oklahoma Health Sciences
   Center and Department of Veterans Affairs
   Medical Center
Oklahoma City, Oklahoma

Michael H. Lehmann, M.D.
Division of Cardiology
Department of Internal Medicine
Wayne State University School of Medicine/
   Harper Hospital
Detroit, Michigan

James W. Leitch, MBBS, FRACP
Department of Medicine
University of Western Ontario
Arrhythmia Service, Cardiac Investigation
   Unit
University Hospital
London, Ontario
Canada

Timothy J. Lessmeier, M.D.
Division of Cardiology
Department of Internal Medicine
Wayne State University School of Medicine/
   Harper Hospital
Detroit, Michigan

Maurice Lev, M.D.
Professor of Pathology
Rush-Presbyterian-St. Lukes Medical Center
Rush Medical College
Chicago, Illinois;
Associate Director
Congenital Heart and Conduction System
   Center
Heart Institute for Children
Christ Hospital and Medical Center
Oak Lawn, Illinois

Teri A. Manolio, M.D., M.H.S.
National Heart, Lung, and Blood Institute
National Institutes of Health
Bethesda, Maryland

Barry J. Maron, M.D.
Cardiovascular Research Center
Minneapolis Heart Institute Foundation
Minneapolis, Minnesota

Jane McHowat, M.D.
Cardiovascular Division
Departments of Internal Medicine and
   Molecular Biology and Pharmacology
Washington University School of Medicine
St. Louis, Missouri

Marc D. Meissner, M.D., C.M.
Assistant Professor of Medicine
Wayne State University
Director, Arrhythmia Service and Cardiac
   Electrophysiology Laboratory
Allen Park VA Medical Center
Associate Director, Arrhythmia Service
Harper Hospital
Detroit, Michigan

John M. Miller, M.D.
Department of Medicine
Division of Cardiology
Temple University Medical Center
Philadelphia, Pennsylvania

Raman L. Mitra, M.D., Ph.D.
Department of Medicine
Cardiology Division
Rush-Presbyterian-St. Lukes Medical Center
Chicago, Illinois

Andrea Mortara
Centro Medico di Montescano
Divisione di Cardiologia
Montescano (PV), Italy

Arthur J. Moss, M.D.
Heart Research Follow-Up Program
University of Rochester Medical Center
Rochester, New York

Robert J. Myerburg, M.D.
Professor of Medicine and Physiology
Director, Division of Cardiology
University of Miami School of Medicine
Miami, Florida

Lisa Naditch, M.D.
Service de Rythmologie et de Stimulation
   Cardiaque
Hôpital Jean Rostand
Ivry, France

Bruce D. Nearing, Ph.D.
Department of Pharmacology
Georgetown University School of Medicine
Washington, D.C.

Imran Niazi, M.D.
Electrophysiology Laboratory
University of Wisconsin Medical School
Milwaukee Clinical Campus
Sinai Samaritan Medical Center
Staff Electrophysiologist
St. Luke's Medical Center
Milwaukee, Wisconsin

Susan O'Donoghue, M.D.
Assistant Professor of Medicine
Georgetown University School of Medicine
Associate Director, Cardiac Arrhythmia Center
Washington Hospital Center
Washington, D.C.

Anil Om, M.D.
Division of Cardiology
Medical College of Virginia
Richmond, Virginia

Sean O'Nunain, M.D.
Harvard Medical School
Cardiac Unit
Massachusetts General Hospital
Boston, Massachusetts

Joseph Ornato, M.D.
Division of Cardiology
Medical College of Virginia
Richmond, Virginia

Robert A. O'Rourke, M.D.
Divison of Cardiology
The University of Texas Health Science Center
San Antonio, Texas

Stefan Osswald, M.D.
E. P. Fellow
Cardiac Arrhythmia Service
Massachusetts General Hospital
Boston, Massachusetts

Patricia A. Penkoske, M.D.
Departments of Surgery and Pediatrics
University of Alberta School of Medicine
Edmonton, Alberta
Canada

Edward V. Platia, M.D.
Director, Cardiac Arrhythmia Center
Washington Hospital Center
Washington, D.C.

Philip J. Podrid, M.D.
Associate Professor of Medicine
Boston University School of Medicine
Section of Cardiology
University Hospital
Boston, Massachusetts

Eric N. Prystowsky, M.D.
Director, Clinical Electrophysiology Laboratory
St. Vincent Hospital
Indianapolis, Indiana;
Consulting Professor of Medicine
Duke University Medical Center
Durham, North Carolina

Shahbudin H. Rahimtoola, M.D., FRCP
George C. Griffith Professor of Cardiology
Professor of Medicine
Chief, Section of Cardiology
University of Southern California
Los Angeles, California

Stephen Remole, M.D.
University of Minnesota Hospital
Minneapolis, Minnesota

Charanjit S. Rihal, M.D.
Fellow in Cardiovascular Disease
Mayo Graduate School of Medicine
Rochester, Minnesota

William C. Roberts, M.D.
Baylor Cardiovascular Institute
Baylor University Medical Center
Dallas, Texas

Jeremy N. Ruskin, M.D.
Associate Professor of Medicine
Harvard Medical School
Director, Cardiac Arrhythmia Service
Massachusetts General Hospital
Boston, Massachusetts

Melvin Scheinman, M.D.
Department of Medicine
Cardiovascular Research Institute
University of California
San Francisco, California

Peter J. Schwartz, M.D.
Professor of Medicine
Dipartimento di Medicina
Universita' di Pavia
Pavia, Italy;
Istituto di Clinica Medica II
Universita' degli Studi di Milano
Milano, Italy

Jasbir S. Sra, M.D.
Assistant Professor
Electrophysiology Laboratory
University of Wisconsin Medical School
Milwaukee Clinical Campus
Sinai Samaritan Medical Center
Staff Electrophysiologist
St. Luke's Medical Center
Milwaukee, Wisconsin

Russell T. Steinman, M.D.
Division of Cardiology
Department of Internal Medicine
Wayne State University/Harper Hospital
Detroit, Michigan

Patrick J. Tchou, M.D.
Director, Cardiac Electrophysiology
University of Pittsburgh School of Medicine
Pittsburgh, Pennsylvania

Wee Siong Teo, M.D.
Department of Medicine
University of Western Ontario
Arrhythmia Service, Cardiac Investigation
  Unit
University Hospital
London, Ontario
Canada

Joelci Tonet, M.D.
Service de Rythmologie et de Stimulation
  Cardiaque
Hôpital Jean Rostand
Ivry, France

Thomas G. Trouton, M.D.
Cardiac Arrhythmia Service
Massachusetts General Hospital and Harvard
  Medical School
Boston, Massachusetts

Emilio Vanoli, M.D.
Istituto di Clinica Medica II
Universita' degli Studi di Milano
Milano, Italy

Petra van Pol, M.D.
Department of Cardiology
University of Limburg
Maastricht, The Netherlands

Richard L. Verrier, Ph.D.
Professor of Pharmacology
Georgetown University School of Medicine
Washington, D.C.

Hein J. J. Wellens, M.D.
Professor and Chairman
Department of Cardiology
Annadal Hospital
Maastricht, The Netherlands

Josef Widerhorn, M.D.
Director of Electrophysiology Laboratory/
  Arrhythmia Services
All Saints Episcopal Hospital
Fort Worth, Texas

Stephen L. Winters, M.D.
Associate Professor of Medicine
The Mount Sinai School of Medicine
Associate Director of Electrophysiology
The Mount Sinai Medical Center
New York, New York

Andrew L. Wit, Ph.D.
Professor
Department of Pharmacology
College of Physicians and Surgeons of
  Columbia University
New York, New York

Francis Witkowski, M.D., FRCP(C)
Associate Professor of Medicine
Division of Cardiology
University of Alberta School of Medicine
Edmonton, Alberta
Canada

Raymond L. Woosley, M.D., Ph.D.
Professor and Chairman
Department of Pharmacology
Georgetown University Medical Center
Washington, D.C.

Raymond Yee, M.D., FRCP(C)
Department of Medicine

University of Western Ontario
Arrhythmia Service, Cardiac Investigation
  Unit
University Hospital
London, Ontario
Canada

Douglas P. Zipes, M.D.
Professor of Medicine
Indiana University School of Medicine
Senior Research Associate
Krannert Institute of Cardiology
Indianapolis, Indiana

Contents

A. General Considerations

1. Epidemiology of Sudden Cardiac Death 3
   Teri A. Manolio, Curt D. Furberg

2. Anatomic Features in Victims of Sudden Coronary Death: Coronary Artery Pathology 21
   Michael J. Davies

3. Interactions Between Structure and Function in Sudden Cardiac Death 32
   Robert J. Myerburg, Kenneth M. Kessler, Agustin Castellanos

B. Knowledge of Sudden Cardiac Death Gathered from Animal Models

4. Role of Ischemia and Infarction in the Genesis of Lethal Arrhythmias 51
   Andrew L. Wit, Michiel J. Janse

5. Biochemical Membrane Mechanisms Underlying Arrhythmias During Myocardial Ischemia and Their Role in Sudden Cardiac Death 82
   Jane McHowat, Peter B. Corr

6. The Autonomic Nervous System and Sudden Cardiac Death: A Rational Basis for Post-Myocardial Infarction Risk Stratification 102
   Peter J. Schwartz, Maria Teresa La Rovere, Andrea Mortara, Emilio Vanoli

7. Critical Mass Hypothesis in the Initiation and Sustenance of Ventricular Fibrillation 124
   Francis K. Witkowski, Patricia A. Penkoske, Katherine M. Kavanagh

8. Myocardial Activation at the Onset of and During Ventricular Fibrillation 128
   Susan M. Blanchard, Eric E. Johnson, Raymond E. Ideker

C. Underlying Substrates in Sudden Cardiac Death

9. Sudden Death Late After a Myocardial Infarction: Substrate and Risk Stratification 147
   Hein J. J. Wellens

10. Sudden Death in Patients with Idiopathic Dilated Cardiomyopathy 155
    Patrick J. Tchou, Stephen G. Keim, Robert Kinn

11. Mechanisms of Sudden Death in Patients with Hypertrophic Cardiomyopathy 163
    Kelley P. Anderson

12. Role of Left Ventricular Ejection Fraction — 190
    J. Thomas Bigger, Jr.

13. Sudden Death in Patients with Structural Heart Disease — 202
    John P. DiMarco

14. Sudden Cardiac Death in the Long QT Syndrome — 209
    Arthur J. Moss

15. Sudden Cardiac Death in the Wolff-Parkinson-White Syndrome — 215
    Wee Siong Teo, George J. Klein, Raymond Yee, James Leitch

16. Arrhythmogenic Right Ventricular Dysplasia: Definition and Mechanism of Sudden Death — 226
    Guy Fontaine, Fabrice Fontaliran, Toru Iwa, Philippe Aouate, Lisa Naditch, Gilles Lascault, Joelci Tonet, Robert Frank

17. Causes and Implications of Sudden Cardiac Death in Athletes — 238
    Barry J. Maron, William C. Roberts

18. Sudden Death in Children — 258
    Arnold L. Fenrich, Jr., Susan W. Denfield, Arthur Garson, Jr.

19. Role of Specialized Conduction System Abnormalities in Sudden Cardiac Death — 274
    Saroja Bharati, Maurice Lev

D. Role of Triggers in Sudden Cardiac Death

20. Role of Acute Myocardial Ischemia in the Pathogenesis of Sudden Cardiac Death — 293
    Charanjit S. Rihal, Bernard J. Gersh

21. Acute-on-Chronic Ischemia in the Genesis of Ventricular Arrhythmias — 318
    Thomas G. Trouton, You-Ho Kim, Hasan Garan

22. Electrolyte Abnormalities as Triggers for Lethal Ventricular Arrhythmias — 327
    Leonard S. Gettes

23. Autonomic Innervation of the Heart and Ventricular Arrhythmias — 341
    Douglas P. Zipes

24. Exercise Testing and Its Role in the Management of Patients with Ventricular Arrhythmias — 350
    Philip J. Podrid

25. Triggers for Sudden Cardiac Death from the Central Nervous System — 367
    Richard L. Verrier, Bruce D. Nearing, Linda W. Dickerson

26. Role of Electrical Triggers in the Causation of Sudden Cardiac Death — 385
    Masood Akhtar, Mohammad R. Jazayeri, Jasbir S. Sra, Anwer A. Dhala, Sanjay S. Deshpande, Imran Niazi

27. Pharmacological Triggers of Sudden Death: Lethal Proarrhythmia — 394
    Ralph Lazzara

28. Mechanisms of Bradyarrhythmic Sudden Death — 407
    Stephen Remole, Ronnell Hansen, David G. Benditt

E. Out-of-Hospital Management Strategies

29. Results of Large-Scale Studies with β-Adrenergic Blocking Drugs and Other Nonantiarrhythmic Agents for the Prevention of Sudden Cardiac Death 419
    Josef Widerhorn, Shahbudin H. Rahimtoola

30. Results of the Cardiac Arrhythmia Suppression Trial 439
    Robert L. Woosley

31. Community Experience in Treating Out-of-Hospital Cardiac Arrest 450
    Joseph P. Ornato, Anil Om

F. Work-up and Assessment of Risk for Sudden Cardiac Death

32. Patients with Cardiac Arrest and Documented Ventricular Fibrillation 465
    Stefan Osswald, Thomas G. Trouton, Sean O'Nunain, Jeremy N. Ruskin

33. Patients with Nonsustained Ventricular Tachycardia 486
    Alfred E. Buxton

34. Hemodynamically Tolerated Sustained Ventricular Tachycardia: Clinical Features and Risk of Sudden Death During Follow-up 496
    Marc D. Meissner, Timothy J. Lessmeier, Russell T. Steinman, Michael H. Lehmann

35. Post-infarction High Risk of Sudden Death 513
    J. Anthony Gomes, Stephen L. Winters, John Ip

G. Therapeutic Options and Assessment of Efficacy

36. Coronary Artery Surgery for the Prevention and Treatment of Sudden Cardiac Death 531
    Robert A. O'Rourke

37. Role of Noninvasive Techniques to Guide Drug Therapy in High-Risk Cases 541
    Susan O'Donoghue, Edward Platia

38. Serial Electrophysiological-Electropharmacological Testing in Survivors of Cardiac Arrest 554
    Eric N. Prystowksi, Timothy K. Knilans

39. Results of Surgery for Ventricular Tachycardia 562
    Raman L. Mitra, Petra van Pol, John M. Miller, W. Clark Hargrove, Mark E. Josephson

40. Role of Catheter Ablation 574
    Melvin M. Scheinman

41. Role of Implantable Cardioverter-Defibrillators in the Management of Patients with Ventricular Tachycardia and Ventricular Fibrillation 588
    Masood Akhtar, Mohammad Jazayeri, Jasbir Sra, Anwer Dhala, Sanjay Deshpande, Zalmen Blanck, Kathi Axtell

42. Comparison of Therapeutic Modalities for Preventing Sudden Cardiac Death in Patients with Sustained Ventricular Tachyarrhythmias 600
    Michael H. Lehmann, Russell T. Steinman, Marc D. Meissner

A
General Considerations

1

Epidemiology of Sudden Cardiac Death

TERI A. MANOLIO
CURT D. FURBERG

Sudden cardiac death (SCD) is the most common and arguably the most dramatic manifestation of coronary artery disease. In an estimated one in five people who develop coronary disease, SCD is the first and only symptom.[1] Sudden death may also be the first manifestation of several other types of congenital and structural heart disease. Fortunately, the incidence of SCD is declining in parallel with a declining mortality from all forms of coronary heart disease (CHD).[2,3] It also appears to be increasingly detectable and treatable as new forms of antiarrhythmic therapy and risk detection become available.

Every presentation of data on sudden death should begin with a definition. Regrettably, there is no universally accepted definition of sudden death. Implicit in all suggested definitions is that deaths are of cardiovascular origin and are natural (as opposed to accidental or deliberate), unexpected, and occur within a short time from the onset of acute symptoms (if any occurred).

In his "De Subitaneis Mortibus," published in 1707, Giovanni Maria Lancisi described many of the features implicit in modern definitions of sudden death.[4] Indeed, little of his philosophy has changed with time:

> . . . I have known of no death except as sudden or as happening in a moment of time, and it stands to reason, that, . . . when something necessary unto life is most consistently missing, then the end of life comes always suddenly, that is at a specific point in time. . . . Some of them [deaths] nevertheless, are inflicted upon us foreseen in fear and sorrow, and felt . . . long before hand. Others, however, come quietly, as with sudden stealth, unexpected as it were.

Lancisi further recognized an element of untimeliness in sudden death, that it came often to those "who in every other respect are healthy and vigorous." Even more impressive, he considered that by diligent research and study, some instances of sudden death might be "foreseen through some sort of a hidden and extraordinary symptom, and then delayed for some while through the administration of a medicament."

In the three centuries since Lancisi's work, no author has provided one succinct statement that clearly defines sudden death. Similarly, any literature review comparing rates of sudden death is limited by variations in definitions as well as by factors such as missing information, lack of autopsy verification, and differences in classifying causes of death. In spite of these limitations, however, a review of the epidemiology of sudden death provides an important foundation for clinicians, scientists, and health care planners attempting to understand and manage this syndrome.

INCIDENCE

U.S. Data

Standardized data on SCD are difficult to come by because of the lack of a standard definition and coding system for the condition. Using deaths occurring out of hospital or in emergency rooms as an indicator of sudden death, Gillum[5] has estimated that more than 350,000 people die suddenly each year from cardiovascular causes. Sudden deaths due to atherosclerotic heart disease almost always occur in persons with severe, diffuse coronary atherosclerosis,[6] even though the disease may be unrecognized. The proportion of first coronary events that are sudden deaths varied from 19 to 26% in a series of studies reviewed in 1966.[7] Approximately half of all deaths attributed to CHD occur suddenly, with this proportion being somewhat higher in men than in women.[8] Though sudden death may occur in persons without any prior cardiac history, and thus may be the initial manifestation of CHD, the risk of sudden death is several times higher in those with known CHD than in those without it. Almost half of all sudden deaths occur in persons with known disease.[8]

Standardized data on regional variations in SCD mortality are also scant but can be estimated from National Center for Health Statistics (NCHS) data on ischemic heart disease (IHD) deaths occurring out of hospital or in emergency rooms.[9] Limiting analysis to deaths classified by the ninth revision of the International Classification of Diseases (ICD-9)[10] as due to IHD (ICD-9 410-414) in white men aged 55–64 years from 42 states, Gillum showed that northern Rocky Mountain states and states surrounding Lake Michigan had the highest proportions of deaths occurring out of hospital or in emergency rooms (Fig. 1–1).[11] These trends were inconsistent, however, in that two southern mountain states were among the ten states with the lowest proportions, and neighboring states were sometimes at opposite extremes in ranking. Nonmetropolitan counties had higher proportions of IHD deaths occurring out of hospital or in emergency rooms than did metropolitan counties. Though some of these differences may be due to variations in coding of place of death, they are undoubtedly also due to differences in availability of emergency medical care. Time to initiation of cardiopulmonary resuscitation and time to definitive care as provided by advanced paramedic-type emergency medical systems were

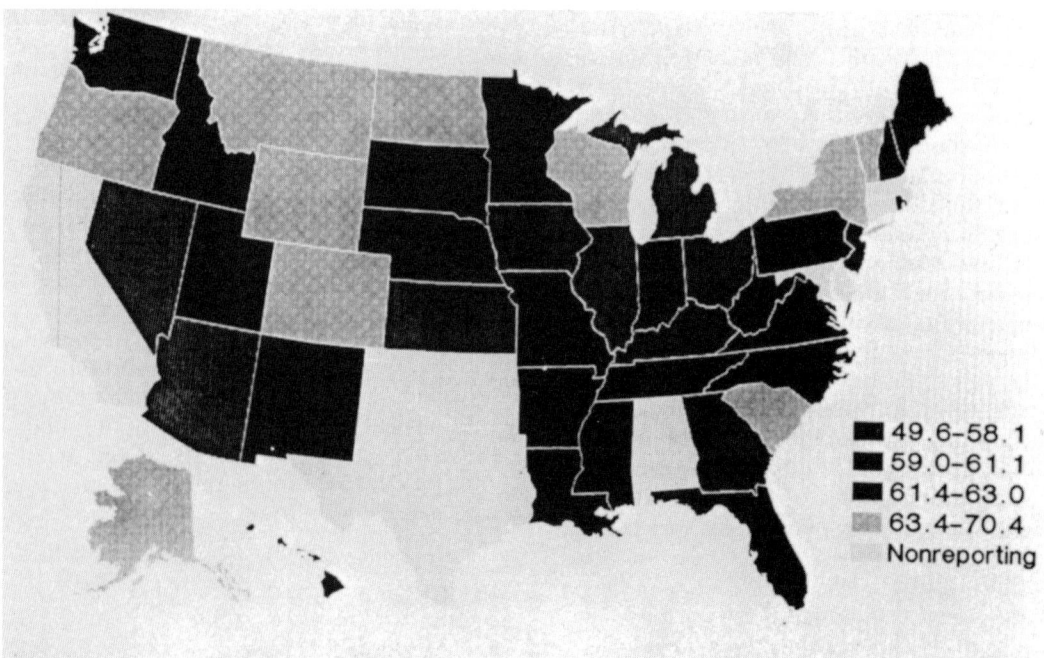

Fig. 1–1. Percent of deaths from ischemic heart disease occurring out of hospital or in emergency rooms in white men aged 55–64 years: 42 states, 1984–1986. (Reprinted with permission from Gillum RF: Geographic variation in sudden coronary death. Am Heart J *119*:380–389, 1990.)

strongly associated with successful resuscitation from out-of-hospital cardiac arrest.[12] Although overall IHD risk may be lower, less urbanized areas are more likely to have longer ambulance response times, which would increase the proportion of IHD deaths occurring out of hospital or in emergency rooms.

The annual incidence of sudden death, defined as death occurring out of hospital or in emergency rooms, in people between the ages of 35 and 74 years in the 40 states reported by Gillum[5] was 1.91/1000 for white men, 1.91/1000 for nonwhite men, 0.57/1000 for white women, and 0.90/1000 for nonwhite women. Approximately 60% of deaths in males and 50% of deaths in females with IHD occurred out of hospital or in emergency rooms, and 56% of those dying out of hospital or in emergency rooms had known prior CHD. Regional data from selected areas suggest similar rates for SCD (Table 1–1),[5,7,13–20] though definitions, populations studied, and time periods vary. Rates in women are consistently a half to a third those in men, with rates falling in the past two to three decades. The proportion of IHD deaths that are sudden is fairly constant at 50–60%, except in the Framingham study, in which the proportion was 22–23%.[13] This lower rate is probably due to persons with known CHD not being considered at risk for sudden death. The proportion of sudden deaths in people with known prior CHD is also constant in regional data at roughly one half, and approximately half of these have had prior documented myocardial infarction (MI).

Table 1–1
Regional U.S. Studies of Sudden Death

Location/Study	Years	Definition of SCD	Population Studied	Annual Incidence (per 1000)	Proportion of IHD Deaths	Proportion with Known CHD
Framingham/Schatzkin et al[13]	1948–74	1 hr	M/F, 30–62 yr, excluding prior CHD	M: 1.51 W: 0.53 (excl. CHD)	M: 22% F: 23%	—
Rochester/Elveback et al[14]	1950–75	Not defined	Excluding prior CHD	1950: 1.26 1955: 1.32 1960: 1.12 1965: 0.96 1970: 0.79	—	—
Tecumseh/Chiang et al[15]	1959–65	1 hr	M/F ≥30 yr	2.00	45.9	40.0
Baltimore/Kuller et al[7,16]	1964–65	24 hr	M/F, 40–64 yr	By age, race, sex	60.2	50.9
Nashville/Hagstrom et al[17]	1967–68	24 hr	M/F, ≤75 yr	1.55	—	29.5 (MI only)
Minn-St. Paul/Gillum et al.[18]	1970	OOH/ER	M/F, 30–74 yr	M: 3.11 F: 0.96	M: 61.2 F: 55.5	M: 25.5 F: 13.1 (MI only)
Albany-Framingham/Kannel et al.[19]	1975	1hr	M, 45–74 yr	2.35	46.6	43.1
Worcester/Goldberg et al[20]	1975–84	OOH/ER	M/F, ≥25 yr	1975: 2.65 1978: 1.74 1981: 1.70 1984: 1.48	—	—
Minn-St. Paul/Gillum et al[18]	1980	OOH/ER	M/F, 30–74 yr	M: 2.44 F: 0.70	M: 66.7 F: 59.8	M: 26.0 F: 15.5 (MI only)
40 states/Gillum[5]	1985	OOH/ER	M/F, 35–74 yr, white	M: 1.91 F: 0.57	M: 59.7 F: 49.6	56.1

Abbreviations: OOH, out of hospital; ER, emergency room; MI, myocardial infarction; IHD, ischemic heart disease; CHD, coronary heart disease; SCD, sudden cardiac death.

International Data

Sudden death in countries outside the United States is less well documented but has been compiled by the World Health Organization (WHO) from death certificates meeting ICD-9 codes 798, 798.1, and 798.2.[21] Rates of sudden death in industrial countries are fairly consistent with those in the United States, while rates in developing countries are considerably lower, paralleling the rates of IHD mortality as a whole.

Regional data from selected studies show the same patterns, except that rates in Finland are considerably higher than those in the United States, again paralleling the rates of IHD mortality (Table 1–2).[21–26] Rates in China are much lower, even when examined in age-specific strata, consistent with the lower IHD rates currently observed in that population. The substantial differences in proportions of sudden death victims with known CHD (15–75%) are primarily due to differences in the definition and diagnosis of CHD among studies.

International data on sudden death incidence are available from the World Health Organization Myocardial Infarction Community Registers, a surveillance study of more than 3.5 million men and women aged 20–64 years.[21] Thirty-eight percent of all reported deaths in this study occurred within 1 hour of onset of symptoms. Difficulties in obtaining complete and accurate information varied among the communities. In the centers with the most complete information on time of death, the proportion of patients dying within the first hour was 45–50%. International patterns in rates of sudden death are similar to those for CHD, with U.S. rates near the median for 29 industrialized countries (Fig. 1–2).

Associations with Age, Sex, and Race

The relationships between sudden death and major demographic risk factors are similar to those between IHD and these risk factors. The incidence of sudden death increases markedly with age in all studies cited and is two to three times higher in men than in women in all studies that included both, paralleling the male/female difference in rates of IHD as a whole (Fig. 1–3). The proportion of IHD deaths that occur out of hospital or in emergency rooms, however, declines with age, from approximately 75%

Table 1–2
Regional International Studies of Sudden Cardiac Death

Location/Study	Years	Definition of SCD	Population Studied	Annual Incidence (per 1000)	Proportion of IHD Deaths	Proportion with Known CHD
Finland/Suhonen et al[22]	1966–79	1 hr	M, 40–59 yr	4.2	64.1	23.3 (MI only)
N. Karelia/Salonen et al[23]	1972–78	1 hr	M/F, 35–64 yr	1975 M: 3.2 1975 F: 0.4 1978 M: 2.8 1978 F: 0.3	M: 57.9 F: 46.2	—
Beijing/Xiang-gu et al[24]	1974–80	6 hr	M/F, ≥30 yr	0.2*	—	37.1
Auckland/Beaglehole et al[25]	1981–82	24 hr	M/F, 25–69 yr	M: 1.90 F: 0.49	—	15.5 (MI only)
Denmark/Madsen[26]	1982	24 hr	M/F, ≥25 yr	M: 2.12* F: 1.12*	—	74.6 (CHD, CHF, HTN)
WHO[21]	1985	OOH/ER	M/F, 35–74 yr, white	M: 1.91 F: 0.57	M: 59.7 F: 49.6	56.1

Abbreviations: SCD, sudden cardiac death; IHD, ischemic heart disease; CHD, coronary heart disease, CHF, congestive heart failure; HTN, hypertension; MI, myocardial infarction.
* Not adjusted for age.

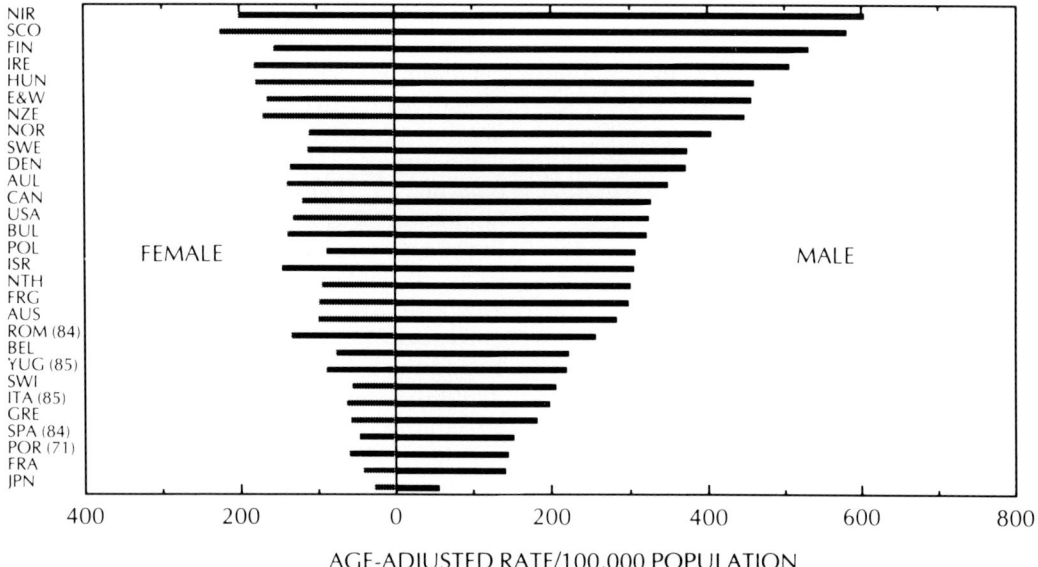

Fig. 1–2. Death rates for coronary heart disease, ages 35–74 years, by sex and country, 1986. (World Health Organization, Geneva: *World Health Statistics Annual*, issues dated 1988, 1987, 1983, 1982, 1981, 1970, 1969. Reprinted from *Morbidity and Mortality Chartbook on Cardiovascular, Lung, and Blood Disease/1990*, National Heart, Lung, and Blood Institute, U.S. Department of Health and Human Services.)

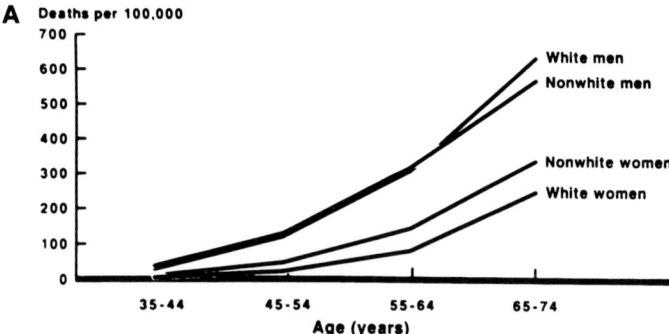

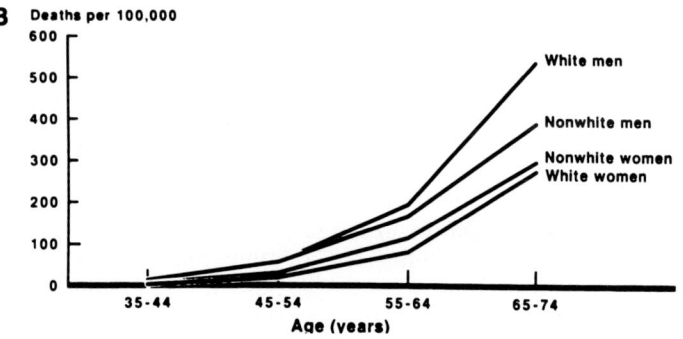

Fig. 1–3. Plots of mortality rates (deaths per 100,000) for ischemic heart disease occurring out of hospital or in emergency room (**A**) and occurring in hospital (**B**), by age, sex, and race in 40 states during 1985. (Data from National Center for Health Statistics. Reprinted with permission from Gillum RF: Sudden coronary death in the United States: 1980–1985. Circulation 79:756–765, 1989.)

at ages 35–44 years to approximately 50% at ages 75–84 years.[5]

Data on racial differences in sudden death, though sparse and somewhat conflicting, suggest that blacks are more likely than whites to suffer sudden death in excess of their risk of CHD mortality.[27] Interpretation of data on all types of CHD in blacks is complicated by several factors, as described in detail by Gillum.[28] These factors include (1) a younger age distribution of black populations, so that crude rates give the impression of lower rates of CHD even though age-specific rates are similar; (2) greater inaccuracy of death certificate data in blacks; (3) a greater impact on black populations of changes in classification, particularly abandonment of the term "myocardial degeneration" and a decrease in use of the term "hypertensive heart disease"; and (4) frequent failure to report data in minorities separately from whites and to distinguish blacks from other minority groups such as Hispanics, Asians, and American Indians, which have widely varying rates of IHD.

Rates of CHD mortality (ICD-9 410-414) are similar in black men and white men, but are 1.5 to 2 times higher in black women than white women.[29] Hagstrom et al[17] showed approximately similar black/white ratios for sudden death in Nashville. Kuller et al[7] in Baltimore showed lower rates of sudden death in black men than in white men, and slightly higher rates in black women than in white women. Blacks in that study were more likely than whites to suffer unwitnessed sudden death or death within 2 hours, while whites were more likely to die within 2–24 hours of onset of symptoms. In contrast, Keil showed a threefold higher sudden death rate among black men compared to white men, and a 1.5-fold increased rate among black women compared to white women.[30] Gillum[5] documented greater proportions of IHD deaths occurring out of hospital and in emergency rooms in blacks than in whites: 66% of IHD deaths in black men and 56% in black women aged 55–64 years occurred out of hospital or in emergency rooms, compared to 61% of IHD deaths in white men and 50% in white women (Fig. 1–4). The excess mortality was due to deaths out of hospital, with emergency room deaths tending to be lower in blacks except in older women.

Gillum[5] has proposed several possible explanations for the higher proportion of IHD deaths occurring out of hospital or in emergency rooms among younger persons, men, and blacks. These include the increased likelihood of these groups to deny or attempt self-medication for prodromal symptoms, to delay summoning emergency services, or to work or play in areas where emergency medical response is less prompt. In addition, these groups in general are less likely to use preventive services or to have a source of regular medical care, and may be less likely to have underlying heart disease detected and treated. Blacks are also more likely than whites to be using diuretics, which may promote hypokalemia and provoke sudden death.[31,32] They also have a higher prevalence of left ventricular hypertrophy and electrocardiographic repolarization abnormalities, which may further increase their risk of sudden death.[33] The lower proportions of blacks dying in emergency rooms suggests that access to or use of emergency services may be an important component of racial differences in sudden death.[5] Issues of access to care and prehospital delay in blacks in particular need further evaluation and intervention.

Temporal Trends

Examination of the data in Table 1–1 shows declining incidences of sudden death for all studies that reported time trends.[14,18,20,22] This decline has paralleled the decline in CHD death which began in the mid-1960s (Fig. 1–5).[34] Reasons for the decline in CHD death are complex and could include improvements in risk factor profiles, prehospital care, in-hospital treatment, and postdischarge secondary prevention.[35] Studies in Minnesota, Chicago, Massachusetts, and in DuPont Company employees have noted declines in sudden death or death within the first 24 hours with little change in incidence rates of MI.[2] Faster declines have been noted for sudden death than for other CHD deaths in the two Minnesota studies.[18,36]

Gillum has demonstrated a nationwide decline in the combined proportion of IHD deaths occurring out of hospital or in emergency rooms, although the proportion oc-

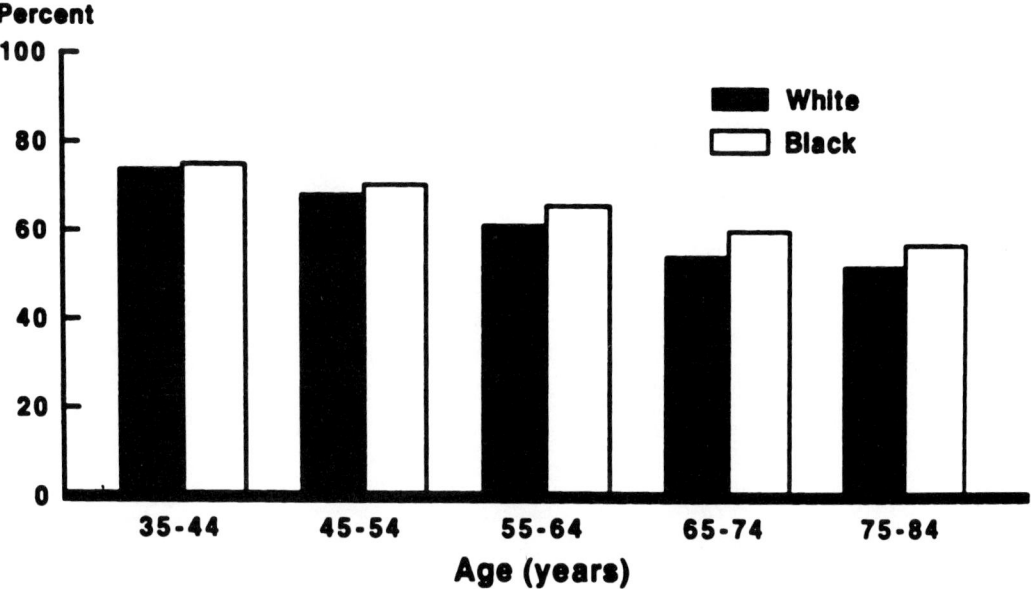

Fig. 1–4. Bar graph of percent distribution of place of death of white and black men aged 55–64 years dying of ischemic heart disease in 40 states during 1980 and 1985. OUT, out of hospital; ER, emergency room; IN, in hospital. (Data from National Center for Health Statistics. Reprinted with permission from Gillum RF: Sudden coronary death in the United States: 1980–1985. Circulation 79: 756–765, 1989.)

curring in emergency rooms alone has increased substantially.[5] He suggests several possible explanations for the decline in out-of-hospital deaths, including (1) a decreased incidence of sudden death in persons without known CHD, owing to population-wide reductions in CHD risk factors; (2) a decreased incidence of sudden death in persons with known CHD, owing to improved secondary prevention; (3) a decreased prehospital case fatality rate, owing to improved emergency medical services or patient awareness; (4) a decreased incidence of sudden death, owing to improved resuscitation of persons with out-of-hospital cardiac arrest; or (5) any combination of the above. The rise in deaths in emergency rooms suggests that the fourth proposed mechanism is certainly having an effect, but the relative contributions of each of these mechanisms cannot be determined. A decline in the proportion of CHD deaths classified as "dead on arrival" probably reflects a temporal trend toward increased resuscitative attempts and prehospital emergency treatment,[37] but could also be related to changes in hospital reimbursement, or "DRG creep."[38]

Circadian, Daily, and Seasonal Variation

Following the reports of an increased likelihood for acute MI to occur in the morning,[39] several studies have reported similar circadian variations in sudden death.[40–43] A study of 2203 persons dying out of hospital from acute MI (ICD-410) within 1 hour of onset of symptoms in Massachusetts in 1983 showed a significant primary peak in time of death at 10 to 11 A.M. and a secondary peak from 5 to 6 P.M. (Fig. 1–6).[40] This rhythm was quite similar to that reported for nonfatal MI.[39] Review of other studies of circadian variation in sudden deaths showed a significantly lower proportion occurring during sleep (12% vs. 29% expected if deaths were evenly distributed throughout the day). The Framingham Heart Study investigators showed a 70% increased risk of sudden death from 7 to 9 A.M., compared to all other times, and a decreased incidence from 9 A.M. to 1 P.M. The Beta-Blocker Heart Attack Trial investigators demon-

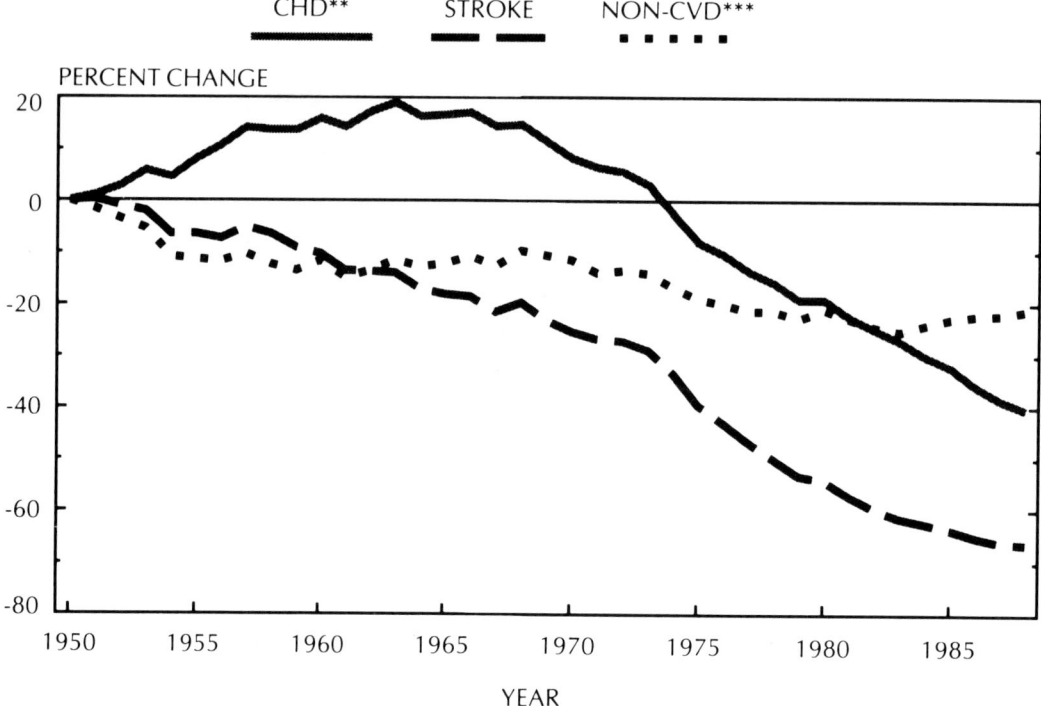

Fig. 1–5. Percent change in age-adjusted death rates since 1950. CHD, coronary heart disease; non-CVD, total mortality minus cardiovascular disease. (Reprinted from *Morbidity and Mortality Chartbook on Cardiovascular, Lung, and Blood Disease/1990,* National Heart, Lung, and Blood Institute, U.S. Department of Health and Human Services.)

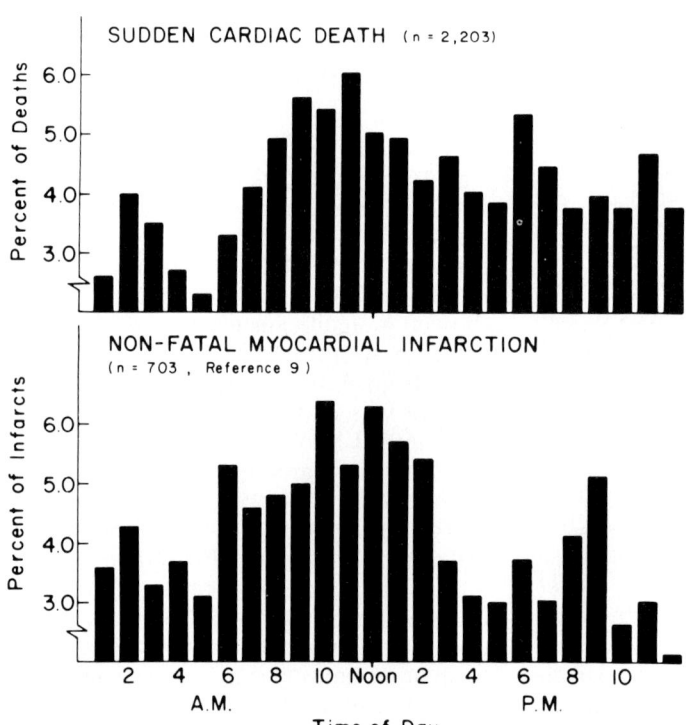

Fig. 1–6. Comparison between the circadian rhythm of sudden cardiac death and the circadian rhythm of nonfatal myocardial infarction. The percent of total events occurring during each hour of the day for the 24-hour period is plotted. Both rhythms show a trough during the night (midnight to 4 A.M.), a primary peak between 6 A.M. and noon, and a secondary peak between 5 and 9 P.M. (Reprinted with permission from Muller JE, et al: Circadian variation in the frequency of sudden cardiac death. Circulation 75:131–138, 1987.)

strated a peak at 8 to 11 a.m. in both propranolol- and placebo-treated patients, but the peak was less prominent in the propranolol group, suggesting that propranolol may affect the mechanism of the circadian variation.[42]

Proposed mechanisms for the increased morning incidence of sudden death include increases in sympathetic tone associated with awakening and assumption of an upright posture.[39] Such changes could be associated with increased platelet aggregation on atherosclerotic coronary plaques, increased coronary vasomotor tone, increased myocardial oxygen demands, or increased electrical instability and tendency to primary arrhythmic events.[44,45]

An increased frequency of death within 24 hours of onset on Saturdays has been suggested in data from Rochester, Minnesota,[46] and Newcastle-upon-Tyne, England,[47] but these differences were not significant. Other studies have not shown such a relationship or have suggested a slight increase on Mondays.[16,48,49] Sudden death rates have consistently been reported as highest in winter and lowest in summer, but these trends are also not different from what would be expected by chance.[16,46,49]

ISSUES IN INTERPRETING EPIDEMIOLOGICAL DATA ON SUDDEN DEATH

Epidemiological studies of SCD are complicated by lack of standard definitions and lack of classification systems for sudden death. Epidemiological data on sudden death cannot be properly evaluated without an understanding of the potential pitfalls and biases associated with the lack of ICD codes for sudden death, the variations in definitions of sudden death, and the collection and use of data on prodromal symptoms.

Lack of ICD Codes

The International Classification of Diseases has no code for SCD, making national and international comparisons difficult. While there is a code 798 for "sudden death, cause unknown" (including 798.1, "instantaneous death"; 798.2, "death occurring in less than 24 hours from onset of symptoms, not otherwise explained"; and 798.9, "unattended death"), these are intended for deaths in which no cause could be discovered. Deaths that can be ascribed to coronary disease are more often classified under codes for ischemic heart disease (410–414), particularly code 410, "acute myocardial infarction." Code 427.5, "cardiac arrest," is infrequently applied to cases of SCD. The tenth revision of the International Classification of Diseases, due to be released in 1994, will include a code for SCD, making data collected after that time more available for analysis and comparison.

Biases Associated with Varying Definitions

In addition to lack of standardization in death certificate coding, different authors use different definitions of sudden death. These involve differences in the length of time between symptom onset and death, use of data on location of death, inclusion or exclusion of unwitnessed deaths, and consideration of the unexpected nature of the death.

Time intervals used for defining sudden death have varied from 1 to 24 hours, as shown in Tables 1–1 and 1–2. The time of death is generally approximated by the time of collapse and loss of vital signs.[50] Time of onset of symptoms is more difficult to define, as many patients dying "suddenly" have been unwell for days or weeks prior to death.[51] Kuller[50] has recommended defining onset as "the time when the victim was required to change or substantially modify his/her activity," and prodromata as "the constellation of signs and symptoms not interfering with the individual's usual activities." Studies using a shorter time period (i.e., 1 hour) will necessarily report lower incidences of sudden death than studies using a broader definition (i.e., up to 24 hours), but more of these deaths may be classified clinically as due to CHD.[52] Accurate pathologic classification of deaths occurring shortly after onset of symptoms may be difficult, however, since pathologic changes are rarely detected in such subjects.[53] Patients surviving minutes to 24 hours after onset often have evidence of hemorrhage, plaque rupture, coronary thrombosis, or acute MI.[50]

Some authors, notably Gillum,[5,18] avoid use of time intervals altogether because of the unavailability of reliable data and depend instead on location of death. Most investigators accept that sudden and unexpected deaths occur outside the hospital, and exclude deaths occurring in hospital. In recent years, however, this definition has been extended to include deaths occurring in the emergency room, because of the increased use of emergency services and the reluctance to declare death until advanced life support efforts have been attempted. The declining proportion of IHD deaths occurring out of hospital and the concomitant rise in the proportion of emergency room deaths are evidence of this trend.[5] The availability of emergency medical services also influences the proportion of deaths occurring out of hospital or in emergency rooms, as demonstrated by the high rates of such deaths in nonmetropolitan areas.[11] Individual preference and local practice may also affect whether deaths in the emergency room are coded as occurring in hospital. Thus, using location of death may induce some biases in measuring SCD, but it has the advantage of being available for interstate and international comparisons over a long period of time.

Although up to one third of all sudden and unexpected deaths may be unwitnessed, many studies exclude unwitnessed death because time of symptom onset and of death cannot be determined reliably.[50] The probability of death being unwitnessed is related to the length of survival from symptom onset, with patients surviving for shorter periods being more likely to die unwitnessed. Unwitnessed deaths are also more likely in persons living alone or having unreliable witnesses, and in deaths occurring at home. Sudden deaths in persons without a history of heart disease are also more likely to be unwitnessed than deaths in those with known heart disease.[50] The elderly, especially elderly women, are particularly likely to be living alone, at home, or with unreliable witnesses. Women are also more likely not to have a prior history of heart disease. Exclusion of unwitnessed deaths will thus seriously bias a study by under-representing those with shorter survival, without known heart disease, or living alone, as well as deaths occurring at home, in the elderly, and in women. Inclusion of such deaths in studies of sudden death should be predicated on efforts to obtain detailed postmortem examinations and to interview physicians and next of kin on prior illnesses and symptoms. Because sudden unwitnessed death may also be the result of heavy alcohol intake, homicide, or suicide, these possibilities should be explored as fully as possible. Studies of sudden death should include evaluation, if feasible, to exclude death due to these causes.

The degree of unexpectedness of death may also cause differences in definitions of SCD. Most authors exclude deaths occurring in hospitals or in persons who are severely disabled as not being truly sudden or unexpected. Up to half of persons suffering sudden and unexpected deaths in community samples may have a prior clinical history of heart disease, and physicians are often likely to ascribe such deaths to coronary disease without further investigation.[50] Sudden deaths in persons without heart disease are more likely to be referred for autopsy, so medical examiners' and autopsy series tend to under-represent persons with known heart disease. Use of such data for projecting the incidence of sudden death and the need for emergency services is likely to underestimate the actual number of persons who might benefit from out-of-hospital emergency care.

Prodromal Symptoms in Sudden Death Victims

As discussed by Kuller,[50] few situations in medical practice are more distressing than the sudden death of an apparently healthy person who has recently received a clean bill of health from his or her physician. Although some sudden deaths are truly unexpected and totally without warning, many victims have had some kind of prodrome, and a surprising proportion have recently seen their physician. Autopsy studies have demonstrated that the majority of persons dying suddenly from coronary disease have severe diffuse atherosclerosis, and many have scars consistent with prior MI.

Of 666 persons aged 40–64 years who died suddenly of atherosclerotic disease in Baltimore, 24% had seen a physician within 7 days of death; 32% of those had a history of heart disease and 17% had no prior history. This is compared to only 7.5% of a community sample of white men of the same ages.[7] The reasons why these persons saw their physicians were not reported. In a study of prodromal symptoms, white men without heart disease who died suddenly were twice as likely as living controls to have reported chest pain in the preceding 2 weeks, 1.4 times as likely to have reported shortness of breath, and 2.7 times as likely to have reported fatigue in the 2 weeks preceding the fatal events.[54] Similar associations were seen in men with a history of heart disease, but little difference in symptoms was found between female cases and controls.

Types of prodromal symptoms in victims of sudden death appear to be similar to prodromes of acute MI, but frequency of symptoms may vary. Chest pain is the most common prodromal symptom in acute MI[55] but is reported only half as frequently in sudden death victims.[51] Fatigue is a more common symptom, but it is reported at a frequency similar to that in infarction patients, as is dyspnea.

UNDERLYING CONDITIONS

Atherosclerotic Coronary Disease

Because death ensues rapidly after loss of cardiac function, any condition producing abrupt cessation of cardiac output can produce sudden death. Although there are some distinguishing features, few characteristics have been identified as being predictive of the "suddenness" of death.[1] Causes of SCD thus tend to mirror, in risk factors and prevalence, the predominant cardiac causes of death (sudden or otherwise) in a given population. In developed countries, the majority (80%) are estimated to be due to coronary artery disease, a further 10–15% to cardiomyopathies, and 5% to valvular heart disease.[56] These proportions have remained relatively constant with time; in Kuller's series from the 1960s, 88% of SCDs occurring within 2 hours of onset of symptoms were attributed to atherosclerotic heart disease, 6–8% to hypertensive heart disease, and 4–5% to rheumatic heart disease.[16]

Coronary disease can produce sudden death by several routes, the most common believed to be complications of sudden coronary occlusion by spasm, hemorrhage, or thrombosis at the site of an existing atherosclerotic plaque. Acute coronary occlusion can induce sudden death by provoking lethal ventricular arrhythmias or, probably less commonly, by producing the rapid onset of acute severe left ventricular dysfunction and death due to hypoperfusion. Acute ischemia can also lead to ventricular septal, ventricular free wall, or coronary artery rupture with acute hemopericardium and pericardial tamponade.

Autopsy studies have demonstrated fresh thrombotic occlusion in approximately 40% of persons dying suddenly of atherosclerotic coronary disease.[56,57] Although fresh infarction is often difficult to detect in sudden death victims (requiring approximately 6 hours to become evident pathologically), an estimated 20–30% of sudden deaths studied at autopsy have demonstrable infarction.[58] This figure varies from 0 to 46% in published series, with the highest incidence in patients dying at 24 hours.[56] A series of 151 SCD victims (death within 24 hours of onset of symptoms) from Helsinki showed recent definite or early MI in 77%,[59] although this high proportion may be related to case selection and a broader definition of infarction. This is in contrast to a proportion of demonstrable infarctions of 13–17% of persons resuscitated from cardiac arrest.[60,61] Whether this latter group represents a subset with a less severe cardiac insult or simply one that has had more rapid or successful medical intervention is difficult to determine. What seems clear, however, is that SCD may occur in the absence of infarction but almost always occurs in the presence of severe diffuse coronary atherosclerosis.[2]

Nonatherosclerotic Coronary Disease

While coronary atherosclerosis is believed to cause or contribute to the vast majority of SCDs, nonatherosclerotic coronary anomalies can also produce the syndrome. Among these are anomalous origins of the coronary arteries or deep myocardial bridges interfering with coronary flow.[62] Such conditions are rare, but the risk of sudden death associated with them is high, and they account for a disproportionately large share of sudden deaths in the young.

Other Cardiac Causes of Sudden Death

Noncoronary cardiac causes of sudden death are legion, as shown in Figure 1–7.[62] Cardiomyopathy and valvular heart disease account for the largest proportion of nonatherosclerotic SCDs. Recognition of persons at risk for these conditions may permit effective therapeutic interventions. Hypertension, especially among blacks,[63] heavy alcohol use, and familial hypertrophic obstructive cardiomyopathy are common and easily recognized conditions that can lead to cardiomyopathies associated with a high risk of sudden death. Aortic stenosis is the classic valvular lesion associated with sudden death, but sudden death has also been associated with mitral valve prolapse, a much more common condition. Fortunately, the risk of sudden death associated with mitral valve prolapse is quite low.[64]

Congenital heart diseases associated with sudden death include congenital aortic stenosis, Eisenmenger's syndrome, and postsurgical repair of complex lesions such as tetralogy of Fallot.[65] The long QT syndrome[66] is a rare cause of sudden death in persons under the age of 20. Families are usually identified after a proband suffers a syncopal episode or cardiac arrest during childhood or the teenage years. The conventional electrocardiographic definition is a QT interval greater than 0.44 sec. Other features of the syndrome are congenital deafness (present in approximately 7% of cases) and history of ventricular tachyarrhythmia (approximately 47%). Other electrophysiological abnormalities such as the pre-excitation syndromes are also associated with an increased risk of sudden death.

Noncardiac Causes of Sudden Death

The importance of these conditions in the epidemiology of SCD relates primarily to the need to rule them out if at all possible. Although this can be difficult without an autopsy, prior history and examination after death may provide some helpful clues. Ruptured abdominal aortic aneurysm is associated with advanced age (>70 years), hypertension, and smoking; it may be preceded by abdominal or back pain, and discoloration of the flanks after death may be noticeable. Thoracic aortic aneurysms are associated with syphilis, now quite rare in

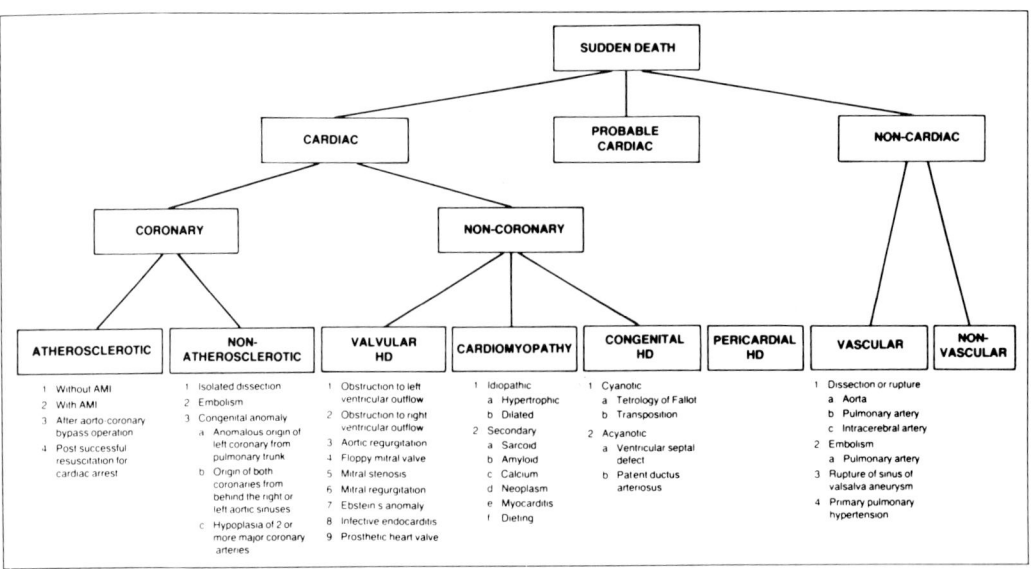

Fig. 1–7. Various causes of sudden death. HD, heart disease. (Reproduced with permission from Roberts WC: Sudden cardiac death: A diversity of causes with focus on atherosclerotic coronary artery disease. Am J Cardiol 65:13B–19B, 1990.)

developed countries, and with Marfan's syndrome, both of which may be detectable after death but without an autopsy. Intracranial hemorrhage may be secondary to hypertension or intracranial aneurysm, histories of which may be obtained from next of kin; it may also be preceded by acute severe headache. In addition, victims of intracranial catastrophes generally lose consciousness *before* they lose a detectable pulse. Victims of SCD generally have no obtainable pulse at the time of loss of consciousness. Without an astute observer at the time of collapse, however, this distinction may not be possible. Finally, massive pulmonary embolism can cause death almost instantaneously, but with signs and symptoms almost identical to those of SCD. A preceding history of venous thrombosis, thrombophlebitis, or transient episodes of pulmonary embolism may be suggestive, but confident ascertainment of this cause (as with the other causes listed above) often requires an autopsy.

The proportion of sudden deaths in coroners' series due to these noncardiac causes is shown in Table 1–3. Owing to the low rate of autopsy or coroner's investigation into nonviolent deaths in the United States, data from American studies are limited and considerably dated. Kuller reviewed studies reported during the 1930s through 1950s, which included only one U.S. study.[52] Approximately 59% of the nearly 21,000 autopsies attributed death to diseases of the heart and aorta, followed by 9% pulmonary and 11% cerebral causes. The majority (91% in men and 52% in women) of sudden deaths occurring within 1 hour of onset of symptoms were attributed to coronary disease. These proportions dropped by approximately one third with longer periods of time from onset to death.

The proportion of sudden deaths attributed to heart disease in autopsy and coroners' series is fairly constant over time and across the developed world (Table 1–3). Approximately 60% of sudden deaths are considered to be of cardiac origin, with this proportion perhaps drifting slightly higher in later years. The 77% figure from Glasgow may reflect the small size or selected nature of this sample.[70] Pulmonary and cerebral disease each account for another 10–15% of sudden deaths.

Table 1–3
Proportion of Sudden Atraumatic Deaths Due to Various Causes in Autopsy and Coroners' Series

Location	Years	No. of Deaths	Heart	Aorta	Respiratory	Cerebral	Digestive*	Other
Brighton	1944–54	2,000	59.4†		15.0	14.6	7.0	4.0
New York	1948	2,030	44.9†		23.1	17.9	9.9	4.4
Scandinavia	1937	403	51.0†		15.0	9.0	13.0	
London	1947	6,267	58.8†		5.7	12.8	—	23.7
Germany	1939	6,481	66.3†		—	—	—	—
Tokyo	1952–56	3,800	56.0†		16.8	18.5	6.3	2.4
Combined/Kuller[52]	1937–56	20,981	59.2†		8.6	10.6	2.9	8.6
Baltimore/Kuller et al[16]	1964–65	407	63.9		5.9	11.5	—	17.9
Gothenburg/Wennerblom et al[67]	1975–76	1,073	64/5.8‡	1.2	11	3.8	2.7	11.5
Wandsworth/Thomas et al[68]	1980s	350	59/7.5‡	3.4	17.7	4.3	2.2	6.2
Denmark/Madsen[26]	1982	218	76.6	2.3	7.8	9.6	1.8	2.3
Osaka/Matoba et al[70]	1982–86	1,230	66	4	6	16	5	2
Glasgow/Fawal et al[71]	1987	130	77/1.5‡	—	4.6	1.5	—	12.3

* For studies reported by Kuller,[53] digestive diseases are combined with diseases of the urogenital system.
† Deaths due to aortic aneurysm were reported with heart diseases in these six studies.
‡ Where available, proportions of heart disease considered to be ischemic and nonischemic are listed separately.

PREDISPOSING FACTORS

Standard CHD Risk Factors

Given that 80% of SCDs are attributable to CHD, at least in developed countries, the risk factors for SCD closely parallel those of coronary disease. Standard risk factors include male sex, age, cigarette smoking, hypertension, hypercholesterolemia, and left ventricular hypertrophy. The latter five factors were combined to produce a multivariate model of probability of sudden death in 4120 middle-aged men in a combined analysis of the Albany and Framingham studies.[19] The investigators showed a 16-fold gradation in incidence of sudden death from the lowest to the highest decile of this risk score (Table 1–4). While this score isolates a group at high risk of sudden death, prediction in the individual remains problematic; only 32 of the approximately 400 men in the highest decile died suddenly, and they were not readily distinguishable from the 368 who did not.[19]

Factors related to the suddenness of death can be evaluated by comparing the proportion of CHD deaths that were sudden in persons with and without the risk factors listed above.[1] Prior known CHD, a powerful risk factor for sudden death,[8] was associated with an increased proportion of CHD deaths occurring suddenly in a study of Finnish men (67% vs. 60%)[22] but with a decreased proportion in the combined Albany-Framingham studies (41% vs. 53%),[1] although in neither case was the difference significant.

Left ventricular hypertrophy on electrocardiography, serum cholesterol levels, and blood pressure levels were not consistently related to the proportion of deaths occurring suddenly in the combined Albany-Framingham studies.[1] A suggestive relationship was noted for cigarette smoking: CHD deaths in nonsmokers were less likely to be sudden than in smokers, but a relationship with number of cigarettes smoked could not be identified. Increasing age and obesity were both related to an increased proportion of CHD deaths occurring suddenly, but only in the Framingham cohort of the combined Albany-Framingham studies.[1] In the male Finnish cohort described by Suhonen et al,[22] smoking appeared to be a more important predictor of SCD than of nonsudden cardiac death, while other standard CHD risk factors seemed to predict sudden and nonsudden death more or less equally. Obesity was not an independent risk factor for sudden death in this study. Other investigators have found strong relationships between smoking and SCD.[71,72] Kuller[2] be-

Table 1–4
Incidence of Sudden Death According to Decile of Multivariate Risk: Framingham-Albany Combined Analysis

Decile of Multivariage Risk	No. of Sudden Deaths			2-Year Incidence of Sudden Death/1000
		Prior CHD?		
	Total	Yes	No	
1	2	1	1	0.89
2	2	2	0	0.89
3	2	0	2	0.89
4	6	3	3	2.69
5	8	2	6	3.58
6	6	1	5	2.69
7	12	5	7	5.37
8	10	4	6	4.48
9	17	6	11	7.61
10	32	13	19	14.32
Total	97	37	60	4.34

SOURCE: Kannel WB, et al: Circulation 51:606–613, 1975.[19] Reproduced with permission.

lieves that smoking is probably the most important precipitating factor for SCD.

Other risk factors for sudden death have included vital capacity (which may also be related to an increased proportion of deaths occurring suddenly),[72] diabetes,[15] rapid heart rate (in men only),[72] and possibly increased physical activity. The relationship with physical activity is complex because increased activity decreases overall CHD risk, but death, when it does occur, may be more likely to be sudden.[73] This supposition is supported by the data of Friedman et al,[53] who showed that a substantial number of sudden deaths occurred during or shortly after strenuous exercise. Other studies have showed either no relationship[74] or a protective effect[75] of physical activity on the risk of sudden death.

Psychosocial Factors

Psychosocial factors such as social isolation and recent life change have been associated with SCD.[76,77] An increased risk of coronary events has been reported in those with an increased life-change score in the preceding 6 months and was especially notable for sudden death.[76] A study of sudden death in women[77] showed increased risk among those who were not married, had fewer children, and had greater differences in education level from their spouses. Prior psychiatric treatment, alcohol use, and cigarette smoking were also associated with increased risk.[77] A study of 2320 men surviving MI showed increased risks of sudden and total deaths associated with social isolation and high life stress, both of which were also associated with low education levels.[78] Type A personality has also been associated with an increased incidence of sudden death, as with many other manifestations of coronary disease.[79]

Electrocardiographic Abnormalities

Electrocardiographic abnormalities such as intraventricular conduction disturbance, ventricular premature contractions, and nonspecific ST- and T-wave changes have also been associated with sudden death in persons with known CHD in the 30-year follow-up of the Framingham cohort.[8] In addition, intraventricular conduction delay may be related to an increased proportion of CHD deaths occurring suddenly.[72] As mentioned above, pre-excitation syndromes and prolongation of the QT interval are also associated with sudden death.

Sex Differences in Risk of Sudden Death

Further analyses of data from the Framingham study indicate substantial differences in risk factors for sudden death in women compared to men. Hematocrit, for example, was associated with sudden death incidence in women with or without prior CHD, while no relationship was found in men. Vital capacity, serum cholesterol levels, and serum glucose levels were all associated with sudden death in women without prior CHD, but not in those with prior CHD. Systolic blood pressure, weight, and cigarette smoking were not associated with sudden death incidence in women. The lack of relationship with smoking may be due to the inclusion of factors such as hematocrit and vital capacity, which may more accurately reflect the physiological effects of smoking than does a simple yes/no variable. Other investigators have noted weak associations between smoking and sudden death in women.[71,80] As mentioned earlier, psychosocial factors and educational level appear to play an important role in sudden death risk in women. Few studies, however, have encountered sufficient numbers of CHD deaths in women to permit accurate estimates of risk.

SUMMARY

Sudden cardiac death is a distressingly common outcome of established CHD, accounting in many studies for close to half of all CHD deaths. In a smaller proportion (20–25% in older series), sudden death may the first and only manifestation of CHD. Prodromal symptoms such as fatigue, dyspnea, and chest pain may occur in a large proportion of patients without being recognized as such. Prehospital delay may contribute to the risk of sudden death, particularly among men.

The risk of SCD increases with age, is greater in men than in women, and appears to be greater in blacks than in whites, especially black women. Incidence, risk factors, geographic distribution, circadian variation, and temporal trends parallel closely those for other forms of CHD. Declines in SCD appear to account for a large proportion of the decline in CHD mortality evident since the mid-1970s.

Epidemiological studies of SCD are hampered by a lack of standard definitions and by the need to rely on death certificate data for many national and international comparisons. Autopsy data are most useful in ruling out competing causes of death but are available in only a selected subset. Since most patients are stricken outside the hospital, primary prevention may be the only effective method for reducing the incidence of sudden death. Much of the recent decline in sudden death is attributed to improvements in cardiovascular risk factors such as hypertension and smoking. Rapid response emergency systems may also have played a role, particularly in urban areas.

REFERENCES

1. Doyle JT, Kannel WB, McNamara PM, Quickenton P, Gordon T: Factors related to suddenness of coronary death: Combined Albany-Framingham studies. Am J Cardiol 37:1073–1078, 1976.
2. Kuller LH, Perper JA, Dai WS, Rutan G, Traven N: Sudden death and the decline in coronary heart disease mortality. J Chronic Dis 39:1001–1019, 1986.
3. Goldberg RJ: Declining out-of-hospital sudden coronary death rates: Additional pieces of the epidemiologic puzzle [editorial]. Circulation 79:1369–1373, 1989.
4. Lancisi GH: De Subitaneis Mortibus, 1707, transl. by PD White and AV Boursy: On Sudden Deaths. New York, St. John's University Press, 1981.
5. Gillum RF: Sudden coronary death in the United States: 1980–1985. Circulation 79: 756–765, 1989.
6. Perper JA, Kuller LH, Cooper M: Arteriosclerosis of coronary arteries in sudden, unexpected death. Circulation 51:27–33, 1975.
7. Kuller L, Lilienfeld A, Fisher R: Epidemiological study of sudden and unexpected deaths due to arteriosclerotic heart disease. Circulation 34:1056–1068, 1966.
8. Kannel WB, Cupples LA, D'Agostino RB: Sudden death risk in overt coronary heart disease: The Framingham study. Am Heart J 113:799–804, 1987.
9. National Center for Health Statistics: Vital Statistics of the United States, 1984. Vol. II. Mortality Part A. Department of Health and Human Services publication No. (PHS) 87-1122. Public Health Service, Washington, D.C., U.S. Government Printing Office, 1987.
10. World Health Organization: Manual of the International Statistical Classification of Diseases, Injuries, and Causes of Death. Geneva, World Health Organization, 1977, pp 259–271.
11. Gillum RF: Geographic variation in sudden coronary death. Am Heart J 119:380–389, 1990.
12. Eisenberg M, Bergner L, Hallstrom A: Paramedic programs and out-of-hospital cardiac arrests: I. Factors associated with successful resuscitation. Am J Public Health 69:30–38, 1979.
13. Schatzkin A, Cupples LA, Heeren T, Morelock S, Mucatel M, Kannel WB: The epidemiology of sudden unexpected death: Risk factors for men and women in the Framingham Heart Study. Am Heart J 107: 1300–1306, 1984.
14. Elveback LR, Connolly DC, Kulrand LT: Coronary heart disease in residents of Rochester, Minnesota: II. Mortality, incidence, and survivorship, 1950–1975. Mayo Clin Proc 56:655–672, 1981.
15. Chiang BN, Perlman LV, Fulton M, Ostrander LD, Epstein FH: Predisposing factors in sudden cardiac death in Tecumseh, Michigan. Circulation 41:31–37, 1970.
16. Kuller LH, Lilienfeld AM, Fisher R: An epidemiological study of sudden and unexpected deaths in adults. Medicine 46: 341–361, 1967.
17. Hagstrom RM, Federspiel CF, Ho YC: Incidence of myocardial infarction and sudden death from coronary heart disease in Nashville, Tennessee. Circulation 44:884–890, 1971.
18. Gillum RF, Folsom A, Luepker RV, et al: Sudden death and acute myocardial infarction in a metropolitan area, 1970–1980. N Engl J Med 309:1353–1358, 1983.
19. Kannel WB, Doyle JT, McNamara PM, Quickenton P, Gordon T: Precursors of sudden coronary death. Circulation 51:606–613, 1975.
20. Goldberg RJ, Gore JM, Alpert JS, Dalen JE: Incidence and case fatality rates of acute myocardial infarction (1975–1984): The Worcester Heart Attack Study. Am Heart J 115:751–767, 1988.
21. Myocardial Infarction Community Registers: Public Health in Europe 5. Copenhagen, Regional Office for Europe, World Health Organization, 1976.

22. Suhonen O, Reunanen A, Knekt P, Aromaa A: Risk factors for sudden and nonsudden coronary death. Acta Med Scand 223:19–23, 1988.
23. Salonen JT: Primary prevention of sudden coronary death: A community-based program in North Karelia, Finland. Ann NY Acad Sci 382:423–437, 1982.
24. Xiang-gu Z, Shou-qi T, Shu-yu W: A community study of acute myocardial infarction and coronary sudden death. Chinese Med J 96:495–498, 1983.
25. Beaglehole R, Bonita R, Jackson R, Stewart A, et al: Trends in coronary heart disease event rates in New Zealand. Am J Epidemiol 120:225–235, 1984.
26. Madsen AK: Ischaemic heart disease and prodromes of sudden cardiac death. Br Heart J 54:27–32, 1985.
27. Gillum RF: Coronary heart disease mortality in United States blacks, 1940–1978: Trends and unanswered questions. Am Heart J 108:728–731, 1984.
28. Gillum RF: Coronary heart disease in black populations: I. Mortality and morbidity. Am Heart J 104:839–851, 1982.
29. Report of the Secretary's Task Force on Black and Minority Health. Volume IV: Cardiovascular and Cerebrovascular Disease, Part 1. U.S. Department of Health and Human Services, January 1986, p 97.
30. Keil JE, Loadholt CB, Weinrich MC, Sandifer SH, Boyle E: Incidence of coronary heart disease in blacks in Charleston, South Carolina. Am Heart J 108:779–786, 1984.
31. Kannel WB, Schatzkin A: Sudden death: Lessons from subsets in population studies. J Am Coll Cardiol 5(suppl):141B–149B, 1985.
32. Multiple Risk Factor Intervention Trial Research Group: Multiple Risk Factor Intervention Trial. JAMA 248:1465–1477, 1982.
33. Gillum RF, Grant CT: Coronary heart disease in black populations: II. Risk factors. Am Heart J 104:852–864, 1982.
34. Havlik RJ, Feinleib M (eds): Proceedings of the Conference on the Decline in Coronary Heart Disease Mortality. U.S. Department of Health, Education, and Welfare, NIH publication No. 79–1610, May 1979, pp xxiii–xxvii.
35. Higgins MW, Luepker RV (eds): Trends in Coronary Heart Disease Mortality. New York, Oxford University Press, 1988, pp vii–x.
36. Elveback LR, Connally DC: Coronary heart disease in Rochester, Minnesota: V. Prognosis in coronary heart disease by initial manifestation. Mayo Clin Proc 60:305–311, 1985.
37. Higgins MW, Luepker RV (eds): Trends in Coronary Heart Disease Mortality. New York, Oxford University Press, 1988, p 293.
38. Hsia DC, Krushat WM, Fagan AB, Tebbutt JA, Kusserow RP: Accuracy of diagnostic coding for Medicare patients under the prospective-payment system. N Engl J Med 318:352–355, 1988.
39. Muller JE, Stone PH, Turi ZG, et al: Circadian variation in the frequency of onset of acute myocardial infarction. N Engl J Med 313:1315–1322, 1985.
40. Muller JE, Ludmer PL, Willich SN, et al: Circadian variation in the frequency of sudden cardiac death. Circulation 75:131–138, 1987.
41. Willich SN, Levy D, Rocco MB, Tofler GH, Stone PH, Muller JE: Circadian variation in the incidence of sudden cardiac death in the Framingham Heart Study population. Am J Cardiol 60:801–806, 1987.
42. Peters RW: Propranolol and the morning increase in sudden cardiac death: The Beta-Blocker Heart Attack Trial experience. Am J Cardiol 66:57G–59G, 1990.
43. Willich SN: Epidemiologic studies demonstrating increased morning incidence of sudden cardiac death. Am J Cardiol 66:15G–17G, 1990.
44. Tofler GH, Brezinski D, Schafer AI: Concurrent morning increase in platelet aggregability and the risk of myocardial infarction and sudden cardiac death. N Engl J Med 316:1514–1518, 1987.
45. Turton MB, Deegan T: Circadian variations of plasma catecholamines, cortisol, and immunoreactive insulin concentrations in supine subjects. Clin Chim Acta 55:389–397, 1974.
46. Beard CM, Fuster V, Elveback LR: Daily and seasonal variation in sudden cardiac death, Rochester, Minnesota, 1950–1975. Mayo Clin Proc 57:704–706, 1982.
47. Myers A, Dewar HA: Circumstances attending 100 sudden deaths from coronary artery disease with coroner's necropsies. Br Heart J 37:1133–1143, 1975.
48. Rabkin SW, Mathewson FAL, Tate RB: Chronobiology of cardiac sudden death in men. JAMA 244:1357–1358, 1980.
49. Rogot E, Fabsitz R, Feinleib M: Daily variation in USA mortality. Am J Epidemiol 103:198–211, 1976.
50. Kuller L: Sudden death: Definition and epidemiologic considerations. Prog Cardiovasc Dis 23:1–12, 1980.
51. Feinleib M, Simon AB, Gillum RF, et al: Prodromal symptoms and signs of sudden death. Circulation 52(6 Suppl 3):155–159, 1975.

52. Kuller L: Sudden and unexpected non-traumatic deaths in adults: A review of epidemiological and clinical studies. J Chronic Dis 19:1165–1192, 1966.
53. Friedman M, Manwaring JH, Rosenman RH, et al: Instantaneous and sudden deaths: Clinical and pathological differentiation in coronary artery disease. JAMA 225:1319–1328, 1973.
54. Kuller LH: Prodromata of sudden death and myocardial infarction. Adv Cardiol 5:1–14, 1979.
55. Simon AB, Feinleib M, Thompson HK: Components of delay in the pre-hospital phase of acute myocardial infarction. Am J Cardiol 30:476–482, 1972.
56. Virmani R, Roberts WC: Sudden cardiac death. Hum Pathol 18:485–492, 1987.
57. Myerburg RJ, Kessler KM, Bassett AL, Castellanos A: A biological approach to sudden cardiac death: Structure, function and cause. Am J Cardiol 63:1512–1516, 1989.
58. Davies MJ, Thomas A: Thrombosis and acute coronary-artery lesions in sudden cardiac ischemic death. N Engl J Med 310:1137–1140, 1984.
59. Rissanen V, Romo M, Siltanen P: Prehospital sudden death from ischaemic heart disease: A postmortem study. Br Heart J 40:1025–1033, 1978.
60. Schaffer WA, Cobb LA: Recurrent ventricular fibrillation and modes of death in survivors of out-of-hospital ventricular fibrillation. N Engl J Med 293:259–262, 1975.
61. Baum RS, Alvares H, Cobb LA: Survival after resuscitation from out-of-hospital ventricular fibrillation. Circulation 50:1231–1235, 1974.
62. Roberts WC: Sudden cardiac death: A diversity of causes with focus on atherosclerotic coronary artery disease. Am J Cardiol 65:13B–19B, 1990.
63. Koren MJ, Devereux RB, Casale PN, Savage DD, Laragh JH: Relation of left ventricular mass and geometry to morbidity and mortality in uncomplicated essential hypertension. Ann Intern Med 114:345–352, 1991.
64. Chesler E, King RA, Edwards JE: The myxomatous mitral valve and sudden death. Circulation 67:632, 1983.
65. Myerburg RJ, Castellanos A: Cardiac arrest and sudden cardiac death. In Braunwald E (ed): Heart Disease, 3rd ed. Philadelphia, WB Saunders, 1988.
66. Moss AJ, Schwartz PJ. Sudden death and the idiopathic long Q-T syndrome. Am J Med 66:6–7, 1979.
67. Wennerblom B, Holmberg S. Death outside hospital with special reference to heart disease. Eur Heart J 5:266–274, 1984.
68. Thomas AC, Knapman PA, Krikler DM, Davies MJ: Community study of the causes of "natural" sudden death. Br Med J 297:1453–1456, 1988.
69. Matoba R, Shikata I, Iwai K, et al: An epidemiologic and histopathological study of sudden cardiac death in Osaka Medical Examiner's Office. Jpn Circ J 53:1581–1588, 1989.
70. Fawal ME, Berg GA, Wheatley DJ, Harland WA: Sudden coronary death in Glasgow: Nature and frequency of acute coronary lesions. Br Heart J 57:329–335, 1987.
71. Talbott E, Kuller LH, Perper J, et al: Sudden unexpected death in women: Biologic and psychosocial origins. Am J Epidemiol 114:671–682, 1981.
72. Kannel WB, Thomas HE Jr: Sudden coronary death: The Framingham study. Ann NY Acad Sci 382:3, 1982.
73. Kannel WB, Sorlie PD: Some health benefits of physical activity: The Framingham study. Arch Intern Med 139:857, 1979.
74. Paffenbarger RS, Wing AL, Hyde RT: Physical activity as an index of heart attack risk in college alumni. Am J Epidemiol 108:161, 1978.
75. Siscovick DS, Weiss NS, Hallstrom AP, et al: Physical activity and primary cardiac arrest. N Engl J Med 248:3113, 1982.
76. Rahe RH, Romo M, Bennett L, Siltman P: Recent life changes, myocardial infarction, and abrupt coronary death. Arch Intern Med 133:221, 1974.
77. Talbott E, Kuller LH, Detre K, Perper J: Biologic and psychosocial risk factors of sudden death from coronary disease in white women. Am J Cardiol 39:858, 1977.
78. Ruberman W, Weinblatt, Goldberg JD, Chaudhary BS: Psychosocial influences on mortality after myocardial infarction. N Engl J Med 311:552, 1984.
79. Friedman M, Rosenman RH: Association of specific overt behavior patterns with blood and cardiovascular findings. JAMA 169:1286, 1959.
80. Krueger DE, Ellenberg SS, Bloom S, et al: Risk factors for fatal heart attack in young women. Am J Epidemiol 113:357–370, 1981.

2

Anatomical Features in Victims of Sudden Coronary Death: Coronary Artery Pathology

MICHAEL J. DAVIES

DEFINITIONS

It is ostensibly a simple task to describe the morphology of the lesions found in the coronary arteries in victims of sudden ischemic death; there are, after all, 350,000 deaths per annum in the United States from this cause, and for legal reasons many are subject to autopsy.[1] Pathological studies are remarkable for their lack of uniformity concerning the nature of the lesions present in the coronary arteries. For example, a review of 17 papers that looked for the presence of occluding coronary thrombi at autopsy in sudden ischemic death found a range of 4–64% of cases.[2] The explanation for such divergent data probably lies in the use of different definitions. In 1895 Humpty Dumpty was reported by Lewis Carroll to expound the view, in conversation with Alice, that, "When I use a word it means just what I choose it to mean, neither more nor less." This is a paradigm of the use of definitions for each and every component of sudden ischemic death, definitions so different that authors are seldom writing about equivalent groups of subjects. Different selection criteria for entry into any study will predetermine the type of morphological lesion found at autopsy.

Despite the difficulties concerning definitions, a common theme has emerged from both pathological and clinical studies. This view, stated in its simplest form, is that sudden ischemic death is not a homogeneous phenomenon affecting one subset of patients with new acute myocardial ischemia and another subset of patients without acute ischemia but with an arrhythmogenic substrate based on left ventricular (LV) scarring and hypertrophy. This concept has been expressed by a number of terms, including myocardial ischemia versus ventricular dysfunction[3] and as acute versus chronic arrhythmogenic myocardial tissue.[4] Attempts have been made to relate the timing and clinical manifestations of sudden death with the mechanisms involved. It has been assumed that instantaneous death equates with an arrhythmia arising on the basis of chronic myocardial scarring, while deaths after a longer period of symptoms were associated with significant areas of acute infarction and mechanical contractile dysfunction (nonarrhythmic death).[5,6] Classification of death as sudden or nonsudden has not, however, proved a sensitive means of distinguishing the two forms of sudden ischemic death.[3,6,7] The difficulties encountered by these clinical studies highlight yet again the problem of definitions. Every component of the term *sudden ischemic death* is subject to a different interpretation.

Sudden has been defined as time intervals of less than 1 minute (instantaneous) up to 24 hours from the onset of symptoms before death.[8] A period of 24 hours significantly influences the pathology present at autopsy and will include many deaths from in-hospital cardiogenic shock due to established infarction. Periods of time of less than 6 hours between onset of symptoms and death are more usually accepted, with a subdivision into deaths that are instantaneous, those occurring in less than 1 hour, and those occurring between 1 and 6 hours after the onset of symptoms. Many studies are of subjects who have been well, leading a normal life outside the hospital, and who are not expected to die by relatives or the medical practitioner. Some studies have focused specifically on sudden death in patients with heart failure and ischemic heart disease and who thus have radically different underlying pathology. Studies may not be comparable in the number of subjects who die suddenly without a previous known history of ischemic heart disease (IHD) and those known to have recovered from an infarct in the past. Further problems are created by cases in which, although the death was witnessed as instantaneous, questions asked of a partner or spouse indicate that episodes of prodromal chest pain unrecognized as cardiac had occurred in the few days preceding death. Such cases would be included as sudden within some series, rejected from others.

Whether death was truly due to coronary artery disease can best be decided on the negative side by exclusion of any other possible cause of death by a careful autopsy. The positive side is that evidence of significant coronary atherosclerosis should be present. The question arises as to the threshold at which coronary atherosclerosis can be considered to cause death, given that the background level of arterial disease in Western populations is high. Up to 15% of males under 69 years of age with a clear noncardiac cause of death have at least single-vessel coronary artery stenosis of over 50% by diameter.[9,10] In practice, the dual criteria of the absence of any other cause of death and at least one segment of high-grade stenosis (>50% diameter) are used to categorize death as "ischemic." It is, however, a diagnosis based on probability, not certainty. Very few pathologists measure the degree of stenosis or carry out postmortem angiography; whether coronary atherosclerosis at autopsy is "significant" becomes a subjective opinion in many cases. Even death is now a qualified term, with electrophysiological studies being reported on survivors of out-of-hospital cardiac arrest. These survivors of sudden death are often taken as representative of the original group before cardiac arrest occurred; in truth, the survivors are highly selected.

In comparing studies of sudden ischemic death it must always be asked, therefore, how these different definitions and selection factors have been applied. When this is done the discrepancies between the reported frequency of new acute myocardial ischemia and arrhythmias arising in a scarred myocardium are far more understandable.

THE PROPORTION OF SUDDEN DEATH DUE TO CORONARY DISEASE

Coronary atherosclerosis is usually considered to be the single most common cause of sudden natural death.

Personal experience of the morphological basis of sudden cardiac death was obtained from a study in the Wandsworth area (population 190,000) of London that was carried out over a 3-year period.[9,10] Autopsies were performed on 322 consecutive subjects (male or female, caucasian, <65 years old) with witnessed sudden death (<6 hours after onset of symptoms) who were dead on arrival or could not be resuscitated in the admission room of the hospital. All the subjects had been well and able to work and had not consulted their doctors in the preceding 3 weeks. No subject with chronic heart failure was included. The study involved quantification of the whole coronary arterial tree after angiography. Death was ascribed to coronary heart disease (CHD) when there was no other cause of death and there was a minimum of one major coronary artery with stenosis of more than 75% by cross-sectional area. Sudden natural death from all causes (cardiac and noncardiac) was more common in men than women—238 (73.9%) vs. 84 (26.1%). In men, IHD accounted for 65.1% of all natural sudden deaths, while it accounted for 40.4% of deaths in women. The proportion of deaths due to IHD in men at time intervals of less than 15 minutes, less than 1 hour, and less than 6 hours after onset of symptoms did not differ. Cardiac nonischemic death occurred in 5.9% of men and 11.9% of women.

This study therefore confirmed that coronary artery disease is numerically the single most common cause of cardiac sudden death in males. This finding is in accord both with other autopsy data[11] and with data obtained from large epidemiological studies[12] using death certification.

The high background level of coronary atherosclerosis in asymptomatic individuals is always a factor that must be considered by pathologists when making decisions on whether sudden death is really due to CHD. Several reports have stressed the high background level of atherosclerosis in individuals who die in war or accidents.[13–15] The control population in our own study of SCD in the Wandsworth area of London was made up of caucasian individuals without any history of IHD who died suddenly of trauma, suicide, or natural diseases such as intracerebral hemorrhage or aortic dissection. In 124 males, coronary arteriography and quantification of the severity of stenosis showed that 15 (10.3%) had single-vessel disease, four (2.8%) had double-vessel disease, and two (1.4%) had triple-vessel disease. Thus, any decision that death is due directly to coronary atherosclerosis must be supported by rigorous exclusion at autopsy of any other possible cause of death.

MORPHOLOGICAL STUDIES OF CORONARY LESIONS IN SUDDEN DEATH

There is agreement that the number and distribution of chronic stenoses found at autopsy in SCD do not significantly differ from that found in patients with stable angina or previous infarction who do not die suddenly. One study of 70 sudden deaths due to coronary artery disease reported 15% to have single-vessel disease, 27% double-vessel disease, 47% triple-vessel disease, and 10% disease of all three vessels plus left main stenosis.[16] Another study of 121 cases of sudden death without previous infarction gave figures of 20%, 32%, and 48%, while in 118 cases with previous infarction the figures were 12%, 26%, and 62% for single-, double-, and triple-vessel disease.[17] A similar study of 205 cases of sudden ischemic death in Wandsworth found the figures to be 26%, 39%, and 33% respectively for single-, double-, and triple-vessel disease.[9] These three studies actually measured the degree of stenosis present, but previous studies in which the lesions were assessed by visual methods gave very similar results.[18–23] One facet of the previously reported studies that highlights the difficulty of comparisons is that in one study,[23] 24% of the cases had no segments of stenosis visually graded as severe (>50% of diameter), and thus the question arises as to whether these patients in reality died of other unrecognized cardiac disease.[23] The number of arterial segments that are significantly narrowed is higher in cases of sudden death in which there is a previous history of angina or infarction.[24] There are no data to suggest that the frequency of eccentric, calcified, or recanalized segments is different in cases of sudden as compared with nonsudden ischemic death.

There is far less agreement on the presence or absence of acute coronary thrombi in sudden ischemic death. Prior to 1980, a number of studies were reported in which major occluding thrombi in the coronary arteries were sought at autopsy by naked eye examination without the benefit of postmortem angiography. Some of these studies used a temporal definition of "sudden" as long as 24 hours and must have included cases with established regional infarction, which would result in a high frequency of thrombi. The overall figures gave a range of 4–64% for the occurrence of major thrombi.[2,25] The time interval did not appear to be the factor behind the variable frequency; one of the largest studies, comprising 220 subjects who died within 15 minutes of onset of symptoms, found coronary thrombi in 58%.[21]

The decade following publication of these studies has seen a realization that thrombosis over a culprit unstable plaque is the major cause of both type B unstable angina and acute regional myocardial infarction (MI). Thrombosis may develop either because of a superficial injury to the plaque with loss of the endothelium or because of deep injury in which a tear or fissure extends from the lumen into the center of the plaque itself.[26–28] Three quarters of major thrombi follow deep intimal injury to a plaque.[27]

Progression of Coronary Thrombosis and Plaque Instability

The initial event that develops following a tear from the lumen into the core of a lipid-rich plaque is entry of blood, followed by thrombus formation within the intima itself, expanding the plaque volume and altering its configuration. A sudden increase in the degree of arterial obstruction may result from this plaque expansion. The thrombus within the plaque is rich in platelets, their numbers suggesting that blood must enter and leave the interior of the plaque over some time. The interior of the plaque contains an intensely thrombogenic surface both because of exposed collagen, which is a potent platelet-activating agonist, and because of tissue factor.[29]

The second stage of the thrombotic process is characterized by a mass of thrombus that projects into the lumen from the torn plaque. This thrombus is initially mural, that is, it does not occlude the vessel, thus allowing antegrade blood flow to continue. Exposed thrombus of this type may act as a nidus for embolization of platelet clumps into the more distal vascular bed. These mural thrombi occurring over fissured plaques give rise to a characteristic angiographic morphology both before and after death.[26,30] The stenosis is eccentric, with ragged or overhanging edges, and there may be an associated intraluminal filling defect (Fig. 2–1). These appearances have been designated type II to distinguish them from the smooth stenoses typical of stable angina (type I). Type II lesions are found in unstable angina, in the artery supplying nontransmural infarcts, and in arteries that have been reopened after fibrinolysis during acute infarction.[31-34] Coronary angioscopy in living patients has confirmed that type II angiographic lesions are torn plaques with overlying thrombus.[35]

Thrombosis that occludes the vessel, preventing all antegrade flow, is the third and final stage of the process. The three stages represent points in a dynamic spectrum: mural thrombus may become occlusive and vice versa over short periods of time. The amount of regional myocardial necrosis that develops after complete occlusion by thrombosis is very variable, depending on the degree of previous collateral formation and the speed and duration of thrombus formation.

Previous studies of the pathology of the coronary arteries in sudden ischemic death have not used postmortem angiography and are likely to have underestimated the frequency of mural thrombosis. The third stage, occlusive thrombus, is more easily identified by dissection techniques in which multiple cross sections of the coronary ar-

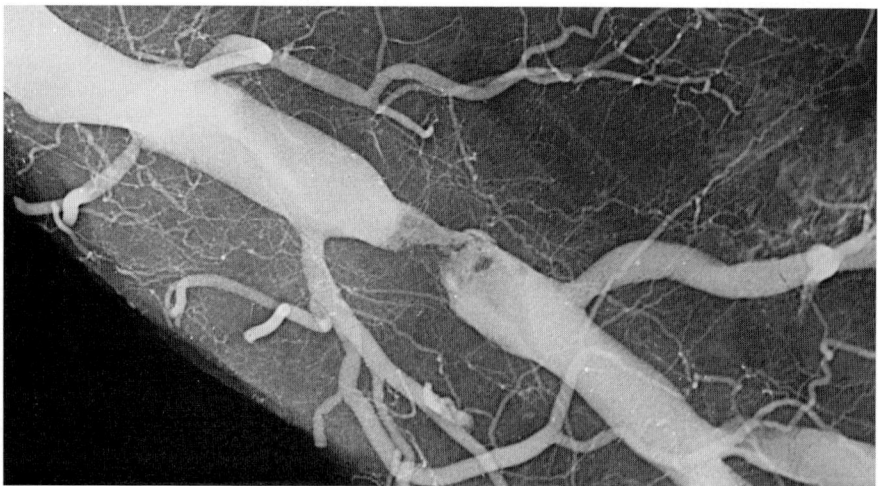

Fig. 2–1. Typical type II stenosis with an eccentric ragged outline and associated intraluminal filling defect. While regarded clinically as the hallmark of unstable angina, on postmortem angiography it is equally the angiogram of sudden cardiac death.

teries are cut by hand and examined by the naked eye.

Coronary Thrombosis in Sudden Ischemic Death

Our own pilot study of 100 cases of sudden ischemic death used postmortem coronary arteriography as a routine method,[36] and it became apparent that type II lesions on postmortem angiograms could be regarded as characteristic of sudden ischemic death, analogous to the way in which they were the hallmark of unstable angina in living patients undergoing angiography. Detailed histological analysis of lesions identified by postmortem angiography showed that a stage I thrombus (intraplaque thrombus only) was found in 21% of individuals dying suddenly from IHD; stage II and III thrombi (intraluminal thrombus with intraplaque thrombus) were found in 74%. Thus, 95% of individuals who died suddenly from coronary artery disease had at least one unstable plaque.

These figures concerning the frequency with which various forms of thrombosis can be found in sudden ischemic death must be considered in the context of what would be found in subjects with coronary atherosclerosis who die suddenly of noncardiac causes, including trauma. Such a series is difficult to collect but can be assembled from records of subjects with hypertension or diabetes, all of whom are likely to have atherosclerosis. In such a series,[10] detailed analysis of the whole coronary artery tree showed an appreciable prevalence of intraplaque thrombi associated with a recently healed plaque fissure. In subjects without hypertension the frequency was 8%; in subjects with hypertension and/or diabetes the figure rose to 16%. These figures suggest that plaque fissuring with the formation of an intraplaque thrombus is a common event in the natural history of plaque growth. It is probably the phenomenon responsible for the intermittent and unpredictable progression of stenoses demonstrated by sequential angiography.[37,38] The greater frequency of recent plaque fissure in control subjects with hypertension and diabetes may indicate a great number of plaques at risk or an increased risk of fissuring. The distinction between plaque tears that are clinically silent and lead only to an episode of plaque growth and those that are expressed clinically as unstable angina, infarction, or sudden death lies in whether intraluminal thrombus is found. A major determinant of whether such intraluminal thrombus will form is the magnitude of injury to the plaque: the larger the tear, the more likely is intraluminal thrombus to develop.

In relation to SCD, the pathologist is therefore not justified in ascribing a recent plaque fissure without overlying intraluminal thrombus as the initiator of ventricular fibrillation; if, however, there is overlying intraluminal thrombus formation, it can be regarded as causative with far greater certainty. Adopting this principle, it is therefore now our experience[10] that a minimum of 73.3% of SCDs are associated with an unstable plaque and intraluminal thrombosis that provide a basis for an episode of acute myocardial ischemia (Table 2–1).

Although a plaque that contains a recent thrombus as a result of fissuring but not an intraluminal thrombus cannot be taken as an incontrovertible cause of death, owing to the frequency of similar lesions in control hearts, some almost certainly do cause acute ischemia. In the 13 cases of plaque fissuring without an intraluminal thrombus but no other cause of death other than coronary atheroma, there was clear histological evidence in 5 of recent myocardial necrosis in the territory supplied by that artery. It is probable that intraluminal thrombus had been present at some time prior to death and had undergone spontaneous fibrinolysis. A further possibility, and one that cannot be excluded by any morphological method, is that plaque fissuring invokes intense local arterial spasm, which in turn causes acute regional ischemia.

Other recent pathological studies have also reported a high frequency of coronary thrombosis in sudden ischemic death,[39,40] while others have not found such a high frequency. In a technically meticulous study that also used coronary stenosis quantification, a figure as low as 20% was reported.[16,17,24] As emphasized by Roberts et al,[17] it is probably meaningless to compare modern data with data reported in earlier decades when detailed quantification was not carried out, but even so, there remains a major discrepancy between recent well-

Table 2–1
Distribution of Vascular Events in Control and Sudden Coronary Death Hearts

	Basal Control		Atheroma-Related Control		Sudden Ischemic Death	
	No.	(%)	No.	(%)	No.	(%)
No acute change in any plaque	63	(91.3)	47	(78.3)	32	(19)
Plaque fissure/intraintimal thrombus	6	(8.7)	10	(16.7)	13	(7.7)
Intraluminal nonocclusive thrombus	0		3	(5)	73	(43.5)
Occulsive thrombus	0		0		50	(29.8)
Total	69	(100)	60	(100)	168	(100)

conducted autopsy studies on the frequency of thrombosis and therefore acute myocardial ischemia in SCD.

The further studies carried out by our group therefore sought to examine the possible factors in case selection that might predetermine the presence or absence of acute coronary thrombi at autopsy (Table 2–2).[10] In a study of 168 subjects who died of CHD within 6 hours of the onset of acute symptoms, the variables of sex, a previous clinical history of IHD, a retrospective history of prodromal chest pain obtained from witnesses, the demonstration of acute or old regional infarction in the myocardium at autopsy, the number of coronary vessels with stenosis, and the LV mass were considered in relation to the presence or absence of intraluminal coronary thrombi at autopsy. Strong positive and negative associations of some of these factors with coronary thrombi were found.

Overall, in the 168 subjects, 123 (73.3%) had recent intraluminal coronary thrombus.[10] Prodromal chest pain and/or the presence of demonstrable MI at autopsy was present in 116 of the 168 subjects, and in this group 84% had coronary thrombosis. In the 52 patients without warning pain or demonstrable MI, only 48% had coronary thrombi. Thus, any autopsy series that uses warning pain or the presence of acute MI as exclusion criteria will of necessity report a lower frequency of coronary thrombosis (see Table 2–2). Conversely, selection of initial cases with old MI and a history of previous IHD will reduce the frequency of coronary thrombosis. In our study the number of vessels involved and the degree of LV hypertrophy were not predictive of the presence or absence of coronary thrombi. The exception was a small number of patients without previous MI and with no acute coronary lesion; in this subgroup an

Table 2–2
Sudden Coronary Death: Correlation of Presence or Absence of Coronary Thrombosis with Clinical Factors

	No Coronary Thrombus ($n = 32$)		Coronary Thrombus Present ($n = 32$)	
	No.	(%)	No.	(%)
Previous known history of ischemic heart disease	22	(69)	50	(41)
Old infarct at autopsy	25	(78)	61	(50)
Prodromal pain prior to collapse	7	(22)	76	(62)
Acute myocardial necrosis at autopsy	4	(13)	59	(50)

increase in LV mass was very striking. The results therefore suggest that the major factor in the apparent variability in the frequency of coronary thrombi in autopsy studies lies in case selection. If it is wished to create a pathology series with a high incidence of coronary thrombi, cases are used without a history of previous IHD, angina, or MI and with prodromal pain prior to death; to create the converse, a series with a low incidence of thrombosis, a series dominated numerically by patients with old infarction who did not have prodromal pain prior to death should be constructed.

MECHANISMS IN THE INDUCTION OF VENTRICULAR FIBRILLATION

The hypothesis that SCD is due either to new acute ischemia or to an arrhythmia arising in a scarred myocardium, and as a subsidiary question, the relative numerical proportion of each group, can be tested indirectly by pathological studies of the myocardium, by ambulatory monitoring of subjects with coronary atherosclerosis who happen by chance to die suddenly, and by consideration of the clinical, angiographic, electrocardiographic (ECG), and electrophysiological characteristics of subjects resuscitated from out-of-hospital cardiac arrest.

Pathological Studies of the Myocardium in Sudden Ischemic Death

The myocardial lesions present in sudden ischemic death are considered more fully in another section of this book, but some principles must also be considered here. It is often assumed that "acute myocardial infarction" has an absolute meaning. There are, however, problems for the pathologist, for the common form of coagulative necrosis found in regional transmural infarction does not become apparent histologically until the patient has lived for at least 6 hours following the event. It is thus entirely possible for a subject to have regional infarction by clinical criteria that cannot be confirmed pathologically. Contraction band necrosis is recognized earlier but occurs to some extent in ventricular fibrillation (VF) from any cause, and thus can be an agonal phenomenon; in such cases to call the morphological change infarction is inappropriate, and sensitivity has far outstripped specificity.

Nonoccluding intraluminal coronary thrombi are associated with emboli of platelet aggregates in the distal microvascular bed. These emboli, which occlude intramyocardial arterioles and capillaries up to 200 μm in external diameter, are more prevalent in the subepicardial zone than the subendocardial zone and are confined to the region of myocardium supplied by an artery containing a nonocclusive mural thrombus. Multifocal small areas of myocardial necrosis are a constant accompanying feature of platelet emboli. Autopsy studies have consistently showed that up to 50% of subjects dying suddenly have myocardial platelet emboli when these are specifically sought.[41,42] One series[42] found that the frequency of microemboli was doubled in patients with premonitory chest pain than in those who had no chest pain. Earlier studies had also emphasized the presence of platelet microthrombi in the myocardium[43,44] but had regarded them as indicative of an overall hypercoagulation state.

Ambulatory Monitoring at the Time of Death

Ambulatory sudden death, defined as unexpected sudden death from natural causes in a patient whose cardiac state is stable outside the hospital, has been recorded by Holter monitoring, and the cases reported up to 1988 in the literature have been reviewed by de Luna et al[45] In the 157 cases, VF developed in 62.4% following ventricular tachycardia (VT), primary developed in 8.3%, 16.5% had bradyarrhythmia, and 12.7% had torsades de pointes. Ischemic ST-segment changes preceding the arrhythmia were not common; overall, in the five series in which ST-segment changes were specifically looked for, the figure was 12.6%, with the highest being 26%. The low incidence of ischemia as demonstrated by ST-segment changes may not reflect the real frequency of acute ischemia as a factor precipitating sudden death. The sample is highly biased, for it included only patients undergoing monitoring for a clinical indication and therefore cannot reflect the generality of patients with coronary atherosclerosis. There are no patients in whom sudden death is the initial presentation, whereas such patients may account for as many as 40–50% of sudden deaths in the community. Finally, the ECG leads used are not those usually designed to detect ST-segment changes. Nevertheless, the results of ambulatory monitoring have been used as evidence to diminish the role of acute ischemia in sudden death.

Clinical Investigations of Subjects Resuscitated from Out-of-Hospital Cardiac Arrest

The proportion of patients resuscitated from out-of-hospital cardiac arrest and who are found subsequently to have developed acute infarction as judged by the appearance of new Q waves ranges from 19% to 44%.[21,46–49] If those patients who have elevated cardiac enzyme levels are included, the figures rise to 36% to 78%. Resuscitation itself, however, may cause increases in cardiac enzyme levels. The difficulty thus lies in adjusting the sensitivity of the method of detecting infarction clinically. Pathological studies show that many subjects who die suddenly have small foci of myocardial necrosis. It is uncertain whether this would be detected by current clinical methods, although more sensitive enzyme assays may do so in the future.

Coronary arteriography after resuscitation has provided some evidence of the presence of unstable plaques in a proportion of subjects who die suddenly from IHD. In a study of 49 survivors of out-of-hospital ischemic cardiac arrest without acute infarction, type II angiographic lesions were found in 16 (32.6%). When the 22 subjects without an inducible tachycardia were compared with the 27 subjects with an inducible tachycardia, the frequency of type II lesions was 50% vs. 19% ($p < 0.05$). These results have suggested that thrombosis played a part in causing ischemia and thus sudden death in subjects who do not have a chronic arrhythmogenic substrate.[50] Similar results were obtained in a study of 19 survivors of out-of-hospital cardiac arrest.[51]

CAUSES OF LATE SUDDEN DEATH AFTER ACUTE MYOCARDIAL INFARCTION

Patients who previously suffered an acute MI and recovered well, then die unexpectedly out of hospital, have been studied intensively, both clinically and pathologically. Such patients would be expected to exhibit a preponderance of sudden deaths due to primary VF since they already have a scar-determined substrate for VT. A clinical study of 867 survivors of acute MI found that 144 (17%) had died within 4 years.[7] Of these deaths, 107 were witnessed; 57 were judged to be arrhythmic in that the subject lost consciousness abruptly and the pulse ceased without prior circulatory collapse. Of these 57, 33 (58%) had chest pain, which was thought to indicate new ischemia just prior to death. Two autopsy studies of survivors of acute MI who subsequently died outside of a hospital support this proportion of deaths (approximately 60%) as being due to new ischemia. In a 2-year follow-up of 359 males, 35 died suddenly; 33 of these underwent autopsy and 23 (69.7%) were found to have new acute ischemic changes.[52] In another study of 28 out-of-hospital deaths later after infarction, 19 (68%) had evidence of new myocardial ischemia at autopsy.[53] Thus, in sudden death in patients with a healed infarct, new ischemia is still the predominant cause of a sudden ventricular arrhythmia.

NEW ISCHEMIA VERSUS CHRONIC NONISCHEMIC TACHYARRHYTHMIA IN SUDDEN ISCHEMIC DEATH

It is clear that new acute ischemia, irrespective of whether it progresses to acute infarction, plays a major role in the precipitation of sudden VF. The demonstration, however, of an acute lesion in the coronary artery acting as a putative cause of new ischemia can only be part of the story. The majority of patients who develop coronary thrombosis probably survive; new acute ischemia therefore represents a substrate on which other arrhythmogenic factors act. These factors range through circadian variation in vascular and sympathetic tone[54] to coexisting hypertrophy,[55] autonomic imbalance,[56,57] and electrolyte disturbances[58,59] that may alter myocardial electrical stability.

It is equally clear that a substantial group of patients with sudden ischemic death have a ventricular tachyarrhythmia in the presence of myocardial scarring and/or hypertrophy in the absence of acute ischemia. This group may make up 20-40% of all sudden ischemic deaths,[60] although, as discussed above, the series on which such figures are based comprise survivors of out-of-hospital cardiac arrest,[61,62] a highly selected subgroup.

What is perhaps important is to realize the complexity of the factors that interact to produce sudden ischemic death. In an individual, multiple mechanisms may coexist or even act synergistically.[60]

REFERENCES

1. Gillum R: Sudden coronary death in the United States, 1980-1985. Circulation 79: 756-765, 1989.
2. Davies M: Pathological view of sudden cardiac death. Br Heart J 45:88-96, 1981.
3. Goldstein S: Toward a new understanding of the mechanism and prevention of sudden death in coronary heart disease. Circulation 82:284-288, 1990.
4. Breithardt G, Borggrefe M, Podezeck A, Martinez-Rubio A: Mechanisms of syncope and of sudden death due to ventricular tachyarrhythmias. In Refsum H, Sulg I, Rasmussen K (eds): Heart and Brain. New York, Springer-Verlag, 1989, pp 165-184.
5. Hinkle L, Thaler H: Clinical classification of cardiac deaths. Circulation 65:457-464, 1982.
6. Greene H, Richardson D, Barker A, et al: Classification of deaths after myocardial infarction as arrhythmic or nonarrhythmic (The Cardiac Arrhythmia Pilot Study). Am J Cardiol 63:1-6, 1989.
7. Marcus F, Cobb L, Edwards J, et al: Mechanism of death and prevalence of myocardial ischemic symptoms in the terminal event after acute myocardial infarction. Am J Cardiol 61:8-15, 1988.
8. Goldstein S: The necessity of a uniform definition of sudden coronary death: Witnessed death within 1 hour of the onset of acute symptoms. Am Heart J 103:156-159, 1982.
9. Thomas A, Knapman P, Krikler D, Davies M: Community study of the causes of "natural" sudden death. Br Med J 297:1453-1456, 1988.
10. Davies M, Bland J, Hangartner J, Angelini A, Thomas A: Factors influencing the presence or absence of acute coronary artery thrombi in sudden ischemic death. Eur Heart J 10:203-208, 1989.
11. Wennerblom B, Homberg B: Death outside hospital with special reference to heart disease. Eur Heart J 5:266-274, 1984.
12. Kuller L: Sudden death: Definition and epidemiologic considerations. Prog Cardiovasc Dis 23:1-12, 1980.
13. Stary H: Evolution and progression of atherosclerotic lesions in coronary arteries of children and young adults. Arteriosclerosis 9:1-19, 1989.
14. Enos W, Holmes R, Beyer J: Coronary disease among United States soldiers killed in action in Korea. JAMA 152:1090-1093, 1953.
15. McNamara J, Molot M, Stremple J, Cutting R: Coronary artery disease in combat casualties in Vietnam. JAMA 216:1185-1187, 1971.
16. Warnes C, Roberts W: Sudden coronary death: Relation of amount and distribution of coronary narrowing at necropsy to previous symptoms of myocardial ischemia, left ventricular scarring and heart weight. Am J Cardiol 54:65-73, 1984.
17. Roberts W, Potkin B, Solus D, Reddy S: Mode of death, frequency of healed and acute myocardial infarction, number of major epicardial coronary arteries severely narrowed by atherosclerotic plaque, and heart weight in fatal atherosclerotic coronary artery disease: Analysis of 889 patients studied at necropsy. J Am Coll Cardiol 15: 196-203, 1990.
18. Kuller L, Perper J: Myocardial infarction and sudden death in an urban community. Bull NY Acad Med 49:532-543, 1973.
19. Friedman M, Manwaring J, Rosenman R, Dolan G, Ortega P, Grube S: Instantaneous and sudden deaths: Clinical and pathological differentiation in coronary artery disease. JAMA 225:1319-1328, 1973.
20. Liberthson R, Nagel E, Hirschman J, Nussenfeld S: Prehospital ventricular defibrillation: Prognosis and follow-up course. N Engl J Med 291:317-321, 1974.
21. Liberthson R, Nagel E, Hirschman J, Nussenfeld S, Blackbourne B, Davies J: Pathophysiologic observations in prehospital ventricular fibrillation and sudden cardiac death. Circulation 49:790-798, 1974.
22. Perper J, Kuller L, Cooper M: Arteriosclerosis of coronary arteries in sudden, unexpected death. Circulation 52:27-33, 1975.
23. Baroldi G, Falzi G, Mariani F. Sudden coronary death: A post mortem study in 298 selected cases compared to 97 "control" subjects. Am Heart J 98:20-31, 1979.
24. Warnes C, Roberts W: Sudden coronary death: Comparison of patients with those without coronary thrombus at necropsy. Am J Cardiol 54:1206-1211, 1984.

25. Thomas A, Davies M: Post mortem investigation and quantification of coronary artery disease. Histopathology 9:959–976, 1985.
26. Davies M, Thomas A: Plaque fissuring—the cause of acute myocardial infarction, sudden ischaemic death and crescendo angina. Br Heart J 53:363–373, 1985.
27. Davies M: A macroscopic and microscopic view of coronary thrombi. Circulation 82:1138–1146, 1990.
28. Constantinides P: Plaque fissures in human coronary thrombosis. J Atheroscl Res 6:1–17, 1966.
29. Wilcox J, Smith K, Schwartz S, Gordon D: Localization of tissue factor in the normal vessel wall and in the atherosclerotic plaque. Proc Natl Acad Sci USA 86:2839–2843, 1989.
30. Levin D, Fallon J: Significance of the angiographic morphology of localized coronary stenosis: Histopathologic correlations. Circulation 66:316–320, 1982.
31. Fuster V, Stein B, Badimon L, Chesebro J: Antithrombotic therapy after myocardial reperfusion in acute myocardial infarction. J Am Coll Cardiol 12A:78–84, 1988.
32. Gorlin R, Fuster V, Ambrose J: Anatomic-physiologic links between acute coronary syndromes. Circulation 74:6–9, 1986.
33. Ambrose J, Winters S, Arora R, et al: Coronary angiograph morphology in acute myocardial infarction: Link between the pathogenesis of unstable angina and myocardial infarction. J Am Coll Cardiol 6:1233–1238, 1985.
34. Ambrose J, Winters S, Stern A: Angiographic morphology and the pathogenesis of unstable angina. J Am Coll Cardiol 5:609–616, 1985.
35. Sherman C, Litvack F, Grundfest W: Coronary angioscopy in patients with unstable pectoris. N Engl J Med 315:913–919, 1986.
36. Davies M, Thomas A: Thrombosis and acute coronary artery lesions in sudden cardiac ischaemic death. N Engl J Med 310:1137–1140, 1984.
37. Bruschke A, Kramer J, Bal E, Haque I, Detranto R, Goormastic M: The dynamics of progression of coronary atherosclerosis studied in 168 medically treated patients who underwent coronary arteriography three times. Am Heart J 117:296–305, 1989.
38. Ambrose J, Tannenbaum M, Alexopoulos D, et al: Angiographic progression of coronary artery disease and the development of myocardial infarction. J Am Coll Cardiol 12:56–62, 1988.
39. El-Fawal M, Berg G, Whealey D, Harland W: Sudden coronary death in Glasgow: Nature and frequency of acute coronary lesions. Br Heart J 57:329–335, 1987.
40. van Dantzig J, Becker A: Sudden cardiac death and acute pathology of coronary arteries. Eur Heart J 7:987–991, 1986.
41. Falk E: Unstable angina with fatal outcome: Dynamic coronary thrombosis leading to infarction and/or sudden death. Circulation 71:699–708, 1985.
42. Davies M, Thomas A, Knapman P, Hangartner R: Intramyocardial platelet aggregation in patients with unstable angina suffering sudden ischemic cardiac death. Circulation 73:418–427, 1986.
43. Haerem J: Mural platelet microthrombi and major acute lesions of main epicardial arteries in sudden coronary death. Atherosclerosis 19:529–541, 1974.
44. El-Maraghi N, Genton E: The relevance of platelet and fibrin thromboembolism of the coronary microcirculation with special reference to sudden cardiac death. Circulation 62:936–944, 1980.
45. de Luna A, Coumel P, Leclercq J: Ambulatory sudden cardiac death: Mechanisms of production of fatal arrhythmia on the basis of data from 157 cases. Am Heart J 117:151–159, 1989.
46. Myerburg R, Conde C, Sung R: Clinical, electrophysiologic and hemodynamic profile of patients resuscitated from prehospital cardiac arrest. Am J Med 68:568–576, 1980.
47. Baum R, Alvarez H, Cobb L: Survival after resuscitation from out-of-hospital ventricular fibrillation. Circulation 50:1231–1235, 1974.
48. Goldstein S, Landis J, Leighton R, et al: Characteristics of the resuscitated out-of-hospital cardiac arrest victim with coronary heart disease. Circulation 64:977–984, 1981.
49. Schaffer WA, Cobb LA: Recurrent ventricular fibrillation and modes of death in survivors of out-of-hospital fibrillation. N Engl J Med 293:259–262, 1975.
50. Lo Y-SA, Cutler J, Blake K, Wright A, Kron J, Swerdlow C: Angiographic coronary morphology in survivors of cardiac arrest. Am Heart J 115:781–785, 1988.
51. Stevenson W, Wiener I, Yeatman L, Wohlgelernter D, Weiss J: Complicated atherosclerotic lesions: A potential cause of ischemic ventricular arrhythmias in cardiac arrest survivors who do not have inducible ventricular tachycardia? Am Heart J 116:1–6, 1988.
52. Vedin A, Willhelmsson C, Elmfelot D, Save-Doderbergh J, Tibblin G, Willhelmsen L: Deaths and non-fatal reinfarctions during two years' follow-up after myocardial infarction. Acta Med Scand 198:353–364, 1975.
53. Stevenson W, Linssen G, Havenith M, Brugada P, Wellens H: The spectrum of death

after myocardial infarction: A necropsy study. Am Heart J *118*(1182), 1989.
54. Panza JA, Epstein SE, Quyyumi AA: Circadian variation in vascular tone and its relation to α-sympathetic vasoconstrictor activity. N Engl J Med *325:*986–990, 1991.
55. Anderson HP: Sudden death, hypertension, and hypertrophy. J Cardiovasc Pharmacol *6(suppl III):*III-498–III-503, 1984.
56. Randall WC, Kaye MP, Hageman GR, Jacobs HK, Euler DE, Wehrmacher W: Cardiac dysrhythmias in the conscious dog after surgically induced autonomic imbalance. Am J Cardiol *38:*178–183, 1976.
57. Schwartz PJ, Stone HL: Left stellectomy in the prevention of ventricular fibrillation caused by acute myocardial ischemia in conscious dogs with anterior myocardial infarction. Circulation *62:*1256–1265, 1980.
58. Garan H, McGovern BA, Canzanello VJ, et al: The effect of potassium ion depletion on postinfarction canine cardiac arrhythmias. Circulation *77:*696–704, 1988.
59. Teo KK, Yusuf S, Collins R, Held PH, Peto R: Effects of intravenous magnesium in suspected acute myocardial infarction: Overview of randomized trials. Br Med J *303:* 1499–1503, 1991.
60. Meissner MD, Akhtar M, Lehmann MH: Nonischemic sudden tachyarrhythmic death in atherosclerotic heart disease. Circulation *84:*905–912, 1991.
61. Furukawa T, Rozanski JJ, Nogami A, Moroe K, Gosselin AJ, Lister JW: Time-dependent risk of and predictors for cardiac arrest recurrence in survivors of out-of-hospital cardiac arrest with chronic coronary artery disease. Circulation *80:*599–608, 1989.
62. Wilber DJ, Garan H, Finkelstein D, et al: Out-of-hospital cardiac arrest: Use of electrophysiologic testing in the prediction of long-term outcome. N Engl J Med *318:* 19–24, 1988.

3

Interactions Between Structure and Function in Sudden Cardiac Death

ROBERT J. MYERBURG
KENNETH M. KESSLER
AGUSTIN CASTELLANOS

The recognition of sudden cardiac death (SCD) as a major public health problem has evolved in the past three decades as epidemiologists, clinicians, and basic scientists began to focus efforts on understanding, managing, and preventing potentially fatal arrhythmias. As a result of these efforts, ventricular fibrillation (VF) and some forms of ventricular tachycardia (VT), that were almost uniformly fatal in all clinical settings (including in-hospital) 30 years ago can now be survived with appropriate interventions in many clinical settings. A major remaining limitation is the difficult chore of identifying potential victims *before* they enter into a clinical circumstance that predicts a fatal outcome in a very short time. Clinical prodromes, as currently understood, have not been generally helpful, and the time from onset of an acute clinical change that is predictive of a transition to cardiac arrest is too short to permit interventions in most individuals (Fig. 3–1). Therefore, the next major advance against the problem of SCD will have to come from the refinement and application of newer concepts of the pathophysiology of sudden death, which may allow the required forewarnings for prevention of initiating events. To this end, it is increasingly recognized that the abnormal electrophysiology operative in the genesis of potentially fatal arrhythmias is not unidimensional: predisposing electrophysiological factors interact with triggering events, and neither is independent of nonelectrophysiological factors.[1-3]

PATHOPHYSIOLOGICAL LIMITATIONS OF THE PVC HYPOTHESIS

The premature ventricular contraction (PVC) hypothesis states that there is a causal relationship between chronic PVCs and potentially fatal VT or VF. The hypothesis assumes that PVCs serve a triggering function under conditions that make ventricular muscle capable of sustaining VT or disorganizing into VF. The premise that PVC suppression protects against sudden death by eliminating the electrical triggering events derives from this hypothesis. However, clinical application of the PVC hypothesis, and the derived suppression theory, are limited by the fact that patients who are easily inducible into sustained arrhythmias during programmed electrical stimulation and have frequent and/or repetitive forms of PVCs, still require special circumstances to initiate spontaneous clinical events. These circumstances, which usually are not foreseen and may not be recognized

---

Supported in part by NHLBI research grants No. HL-28130 and No. HL-21735 (R.J.M.) and by the Florida Affiliate of the American Heart Association, Palm Beach Chapter, grant No. 89G1A85.

TIME REFERENCES IN SUDDEN CARDIAC DEATH

PRODROMES	ONSET OF TERMINAL EVENT	CARDIAC ARREST	BIOLOGICAL DEATH
NEW OR WORSENING CARDIOVASCULAR SYMPTOMS: CHEST PAIN PALPITATIONS DYSPNEA WEAKNESS FATIGUABILITY	ABRUPT CHANGE IN CLINICAL STATUS: ARRHYTHMIAS HYPOTENSION CHEST PAIN DYSPNEA LIGHTHEADEDNESS	SUDDEN COLLAPSE ----- LOSS OF EFFECTIVE CIRCULATION LOSS OF CONSCIOUSNESS	FAILURE OF RESUSCITATION - OR - FAILURE OF ELECTRICAL, MECHANICAL, OR CNS IMPROVEMENT AFTER INITIAL RESUSCITATION

INSTANTANEOUS TO 1 HOUR

Fig. 3–1. Time factors in sudden cardiac death. The interval between the onset of an acute change in cardiovascular status leads to a cardiac arrest is generally defined as ≤1 hour, too short to permit effective preventive measures. Clinical prodromes extending over longer periods of time, however, lack specificity. Preventive measures require new ways to forewarn of the terminal event. See text for details. (Modified and reproduced by permission from Myerburg RJ, et al.[6])

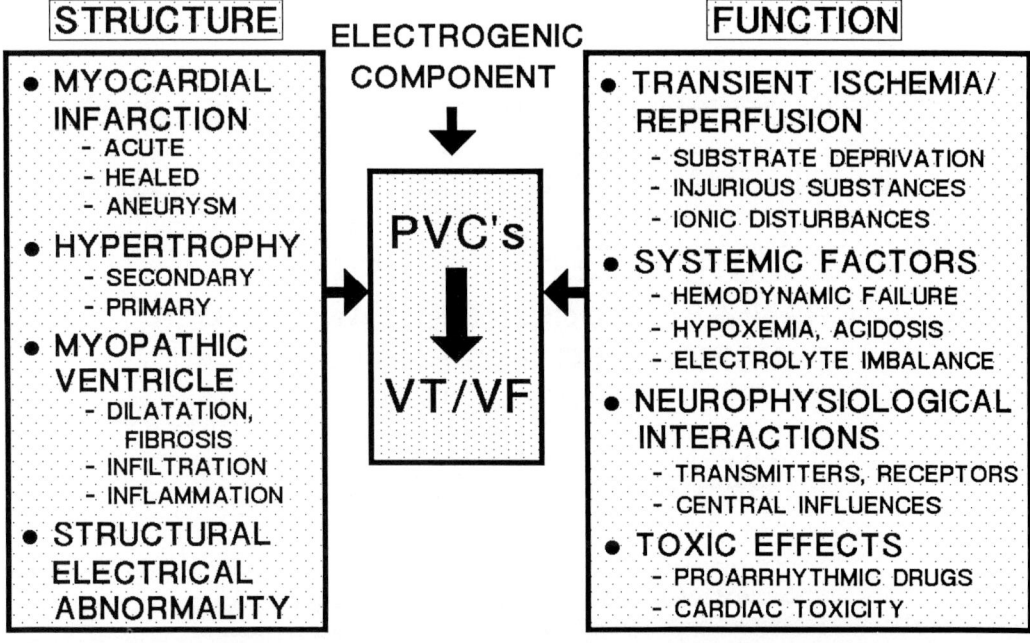

Fig. 3–2. Structure, function, and sudden death. Pathophysiological relationships between PVCs and potentially fatal ventricular tachycardia/fibrillation (VT/VF) (i.e., the electrogenic component of risk) require the interaction of two factors: (1) structural abnormalities, which serve as the substrate for sustained arrhythmias, and (2) transient functional changes, which are necessary for triggering an arrhythmia at a specific point in time. See text for details. (Modified and reproduced by permission from Myerburg RJ, et al: Am J Cardiol 63:1512–1516, 1989.[1])

even immediately prior to an event, may result from functional modulation of a pre-existing structural abnormality, serving as the link between the trigger and the clinical event. The PVC hypothesis is further questioned by results of clinical intervention studies, such as the Cardiac Arrhythmia Suppression Trial (CAST).[4] The fact that suppression of PVCs by two of the antiarrhythmic drugs in the study was associated with increased risk emphasizes the absence of a simple relationship between PVC and VT/VF. The PVC-VT/VF relationship is likely modified by other factors that influence the response of the ventricular myocardium to drugs.[5] A structure/function concept[1] explains many of these interactions. It states that the initiation of sustained tachyarrhythmias requires both a pre-existing structural abnormality that provides the condition for establishing pathways or foci responsible for sustained arrhythmias, and a modification of the pre-existing abnormality by functional changes at a specific point in time. The diagram in Figure 3-2 illustrates the elements that may participate in a relationship between structure/function and electrogenic factors. Furthermore, the cascade hypothesized by Figure 3-3 suggests that functional changes alter a stable electrophysiological abnormality, converting it to an unstable state because of transient changes in electrophysiology.

THE STRUCTURE/FUNCTION CONCEPT

References to causes of cardiac arrest or SCD often fail to distinguish between defined structural cardiac abnormalities and transient functional changes. Coronary heart disease (CHD) and ischemic mechanisms, or cardiomyopathy and heart failure, have been used interchangeably. As new information has become available, however,

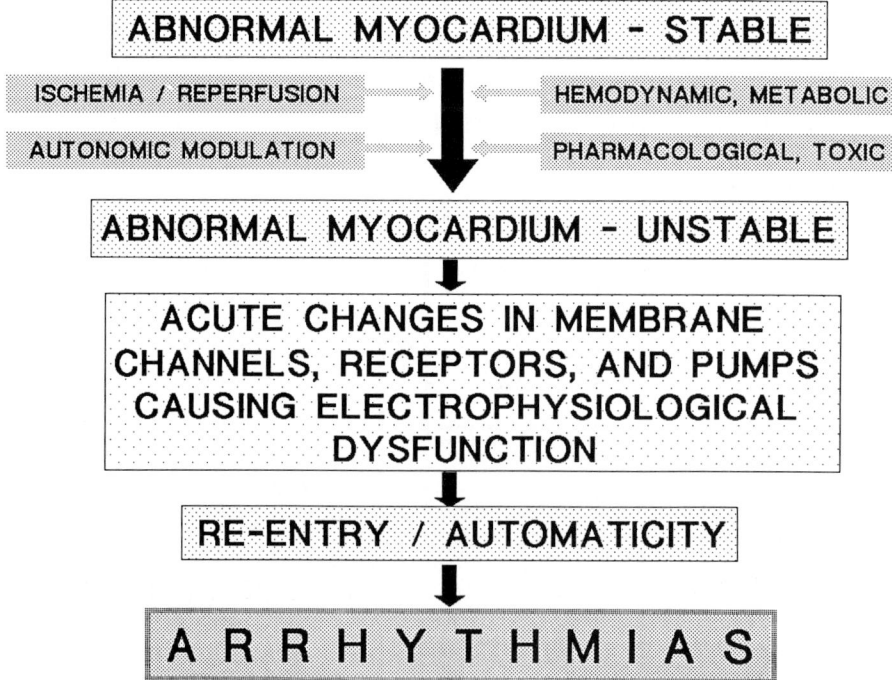

Fig. 3-3. Functional modulations responsible for destabilizing a structurally abnormal heart—An arrhythmic cascade. The abnormal heart has steady-state electrophysiological abnormalities that are stable until modifying influences cause changes that destabilize the myocardium. Acute or subacute changes in membrane channels, receptors, effectors, and pumps then cause electrical dysfunction, leading to the genesis of arrhythmias. (Reproduced with permission from Myerburg RJ, et al: PACE 14:935-943, 1991.[3])

it has become evident that pre-existing structural alterations and acute functional events are interactive, not physiologically or clinically synonymous.

The more common structural abnormalities identified in victims of SCD or survivors of cardiac arrest include the cardiac structural consequences of coronary artery disease, ventricular hypertrophy, myopathic ventricles (including inflammation and infiltration), and structural electrical abnormalities such as atrioventricular bypass tracts. Clinical and experimental evidence supports a role for each of these groups of abnormal structures in establishing a precondition for the generation of potentially fatal arrhythmias. Functional factors that can modulate the structurally based pathophysiology include the consequences of transient ischemia and reperfusion, hemodynamic and metabolic abnormalities, autonomic nervous system fluctuations, and the effects of toxic substances on the heart. Within each of these categories, common clinical experience and existing investigative data both suggest that one or more modulating influences can alter susceptibility to potentially fatal arrhythmias in the abnormal but otherwise stable heart. However, we have only limited insight into the *mechanisms* by which modifying functional factors contribute to the initiation of arrhythmias in structurally susceptible hearts. Such investigative efforts are beginning, and provocative information is emerging.

STRUCTURAL ABNORMALITIES PREDISPOSING TO POTENTIALLY FATAL ARRHYTHMIAS

Nearly all structural heart diseases are associated with the risk of SCD.[6] However, the risk appears to be largely nonspecific, in the sense that approximately 50% of all cardiac deaths are sudden among most disease categories. Thus, other than the few exceptions discussed in this section, the identification of specific structural causes is not discriminatory with respect to risk of SCD. Moreover, approximately 80% of all SCDs in the Western hemisphere are due to the structural consequences of one disease—atherosclerotic coronary artery disease—and another 10–15% are due to the various cardiomyopathies. The statistics reflect the general prevalence of these diseases among the population.

Coronary Heart Disease and Its Structural Consequences

The specific structural abnormalities in CHD can be categorized into acute and chronic processes involving coronary arteries and the ventricular muscle (Table 3–1) and include acute, healing, and healed myocardial infarction (MI), patchy fibrosis, discrete ventricular aneurysms, and acute and chronic lesions of the coronary arteries.

Chronic atherosclerotic lesions in multiple coronary arteries is the dominant structural finding in the coronary arteries of victims of SCD. Among 169 hearts studied by Perper et al,[7] lesions causing ≥75% stenosis were found in three or four of the major coronary vessels in 61% of hearts. Such lesions were found in two vessels in another 15% of hearts, and only 24% of the hearts had single-vessel disease or no vessels with 75% or greater stenosis. No specific pattern of vessel involvement was identified, and there were no quantitative differences between disease in the proximal and distal portions of the vessels studied. Kuller et al[8] noted ≥90% stenosis in at least one coronary artery among 77% of sudden death victims studied at autopsy. This finding was observed in only 8% of victims of sudden

Table 3–1
Structural Abnormalities in Sudden Death due to Coronary Heart Disease

Abnormalities of the Coronary Arteries
Chronic atherosclerosis
Acute lesions
Acute thrombus
Hemorrhage into plaque
Platelet aggregates
Plaque fissuring
Organizing thrombus
Abnormalities of Ventricular Myocardium
Healed infarction ± aneurysm
LV hypertrophy
Subacute infarction
Acute infarction

SOURCE: Myerbury et al.[6] Modified and reproduced with permission.

death due to other causes. Roberts and Jones[9] studied the full length of the major epicardial coronary arteries in 5-mm intervals in order to estimate the cumulative loss of coronary cross-sectional area in sudden death victims. Thirty-six percent of the segments of coronary arteries from a group of sudden death victims had ≥75% cross-sectional area reductions, compared to only 3% in controls. An additional 34% of the sections had area reductions between 51% and 75%, and only 7% of the sections from sudden death victims had <25% reductions in cross-sectional area. Again, there was no specific vessel predilection. These studies and others indicate that SCD due to CHD is accompanied by extensive coronary atherosclerosis that tends to be generalized, and that no specific pattern of vessel involvement provides predictive information.

The characteristics of *acute* coronary lesions in postmortem examinations of sudden death victims have also been studied. Friedman et al[10] observed an association between acute coronary artery abnormalities, such as hemorrhage into plaques and thrombosis, and *instantaneous* sudden death. More recently, Davies and Thomas[11] provided further insight into the role of acute coronary lesions. Among 100 consecutive SCD victims, 95 were found to have acute coronary lesions at postmortem examination; the lesions consisted of plaque fissuring and/or platelet aggregation and/or acute thrombosis. Recent acute thrombi were present in 74%, while 21% had only plaque fissuring. Sixty-five percent of the thrombi were at the sites of pre-existing high-grade stenoses and 19% were at the sites of stenoses of less than 50%. More important, only 44% of the hearts had evidence of >50% luminal occlusion by recent thrombi, and the remaining 51% had only minor occlusive thrombi or plaque fissuring alone. These observations suggest that the acute lesions may play a role beyond direct thrombotic or hemorrhagic occlusion. Specifically, coronary spasm at the site of acute thrombosis or distal to it may be an intermediate factor between the structural changes associated with plaque fissuring and thrombosis and the myocardial electrophysiological disturbance causing fatal tachyarrhythmias.

The myocardial pathology in SCD victims parallels the extent of disease in the coronary arteries. Prior healed MIs are common, frequently multiple, and tend to cause significant losses of myocardial mass, as reflected in the clinical association between low ejection fractions and sudden death. Healed MI has been reported in 40% to more than 70% at autopsy[6]; and in one study, 72% of males who died suddenly within 24 hours of the onset of symptoms with no prior history of CHD had healed MIs.[12,13] Sixty-three percent of these had large infarctions and 9% had small infarctions. In this study, only 20% of the hearts had evidence of recent acute MI, consistent with reports from other studies of SCD victims. The low rate of acute MI among sudden death victims is not in conflict with the Davies and Thomas data on the frequency of acute coronary lesions.[11] It likely attests to the acuteness of the lesions in the coronary arteries and their ability to participate in the generation of fatal arrhythmias.

The well-known clinical association between discrete ventricular aneurysms and sustained VT is not necessarily related specifically to SCD. Sustained monomorphic VT is commonly cited as a potentially fatal arrhythmia; but it is not clear that, in the presence of a chronic stable left ventricular (LV) aneurysm, this association carries any more excess risk than any other anatomic form of healed MI. Aneurysms are often associated with stable, hemodynamically well-tolerated, sustained monomorphic VT. However, the latter may degenerate to rapid unstable VT or VF when accompanied by other factors, such as ischemia or heart failure. The regional distribution of the disease process is considered the basis for reentrant arrhythmias and explains many clinical observations and approaches to management. Furthermore, CHD may be accompanied by other structural abnormalities associated with risk of cardiac arrest, such as regional LV hypertrophy.[14,15]

Hypertrophy

The second structural category, ventricular hypertrophy, has received increasing attention. Early epidemiological and pathologic data suggested that LV hypertrophy is an independent risk factor for SCD,[16] both in the presence and in the absence of concomitant coronary artery disease.[17] Patients with secondary LV hypertrophy (usually due to hypertension) and patients with primary hypertrophic cardiomyopathies both are at increased risk for sudden death, and LV hypertrophy is a common pathologic finding in victims of SCD due to coronary artery disease. In fact, as many as 75% of SCD victims with coronary artery disease have coexisting LV hypertrophy, with the severity of the hypertrophy independent of the severity of the coronary artery disease.[6,7] Clinically, several studies have demonstrated that LV hypertrophy predisposes to advanced forms of ambient PVCs,[18,19] and that hearts with LV hypertrophy may be inducible into sustained VT or VF, both in the presence and in the absence of prior clinical arrhythmic events.[20,21] Associations between LV hypertrophy and strain patterns on ECG, an increased LV mass identified echographically, and various patterns of advanced ambient ectopy have been reported.[18,19] Finally, recent experimental data have demonstrated that the membrane electrophysiology of hypertrophied myocytes is abnormal. A combination of delayed inactivation of the slow inward Ca^{2+} current (I_{si}) and delayed onset of activation of the delayed rectifier current (I_k), a major repolarizing K^+ current, accounts for prolonged recovery of excitability.[22] The regional hypertrophy observed in healed MI[14,15] may therefore contribute to electrophysiological heterogeneity. Other cellular abnormalities, especially in response to transient ischemia and reperfusion,[23] also may make hypertrophied cells susceptible to afterdepolarizations and triggered arrhythmias.

Ventricular Myopathies

The third structural category, the nonischemic myopathic ventricle, also predisposes to cardiac arrest and SCD. The risk is not limited to dilated cardiomyopathy but includes various infiltrative and inflammatory abnormalities such as myocarditis and the infiltrative restrictive myopathies.[6] The dilated myopathy category has recently been recognized to have a proportionate risk of 50% of sudden deaths,[24] and it is likely that the initiating functional factors that occur in myopathic ventricles are different from those that relate to the ventricles with MI or LV hypertrophy (Fig. 3–4).

Structural Electrophysiological Abnormalities

The fourth structural category, abnormalities of conducting tissue, is highlighted by the high-risk subgroup of patients with Wolff-Parkinson-White syndrome who have short refractory period bypass tracts and a propensity to VF during atrial flutter/fibrillation. While accurate risk estimates are not available because of the absence of a valid denominator for high-risk subgroups, the risk is phenomenologically well established.[25] The risk associated with other structural electrophysiological abnormalities, such as disease of the His-Purkinje system, is even less clearly defined. It may function independently of coexisting coronary artery disease or cardiomyopathy, but limited data suggest that specialized conducting system disease may increase the risk of sudden death due to ventricular tachyarrhythmias[26,27] rather than fatal bradyarrhythmic events.

Each of these structural categories provides identifiable electrophysiological abnormalities that predispose to the initiation of VT or VF. The most extensively studied structural subgroup is hearts with prior coronary events, in which re-entrant pathways can be inferred from electrophysiological testing and mapping techniques. Studies of methods of VT induction, entrainment, and tachycardia cycle lengths have contributed to the understanding of VT/VF in this category. These electrophysiological parameters differ between stable VT, rapid unstable VT, and VF. Less well understood is the structural basis for arrhythmias in the myopathic ventricle (Fig. 3–4), in which defined anatomic patterns in the myocardium are not apparent. A possible exception may be the role of specialized conducting tissue in relation to the clinical observation of bundle-branch re-entry in cardiomyopathies.[28,29] Each structural abnormality may be viewed as a "stable" abnormality that preconditions the heart to the generation of a potentially fatal arrhythmia when other factors alter the stable state (Fig. 3–3).

MECHANISMS OF VT/VF IN CARDIOMYOPATHIES

• ISCHEMIC CARDIOMYOPATHY

STRUCTURE:
- RE-ENTRANT PATHWAYS
- DILATED VENTRICLE
- REGIONAL HYPERTROPHY

FUNCTIONAL:
- TRANSIENT ISCHEMIA/REPERFUSION
- AUTONOMIC DYSFUNCTION
- HEMODYNAMIC VARIATIONS
- METABOLIC / TOXIC

• NON-ISCHEMIC DILATED CARDIOMYOPATHY

STRUCTURE:
- DILATED VENTRICLE
- PATCHY FIBROSIS / NECROSIS
- BUNDLE BRANCHS - RE-ENTRY

FUNCTIONAL:
- HEMODYNAMIC VARIATIONS
- METABOLIC / TOXIC
- AUTONOMIC DYSFUNCTION

• HYPERTROPHIC CARDIOMYOPATHY

STRUCTURE:
- HYPERTROPHIED MUSCLE
- VASCULAR MISMATCH
- REGIONAL FIBER DISARRAY

FUNCTIONAL:
- RELATIVE ISCHEMIA
- HEMODYNAMIC VARIATIONS
- AUTONOMIC DYSFUNCTION

Fig. 3–4. The structure function concept applied to myopathic ventricles. Myopathies of different causes have different structural properties and functional modifiers that invoke structure/function by different means. The common denominator is the genesis of potentially fatal arrhythmias. (Reproduced with permission from Myerburg RJ, et al: PACE 14:935–943, 1991.[3])

FUNCTIONAL MODULATION OF STRUCTURAL ABNORMALITIES

Dynamic changes in systemic or cardiovascular status serve as conditioning events to convert a structural abnormality from a stable to an unstable state, thereby allowing the initiation of a fatal arrhythmia. Functional factors that may contribute to this change may be grouped into four categories: (1) transient myocardial ischemia and reperfusion; (2) systemic alterations in hemodynamics, metabolic status, and biochemical fluctuations; (3) neurophysiological modulations; and (4) toxic cardiac effects such as cardiotoxic substances or drug effects (Fig. 3–2). Each of these functional modifiers may interact with one or more of the structural abnormalities to generate specific responses that serve as the initiating condition for fatal arrhythmias. For most, a functional factor alone (e.g., transient ischemia), if of sufficient severity or intensity, may itself initiate a fatal arrhythmia in the absence of structural heart disease. However, the more common circumstance is the interaction with pre-existing structural changes.

Transient Ischemia and Reperfusion

The role of ischemia as an initiating factor for potentially fatal arrhythmias has received a great deal of attention in the past 20 years from both clinicians and investigators.[29]

The electrophysiological effects of acute ischemia have been studied in both normal hearts and superimposed on prior MI, largely in experimental studies.[30,31] Clinically, the role of ischemia has been widely appreciated and speculated upon, but its transient nature has defied controlled clinical studies. An important pathology study by Davies and Thomas,[11] however, has suggested a potentially major role for *transient* ischemia in the mechanism of many sudden deaths. The investigators identified acute coronary lesions in many victims. The lesions included plaque fissuring, platelet aggregation, and acute thrombosis (not always occlusive), suggesting a role for acute lesions in the pathogenesis of terminal events. Spasm overlying those acute lesions that are not occlusive may also participate in the initiation of the fatal events.

Ischemia causes immediate acute electrophysiological changes at a cellular level that may alter regional conduction velocity. The resulting dispersion of both conduction patterns and refractoriness establishes the environment for the initiation of re-entrant arrhythmias.[32] It likely also generates some forms of abnormal automatic activity. Using an experimental model consisting of an isolated left ventricle, Kimura et al[33,34] demonstrated endocardial/epicardial heterogeneities in the time course of repolarization during acute ischemia (Fig. 3-5), and studied the evolution of these changes as a function of duration of ischemia, as well as relating them to arrhythmias. Within the first 5 to 10 minutes after cessation of coronary blood flow, shortening of action potential duration (APD) in the ischemic region was much greater in the epicardium than in the endocardium, and this difference was accompanied by greater shortening of refractory periods in the epicardium. The epicardial/endocardial differences in APD decreased during the next 20 minutes of ischemia, and this was accompanied by the development of greater postrepolarization refractoriness in the epicardium by 30 minutes of ischemia. At that time, epicardial refractory periods exceed endocardial refractory periods. This combination of events resulted in recovery of excitability, which was heterogeneous at 10 minutes and 30 minutes of ischemia but was uniform at 20 minutes (Figs. 3-5 and 3-6). The frequency of spontaneous and induced arrhythmias was greater during the time periods of greater heterogeneity (Fig. 3-6). The mechanisms for the endocardial/epicardial differences during acute ischemia are not well understood, but several clues have developed. One is the observation that specific membrane channels respond differently in endocardial and epicardial cells. The adenosine triphosphate (ATP)-sensitive potassium channel is closed in the presence of ATP and opens as ATP fails to low levels, as in the presence of ischemia. Accordingly,

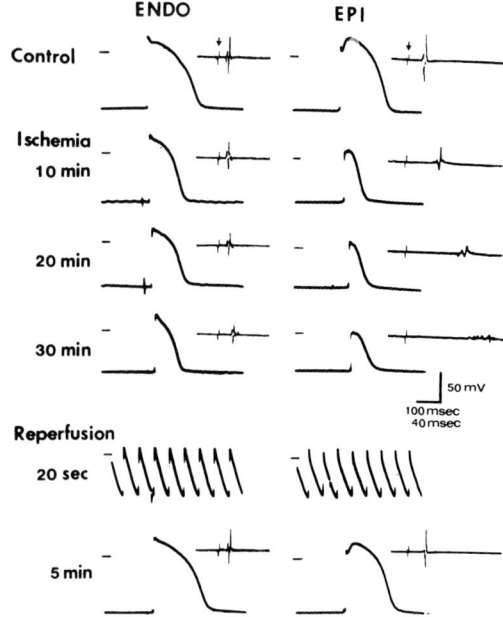

Fig. 3-5. Changes in transmembrane action potential and bipolar electrograms recorded simulaneously from endocardial and epicardial muscle cells during ischemia and reperfusion. Action potential amplitude and duration are reduced, and conduction time is prolonged, to a greater extent in epicardial (EPI) cells than endocardial (ENDO) cells during 30 minutes of ischemia. During subsequent reperfusion, rapid runs of extrasystolic impulses (VT/VF) developed 20 seconds after reperfusion was started and lasted for 1 minute before stopping spontaneously. Action potentials and bipolar electrograms of both endocardial and epicardial cells returned to normal 5 minutes after reperfusion. Horizonal bars represent zero potentials; arrows indicate the stimulation artifact on the bipolar electrogram traces. (Reproduced with permission from Kimura S, et al: Circulation 64:401-409, 1986.[34])

the observation that ATP-sensitive K^+ channels are more sensitive to ischemia in epicardial than endocardial cells[35] (Fig. 3-7) is consistent with the excessive shortening of APD in the epicardium during ischemia. Another recent experimental study[31] quantitated the effects of partial reductions of coronary blood flow in the presence and absence of healed MI. In normal hearts (Table 3-2), the spontaneous occurrence of VF or the induction of sustained VT (always polymorphic) required 100% reduction of flow, but in the presence of healed infarction, as

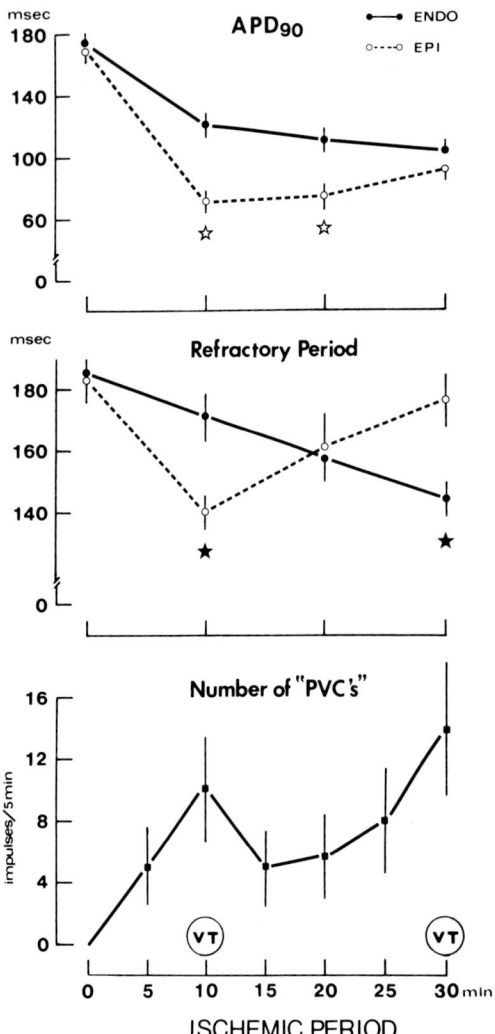

Fig. 3–6. Relationship between action potential duration at 90% repolarization (APD_{90}), refractory periods, and extrasystolic impulses during ischemia. The mean frequency of single extrasystolic impulses or couplets (PVCs) is maximal at approximately 10 minutes and again at 30 minutes of ischemia. At 10 minutes of ischemia, the refractory period, as well as APD_{90} of EPI muscle cells, are shorter than those of ENDO muscle cells. At 30 minutes of ischemia, the refractory period of EPI muscle cells is longer than that of ENDO muscle cells because of the development of greater postrepolarization refractoriness in EPI. At 10 minutes and 30 minutes of ischemia, rapid runs of extrasystolic impulses (VT) are induced by extrastimuli. (Reproduced with permission from Kimura S, et al: Circulation 64:401–409, 1986.[34])

little as a 50% reduction in blood flow significantly increased the probability of inducing VT. Spontaneous VF, in both the presence and the absence of prior infarction, required a greater total ischemic mass (i.e., healed infarction plus acute ischemia) than did the induction of sustained VT. Clinically, marked transient ischemia is associated with the risk of VF, flutter, or rapid polymorphic VT. Slow or stable monomorphic VT is usually associated with a conditioning anatomical substrate (e.g., healed infarction), although lesser degrees of transient ischemia may be responsible for initiation of the VT event.

The electrophysiological consequences of reperfusion are less emphasized but possibly of equal importance. Three points must be appreciated: (1) reperfusion events may be as common as transient ischemic events; (2) electrophysiologically, reperfusion is not simply the reversal of ischemia; and (3) reperfusion arrhythmias can generate in a much smaller mass of tissue than is required for re-entry. Patterns of collateral blood flow and vasospastic mechanisms of transient ischemia both set the stage for reperfusion arrhythmias, either concomitant with ongoing ischemia (e.g., collateralization) or subsequent to ischemia as vasospastic vessels dilate or thrombi are lysed. While reversal of the reductions in transmembrane action potential amplitude and duration that accompany the onset of ischemia may occur sequentially during reperfusion, additional specific patterns of membrane disturbance occur during reperfusion that are not simply a reversal of the pathophysiology of ischemia.[33,36] It has been demonstrated during experimental ischemia and reperfusion that an inward flux of Ca^{2+} occurs,[37] resulting in Ca^{2+} overload, and that this influx correlates in time with bursts of spontaneous ventricular ectopy (Fig. 3–5) that are rapid, self-limited, blocked or prevented by Ca^{2+} entry-blocking agents, and may be due to some form of automaticity, possibly triggered activity.[33] These bursts of activity, which have been observed experimentally in several different models and may also occur clinically, may be initiating events for sustained VT or VF. Interestingly, the clinical and experimental consequences of reperfusion appear to be related to the duration of the conditioning ischemic

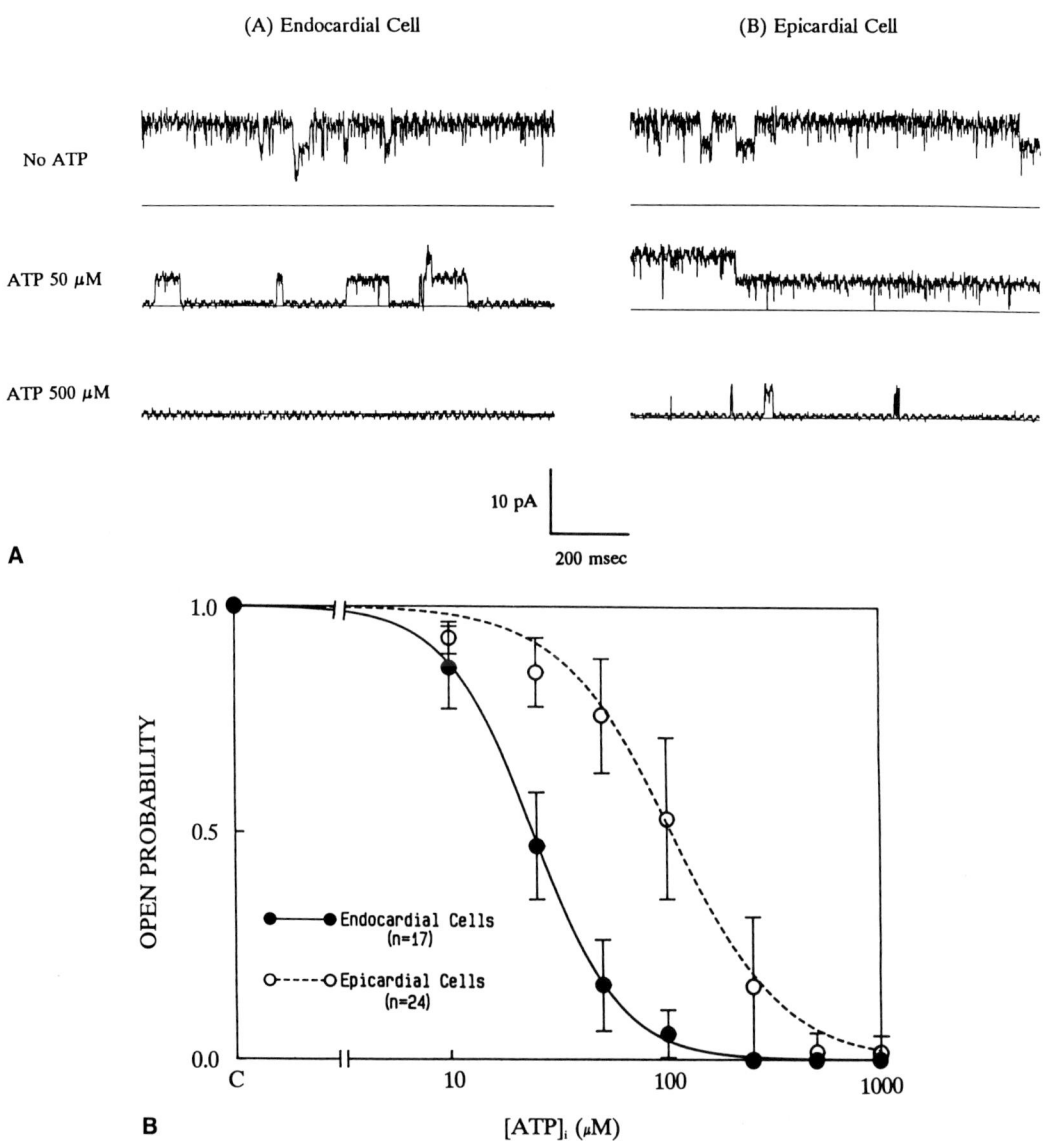

Fig. 3–7. Differential endocardial/epicardial sensitivity of ATP-sensitive K$^+$ channels to stimulated ischemia. **A.** Representative tracings of single channel currents during exposure of the intracellular membrane surface to solutions containing no ATP, 50 μM ATP, and 500 μM ATP, in an endocardial *(left)* and an epicardial *(right)* patch are shown. Membrane potential was held at 80 mM positive to the reversal potential. Solid lines indicate the closed state of the channel; outward currents are shown as upward deflections. The currents were displayed through a 1-kHz low-pass filter. **B.** Dose-response relationships between ATP concentration and open-state probability of ATP-K$^+$ channels for endocardial (solid circles) and epicardial (open circles) membrane patches. Open-state probability of a channel was calculated using data obtained at a membrane potential of 80 mV positive to the reversal potential. ATP concentration for half-maximal inhibition of channel activity was 23.6 ± 21.9 mM for endocardial cells and 97.6 ± 48.1 mM for epicardial cells ($p < 0.01$). (Reproduced with permission from Furukawa T, et al: Circ Res 68:1693–1702, 1991.[35])

Table 3-2
Ventricular Arrhythmias After Graded Circumflex Artery Flow Reductions in Hearts with Healed Myocardial Infarction

	Normal Flow	Flow ↓ 25%	Flow ↓ 50%	Flow ↓ 75%	No Flow
Sham-Operated Controls					
VF (spon)	0	0	0	0	1/10 (10%)
VT (ind)	0	0	0	0	2/9 (22%)
Healed Myocardial Infarction					
VF (spon)	0	0	0	6/22	10/21
VT (ind)	5/24 (21%)	5/23 (22%)	12/24 (50%)	9/16 (56%)	6/11 (55%)

SOURCE: Furukawa T, et al: Circulation 84:363–377, 1991. Modified and reproduced with permission.
Abbreviations: spon, spontaneous; ind, induced; VT, ventricular tachycardia; VF, ventricular fibrillation; flow ↓, reduction in circumflex artery flow.

event (Fig. 3–8).[38] After short periods of ischemia, such as occur with spontaneous coronary artery spasm or transient occlusion experimentally and last for 5 to 30 minutes, reperfusion is associated with the self-terminating bursts of the rapid activity described above. With yet shorter periods of ischemia (<5 minutes), these reperfusion-induced bursts of rapid electrical activity are not seen. Moreover, with longer periods of ischemia, such as ischemia during the acute phase of MI and its reversal by thrombolysis (1–6 hours), the rapid bursts of activity are also less common and

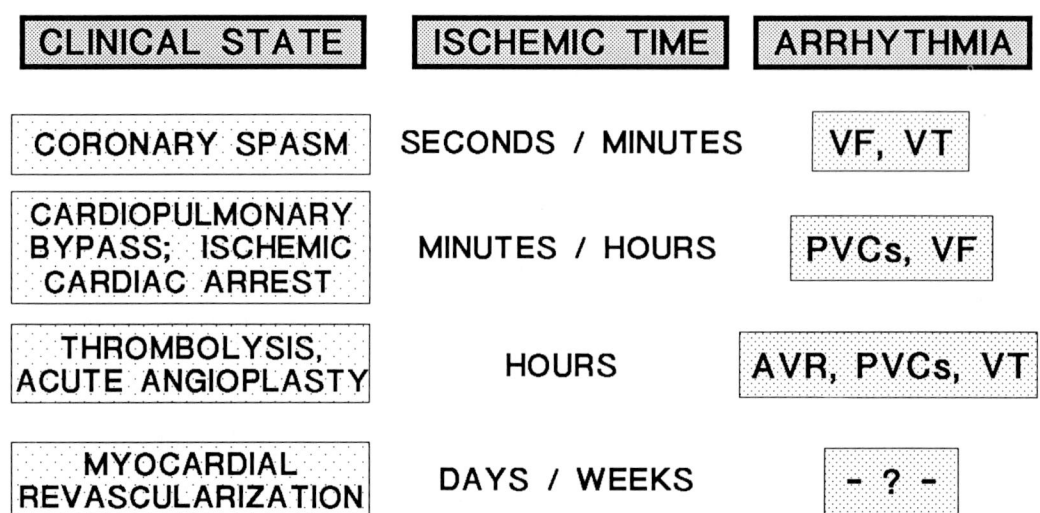

Fig. 3–8. Reperfusion arrhythmias as a function of duration of preceding ischemia. The duration of ischemia appears to determine both the probability and the form of reperfusion arrhythmias. Of particular interest is the reperfusion arrhythmia that occurs after only minutes of ischemia, since this circumstance generates rapid polymorphic tachycardias that may induce VF. (Modified from Manning AS, et al,[38] and reproduced with permission from Myerburg RJ, et al: PACE 14:935–943, 1991.[3])

reperfusion is associated clinically with enhanced automaticity and accelerated ventricular rhythms and PVCs. With yet longer periods of ischemia, the arrhythmias are not as clearly defined. Thus, the most ominous pattern of reperfusion arrhythmias are those associated with short episodes of ischemia; but if they are too short, reperfusion arrhythmias do not occur.[38]

Systemic Factors

Many of the systemic factors that modulate structural abnormalities may be reversible with prompt attention. Although severe acute or subacute hemodynamic deterioration may precipitate a *secondary* cardiac arrest, which carries a very high short-term risk of death, the relationships between chronically impaired LV function and the worsening of arrhythmias or predisposition to VT/VF are less well defined. The risk of SCD increases as ejection fraction decreases, with the greatest rate of change of risk in the 30–40% range.[39] The high risk of SCD among patients with dilated cardiomyopathy also suggests a relationship between hemodynamics and sudden death, and the propensity to worsening arrhythmias during periods of hemodynamic deterioration supports this concept.[40,41] Although it has been reported that an acute reduction in afterload by vasodilators does not reverse inducibility of VT in patients who have had sustained VT/VF, insufficient clinical research has been done to clarify the mechanisms by which hemodynamic factors interact with electrophysiology, and how they may be reversed. Experimentally, however, volume loading studies carried out in isolated perfused canine ventricles have demonstrated that increasing ventricular volume shortens refractory periods[42]—the contraction-excitation feedback. Moreover, such changes in response to acute volume loads may be regionally disparate in hearts with MI.[43]

Hypoxemia and acidosis also contribute to destabilization (Fig. 3–3),[24] are generally recognizable clinically, and are reversible with appropriate interventions. Chronic electrolyte disturbances, especially hypokalemia associated with long-term diuretic use, may be responsible for an increased risk of sudden and total cardiovascular mortality.[44] Hypokalemia may play a special role because of its relationship to torsade de pointes/rapid polymorphic VT, especially in the presence of Class IA antiarrhythmic agents. Hypokalemia prolongs repolarization of ventricular muscle, followed by emergence of early afterdepolarizations, a possible mechanism for torsade and some polymorphic VTs.

Autonomic Nervous System and Sudden Death

Neurophysiological factors—both systemic and local cardiac—are receiving increasing attention, both as markers for identifying subgroups of patients at risk for SCD and for understanding mechanisms of potentially fatal arrhythmias. Disturbances of autonomic function may occur at several levels. An increasing body of experimental information[45–49] and a limited amount of clinical information[50–55] suggest that cardiac abnormalities that predispose to the risk of SCD are accompanied by regional changes in autonomic function within the heart itself. Several different patterns of regional changes in response to sympathetic stimulation have been reported in different MI models.[45–47] Alterations in β-adrenergic receptor content, coupling proteins, and adenylate cyclase activity have been observed regionally in hearts with healed MI in one study.[48] In this study, the regions affected were the same ones that showed altered responses to cardiac sympathetic nerve stimulation in an in-situ healed MT preparation, the latter alterations measured as local differences in epicardial refractory period shortening during sympathetic nerve stimulation.[46] Experimental and clinical imaging studies of cardiac nerves have shown a disruption of myocardial sympathetic innervation after acute MI, with apparent healing during the convalescent phase.[49] Clinical data, on the other hand, have shown that isoproterenol infusion during programmed electrical stimulation studies may sensitize the heart to inducibility of sustained VT or VF not present in the absence of isoproterenol among patients who have had clinical sustained tachyarrhythmias or cardiac arrest.[50] In addition, both isoproterenol-sensitized induction of ventricular tachycardia and induction of unstable ventricular arrhythmias, particularly among cardiac arrest survivors, may respond to β-adrenergic blockade.[50,54] The extent to which these clinical observations reflect regional abnormalities in cardiac sympathetics has not yet been determined. However, these experimental and clinical observations suggest a potential role for regional alteration in sympathetic receptors and effectors at a cardiac level.

Several recent studies have also shown that changes in a more general neurophysiological modulation of cardiac activity may identify subgroups at increased risk for SCD. Cardiac responses to alterations in systemic autonomic balance, measured as heart rate variability or baroreceptor sensitivity, have been studied in selected subgroups of patients. Among MI survivors[51] and survivors of out-of-hospital cardiac arrest,[52] altered heart rate variability has been suggested as a marker for risk of sudden death. The normal diurnal variations are not lost in the high-risk subgroups, but the variability is blunted, especially during the early morning hours, when risk is highest. A study employing spectral analysis has suggested that loss of the high-frequency components of variability, reflecting blunted parasympathetic modulations, is more prominent than changes in low-frequency components of heart rate variability among survivors of out-of-hospital cardiac arrest, compared to age- and disease-matched controls.[52] Another approach has been the use of a measure of baroreceptor sensitivity to identify high-risk patients. Using a technique of phenylephrine infusion and beat-to-beat analysis of R-R interval responses to increases in blood pressure, a depressed baroreceptor response (<3 msec of R-R interval lengthening/mm Hg change in blood pressure) has identified a subgroup of patients at increased risk for sudden death and documented for ventricular arrhythmias after MI. In both the heart rate variability studies and baroreceptor sensitivity studies, the neurophysiological defect appears to be blunted parasympathetic modulation, possibly leaving an abnormally elevated sympathetic activity unbalanced. In addition, alterations in autonomic responses have been suggested as one possible mechanism contributing to hemodynamic instability during induced VT,[54] and the post-MI β-blocker studies have suggested an improved outcome (including improved risk for fatal arrhythmic events) in patients so treated.[55-57] At the present level of knowledge, the autonomic influences can be viewed as systemic variations that may be primary (identifying an inherently high-risk subset), or secondary to a cardiac event (proposed altered autonomic reflexes in the post-MI patient), interacting with regionally altered myocardial responses to autonomic variations. The latter causes a dispersion of the quantitative and qualitative responses to sympathetic stimulation in the abnormal heart and may interact with structural abnormalities such as healed MI or LV hypertrophy in predisposing to the genesis of potentially fatal arrhythmias.

Toxic and Proarrhythmic Effects

The first recognized relationship between a clinically used substance and VT was the risk of VF during chloroform anesthesia. Although the mechanism is not fully clarified, a relationship to catecholamine stimulation may favor its development. Today, the toxic causes of functional perturbations are primarily the various substances with known proarrhythmic properties. The classic proarrhythmic response to quinidine—torsade de pointes—may occur with any of the Class IA antiarrhythmics, the Class III drugs, and less frequently with an enlarging number of unrelated substances, such as psychotropic drugs, seldane, erythromycin, and pentamidine. The mechanism, at least for the Class IA and Class III antiarrhythmic drugs, may be the evolution of early afterdepolarizations because of prolonged action potential durations.[58] These responses may occur in any of the structural abnormalities and may contribute in an additive way to other functional abnormalities such as transient ischemia or hemodynamic dysfunction. LV hypertrophy, which itself tends to prolong APDs, may interact with ischemia/reperfusion or toxic substances to generate even greater prolongation of APD. The increased risk of sudden death related to the use of flecainide or encainide in the CAST study[4] appears to result from a different form of "proarrhythmia,"[5] possibly related to the increased risk of ischemic arrhythmias when the drugs are present during acute ischemia in a heart with prior infarction. An observation of current interest is the increased risk of SCD in persons using cocaine and alcohol concomitantly. The combination results in the generation of a unique toxic metabolite, cocaethylene,[59] which is produced in the liver and has been proposed to have enhanced cardiotoxicity.

SUMMARY

A hypothetical cascade involved in the transition from a chronic stable abnormality to a potentially fatal arrhythmic event is depicted in Figure 3–3. The cascade integrates the range of structure/function alterations with membrane physiology and mechanisms of arrhythmias as they are currently understood. With further investigative efforts, the many gaps remaining in this basic design should be filled in in the future.

REFERENCES

1. Myerburg RJ, Kessler KM, Bassett AL, Castellanos A: A biological approach to sudden cardiac death: Structure, function, and cause. Am J Cardiol 63:1512–1516, 1989.
2. Myerburg RJ, Kessler KM, Castellanos A: Sudden cardiac death: Structure, function and time dependence of risk. Circulation 85(suppl 1):I-2–I-10, 1992.
3. Myerburg RJ, Kessler KM, Castellanos A: Pathophysiology of sudden cardiac death. PACE 14(II):935–943, 1991.
4. Echt DS, Liebson PR, Mitchell B, et al: Mortality and morbidity in patients receiving encainide, flecainide, or placebo: The Cardiac Arrhythmia Suppression Trial. N Engl J Med 324:781–788, 1991.
5. Akhtar M, Breithardt GM, Coumel P, et al: CAST and Beyond: Implications of the Cardiac Arrhythmia Suppression Trial. Circulation 81:1123–1127, 1990.
6. Myerburg RJ, Castellanos A: Cardiac arrest and sudden cardiac death. In Braunwald E (ed): Heart Disease: A Textbook of Cardiovascular Medicine, 3rd ed. New York, WB Saunders, 1987, pp 742–777.
7. Perper JA, Kuller LH, Cooper M: Arteriosclerosis of coronary arteries in sudden, unexpected deaths. Circulation 52(suppl III): 27–33, 1975.
8. Kuller L, Cooper M, Perper J: Epidemiology of sudden death. Arch Intern Med 129: 714–719, 1972.
9. Roberts WC, Jones AA: Quantitation of coronary arterial narrowing at necropsy in sudden coronary death: Analysis of 31 patients and comparison with 25 controls. Am J Cardiol 44:39–45, 1979.
10. Friedman M, Manwaring JH, Rosenman RH, Donlon G, Ortega P, Grube SM: Instantaneous and sudden deaths: Clinical and pathological differentiation in coronary artery disease. JAMA 225:1319–1328, 1973.
11. Davies MJ, Thomas A: Thrombosis and acute coronary artery lesions in sudden cardiac ischemic death. N Engl J Med 310: 1137–1140, 1984.
12. Newman WP, Strong JP, Johnson WD, Oalmann MC, Tracy RE, Rork WA: Community pathology of atherosclerosis and coronary heart disease in New Orleans: Morphologic findings in young black and white men. Lab Invest 44:496–501, 1981.
13. Newman WP, Tracy RE, Strong JP, Johnson WD, Oalmann MC: Pathology of sudden cardiac death. Ann NY Acad Sci 382:39–49, 1982.
14. Ginzton LE, Conant R, Rodrigues DM, Laks MM: Functional significance of hypertrophy of the non-infarcted myocardium after myocardial infarction in humans. Circulation 80:816–822, 1989.
15. Cox MM, Berman I, Myerburg RJ, Smets MJD, Kozlovskis PL: Morphometric mapping of regional myocyte diameters after healing of myocardial infarction in cats. J Mol Cell Cardiol 23:127–135, 1991.
16. Kannel WB, Thomas HE: Sudden coronary death: The Framingham study. Ann NY Acad Sci 38:3–21, 1982.
17. Rissanen V, Romo M, Siltanen P: Prehospital sudden death from ischaemic heart disease: A postmortem study. Br Heart J 40: 1025–1033, 1978.
18. Messerii FH, Ventura HO, Elizardi DJ, Dunn FG, Froelich ED: Hypertension and sudden death: Increased ventricular ectopic activity in left ventricular hypertrophy. Am J Med 77:18–22, 1984.
19. McLenachan JM, Henderson E, Morris Kl, Dajgie HJ: Ventricular arrhythmias in patients with hypertensive left ventricular hypertrophy. N Engl J Med 317:787–792, 1987.
20. Anderson KP: Sudden death, hypertension, and hypertrophy. J Cardiovasc Pharmacol 6(suppl III):S498–S503, 1984.
21. Fanspazir L, Tracy CM, Leon MB, et al: Electrophysiologic abnormalities in patients with hypertrophic cardiomyopathy: A consecutive analysis of 155 patients. Circulation 80:1259–1268, 1989.

22. Furukawa T, Myerburg RJ, Furukawa N, Kimura S, Bassett AL: The responses to metabolic inhibition of Ca^{++} current and K^+ currents in feline left ventricular hypertrophy. Am J Physiol [submitted].
23. Furukawa T, Bassett AL, Kimura S, Furukawa N, Myerburg RJ: "Reperfusion" early afterdepolarizations (EAD) in hypertrophied feline myocytes: Role of membrane currents. Circulation 82(suppl III):III-100, 1990.
24. Packer M: Sudden unexpected death in patients with congestive heart failure: A second frontier. Circulation 72:681–685, 1985.
25. Klein GJ, Bashore TM, Sellers TD, Pritchett EL, Smith WM, Gallagher JJ: Ventricular fibrillation in the Wolff-Parkinson-White syndrome. N Engl J Med 301:1080–1085, 1979.
26. Myerburg RJ, Conde CA, Sung RJ, et al: Clinical, electrophysiologic, and hemodynamic profile of patients resuscitated from prehospital cardiac arrest. Am J Med 68:568–576, 1980.
27. Lie KI, Liem KL, Schuilenberg RM, David GK, Durrer D: Early identification of patients developing late in-hospital ventricular fibrillation after discharge from the coronary care unit. Am J Cardiol 41:674–677, 1978.
28. Caceres J, Jazayeri M, McKinnie J, et al: Sustained bundle branch reentry mechanism of clinical tachycardia. Circulation 79:256–270, 1989.
29. Furukawa T, Myerburg RJ: Mechanisms of arrhythmias in chronic ischemic heart disease. In Waxman HL, Greenspon A (eds): Contemporary Management of Ventricular Arrhythmias. Philadelphia, F.A. Davis, 1991, pp 351–373.
30. Myerburg RJ, Epstein K, Gaide MS, et al: Electrophysiologic consequences of experimental acute ischemia superimposed upon healed myocardial infarction in cats. Am J Cardiol 49:323–330, 1982.
31. Furukawa T, Moroe K, Mayrovitz HN, Sampsell R, Furukawa N, Myerburg RJ: Arrhythmogenic effects of graded coronary blood flow reduction superimposed upon prior myocardial infarction in dogs. Circulation 84:368–377, 1991.
32. Janse MJ, Downer E: The effect of acute ischemia on transmembrane potentials in the intact heart: Relation to reentry mechanisms. In Kulburtus HE (ed): Reentrant Arrhythmias. Lancaster, PA, MTP Press, 1977, pp 195–209.
33. Kimura S, Bassett AL, Saoudi NC, Cameron JS, Kozlovskis PL, Myerburg RJ: Cellular electrophysiologic changes and "arrhythmias" during experimental ischemia and reperfusion in isolated cat ventricular myocardium. J Am Coll Cardiol 7:833–842, 1986.
34. Kimura S, Bassett AL, Kohya T, Kozlovskis PL, Myerburg RJ: Simultaneous recording of action potentials from endocardium and epicardium during ischema in the isolated cat ventricles. Circulation 64:401–409, 1986.
35. Furukawa T, Kimura S, Furukawa N, Bassett AL, Myerburg RJ: Role of cardiac ATP-regulated potassium channels in differential responses of endocardial and epicardial cells to ischemia. Circ Res 68:1693–1702, 1991.
36. Manning AS, Coltart DJ, Hearse DJ: Ischemia and reperfusion induced arrhythmias in the rat: Effects of xanthine oxidase inhibition with allopurinol. Circ Res 55:545–548, 1984.
37. Clusin WT, Buchbinder M, Harrison DC: Calcium overload "injury current" and early ischemic cardiac arrhythmias: A direct connection. Lancet ii:272–274, 1983.
38. Manning AS, Hearse DJ: Reperfusion-induced arrhythmias: Mechanisms and prevention. J Mol Cell Cardiol 16:497–518, 1984.
39. Bigger JT, Fleiss JL, Kleiger R, Miller JP, Rolnitzky LM, the Multicenter Post-Infarction Research Group: The relationship among ventricular arrhythmias, left ventricular dysfunction, and mortality in the 2 years after myocardial infarction. Circulation 69:250–258, 1983.
40. Meinertz T, Hoffman T, Kasper W, et al: Significance of ventricular arrhythmias in idiopathic dilated cardiomyopathy. Am J Cardiol 53:902–907, 1984.
41. Chakko CS, Gheorghiade M: Ventricular arrhythmias in severe heart failure: Incidence, significance, and effectiveness of antiarrhythmic therapy. Am Heart J 109:497–504, 1985.
42. Lab MJ: Contraction-excitation feedback in myocardium: Physiologic basis and clinical relevance. Circ Res 50:757–766, 1982.
43. Calkins H, Maughan WL, Weissman HF, Sugiura S, Sagawa K, Levine JH: Effect of acute volume load on refractoriness and arrhythmia development in isolated chronically infarcted canine hearts. Circulation 79:687–697, 1989.
44. Multiple Risk Factor Intervention Trial Research Group: Multiple-Risk Factor Intervention Trial: Risk factor changes in mortality results. JAMA 248:1465, 1982.
45. Barber MJ, Mueller TM, Henry DF, Felton SJ, Zipes DP: Transmural myocardial infarction in the dog produces sympathectomy in non-infarcted myocardium. Circulation 67:787–796, 1982.

46. Gaide MS, Myerburg RJ, Kozlovskis PL, Bassett AL: Elevated sympathetic response of epicardium proximal to healed myocardial infarction. Am J Physiol *14*:646–652, 1983.
47. Kammerling JJ, Green FJ, Watanabe AM, et al: Denervation supersensitivity of refractoriness in non-infarcted areas apical to transmural myocardial infarction. Circulation *76*:383–393, 1987.
48. Kozlovskis PL, Smets MJD, Duncan RC, Bailey BK, Bassett AL, Myerburg RJ: Regional beta-adrenergic receptors and adenylate cyclase activity after healing of myocardial infarction in cats. J Mol Cell Cardiol *22*:311–322, 1990.
49. Tuli M, Minardo J, Mock BH, et al: SPECT with high purity I-123-MIBG after transmural myocardial infarction (TMI), demonstrating sympathetic denervation followed by reinnervation in a dog model. J Nucl Med *28*:669, 1987.
50. Interian A, Fernandez P, Robinson E, et al: Long-term effect of propranolol in ventricular tachycardia/fibrillation patients with isoproterenol dependent inducibility. Circulation *82(suppl III)*:435, 1990.
51. Kleiger RE, Miller JP, Bigger JT, Moss AJ, the Multicenter Post-Infarction Research Group: Decreased heart rate variability and its association with increased mortality after acute myocardial infarction. Am J Cardiol *59*:256–262, 1987.
52. Huikuri HV, Linnaluoto MK, Valkama JO, Kessler KM, Takkunen JT, Myerburg RJ: Heart rate variability and its circadian rhythm in survivors of cardiac arrest. Circulation *82(suppl III)*:III-237, 1990.
53. La Rovere MT, Specchia G, Mortara A, Schwartz PJ: Baroreflex sensitivity, clinical correlates and cardiovascular mortality among patients with a first myocardial infarction: A prospective study. Circulation *78*:816–824, 1988.
54. Huikuri HV, Zaman L, Castellanos A, et al: Changes in spontaneous sinus node rate as an estimate of cardiac autonomic tone during stable and unstable ventricular tachycardia. J Am Coll Cardiol *13*:646–652, 1989.
55. Huikuri HV, Cox M, Interian A Jr, Kessler KM, Castellanos A, Myerburg RJ: Efficacy of intravenous propranolol for suppression of inducibility of ventricular tachyarrhythmias with different electrophysiologic characteristics in coronary artery disease. Am J Cardiol *64*:1305–1309, 1989.
56. Beta-Blocker Heart Attack Research Group: A randomized trial of propranolol in patients with acute myocardial infarction: I. Mortality results. JAMA *247*:1707–1714, 1982.
57. Pederson TR, The Norwegian Multicenter Study Group: Six-year follow-up of the Norwegian multicenter study on timolol after acute myocardial infarction. N Engl J Med *313*:1055–1058, 1985.
58. Jackman WM, Friday KJ, Anderson JL, Aliot EM, Clark M, Lazzara R: The long QT syndrome: A critical review, new clinical observations, and a unifying hypothesis. Prog Cardiovasc Dis *31(2)*:115–172, 1988.
59. Hearn WL, Flynn DD, Hine GW, et al: Cocaethylene: A unique cocaine metabolite displays high affinity for the dopamine transporter. J Neurochem [in press].

B
Knowledge of Sudden Cardiac Death Gathered from Animal Models

4

Role of Ischemia and Infarction in the Genesis of Lethal Arrhythmias

ANDREW L. WIT
MICHIEL J. JANSE

Coronary artery disease resulting in myocardial ischemia and infarction is a primary cause of sudden death (SCD) because of the marked effects on the electrophysiological properties of the affected myocardium. Abnormalities in the electrophysiology of ischemic myocardium lead to the occurrence of lethal arrhythmias. Much of our knowledge concerning these abnormalities has come from studies in experimental animal models. This chapter discusses the effects of ischemia and infarction on the electrophysiology of the ventricles.

VENTRICULAR ARRHYTHMIAS IN THE ACUTE PHASE OF MYOCARDIAL ISCHEMIA AND INFARCTION

The term *acute phase of myocardial ischemia* refers to events occurring within the first 2–4 hours after the sudden onset of a reduction in blood flow through a coronary artery. Acute ischemia in humans may result from a transient coronary occlusion as a consequence of vasospasm or the formation of a reversible platelet plug. When coronary artery occlusion is not transient but persists (because of, for example, occlusive thrombi), ischemic cells become irreversibly damaged and myocardial infarction (MI) results. The relationship between total occlusion of a coronary artery in humans and infarction has been documented in both clinical and postmortem pathological studies.[1,2]

Electrophysiological changes in cardiac muscle and the mechanisms of arrhythmias caused by acute ischemia and infarction cannot easily be studied in patients, and therefore experimental animal models are used. The majority of studies in these models involve obstructing flow through a coronary artery to cause ischemia. In hearts of large animals such as the dog or pig, coronary artery occlusion rapidly results in the kinds of arrhythmias sown in Figure 4–1. In this figure, 60-DC extracellular electrograms are shown that were simultaneously recorded from the anterior surface of the left ventricle of an isolated pig heart, before occlusion of the left anterior descending coronary artery (left of figure) and 3–4 minutes after occlusion (center and right of figure). Under control conditions (left), the area under the electrodes is almost synchronously excited, and on the time scale shown, no differences in timing of the intrinsic (negative) deflections can be distinguished. (In reality the difference between earliest and latest activated electrode site is 15 msec.) Three minutes after coronary occlusion, there is TQ-segment depression and ST-segment elevation in many of the complexes, and the configuration of the electrograms is drastically altered (center). Initially there still is sinus rhythm (left side of center panel), but at the end of the tracing spontaneous premature beats appear (right side of center panel) that form the beginning of a period of ventricular tachycardia (VT).

51

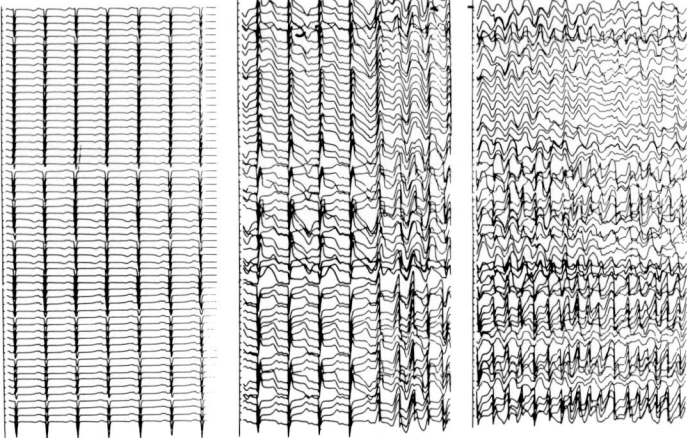

Fig. 4–1. Direct current extracellular electrograms simultaneously recorded from the epicardial surface of the left ventricle of a pig heart before (left panel) and 3 to 4 minutes after occlusion of the left anterior descending coronary artery (middle and right panel). (Modified and reproduced with permission from Janse.[164])

Tachycardia eventually degenerates into ventricular fibrillation (VF; right panel). The next sections of this chapter are devoted to the electrophysiological changes that lead to these dramatic disturbances of the cardiac rhythm.

Electrophysiological Effects of Acute Myocardial Ischemia

Myocardial ischemia that results from coronary artery occlusion has a profound effect on the electrophysiological properties of cardiac cells which eventually results in the rhythm disturbance described for Figure 4–1. Changes in resting membrane potential and in inward and outward currents during the action potential lead to alterations in conduction, refractoriness, and ability to initiate impulses, all of which contribute to the occurrence of ventricular arrhythmias. In addition to changes in active membrane properties, passive electrical properties are changed as well, and these changes also influence propagation in ischemic myocardium and contribute to arrhythmogenesis.

Resting Membrane Potential

The resting potential of myocardial cells in the ischemic region begins to depolarize within minutes following experimental coronary artery occlusion.[3–7] This fall in resting potential has been linked at least partly to alterations in the distribution of potassium ions (K^+) across the cell membrane. Increases in extracellular K^+ have been measured with ion-selective electrodes soon after coronary occlusion both in vivo during regional ischemia and in isolated perfused hearts during global ischemia.[6,8–16] A close association between the rise in extracellular K^+ and the decrease in resting membrane potential has been described. The accumulation of extracellular K^+ occurs in two phases. The first phase is rapidly reversible when reperfusion occurs within 15 minutes,[9,15,16] and resting potential also quickly returns to normal.[4] Following this first phase of increased extracellular K^+ during maintained occlusion, the potassium concentration remains nearly constant for 10–20 minutes, and sometimes even decreases somewhat before a second increase in extracellular K^+ begins that is not reversed by reperfusion.[9,16] This second phase is most likely due to irreversible cell damage. The increase in extracellular K^+ in the first 10 minutes is substantial; measurements have shown an average rate of increase of 1.5 mM/min.[6,9,15] However, it represents only a relatively small decline in intracellular K^+ concentration (from about 140 to 135 mM) because the ions are transferred from an intracellular space that is three times larger than the extracellular space.[17] However, eventually there may also be a significant loss of intracellular K^+ that contributes to a decrease in the K^+ equilibrium potential and resting potential.[18,19]

To account for the K^+ loss from the myocardial cells during the early period of ischemia there is an increase in K^+ efflux as well as a decrease in K^+ influx back into the cell after each action potential. One possible mechanism for the increased K^+ efflux involves an increase in membrane permeability to anions caused by ischemia, which depolarizes the cell membrane. K^+ then is passively redistributed. However, at least part of the cellular K^+ loss is not related to anion efflux and probably results from an increase in membrane conductance for K^+.[20] An increased conductance of K^+ channels might result from the effects of adenosine triphosphate (ATP) depletion on ATP-sensitive K^+ channels.[21-23] It has also been proposed that K^+ loss from cells and accumulation in the extracellular space during ischemia might be linked to be development of intracellular acidosis.[6,24] Net K^+ efflux is proposed to be secondary to electrogenic lactate efflux at a low extracellular pH, similar to that occurring in fatigued skeletal muscle.[25] Intracellular acidification also increases a time-independent outward K^+ current, supporting the proposal that K^+ loss is linked to acidosis.[26]

Other causes for depolarization besides extracellular K^+ accumulation might also occur concomitantly. It has been proposed that some of the depolarization occurs as a direct consequence of intracellular calcium overload in ischemic myocardium that increases an inward (depolarizing) membrane current.[27-29] A class of metabolites that accumulates in ischemic myocardium and that has been implicated as a cause of depolarization of the membrane potential is the lysophosphoglycerides, among which lysophosphatidylcholine and lysophosphatidylethanolamine are the most important.[30,31]

The Na^+/K^+ pump is still functioning within the first 10–15 minutes of ischemia, although experimental evidence shows that energy-rich phosphate compounds rapidly decline during the early phases of hypoxia and ischemia.[32,33] It appears that a moderate decrease in Na^+/K^+ ATP-ase activity is compatible with maintenance of at least some active Na^+/K^+ pumping. Some pump suppression, however, may contribute to the rise in extracellular K^+, since K^+ is not transferred back into cells at a normal rate. Another consequence of Na^+/K^+ pump suppression is a moderate increase in intracellular Na^+ although not until after 15 minutes or more.[6,34] Although depression of the Na^+/K^+ pump might be expected to result in a more severe rise in intracellular Na^+, depolarization of the membrane potential during acute ischemia decreases the electrical gradient for movement of Na^+ into the cell, probably accounting for the negligible increase in Na^+ during the initial minutes of acute ischemia.

Changes in Intracellular and Extracellular Potentials

Microelectrode recordings from the epicardial surface of intact hearts (either in open-chest animals or in the Langendorff perfused heart model) have shown that within a few minutes after coronary artery occlusion, the amplitude, upstroke velocity, and duration of ventricular muscle action potentials decrease along with the depolarization of the resting membrane potential. After depolarization to resting membrane potentials of around -60 to -65 mV, the cells become unresponsive.[3-5] Figure 4–2 shows recordings made in an isolated perfused pig heart. The upper traces in each panel are transmembrane potentials recorded with a microelectrode. The lower traces are unipolar direct-current extracellular electrograms recorded from the same site as the microelectrode on the anterior aspect of the left ventricle. In the control situation, the resting membrane potential was -97 mV, and action potential amplitude was 118 mV. The TQ and ST segments of the extracellular electrograms are isoelectric. The intrinsic deflection (rapid negative deflection) corresponds to the upstroke of the transmembrane action potential. Following coronary artery occlusion, the first change is a decrease in resting membrane potential without much change in action potential configuration, except for a reduction in upstroke velocity (top right panel, 2½ min occlusion). The loss of resting membrane potential is reflected in the direct-current electrogram by a negative displacement of the TQ segment (TQ depression). Between 2 and 4 minutes following onset of ischemia, resting membrane potential further decreased from -86 to -75 mV, with a concomitant increase in TQ depression from -2 to -11 mV (lower left panel, 4 min occlusion). After 4 minutes, the action potential upstroke has become slow and slurred and two components are evi-

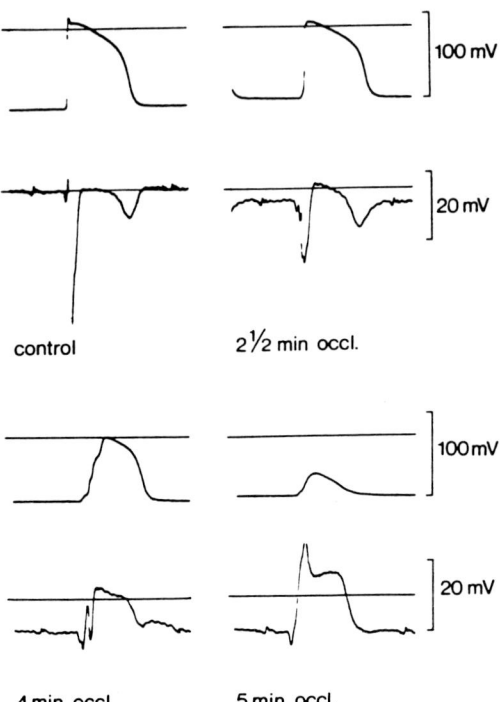

Fig. 4–2. Transmembrane potentials (top trace) and local direct current (DC) extracellular electrograms (lower trace) recorded from an isolated, perfused pig heart before (control) and 2½, 4, and 5 minutes after occlusion of the left anterior descending coronary artery. (Reproduced with permission from Janse MJ: Can J Cardiol 00:46A–52A, 1986.[164])

dent. Action potential amplitude decreased, and the moment of activation of the ischemic cell was delayed. After 5 minutes, the action potential was reduced to a very small-amplitude response, which was probably unable to propagate (bottom right panel, 5 min occlusion). In the extracellular electrograms, true ST-segment elevation is apparent. There still is a small negative deflection ("intrinsic deflection") that coincides with the small-amplitude response. After 5–8 minutes of ischemia, cells in the center of the ischemic zone fail to produce action potentials. With maintained coronary occlusion, transmembrane potentials can again be recorded in previously unresponsive cells after about 15–30 minutes. The action potentials at that time are abnormal; they have a short duration, a low amplitude, and a reduced upstroke velocity, yet they are able to propagate. After 40–60 minutes, these action potentials disappear and the cells in the center of the ischemic zone become inexcitable and remain so. The decrease in amplitude and upstroke velocity of action potentials of ischemic cells cannot be attributed solely to inactivation of Na^+ channels resulting from the decreased resting potential.[35,36] Other components of the ischemic environment probably contribute to the decrease in depolarizing inward current, perhaps by acting on the Na^+ channels. The question of whether action potentials with upstrokes dependent on the slow inward calcium current (slow responses)[37] occur in the ischemic environment has not yet been answered.

The duration of the ventricular muscle action potential has been shown to undergo a biphasic change after coronary artery occlusion in experiments in which action potentials have been recorded from the epicardial surface of whole hearts. Initially, it lengthens slightly[4,38] because of a slight reduction in the temperature in the subepicardial muscle layers. Subepicardial temperature decreases after a coronary occlusion since the normal blood flow serves to warm the muscle. The duration of the refractory period during the first 2 minutes following coronary artery occlusion increases concomitantly with the lengthening of the action potential.[4,39] Subsequently, action potential duration (APD) shortens, mainly because of a shortening of the plateau phase. The shortening of the APD is a result of the combined effects of a number of the components of the ischemic environment. Hypoxia has been shown to shorten APD in the absence of the other components of ischemia and undoubtedly contributes to this effect of ischemia.[40] Likely causes for APD shortening during hypoxia are a decrease in the inward L-type calcium current and an increase in a time-independent outward K^+ current. The increase in K^+ conductance results from the effects of ATP depletion on ATP-sensitive K^+ channels.[22,23] After coronary occlusion, shortening of the APD parallels the decrease in resting potential and action potential amplitude. Therefore, the decrease in resting potential may also contribute to the shortening of the APD. Other components of the ischemic environment (high K^+, metabolic products, etc.) may shorten APD as well. Refractory periods of ischemic myocardium shorten along with the APD after the first 2 minutes following complete coronary artery occlusion.[41,42]

The refractory period of ischemic ventricular cells is not simply determined by the APD as it is in normally polarized myocardium and Purkinje cells; ischemic fibers may remain inexcitable even after completely repolarizing.[4,43] As a result, after an initial shortening, the refractory period may actually be prolonged despite the shorter APD. This "postrepolarization refractoriness" is probably related to depolarization of the myocardial cell. In partially depolarized fibers, recovery from inactivation of both fast Na^+ and slow Ca^{2+} inward currents has been shown to be markedly delayed until many milliseconds after completion of repolarization.[44,45] The postrepolarization refractoriness that occurs in ischemic cells is unlike the response to hypoxia alone, where refractory periods shorten along with APD, and the upstroke of stimulated premature action potentials is already maximal following complete repolarization.[46] Figure 4–3 shows some of the changes in APD and refractory period described above. Two simultaneously recorded action potentials from sites 2.5 cm apart in the isolated perfused pig heart are displayed. Premature stimuli were applied to the ischemic regions, as indicated by arrows. The top panel shows the control effective refractory period, which was determined to be 260 msec. There is initial lengthening of the APD and refractory period to 290 msec by 1½ minutes after the coronary occlusion. At 6 minutes, marked alternation developed in the upper cell, with a 60-msec difference in refractory period between the short (240 msec) and the long (300 msec) action potential. There is also a long latency between premature stimulus and response that is evident in the records.

Inhomogenetics in electrophysiological properties within the ischemic zone, largely caused by local differences in extracellular K^+, are crucial in setting the stage for reentrant arrhythmias. Inhomogeneities in extracellular K^+ are found at the borders of

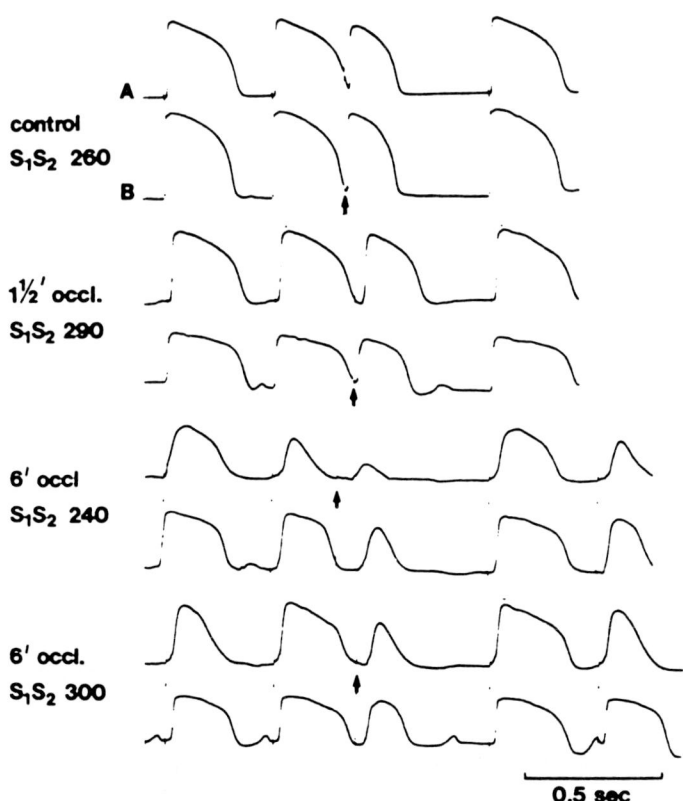

Fig. 4–3. Changes in local excitability following coronary artery occlusion. In each panel simultaneous recordings of two action potentials from the epicardial surface of the pig heart are shown during control and after coronary occlusion. Arrows indicate the earliest coupling interval of a premature stimulus (S_2) that elicited a response. (Reproduced with permission from Downar E, et al: Circulation 56:217–224, 1977.[4])

ischemic and normal myocardium where K^+ moves from the ischemic zone toward the normal zone. The movement of K^+ is probably caused by a combination of diffusion and mixing of the extracellular space because of the contractions of the heart. As described earlier, recovery of excitability of acutely ischemic myocardium is delayed ("postrepolarization refractoriness") and this results in a lengthening rather than a shortening of the refractory period. However, in regions toward the border, refractory periods may not be prolonged as much as in the central ischemic region or they may even be shorter than normal, resulting in significant inhomogeneities.[47,48]

The changes in the resting membrane potential, the depolarization phase of the action potential, the APD, and the time course of recovery of excitability have important effects on conduction in the ischemic region. After 2 minutes of coronary occlusion, delays in activation of ischemic myocardium on the order of 200–300 msec after the onset of ventricular activation, caused by slowing of conduction, have been found (normally the ventricles are activated within 80–100 msec).[49–51] Delayed activation is especially prominent in ischemic subepicardium, whereas activation of subendocardial layers is relatively unaffected.[52] Epicardial conduction delay increases when the heat rate is increased as expected if the time course for recovery of excitability after an action potential is prolonged.[53] An increase in sinus rate, for example, caused by enhanced sympathetic activity, may unmask the inhomogeneity in recovery of excitability in the ischemic zone and produce unidirectional block and re-entry even in the absence of an initiating premature impulse. The large delays in epicardial activation cannot be accounted for only by a decrease in conduction velocity. In addition, they are caused by irregular conduction from endocardium to epicardium at reduced speed around multiple sites of intramural conduction block. After 10–30 minutes of coronary occlusion, activation delay in the subepicardium diminishes and the amplitude of bipolar extracellular complexes increases.[54,55] This improvement in conduction is related to the appearance of transmembrane potentials in previously unresponsive cells, which we have described elsewhere.[5,56] However, intramural cells may die, leading to an absence of conduction through these regions of the developing infarct.

In addition to the decrease in the inward depolarizing current, changes in passive electrical properties may be important in causing the decrease in conduction velocity and conduction block that occurs during acute ischemia. By decreasing membrane conductance for Na^+, conduction velocity can only be reduced to about one third of its normal value, whereas by increasing the degree of cellular uncoupling it can be reduced by a factor of 20 before block occurs.[57] Intracellular resistance remains unchanged during the initial phase of ischemia (from 12 to 23 minutes), suggesting that cell coupling is fairly normal. Afterward, rapid cellular uncoupling occurs to cause an increase in intracellular resistance.[58] This sudden increase in intracellular resistance is in agreement with the results of a morphological study in which it was found that after 24 minutes of ischemia the majority of gap junctions became dissociated.[59] Focal pathological separation of intercalated disk membranes has been observed after 30 minutes of hypoxia, whereas after 1 hour of hypoxia gap junction surface density was reduced by 45%.[60] Cellular uncoupling heralds the onset of irreversible damage. It coincides with the second phase of extracellular K^+ accumulation.[61] During the initial phase, when intracellular coupling resistance is unchanged, the decrease in conduction velocity is a consequence of the decrease in action potential upstroke and an increase in extracellular resistance (probably related to osmotic swelling). The rapid cellular uncoupling that occurs later causes conduction to become slow and discontinuous and eventually leads to complete conduction block.[58] The reasons for electrical uncoupling have not been completely established. It is more than likely that the increase in intracellular calcium that occurs after 15–20 minutes of ischemia[62,63] plays a major role, as well as intracellular acidosis, since it is known that both factors increase coupling resistance.[64,65]

Mechanisms of Arrhythmias During Acute Ischemia

During the first 30 minutes following experimental complete coronary artery occlusion, ventricular arrhythmias (ventricular premature depolarizations, VT, and VF) occur in two distinct phases. The first phase, called phase 1a, or "immediate ventricular arrhythmias," usually occurs between 2 and 10 minutes after occlusion, with the highest incidence of arrhythmias at around 5–6 minutes (see Fig. 4–1); the second phase, called phase 1b, or "delayed ventricular arrhythmias," occurs after approximately 12–30 minutes after occlusion, with a peak at 15–20 minutes. Sinus rhythm may be present between the two phases. This bimodal distribution of early arrhythmias has been demonstrated in the dog,[66,67] pig,[16] sheep,[68] and rat.[69] Individual animals may sometimes exhibit only 1a or 1b arrhythmias, but both phases may occur in the same animal.[67] No information is available about whether arrhythmias also occur in humans with a similar bimodal distribution during the first 30 minutes of a developing MI.

The experimental evidence suggests that the mechanism and/or site of origin of 1a and 1b arrhythmias is different. Phase 1a arrhythmias occur when there is a high degree of conduction slowing and delayed activation in the subepicardial muscle of the ischemic region. At this time, extracellular subepicardial electrograms are highly abnormal and consist of multiple components. A change in the extracellular electrogram from a smooth high-amplitude, biphasic deflection to a low-amplitude, multicomponent deflection is often interpreted to be caused by membrane depolarization, and slow and inhomogeneous conduction. On the basis of these electrogram characteristics it was proposed that 1a arrhythmias are caused by re-entry.[49,51,54,70,71] Phase 1b arrhythmias often occur in the absence of evidence of abnormal epicardial conduction. Subepicardial electrograms recorded during the 1b phase are not as abnormal as during the 1a phase, and there may be less spatial inhomogeneity of subepicardial activation delay during the 1b phase than during the 1a phase.[66–68] Also, the arrhythmias of phase 1a are related to a marked increase in refractory period, conduction delay, and threshold for excitation, whereas during the 1b phase there is a partial recovery of these parameters.[72] It has therefore been implied that mechanisms other than re-entry might be the cause for 1b arrhythmias. However, it is still possible that electrophysiological abnormalities associated with re-entry occur in regions of the ventricular wall other than the subepicardium and have not been detected.

Mapping experiments using simultaneous recordings from multiple sites have demonstrated that circus movement re-entry occurs during the 1a phase of ischemic arrhythmias.[73–75] Figure 4–4 demonstrates the excitation pattern during VT in the pig heart after a coronary occlusion. Activation sequences are shown for beats 27 to 35 of the tachycardia. Most often, a single circus movement is responsible for continuation of the arrhythmia, as shown in beat 27 (upper left panel); activation begins at the 20 msec isochrone and moves in a large circular pattern shown by the arrow, returning to its origin after 220 msec. It continues from this point at 230 msec during beat 28 and follows a somewhat larger circular pathway (arrow), again returning to its origin at 410 msec. Once again, during beat 29, it follows a similar circular pathway beginning at the 420 msec isochrone and ending at the 600 msec isochrone. However, additional wave fronts, possibly originating from re-entrant circuits elsewhere, also occurred (isochrone at 500 msec in the lower right part in beat 29). Furthermore, no continuity of activity between beats 29 and 30 was detected; a new wave front appears in a small area indicated by the 720 msec in beat 30, 120 msec after activation during beat 29 ended. This could be an offspring of an intramurally located re-entrant circuit, but it might also be caused by some sort of focal activity. In beats 30 and 31, a figure-of-eight type of circus movement is present where two wave fronts propagate around an area of block, one clockwise, the other counterclockwise, and fuse in a final common pathway. To form this pattern, activity during beat 31 moves from the 870 msec isochrone to the 940 msec isochrone and the wave front splits, with one front moving upward around the base and the other moving downward around the apex. The two wave fronts merge after the 1020 msec isochrone. This figure-of-eight configuration is present also in beat 32 beginning at the 1080 msec isochrone, but one wave front blocks at 1200 msec toward the base, whereas the other

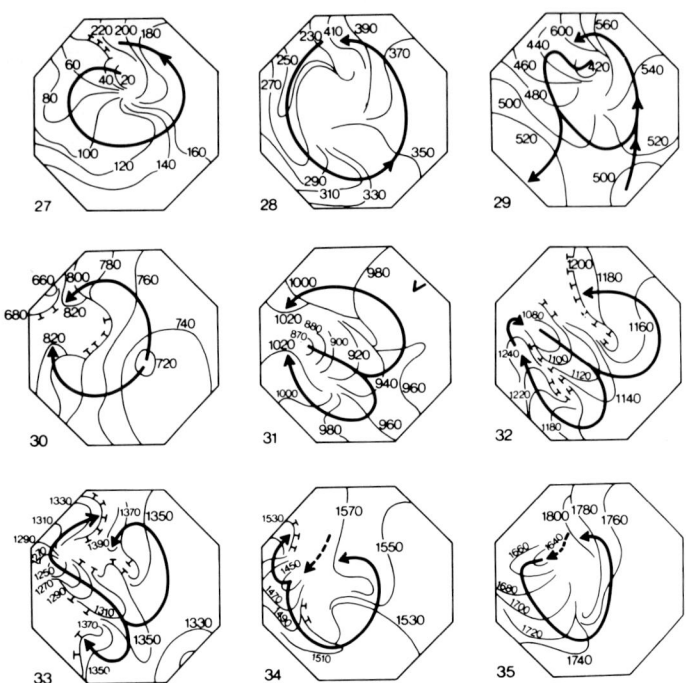

Fig. 4–4. Patterns of activation during a ventricular tachycardia after acute coronary artery occlusion in the pig heart. Note that basically one circus movement of fairly large dimensions is responsible for continuation of the tachycardia, although both dimension and position of the reentrant circuit changes from beat to beat. (Reproduced with permission from Janse MJ, et al: Circ Res 47: 151–165, 1980.[73])

toward the apex continues to complete a single re-entrant loop after 1240 msec. The activation pattern in beat 33 is rather complex, but it seems that the wave front ending at 1390 msec continues in beat 34 at 1450 msec to create a new, single circus movement. Since relatively few electrodes were present in this area, we drew a dotted line connecting activity between 1390 and 1450 msec (beat 33 to 34) and between 1570 and 1640 (beat 34 to 35) to indicate our uncertainty. Intramural re-entry might occur as well.

Whereas re-entry is responsible for maintenance of tachycardia and fibrillation, there is some doubt whether the initiating premature beats are always caused by reentry. Nonre-entrant mechanisms may also be operative during the acute ischemic period. Ventricular premature depolarizations can originate from the normal side of the ischemic border, which frequently is separated from the ischemic zone displaying delayed activity by an inexcitable zone.[73,76] Some ectopic activity in the early phase of ischemia might also originate from Purkinje fibers because Purkinje activity sometimes may precede ventricular muscle activity during spontaneous premature ventricular depolarizations.[77,78] The exact mechanism underlying the nonre-entrant ectopic activity is unknown. Triggered activity induced by either early or delayed afterdepolarizations is a possibility. Either early or delayed afterdepolarizations may occur in Purkinje fibers in the subendocardium adjacent to ischemic myocardium that are exposed to lysophosphoglycerides leaking out of the ischemic myocardium, as well as to protons, but to lower concentrations of K^+ ions than in the ischemic core (high concentrations of K^+ can suppress afterdepolarizations).[79] Another factor that may cause afterdepolarizations during early ischemia is stretch, caused by the paradoxical movements of the ischemic part of the ventricular wall.[80] The flow of injury current across the ischemic border is another possible nonre-entrant mechanism for phase 1a arrhythmias.[56,73,76] Such current flow should be generated by the differences in membrane potential between closely adjacent regions either during diastole or during the action potential, the differences in membrane potential being caused by injury to the ischemic region.[5] It has been proposed that this current flowing between the ischemic cells with delayed activity and the normal cells that have repolarized or are repolarizing, through an inexcitable segment of depolarized cells interposed between the two, re-excites the normal cells to cause premature depolarizations.[73]

Reperfusion Arrhythmias

Ventricular fibrillation may occur within seconds after restoration of blood flow to myocardium made ischemic by a period of coronary occlusion (reperfusion). In fact, VF may occur more frequently following reperfusion than after coronary artery ligation.[81] There is a relationship between the length of the ischemic period during the occlusion and the occurrence of reperfusion arrhythmias.[82,83] At least a 3-minute ischemic period during occlusion is necessary before reperfusion arrhythmias occur in dogs.[84] The incidence of reperfusion-induced VF increases when occlusion periods are lengthened from 5 minutes to 20 or 30 minutes. The onset of irreversible injury during ischemia is related to a decrease in reperfusion arrhythmias that occurs after 20–30 minutes,[85,86] since the arrhythmias must arise in viable cells. During relatively brief periods of ischemia (i.e., no longer than 20 minutes) there is marked depression of transmembrane action potentials, and even inexcitability, as we have described. Sudden reperfusion results within seconds in a very rapid restoration of action potentials to this ischemic myocardium,[4,87,88] although the return of electrical activity is not equally rapid for all cells.[4] These restored action potentials have reduced upstroke velocities and low amplitudes, and the duration and amplitude often alternate between high amplitude and long duration and low amplitude and short duration. After 20–30 seconds, action potential configuration has returned to normal.[4] During the first 30 seconds of reperfusion, there is a marked inhomogeneity in the action potentials within the ischemic area and at the border. Action potentials of different cells within the ischemic zone often alternate out of phase, some showing relatively high amplitudes and long durations while others at the same time show little more than local responses. The APD of cells close to the ischemic border may be shortened by as much as 60–100 msec during reperfusion.[48,89] It is quite possible that the increased inhomogeneity in APD in and around the previously ischemic zone immediately after abrupt reperfusion is a major factor contributing to the occurrence of fibrillation by enhancing the likelihood for re-entry. Studies in which activation has been mapped with simultaneous extracellular recordings have demonstrated the presence of multiple re-entrant circuits in the ischemic area during reperfusion-induced fibrillation.[90] However, some reperfusion arrhythmias might be a result of non-re-entrant mechanisms such as enhanced abnormal automaticity or triggered activity, based on the results of experiments on isolated superfused tissues. Delayed afterdepolarizations have been shown to occur during reoxygenation of isolated hypoxic papillary muscles[91] or Purkinje fibers.[92] It has indeed been shown that reperfusion, or restarting of oxidative metabolism after a period of metabolic blockade, results in intracellular calcium overload, which may cause the afterdepolarizations.[93] Early afterdepolarizations and the triggered activity that they cause have also been described in isolated superfused rabbit Purkinje fibers when returned from an ischemic solution to a normal Tyrodes solution, simulating reperfusion.[94]

DELAYED VENTRICULAR ARRHYTHMIAS IN THE SUBACUTE PHASE OF MYOCARDIAL INFARCTION

The acute ischemic phases (1a and 1b) of arrhythmias in the experimental canine model is followed by a period of 3–6 hours during which the predominant rhythm is sinus rhythm.[95] Occasional ventricular premature depolarizations may occur during this time. There is then a gradual increase in the frequency of ventricular premature depolarizations as an infarct develops, and by 8 hours numerous ventricular ectopic beats coexist with sinus beats. After 12–24 hours (the subacute phase of infarction), most or all beats can be of ventricular origin. The progressive increase in frequency of arrhythmias is shown in Figure 4–5, which displays continuous ECG recordings taken at various time periods after a coronary artery occlusion in the dog. The re-

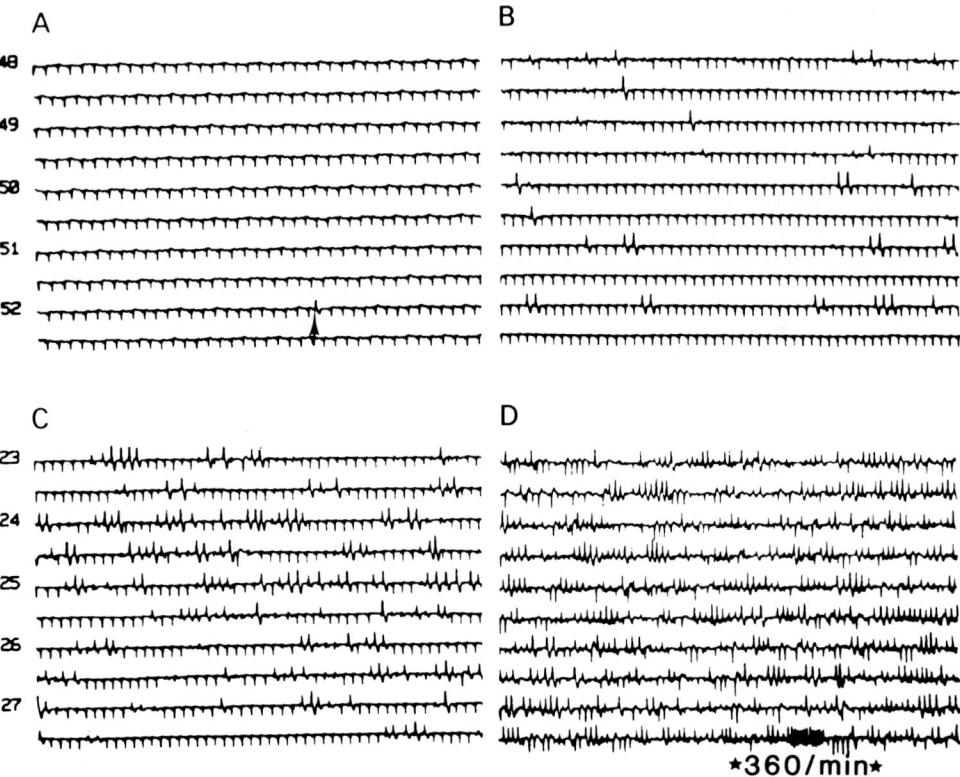

Fig. 4–5. The time course of appearance of ventricular arrhythmias as seen in portions of the 24-hour ECG recordings from a dog with acute myocardial infarction 1–5 hours (**A**), 7 hours (**B**), 12 hours (**C**), and 18 hours (**D**) after left anterior descending coronary artery ligation. The onset of multiform ventricular ectopic beats and tachycardia tended to be about 12 hours after coronary artery ligation (**C**) and persisted throughout the remainder of the 24-hour recording period. Occasional runs of monomorphic ventricular tachycardia at rates between 300 and 400/min (**D**) were seen in those dogs that died suddenly. (Reproduced with permission from Scherlag.[98])

cordings in panel A show only a single ectopic ventricular beat during the early time period, 1–5 hours after the occlusion. A greater frequency of ventricular beats is seen at 7 hours (panel B), a still greater frequency at 12 hours (panel C), while at 18 hours (panel D) most beats are ventricular in origin. The experimental delayed ventricular arrhythmias persist for 24–72 hours, after which time the rate decreases, as does the frequency of ventricular premature depolarizations.[95] Sinus rhythm is usually restored after 3 days, but inhibition of supraventricular activation of the ventricles (such as by stimulation of the vagus) may still reveal some enhanced ventricular firing at this time. The time course of occurrence of a delayed arrhythmic phase in humans is sometimes similar to the time course of occurrence of the experimental arrhythmias depicted in Figure 4–5.[96,97] During the time period in which there is an increase in frequency of ventricular arrhythmias, sudden death can occur because of VF.[98]

Characteristics of the Delayed Arrhythmias

The ECG characteristics of the delayed arrhythmias in the canine heart are those of an accelerated idioventricular rhythm or idioventricular tachycardia which are likely caused by arrhythmogenic mechanisms involving abnormal impulse initiation. Some of the arrhythmias during the delayed phase in humans have ECG characteristics identical to those that occur in the experimental models. Paroxysmal VT also occurs in both.[99]

That the frequency of ventricular ectopic beats increases when the sinus node is slowed by vagal stimulation, and that an abnormally rapid ventricular rate ensues when the sinus node is stopped,[55,100,101] are consistent with the expected characteristics of an automatic mechanism rather than triggered activity. When the dominance of the sinus node is removed, the pacemakers in the ventricles can fire uninhibited from overdrive by the more rapid supraventricular pacemaker. Normal automaticity (automaticity at normal levels of diastolic potentials), however, does not appear to be the primary cause of accelerated idioventricular tachycardia. Twenty-four hours after coronary occlusion, there is little or no evidence for the overdrive suppression[101,102] that is characteristic of normal pacemakers.[103] A lack of prominent overdrive suppression is characteristic of abnormal automaticity, which occurs in cells with partially depolarized membrane potentials.[104] Although abnormal automaticity is the dominant arrhythmogenic mechanism, some of the arrhythmic beats are probably caused by triggered activity[105] or re-entrant excitation.[106,107] The rapid tachycardias that occasionally begin with a closely coupled premature ventricular beat at 24 hours after coronary occlusion or those that cause sudden death at 12–18 hours are probably caused by re-entry.

The Development of an Infarct and Its Relationship to the Origin of the Delayed Ventricular Arrhythmias

When myocardial fibers survive in an area of ischemia, they may develop unusual electrophysiological properties because of the continued ischemia, and may cause arrhythmias at a later time. Such surviving fibers are the cause of the delayed phase of ventricular arrhythmias. The delayed arrhythmias arise for the most part in the Purkinje system, which survives on the endocardial surface of transmural infarcts.[55,100,106,108,109] However, it takes many hours for ischemia to alter its electrophysiological properties. After a coronary occlusion, cell death progresses as a "wave front" from the necrosing core in the subendocardium toward the subepicardium and toward the epicardial surface,[110,111] moving more slowly toward the endocardial surface than toward the epicardial surface. After 1 hour, the necrotic wave front moves into the midmyocardial wall, where electrograms become smaller with time (Fig. 4–5).[112] At 1 hour there still are several millimeters of viable muscle cells separating the necrotic region from the Purkinje fibers on the subendocardial surface. In the electrograms recorded at the endocardial surface both ventricular muscle and Purkinje deflections still occur (Fig. 4–5, 1 hour). At 18–24 hours mostly Purkinje fibers remain electrically active on the endocardial surface of the infarct and form and endocardial border zone, while the subendocardial muscle has died (Fig. 4–5, 18 hours).[111] At the time when delayed arrhythmias reach their maximum intensity, at around 24 hours after occlusion, electrical activity is not evident in most of the infarcted ventricular wall.[100,108,109,113] The surviving subendocardial Purkinje fibers are shown in the photomicrograh in Figure 4–6. They are the initiators of most of the delayed arrhythmias. The "wave front" of cell death that proceeds toward the epicardial region also stops short of the epicardial surface, and there is a surviving rim of epicardial muscle, called the epicardial border zone.[114,115]

There are no studies locating the origin of delayed spontaneous arrhythmias in humans. Pathological anatomical studies show that Purkinje fibers on the endocardial surface of transmural human infarcts often remain structurally intact and therefore may be viable.[116] They therefore may be the site of origin of some VTs.

Electrophysiological Properties of Surviving Purkinje Fibers

Microelectrode recordings from Purkinje fibers surviving in transmural canine infarcts have provided important additional information on the mechanisms causing the delayed arrhythmias. Purkinje fiber transmembrane potentials toward the center and apex of the infarcted region may be very depressed; the maximum diastolic potential of many fibers may be -60 mV to -70 mV, and the upstrokes are slow. An example of recordings from these subendocardial Purkinje fibers is shown in Figure 4–7. The action potentials shown were recorded by

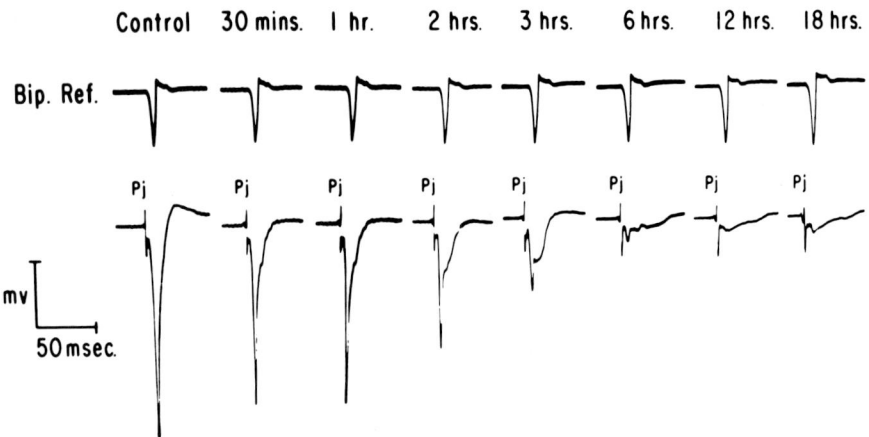

Fig. 4–6. Electrograms recorded from ventricular muscle in a normal region (Bip. Ref.) and from the subendocardium of the left ventricle in an infarcting region of the canine heart. The times listed above the electrograms represent the duration of coronary artery occlusion. No change in the amplitude of the Purkinje complex (P_j) occurred despite its immediate proximity to a severe localized subendocardial infarction. The progressive loss of the negative bipolar electrogram following the Purkinje deflection, which represents subendocardial muscle activity, with time after the coronary artery occlusion was caused by the subendocardial infarction. (Reproduced with permission from Cox JL, et al: Circulation 48:971–983, 1973.[112])

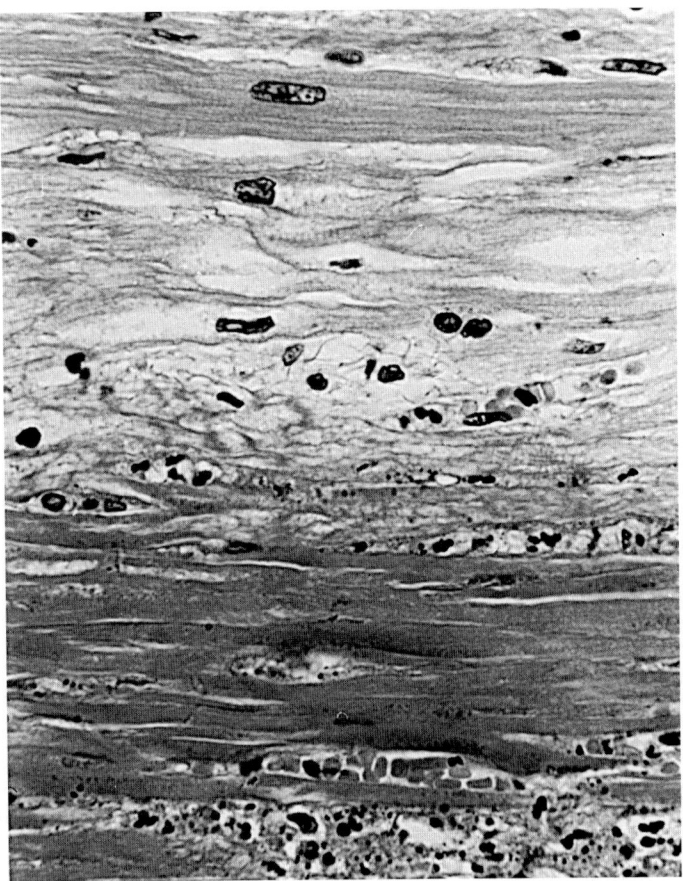

Fig. 4–7. Purkinje fibers in the subendocardial border zone. A histologic section from a 24-hour-old canine infarct caused by LAD occlusion is shown. At the top is the endocardial surface and left ventricular cavity. The first two cell layers beneath the surface are surviving Purkinje fibers characterized by centrally located nuclei, well-defined myofibrils, and intercalated disks. Beneath the Purkinje fibers and the expanded extracellular space caused by edema is the infarcted ventricular muscle, characterized by a lack of well-defined myofibrils and eccentrically located nuclei.

moving the microelectrode laterally from the noninfarcted tip of the papillary muscle (control), across the border of the infarct (represented by the dashed line), into the infarcted region. The control action potential is normal, whereas the maximum diastolic potential and the action potential upstroke and amplitude diminish as the recording site moves further into the infarct. Spontaneous diastolic depolarization is also a prominent characteristic of the Purkinje cells in the infarct, as is illustrated in the records at the bottom in Figure 4–7. Figure 4–8 shows a transmembrane potential recorded from a Purkinje fiber in the infarcted region with spontaneous diastolic depolarization (top trace). The action potential in the bottom trace was recorded from an adjacent noninfarcted region. Because of the enhanced automaticity of these peripheral Purkinje fibers, they act as pacemakers. Automaticity in Purkinje cells that have low maximum diastolic potentials (about −60 mV), such as the one shown in Figure 4–8, is classified as abnormal automaticity, as mentioned before. Delayed afterdepolarizations occur in some Purkinje fibers in the infarcts and can cause triggered activity.[102,105,117] The occurrence of delayed afterdepolarizations suggests that intracellular calcium levels in the Purkinje fibers are elevated. The APD of Purkinje fibers surviving in infarcts 24 hours after coronary occlusion is also prolonged.[108,113] When premature impulses arising at the borders of the infarct propagate into these areas with long APDs and long refractory periods before complete recovery of responsiveness, conduction is markedly slowed. This can lead to conduction block and reentry.[108]

As was mentioned earlier, the spontaneously occurring ventricular tachycardias diminish in frequency by 48 hours, and by 72 hours sinus rhythm is usually restored. The abatement of arrhythmias can be correlated with the gradual return toward normal of the transmembrane potential of the sur-

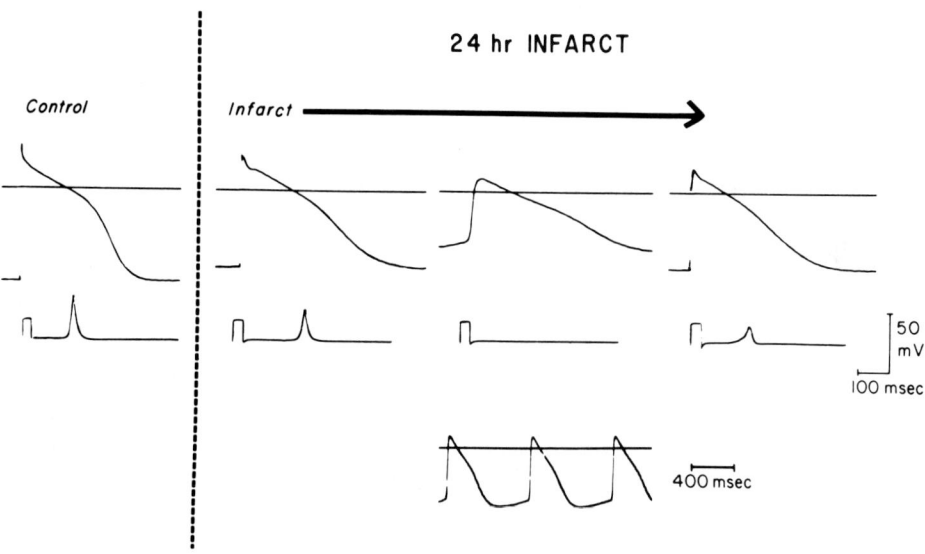

Fig. 4–8. Depression of transmembrane potentials of subendocardial Purkinje fibers within an infarct. Action potentials shown were recorded by moving the microelectrode laterally from the noninfarcted tip of the papillary muscle (control) across the border of the infarct represented by the broken line into the infarcted region. The top trace is the transmembrane action potential and is shown with a horizontal line denoting the zero reference potential. The bottom trace for the control data and the middle trace for the infarct data are the differentiated signal of a 100-mV sawtoothed pulse with a 200 V/sec slope of depolarization (square pulse) and the depolarization phase of the action potential. The bottom trace for the infarct data shows action potentials from the fiber in the middle section recorded at a slower sweep speed. (Reproduced with permission from Friedman PL, et al: Circ Res 33:597–611, 1973.[108])

viving Purkinje cells. There is a significant increase in the resting membrane potential, action potential amplitude, and V_{max} by 3 days after coronary artery occlusion, and spontaneous diastolic depolarization is no longer prominent.[118,119] Delayed afterdepolarizations can sometimes be induced by stimulating the cells at rapid rates. APD, however, remains prolonged. The prolonged action potential of a Purkinje fiber in a 72-hour-old infarct is illustrated in Figure 4–9; below, this recording is superimposed on a normal action potential, indicated by the dashed line. After 3 days, there is also a progressive decline in APD. Although the resting potential and the upstroke of the action potential are normal by about 10 days after the coronary occlusion, the APD decreases to less than normal before it finally returns to normal during the next few weeks (Fig. 4–10).[118,119]

There are several possible reasons that might explain why subendocardial Purkinje fibers survive within the infarcted region and go on to develop abnormal electrical activity that lasts for several days. Normally, coronary flow brings oxygen and nutrients to the subendocardial fibers through a capillary network. In addition, there may be some retrograde flow from the cavity into subendocardial layers, offering an additional or alternative source of oxygen and nutrients.[120] The functional significance[121] or even the existence of such flow is controversial.[122] After a coronary occlusion, this retrograde flow may remain and be sufficient to maintain viability of the subendocardial Purkinje system. Another possible source of oxygen and nutrients is physical diffusion from the ventricular cavity into the subendocardial layers, which would also persist after coronary occlusion.[123] Diffusion of oxygen and nutrients from the ventricular cavity to the surviving Purkinje cells is probably not sufficient to maintain normal electrophysiological properties although it is adequate to keep them alive. The diffusion only keeps the muscle fibers alive for a limited period of time. During this time the muscle is also electrophysiologically abnormal.

The transient abnormal electrophysiology prior to death of the muscle and the longer-lasting electrophysiological abnormalities in the Purkinje fibers are likely to be caused by ischemic alterations in cellular metabolism. Alterations in metabolism of Purkinje fibers in the subendocardial border zone of canine infarcts are indicated by a progressive increase in intracellular lipid deposits in the cytoplasm that parallels the progressive changes in transmembrane potentials during the first 24 hours after occlusion.[111,118] Intracellular accumulation of free fatty acids and lipids may lead to changes in the structure and function of membrane systems in the cardiac cell that have a profound effect on ionic currents. For example, it may be responsible for depolarization of the resting potential that is progressive during the first 24 hours. There is a substantial loss of K^+ (approximately 50 mM) from the Purkinje fibers during this time period.[124,125] On account of this loss, the K^+ equilibrium potential is decreased to about 82 mV. The reduction in the K^+ equilibrium potential accounts for only about one-half the reduction in the maximum diastolic potential. Therefore, membrane conductance changes must also occur to account for part of the depolarization. The decrease in intracellular K^+ may itself lead to a change in the membrane conductance that contributes to the depolarization, by virtue of its effects on the inwardly rectifying K^+ channels.[126] It is possible that the

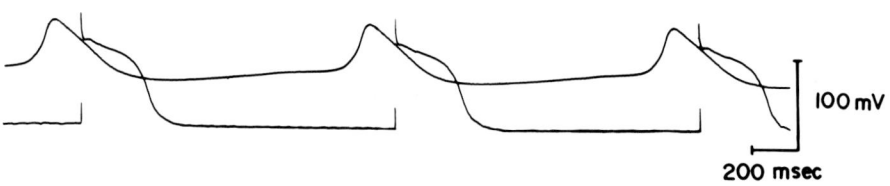

Fig. 4–9. Action potentials recorded from a Purkinje fiber in the endocardial border zone of a 24-hour-old infarct (top trace), and from an adjacent, noninfarcted region. (Modified and reproduced with permission from Friedman PL, et al: Circ Res 33:612–626, 1973.[109])

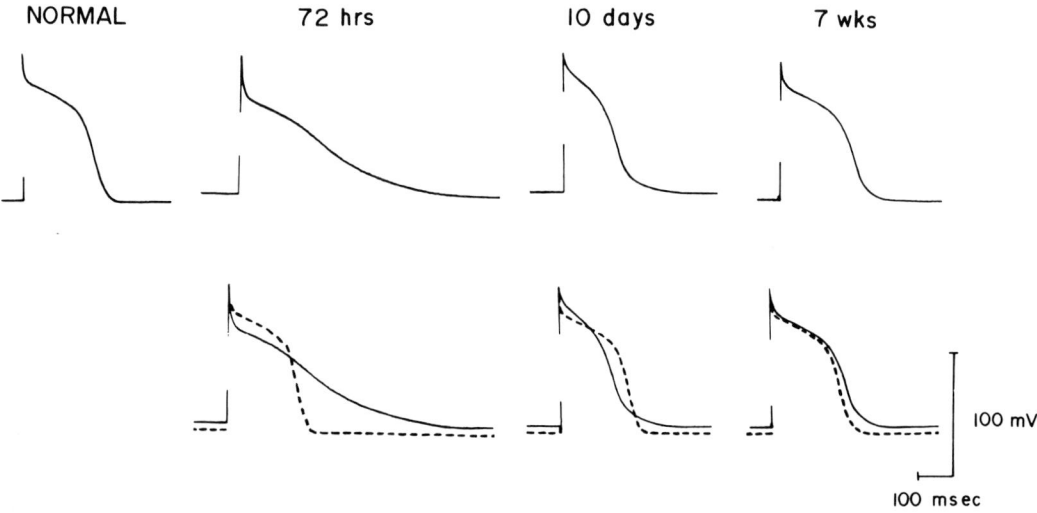

Fig. 4-10. Change in action potential duration of Purkinje fibers in the subendocardial border zone with time after a coronary occlusion. At the top left is the action potential of a Purkinje fiber in a noninfarcted (normal) myocardium. To the right of this record are action potentials of Purkinje fibers in infarcts of the ages shown above each recording. Below each of these traces the action potential of the Purkinje fiber in the infarct (solid trace) is superimposed on the action potential of the normal Purkinje fiber (dashed trace).

same increase in K^+ channel conductance and passive K^+ efflux that has been proposed for ventricular muscle occurs. K^+ loss from the Purkinje cells during the early hours of ischemia cannot all be pumped back into the cells because of a depression in the activity of the Na^+/K^+ exchange pump. This depression is evident by 3 hours after the coronary occlusion[127] and also may be related to the abnormal lipid metabolism. Depression of the Na^+/K^+ pump by free fatty acids[128,129] would be expected to cause some depolarization as well as prolongation because of a decrease in outward pump current.[130]

There is some evidence that 24 hours after coronary occlusion, occasional ventricular beats might also arise in epicardial muscle over the infarct (the epicardial border zone). At 24 hours, epicardial border zone muscle cells studied in vitro in isolated superfused tissue preparations have low resting potentials (-60 to -80 mV),[115,131] at least partly a result of a significant decrease in intracellular K^+.[132] Spontaneous diastolic depolarization causing abnormal impulse initiation has been recorded in these cells, most often after exposure to catecholamines.[131]

LATER PHASES OF VENTRICULAR ARRHYTHMIAS

Arrhythmias may continue to occur after the early acute and subacute periods in patients who have had an infarction.[133] Both clinical and experimental evidence shows that these later phases of arrhythmias have still different underlying electrophysiology than the earlier phases. The later phases of clinical arrhythmias can be subdivided into "late hospital" arrhythmias, which are arrhythmias documented just prior to hospital discharge, when the infarct is healing, and post-hospital arrhythmias, also referred to as chronic arrhythmias, when the infarct is healed. The results of a large number of clinical electrophysiological studies, beginning with Wellens' initial investigation in 1972,[134] have provided data strongly suggesting that re-entrant excitation is the principal causative mechanism of the ventricular arrhthymias. Experimental studies on animal models have confirmed this conclusion and have provided additional information on the properties and characteristics of the re-entrant circuits.

One of the characteristics of the clinical arrhythmias is that they can often be in-

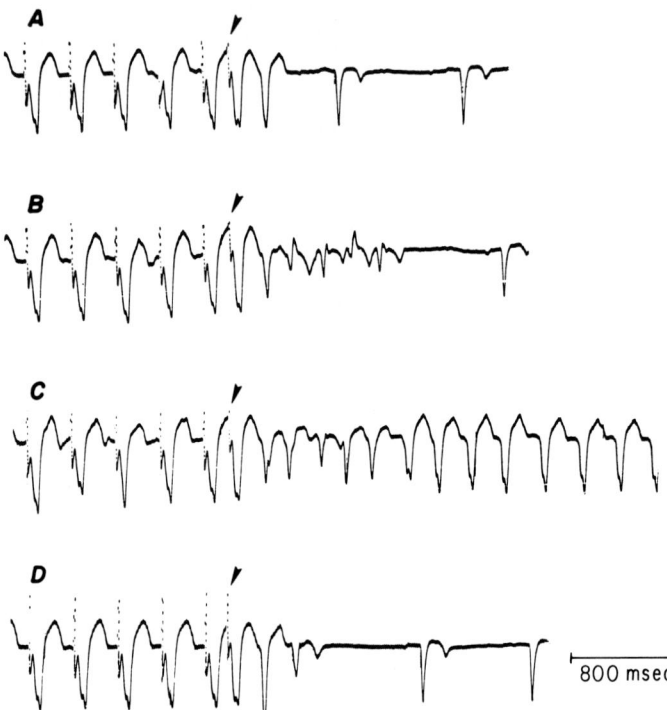

Fig. 4–11. Initiation of ventricular tachycardia in a dog on the third day after occlusion of the left anterior descending coronary artery for 2 hours followed by reperfusion. The ECG is shown in each panel. Panels **A–D** show records in which the ventricles were driven at a cycle length of 350 msec, and a single stimulated premature impulse (arrows) was stimulated. (Reproduced with permission from Karagueuzian HS, et al: Circ Res 44:833–846, 1979.[135])

duced by programmed electrical stimulation. Similarly, as shown in Figure 4–11, ventricular arrhythmias can be induced by programmed stimulation of the canine heart with a healing infarct. A single nonstimulated ventricular depolarization follows the stimulated premature ventricular depolarization delivered at a coupling interval of 205 msec (Fig. 4–11A, arrow). As the coupling interval of the premature stimulus was decreased (to 195 msec in Fig. 4–11B), the number of nonstimulated impulses that it induced increased, resulting in nonsustained tachycardia. At shorter premature stimulus coupling intervals sustained tachycardia occurred, as shown in Figure 4–11C, where the premature stimulus was applied with a coupling interval of 190 msec. The initiation of tachycardia by electrical stimulation is very important evidence supporting a re-entrant mechanism and excluding an automatic mechanism.

Location of Re-entrant Circuits Causing Ventricular Tachyarrhythmias

The site of arrhythmia origin is dependent on the location of surviving myocardial cells in and around the infarcted region. These cells may have electrophysiological properties that are favorable for the occurrence of re-entry as a result of being exposed to the trauma of the ischemic environment for a long period of time, or the geometric arrangement of the cells that survive may be favorable for the formation of re-entrant circuits, or a combination of the two may be operating. The location of the surviving cells in the infarct region is influenced by the particular coronary artery that is occluded, by the location of the occlusion along the length of the coronary artery (proximal or distal), by the presence and location of collateral blood supply, and by the duration of the occlusion (permanent vs. temporary with reperfusion). In the experimental animal models in which the effects of prolonged ischemia and infarction have been studied, myocardial fibers may survive on either on both of the epicardial or endocardial surfaces of healing and healed infarcts, even when the coronary artery is occluded near its origin and the infarct is transmural.[113,114,118,135–139] These regions of surviving myocardial cells are called the epicardial and endocardial border zones.[140] Muscle fibers may also survive in intramural regions of the infarct, particularly if there is reperfusion of the ischemic region before intramural cell death is complete.[135,141] Both epicardial and endocardial border zones as well as the intramural fibers are important sites of arrhythmogenesis. Similar patterns of cell survival also occur in human infarcts.[142,143]

The epicardial border zone is an important site of arrhythmia origin in healing canine infarcts[139,140,144] and is also a site of arrhythmia origin in human infarcts.[145,146] Muscle fibers on the epicardial surface of transmural anteroseptal canine infarcts caused by permanent occlusion of the left anterior descending coronary artery (LAD) near its origin survive because they still receive blood flow from epicardial branches of the circumflex artery or from collaterals of the LAD that anastomose with the patent circumflex. The surviving epicardial muscle-fiber bundles are arranged parallel to one another during the healing phase (first 2 weeks) after infarction. The muscle fibers may be either tightly packed together, as they are in the normal subepicardium (Fig. 4-12B), or they may be separated by edema, which is commonly seen in a healing infarct (Fig. 4-12A). Despite the normal histological appearance, the presence of lipid in the surviving muscle indicates that ischemia has altered cellular metabolism, which in turn might be related to some of the changes in transmembrane action potentials during the healing phase.[115] As the infarct continues to heal, there are further changes in the structure of the epicardial border zone, as determined by studies in canine models. Figure 4-13 shows that the muscle cells become trapped in the dense scar tissue formed from the infarct below and the pericarditis above. Parallel-oriented fibers are separated by increased connective tissue in regions where they are present in relatively large numbers (20-30 cell layers).[115] In regions with fewer cell layers, myocardial fibers become markedly separated from each other along their length, to such an extent that side-to-side connections between bundles are not always apparent.[115,147] The individual cells and their orientation are also

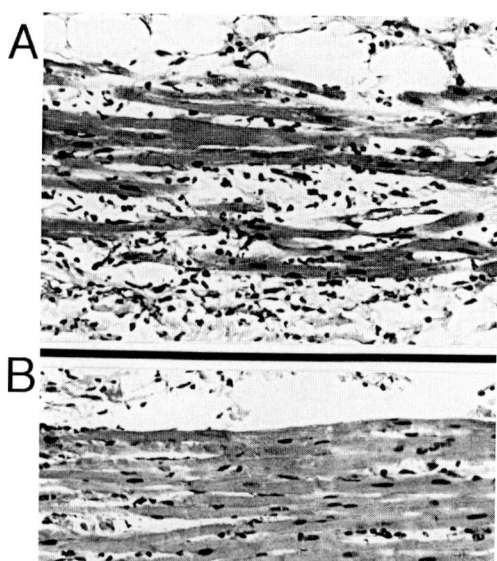

Fig. 4-12. Photomicrographs of the parallel surviving muscle fibers in the epicardial border zone of a healing canine infarct. In some regions (A) muscle fibers are widely separated, while in others (B) they are packed more closely together. However, in both cases the fibers are oriented parallel to each other. (Reproduced with permission from Dillon SM, et al: Circ Res 63:182-206, 1988.[152])

deformed by the growth of fibrous tissue (Figs. 4-13C and D).

Myocardial fibers survive on the endocardial surface of even extensive transmural infarcts in the canine heart, as we discussed earlier. The endocardial border zone that these muscle fibers comprise is an important site of arrhythmia origin in human infarcts.[148] Subendocardial ventricular muscle rarely survives after permanent occlusion near the origin of the LAD in the canine heart, but it may survive if the infarcts are reperfused after a several-hour period of occlusion or if the occlusion is below one or more of the diagonal branches.[136] Reperfusion restores coronary blood flow before the wave front of necrosis reaches the subendocardial muscle. More distal occlusions may spare some branches of the LAD that supply the subendocardial muscle. Subendocardial muscle and Pur-

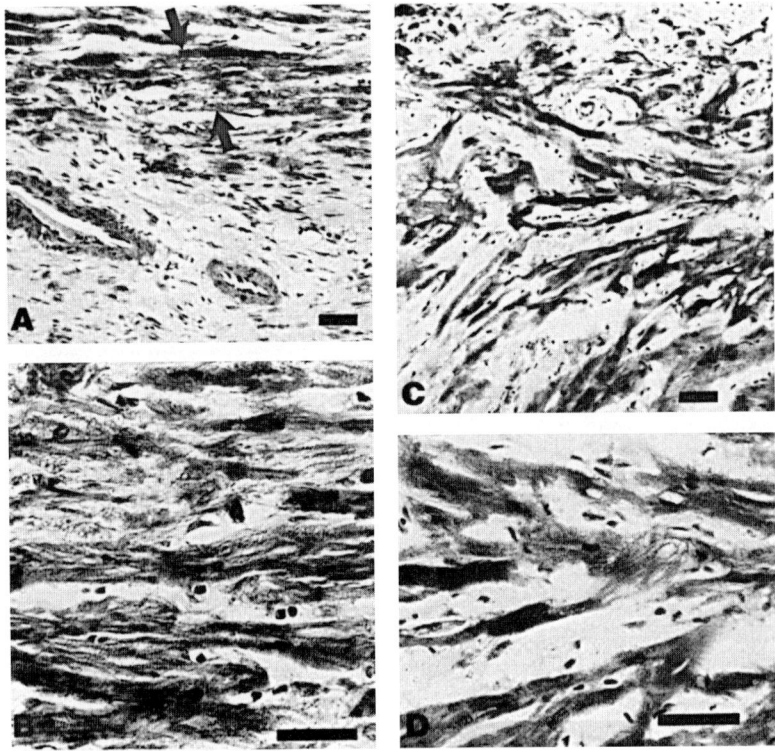

Fig. 4–13. Surviving epicardial muscle fibers in a 2-week-old canine infarct (**A** and **B**) and in a 2-month-old canine infarct (**C** and **D**). In **A**, the thin surviving rim at 15 days (arrows) consists of several layers of ventricular muscle cells between the epicardium and the granulation tissue of the healing infarct. These surviving cells are separated by fibrous tissue, especially adjacent to the infarct. The parallel orientation of the fibers, however, is generally retained. At high magnification (**B**), these myocardial cells appear to be intact, with distinct cross-striations. In C, the disorganization of the surviving myocardial cells in the thin rim at 2 months is evident. The cells are widely separated and disoriented because of the ingrowth of fibrous tissue from the adjacent infarct. At high magnification (**D**), the myocardial cells have distinct cross-striations and central nuclei. Scale bars = 50 μm. (Reproduced with permission from Ursell PC, et al: Circ Res 56:436–451, 1985.[115])

kinje fibers survive after occlusion of the ventrolateral coronary artery in feline hearts.[138] By 1–2 months, the ultrastructure of Purkinje cells that form the subendocardial border zone is normal, as are the transmembrane potentials of these cells.[118] However, other structural changes that occur in this region during healing are similar to the changes in the epicardial border zone. When there is surviving subendocardial muscle, subendocardial fibrosis has similar effects on geometric arrangement and intercellular connections as in the epicardial border zone, separating the muscle fibers and sometimes distorting their orientation.

Viable muscle bundles may protrude into the infarct from its lateral edge and interdigitate with scar tissue in canine infarcts caused by either permanent occlusion of the LAD or by occlusion and reperfusion, and these muscle bundles may be an important factor in arrhythmogenesis.[135,141,149] The muscle bundles may extend as far as the center of the infarcted wall and appear as surviving intramural muscle. Intramural muscle bundles may form part of re-entrant circuits in the animal models and in human infarcts.[150,151]

The changes in morphology in the epicardial and endocardial border zones of canine infarcts that occur as the infarcts heal are representative of changes that occur in other infarct regions where myocardial cells survive, and show the changes in the anatomical substrate of tachyarrhythmias that occur during infarct healing. As we discuss later, where there is parallel orientation of the muscle fibers, the epicardial border zone has the conduction properties of a non-uniform anisotropic structure, which may be important for re-entry.[152] Where the parallel orientation is lost, these conduction properties change drastically, but the structure may still contribute to the slow conduction that causes re-entry.[115,147] Therefore, changes in the anatomical substrate during healing influence electrophysiological properties, which in turn may influence properties of the re-entrant circuits and tachycardia.

As described in Figure 4-11, one of the hallmarks of tachyarrhythmias in human and canine hearts with healing or healed infarcts is their initiation by electrical stimulation of the ventricles, which acts as a trigger. Spontaneous initiation of arrhythmias may sometimes be triggered by premature beats, although often the initiating impulse has a long coupling interval (unlike the initiating stimulated impulse).[153] The initiation of tachyarrhythmias by such a trigger indicates that the re-entrant circuit either is not present or is not functioning until this initiating event occurs. Activation maps of the epicardial border zone in the canine model have shown exactly how premature stimuli initiate arrhythmias. An example is shown in Figure 4-14. Activation times measured simultaneously at 196 sites within a 4 × 5-cm region went into the construction of these maps. The upper left panel shows that the basic drive stimuli, applied on the epicardial surface of the right ventricle adjacent to the LAD (pulse symbol) at a cycle length of 280 msec, initiated excitation wave fronts that spread over the epicardial border zone from this margin toward the opposite margin at the apex of the lateral free wall (arrows). The isochrones progress in sequence from 0 to 90 msec. There is no evidence of a re-entrant circuit in this region. The prematurely stimulated impulses that initiate arrhythmias have very different activation patterns. Stimulated premature impulses that initiate tachycardias propagate into the epicardial border zone and block.[137,144,152,154] The region of conduction block forms a line that extends for several centimeters, called the arc of conduction block by El-Sherif.[144] Conduction block of a premature impulse with a coupling interval of 150 msec to the last basic drive impulse that resulted in re-entry is shown in the activation map in the lower left panel in Figure 4-14. Activation of the epicardial border zone by this premature impulse occurred from the LAD margin, where it was initiated (pulse symbol), to the 60 msec isochrone, about one third of the distance into the border zone before the block occurred. Conduction block is indicated by the thick black line. Re-entry occurs when stimulated wave fronts propagate around the extremities of the arc of conduction block and activate myocardium on the distal side of the block after myocardium on the proximal side has recovered excitability. These wave fronts can then re-excite the myocardium on the proximal side. This pattern of activation is shown by the arrows in Figure 4-14 (lower left panel). The region on the distal side of the line of block was activated at between 150 and 160 msec by wave fronts propagating around both ends of the line of block. Activation on the distal side of the line of block occurred about 100 msec after block occurred at the proximal side (at 60 msec). This time lapse of 100 msec allowed the proximal side time to recover excitability. The map in the lower right panel of Figure 4-14 shows the wave front from the distal side of the line of block (asterisk) propagating retrogradely across it to re-excite the proximal side (isochrones 10 to 30). The wave front returned to the LAD margin (40 msec isochrone), where it exited the border zone to excite the ventricles as the first tachycardia impulse (T1). A functional re-entrant circuit was therefore formed by the premature activation. If the length of the line of block is too short, activation of the distal side may occur too quickly, before the proximal side has recovered excitability. The proximal side of the region of block cannot then be re-excited and re-entry cannot occur. Failure of a premature impulse to cause a sufficiently long arc of block and initiate re-entry may occur if the coupling interval of the premature stimulus to the basic drive stimulus is too long. The arc of block lengthens as the premature coupling interval is decreased. In addition, conduction around the arc of block may be too rapid at long coupling intervals and may

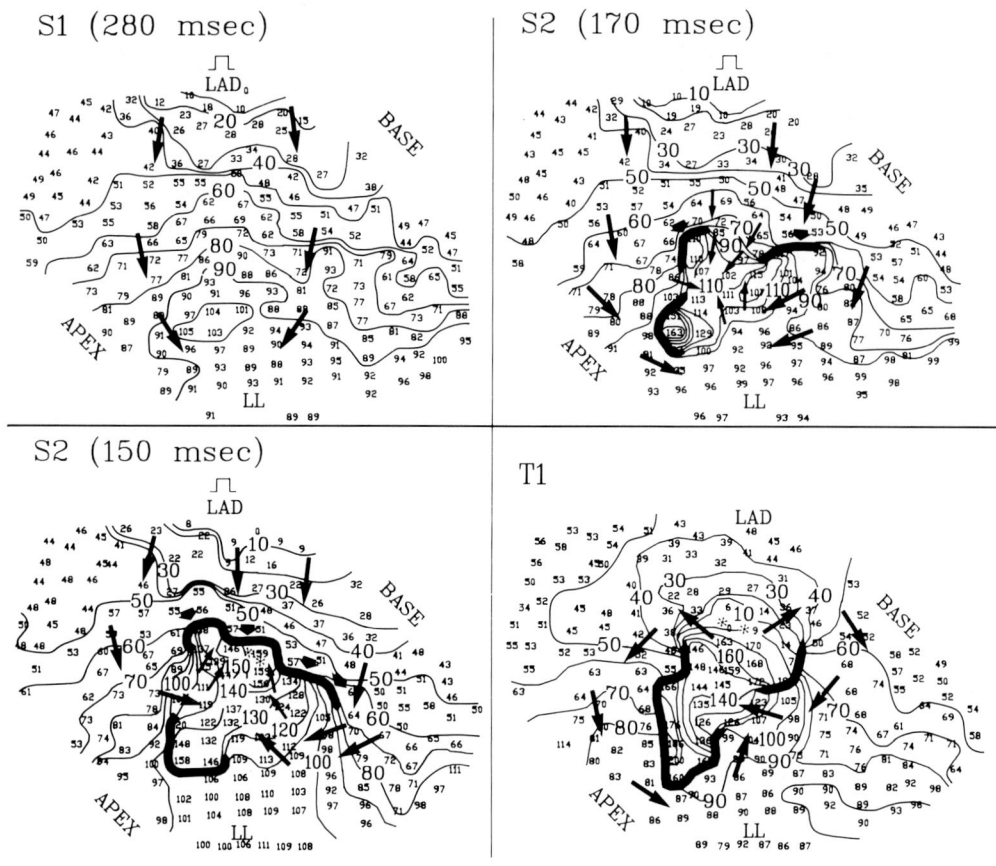

Fig. 4–14. Activation maps of the epicardial border zone showing the initiation of re-entrant ventricular tachycardia by a premature stimulus in a canine heart with a 4-day-old infarct. In each panel, the border of the electrode array adjacent to the left anterior descending coronary artery (LAD) is at the top, and the border of the electrode array on the lateral left ventricle (LL) is at the bottom. The base of the heart is to the right and the apex to the left. Activation times are plotted at each of the recording sites. The ventricles were driven at a regular cycle length (280 msec) by basic drive stimuli (S_1) applied through electrodes along the LAD margin of the epicardial border zone at the top of each map. The activation pattern of the epicardial border zone during the basic drive is shown in the top left panel (S_1—280 msec). The arrows indicate the direction of activation. The top right panel shows the activation pattern of a single premature impulse (S_2) elicited from the same stimulation site at the LAD margin at the coupling interval of 170 msec. This premature impulse did not initiate re-entry, although there were local areas of conduction block indicated by the thick black lines (see text). The bottom left panel shows activation by another premature impulse elicited with a coupling interval of 150 msec. Conduction of this premature impulse blocked along the region indicated by the horizontal, thick black line (short thick arrow). Conduction around the line of block (large arrows) initiated re-entry. The bottom right panel shows the re-entrant excitation pattern of the first impulse of the tachycardia. Activation in this time window begins at the asterisk within the 10 msec isochrone, the point where the activation in the previous map and time window (lower left panel) ended. (Modified and reproduced with permission from Wit.[157])

slow as the premature coupling interval is decreased, facilitating the occurrence of re-entry. These effects of prematurity explain why tachycardias are initiated only by appropriately timed stimulated premature impulses during programmed electrical stimulation. The top right panel in Figure 4–14 shows the activation pattern of a premature impulse, stimulated at a longer coupling interval of 170 msec, which did not induce tachycardia (compared to the premature impulse with a coupling interval of 150 msec, which did). Activation spread away from the LAD stimulation site, and several small areas of conduction block developed, as indicated by the thick black lines. The distal sides of the lines of block were activated with a delay of 20–50 msec beyond the activation time proximal to the lines of block, which was not sufficient to allow re-entry to occur.

Block of premature impulses depends to a significant extent on dispersions of refractoriness of the surviving epicardial muscle fibers.[155] Stimulated impulses block when they run into a region of increased effective refractory period. Slow conduction around the zone of conduction block may be attributed at least partly to propagation in regions with prolonged refractoriness that have partially recovered excitability.[155,156] The anisotropic structure of the epicardial border zone in the canine model may also provide an additional mechanism for the block and slow conduction.[152,157] Most of the arc of conduction block during initiation of tachycardia is usually oriented transverse to the long axis of the myocardial fibers that compose the epicardial border zone, meaning that the blocked activation wave propagates in the same direction as the long axis of the myocardial fibers. In nonuniformly anisotropic myocardium, the safety factor for conduction in this direction is low and can lead to block of prematurely stimulated impulses without the necessity for a prolonged refractory period.[158] The wave front propagating around the line of block must also propagate for a time in a direction transverse to the long axis of the myocardial fibers. Propagation in this direction is slow even in completely recovered myocardium.[157]

Excitation maps of the epicardial border zone in the canine infarct have shown that once the stimulated impulse that initiates re-entry re-excites the region proximal to the arc of conduction block (Fig. 4–14, lower right panel), the excitation wave may continue to propagate in a circular pattern to form a re-entrant circuit that causes tachycardia or, possibly, fibrillation. The location, size, and shape of the circuit are not usually the same as for the circuit traversed by the initiating impulse.[137,139,144,152,154,157]

Figure 4–15 shows an activation map of re-entrant circuit in the epicardial border zone, obtained during one beat of a sustained and stable monomorphic VT. In the time window that is shown, activation begins within the 10 msec isochrone (asterisk) and moves toward the LAD margin, where the wave front divides in two (black arrows). One wave front moves to the left on the map, which is the direction toward the apex of the left ventricle, and the other moves toward the right, which is the direction toward the base. Activation by both wave fronts then moves toward the lateral left margin, where the two wave fronts coalesce at around the 120 msec isochrone and then progress back toward the LAD margin to the region where activation began. This sequence is illustrated by the black arrows. The re-entrant circuit is completed after 183 msec, the cycle length of the tachycardia. The sequence of activation shown in this map repeated itself exactly for each beat of the tachycardia. Electrograms from sites in the re-entrant circuit that are circled are shown to the right of the activation map.

The activation sequence shown in Figure 4–15 during re-entry is around two long lines of conduction block (the two thick black lines in the figure) which are arranged parallel to each other and parallel to the long axis of the myocardial fibers. These are not the same lines of block that occurred during initiation of tachycardia by the premature impulse. The lines of block around which re-entrant excitation circulates are not caused by any grossly visible anatomical obstacle, nor are there well-defined, gross anatomical pathways that form the re-entrant circuit. The regions of block and the re-entrant circuits are not evident in the absence of tachycardia such as during sinus beats or ventricular pacing. Therefore, these are functional re-entrant circuits.

In Figure 4–15 there are actually two re-entrant circuits causing the tachycardia. Each one is in the form of an oval that is characteristic of re-entry in an anisotropic medium.[152,157] One is rotating clockwise and the other counterclockwise around the long lines of apparent block, and they share a common central pathway of conduction. This is the so-called figure-of-eight pattern, named as such by El-Sherif.[144] Complete re-entrant circuits have also been mapped in

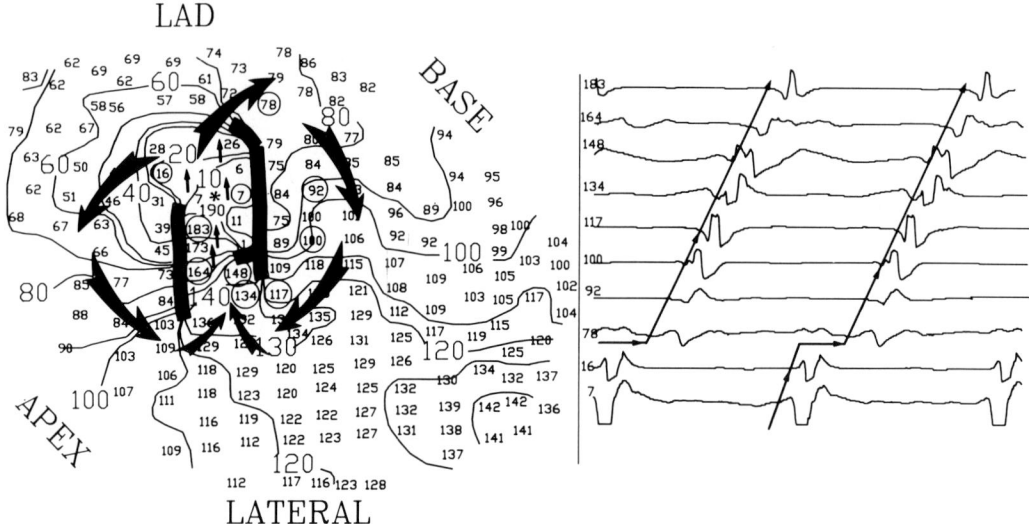

Fig. 4–15. Activation map of a re-entrant circuit in the epicardial border zone of a canine heart with a 4-day-old infarct. The margins of the electrode array are adjacent to the left anterior descending coronary artery (LAD), base, lateral left ventricle, and apex. Activation times at each of the recording sites are plotted for one impulse of tachycardia (small numbers). Isochrones are drawn at 10-msec intervals and labeled with large numbers. Arrows point out the direction of activation. At the right are selected electrograms recorded at sites in the reentrant circuit indicated by the circles on the activation map. The numbers at the left of the electrogram traces are the activation times on the map. (Reproduced with permission.)

the epicardial and endocardial border zones in patients. The figure-of-eight re-entrant activation pattern has been documented.[145,159,160]

Electrophysiological Properties of Myocardial Fibers Causing Ventricular Arrhythmias

The characteristics of the transmembrane potentials of the cardiac cells that survive the acute ischemic insult and that form the re-entrant circuits in the experimental animal models have been determined by microelectrode recordings from isolated tissue superfused with a physiological solution.[115,161,162] As the surviving myocardial cells recover from the acute ischemia while the infarct heals, their transmembrane potentials undergo a progression of changes until a stable state is reached in the completely healed infarct. The microelectrode studies have shown that the maximum diastolic potential and action potential amplitude of the surviving ventricular muscle cells in the epicardial border zone during the *first week* after permanent coronary occlusion or coronary occlusion and reperfusion are reduced to a range of -65 to -75 mV, compared with -85 to -90 mV for normal epicardial ventricular muscle cells. Severely depressed (depolarized) diastolic potentials of less than -70 mV sometimes occur.[115,161,162] Along with the decrease in maximum diastolic potential, V_{max} of phase 0 is also decreased.[115,161] However, the maximum diastolic potential and the rate of depolarization during phase 0 are higher than during acute ischemia and represent a partial recovery from the acute ischemic period. Another abnormality in these cells during the first week of infarct healing that is shown in Figure 4–16 is that the action potentials have little plateau phase during repolarization and the action potential duration at the plateau is therefore decreased[115,161] (compare action potential B and C from a 1-day-old and a 5-day-old infarct with action potential A from a noninfarcted heart in Fig. 4–16). This characteristic is similar to the reduction of the plateau during the acute ischemic period.

The maximum diastolic potential, action

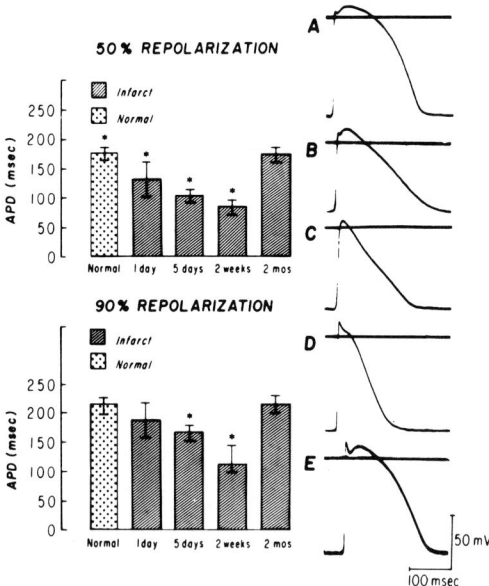

Fig. 4–16. Changes in action potential duration (APD) measured to 50% repolarization (top left) and 90% repolarization (bottom left) of muscle fibers in the epicardial border zone of canine infarcts with increasing time after coronary artery ligation. Column heights represent mean values for the first layer of muscle fibers beneath the epicardial surface in normal noninfarcted left ventricles (stippled columns) and in each group of infarcted left ventricles (cross-hatched columns) studied at the times after coronary occlusion, indicated on the abscissa. Brackets indicate ± standard deviation. Asterisks denote values significantly different from control. At the right are shown representative epicardial muscle fiber transmembrane potential recordings: A is from a noninfarcted heart, B is from a 1-day-old infarct, C is from a 5-day-old infarct, D is from a 2-week-old infarct, and E is from a 2-month-old infarct. (Reproduced with permission from Ursell PC, et al: Circ Res 56:436–451, 1985.[115])

potential amplitude and V_{max} of phase 0 of muscle fibers in the epicardial border zone return to normal by 2 weeks. In contrast, the APD is even shorter at 2 weeks than at 5 days, and there is still little evidence of a plateau phase. (In Fig. 4–16, compare action potential D, recorded at 2 weeks, with action potential C, recorded at 5 days).[115,161] After 2 weeks, the maximum diastolic potential, action potential amplitude and V_{max} of phase 0, and action potential repolarization are not significantly different from normal muscle fibers (Fig. 4–16, action potential E). The recovery of the transmembrane action potentials late in the healing phase of infarction and persistence of this recovery in the healed phase also occur in the subendocardial border zone of healed feline infarcts.[138] Therefore, it seems that the cellular electrophysiological characteristics of the cardiac fibers supporting re-entry may be different, depending on the time of occurrence of the arrhythmias relative to the acute event that causes the infarction.

Slow activation is apparent in the maps of the re-entrant circuits causing VT and is necessary for re-entry to be successful. Depression or reduction of the transmembrane resting potential and the action potential depolarization phase are probably not the only factors or even the most important factors causing the necessary slow conduction for re-entry, as they were for the acute ischemic arrhythmias, since transmembrane potentials are not usually severely depressed in healing infarcts and are nearly normal in healed infarcts. The structure of the infarct, more specifically, the physical arrangement of the surviving myocardial fibers, plays an important role in determining conduction properties. During the healing phase (during the first several weeks after occlusion) when the surviving myocardial fibers are still organized in parallel bundles, conduction in the epicardial border zone of healing canine infarcts is anistotropic, that is, it is influenced markedly by the direction of propagation relative to the orientation of the long axis of the myocardial fiber bundles.[152] In an anisotropic medium, conduction transverse to the long axis of the myocardial fiber bundles can be slow enough to cause re-entry. This influence of myocardial fiber orientation is also likely to apply to other regions of healing infarcts in which there are surviving myocardial cells, such as subendocardial border zone or intramural fiber bundles. In some hearts there may be nearly normal action potentials and slow conduction may result only from anisotropic properties of infarct anatomy. In other hearts transmembrane potentials may be depressed and, along with anisotropy, cause slow conduction. The implication of the variety of mechanisms for slow conduction is that re-entrant circuits causing tachyarrhythmias may have different electrophysiological properties in different hearts. The different conduction properties may influence the rate and stability of the arrhythmia as well as a variable response to drugs.

The conduction properties of healed infarcts as determined from studies on the canine epicardial border zone are still different from those of healing infarcts. Very slow conduction velocities in healed infarcts are dependent on the structural alterations that occur as the infarct heals, rather than on abnormalities in transmembrane potentials. The separation and disorganization of the muscle bundles in the epicardial border zone that occurs as it is invaded by fibrous tissue from the adjacent infarct disrupts intercellular connections, thereby slowing conduction.[147] In regions in which muscle fibers are no longer oriented parallel to one another there are no longer the well-defined anisotropic properties seen in healing infarcts; that is, conduction is slow in all directions rather than just transverse to the long axis of parallel organized muscle bundles.[115] In other regions where the parallel arrangement of the muscle bundles is maintained, conduction properties and anisotropic properties are more similar to those of healing infarcts. These same structural features found in the epicardial border zone of canine infarcts, regions of sparse, poorly connected, myocardial fibers in disarray and regions of parallel-oriented bundles of fibers, also occur in the epicardial and endocardial border zone of human infarcts and in regions of surviving intramural muscle bundles and are expected to affect conduction properties in the same way as they do in the experimental infarcts.

Nonuniform anisotropy[158] is a major cause of slow conduction necessary for re-entry in healing or healed MIs.[152] Activation in the re-entrant circuits is rapid when the re-entrant wave front is moving in the direction of the long axis of the muscle fibers and slow when its is moving transverse to the long axis. This characteristic has been called anisotropic re-entry.[157] In regions where the muscle bundles and fibers are no longer oriented in parallel to one another, conduction is slow, independent of the direction the wave front is moving and despite the presence of mostly normal transmembrane potentials. The kind of anatomical structure also provides an ideal matrix for re-entrant circuits. This is another type of anisotropic re-entry since the slow conduction that enables re-entry to occur results from the nonuniform anisotropic properties, and not from alterations in transmembrane potentials. Conduction might be expected to be slow around the entire circuit, although probably not uniformly slow.

SUMMARY

Re-entrant circuits causing ventricular arrhythmias in healing or healed infarcts may follow anatomical pathways composed of intramural muscle bundles surviving in the infarct. They may also be functional and form only after an appropriately timed premature impulse. Slow conduction, a prerequisite for re-entry, occurs because of the anisotropic properties of the surviving muscle bundles, the depression of the transmembrane potentials during the stages of healing when this occurs, or a combination of the two mechanisms.

REFERENCES

1. DeWood MA, Spores J, Notske R, et al: Prevalence of total coronary occlusion during the early hours of transmural myocardial infarction. N Engl J Med 303:897–902, 1980.
2. Davies MJ, Thomas A: Thrombosis and acute coronary-artery lesions in sudden cardiac ischemic death. N Engl J Med 310: 1137–1140, 1984.
3. Czarnecka M, Lewartowski B, Prokopczk A: Intracellular recordings from the in situ working heart in physiological conditions and during acute ischemia and fibrillation. Acta Physiol Pol 24:331–337, 1973.
4. Downar E, Janse MJ, Durrer D: The effect of acute coronary artery occlusion on sub-epicardial transmembrane potentials in the intact porcine heart. Circulation 56: 217–224, 1977.
5. Kléber AG, Janse MJ, Van Capelle FJL, Durrer D: Mechanism and time course of S-T and T-Q segment changes during acute regional myocardial ischemia in the pig heart determined by extracellular and intracellular recordings. Circ Res 42:603–613, 1978.
6. Kléber AG: Resting membrane potential, extracellular potassium activity, and intra-

cellular sodium activity during acute global ischemia in isolated perfused guinea pig hearts. Circ Res 52:442–450, 1983.
7. Kardesch M, Hogancamp CE, Bing RJ: The effect of complete ischemia on the intracellular electrical activity of the whole mammalian heart. Circ Res 6:715–720, 1958.
8. Kléber AG: Extracellular potassium accumulation in acute myocardial ischemia. J Mol Cell Cardiol 16:389–394, 1984.
9. Hill JL, Gettes LS: Effects of acute coronary artery occlusion on local myocardial extracellular K^+ activity in swine. Circulation 61:768–778, 1980.
10. Coronel R, Fiolet JWT, Wilms-Schopman FJG, Opthof T, Schaapherder AFM, Janse MJ: Distribution of extracellular potassium and electrophysiologic changes during two-stage coronary ligation in the isolated, perfused canine heart. Circulation 80:165–177, 1989.
11. Weiss J, Shine KI: Extracellular potassium accumulation during myocardial ischemia: Implications for arrhythmogenesis. J Mol Cell Cardiol 13:699–704, 1981.
12. Weiss J, Shine KI: Extracellular K^+ accumulation during myocardial ischemia in isolated rabbit heart. Am J Physiol 242:H619–H628, 1982.
13. Weiss J, Shine KI: $[K^+]_o$ accumulation and electrophysiological alterations during early myocardial ischemia. Am J Physiol 243:H318–H327, 1982.
14. Weiss J, Shine KI: Effects of heart rate on extracellular $[K^+]$ accumulation during myocardial ischemia. Am J Physiol 250:H982–H991, 1986.
15. Wiegand V, Gggi M, Meesmann W, Kessler M, Greitschus F: Extracellular potassium activity changes in the canine myocardium after acute coronary occlusion and the influence of beta-blockade. Cardiovasc Res 13:297–302, 1979.
16. Hirche HJ, Franz C, Bs L, Bissig R, Lang R, Schramm M: Myocardial extracellular K^+ and H^+ increase and noradrenaline release as possible cause of early arrhythmias following acute coronary artery occlusion in pigs. J Mol Cell Cardiol 12:579–593, 1980.
17. Polimeni PI: Extracellular space and ionic distribution in rat ventricle. Am J Physiol 227:676–683, 1974.
18. Baumgarten CM, Cohen CJ, McDonald TF: Heterogeneity of intracellular potassium activity and membrane potential in hypoxic guinea pig ventricle. Circ Res 49:1181–1189, 1981.
19. Guarnieri T, Strauss HC: Intracellular potassium activity in guinea pig papillary muscle during prolonged hypoxia. J Clin Invest 69:435–442, 1982.
20. Weiss JN, Lamp ST, Shine KI: Cellular K^+ loss and anion efflux during myocardial ischemia and metabolic inhibition. Am J Physiol 256:H1165–H1175, 1989.
21. Kakei M, Noma A, Shibasaki T: Properties of adenosine-triphosphate-regulated potassium channels in guinea-pig ventricular cells. J Physiol 363:441–462, 1985.
22. Noma A: ATP-regulated K^+ channels in cardiac muscle. Nature 305:147–148, 1983.
23. Noma A, Shibasaki T: Membrane current through adenosine-triphosphate-regulated potassium channels in guinea-pig ventricular cells. J Physiol 363:463–480, 1985.
24. Kléber AG, Riegger CB, Janse MJ: Extracellular K^+ and H^+ shifts in early ischemia: Mechanisms and relation to changes in impulse propagation. J Mol Cell Cardiol 19(suppl V):35–44, 1987.
25. Mainwood GW, Lucier GE: Fatigue and recovery in isolated frog sartorius muscles: The effects of bicarbonate concentration and associated potassium loss. Can J Physiol Pharmacol 50:132–142, 1972.
26. Sato R, Noma A, Kurachi Y, Irisawa H: Effects of intracellular acidification on membrane currents in ventricular cells of the guinea pig. Circ Res 57:553–561, 1985.
27. Blake K, Smith NA, Clusin WT: Rate dependence of ischaemic myocardial depolarization: Evidence for a novel membrane current. Cardiovasc Res 20:557–562, 1986.
28. Blake K, Clusin WT, Franz MR, Smith NA: Mechanism of depolarization in the ischaemic dog heart: Discrepancy between T-Q potentials and potassium accumulation. J Physiol 397:307–330, 1988.
29. Clusin WT, Buchbinder M, Ellis AK, Kernoff RS, Giacomini JC, Harrison DC: Reduction of ischemic depolarization by the calcium blocker diltiazem: Correlation with improvement of ventricular conduction and early arrhythmias in the dog. Circ Res 54:10–20, 1984.
30. Corr PB, Cain ME, Witkowski FX, Price DA, Sobel BE: Potential arrhythmogenic electrophysiological derangements in canine Purkinje fibers induced by lysophosphoglycerides. Circ Res 44:822–832, 1979.
31. Corr PB, Snyder DW, Cain ME, Crafford WA Jr, Gross RW, Sobel BE: Electrophysiological effects of amphiphiles on canine Purkinje fibers: Implications for dysrhythmia secondary to ischemia. Circ Res 49:354–363, 1981.
32. Jennings RB, Reimer KA, Hill ML, Mayer SE: Total ischemia in dog hearts, in vitro:

1. Comparison of high energy phosphate production, utilization, and depletion, and of adenosine nucleotide catabolism in total ischemia in vitro vs. severe ischemia in vivo. Circ Res 49:892–900, 1981.
33. Janse MJ, Cinca J, Morna H, et al: The "border zone" in myocardial ischemia: An electrophysiological, metabolic and histochemical correlation in the pig heart. Circ Res 44:576–588, 1979.
34. Wilde AAM, Kléber AG: The combined effects of hypoxia, high K^+, and acidosis on the intracellular sodium activity and resting potential in guinea pig papillary muscle. Circ Res 58:249–256, 1986.
35. Moréna H, Janse MJ, Fiolet JWT, Krieger WJG, Crijns H, Durrer D: Comparison of the effects of regional ischemia, hypoxia, hyperkalemia and acidosis on intracellular and extracellular potentials and metabolism in the isolated porcine heart. Circ Res 46:634–646, 1980.
36. Nguyen-Thi A, Ruiz-Ceretti E, Schanne OF: Electrophysiologic effects and electrolyte changes in total myocardial ischemia. Can J Physiol Pharmacol 59:876–883, 1981.
37. Cranefield PF: The Conduction of the Cardiac Impulse: The Slow Response and Cardiac Arrhythmias. Mount Kisco, NY, Futura, 1975.
38. Daniel WG, Svenson RH, Masters TN, Robicsek F: Electrophysiologic effects of partial coronary flow reduction in the exposed canine heart: Effects of ischemia and ischemic-induced regional hypothermia on refractoriness and conduction delay. Circulation 58:670–678, 1978.
39. Han J, Goel BG, Hanson CS: Re-entrant beats induced in the ventricle during coronary occlusion. Am Heart J 80:778–784, 1970.
40. Trautwein W, Gottstein U, Dudel J: Der Aktionsstrom der Myocardfaser im Sauerstoffmangel, Pflugers Arch 260:40–60, 1954.
41. Elharrar V, Foster PR, Jirak TL, Gaum WE, Zipes DP: Alterations in canine myocardial excitability during ischemia. Circ Res 40:98–105, 1977.
42. Russell DC, Oliver MF: Ventricular refractoriness during acute myocardial ischaemia and its relationship to ventricular fibrillation. Cardovasc Res 12:221–227, 1978.
43. El-Sherif N, Scherlag BJ, Lazzara R, Samet P: Pathophysiology of tachycardia- and bradycardia-dependent block in the canine proximal His-Purkinje system after acute myocardial ischemia. Am J Cardiol 33:529–540, 1974.
44. Gettes LS, Reuter H: Slow recovery from inactivation of inward currents in mammalian myocardial fibres. J Physiol (London) 240:703–724, 1974.
45. Cranefield PF, Wit AL, Hoffman BF: Conduction of the cardiac impulse: III. Characteristics of very slow conduction. J Gen Physiol 59:227–246, 1972.
46. Kodama I, Wilde AAM, Janse MJ, Durrer D, Yamada K: Combined effects of hypoxia, hyperkalemia and acidosis on membrane action potential and excitability of guinea-pig ventricular muscle. J Mol Cell Cardiol 16:247–259, 1984.
47. Janse MJ, Capucci A, Coronel R, Fabius MAW: Variability of recovery of excitability in the normal canine and the ischaemic porcine heart. Eur Heart J 6(suppl D):41–52, 1985.
48. Janse MJ, Downar E: The effect of acute ischaemia on transmembrane potentials in the intact heart: The relation to reentrant mechanisms. In Kulbertus HE (ed): Reentrant Arrhythmia: Mechanisms and Treatment. Baltimore, University Park Press, 1977, pp 195–209.
49. Boineau JP, Cox JL: Slow ventricular activation in acute myocardial infarction: A source of re-entrant premature ventricular contraction. Circulation 48:702–713, 1973.
50. Durrer D, Formijne P, Van Dam RTh, Büller J, Van Lier AAW, Meyler FL: The electrocardiogram in normal and some abnormal conditions: In revived human fetal heart and in acute and chronic coronary occlusion. Am Heart J 61:303–314, 1961.
51. Waldo AL, Kaiser GA: A study of ventricular arrhythmias associated with acute myocardial infarction in the canine heart. Circulation 47:1222–1228, 1973.
52. Ruffy R, Lovelace DE, Mueller TM, Knoebel SB, Zipes DP: Relationship between changes in left ventricular bipolar electrograms and regional myocardial blood flow during acute coronary artery occlusion in the dog. Circ Res 45:764–770, 1979.
53. Hope RR, Williams DO, El-Sherif N, Lazzara R, Scherlag BJ: The efficacy of antiarrhythmic agents during acute myocardial ischemia and the role of heart rate. Circulation 50:507–514, 1974.
54. Kaplinsky E, Ogawa S, Balke CW, Dreifus LS: Two periods of early ventricular arrhythmia in the canine acute myocardial infarction model. Circulation 60:397–403, 1979.
55. Scherlag BJ, El-Sherif N, Hope RR, Lazzara R: Characterization and localization of ventricular arrhythmias resulting from myocardial ischemia and infarction. Circ Res 35:372–383, 1974.

56. Janse MJ, Kléber AG: Electrophysiological changes and ventricular arrhythmias in the early phase of regional myocardial ischemia. Circ Res 49:1069–1081, 1981.
57. Quan W, Rudy Y: Unidirectional block and reentry of cardiac excitation: A model study. Circ Res 66:367–382, 1990.
58. Kléber AG, Riegger CB, Janse MJ: Electrical uncoupling and increase of extracellular resistance after induction of ischemia in isolated, arterially perfused rabbit papillary muscle. Circ Res 61:271–279, 1987.
59. McCallister LP, Trapukdi S, Neely JR: Morphometric observations on the effects of ischemia in the isolated perfused rat heart. J Mol Cell Cardiol 11:619–630, 1979.
60. Hoyt RH, Cohen ML, Saffitz JE: Distribution and three-dimensional structure of intercellular junctions in canine myocardium. Circ Res 64:563–574, 1989.
61. Cascio WE, Yan G-X, Kléber AG: Passive electrical properties, mechanical activity, and extracellular potassium in arterially perfused and ischemic rabbit ventricular muscle: Effects of calcium entry blockade or hypocalcemia. Circ Res 66:1461–1473, 1990.
62. Marban E, Kitakaze M, Kusuoka H, Porterfield JK, Yue DT, Chacko VP: Intracellular free calcium concentration measured with ^{19}F NMR spectroscopy in intact ferret hearts. Proc Natl Acad Sci USA 84:6005–6009, 1987.
63. Steenbergen C, Murphy E, Levy L, London RE: Elevation in cytosolic free calcium concentration early in myocardial ischemia in perfused rat heart. Circ Res 60:700–707, 1987.
64. Hess P, Weingart R: Intracellular free calcium modified by pH_i in sheep cardiac Purkinje fibres. J Physiol (London) 307:60P–61P, 1980.
65. Reber WR, Weingart R: Ungulate cardiac Purkinje fibres: The influence of intracellular pH on the electrical cell-to-cell coupling. J Physiol (London) 328:87–104, 1982.
66. Kabell G, Scherlag BJ, Hope RR, Lazzara R: Regional myocardial blood flow and ventricular arrhythmias following one-stage and two-stage coronary artery occlusion in anesthetized dogs. Am Heart J 104:537–544, 1982.
67. Kaplinsky E, Ogawa S, Balke CW, Dreifus LS: Two periods of early ventricular arrhythmia in the canine acute myocardial infarction model. Circulation 60:397–403, 1979.
68. Euler DE, Spear JF, Moore EN: Effect of coronary occlusion on arrhythmias and conduction in the ovine heart. Am J Physiol 245:H82–H89, 1983.
69. Parratt JR: Inhibitors of the slow calcium current and early ventricular arrhythmias. In Parratt JR (ed): Early Arrhythmias Resulting From Myocardial Ischemia. New York, Oxford University Press, 1982, pp 329–346.
70. Durrer D, Van Dam RTh, Freud RE, Janse MJ: Reentry and ventricular arrhythmias in local ischemia and infarction of the intact dog heart. Proc Kon Ned Akad Wetensch Series C74:321–334, 1971.
71. Scherlag BJ, Helfant RH, Haft JI, Damato AN: Electrophysiology underlying ventricular arrhythmias due to coronary ligation. Am J Physiol 219:1665–1671, 1970.
72. Horacek TH, Neumann M, von Mutius S, Budden M, Meesmann W: Nonhomogeneous electrophysiological changes and the bimodal distribution of early ventricular arrhythmias during acute coronary artery occlusion. Basic Res Cardiol 79:649–667, 1984.
73. Janse MJ, Van Capelle FJL, Morsink H, et al: Flow of "injury" current and patterns of excitation during early ventricular arrhythmias in acute regional myocardial ischemia in isolated porcine and canine hearts: Evidence for two different arrhythmogenic mechanisms. Circ Res 47:151–165, 1980.
74. Pogwizd SM, Corr PB: Reentrant and nonreentrant mechanisms contribute to arrhythmogenesis during early myocardial ischemia: Results using three-dimensional mapping. Circ Res 61:352–371, 1987.
75. Pogwizd SM, Corr PB: Mechanisms underlying the development of ventricular fibrillation during early myocardial ischemia. Circ Res 66:672–695, 1990.
76. Janse MJ, van Capelle FJL: Electrotonic interactions across an inexcitable region as a cause of ectopic activity in acute regional myocardial ischemia: A study in intact porcine and canine hearts and computer models. Circ Res 50:527–537, 1982.
77. Janse MJ, et al: Electrophysiological basis for arrhythmias caused by acute ischemia: Role of the subendocardium. J Mol Cell Cardiol 18:339–355, 1986.
78. Bagdonas AA, Stuckey JH, Piera J, Amer NS, Hoffman BF: Effects of ischemia and hypoxia on the specialized conducting system of the canine heart. Am Heart J 61:206–218, 1961.
79. Pogwizd SM, Onufer JR, Kramer JB, Sobel BE, Corr PB: Induction of delayed afterdepolarizations and triggered activity in canine Purkinje fibers by lysophosphoglycerides. Circ Res 59:416–426, 1986.
80. Lab MJ: Stress-strain-related depolariza-

tion in the myocardium and arrhythmogenesis in early ischaemia. In Parratt JR (ed): Early Arrhythmias Resulting From Myocardial Ischaemia. New York, Oxford University Press, 1982, pp 81–91.
81. Stephenson SE Jr, et al: Ventricular fibrillation during and after coronary artery occlusion: Incidence and protection afforded by various drugs. Am J Cardiol 5:77–87, 1960.
82. Balke CW, Kaplinsky E, Michelson EL, Naito M, Dreifus LS: Reperfusion ventricular tachyarrhythmias: Correlation with antecedent coronary artery occlusion tachyarrhythmias and duration of myocardial ischemia. Am Heart J 101:449–456, 1981.
83. Battle WE, Naimi S, Avitall B, et al: Distinctive time course of ventricular vulnerability to fibrillation during and after release of coronary ligation. Am J Cardiol 34:42–47, 1974.
84. Corbalan R, Verrier RL, Lown B: Differing mechanisms for ventricular vulnerability during coronary artery occlusion and release. Am Heart J 92:223–230, 1976.
85. Manning AS, Hearse DJ: Reperfusion-induced arrhythmias: Mechanisms and prevention. J Mol Cell Cardiol 16:497–518, 1984.
86. Penny WJ, Sheridan DJ: Arrhythmias and cellular electrophysiological changes during myocardial "ischaemia" and reperfusion. Cardiovasc Res 17:363–372, 1983.
87. Kaplinsky E, Ogawa S, Michelson EL, Dreifus LS: Instantaneous and delayed ventricular arrhythmias after reperfusion of acutely ischemic myocardium: Evidence for multiple mechanisms. Circulation 63:333–340, 1981.
88. Penkoske PA, Sobel BE, Corr PB: Disparate electrophysiological alterations accompanying dysrhythmia due to coronary occlusion and reperfusion in the cat. Circulation 58:1023–1035, 1978.
89. Coronel R, Wilms-Schopman FJG, Opthof T, et al: Reperfusion induced ventricular arrhythmias following regional ischemia in isolated perfused pig hearts: Distribution of extracellular potassium and electrophysiological changes. Circ Res [in press].
90. Janse MJ: Electrophysiological changes in the acute phase of myocardial ischaemia and mechanisms of ventricular arrhythmias. In Parratt JR (ed): Early Arrhythmias Resulting From Myocardial Ischaemia. New York, Oxford University Press, 1982, pp 57–80.
91. Hayashi H, Ponnambalam C, McDonald TF: Arrhythmic activity in reoxygenated guinea pig papillary muscles and ventricular cells. Circ Res 61:124–133, 1987.
92. Ferrier GR, Moffat MP, Lukas A: Possible mechanisms of ventricular arrhythmias elicited by ischemia followed by reperfusion: Studies on isolated canine ventricular tissues. Circ Res 56:184–194, 1985.
93. Smith GL, Allen DG: Effects of metabolic blockade on intracellular calcium concentration in isolated ferret ventricular muscle. Circ Res 62:1223–1236, 1988.
94. Rozanski GJ, Witt RC: Early afterdepolarizations and triggered activity in rabbit cardiac Purkinje fibers recovering from ischemic-like conditions: Role of acidosis. Circulation 83:1352–1360, 1991.
95. Harris AS: Delayed development of ventricular ectopic rhythms following experimental coronary occlusion. Circulation 1:1318–1328, 1950.
96. Campbell RWF, Murray A, Julian DG: Ventricular arrhythmias in the first 12 hours of acute myocardial infarction: Natural history study. Br Heart J 46:351–357, 1981.
97. Northover VJ: Ventricular tachycardia during the first 72 hours after acute myocardial infarction. Cardiology 69:149–156, 1982.
98. Scherlag BJ, Patterson ES, Berbari EJ, Lazzara R: Experimental simulation of sudden cardiac death in humans: Electrophysiological mechanisms and role of adrenergic influences. In Brachmann J, Schömig A (eds): Adrenergic System and Ventricular Arrhythmias in Myocardial Infarction. Berlin, Springer-Verlag, 1989, pp 299–312.
99. de Soyza N, Bissett JK, Kane JJ, Murphy ML, Doherty JE: Association of accelerated idioventricular rhythm and paroxysmal ventricular tachycardia in acute myocardial infarction. Am J Cardiol 34:667–670, 1974.
100. Horowitz LN, Spear JF, Moore EN: Subendocardial origin of ventricular arrhythmias in 24-hour-old experimental myocardial infarction. Circulation 53:56–63, 1976.
101. Spinelli W, Hoffman B, Hoffman BF: Antiarrhythmic drug action in the Harris dog model of ventricular tachycardia. J Cardiovasc Electrophysiol 2:21–33, 1991.
102. Le Marec H, Dangman KH, Danilo P Jr, Rosen MR: An evaluation of automaticity and triggered activity in the canine heart one to four days after myocardial infarction. Circulation 71:1224–1236, 1985.
103. Vassalle M, Levine MJ, Stuckey JH: On the sympathetic control of ventricular automaticity: The effects of stellate ganglion stimulation. Circ Res 23:249–258, 1968.
104. Dangman KH, Hoffman BF: Studies on overdrive stimulation of canine cardiac

Purkinje fibers: Maximal diastolic potential as a determinant of the response. J Am Coll Cardiol 2:1183–1190, 1983.
105. El-Sherif N, Gough WB, Zeiler RH, Mehra R: Triggered ventricular rhythms in 1-day-old myocardial infarction in the dog. Circ Res 52:566–579, 1983.
106. El-Sherif N, Mehra R, Gough WB, Zeiler RH: Ventricular activation patterns of spontaneous and induced ventricular rhythms in canine one-day-old myocardial infarction: Evidence for focal and reentrant mechanisms. Circ Res 51:152–166, 1982.
107. Scherlag BJ, Kabell G, Brachmann J, Harrison L, Lazzara R: Mechanisms of spontaneous and induced ventricular arrhythmias in the 24-hour infarcted dog heart. Am J Cardiol 51:207–213, 1983.
108. Friedman PL, Stewart JR, Fenoglio JJ Jr, Wit AL: Survival of subendocardial Purkinje fibers after extensive myocardial infarction in dogs: In vitro and in vivo correlations. Circ Res 33:597–611, 1973.
109. Friedman PL, Stewart JR, Wit AL: Spontaneous and induced cardiac arrhythmias in subendocardial Purkinje fibers surviving extensive myocardial infarction in dogs. Circ Res 33:612–626, 1973.
110. Reimer KA, Lowe JE, Rasmussen MM, Jennings RB: The wavefront phenomenon of ischemic cell death: 1. Myocardial infarct size vs duration of coronary occlusion in dogs. Circulation 56:786–794, 1977.
111. Fenoglio JJ Jr, Karageuzian HS, Friedman PL, Albala A, Wit AL: Time course of infarct growth toward the endocardium after coronary occlusion. Am J Physiol 236: H356–H370, 1979.
112. Cox JL, Daniel TM, Boineau JP: The electrophysiologic time-course of acute myocardial ischemia and the effects of early coronary artery reperfusion. Circulation 48:971–983, 1973.
113. Lazzara R, El-Sherif N, Scherlag BJ: Electrophysiological properties of canine Purkinje cells in one day old myocardial infarction. Circ Res 33:722–734, 1973.
114. Reimer KA, Jennings RB: The "wavefront" phenomenon of myocardial ischemic cell death: II. Transmural progression of necrosis within the framework of ischemic bed size (myocardium at risk) and collateral flow. Lab Invest 40:633–644, 1979.
115. Ursell PC, Gardner PI, Albala A, Fenoglio JJ Jr, Wit AL: Structural and electrophysiological changes in the epicardial border zone of canine myocardial infarcts during infarct healing. Circ Res 56:436–451, 1985.
116. Fenoglio JJ Jr, Albala A, Silva FG, Friedman PL, Wit AL: Structural basis of ventricular arrhythmias in human myocardial infarction: A hypothesis. Hum Pathol 7: 547–563, 1976.
117. Dangman KH, Hoffman BF: Effects of nifedipine on electrical activity of cardiac cells. Am J Cardiol 46:1059–1067, 1980.
118. Friedman PL, Fenoglio JJ Jr, Wit AL: Time course for reversal of electrophysiological and ultrastructural abnormalities in subendocardial Purkinje fibers surviving extensive myocardial infarction in dogs. Circ Res 36:127–144, 1975.
119. Lazzara R, El-Sherif N, Scherlag BJ: Early and late effects of coronary artery occlusion on canine Purkinje fibers. Circ Res 35: 391–399, 1974.
120. Myers WW, Honig CR: Amount and distribution of Rb^{86} transported into myocardium from ventricular lumen. Am J Physiol 211:739–745, 1966.
121. Wiggers CJ: The functional importance of coronary collaterals. Circulation 5: 609–615, 1952.
122. Moir TW: Study of luminal coronary collateral circulation in the beating canine heart. Circ Res 24:735–744, 1969.
123. Wilensky RL, Tranum-Jensen J, Coronel R, Wilde AAM, Fiolet JWT, Janse MJ: The subendocardial border zone during acute ischemia of the rabbit heart: An electrophysiologic, metabolic, and morphologic correlative study. Circulation 74:1137–1146, 1986.
124. Dresdner KP, Kline RP, Wit AL: Intracellular K^+ activity, intracellular Na^+ activity and maximum diastolic potential of canine subendocardial Purkinje cells from one-day-old infarcts. Circ Res 60:122–132, 1987.
125. Kline RP, Hanna MS, Dresdner KP, Wit AL: Time course of changes in intracellular K^+, Na^+, and pH of subendocardial Purkinje cells during the first 24 hours after coronary occlusion. Circ Res 70:566–575, 1992.
126. Cohen IS, DiFrancesco D, Mulrine N, Pennefather P: Internal and external K^+ help gate the inward rectifier. Biophys 55: 197–202, 1989.
127. Dresdner KP Jr, Hanna MS, Kline RP, Wit AL: Na^+/K^+ pump failure in canine cardiac Purkinje fibers surviving in infarcts. Circulation 78(suppl II):II-637, 1988.
128. Lamers JMJ, and Hülsmann WC: Inhibition of (Na^+/K^+)-stimulated ATPase of heart by fatty acids. J Mol Cell Cardiol 9: 343–346, 1977.
129. Lamers JMJ, Stinis HT, Montfoort A and Hülsmann WC: The effect of lipid interme-

129. diates on Ca^{2+} and Na^+ permeability and $(Na^+ + K^+)$ ATPase of cardiac sarcolemma. Biochim Biophys Acta 774:127–137, 1984.
130. Gadsby DC, Cranefield PF: Electrogenic sodium extrusion in cardiac Purkinje fibers. J Gen Physiol 73:819–837, 1979.
131. Dangman KH, Dresdner KP Jr, Zaim S: Automatic and triggered impulse initiation in canine subepicardial muscle cells from border zones of 24-hour transmural infarcts: New mechanisms for malignant cardiac arrhythmias? Circulation 78:1020–1030, 1988.
132. Hanna MS, Dresdner KP, Kline RP, Wit AL: Characterization of transmembrane potential and intracellular potassium activity in the epicardial border zone 24 hours after myocardial infarction [abstract]. Circulation 76(suppl IV):IV-16, 1987.
133. Bigger JT Jr, Dresdale RJ, Heissenbuttel RH, Weld FM, Wit AL: Ventricular arrhythmias in ischemic heart disease: Mechanism, prevalence, significance, and management. Prog Cardiovasc Dis 19:255–300, 1977.
134. Wellens HJJ, Schuilenburg RM, Durrer D: Electrical stimulation of the heart in patients with ventricular tachycardia. Circulation 46:216–226, 1972.
135. Karagueuzian HS, Fenoglio JJ Jr, Weiss MB, Wit AL: Protracted ventricular tachycardia induced by premature stimulation of the canine heart after coronary artery occlusion and reperfusion. Circ Res 44:833–846, 1979.
136. Karagueuzian HS, Fenoglio JJ Jr, Weiss MB, Wit AL: Coronary occlusion and reperfusion: Effects on subendocardial cardiac fibers. Am J Physiol 238:H581–H593, 1980.
137. Mehra R, Zeiler RH, Gough WB, El-Sherif N: Reentrant ventricular arrhythmias in the late myocardial infarction period: 9. Electrophysiologic-anatomic correlation of reentrant circuits. Circulation 67:11–24, 1983.
138. Myerburg RJ, Gelband H, Nilsson K, et al: Long-term electrophysiological abnormalities resulting from experimental myocardial infarction in cats. Circ Res 41:73–84, 1977.
139. Kramer JB, Saffitz JE, Witkowski FX, Corr PB: Intramural reentry as a mechanism of ventricular tachycardia during evolving canine myocardial infarction. Circ Res 56:736–754, 1985.
140. Wit AL, Allessie MA, Bonke FIM, Lammers W, Smeets J, Fenoglio JJ Jr: Electrophysiologic mapping to determine the mechanism of experimental ventricular tachycardia initiated by premature impulses: Experimental approach and initial results demonstrating reentrant excitation. Am J Cardiol 49:166–185, 1982.
141. Michelson EL, Spear JF, Moore EN: Electrophysiologic and anatomic correlates of sustained ventricular tachyarrhythmias in a model of chronic myocardial infarction. Am J Cardiol 45:583–590, 1980.
142. Bolick DR, Hackel DB, Reimer KA, Ideker RE: Quantitative analysis of myocardial infarct structure in patients with ventricular tachycardia. Circulation 74:1266–1279, 1986.
143. Fenoglio JJ Jr, Albala A, Silva FG, Friedman PL, Wit AL: Structural basis of ventricular arrhythmias in human myocardial infarction: A hypothesis. Hum Pathol 7:547–563, 1976.
144. El-Sherif N: The figure 8 model of reentrant excitation in the canine postinfarction heart. In Zipes DP, Jalife J (eds): Cardiac Electrophysiology and Arrhythmias. New York, Grune & Stratton, 1985, pp 363–378.
145. Littmann L, Svenson RH, Gallagher JJ, et al: Functional role of the epicardium in postinfarction ventricular tachycardia: Observations derived from computerized epicardial activation mapping, entrainment, and epicardial laser photoablation. Circulation 83:1577–1591, 1991.
146. Svenson RH, Littmann L, Gallagher JJ, et al: Termination of ventricular tachycardia with epicardial laser photocoagulation: A clinical comparison with patients undergoing successful endocardial photocoagulation alone. J Am Coll Cardiol 15:163–170, 1990.
147. Gardner PI, Ursell PC, Fenoglio JJ Jr, Wit AL: Electrophysiologic and anatomic basis for fractionated electrograms recorded from healed myocardial infarcts. Circulation 72:596–611, 1985.
148. Josephson ME, Horowitz LN, Farshidi A, Spear JF, Kastor JA, Moore EN: Recurrent sustained ventricular tachycardia: 2. Endocardial mapping. Circulation 57:440–447, 1978.
149. Denniss AR, Richards DA, Waywood JA, et al: Electrophysiological and anatomic differences between canine hearts with inducible ventricular tachycardia and fibrillation associated with chronic myocardial infarction. Circ Res 64:155–166, 1989.
150. Garan H, Fallon JT, Rosenthal S, Ruskin JN: Endocardial, intramural and epicardial activation patterns during sustained monomorphic ventricular tachycardia in late canine myocardial infarction. Circ Res 60:879–896, 1987.

151. De Bakker JMT, van Capelle FJL, Janse MJ, et al: Reentry as a cause of ventricular tachycardia in patients with chronic ischemic heat disease: Electrophysiologic and anatomic correlation. Circulation 77: 589–606, 1988.
152. Dillon SM, Allessie MA, Ursell PC, Wit AL: Influence of anisotropic tissue structure on reentrant circuits in the epicardial border zone of subacute canine infarcts. Circ Res 63:182–206, 1988.
153. Berger MD, Waxman HL, Buxton AE, Marchlinski FE, Josephson ME: Spontaneous compared with induced onset of sustained ventricular tachycardia. Circulation 78:885–892, 1988.
154. Cardinal R, Savard P, Carson DL, Perry J-B, Pagé P: Mapping of ventricular tachycardia induced by programmed stimulation in canine preparations of myocardial infarction. Circulation 70:136–148, 1984.
155. Gough WB, Mehra R, Restivo M, Zeiler RH, El-Sherif N: Reentrant ventricular arrhythmias in the late myocardial infarction period in the dog: 13. Correlation of activation and refractory maps. Circ Res 57: 432–442, 1985.
156. Restivo M, Gough WB, El-Sherif N: Ventricular arrhythmias in the subacute myocardial infarction period: High-resolution activation and refractory patterns of reentrant rhythms. Circ Res 66:1310–1327, 1990.
157. Wit AL, Dillon SM, Coromilas J, Saltman AE, Waldecker B: Anisotropic reentry in the epicardial border zone of myocardial infarcts. In Jalife J (ed): Mathematical Approaches to Cardiac Arrhythmias. Ann NY Acad Sci 591:86–108, 1990.
158. Spach MS, Dolber PC, Heidlage JF: Influence of the passive anisotropic properties on directional differences in propagation following modification of the sodium conductance in human atrial muscle: A model of reentry based on anisotropic discontinuous propagation. Circ Res 62:811–832, 1988.
159. Kaltenbrunner W, Cardinal R, Dubuc M, et al: Epicardial and endocardial mapping of ventricular tachycardia in patients with myocardial infarction: Is the origin of the tachycardia always subendocardially localized? Circulation 84:1058–1071, 1991.
160. Harris L, Downar E, Mickleborough L, Shaikh N, Parson I: Activation sequence of ventricular tachycardia: Endocardial and epicardial mapping studies in the human ventricle. J Am Coll Cardiol 10:1040–1047, 1987.
161. Spear JF, Michelson EL, Moore EN: Cellular electrophysiologic characteristics of chronically infarcted myocardium in dogs susceptible to sustained ventricular tachyarrhythmias. J Am Coll Cardiol 1: 1099–1110, 1983.
162. Lazzara R, Hope RR, El-Sherif N, Scherlag BJ: Effects of lidocaine on hypoxic and ischemic cardiac cells. Am J Cardiol 41: 872–879, 1978.
163. Janse MJ: Electrophysiological changes in the acute phase of myocardial ischaemia and mechanisms of ventricular arrhythmias. In Parratt JR (ed): Early Arrhythmias Resulting From Myocardial Ischaemia. New York, Oxford University Press, 1982, pp 57–80.
164. Janse MJ: Electrophysiology and electrocardiology of acute myocardial ischemia. Can J Cardiol 00(suppl A):46A–52A, 1986.

5
Biochemical Membrane Mechanisms Underlying Arrhythmias During Myocardial Ischemia and Their Role in Sudden Cardiac Death

JANE McHOWAT
PETER B. CORR

Sudden cardiac death (SCD) in patients with coronary artery disease is most often a result of ventricular fibrillation (VF) with or without preceding ventricular tachycardia (VT).[1-4] Autopsy results in patients who have succumbed to SCD demonstrate a high incidence of severe coronary artery disease, but only about half of the patients had evidence of a recent, highly defined myocardial infarct (MI).[5] These results suggest that transient and recent myocardial ischemia secondary to a coronary thrombus leading to the development of malignant ventricular arrhythmias is likely to be the major mechanism responsible for SCD in patients with coronary artery disease.

Myocardial ischemia in vivo leads to dramatic electrophysiological alterations within minutes of cessation of coronary flow.[6] Acute ischemia results in depolarization of the resting membrane potential, a decrease in upstroke velocity of phase 0 depolarization, and a reduction in both action potential amplitude and duration.[6,7] Within minutes of the onset of ischemia, premature ventricular contractions occur commonly and frequently initiate VT, VF, or both.

Work was supported in part by National Institutes of Health grant HL-17646, SCOR in Ischemic Heart Disease, and grants HL-28995 and HL-36773.

Using detailed three-dimensional mapping from 232 simultaneous intramural sites throughout the left ventricle, right ventricle, and septum of the feline heart in vivo, we have shown that ischemia elicits profound and heterogeneous degrees of conduction delay and block within 1–2 minutes.[8] Because of the functional as opposed to anatomical nature of the conduction block, the site and extent of block vary from beat to beat.[8] In 75% of cases, the initiation of premature ventricular complexes (PVCs) or VT after early ischemia occurred by a reentrant mechanism, primarily intramural in origin.[8]

These rapid and heterogeneous electrophysiological alterations seen early after the onset of ischemia are totally reversible if reperfusion occurs within the first 7–10 minutes, leaving no evidence of any cellular damage with the exception of significant depletion of glycogen. These findings suggest that some subtle biochemical alterations within or near the sarcolemma occur in response to brief ischemia and account for the rapidity and reversibility of the electrophysiological derangements. Previous studies have shown that venous blood obtained from the ischemic region in vivo can elicit electrophysiological derangements in normoxic tissue in vitro, which suggests, indirectly, that the ischemic myocardium or vasculature may release a factor or factors that may dramatically alter the electrical activity of the myocardium.[9] Although factors including reduced P_{O_2} (hypoxia), acidosis, and elevated extracellular K^+ contribute to the electrophysiological alterations after ischemia, their presence did not replicate several of the unique changes induced by venous blood obtained from the ischemic regions.[9]

Our laboratory has been investigating the electrophysiological effects of two amphipathic metabolites, long-chain acylcarnitine and lysophosphatidylcholine (LPC), both of which have been shown to increase rapidly in ischemic tissue in vivo and to elicit electrophysiological derangements in vitro (for review see ref. 10). This chapter considers the role of both of these metabolites in ischemic myocardium, potential factors responsible for their accumulation, and the possible mechanisms through which they elicit electrophysiological derangements. The ultimate goal is to develop specific and effective therapeutic approaches to modify the arrhythmias responsible for SCD in patients with ischemic heart disease.

STRUCTURE AND FUNCTION OF THE SARCOLEMMA AND THE EFFECTS OF AMPHIPHILES ON MOLECULAR MEMBRANE DYNAMICS

The sarcolemma is the electrically excitable membrane of individual myocytes and as such maintains a permeability barrier between the myocyte and the extracellular space. The sarcolemma solvates transmembrane ion channels and pumps that determine the electrophysiological function of the cells. The sarcolemma is composed predominantly of phospholipids, cholesterol, and proteins, but it constitutes only 2–4% of the total cellular phospholipid. Phospholipids are amphipathic in nature and are composed of a charged polar headgroup region and a nonpolar long-chain aliphatic hydrocarbon region. To provide maximal thermodynamic stability in aqueous solutions, the individual phospholipids spontaneously form a bilayer where the polar headgroup regions interface with either the aqueous cytosol or extracellular space and the nonpolar hydrocarbon fatty acids are directed inward to form the nonpolar interior of the membrane, the lipid bilayer (Fig. 5–1). The polar headgroup regions consist of glycerol and a phosphoryl base. Phospholipids are classified according to their phosphoryl base and include phosphatidylcholine, phosphatidylethanolamine, phosphatidylinositol, and phosphatidylserine. Two long-chain fatty acids are covalently attached either to the sn-1 or sn-2 position of the glycerol backbone. The hydrocarbon groups at the sn-2 position are covalently bound in the form of o-acyl esters, whereas those of the sn-1 position include o-acyl esters and vinyl ethers (Fig. 5-1). Plasmalogens are phospholipids with a vinyl ether linkage at the sn-1 position and are found to constitute approximately 60% of choline and ethanolamine phospholipids in the sarcolemma of adult cardiac cells.[11] Plasmalogens are not found in inositol or serine phospholipids.

Integral membrane proteins within the sarcolemma determine the metabolic characteristics and the active and passive transport functions. These proteins include ion channels, transport proteins, receptors, proteins involved in signal transduction, structural proteins, surface antigens, and a variety of different enzymes. An example of the structure of ion channels derived from subunit sequence analysis and modeling based primarily on hydrophobicity studies is shown in Figure 5–2. Modulation of the activity of these proteins may arise through interaction with adjacent membrane phospholipids. For example, alterations in the composition of membrane phospholipids result in corresponding alterations in the bulk biophysical properties of the membrane, which may have a profound impact on the functional characteristics of these multiple, integral membrane proteins, including ion channels.

During ischemia, both long-chain acylcarnitine and LPC, because of their amphipathic nature, incorporate into the phospholipid bilayer of the sarcolemma (see below). The effects of these amphiphiles on membrane phospholipid dynamics as well as the conformation of the phospholipids appear to be critical in altering the transmembrane ion channels as well as in modifying ligand-receptor coupling and the activity of membrane-bound enzymes. Modest changes in

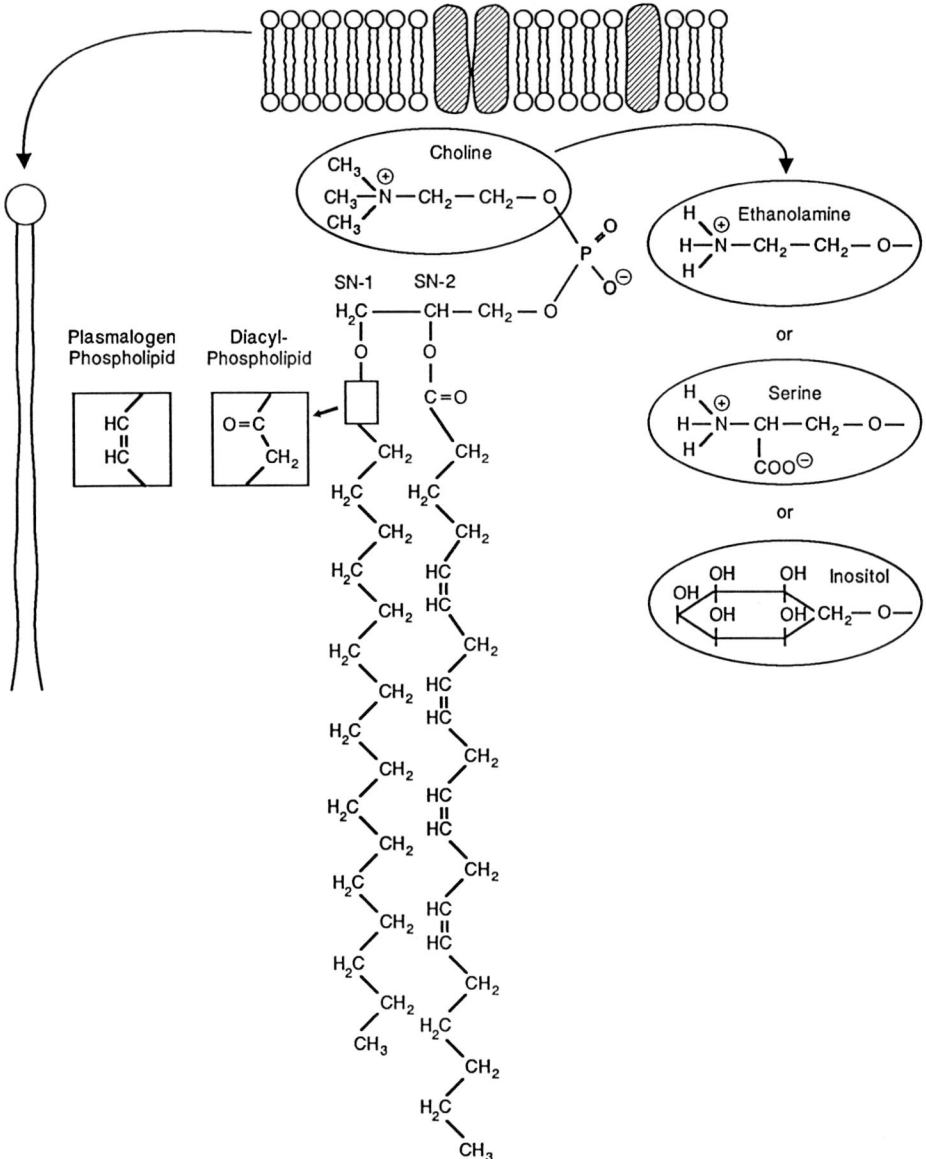

Fig. 5–1. Diagrammatic representation of the structure of the sarcolemma. The packing of membrane phospholipids to form the lipid bilayer together with two integral membrane proteins is shown in the top portion of the figure, with the individual structure of the phospholipids shown below. The structures to the right indicate the different polar headgroups, and the structural variations for the covalent attachment of the sn-1 fatty acid to the phospholipid polar headgroup are shown on the left. (Reproduced with permission from Creer et al.[10])

amphiphile content of the sarcolemma have profound effects on the physical characteristics of the sarcolemma. Electron spin resonance studies on isolated canine myocardial sarcolemma have demonstrated that as little as 1.5 mol % of amphiphile incorporation results in significant changes in the molecular dynamics of the sarcolemmal membrane, with a marked increase in membrane fluidity.[12] Under normoxic conditions, the concentrations of these amphiphilic metabolites within the myocyte are tightly con-

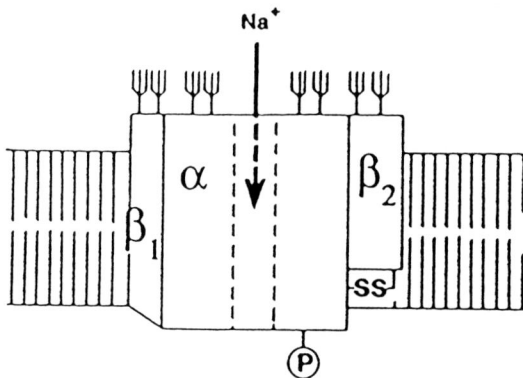

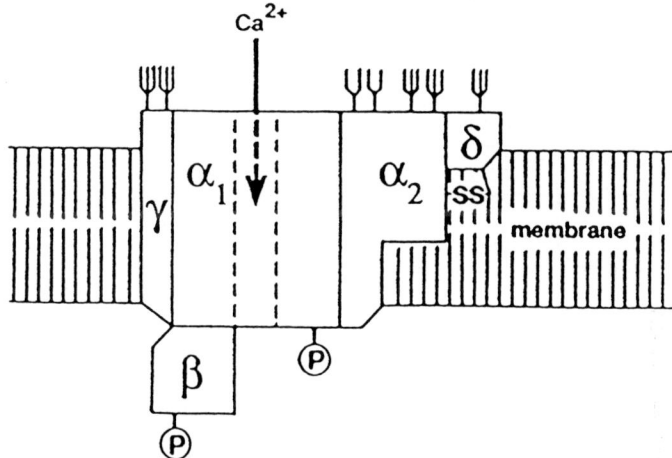

Fig. 5–2. Subunit structure of Na^+ channels and Ca^{2+} channels. Disulfide bonds, glycosylation sites, and phosphorylation sites are illustrated. (Reproduced with permission from Catterhall.[127])

trolled. However, during ischemia, the mechanisms for maintaining low levels of both metabolites are disrupted, leading to an abrupt increase in both long-chain acylcarnitine and LPC.

MECHANISMS RESPONSIBLE FOR THE ACCUMULATION OF LONG-CHAIN ACYLCARNITINE DURING EARLY ISCHEMIA

The myocardium has one of the highest energy requirements of any organ system. Since fatty acids provide more adenosine triphosphate (ATP) on a per-mole basis than any other energy source, it is not surprising that oxidation of fatty acids accounts for 60–80% of the energy requirements of the myocardium.[13] The majority of unesterified free fatty acids in plasma are bound to albumin, with small quantities free in solution that are in equilibrium with albumin-bound free fatty acid. The unbound fatty acid is capable of entering the myocyte by passive diffusion or via a saturable fatty acid transport process involving sarcolemmal proteins.[14] Once within the cytoplasm, the free fatty acid is bound to a cytosolic fatty acid–binding protein that maintains an inward concentration gradient to permit further uptake of free fatty acid into the myocyte.[15–17]

Metabolism of intracellular free fatty acids proceeds initially by thioesterification of fatty acid and free CoA to fatty acid–CoA esters mediated by acyl CoA synthetase, located primarily on the outer membrane of

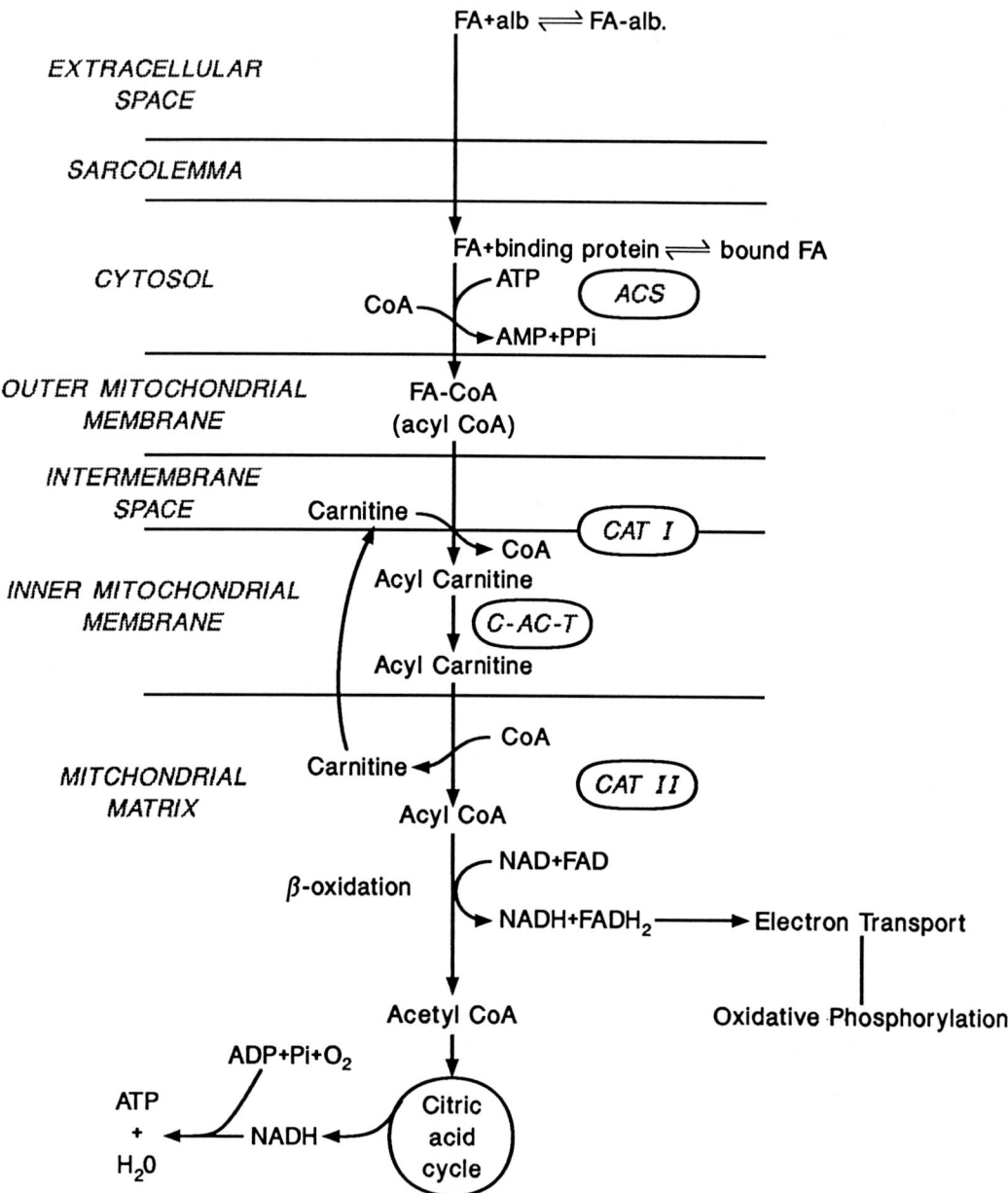

Fig. 5–3. Metabolite pathway for oxidation of free fatty acids (FA) in cardiac myocytes. Abbreviations: alb, albumin; CoA, "free" (nonesterified) coenzyme A; FA-CoA, fatty acyl-CoA; ACS, acyl-CoA synthetase; CAT I, carnitine acyltransferase I; CAT II, carnitine acyltransferase II; C-AC-T, carnitine-acylcarnitine translocase.

the mitochondria (Fig. 5–3).[18] This reaction is coupled to the hydrolysis of ATP to adenosine monophosphate and pyrophosphate. The inner mitochondrial membrane is impermeable to long-chain acyl CoA. To facilitate passage of acyl CoA across the inner mitochondrial membrane to the matrix, acyl CoA is transesterified to free carnitine at the outer portion of the inner mitochondrial membrane to form long-chain acylcarnitine and free CoA by the action of the enzyme carnitine acyltransferase I (CAT I).[19,20]

Long-chain acylcarnitine is then translocated across the inner mitochondrial membrane to the mitochondrial matrix in exchange for free carnitine by carnitine–acylcarnitine translocase.[21,22] At the mitochondrial matrix, long-chain acylcarnitine is transesterified to free CoA to form acyl CoA and free carnitine in a reversible reaction catalyzed by carnitine acyltransferase II (CAT II). Acyl CoA within the mitochondrial matrix is now available for β-oxidation (Fig. 5-3).

The major products of β-oxidation of fatty acids are acetyl CoA and the reduced forms of nicotinamide and flavin adenine dinucleotides (NADH and $FADH_2$). NADH and $FADH_2$ are closely coupled to electron transport and oxidative phosphorylation to maintain high rates of fatty acid oxidation in the mitochondria. Cytochrome oxidase, the terminal enzyme of electron transport, has an absolute requirement for oxygen. During ischemia, the abrupt interruption of coronary flow rapidly lowers the P_{O_2} in the involved tissue to near zero mm Hg. Electron transport is inhibited and results in an increase in NADH and $FADH_2$, which in turn leads to an inhibition of flux through the β-oxidation pathway by a negative feedback mechanism. A marked increase in both acyl CoA and long-chain acylcarnitine occurs.[13,23–26] Long-chain acylcarnitines can readily diffuse back across the mitochondrial membrane to gain access to most myocytic subcellular membrane compartments, including the sarcolemma.[25] Acyl CoA remains predominantly in the mitochondrial matrix during the reversible phase of ischemia because of its inability to traverse the inner mitochondrial membrane.[25]

Two mechanisms contribute to the increase in the cytosolic level of long-chain acylcarnitine. First, as acyl CoA accumulates in the mitochondrial matrix, the free carnitine concentration in the matrix is reduced by reversal of the CAT II reaction. This reduction in free carnitine at the matrix leads to a decrease in the rate of translocation of long-chain acylcarnitine from the cytosol to the matrix by carnitine–acylcarnitine translocase. Second, the activity of the translocase enzyme is decreased under ischemic conditions as a result of modification of protein sulfhydryl groups.[27] Inhibition of carnitine–acylcarnitine translocase and depletion of matrix free carnitine are the critical events responsible for the increase in long-chain acylcarnitine in the cytosol of the ischemic myocyte.

The magnitude of the increase in long-chain acylcarnitine during ischemia is limited by several mechanisms. First, the increase in long-chain acylcarnitine inhibits the CAT I enzyme which catalyzes the formation of long-chain acylcarnitine at the outer portion of the inner mitochondrial membrane.[28] Second, the uptake of free fatty acid decreases rapidly following a reduction in coronary flow.[13] Third, acylcarnitine hydrolase, an enzyme that catalyzes the hydrolysis of long-chain acylcarnitine to form free fatty acid and carnitine, is present in myocardial tissue.[29] Despite these three mechanisms to limit the increase in long-chain acylcarnitines during ischemia, this amphiphile increases markedly within the first 2 minutes of ischemia in vivo.

We and others have demonstrated that long-chain acylcarnitine levels increase in ischemic tissue in vivo[23,25,26,30] and in hypoxic myocytes in vitro.[31–34] For example, regional ischemia in the cat in vivo led to a 3.5-fold increase in long-chain acylcarnitine levels within 2 minutes in the ischemic compared to the corresponding nonischemic region of the left ventricle.[34] This marked increase in long-chain acylcarnitine is rapid enough to contribute, at least in part, to the electrophysiological derangements seen early after the onset of ischemia. We have also shown that long-chain acylcarnitine increases 9-fold within 10 minutes of hypoxia in isolated adult canine myocytes, and that this increase can be reversed by reoxygenation or blocked by pretreatment with the CAT I blocker sodium 2-[5 -(4 -chlorophenyl) -pentyl] -oxirane -2-carboxylate (POCA).[35] Most important, in isolated adult canine myocytes, electron microscopic autoradiography of cells prelabeled with ^{3}H-carnitine demonstrates that hypoxia of only 10 minutes' duration elicits a 100-fold increase in long-chain acylcarnitine content within the sarcolemma, achieving a value of 1 mol % of membrane phospholipid, a concentration sufficient to elicit electrophysiological derangements.[35] These findings are analogous to those shown previously from our laboratory in neonatal rat ventricular myocytes exposed to hypoxia.[31]

MECHANISMS RESPONSIBLE FOR THE ACCUMULATION OF LYSOPHOSPHATIDYLCHOLINE DURING ISCHEMIA

Lysophosphatidylcholine (LPC) is generated by the hydrolytic cleavage of one of the covalently bound aliphatic hydrocarbon groups of diacyl phosphatidylcholine (PC). Removal of the fatty acid at the sn-1 position is catalyzed by either phospholipase A_1[36] or plasmalogenase, which cleaves the ester or the vinyl ether linkage of diacyl or plasmalogen PC, respectively (Fig. 5–4). The product of either enzyme is 2-monoacyl LPC. In contrast, hydrolysis of the sn-2 fatty acid to produce 1-monoacyl-LPC and free fatty acid is catalyzed by at least three distinct classes of phospholipase A_2 in the heart. One PLA_2 is maximally active at acidic pH, is of lysosomal origin, acts on diacyl-PC as the substrate, and exhibits a positive Ca^{2+} dependence.[36] Another PLA_2 is maximally active at neutral pH, is Ca^{2+} dependent, and has been partially purified and characterized in rabbit myocardium and cardiac myocytes obtained from chick embryos.[37] Finally, a plasmalogen-selective PLA_2 has recently been identified in canine myocardium.[38] In contrast to PLA_2 that uses diacyl-PC as a substrate, the activity of this enzyme is not influenced by calcium. This enzyme is active at neutral pH and is present in the cytosol. The majority of LPC in myocardial tissue is derived by hydrolysis of the sn-2 fatty acid of diacyl-PC catalyzed by PLA_2. However, plasmalogens are the predominant species in the sarcolemma, and it is possible that relatively large increases in the concentration of lysoplasmalogens within the sarcolemma per se could occur during ischemia and result in significant electrophysiological alterations without a large change in the total cellular content.

LPC is usually present in small concentrations within cardiac cells because of the relatively high activity of several catabolic enzymes. Catabolism of LPC occurs through three different pathways mediated

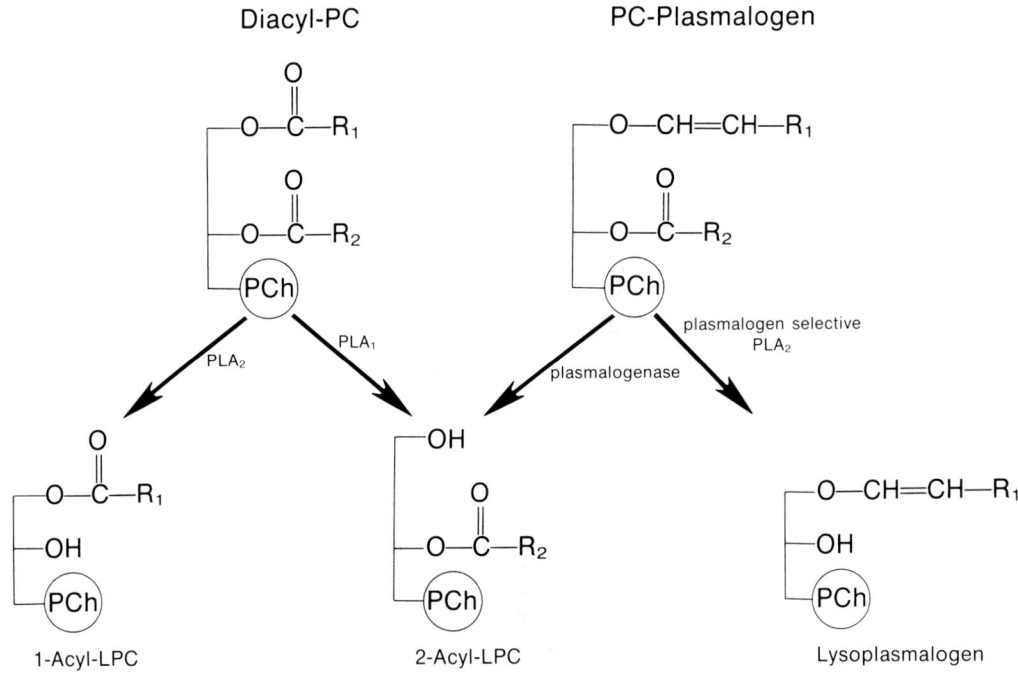

Fig. 5–4. Pathways of synthesis of lysophosphatidylcholine (LPC) and lysoplasmalogen from phosphatidylcholine (PC) and PC plasmalogen, respectively. PCh, phosphorylcholine; R_1 and R_2, long-chain aliphatic hydrocarbon groups at the sn-1 and sn-2 positions, respectively. (Reproduced with permission from Creer et al.[10])

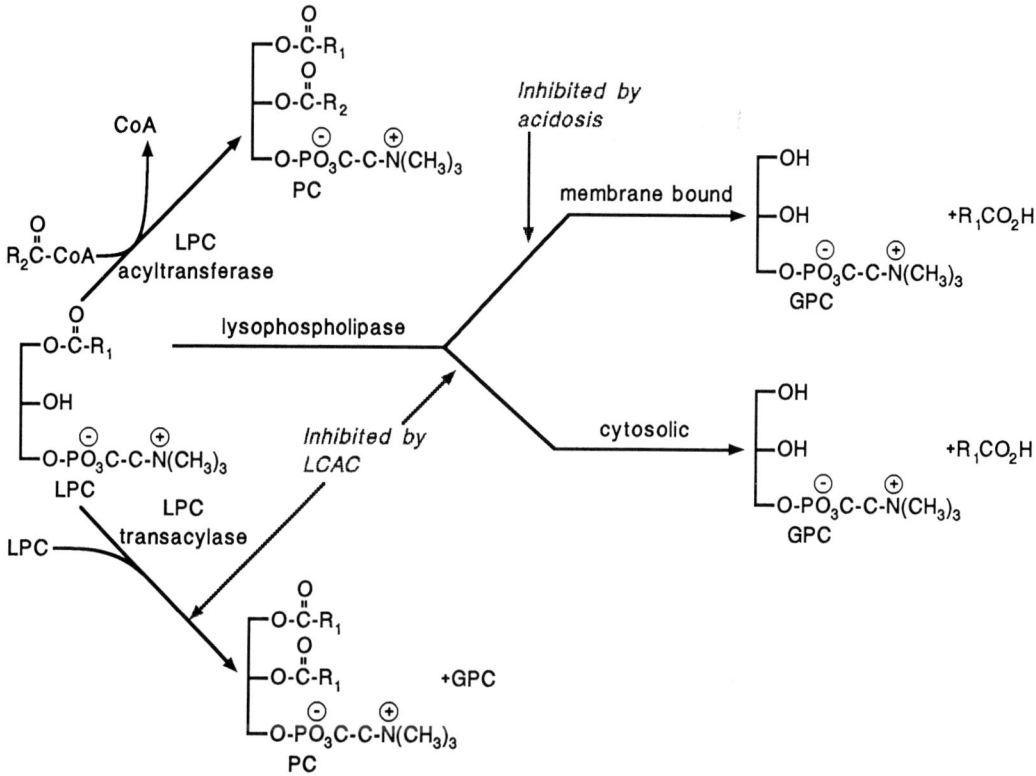

Fig. 5–5. Pathways of catabolism of lysophosphatidylcholine (LPC) to either phosphatidylcholine (PC) or glycerophosphorylcholine (GPC) in heart tissue.

by four separate enzymes (Fig. 5–5). Lysophospholipase catalyzes the hydrolysis of LPC to glycerophosphorylcholine (GPC) and fatty acid. There are at least two distinct lysophospholipases, one found in the cytosol and one membrane-bound, which is highly pH-dependent.[39–41] Coenzyme A-LPC acyltransferase catalyzes the reacylation of LPC with acyl CoA to form diacyl-PC. Lysophospholipase-transacylase catalyzes a disproportionate reaction between two molecules of LPC to form diacyl-PC and GPC. The reactions catalyzed by lysophospholipase and lysophospholipase-transacylase have been shown to account for 70% of the total capacity for catabolism of LPC in homogenates of rabbit myocardium.[42,43] Under normoxic conditions, the capacity for catabolism of LPC is more than 100-fold greater than the capacity for production of LPC through activation of PLA_2.[37,38,42] Thus, the accumulation of LPC is precluded.

During ischemia, intracellular pH falls within minutes to 6.5–6.7. Together with an increase in long-chain acylcarnitine levels, this could lead to inhibition of catabolism of LPC and thus an increase in the concentration of LPC in ischemic myocardium. The membrane-bound lysophospholipase enzyme is almost completely inhibited by a decrease in pH (Fig. 5–5).[42] Cytosolic lysophospholipase and lysophospholipase transacylase are both inhibited by long-chain acylcarnitine at concentrations achieved in ischemic tissue.[42,43]

We have shown a twofold increase in LPC and a threefold increase in long-chain acylcarnitine following 5 minutes of ischemia in the in situ cat heart.[30] The increase in *both* metabolites was prevented by pretreatment with POCA, suggesting that the marked increase in long-chain acylcarnitine is necessary for the net accumulation of LPC.[30]

In addition to inhibition of the catabolism

of LPC during ischemia, several studies have reported that the activity of PLA$_2$ is also increased during ischemia, thereby contributing to the net increase in LPC. Recent evidence suggests that the activity of a membrane-associated, calcium-independent, plasmalogen-selective PLA$_2$ is dramatically increased after very short intervals of ischemia in the isolated perfused rabbit heart.[44,45] This activation of the plasmalogen-selective PLA$_2$ was rapidly reversible during reperfusion following short intervals of ischemia.[44] These findings suggest that activation of this plasmalogen-selective PLA$_2$ may directly enhance the production of lysoplasmalogens within the sarcolemma and thereby contribute directly to the electrophysiological derangements during ischemia (see below).

During short intervals of ischemia, numerous studies have indicated that LPC increases in venular and lymphatic effluents from ischemic tissue.[46,47] Interestingly, recent results from Sedlis and colleagues have shown a marked increase in LPC in the coronary effluent of patients with pacing-induced ischemia but no change in LPC in normal control patients without ischemic heart disease.[48] Although this could be a reflection of increased efflux of LPC from ischemia tissue to the vascular space, these increases are observed very early after the onset of ischemia, before there is evidence of irreversible cell damage and significant disruption of the sarcolemma. In addition to production of LPC by myocytes as described above, there may be extramyocytic sources of LPC in response to ischemia. The appearance of LPC in both blood and lymph would suggest a vascular site of origin, possibly endothelial or smooth muscle cells. Although we and others[49] have shown that isolated platelets produce LPC in response to thrombin stimulation, it is doubtful that the relatively small number of platelets present in the coronary circulation would contribute substantially to the increased extracellular accumulation of LPC during ischemia (unpublished findings).

We have recently demonstrated an increase in LPC production in endothelial cells in response to stimulation with thrombin, an increase that was potentiated by pretreatment with the metabolic inhibitor, iodoacetate.[50] Iodoacetate induces biochemical alterations that stimulate changes in intact ischemic tissue, including activation of phospholipases, selective release of unsaturated free fatty acids and intracellular enzymes, depletion of high-energy phosphate pools, and the development of ultrastructural changes. The increase in LPC in response to thrombin was completely blocked by pretreatment with hirudin.[50] These results suggest that a thrombin-specific stimulation of endothelial cells could contribute to the increase in LPC observed extracellularly in ischemic myocardium. Whether this contribution by endothelial cells is sufficient to account for the twofold increase in LPC in venous and lymphatic effluents from ischemic myocardium remains to be determined. These findings would also suggest that the presence of an interacoronary thrombus with its attendant release of thrombin may be potentially arrhythmogenic through the extracellular production of LPC.

In summary, the increase in LPC in both ischemic myocardium and effluents from ischemic regions may arise by multiple mechanisms. The relative importance of each mechanism remains to be elucidated.

CONTRIBUTION OF LONG-CHAIN ACYLCARNITINE AND LYSOPHOSPHATIDYLCHOLINE TO ARRHYTHMOGENESIS FOLLOWING THE ONSET OF ISCHEMIA

At concentrations similar to those observed in ischemic tissue, LPC and palmitoylcarnitine induce concentration-dependent reductions in maximum diastolic potential, total amplitude, $\dot{V}_{max}$ of phase 0, and action potential duration (APD) in normoxic canine Purkinje fibers.[51] The extent of electrophysiological derangements is enhanced two- to threefold in the presence of acidosis (pH = 6.8), analogous to what occurs in ischemic tissue in vivo.[51] Catabolites of LPC and long-chain acylcarnitine, including free fatty acid, GPC, and carnitine, fail to elicit significant electrophysiological derangements at similar concentrations, suggesting a specific effect of the amphiphiles.[51] LPC and long-chain acylcarnitine in combination induced electrophysiological derangements similar to those induced by comparable concentrations of either amphiphile alone, indicating an additive but not synergistic effect.[51] This, together with the fact that the effects of LPC and long-chain acylcarnitine on membrane molecular dynamics, as determined by electron spin resonance,[12] are additive, would suggest that the pathophysiological effects of the accumulation of these amphiphiles are mediated by alterations in the biophysical properties of the sarcolemmal membrane, including a marked increase in membrane fluidity.

In studies performed several years ago in our laboratory, isolated neonatal rat myocytes exposed to hypoxia developed significant decreases in maximum diastolic potential, total amplitude, and $\dot{V}_{max}$ of phase 0 of the action potential.[31] The severity of electrophysiological derangements was dependent on the magnitude of the increase in long-chain acylcarnitines in these myocytes. With marked elevations in endogenous long-chain acylcarnitine, the cells became unresponsive to stimulation (3.5 mol % of sarcolemmal membrane phospholipid). Most important, exposure of these hypoxic cells to an inhibitor of CAT I, POCA, prior to induction of hypoxia prevented the increase in long-chain acylcarnitine and markedly attenuated but did not completely prevent the associated electrophysiological alterations. These findings suggest that endogenous accumulation of long-chain acylcarnitines in the sarcolemma of hypoxic myocytes may be an important contributor to the associated electrophysiological alterations. Since hypoxia in isolated adult myocytes does not result in a measurable increase in LPC, it is likely that other factors may be involved during ischemia, including the extramyocytic sources discussed in a previous section. In neonatal rat myocytes, the depressant effects of LPC on contractility were found to be potentiated by acidosis and by the presence of superoxide radicals,[52] both of which are prominent in ischemic tissue in vivo.

Although hypoxia does in fact simulate one major component of ischemia in vivo, multiple additional factors are absent in this type of system. Evaluation of the direct arrhythmogenic properties of an amphiphile such as LPC requires assessing its presence in the tissue, its subcellular site of accumulation, and its effects on membrane properties. In addition, cause-and-effect relationships requires inhibition of its accumulation with corresponding effects on modifying arrhythmogenesis.

For example, in isolated rat hearts perfused with low concentrations of LPC (5 μM), a direct relation between the tissue content of LPC and the severity of arrhythmias has been observed.[53] No consistent alteration in total phospholipid, phosphatidylcholine, or cholesterol content was observed, suggesting that the arrhythmogenic effects of the LPC were not mediated through major alterations in lipid components of the heart.[53] Interestingly, the isolated rat heart appears to be more susceptible to the arrhythmogenic effects of LPC than the rabbit or guinea pig heart.[54] Perfusion with radiolabeled LPC indicated that the severity of arrhythmias was directly related to the incorporation of LPC into the microsomal membrane fraction, which includes not only the sarcolemma but other intracellular membranes as well.[54] Therefore, the extent of sarcolemmal incorporation of LPC and its direct relation to arrhythmogenesis in the intact heart has not yet been established.

We have shown that during a 5-minute period of regional ischemia in the in situ cat heart, long-chain acylcarnitine content increased 5-fold and LPC increased 2.5-fold selectively in the ischemic region, associated with a 64% incidence of VF and/or VT.[30] Pretreatment of animals with an inhibitor of CAT I, POCA, resulted in no increase in long-chain acylcarnitine or LPC content in the ischemic region, and none of the animals pretreated with POCA demonstrated VT or VF.[30] The protective effects of POCA during this brief 5-minute ischemic interval were not the result of improved hemodynamic function or enhanced coronary flow.[30] These results provide direct evidence, independent of changes in regional coronary flow or hemodynamic function, for a cause-and-effect relationship between the accumulation of both of these amphipathic metabolites and arrhythmogenesis in vivo in response to ischemia.

In summary, the results from the above studies demonstrate that both the LPC and long-chain acylcarnitine content of myocardium increase rapidly during short periods of ischemia and are capable of contributing to arrhythmogenesis. Studies in vitro demonstrate that both amphiphiles are capable of causing dramatic and reversible alterations in electrophysiological indices. The similarity of the electrophysiological derangements induced by these amphiphiles suggests that the effects are mediated by amphipathic properties common to both compounds.

EFFECTS OF LPC AND LONG-CHAIN ACYLCARNITINES ON INDIVIDUAL IONIC CURRENTS

Our knowledge of the precise mechanisms whereby either of these amphiphiles alters the ionic currents in cardiac cells is incomplete. The voltage-sensitive rapid Na^+ inward current is decreased by both amphiphiles, not only as a result of a direct decrease in the peak magnitude of the current but also secondary to a reduction in the resting membrane potential. Arnsdorf and Sawicki demonstrated that LPC decreased Na^+ conductance, resulting in biphasic effects on excitability, with an initial increase followed by a decrease in excitability, and often the development of complete inexcitability.[55] Interestingly, this type of biphasic response in excitability occurs in ischemic myocardium in vivo. In a recent study by Burnashev and colleagues,[56] LPC actually induced prolonged open times of sodium channels, and a subsequent study by Undrovinas and colleagues[57] demonstrated that this influence of LPC is secondary to a clustering of the Na^+ channels within the membrane, with a marked delay in inactivation of the Na^+ channel. This influence of LPC during ischemia could contribute to the marked slowing in conduction and conduction block, a reduction in resting membrane potential due to a potential increase in intracellular Na^+, and the development of both early and delayed afterdepolarizations, as discussed in detail below. Although long-chain acylcarnitines also decrease the rapid Na^+ inward current, as judged from the marked decrease in V_{max} of phase 0 depolarization,[51] whether the mechanism is similar or identical to that induced by LPC will require further investigation.

The influence of either amphiphile on K^+ currents has not been completely delineated. Clarkson and Ten Eick demonstrated that the reduction in membrane potential in response to LPC was secondary to a decreased potassium conductance at negative membrane potentials.[58] This was confirmed by the studies of Kiyosue and Arita, who reported that LPC decreased conductance through the inward rectifier K^+ channel (I_{K1}) and thereby decreased the resting membrane potential of isolated guinea pig ventricular myocytes.[59]

The voltage-dependent Ca^{2+} current ($I_{Ca(L)}$) in cardiac cells determines the APD,[60] thereby influencing the refractory period in ventricular muscle cells. Also, calcium ions entering the myocyte through these channels are essential for excitation-contraction coupling, since they initiate the normal cardiac contraction by triggering calcium release from the sarcoplasmic reticulum.[61-63] The direct influence of long-chain acylcarnitine and LPC on $I_{Ca(L)}$ has only recently been evaluated. Previous studies have suggested that long-chain acylcarnitines may activate or enhance $I_{Ca(L)}$ not only in cardiac tissue[64] but in smooth muscle cells as well.[65,66] This conclusion was supported by findings wherein palmitoylcarnitine increased the action potential duration, amplitude, and maximal rate of rise in isolated avian ventricular myocytes that were depolarized with elevated extracellular K^+.[64] Likewise, in isolated guinea pig myocytes, Meszaros and Pappano demonstrated that palmitoylcarnitine could induce delayed afterdepolarizations, which suggested indirectly that palmitoylcarnitine increased intracellular Ca^{2+}, thereby activating the transient inward current (I_{ti}).[67] However, we have recently used whole-cell voltage clamp procedures in isolated guinea pig myocytes to assess the direct effects of long-chain acylcarnitine on $I_{Ca(L)}$.[68] Both extracellular and intracellular delivery of long-chain acylcarnitine inhibited rather than stimulated $I_{Ca(L)}$ by approximately 50%.[68] Despite the marked decrease in $I_{Ca(L)}$, long-chain acylcarnitine induced both early and delayed afterdepolarizations with triggered activity, which likely contributes to the arrhythmogenic effect of long-chain acylcarnitines during ischemia.[68] Although the direct effects of LPC on $I_{Ca(L)}$ are not known, LPC has been shown to decrease the magnitude of action potentials dependent solely on $I_{Ca(L)}$ for membrane depolarization, which suggests indirectly that $I_{Ca(L)}$ is decreased.[58] Despite the fact that LPC likely decreases $I_{Ca(L)}$, a simultaneous positive ionotropic effect is associated with an increase in intracellular calcium, although the precise mechanisms are unknown.[58] We have shown that LPC induces delayed afterdepolarizations and triggered rhythms in isolated tissue, an effect that is coupled to an increase in intracellular calcium.[69] Delayed afterdepolarizations induced by LPC persisted even in the presence of acidosis and increased extracellular K^+, analogous to those changes seen in ischemic tissue in vivo.[69]

ACCUMULATION OF AMPHIPHILES AND ALTERATIONS IN INTRACELLULAR CALCIUM

Primary abnormalities in the regulation of intracellular calcium in ischemic myocardium may contribute significantly to arrhythmogenesis, including the development of VF. Several studies have demonstrated that ischemia results in a rapid increase in cytosolic calcium,[70,71] although others have suggested that the increase is delayed for approximately 10 minutes.[72-74] It is possible that either or both of these amphiphiles could have a primary role in the increase in intracellular calcium during early ischemia, despite suppression of $I_{Ca(L)}$. One potential mechanism may involve inhibition of sarcolemmal Na^+/K^+-ATPase. The Na^+/K^+-ATPase pump normally removes sodium ions from cells and returns potassium ions in a 3:2 ($Na^+:K^+$) exchange utilizing the hydrolysis of ATP (for review see ref. 75). The amount of long-term, restorative electrochemical work performed by the cardiac Na^+/K^+-ATPase pump is considerable. The Na^+/K^+-ATPase pump maintains the intracellular Na^+ ion concentration at a low level to maintain a large, inwardly directed electrochemical potential gradient for Na^+ that not only sustains electrical excitability but also supplies the energy for several cotransport and countertransport systems. Among these is Na^+/Ca^{2+} exchanger, which helps maintain the cytoplasmic Ca^{2+} ion concentrations at low levels during diastole (75–150 nM).[76-78]

Palmitoylcarnitine has been shown to inhibit Na^+/K^+-ATPase activity and reduce the binding of [^3H]-ouabain to cardiac membranes.[79] These effects occurred within the concentration range of long-chain acylcarnitine that occurs during acute episodes of ischemia. Na^+/K^+-ATPase is a transmembrane protein that depends on structurally associated phospholipids of the sarcolemma for its activity and for binding of digitalis. Perturbation of the phospholipid bilayer by incorporation of long-chain acylcarnitine into the sarcolemma could thereby result in alterations in enzyme activity and reactivity of the Na^+/K^+-ATPase to digitalis.[80] The opposite findings have been reported by Owens and coworkers, who analyzed the susceptibility of Na^+/K^+-ATPase in highly enriched cardiac sarcolemma to perturbation by LPC, palmitoyl CoA, and palmitoylcarnitine.[81] Palmitoylcarnitine at a ratio of up to 10 μmol/mg of sarcolemmal protein did not produce significant inhibition of Na^+/K^+-ATPase, even after preincubation at 37°C.[81] In contrast, LPC produced a 40% inhibition of Na^+/K^+-ATPase at a concentration of 0.6 μmol/mg protein, a finding confirmed by others at relatively low concentrations of LPC (10–30 μM).[82] At much higher concentrations of LPC (>2 mM), stimulation of Na^+/K^+-ATPase was observed, likely due to the nonspecific detergent effects of the amphiphile.[83] Thus, there is good evidence in isolated membranes that LPC can inhibit Na^+/K^+-ATPase, but the data with long-chain acylcarnitines are to date inconclusive. Most important, future studies will be required wherein the effects of these amphiphiles on the Na^+/K^+-ATPase pump in intact cells are determined. If Na^+/K^+-ATPase is actually inhibited by either or both amphiphiles, there would be a net increase in intracellular Na^+ that could contribute to membrane depolarization, the accumulation of extracellular K^+, and the increase in intracellular Ca^{2+} via enhanced Na^+/Ca^{2+} exchange. Although Bersohn and coworkers reported that high concentrations of LPC (0.3 μmol LPC/mg protein) resulted in a 50% inhibition of Na^+/Ca^{2+} exchange in normal canine sarcolemmal vesicles,[83] the amount of LPC incorporated into the sarcolemma in these experiments was high compared to the range found in ischemic tissue. These findings, together with the fact that the concentration of LPC required to inhibit Na/K-ATPase was lower than those that modulate other membrane-bound enzymes, suggests that inhibition of Na^+/K^+-ATPase may be critical to the electrophysiologic effects of these amphiphiles.

Inhibition of Ca-ATPase activity in the sarcoplasmic reticulum (SR) by amphiphiles may also contribute to an increase in intracellular calcium. This may be a particularly important mechanism since inhibition of SR Ca-ATPase may result in a delay in reuptake of cytosolic Ca^{2+}, leading to activation of I_{ti} and thereby triggered rhythms. Calcium-dependent ATPase from the sarcoplasmic reticulum pumps Ca against a concentration gradient at the expense of hydrolysis of ATP. Palmitoylcarnitine has been shown to produce a concentration-dependent, biphasic effect on SR Ca-ATPase activity with an increase in activity at low concentrations of palmitoylcarnitine and inhibition of Ca-ATPase activity at higher concentrations.[80] In contrast, Pitts and coworkers reported that palmitoylcarnitine inhibited Ca binding and Ca-ATPase activity only in sarcoplasmic reticulum, regardless of concentration.[84] Therefore modulation of Ca-ATPase by either or both amphiphiles may be important in arrhythmogenesis, but assessment in intact cell systems will be required.

Cytosolic protein kinase C (PKC) binds free Ca, causing it to translocate to the cell membrane, where it interacts with phospholipids and binds diacylglycerol with high affinity. Because the enzyme can be active in the absence of diacylglycerol if it is fully integrated into the membrane, simply raising intracellular calcium levels can be sufficient to activate the enzyme. The effects of protein kinase C on cardiac L-type Ca^{2+} channels have not been resolved. For example, phorbol esters (which produce direct, persistent activation of protein kinase C) have been shown to stimulate $I_{Ca(L)}$ in neonatal rat myocytes[85] and canine Purkinje cells and ventricular muscle cells.[86] However, there was no stimulation by the potent phorbol ester, phorbol 12,13-dibutyrate, in guinea pig ventricular myocytes. LPC has been shown to stimulate protein kinase C at low concentrations (<20 μM) and inhibit it at higher concentrations (>30 μM).[87] However, since $I_{Ca(L)}$ appears to be inhibited by both long-chain acylcarnitines and LPC, as discussed earlier, it is unlikely that modulation of the activity of protein kinase C by either amphiphile is critical for the increase in intracellular Ca^{2+} in the intact ventricular muscle cell. Another amphiphile, the plasmalogen metabolite 1-O-alkyl-1'-enyl-2-acyl-sn-glycerol (AAG), has recently been shown to be a potent activator of protein kinase C and to accumulate in ischemic myocardium.[88,89] Accumulation of AAG in ischemic myocardium in conjunction with increases in intracellular free Ca^{2+} may synergistically activate protein kinase C and thereby modulate phosphorylation of other membrane channel proteins that are critical in arrhythmogenesis. However, this sequence of events has not yet been addressed.

The final mechanism potentially responsible for the increase in intracellular Ca^{2+} in response to LPC or long-chain acylcarnitine is the delay in inactivation of the voltage-dependent Na^+ channel,[56,57] leading to an increase in intracellular Na^+. The increase in intracellular Na^+, independent of inhibition of Na^+/K^+-ATPase, could lead to an increase in intracellular Ca^{2+} through Na^+/Ca^{2+} exchange, resulting in enhanced release of Ca^{2+} from the sarcoplasmic reticulum.

Therefore, both long-chain acylcarnitines and LPC are capable of increasing intracellular Ca^{2+} by at least three potential mechanisms: (1) by inhibition of Na^+/K^+-ATPase, leading to an increase in $[Na^+]_i$ and thereby activating Na^+/Ca^{2+} exchange; (2) by inhibition of Ca^{2+}-ATPase activity in the sarcoplasmic reticulum, leading to a reduction in net Ca^{2+} uptake and resulting in an increase in intracellular calcium concentration; and (3) by a delay in inactivation of the Na^+ channel, leading to an increase in intracellular Na^+ and enhanced Na^+/Ca^{2+} exchange.

EXTRACELLULAR POTASSIUM

A very early event during ischemia is a net loss of a small fraction of total intracellular potassium.[90,91] This potassium loss begins within seconds after the onset of ischemia; extracellular potassium gradually increases from about 4 mM to 10–15 mM during the first 4–6 minutes of ischemia.[92-98] Studies of unidirectional K^+ flux indicate that the early K^+ depletion and extracellular accumulation are due to an increased rate of efflux of K^+ out of the cell. Data to date suggest that K^+ influx via the Na^+/K^+-ATPase pump is not a major contributing mechanism and that intracellular Na^+ may not be increased in the earliest phase of ischemia.[94,99,100] An increase in extracellular potassium depolarizes the resting membrane, shifts threshold potential to more positive potentials, reduces the maximum rate of rise of the action potential upstroke ($\dot{V}_{max}$), lowers the action potential amplitude and plateau potential, shortens the plateau duration, accelerates the slope of rapid repolarization, suppresses the oscillatory afterpotentials induced by an increase in intracellular calcium, and decreases the rate of spontaneous diastolic depolarization in Purkinje fibers.[101-103] In brief, an increase in extracellular K^+ can potentially elicit many of the electrophysiological alterations associated with early ischemia. It is also possible that other factors such as LPC or long-chain acylcarnitines could lead to membrane depolarization secondary to an increase in intracelluar Na^+, as discussed earlier, and that K^+ efflux occurs as a result of a new, more positive membrane potential and hence a new equilibrium potential for K^+.

The mechanisms responsible for the enhanced K^+ efflux during early ischemia are not completely understood. It is possible that the extracellular K^+ accumulation is a result of release of potassium from the cell to maintain charge neutrality during ischemia when weak acids accumulating intracellularly are released from the ischemic cell.[97,104] It is also possible that activation of the ATP-dependent potassium channel may contribute to potassium loss from the myocyte.[105] The channel is activated by a fall in ATP. However, the total intracellular level of ATP does not fall rapidly during early ischemia to a level sufficient to activate this channel at a time when extracellular K^+ increases markedly.[106] It is possible that activation of only a small percentage of the ATP-dependent channels, as may occur with modest falls in ATP, could be sufficient to account for the increase in extracellular K^+ and thereby elicit the electrophysiological effects indicated earlier.[107] Subcellular sites near the membrane ATP-dependent K^+ channel may sense a different pool of ATP than the rest of the cytoplasm, and this may be sufficient to activate this channel and thereby increase extracellular K^+.[108-112] Although LPC or long-chain acylcarnitines may activate the ATP-sensitive K^+ channel during ischemia, initial evidence suggests that LPC actually suppresses rather than activates the ATP-sensitive K^+ channel.

ACCUMULATION OF AMPHIPATHIC METABOLITES AND THEIR INFLUENCE ON CELL COUPLING

Gap junctions form low-resistance pathways between adjacent myocytes that permit the rapid and uniform flow of current from cell to cell and thereby uniform and rapid conduction of the wave front of electrical propagation.[113-115] These gap junctions are found primarily at the intercalated disks, structures that connect individual myocytes. A reduction in gap junctional conductance could contribute to slow conduction and ultimately conduction block, particularly in the presence of altered active membrane properties.

Internal longitudinal resistance and intracellular resistivity increase markedly in ischemic myocardium.[116-120] The specific cause of this increase is generally considered to be cellular uncoupling at gap junctions, mediated by decreases in intracellular pH and/or an increase in the intracellular Ca^{2+} concentration.[121,122] In canine myocardium, irreversible cellular uncoupling was observed after 30 minutes of hypoxia, probably owing to a decrease in the number of open gap junctional channels.[123] More extensive cellular uncoupling occurs after 60 minutes of hypoxia, which is likely due to irreversible damage to cell membranes and a quantitative reduction in the number of gap junction channels. In the isolated blood-perfused rabbit papillary muscle, Kléber and coworkers have shown rapid cellular uncoupling after 15–20 minutes of ischemia.[98,118] Coincident with cellular uncoupling was the development of ischemic contracture and a secondary rise in extracellular K^+.[98] A recent study using neonatal rat myocytes has demonstrated that free fatty acids can cause uncoupling between cell pairs.[124] The mechanism of uncoupling appears to involve destabilization of the channel through a disordering effect of the fatty acid. However, in a more recent preliminary study in adult rather than neonatal myocytes, the effect of free fatty acids was much less marked and required much higher concentrations to produce a similar uncoupling response.[125]

In isolated pairs of adult canine myocytes, and using double whole-cell voltage clamp procedures, we recently demonstrated that palmitoylcarnitine (5 μM) induced a rapid and progressive decrease in gap junctional conductance by almost 70%, an effect that was reversible after washout of the amphiphile.[126] Most important, electron microscopic autoradiographic studies in isolated canine ventricular myocytes exposed to hypoxia demonstrated a sevenfold preferential incorporation of endogenous long-chain acylcarnitines into the junctional as opposed to nonjunctional regions of the sarcolemma and composed 4 mol % of the total phospholipid content in the junctional region within 10 minutes of hypoxia.[126] These results suggest that during early ischemia, selective accumulation of long-chain acylcarnitines in junctional regions of the sarcolemma contributes to a reduction in cellular coupling between adjacent myocytes. A reduction in cellular coupling could contribute to slowed conduction and thereby the development of re-entrant arrhythmias, particularly in the presence of depressed active membrane properties, including decreased I_{Na}.

SUMMARY

At least two membrane-active amphiphiles, long-chain acylcarnitine and LPC, contribute to membrane dysfunction early after ischemia and thereby contribute to the development of both re-entrant and nonreentrant arrhythmias. Further work will be required to ascertain the precise role of these amphiphiles in arrhythmogenesis and the dominant cellular and subcellular mechanisms whereby these moieties influence the electrophysiological behavior of the heart. Therapeutic inhibition of the accumulation of these amphiphiles in response to ischemia in the intact heart may offer a specific approach to preventing sudden cardiac death in patients with ischemic disease.

REFERENCES

1. Nikolic G, Bishop RL, Singh JB: Sudden death during Holter monitoring. Circulation 66:218–225, 1982.
2. Panidis IP, Morganroth J: Sudden death in hospitalized patients: Cardiac rhythm disturbances detected by ambulatory electrocardiographic monitoring. J Am Coll Cardiol 2:798–805, 1983.
3. Wang FS, Lien WP, Fong TE, et al.: Terminal cardiac electrical activity in adults who die without apparent cardiac disease. Am J Cardiol 58:491–495, 1986.
4. Bayés de Luna A, Coumel P, Leclercq JF: Ambulatory sudden cardiac death: Mechanisms of production of fatal arrhythmia on the basis of data from 157 cases. Am Heart J 117:151–159, 1989.
5. Lie JT, Titus JL: Pathology of the myocardium and the conduction system in sudden coronary death. Circulation 52(Suppl III): 41–52, 1975.
6. Downar E, Janse MJ, Durrer D: The effect of acute coronary artery occlusion on subepicardial transmembrane potentials in the intact porcine heart. Circulation 56: 217–224, 1977.
7. Kléber AG, Janse MJ, van Capelle FJL, Durrer D: Mechanism and time course of S-T and T-Q segment changes during acute regional myocardial ischemia in the pig heart determined by extracellular and intracellular recordings. Circ Res 42:603–613, 1978.
8. Pogwizd SM, Corr PB: Reentrant and non-reentrant mechanisms contribute to arrhythmogenesis during early myocardial ischemia: Results using three-dimensional mapping. Circ Res 61:352–371, 1987.
9. Downar E, Janse MJ, Durrer D: The effect of "ischemic" blood on transmembrane potentials of normal porcine ventricular myocardium. Circulation 55:455–462, 1977.
10. Creer MH, Dobmeyer DJ, Corr PB: Amphipathic lipid metabolites and arrhythmias during myocardial ischemia. In Zipes DP, Jalife J (eds): Cardiac Electrophysiology: From Cell to Bedside. Philadelphia, WB Saunders, 1990, pp 417–433.
11. Gross RW: High plasmalogen and arachi-

donic acid content of canine myocardial sarcolemma: A fast atom bombardment mass spectroscopic and gas chromatography-mass spectroscopic characterization. Biochemistry 23:158–165, 1984.
12. Fink KL, Gross RW: Modulation of canine myocardial sarcolemmal membrane fluidity by amphiphilic compounds. Circ Res 55: 585–594, 1984.
13. Whitmer JT, Idell-Wenger JA, Rovetto MJ, Neely JR: Control of fatty acid metabolism in ischemic and hypoxic hearts. J Biol Chem 253:4305–4309, 1978.
14. Stein O, Stein Y: Lipid synthesis, intracellular transport, and storage: III. Electron microscopic radioautographic study of the rat heart perfused with tritiated oleic acid. J Cell Biol 36:63–77, 1968.
15. Ockner RK, Manning JA, Poppenhausen RB, Ho WKL: A binding protein for fatty acids in cytosol in intestinal mucosa, liver, myocardium and other tissues. Science 177:56–58, 1972.
16. Fournier N, Geoffroy M, Deshusses J: Purification and characterization of a long chain, fatty-acid-binding protein supplying the mitochondrial β-oxidative system in the heart. Biochim Biophys Acta 533:457–464, 1978.
17. Fournier NC, Zuker M, Williams RE, Smith ICP: Self-association of the cardiac fatty acid binding protein: Influence on membrane-bound, fatty acid-dependent enzymes. Biochemistry 22:1863–1872, 1983.
18. Oram JF, Wenger JI, Neely JR: Regulation of long chain fatty acid activation in heart muscle. J Biol Chem 250:73–78, 1975.
19. Haddock BA, Yates DW, Garland PB: The localization of some coenzyme A-dependent enzymes in rat liver mitochondria. Biochem J 119:565–573, 1970.
20. Brosnan JT, Fritz IB: The permeability of mitochondria to carnitine and acetylcarnitine. Biochem J 125:94P–95P, 1971.
21. Pande SV: A mitochondrial carnitine acylcarnitine translocase system: Carnitine acylcarnitine transport/exchange diffusion/acyl(+)carnitine inhibition/fatty acyl transport. Proc Natl Acad Sci USA 72:883–887, 1975.
22. Ramsey RR, Tubbs PK: The mechanism of fatty acid uptake by heart mitochondria: An acylcarnitine-carnitine exchange. FEBS Lett 54:21–25, 1975.
23. Shug AL, Thomsen JH, Folts JD, et al: Changes in tissue levels of carnitine and other metabolites during myocardial ischemia and anoxia. Arch Biochem Biophys 187:25–33, 1978.
24. Hochachka PW, Neely JR, Driedzic WR: Integration of lipid utilization with Krebs cycle activity in muscle. Fed Proc 36: 2009–2014, 1977.
25. Idell-Wenger JA, Grotyohann LW, Neely JR: Coenzyme A and carnitine distribution in normal and ischemic hearts. J Biol Chem 253:4310–4318, 1978.
26. Liedtke AJ, Nellis S, Neely JR: Effects of excess free fatty acids on mechanical and metabolic function in normal and ischemic myocardium in swine. Circ Res 43: 652–661, 1978.
27. Pauly DF, Yoon SB, McMillin JB: Carnitine-acylcarnitine translocase in ischemia: Evidence for sulfhydryl modification. Am J Physiol 253:H1557–H1565, 1987.
28. Kopec B, Fritz IB: Properties of a purified carnitine palmitoyltransferase, and evidence for the existence of other carnitine acyltransferases. Can J Biochem 49: 941–948, 1971.
29. Moore KH, Bonema JE, Solomon FJ: Long-chain acyl-CoA and acylcarnitine hydrolase activities in normal and ischemic rabbit heart. J Mol Cell Cardiol 16:905–913, 1984.
30. Corr PB, Creer MH, Yamada KA, Saffitz JE, Sobel BE: Prophylaxis of early ventricular fibrillation by inhibition of acylcarnitine accumulation. J Clin Invest 83: 927–936, 1989.
31. Knabb MT, Saffitz JE, Corr PB, Sobel BE: The dependence of electrophysiological derangements on accumulation of endogenous long-chain acylcarnitine in hypoxic neonatal rat myocytes. Circ Res 58: 230–240, 1986.
32. Heathers GP, Yamada KA, Kanter EM, Corr PB: Long-chain acylcarnitines mediate the hypoxia-induced increase in α_1-adrenergic receptors on adult canine myocytes. Circ Res 61:735–746, 1987.
33. Priori SG, Yamada KA, Corr PB: Influence of hypoxia on adrenergic modulation of triggered activity in isolated adult canine myocytes. Circulation 83:248–259, 1991.
34. DaTorre SD, Creer MH, Pogwizd SM, Corr PB: Amphipathic lipid metabolites and their relation to arrhythmogenesis in the ischemic heart. J Mol Cell Cardiol 23(suppl I):11–22, 1991.
35. McHowat J, Yamada KA, Saffitz JE, Corr PB: Rapid and selective accumulation of long-chain acylcarnitines in the sarcolemma of adult myocytes. Circulation 84(suppl II):495, 1991.
36. Franson R, Waite M, Weglicki W: Phospholipase A activity of lysosomes of rat myocardial tissue. Biochemistry 11: 472–476, 1972.

37. Franson RC, Weir DL, Thakkar J: Solubilization and characterization of a neutral-active, calcium-dependent, phospholipase A_2 from rabbit heart and isolated chick embryo myocytes. J Mol Cell Cardiol 15:189–196, 1983.
38. Wolf RA, Gross RW: Identification of neutral active phospholipase C which hydrolyzes choline glycerophospholipids and plasmalogen selective phospholipase A_2 in canine myocardium. J Biol Chem 260: 7295–7303, 1985.
39. Gross RW: Purification of rabbit myocardial cytosolic acyl CoA hydrolase, identity with lysophospholipase, and modulation of enzymic activity by endogenous cardiac amphiphiles. Biochemistry 22:5641–5646, 1983.
40. Gross RW, Sobel BE: Lysophosphatidylcholine metabolism in the rabbit heart: Characterization of metabolic pathways and partial purification of myocardial lysophospholipase-transacylase. J Biol Chem 257:6702–6708, 1982.
41. Gross RW, Ahumada GG, Sobel BE: Cytosolic lysophospholipase in cardiac myocytes and its inhibition by L-palmitoyl carnitine. Am J Physiol 246:C266–C270, 1984.
42. Gross RW, Sobel BE: Rabbit myocardial cytosolic lysophospholipase: Purification, characterization, and competitive inhibition by L-palmitoyl carnitine. J Biol Chem 258:5221–5226, 1983.
43. Gross RW, Drisdel RC, Sobel BE: Rabbit myocardial lysophospholipase-transacylase: Purification, characterization and inhibition by endogenous cardiac amphiphiles. J Biol Chem 258:15165–15172, 1983.
44. Ford DA, Hazen SL, Saffitz JE, Gross RW: The rapid and reversible activation of a calcium-dependent plasmalogen-selective phospholipase A_2 during myocardial ischemia. J Clin Invest 88:331–335, 1991.
45. Hazen SL, Ford DA, Gross RW: Activation of a membrane-associated phospholipase A_2 during rabbit myocardial ischemia which is highly selective for plasmalogen substrate. J Biol Chem 266:5629–5633, 1991.
46. Snyder DW, Crafford WA Jr, Glashow JL, Rankin D, Sobel BE, Corr PB: Lysophosphoglycerides in ischemic myocardium effluents and potentiation of their arrhythmogenic effects. Am J Physiol 243: H700–H707, 1981.
47. Akita H, Creer MH, Yamada KA, Sobel BE, Corr PB: Electrophysiologic effects of intracellular lysophosphoglycerides and their accumulation in cardiac lymph with myocardial ischemia in dogs. J Clin Invest 78:271–280, 1986.
48. Sedlis SP, Sequeira JM, Altszuler HM: Coronary sinus lysophosphatidylcholine accumulation during rapid atrial pacing. Am J Cardiol 66:695–698, 1990.
49. Broekman MJ, Ward JW, Marcus AJ: Phospholipid metabolism in stimulated human platelets: Changes in phosphatidylinositol, phosphatidic acid, and lysophospholipids. J Clin Invest 66:275–283, 1980.
50. McHowat J, Corr PB: Thrombin induced increases in lysophosphatidylcholine derived from endothelial cells. Circulation 84(suppl II):274, 1991.
51. Corr PB, Snyder DW, Cain ME, Crafford Jr WA, Gross RW, Sobel BE: Electrophysiological effects of amphiphiles on canine Purkinje fibers: Implications for dysrhythmia secondary to ischemia. Circ Res 49: 354–363, 1981.
52. Sedlis SP, Sequeira JM, Altszuler HM: Potentiation of the depressant effects of lysophosphatidylcholine on contractile properties of cultured cardiac myocytes by acidosis and superoxide radical. J Lab Clin Med 115:203–216, 1990.
53. Man RYK: Lysophosphatidylcholine-induced arrhythmias and its accumulation in the rat perfused heart. Br J Pharmacol 93: 412–416, 1988.
54. Giffin M, Arthur G, Choy PC, Man RYK: Lysophosphatidylcholine metabolism and cardiac arrhythmias. Can J Physiol 66: 185–189, 1988.
55. Arnsdorf MF, Sawicki GJ: The effects of lysophosphatidylcholine, a toxic metabolite of ischemia, on the components of cardiac excitability in sheep Purkinje fibers. Circ Res 49:16–30, 1981.
56. Burnashev NA, Undrovinas AI, Fleidervish IA, Makielski JC, Rosenshtraukh LV: Modulation of cardiac sodium channel gating by lysophosphatidylcholine. J Mol Cell Cardiol 23(suppl I):23–30, 1991.
57. Undrovinas AI, Fleidervish IA, Makielski JC: Maintained Na^+ current at all potentials induced by ischemic metabolite lysophosphatidylcholine. Circulation 84(suppl II):174, 1991.
58. Clarkson CW, Ten Eick RE: On the mechanism of lysophosphatidylcholine-induced depolarization of cat ventricular myocardium. Circ Res 52:543–556, 1983.
59. Kiyosue T, Arita M: Effects of lysophosphatidylcholine on resting potassium conductance of isolated guinea pig ventricular cells. Pflugers Arch 406:296–302, 1986.
60. Dörr T, Denger R, Dörr A, Trautwein W: Ionic currents contributing to the action potential in single ventricular myocytes of the guinea pig studied with action potential clamp. Pflugers Arch 416:230–237, 1990.

61. Fabiato A: Rapid ionic modification during the aequorin-detected calcium transient in a skinned canine cardiac Purkinje cell. J Gen Physiol 85:189–246, 1985.
62. Fabiato A: Time and calcium dependence of activation and inactivation of calcium-induced release of calcium from the sarcoplasmic reticulum of a skinned canine cardiac Purkinje cell. J Gen Physiol 85:247–290, 1985.
63. Fabiato A: Stimulated calcium current can both cause calcium loading in and trigger calcium release from the sarcoplasmic reticulum of a skinned canine Purkinje cell. J Gen Physiol 85:291–320, 1985.
64. Inoue D, Pappano AJ: L-palmitylcarnine and calcium ions act similarly on excitatory ionic currents in avian ventricular muscle. Circ Res 52:625–634, 1983.
65. Spedding M, Mir AK: Direct activation of Ca^{++} channels by palmitoyl carnitine, a putative endogenous ligand. Br J Pharmacol 92:457–468, 1987.
66. Spedding M: Activators and inactivators of Ca^{++} channels: New perspectives. J Pharmacol 16:319–343, 1985.
67. Meszaros J, Pappano AJ: Electrophysiological effects of L-palmitoylcarnitine in single ventricular myocytes. Am J Physiol 258:H931–H938, 1990.
68. Wu J, Corr PB: Influence of long chain acylcarnitines on the voltage dependent calcium current in adult ventricular myocytes. Am J Physiol (Heart Circ Physiol) [in press].
69. Pogwizd SM, Onufer JR, Kramer JB, Sobel BE, Corr PB: Induction of delayed afterdepolarizations and triggered activity in canine Purkinje fibers by lysophosphoglycerides. Circ Res 59:416–426, 1986.
70. Lee HC, Smith N, Mohabir R, Clusin WT: Cytosolic calcium transients from the beating mammalian heart. Proc Natl Acad Sci USA 84:7793–7797, 1987.
71. Lee HC, Mohabir R, Smith N, Franz MR, Clusin WT: Effect of ischemia on calcium-dependent fluorescence transients in rabbit hearts containing Indo-1: Correlation with monophasic action potentials and contraction. Circulation 78:1047–1059, 1988.
72. Marban E, Kitakaze M, Koretsune Y, Yue D, Chacko VP, Pike MM: Quantification of $[Ca^{2+}]_i$ in perfused hearts: Critical evaluation of the SF-BAPTA and nuclear magnetic resonance method as applied to the study of ischemia and reperfusion. Circ Res 66:1255–1267, 1990.
73. Marban E, Kitakaze M, Kusuoka H, Porterfield JK, Yue DT, Chacko VP: Intracellular free calcium concentration measured with 19F NMR spectroscopy in intact ferret hearts. Proc Natl Acad Sci USA 84:6005–6009, 1987.
74. Steenbergen C, Murphy E, Levy L, London RE: Elevation in cytosolic free calcium concentration early in myocardial ischemia in perfused rat heart. Circ Res 60:700–707, 1987.
75. Gadsby DC: The Na/K pump of cardiac myocytes. In Zipes DP, Jalife J (eds): Cardiac Electrophysiology: From Cell to Bedside. Philadelphia, WB Saunders, 1990.
76. Mullins LJ: Ion Transport in Heart. New York, Raven Press, 1981.
77. Reuter H: Na-Ca countertransport in cardiac muscle. In Martonosi AN (ed): Membranes and Transport. Vol 1. New York, Plenum Press, 1982.
78. Reeves JP: The sarcolemmal sodium-calcium exchange system. In Shamoo A (ed): Regulation of Calcium Transport Across Muscle Membranes. New York, Academic Press, 1985.
79. Adams RJ, Pitts BJR, Wood JM, Gende DA, Wallick ET, Schwartz A: Effect of palmitoylcarnitine on ouabain binding to Na, K-ATPase. J Mol Cell Cardiol 11:941–959, 1979.
80. Adams RJ, Cohen DW, Gupte S, et al: In vitro effects of palmitoylcarnitine on cardiac plasma membrane Na,K-ATPase, and sarcoplasmic reticulum Ca^{2+}-ATPase and Ca^{2+} transport. J Biol Chem 254:12404–12410, 1979.
81. Owens K, Kennett FF, Weglicki WB: Effects of fatty acid intermediates on Na^+-K^+-ATPase activity of cardiac sarcolemma. Am J Physiol 242:H456–H461, 1982.
82. Karli JN, Karikas GA, Hatzipavlov PK, Levis GM, Moulopoulos SN: The inhibition of Na^+ and K^+ stimulated ATPase activity of rabbit and dog heart sarcolemma by lysophosphatidylcholine. Life Sci 24:1869–1876, 1979.
83. Bersohn MM, Philipson KD, Weiss RS: Lysophosphatidylcholine and sodium-calcium exchange in cardiac sarcolemma: Comparison with ischemia. Am J Physiol 260:C433–C438, 1991.
84. Pitts BJR, Tate CA, Van Winkle B, McMillin Wood J, Entman ML: Palmityl-carnitine inhibition of the calcium pump in cardiac sarcoplasmic reticulum: A possible role in myocardial ischemia. Life Sci 23:391–402, 1978.
85. Dosemeci A, Dhallan RS, Cohen NM, Lederer WJ, Rogers TB: Phorbol ester increases calcium current and stimulates the effects of angiotensin II on cultured neo-

85. natal rat heart myocytes. Circ Res 62: 347–357, 1988.
86. Tseng GN, Boyden PA: Different effects of intracellular calcium and protein kinase C on the cardiac T and L Ca currents. Am J Physiol.
87. Oishi K, Raynor RL, Charp PA, Kuo JF: Regulation of protein kinase C by lysophospholipids. J Biol Chem 263:6865–6871, 1988.
88. Ford DA, Gross RW: Activation of myocardial protein kinase C by plasmalogenic diglycerides. Am J Physiol 258:C30–C36, 1990.
89. Ford DA, Miyake R, Glaser PE, Gross RW: Activation of protein kinase C by naturally occurring ether-linked diglycerides. J Biol Chem 264:13818–13824, 1989.
90. Case RB: Ion alterations during myocardial ischemia. Cardiology 56:245–262, 1971.
91. Harris AS: Potassium and experimental coronary occlusion. Am Heart J 71: 797–802, 1966.
92. Hill JL, Gettes LS: Effect of acute coronary occlusion on local myocardial extracellular K^+ activity in swine. Circulation 61:768–778, 1980.
93. Weiss J, Shine KI: Extracellular K^+ accumulation during myocardial ischemia in isolated rabbit heart. Am J Physiol 242: H619–H628, 1982.
94. Kléber AG: Resting membrane potential, extracellular potassium activity, and intracellular sodium activity during acute global ischemia in isolated perfused guinea pig hearts. Circ Res 52:442–450, 1983.
95. Wiegand V, Güggi M, Meesmann W, Kessler M, Greitschuss F: Extracellular potassium activity changes in the canine myocardium after acute coronary occlusion and the influence of beta-blockade. Cardiovasc Res 13:297–302, 1979.
96. Kléber AG: Extracellular potassium accumulation in acute myocardial ischemia. J Mol Cell Cardiol 16:389–394, 1984.
97. Kléber AG, Riegger CB, Janse MJ: Extracellular K^+ and H^+ shifts in early ischemia: Mechanisms and relation to changes in impulse propagation. J Mol Cell Cardiol 19(suppl V):35–44, 1987.
98. Cascio WE, Yan G-X, Kléber AG: Passive electrical properties, mechanical activity, and extracellular potassium in arterially perfused and ischemic rabbit ventricular muscle: Effects of calcium entry blockade or hypocalcemia. Circ Res 66:1461–1473, 1990.
99. Goerke J, Page E: Cat heart muscle in vitro: VI. Potassium exchange in papillary muscles. J Gen Physiol 48:933–948, 1965.
100. Rau EE, Shine KI, Langer GA: Potassium exchange and mechanical performance in anoxic mammalian myocardium. Am J Physiol 232:H85–H94, 1977.
101. Gettes LS, Surawicz B, Shiue JD: Effect of high K^+, low K^+ and quinidine on QRS duration and ventricular action potential. Am J Physiol 203:1135–1140, 1963.
102. Weidmann S: The effect of the cardiac membrane potential on the rapid availability of the sodium-carrying system. J Physiol 127:213–224, 1955.
103. Weidmann S: Shortening of the action potential due to brief injections of KCl following the onset of activity. J Physiol 132: 156–163, 1956.
104. Skinner Jr RB, Kunze DL: Changes in extracellular potassium activity in response to decreased pH in rabbit atrial muscle. Circ Res 39:678–683, 1976.
105. Noma A: ATP-regulated K^+ channels in cardiac muscle. Nature 305:147–148, 1983.
106. Elliott AC, Smith GL, Allen DG: Simultaneous measurements of action potential duration and intracellular ATP in isolated ferret hearts exposed to cyanide. Circ Res 64:583–591, 1989.
107. Nichols CG, Ripoll C, Lederer WJ: ATP-sensitive potassium channel modulation of the guinea pig ventricular action potential and contraction. Circ Res 68:280–287, 1991.
108. Baumgarten CM, Cohen CJ, McDonald TF: Heterogeneity of intracellular potassium activity and membrane potential in hypoxic guinea pig ventricle. Circ Res 49: 1181–1189, 1981.
109. Mercer RW, Dunham PB: Membrane-bound ATP fuels the Na/K pump. J Gen Physiol 78:547–568, 1981.
110. Paul RJ: Functional compartmentation of oxidative and glycolytic metabolism in vascular smooth muscle. Am J Physiol 244: C399–C409, 1983.
111. Jones DP: Intracellular diffusion gradients of O_2 and ATP. Am J Physiol 250: C663–C675, 1986.
112. Weiss JN, Lemp ST: Cardiac ATP-sensitive K^+ channels. J Gen Physiol 94: 911–937, 1989.
113. Weidmann S: The diffusion of radiopotassium across intercalated disks of mammalian cardiac muscle. J Physiol 187:323–342, 1966.
114. Weidmann S: Electrical constants of trabecular muscle from mammalian heart. J Physiol 210:1041–1054, 1970.
115. Cranefield PF: The Conduction of the Cardiac Impulse. Mount Kisco, NY, Futura, 1975.

116. Hiramatsu Y, Buchanan JW, Krisley SB, Gettes LS: Rate-dependent effects of hypoxia on internal longitudinal resistance in guinea pig papillary muscles. Circ Res 63: 923–929, 1988.
117. Ikeda K, Hiraoka M: Effects of hypoxia on passive electrical properties of canine ventricualr muscle. Pflugers Arch 393:45–50, 1982.
118. Riegger CB, Alperovich G, Kléber AG: Effect of oxygen withdrawal on active and passive electrical properties of arterially perfused rabbit ventricular muscle. Circ Res 64:532–541, 1989.
119. Streit J: Effects of hypoxia and glycolytic inhibition on electrical properties of sheep cardiac Purkinje fibers. J Mol Cell Cardiol 19:875–885, 1987.
120. Wejtczak J: Contractures and increase in internal longitudinal resistance of cow ventricular muscle induced by hypoxia. Circ Res 44:88–95, 1979.
121. DeMello WC: Intercellular communication in cardiac muscle: Physiological and pathological implications. In Zipes DP (ed): Cardiac Electrophysiology and Arrhythmias. New York, Grune & Stratton, 1985.
122. Reber WR, Weingart R: Ungulate cardiac Purkinje fibers: The influence of intracellular pH on the electrical cell-to-cell coupling. J Physiol 328:87–104, 1982.
123. Hoyt RH, Cohen ML, Corr PB, Saffitz JE: Alterations of intercellular junctions induced by hypoxia in canine myocardium. Am J Physiol 258:H1439–H1448, 1990.
124. Burt JM, Massey KD, Minnich BN: Uncoupling of cardiac cells by fatty acids: Structure-activity relationships. Am J Physiol 260:C439–C448, 1991.
125. Ovadia M, Burt JM: Developmental modulation of susceptibility to arrhythmogenesis in myocardial ischemia: Reduced sensitivity of adult vs. neonatal heart cells to uncoupling by lipophilic substances. Circulation 84(suppl II):II-324, 1991.
126. Wu J, McHowat J, Corr PB: Long-chain acylcarnitines induce reversible uncoupling in adult canine myocytes. Circulation 84(suppl II):325, 1991.
127. Catterall WA: Molecular properties of voltage-gated ion channels in the heart. In Fozzard HA, Haber E, et al (eds): The Heart and Cardiovascular System. New York, Raven, 1991, pp 945–962.

6

The Autonomic Nervous System and Sudden Cardiac Death: A Rational Basis for Post-Myocardial Infarction Risk Stratification

PETER J. SCHWARTZ
MARIA TERESA LA ROVERE
ANDREA MORTARA
EMILIO VANOLI

The combined efforts of several groups of investigators over the last 20 years have provided compelling evidence linking the autonomic nervous system and the problem of sudden cardiac death (SCD).[1-5] There is now a general consensus that, in the setting of acute myocardial ischemia, sympathetic hyperactivity facilitates the onset of malignant arrhythmias, whereas vagal activation can exert an antifibrillatory effect. The knowledge that became available made it logical to examine the possibility that analysis of some functional aspects of cardiac innervation might contribute to a more refined post-myocardial infarction (MI) risk stratification.

This chapter reviews some of the more recent experimental and clinical observations that have suggested new perspectives on the neural pathophysiological mechanisms underlying the onset of lethal arrhythmias, on developing a more accurate identification of the individuals at high risk, and on the concept of novel therapeutic strategies for the prevention of SCD.

BARORECEPTIVE REFLEXES: EXPERIMENTAL STUDIES

Background

A first and essential step was the development of an experimental model for SCD that would allow reasonable clinical extrapolations and the reproducible induction of ventricular fibrillation (VF) by clinically relevant stimuli.

This conscious animal preparation, described in detail elsewhere,[6,7] combines three elements highly relevant to the genesis of malignant arrhythmias in man: a healed MI, acute myocardial ischemia, and physiologically elevated sympathetic activity. Briefly, 30 days after an anterior wall MI, chronically instrumented dogs perform a submaximal exercise stress test. When heart rate reaches approximately 210–220 beats/min, a 2-minute occlusion of the circumflex coronary artery is performed by means of a hydraulic occluder previously positioned around the vessel. After 1 minute exercise ends but the occlusion continues for 1 additional minute. This exercise and ischemia test elicits VF in slightly more than 50% of animals. The animals run with steel paddles ligated to the chest to enable very rapid and effective defibrillation. The outcome of the test is highly reproducible over time in the same animal and has allowed the clear separation of two groups. Animals that develop VF are defined as susceptible (to sudden death) and those that survive are defined as resistant.

A serendipitous but critical observation was that among resistant dogs, acute myocardial ischemia often elicited a surprising reduction in heart rate despite continuation of exercise. This was in clear contrast to the response pattern shown by the susceptible dogs, which consisted of a marked increase in heart rate prior to the onset of VF. The latter response could be explained by a combination of the baroreflex response to the decline in arterial blood pressure and the excitatory cardiocardiac sympathetic reflex

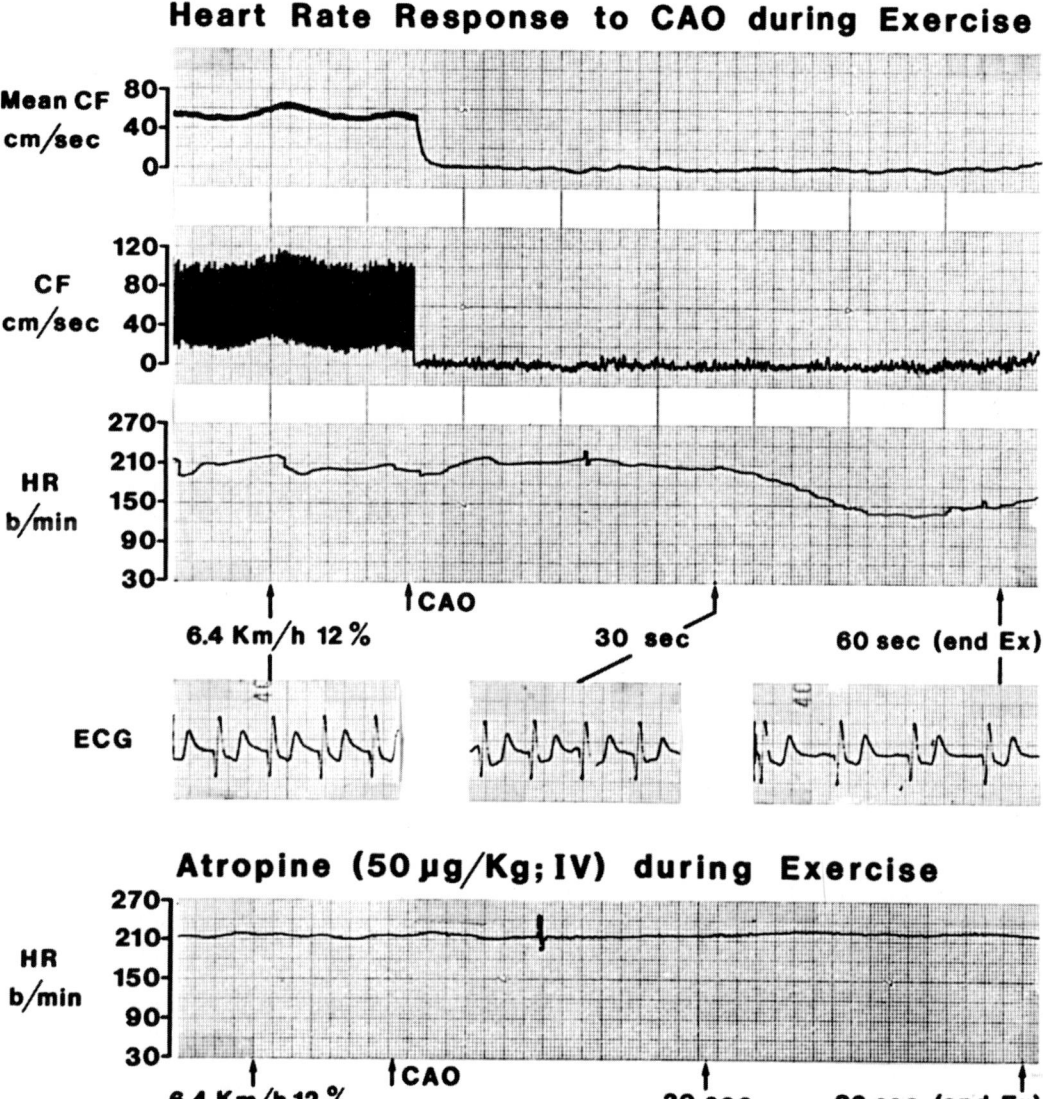

Fig. 6–1. The three upper panels show the circumflex coronary flow velocity, heart rate, and ECG during occlusion of the circumflex coronary artery performed during exercise in a dog with a 1-month-old anterior myocardial infarction. The occlusion was initiated after 15 minutes of exercise when the speed reached was 6.4 km/hr, and the inclination of the treadmill was 12%. The figure shows, without interruptions, the first minute of occlusion and the moment of cessation of exercise. For the first 30 seconds, heart rate oscillated around 210 beats/min, and then strikingly decreased to 130 beats/min while the animal continued to run. When the treadmill stopped (end Ex) and occlusion continued, there were no arrhythmias. The fourth panel shows the repetition of the exercise and ischemia test after pretreatment with atropine. It is evident that the reduction in heart rate during coronary occlusion is fully prevented.

that we had described in 1969.[8] However, in susceptible dogs the reflex tachycardia could not be attributed to a greater hemodynamic impairment, since mean blood pressure just before the occurrence of VF was not different from that in resistant dogs at the same moment. The unexpected heart rate reduction induced by myocardial ischemia in the resistant dogs was clearly dependent on a vagal reflex, as it could be prevented by atropine (Fig. 6–1). Given the preferential distribution of vagal sensory endings in the inferior ventricular wall,[9] the manifestation of a vagal reflex following occlusion of the circumflex coronary artery would have been expected at rest, but its overriding nature during exercise and in the presence of a prior MI was surprising and indicated a very powerful reflex.

The critical issue was that among the two groups of dogs, resistant and susceptible, the dominant autonomic reflex responses were opposite. This represented the starting point and the rationale for a series of further investigations in this model, which ultimately led to clinically relevant findings. Indeed, it became conceivable that analysis of cardiac reflexes at rest might have provided information useful for the early recognition of animals more or less likely to develop VF during an acute ischemic episode. If this hypothesis is confirmed, it might represent a new approach for risk stratification of patients with coronary artery disease. The possibility of determining the moment when the high-risk situation (acute myocardial ischemia during exercise) will occur, and of planning in advance the individual characterization and analysis of risk factors, is one of the advantages of experimental research.

Baroreflex Sensitivity, Myocardial Infarction, and Sudden Death

As a marker of vagal reflexes to the heart, we chose the measurement of baroreflex sensitivity (BRS). As indicated in Figure 6–2, this is something of an oversimplification, because the changes at the sinus node level reflect not only vagal activity but also, if to a much lesser extent, sympathetic activity. The method used was the one described by Sleight's group.[10] Basically, BRS is expressed by the slope of the regression line correlating R-R interval lengthening

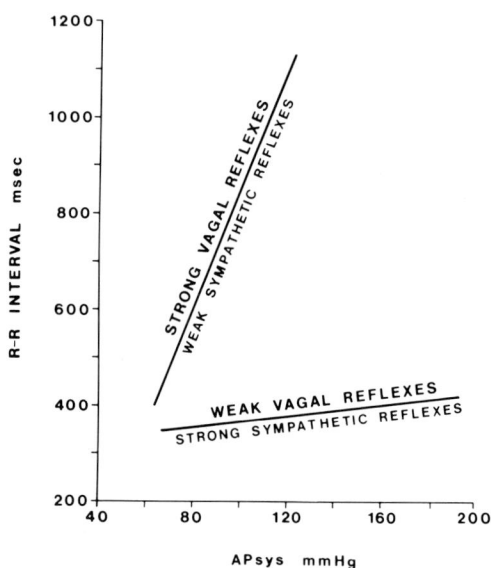

Fig. 6–2. Example of the relationship between R-R interval or heart rate and arterial blood pressure. The upper curve would represent a response primarily characterized by an increase in efferent vagus nerve activity to the sinoatrial node; the lower curve would be the opposite. Sympathetic neural activity may be altered in an opposite direction to vagus nerve activity, but does not contribute greatly to heart rate control under these conditions.

with blood pressure increases induced by the pressor agent phenylephrine. Among the methods usually employed in experimental as well in clinical research, we favored the use of phenylephrine because it was our primary interest to challenge the vagal component of the baroreflex. Nitroglycerin or nitroprusside, also used in our initial study,[11] explore more the sympathetic component.

Three sets of observations made with this methodology will be summarized here: the effect of MI on BRS, the prognostic value of BRS measured after MI, and the prognostic value of BRS measured before MI. These studies were all done in conscious animals, thus avoiding the limitations and confounding effects of anesthesia.

BRS was significantly lower in 192 dogs studied 30 days after an anterior wall MI than in a group of 86 dogs studied in control conditions (12.9 ± 7.6 vs. 19.6 ± 7.9 msec/mm Hg, $p < 0.001$).[12] Even if these data were strongly suggestive, the evidence that MI could impair vagal reflexes was definitively provided by the internal control analysis in a subgroup of 55 dogs in which BRS was measured both before and 30 days after MI.[12] In these animals, BRS was reduced after the infarction from 17.8 ± 6.6 to 13.5 ± 6.7 msec/mm Hg ($p < 0.001$). It is important to note that, as illustrated in Figure 6–3, a reduction in BRS occurred in 73% of the dogs, while in 20% BRS did not change and in 7% it increased. It is equally important to note that in many animals, despite even large reductions, the BRS values after MI were still higher than the BRS values of other animals prior to MI. These observations, together with the wide distribution of BRS values, call for caution in the interpretation of clinical studies based on group comparisons of relatively small populations of patients.

The finding most relevant to the question of early recognition of individuals at high risk for sudden death was that BRS was significantly lower in susceptible dogs than in resistant dogs. This observation was originally made in a small group of animals[11] and was subsequently confirmed in a much larger population.[12] In the latter study, which included 192 dogs, BRS was 17.7 ± 6.0 msec/mm Hg in the resistant group compared to only 9.1 ± 6.5 msec/mm Hg in the susceptible group ($p < 0.001$). This indicated that the capability of reflexly increasing vagal activity was significantly lower in those dogs that were at higher risk for developing VF. Figure 6–4 provides the individual data for each dog studied and allows not only a clear visualization of the relationship between level of BRS and the likelihood of being in the resistant or the susceptible group, but also the calculation of the risk according to a given BRS value. For example, the risk of sudden death during the exercise and ischemia test increased from 12% for a BRS > 20 msec/mm Hg to 91% for a

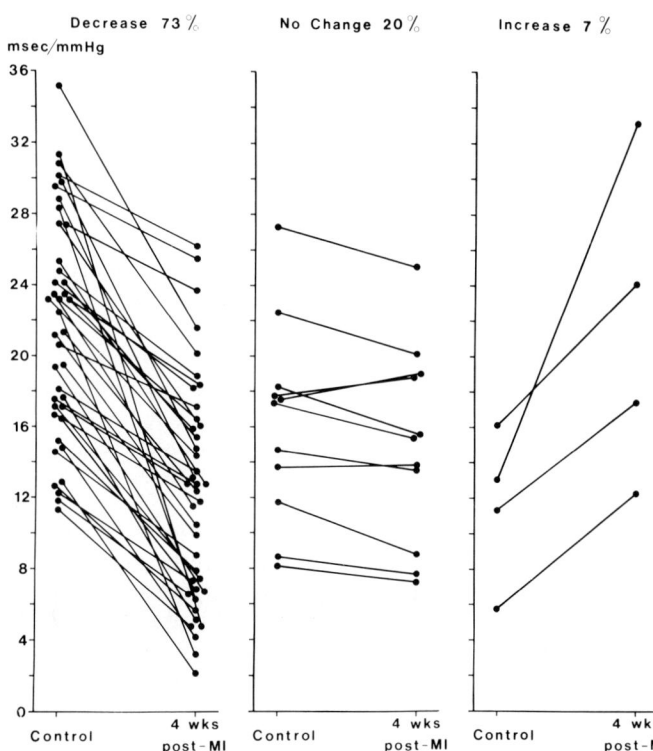

Fig. 6–3. Plots of individual changes in baroreflex sensitivity produced by myocardial infarction in 55 dogs. Baroreflex sensitivity is considered changed if a difference greater than 3 msec/mm Hg occurs. (Reproduced with permission from Schwartz PJ, et al: Circulation 78:969–973, 1988.[12])

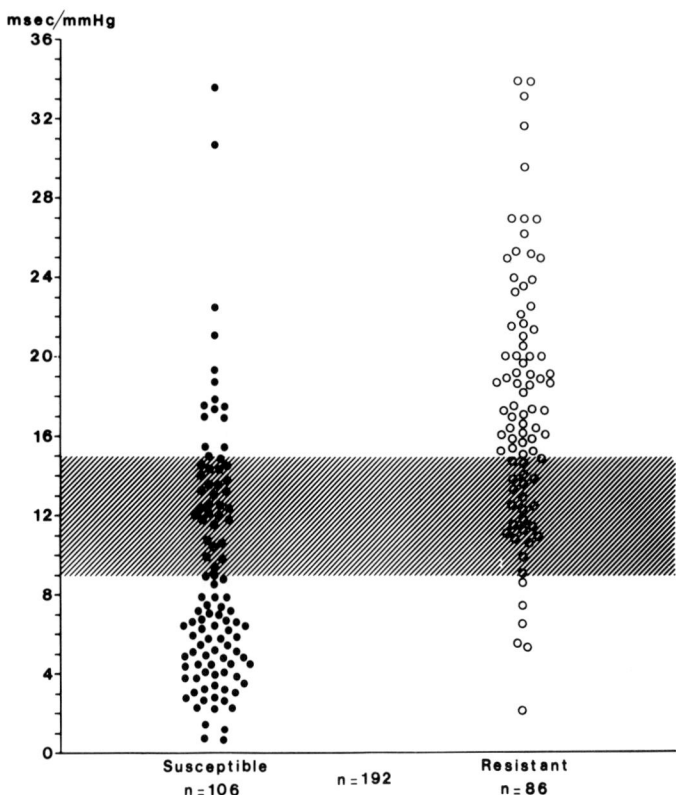

Fig. 6–4. Plot of baroreflex sensitivity in 192 dogs after infarction, and its relation to susceptibility to sudden death. Hatched area is an arbitrary gray zone. At <9 msec/mm Hg, 91% of dogs were susceptible to sudden death, whereas at >15 msec/mm Hg, 80% of dogs survived the exercise and ischemia test. Note the large number of animals with baroreflex sensitivity <9 msec/mm Hg. (Reproduced with permission from Schwartz PJ, et al: Circulation 78:969–973, 1988.[12])

BRS < 9 msec/mm Hg. Both specificity and predictive value were in excess of 85%.

A completely unexpected finding emerged on further analysis of the group of dogs in which BRS was assessed before and after MI. Contrary to our expectations, the reductions in BRS after MI were not significantly different between resistant and susceptible dogs, and we then realized that the difference in BRS between the two groups was already largely present before the MI. Indeed, Figure 6–5 shows that, of 68 dogs studied *prior to* the MI, those that would have died either during the recovery phase after the anterior MI or during the exercise and ischemia test already had a lower BRS than the dogs that would have survived.

Several conclusions can be drawn from these sets of data.

1. It has been demonstrated that MI reduces ability to increase vagal activity in the majority of animals.

2. The correlation between BRS assessed at rest and survival during the exercise and ischemia test suggests that the magnitude of the neural response to a blood pressure increase may be largely predictive of the neural response to acute myocardial ischemia, at least of the inferior ventricular wall. This concept is supported by the earlier observation that the resistant dogs were more capable of responding to acute myocardial ischemia with vagally mediated reductions in heart rate.

3. The evidence that a depressed BRS accurately identifies a group of animals at very high risk for sudden death is the first example of the use of autonomic nervous system functions with the goal of a more accurate post-MI prognosis.

Prior to this study, the possibility that analysis of autonomic reflexes in normal individuals might identify a subgroup at increased risk for sudden death after an MI had not been considered. The intriguing new concept is that already in normal conditions the individual autonomic makeup is characterized by such a wide range of reflex

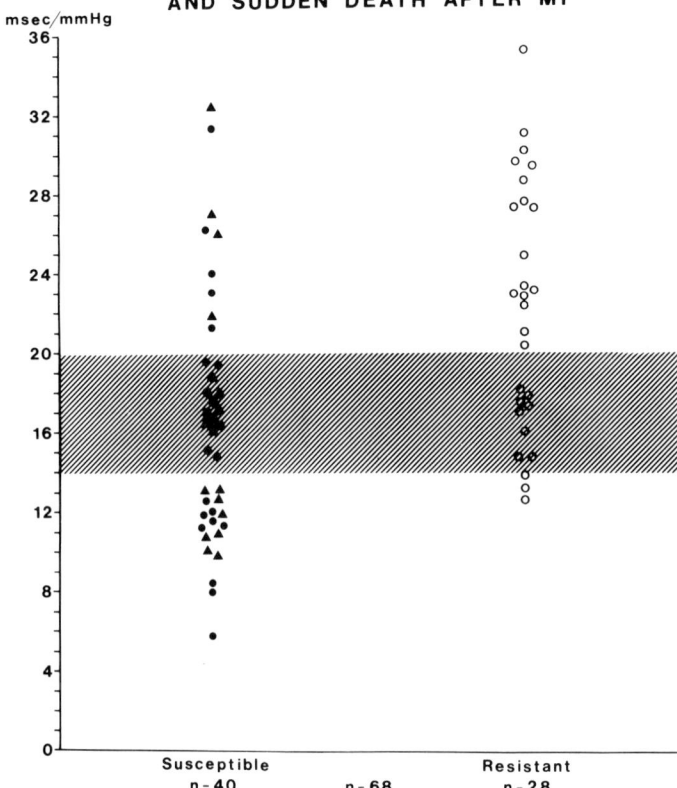

Fig. 6–5. Plot of baroreflex sensitivity before myocardial infarction (MI) in 68 animals, and its relation to susceptibility to sudden death after MI. In this case, the arbitrary gray zone extends from 14 to 20 msec/mm Hg. ●, Animals susceptible to sudden death during the exercise and ischemia test. ▲, Animals that died suddenly during the first 4 weeks after MI. ○, Animals that survived during the exercise and ischemia test. Note how few animals had baroreflex sensitivity <9 msec/mm Hg. (Reproduced with permission from Schwartz PJ, et al: Circulation 78:969–973, 1988.[12])

responses, exemplified by the large differences in BRS, that prognostic inferences can be made. MI, besides creating an arrhythmogenic substrate, displaces the entire range of vagal responses (BRS) toward lower values, thus increasing the chances for a condition associated with a higher risk. Individuals who, because of personal characteristics, are already at the lower end of the normal distribution of baroreflex responses, will find themselves, after an MI, with very low BRS values and thus at very high risk for sudden death.

BARORECEPTIVE REFLEXES: CLINICAL STUDIES

The findings just described raise the question of applicability to the clinical reality of post-MI patients.

We first sought to determine if patients with 2- to 3-week-old MIs had BRS values different from those of age- and sex-matched normal subjects.[13] As in the experimental study,[12] BRS values were significantly lower in patients with a prior MI (8.2 ± 3.7 vs. 12.3 ± 2.9 msec/mm Hg, $p = 0.0001$). Despite considerable overlap, 40% of the patients had a BRS value more than 2 SD below the mean of the control group, where no normal subjects were found (Fig. 6–6). However, this alteration in BRS was transient. At 3 and 12 months after MI the differences between the two groups had disappeared, as BRS increased in most patients.

Two additional observations were made. Five patients whose MI was complicated by early occurrence of VF had a BRS lower than that of the remaining 27 patients (5.2 ± 2.4 vs. 8.8 ± 3.6 msec/mm Hg, $p < 0.01$); this is interesting in light of evidence that patients with an anterior MI complicated, in the early phase, by VF are at increased risk for subsequent sudden death.[14,15] Two patients without an MI who had out-of-hos-

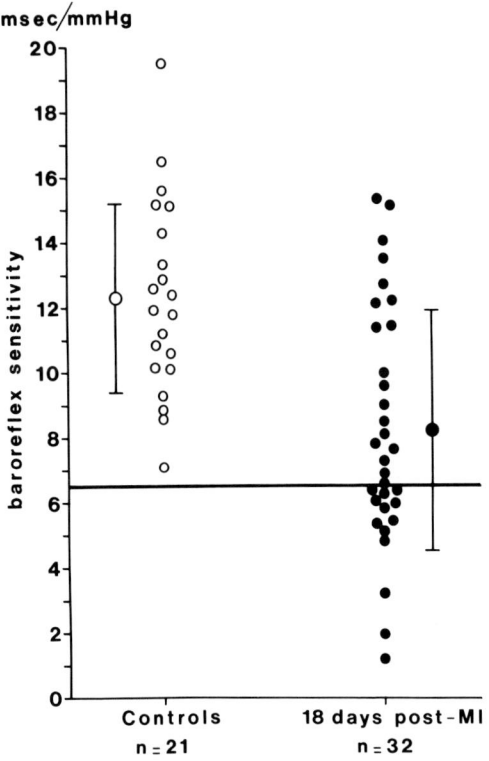

Fig. 6–6. Individual values for baroreflex sensitivity in 21 control subjects and 32 patients, 18 days after myocardial infarction (post-MI). The horizontal line at 6.5 msec/mm Hg represents 2 SD below the mean value for the control subjects. Mean values ± SD are indicated. (Reproduced with permission from Schwartz PJ, et al: J Am Coll Cardiol 12:629–636, 1988.[13])

pital VF had BRS values of 4.6 and 3.6 msec/mm Hg, far below the average of the post-MI patients.

The observation of the transient nature of the depression in BRS is in agreement with the report by Lombardi et al[16] indicating that 2 weeks after MI the high-frequency (vagal) spectral component of heart rate variability is depressed and that it returns to normal values by 6 to 12 months after infarction. In a subsequent study,[17] Bigger et al found that all components of spectral analysis of heart rate variability (from the ultralow to the high-frequency bands) significantly increased over 12 months after MI. Two aspects of this latter study deserve specific comment. First, heart rate variability, did not change significantly between 3 and 12 months, i.e., by 3 months post MI the recovery seemed already to have reached a plateau, but not quite the values observed in a population of control subjects. This finding is at variance with the work by Lombardi et al.[16] Second, the standard deviation of the means of all but the ultralow band were greater than the means, both in control and in post-MI subjects. This indicates that, despite the general trend toward a recovery of autonomic control of the heart, some subjects may not actually recover from the MI-dependent autonomic imbalance. These patients are at greater risk for later mortality, as shown by a more recent work by Bigger's group.[18] More intriguing is the same consideration when applied to patients without evidence of coronary artery disease. In this setting, the large standard deviations observed by Bigger et al[17] might support the speculation, generated in our animal model for sudden death, that the analysis of autonomic balance prior to the manifestation of any cardiovascular disease might already identify subjects at greater risk. Relevant here is the observation that resistant and susceptible dogs have a similar reduction in heart rate variability at 3 days after the creation of an anterior MI. However, by day 10, resistant dogs show a return to an almost normal heart rate variability, while in susceptible dogs cardiac vagal activity remains depressed for several weeks.[19] These studies[13,16,19] taken together may suggest a correlation between the reduction in risk for sudden death in the 6 to 12 months following an MI and the progressive resumption of vagal activity and normalization of the autonomic balance.

A prospective clinical study was then designed with the aim of assessing whether or not BRS correlated with cardiac mortality in patients.[20] BRS was evaluated in 78 patients with a 1-month-old MI. During an average follow-up period of 2 years there were seven cardiac deaths, four of which were sudden. The rather low (9%) 2-year mortality for the entire group reflects the entry criteria, which required all patients to be less than age 65, to have had a first MI, and to be able to perform a maximal exercise stress test in pharmacological washout; thus, they constituted a low-risk group. Nonetheless, within this group, analysis of BRS allowed the identification of a subgroup at very high

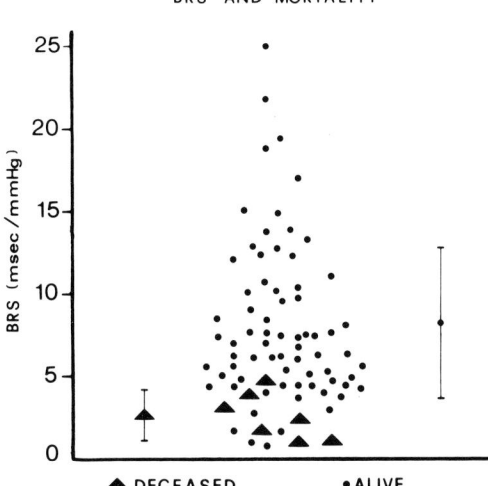

Fig. 6–7. Plot of relation between baroreflex sensitivity (BRS) and cardiovascular mortality. Besides the clear difference in BRS ($p = 0.004$) between deceased patients and survivors, it is noteworthy that, while all decreased patients had a reduced BRS, four were at the extreme lower end of the distribution of BRS for the entire population. (Updated and modified with permission from La Rovera MT, et al: Circulation *78:* 816–824, 1988.[20])

risk. Figure 6–7 provides the individual BRS values for all the patients and shows that BRS was markedly lower in the seven decreased patients than in the 71 survivors (2.4 ± 1.5 vs. 8.2 ± 4.8 msec/mm Hg, $p = 0.004$). When mortality was calculated in respect to the absence or presence of a markedly depressed BRS (≤ 3 msec/mm Hg, i.e., 1 SD below the mean of the entire group), a striking difference became evident, as mortality increased from 3% to 50% (Table 6–1). Even if the number of patients who died ($n = 7$) and who had a markedly depressed BRS ($n = 10$) was relatively small, the difference in mortality is sufficiently large to exclude a mere dependence on the numbers involved.

In the experimental study[12] the site of infarction was always anterior; in this clinical study[20] as well as in another[21] the relationship between BRS and subsequent mortality was independent of the site of infarction.

Depressed cardiac vagal activity and increased sympathetic activity have been documented in patients with congestive heart failure.[22] However, the possibility that a reduced BRS represents nothing more than reduced left ventricular function is ruled out by the complete lack of correlation between BRS and left ventricular ejection fraction (LVEF), assessed during left ventriculography (Fig. 6–8). Figure 6–9 shows the relationship between BRS, LVEF, and mortality. It is evident that, within the group of patients with reduced LVEF, the risk of death was increased with the coexistence of a depressed BRS. This suggests that a depressed pump function represents an important substrate on which an unfavorable alteration of the autonomic balance (i.e., reduced vagal activity and increased sympathetic activity) could more easily act as a trigger for lethal arrhythmias. If so, these two parameters would act synergistically to create a quite dangerous condition. Should this hypothesis be confirmed, new and interesting perspectives for post-MI risk stratification would be opened.

This prospective clinical study raises the possibility that the analysis of baroreceptive reflexes in patients after MI may contribute to a more accurate identification of individuals at high risk for subsequent mortality.

Support for this concept has already been provided by a study by Farrell et al.[21] Using the same methodology described by us,[20] they measured BRS and heart rate variability in 68 patients who had suffered an MI 7 to 10 days earlier. They also assessed the presence of late potentials and used programmed ventricular stimulation to evaluate the inducibility of sustained monomorphic ventricular tachycardia (VT). A first point to be noted, important and reassuring from a methodological point of view, is the striking similarity of the correlations between BRS and age ($r = -0.57, p < 0.001$ vs. $r = -0.53, p < 0.001$) and between BRS

Table 6–1
Baroreflex Sensitivity (BRS) and Mortality

	n	Mortality (%)
Whole population	78	8.9
BRS > 3.0 msec/mm Hg	68	2.9
BRS ≤ 3.0 msec/mm Hg	10	50.0

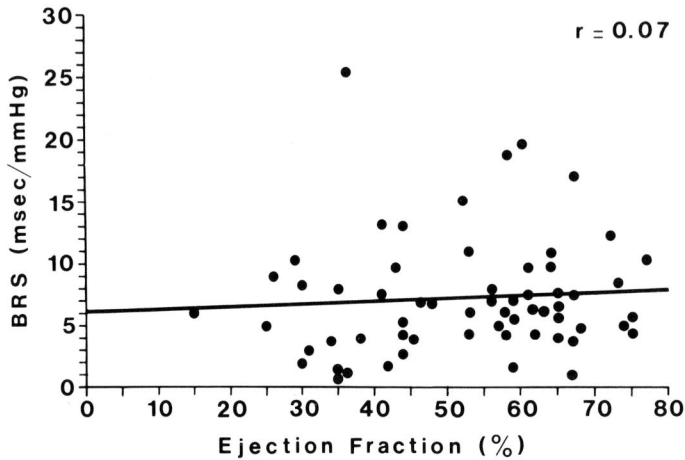

Fig. 6-8. Plot of relation between baroreflex sensitivity (BRS) and left ventricular ejection fraction at rest. (Reproduced with permission from La Rovera MT, et al: Circulation 78:816–824, 1988.[20])

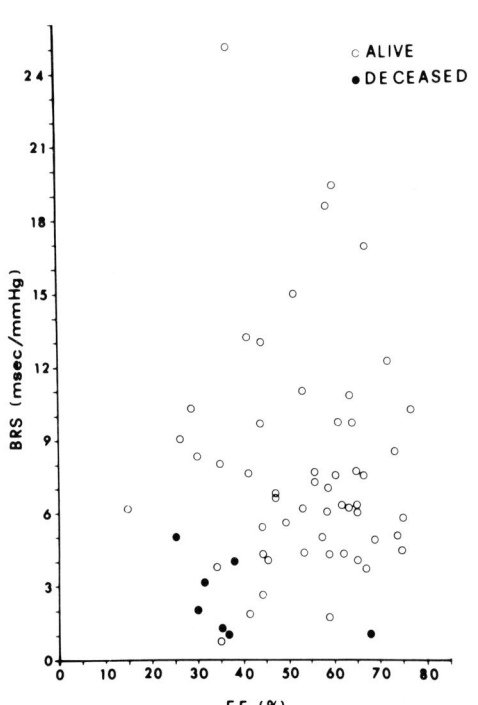

Fig. 6-9. Plot of relation between baroreflex sensitivity (BRS), left ventricular ejection fraction (EF), and cardiovascular mortality. It is evident that, among patients with depressed LVEF, the prediction of mortality is enhanced by the analysis of BRS. (Updated and modified with permission from La Rovere MT, et al: Circulation 78:816–824, 1988.[20])

and LVEF ($r = 0.07$ [NS] vs. $r = 0.035$ [NS]) observed in the two studies. BRS was found to be the most significant predictor of induction of sustained monomorphic VT during programmed ventricular stimulation. During follow-up there were five major arrhythmic events (clinical VT with and without sudden death); they were all correctly identified by depressed BRS and by inducibility during electrical testing. There was a striking difference in BRS when the patients with major arrhythmic events during follow-up were compared with those without events (0.9 ± 0.8 vs. 7.4 ± 4.6 msec/mm Hg, $p = 0.002$). Farrell et al conclude that their study "confirms that depressed BRS identifies a subgroup at high risk for arrhythmic events following myocardial infarction" and interestingly add that "programmed electrical stimulation may be safely limited to this group without any loss of predictive accuracy." The initial observations by Farrell et al have been now extended,[23] and during 1-year follow-up there were ten major arrhythmic events among the 122 patients, including five sudden deaths. The striking feature of this second study was that patients with a depressed BRS (<3 msec/mm Hg) had a relative risk for arrhythmic events during the follow-up of 23.1, superior to any other variable including the different measures of heart rate variability (10.4) or other conventional investigations like LVEF < 40% (10.4) or the presence of frequent ventricular extrasystoles (20.6).

HEART RATE VARIABILITY: CLINICAL AND EXPERIMENTAL STUDIES

Beat-to-beat variability of heart rate depends on instantaneous variations in the balance of the two limbs of the autonomic nervous system and is thought to represent a reliable marker of cardiac vagal tone.[24,25]

The increasing interest in heart rate variability, and the realization that when depressed it is associated with an increased risk for cardiac mortality, in combination with a flourishing of scientific publications, has led to a relatively frequent phenomenon in contemporary medicine: obliviousness to pioneering observations. In 1973 Stewart Wolf and colleagues had already called attention to a potential relationship between heart rate variability and life-threatening arrhythmias.[26] Indeed, even though Wolf was apparently approaching the problem from a different angle and with a different perspective, he concluded, "The study of the behavior of sinus arrhythmia may offer a way to anticipate the occurrence of dangerous cardiac dysarrhythmias and sudden death." In a somewhat unexpected way, the study of what Wolf had called "rhythmic heart rate variability" did eventually provide important information. A few years later, another Wolf proposed a correlation between reduced sinus arrhythmia and an increased risk for cardiac mortality. In this study[27] sinus arrhythmia was calculated, according to Stewart Wolf's method, from a few seconds of chart recording in 72 patients at the time of admission to the ICU. The novel information was that a lack of sinus arrhythmias was associated with an increased incidence of cardiac mortality in the first few days after MI. This was independent of the hemodynamic status of the patient as it was quantified by the Norris index.

After these initial observations, several new techniques to measure heart rate variability were developed.[28-33] Kleiger et al[34] found in a large population of post-MI patients that depressed heart rate variability, measured as the standard deviation of R-R intervals over 24 hours, was significantly correlated with mortality. Indeed, the relative risk for mortality was five times higher in patients with a heart rate variability lower than 50 msec, compared to patients with values greater than 100 msec. The predictive value of heart rate variability analysis has been significantly improved by the use of spectral analysis of its different components, as documented by the most recent work published by the same group.[35] Thus, these studies too contribute to the concept of an inverse relationship between cardiac vagal activity and cardiovascular mortality after an MI.

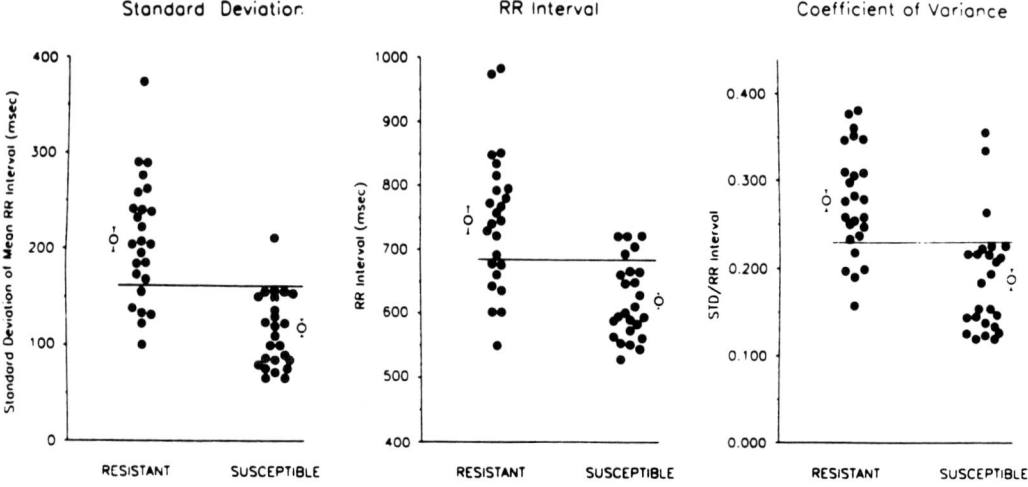

Fig. 6–10. Scattergrams of the standard deviation of the mean, R-R interval, and coefficient of variance in 25 resistant and 25 susceptible animals. Group mean values (± SEM) are displayed adjacent to scatter data; discriminator is placed at the midpoint of group mean values ($p < 0.05$). (Reproduced with permission from Hull SS, et al: J Am Coll Cardiol 16:978–985, 1990.[36])

In our conscious animal model for SCD[6] we examined the prognostic value of heart rate variability, measured in a 30-minute period, taking advantage of the ability to perform the study both before and after an MI.[36] The study was performed in 25 dogs identified during the exercise and ischemia test as susceptible and in 25 identified as resistant to sudden death. There were two main findings of the study. Thirty days after MI, heart rate variability was significantly lower in the susceptible dogs than in the resistant ones (106 ± 9 msec vs. 209 ± 13 msec, $p < 0.001$). This difference was largely independent of the difference in heart rate, for analysis of the coefficient of variance, which corrects for heart rate, provided a similar result (Fig. 6–10). This would simply confirm, in the more controlled environment of the experimental laboratory, the observation made by Kleiger et al[34] in patients. The novel observation comes from the internal control analysis performed in 18 resistant and 15 susceptible dogs studied before and after MI. It was found that before MI, susceptible and resistant dogs had almost an identical heart rate variability (226 ± 30 msec vs. 233 ± 30 msec) and that the MI produced a significant reduction in the susceptible but not in the resistant dogs (Fig. 6–11).

Thus, although heart rate variability effectively distinguishes between individuals at high and low risk after MI, its analysis *before* MI could not predict the outcome during an ischemic episode occurring *after* MI. This represents a major difference in respect to what we had observed with analysis of the BRS.

QUESTIONS, ANSWERS, AND SPECULATIONS

The data presented so far raise a host of questions and implications. To some of them we have already attempted to provide either an answer or an interpretation.

1. Why Does Myocardial Infarction Alter Baroreflex Sensitivity?

The mechanism by which BRS is reduced after MI and by which a depressed BRS is predictive of the neural response to acute MI is not yet defined, but it is likely to involve derangements in the neural activity of cardiac origin. Of the various possibilities,[12] the more tenable seems the one that involves a cardiocardiac sympathovagal reflex.[37] The changes in the geometry of a beating heart secondary to the presence of a necrotic and noncontracting segment may conceivably increase beyond normal the firing of sympathetic afferent fibers by mechanical distortion of their sensory end-

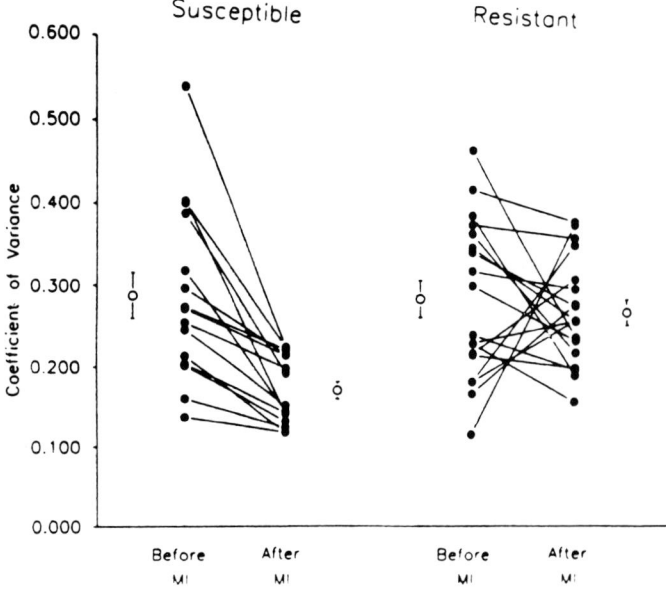

Fig. 6–11. Scatter plots of the coefficient of variance in 15 susceptible dogs and 18 resistant dogs before and 1 month after myocardial infarction. (Reproduced with permission from Hull SS, et al: J Am Coll Cardiol *16*:978–985, 1990.[36])

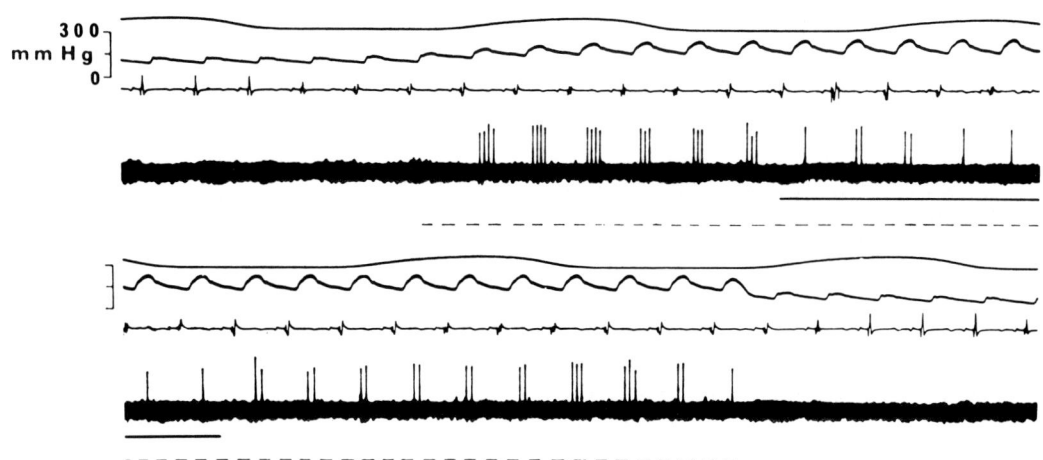

Fig. 6–12. Effects of blood pressure increase by aortic occlusion and of sympathetic afferent activation by electrical stimulation of the cut central end of the left inferior cardiac nerve, on the discharge of a single efferent vagal fiber in an intact, anesthetized cat. Broken line indicates stenosis of the aorta, solid line indicates sympathetic stimulation. The two strips are continuous recordings. The tracings in each section from top to bottom are: respiration, systemic arterial blood pressure, electrocardiogram, and neural activity. This vagal fiber begins to fire only in response to blood pressure elevation (baroreceptor reflex), and the concurrent afferent sympathetic stimulation is able to interfere with this response. (Modified and reproduced with permission from Schwartz PJ, et al: Circ Res 32: 215–220, 1973.[37])

ings.[38] Such a sympathetic excitation affects and impairs the baroreceptor reflex, that is, it interferes with the physiological increase in the activity of vagal fibers directed to the sinus node.[39–41] Figure 6–12 shows the demonstration of this phenomenon with the use of single fiber recording. In a more recent series of experiments we recorded vagal efferent activity before and after removal of the left stellate ganglion.[40] After left stellectomy, not only was tonic vagal activity higher, but the reflex increase following the rise in blood pressure was significantly potentiated. In 16 anesthetized cats removal of the left stellate ganglion increased the resting level of vagal activity from 1.2 ± 0.2 to 2.1 ± 0.3 impulses/sec ($+75\%$, $p < 0.01$) (Fig. 6–13). In the same cats, vagal activity during similar blood pressure increases induced by phenylephrine was also higher after left stellectomy (4.7 ± 0.7 vs. 2.2 ± 0.4 impulses/sec, $p < 0.001$), with an increment of $134 \pm 24\%$ vs. $86 \pm 18\%$ ($p < 0.05$) versus the resting level (Fig. 6–14).

2. Is It Possible to Increase a Depressed BRS, and Would This Affect Survival?

The correlation between depressed BRS and susceptibility to sudden death made it logical to attempt a modification of BRS as a potential physiological means of reducing the risk of VF. In theory, this could be achieved either by increasing vagal efferent activity or, to a lesser extent, by antagonizing sympathetic activity. Relevant to this latter issue is the observation that β-blockade increases baroreflex sensitivity in patients with a prior MI in 40% of the cases.[42]

As an alternative to antiadrenergic interventions, it might be possible to increase vagal activity. One physiological way to achieve this end may be exercise training, as discussed elsewhere.[41] This possibility was specifically tested in our animal model of sudden death.[43]

Three groups of dogs—one of resistant and two of susceptible dogs—with a 1-month-old MI were studied. The resistant dogs and one group of susceptible dogs were treated with daily exercise for a 6-week period, while the other group of susceptible dogs was rested in a cage for the same length of time. This technique allowed us to rule out time as a potential confounding factor for possible changes in the exercising group. Daily exercise produced a marked and significant increase in the BRS of the susceptible animals and, more important, dramati-

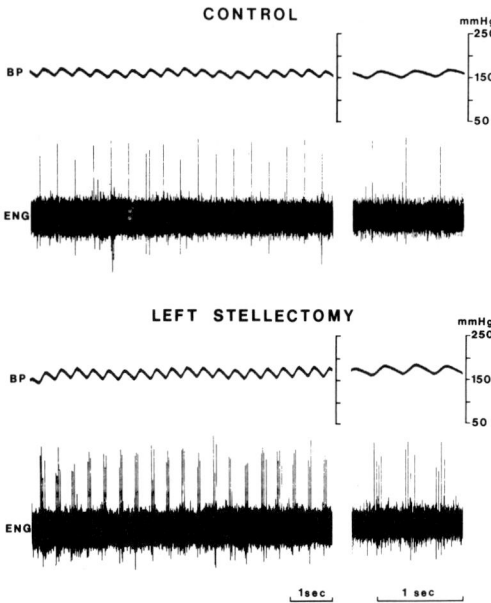

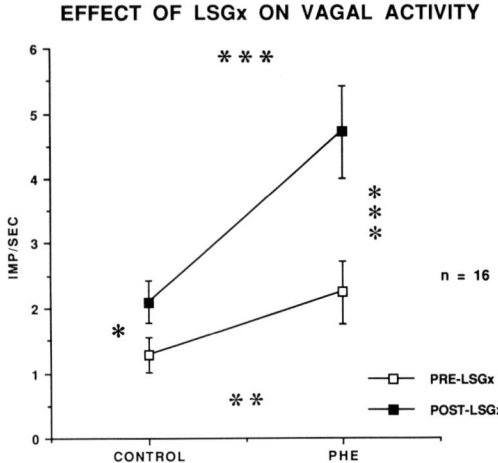

Fig. 6–13. Tracings showing activity of a single cardiac vagal efferent fiber at the same blood pressure (BP) levels induced by phenylephrine before (top panel) and after (bottom panel) left stellectomy. The fiber shows a pulse-synchronous activity. In each panel the upper tracing shows the blood pressure and the lower tracing shows the electroneurogram. (Reproduced with permission from Cerati D, et al: Circ Res 69: 1389–1401, 1991.[40])

Fig. 6–14. Effects of left stellectomy (LSGx) on cardiac vagal activity (impulses/sec) in control conditions and after phenylephrine (PHE) injection. PRE-LSGx, before left stellectomy; POST-LSGx, after left stellectomy. *$p < 0.01$; **$p < 0.005$; ***$p < 0.001$. (Reproduced with permission from Cerati D, et al: Circ Res 69: 1389–1401, 1991.[40])

cally affected their outcome during the exercise and ischemia test. As shown in Figure 6–15, all the exercise-trained susceptible animals survived the second test, whereas all but one of the susceptible, cage-rested dogs again developed VF. Of interest, the only cage-rested susceptible dog that survived the exercise and ischemia test was also the only one that, for unknown reasons, had a baroreflex slope that had increased spontaneously to reach the resistant range (from 4.4 to 16.7 msec/mm Hg). This study indicated the possibility of improving the BRS nonpharmacologically and of obtaining a striking alteration in the probability of survival during an episode of acute myocardial ischemia. A currently ongoing study in conscious dogs without MI further supports the concept that exercise training concomitantly increases cardiac vagal activity and the electrical stability of the myocardium.[44] In 12 dogs, 6 weeks of daily exercise increased BRS and heart rate variability by 18% and 21%, respectively. In the same dogs the threshold current to induce repetitive ventricular responses, the RET,[45] a marker of the propensity of the heart to develop malignant arrhythmias, increased from 33 ± 3 mA to 41 ± 5 mA.

Whether exercise training could increase BRS in patients has been recently evaluated. BRS was measured in 97 patients 1 month after a first MI. The patients were then randomized to enter or not to enter a 4-week endurance program.[46] Among them, 35 cases and 35 controls of the same age were matched for BRS (± 1 msec/mm Hg) and site of infarction. At 2 months post-infarction BRS had increased by 27% (from 7.8 ± 4.0 to 10.4 ± 5.3 msec/mm Hg, $p < 0.001$) among the exercise-trained patients, whereas it did not change (+1.5%) among the controls. This study showed that in humans as well, a nonpharmacological intervention, such as exercise, can improve the autonomic balance, as indicated by the increase in BRS.

Markers of vagal control of heart rate can also be augmented by pharmacological interventions. Low doses of atropine or other muscarinic antagonists have been shown to

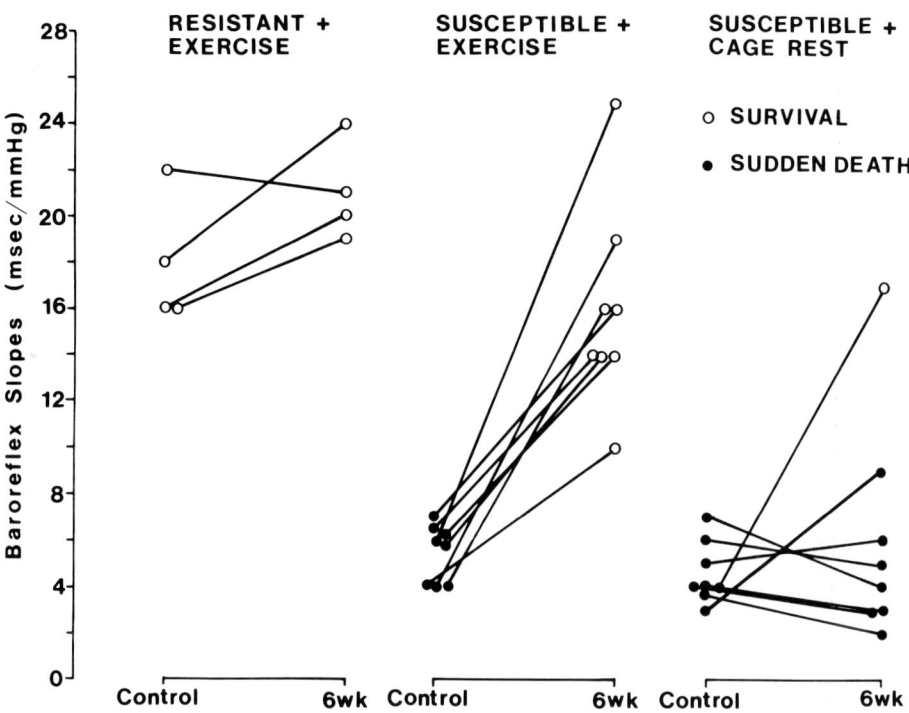

Fig. 6–15. Baroreflex slopes before and after 6 weeks of either daily exercise or cage rest. All animals underwent exercise and ischemia test at these two times. Sudden death on the treadmill is indicated by the closed circles, survival by the open circles. (Reproduced with permission from Billman GE, et al: Circulation 69:1182–1189, 1984.[43])

produce paradoxical vagomimetic effects. Dibner-Dunlap et al[47] observed that transdermal administration of the muscarinic antagonist scopolamine in healthy young men increased mean R-R interval and its standard deviation and baroreceptor responses to graded neck suction. The relevance of this information to the situation of post-MI patients has been recently tested.[48] In 20 patients with 15-day-old MIs a placebo patch had no effects on heart rate variability and BRS. A scopolamine patch in the same group increased R-R interval by 7%, SD of the R-R interval by 25%, MSSD by 38%, and pNN50 by 100%. Spectral analysis of heart rate variability components revealed a 24% decrease after scopolamine of the ratio between low- and high-frequency components, thus indicating a shifting in the autonomic balance toward a vagal prevalence. In the same group BRS after scopolamine increased by 42%. Also, low doses of scopolamine IV significantly blunts the sympathetically mediated reflex in heart rate increase during acute myocardial ischemia in dogs susceptible to sudden death. Thus, pharmacological modulation of autonomic balance might be considered as a promising approach to reduce risk after MI.

3. Does Augmented Vagal Activity During Acute Myocardial Ischemia Really Have an Antifibrillatory Effect?

Despite evidence supporting the existence of a relationship between reduced vagal activity and susceptibility to VF, a protective effect of augmented vagal activity was still to be definitively proved. Previous reports[4,49,50] on the antifibrillatory potential of vagal stimulation were in part limited by the use of anesthesia in most experiments, by the lack of an effective cardioselective muscarinic agonist, and by the widely held view that electrical vagal stimulation in conscious animals was not feasible. We have developed a chronically implantable device to be placed around the cervical right vagus that allows effective stimulation without producing discomfort.[51] One month after MI, 54 dogs were identified as susceptible during an exercise and ischemia test, i.e., they all developed VF. They were then allocated to repeat the exercise and ischemia test in control conditions or after implantation of the vagal device.[52] In the latter group, vagal stimulation was initiated shortly after occlusion of the circumflex coronary artery, while the dogs were performing the submaximal exercise stress test. In the control group, 22 (92%) of 24 dogs again developed VF during the second exercise and ischemia test; this confirmed the high reproducibility of the outcome in this animal model. By contrast, during vagal stimulation VF occurred again in only 3 (10%) of 30 dogs and recurred in 26 (87%) during an additional exercise and ischemia test performed once more in the control condition, i.e., without vagal stimulation. The difference in the incidence VF was significant ($p < 0.001$) by both group comparisons and internal control analysis. In 9 dogs protected by vagal stimulation the exercise and ischemia test was repeated by combining vagal activation with atrial pacing to keep the heart rate at the same level attained just prior to VF in the control test; 5 (55%) of these 9 animals survived again (Fig. 6–16), indicating that a decrease in heart rate is an important but not always essential mechanism underlying the vagally mediated protection from VF.

The antiarrhythmic potential of vagal activation has also been tested by using pharmacological interventions. The effects of the muscarinic agonist oxotremorine has been evaluated in conscious dogs and in experimental preparation involving anesthetized cats. In the cat model, life-threatening arrhythmias are consistently induced by the interaction between acute myocardial ischemia and sympathetic hyperactivity generated by left stellate ganglion stimulation.[53,54] In this preparation several Class 1 antiarrhythmic drugs failed to provide protection, whereas positive results have been

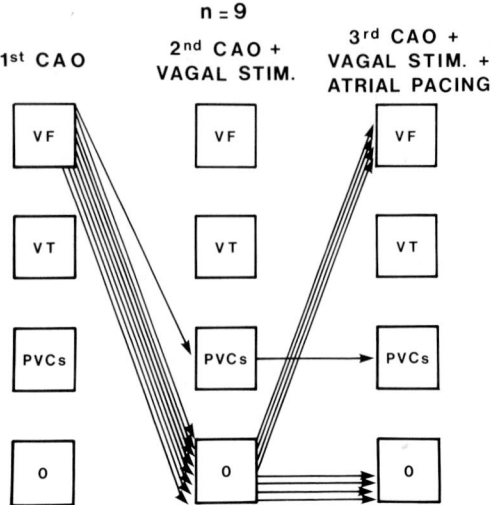

Fig. 6–16. Overall incidence of ventricular arrhythmias in nine dogs during three different coronary artery occlusions (CAO): the first in control condition, the second associated with vagal stimulation, the third when heart rate was kept constant during vagal stimulation by atrial pacing. Each arrow represents one animal. VF, ventricular fibrillation; VT, ventricular tachycardia; PVCs, premature ventricular contractions; O, no ventricular arrhythmias. (Reproduced with permission from Vanoli E, et al: Circ Res 69: 1471–1481, 1991.[52])

obtained by α- and β-adrenergic blocking agents; excellent protection was conferred by amiodarone and several calcium entry blockers.[54–56] Oxotremorine afforded complete protection in 17 cats in which, in control trials, malignant arrhythmias were consistently induced. Of 15 cats that had VF or VT in control trials, only two showed recurrence of VT after oxotremorine administration.[57] The protective effect of muscarinic activation in these experiments was largely independent of the attendant reduction in heart rate since when heart rate was kept by atrial pacing at the same level attained during the control trials, 73% of the animals remained protected from VF or VT.

In the animal model in conscious dogs, oxotremorine prevented the occurrence of VF in 5 (63%) of the 8 susceptible dogs in which it was tested. In the same study propranolol provided protection in 9 of 10 dogs studied. However, the reduction of dP/dt_{max} consequent on acute myocardial ischemia was significantly greater in the propranolol than in the oxotremorine or saline trials. This information is of interest because of the limitations inherent in the use of β-adrenegic blockers in patients with prior MI and depressed LV function.

The effect of vagal activation can also be potentiated by the use of the acetylcholinesterase inhibitor edrophonium. Figure 6–17 shows the different effects of pharmacological interventions in our conscious canine model for sudden death. In this dog a long run of VT occurred after 1 minute of acute myocardial ischemia, a few seconds following cessation of exercise. After administration of edrophonium only one couple of premature ventricular beats occurred during occlusion. After administration of propranolol, despite a lower heart rate at the onset of ischemia, several runs of VT occurred during myocardial ischemia and also at release of occlusion. In this animal protection from life-threatening arrhythmias was conferred by a pharmacological intervention that potentiates the effect of neurally mediated release of acetylcholine, and not by β-adrenergic blockade.

Overall, these studies showed that vagal activation during an acute ischemic episode can effectively prevent VF. This result probably depends on several mechanisms having a synergistic action. Heart rate reduction is an important factor, but the electrophysiological effects secondary to the vagally mediated antagonism of the sympathetic activity on the heart are likely to play a critical role.

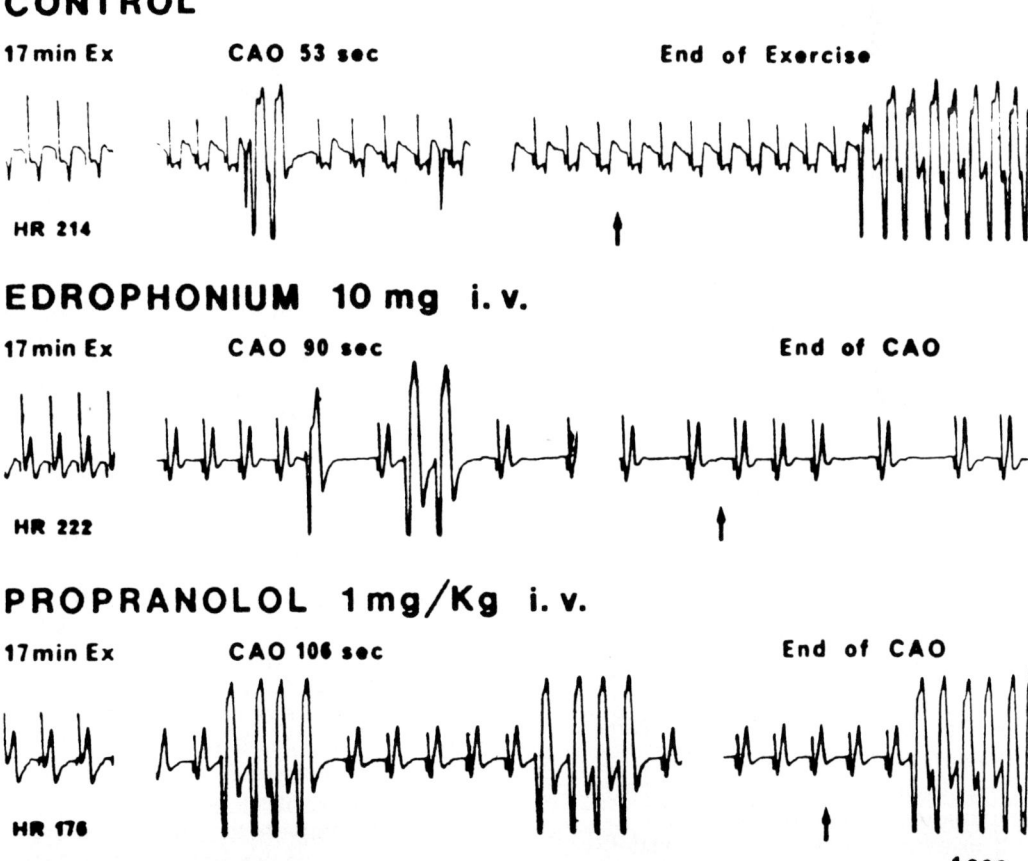

Fig. 6–17. Dog with a 1-month-old myocardial infarction. Response to exercise and ischemia test on different days and with different treatments. The somewhat different ECG morphology reflects different lead positions (chest leads and epicardial leads). For details see text.

4. Among Low-Risk Individuals, Does Removal of the Vagal Effects on the Heart Increase the Risk for Ventricular Fibrillation?

Although several lines of evidence, as indicated above, support the concept of an antifibrillatory influence of vagal activity during acute myocardial ischemia, they do not provide direct evidence for the actual role of spontaneous vagal tone and reflexes. Accordingly, we investigated in a group of resistant dogs the effect of muscarinic receptor blockade by atropine.[58]

A second exercise and ischemia test, after atropine administration, was performed in 45 dogs that had survived the first test in control conditions. In this second test 23 (51%) of 45 dogs showed an arrhythmia worsening and 11 (24%) of 45 developed VF (Fig. 6–18). These 11 animals were characterized by powerful vagal reflexes during the control episode of acute myocardial ischemia, as indicated by a marked heart rate reduction that was almost absent in the remaining animals. When the exercise and ischemia test was repeated and the heart rate was raised by atrial pacing to the same level produced by atropine, 71% of the animals still developed VF. This indicated that a large component of the detrimental effect of atropine is secondary to its effects on heart rate. This study indicates that the main characteristic of the resistant dogs is that they respond to acute myocardial ischemia with only weak or moderate increases in sympathetic activity, and that for them the presence or absence of vagal reflexes is relatively unimportant. However, this study also indicates that in approximately 25% of the resistant animals the ability to activate powerful vagal reflexes, thus reducing heart rate, effectively counteracts a concomitant reflex sympathetic hyperactivity and constitutes the main determinant for survival.

5. Does Direct Recording of Cardiac Vagal Activity Substantiate the Hypotheses Generated by the Analysis of Its Indirect Markers, Baroreflex Sensitivity and Heart Rate Variability?

BRS and heart rate variability are considered markers of reflex and of tonic vagal activity, respectively. The data discussed earlier suggested that no difference existed

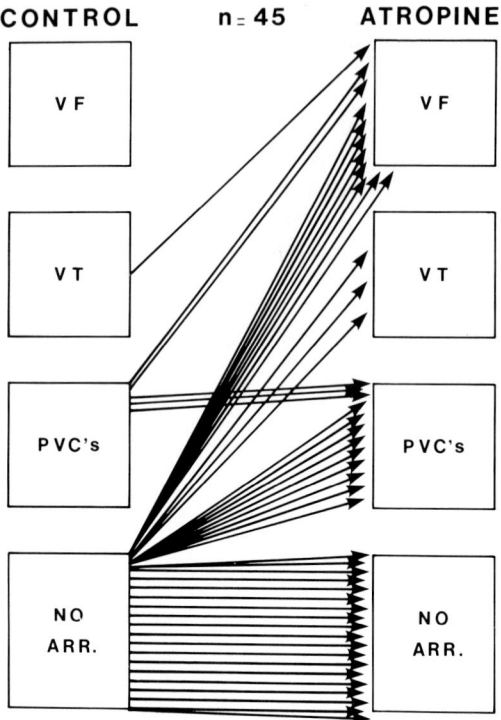

Fig. 6–18. Effect of atropine on the incidence of arrhythmias during the exercise and ischemia test. In control conditions one animal had a single episode of three premature ventricular beats and was assigned to the ventricular tachycardia group (VT), five had scattered isolated premature ventricular beats (less than 10 PVCs), and the remaining had no arrhythmias (NO ARR.). Atropine caused a worsening in 23 (51%) of 45 dogs. (Reproduced with permission from De Ferrari GM, et al: Am J Physiol 261:H63–H69, 1991.[58])

in "tonic" vagal activity *prior to* an MI, i.e., in normal hearts, between resistant and susceptible animals; by contrast, differences were thought to exist in reflex vagal activity.

The only way to study vagal activity directly, and not its markers, is to record the activity of single vagal fibers mostly directed to the sinus node.[37,59] Efferent vagal activity in these fibers is modulated by both vagal and sympathetic afferent activity[59] and receives a major input by the carotid sinus nerve, thus representing the efferent part of the baroreceptive reflex. By means of this experimental preparation we have assessed directly the relationship between tonic and reflex vagal activity and susceptibility to sudden death.[40]

In 17 anesthetized cats, cardiac vagal activity (single fiber recording only) was recorded in control conditions, during blood pressure increases due to phenylephrine, and during a 60-minute occlusion of the left anterior descending coronary artery. VF occurred within 3 minutes of occlusion in 9 cats, defined as susceptible, whereas the remaining 8 survived and were defined as resistant. The analysis of vagal activity prior to coronary occlusion revealed that whereas resting activity (tonic) was similar in the two groups (1.48 ± 0.30 vs. 1.58 ± 0.35), the reflex increase following the blood pressure elevation was markedly smaller in the susceptible animals (80 ± 14% vs. 246 ± 66%, $p < 0.05$). Also, the neural response during the first 2 minutes of coronary occlusion was clearly different among the two groups. In susceptible cats vagal activity was slightly reduced (-18%) by the second minute of occlusion; by contrast, at the same time vagal activity was markedly increased in the resistant animals ($+48\%$) ($p < 0.01$) (Fig. 6–19).

This and other studies[60] support the concept that MI can affect and sometimes impair reflexes of cardiac origin.

These data in anesthetized animals are in agreement with the observations that we had made in conscious dogs by means of markers of vagal activity. Indeed, this study showed that the animals that survive coronary artery occlusion are those capable of reflexly increasing vagal activity during acute myocardial ischemia, and that their outcome could be predicted by analysis of the reflex response to a baroreceptive stimulus and not by analysis of the tonic activity. It is fair to note that "tonic" vagal activity, as defined here, is the resting activity in anesthetized animals and thus only with caution can be extrapolated to the conscious state. This study, as discussed ear-

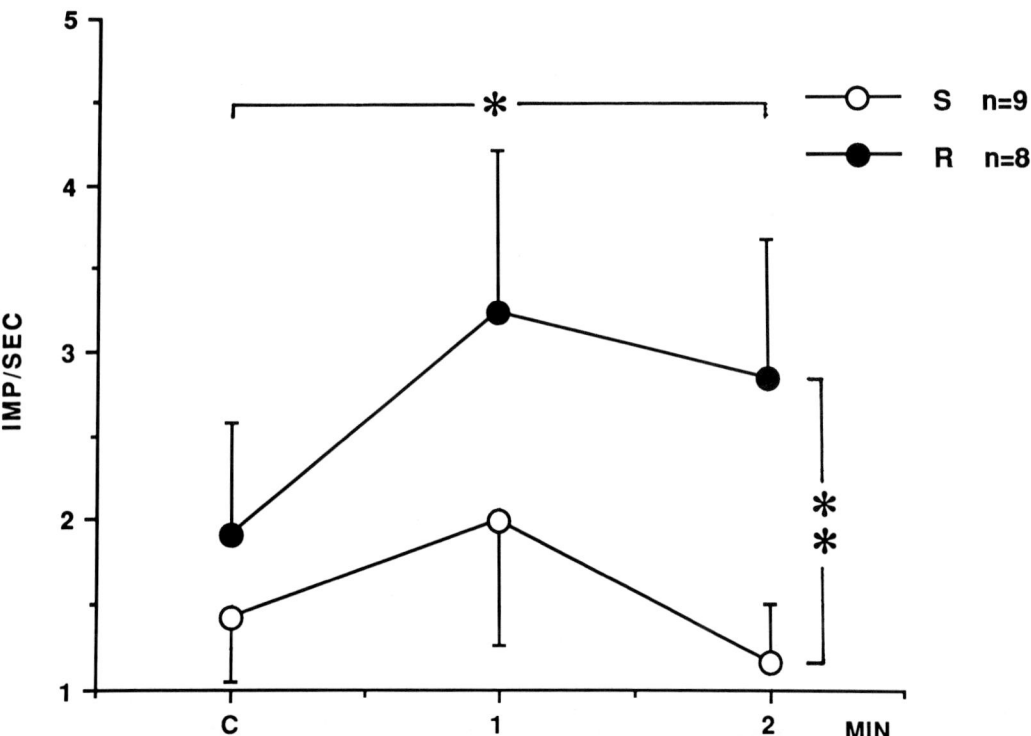

Fig. 6–19. Effect of coronary artery occlusion on vagal activity. The bar shows cardiac vagal activity in 17 cats, in control conditions and during the first 2 minutes of coronary artery occlusion. Data are expressed as impulses/sec. (Reproduced with permission from Cerati D, et al: Circ Res 69:1389–1401, 1991.[40])

lier, has also demonstrated that cardiac afferent sympathetic activity produces a tonic constraint on vagal efferent activity and blunts the reflex increases secondary to blood pressure rises. This finding strongly supports the possibility that the depression in BRS often observed after an MI[12,13] depends largely on an increase in afferent sympathetic traffic of cardiac origin.

6. Does Heart Rate Variability Predict Baroreflex Sensitivity?

The evidence that after MI both BRS[20,21] and heart rate variability[34] are of prognostic value made it important to test whether or not one measure would predict the other. If BRS correlates strictly with heart rate variability, then analysis of reflex vagal activity would add little, if anything, to analysis of tonic vagal activity.

To test this possibility, the two variables were evaluated and compared in 32 patients with a prior MI.[61] BRS was assessed by the phenylephrine method and heart rate variability was assessed by four methodologies, three in the time domain and one in the frequency domain. These variables were the standard deviation of the R-R interval;[34] pNN50, the percentage of R-R (N-N) intervals exceeding by at least 50 msec the preceding R-R interval;[29] MSSD, the mean square root of the difference of successive R-R intervals;[29] and the high-frequency peak of the power spectrum of heart rate variability.[30,62] Interestingly, the three more sophisticated methods for measuring heart rate variability were highly correlated between each other ($r = 0.94$–0.97), but they weakly ($r = 0.55$–0.56) correlated with the standard deviation of the R-R intervals, the only such parameter documented to predict risk for sudden death after MI. The main finding was that although BRS was significantly ($p < 0.01$) correlated with the various measures of heart rate variability, this correlation was weak ($r = 0.57$–0.63); it is stronger at night than during the day ($r = 0.63$ vs. $r = 0.44$) (Fig. 6–20), as expected, since vagal activity is higher during the night.

The implication of this study is that the two methodologies explore different aspects of the autonomic control of heart rate. The information derived from ambulatory ECG recording concerns primarily vagal tone, whereas the phenylephrine test discloses the capability of the parasympathetic nervous system to react to a gross stimulus and thus concerns primarily vagal reflexes. The main conclusion is that the two types of measures are not redundant and cannot be used to accurately predict each other.

ATRAMI

The experimental and clinical data discussed in this chapter represented a suffi-

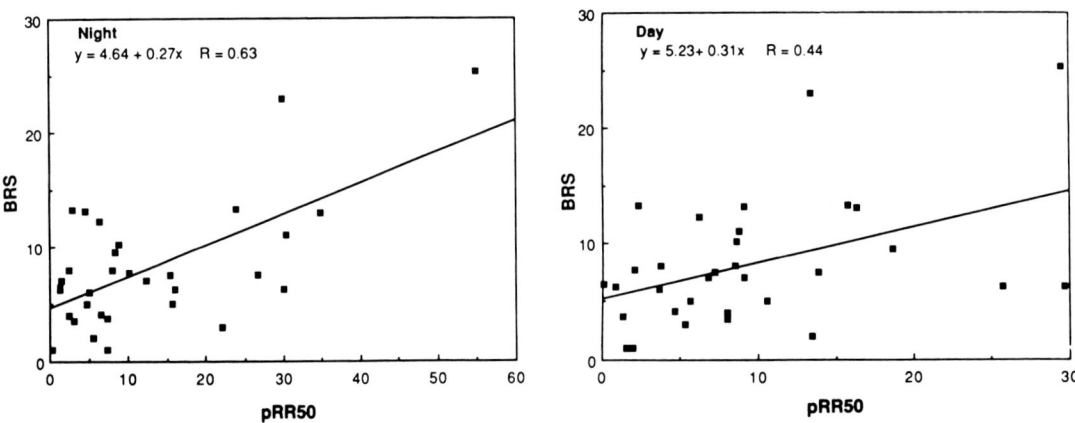

Fig. 6–20. Correlation between baroreflex sensitivity (BRS) in msec/mm Hg and the percent of successive normal R-R intervals differing by more than 50 msec (pRR50), plotted separately for day and night. (Reproduced with permission from Bigger JT Jr, et al: J Am Coll Cardiol 14:1511–1518, 1989.[61])

ciently strong rationale for the design of a large prospective study with the goal of acquiring definitive data on the predictive value in post-MI patients of various methodologies for the study of the autonomic neural control of the heart. ATRAMI (Autonomic Tone and Reflexes After Myocardial Infarction) is a multicenter prospective study that is targeted to involve 1200 patients with a recent MI, who will undergo analysis of BRS and heart rate variability, in addition to evaluation of the traditional clinical variables for risk stratification. The enrollment began in May 1991 and is taking place in over 25 centers in Europe, the United States, and Japan. Regardless of its final results, the mere existence of ATRAMI constitutes a significant clinical evolution of concepts that originated entirely in experimental studies.

REFERENCES

1. Schwartz PJ, Brown AM, Malliani A, Zanchetti A (eds): Neural Mechanisms in Cardiac Arrhythmias. New York, Raven Press, 1978, 442 pp.
2. Lown B: Sudden cardiac death: The major challenge confronting contemporary cardiology. Am J Cardiol 43:313–320, 1979.
3. Corr PB, Yamada KA, Witkowski FX: Mechanisms controlling cardiac autonomic function and their relation to arrhythmogenesis. In Fozzard HA, Haber E, Jennings RB, Katz AM, Morgan HE (eds): The Heart and Cardiovascular System. Vol II. New York, Raven Press, 1986, pp 1343–1403.
4. Schwartz PJ, Stramba-Badiale M: Parasympathetic nervous system and cardiac arrhythmias. In Kulbertus HE, Frank G (eds): Neurocardiology. Mount Kisco, NY, Futura, 1988, pp 179–200.
5. Schwartz PJ, Priori SG: Sympathetic nervous system and cardiac arrhythmias. In Zipes DP, Jalife J (eds): Cardiac Electrophysiology: From Cell to Bedside. Philadelphia, WB Saunders, 1990, pp 330–343.
6. Schwartz PJ, Billman GE, Stone HL: Autonomic mechanisms in ventricular fibrillation induced by myocardial ischemia during exercise in dogs with a healed myocardial infarction: An experimental preparation for sudden cardiac death. Circulation 69:780–790, 1984.
7. Billman GE, Schwartz PJ, Gagnol JP, Stone HL: The cardiac response to submaximal exercise in dogs susceptible to sudden cardiac death. J Appl Physiol 59:890–897, 1985.
8. Malliani A, Schwartz PJ, Zanchetti A: A sympathetic reflex elicited by experimental coronary occlusion. Am J Physiol 217:703–709, 1969.
9. Thames MD, Klopfenstein HS, Abbound FM, Mark AL, Walker JL: Preferential distribution of inhibitory cardiac receptors with vagal afferents to the inferoposterior wall of the left ventricle activated during coronary occlusion in the dog. Circ Res 43:512–519, 1978.
10. Smyth HS, Sleight P, Pickering GW: Reflex regulation of arterial pressure during sleep in man. Circ Res 24:109–121, 1969.
11. Billman GE, Schwartz PJ, Stone HL: Baroreceptor reflex control of heart rate: A predictor of sudden cardiac death. Circulation 66:874–880, 1982.
12. Schwartz PJ, Vanoli E, Stramba-Badiale M, de Ferrari GM, Billman GE, Foreman RD: Autonomic mechanisms and sudden death: New insight from the analysis of baroreceptor reflexes in conscious dogs with and without a myocardial infarction. Circulation 78:969–973, 1988.
13. Schwartz PJ, Zaza A, Pala M, Locati E, Beria G, Zanchetti A: Baroreflex sensitivity and its evolution during the first year after a myocardial infarction. J Am Coll Cardiol 12:629–636, 1988.
14. Schwartz PJ, Zaza A, Grazi S, Lombardo M, Lotto A, Sbressa C, Zappa P: Effect of ventricular fibrillation complicating acute myocardial infarction on long term prognosis importance in the site of infarction. Am J Cardiol 56:384–389, 1985.
15. Schwartz PJ, Motolese M, Pollavini G, et al, and The Sudden Death Italian Prevention Group: Prevention of sudden cardiac death after a first myocardial infarction by pharmacological or surgical antiadrenergic interventions. J Cardiol Electrophysiol 3:2–16, 1992.
16. Lombardi F, Sandrone G, Pernpruner S, et al: Heart rate variability as an index of sympathovagal interaction after acute myocardial infarction. Am J Cardiol 60:1239–1245, 1987.
17. Bigger JT Jr, Fleiss JL, Rolnitzky LM, Steinman RC, Schneider WJ: Time course of recovery of heart period variability after myocardial infarction. J Am Coll Cardiol 18:1643–1649, 1991.
18. Bigger JT Jr, Fleiss JL, Rolnitzky LM, Steinman C: Frequency domain measures of heart period variability and death in chronic coronary heart disease (1 year after infarction). Circulation 86(suppl I):660, 1992.
19. Hull SS Jr, Adamson PB, Albert DE, Huang

MH: Periodic assessment of heart rate variability in dogs at high and low risk for sudden death after myocardial infarction. Circulation 80(suppl II):II-146, 1989.
20. LaRovere MT, Specchia G, Mortara A, Schwartz PJ: Baroreflex sensitivity, clinical correlates and cardiovascular mortality among patients with a first myocardial infarction: A prospective study. Circulation 78:816–824, 1988.
21. Farrell TG, Paul V, Cripps TR, et al: Baroreflex sensitivity and electrophysiological correlates in patients after acute myocardial infarction. Circulation 83:945–952, 1991.
22. Saul JP, Arai Y, Berger R, et al: Assessment of autonomic regulation in chronic congestive heart failure by heart rate spectral analysis. Am J Cardiol 61:1292–1299, 1988.
23. Farrell TG, Odemuyiwa O, Bashir Y, et al: Prognostic value of baroreflex sensitivity testing after acute myocardial infarction. Br Heart J 66:129–137, 1992.
24. Katona PG, Jih F: Respiratory sinus arrhythmia: Noninvasive measure of parasympathetic cardiac control. J Appl Physiol 39:801–805, 1975.
25. Ewing DJ: Cardiovascular reflexes and autonomic neuropathy. Clin Sci Mol Med 55:321–327, 1978.
26. Bond WC, Bohs C, Ebey J Jr, Wolf S: Rhythmic heart rate variability (sinus arrhythmia) related to stages of sleep. Conditional Reflex 8(2):98–107, 1973.
27. Wolf MM, Varigos GA, Hunt D, Sloman JG: Sinus arrhythmia in acute myocardial infarction. Med J Aust 15:52–53, 1978.
28. Ewing DJ, Neilson JMM, Travis P: New method for assessing cardiac parasympathetic activity using 24-hour electrocardiograms. Br Heart J 52:396–402, 1984.
29. Bigger JT Jr, Kleiger RE, Fleiss JL, Rolnitzky LM, Steinman RC, Miller JP, the Multicenter Post-Infarction Research Group: Components of heart rate variability measured during healing of acute myocardial infarction. Am J Cardiol 61:208–215, 1988.
30. Berger RD, Akselrod S, Gordon D, Cohen RJ: An efficient algorithm for spectral analysis of heart rate variability. IEEE Trans Biomed Eng 9:900–904, 1986.
31. Kay SM, Marple SL: Spectrum analysis: A modern perspective. Proc IEEE 69:1380–1419, 1981.
32. Pagani M, Lombardi F, Guzzetti S, et al: Power spectral analysis of heart rate and arterial pressure variabilities as a marker of sympatho-vagal interaction in man and conscious dog. Circ Res 59:178–193, 1986.
33. Malliani A, Pagani M, Lombardi F, Cerutti S: Cardiovascular neural regulation explored in the frequency domain. Circulation 84:482–492, 1991.
34. Kleiger RE, Miller JP, Bigger JT Jr, Moss AJ, the Multicenter Post-Infarction Research Group: Decreased heart rate variability and its association with increased mortality after acute myocardial infarction. Am J Cardiol 59:256–262, 1987.
35. Bigger JT Jr, Fleiss JL, Steinman RC, Rolnitzky LM, Kleiger RE, Rottman JN: Frequency domain measures of heart period variability and mortality after myocardial infarction. Circulation 85:164–171, 1992.
36. Hull SS, Evans AR, Vanoli E, et al: Heart rate variability before and after myocardial infarction in conscious dogs at high and low risk of sudden death. J Am Coll Cardiol 16:978–985, 1990.
37. Schwartz PJ, Pagani M, Lombardi F, Malliani A, Brown AM: A cardiocardiac sympatho-vagal reflex in the cat. Circ Res 32:215–220, 1973.
38. Malliani A, Recordati G, Schwartz PJ: Nervous activity of afferent cardiac sympathetic fibres with atrial and ventricular endings. J Physiol 229:457–469, 1973.
39. Gnecchi Ruscone T, Lombardi F, Malfatto G, Malliani A: Attenuation of baroreceptive mechanisms by cardiovascular sympathetic afferent fibers. Am J Physiol 253:H787–H791, 1987.
40. Cerati D, Schwartz PJ: Single cardiac vagal fiber activity, acute myocardial ischemia, and risk for sudden death. Circ Res 69:1389–1401, 1991.
41. Schwartz PJ: Manipulation of the autonomic nervous system in the prevention of sudden cardiac death. In Brugada P, Wellens HJJ (eds): Cardiac Arrhythmias: Where to Go From Here? Mount Kisco, NY, Futura, 1987, pp 741–765.
42. La Rovere MT, Mortara A, Capomolla S, Cobelli F, Schwartz PJ: Autonomic reflexes and beta blockade in post-MI patients [abstr]. Eur Heart J 11:267, 1991.
43. Billman GE, Schwartz PJ, Stone HL: The effects of daily exercise on susceptibility to sudden cardiac death. Circulation 69:1182–1189, 1984.
44. Hull SS, Vanoli E, Reynolds CM, Foreman RD, Verrier RL, Schwartz PJ: Effect of exercise training on autonomic balance and cardiac electrical stability in conscious dogs. Circulation 84(suppl II):267, 1991.
45. Matta RJ, Verrier RL, Lown B: Repetitive extrasystole as an index of vulnerability to ventricular fibrillation. Am J Physiol 230:1469–1473, 1976.
46. La Rovere MT, Mortara A, Cobelli F, Specchia G, Schwartz PJ: Baroreflex sensitivity

improvement after physical training in post myocardial infarction patients [abstr]. Eur Heart J 10:126, 1989.
47. Dibner-Dunlap ME, Eckberg DL, Magid NM, Cintron-Trevino NM: The long-term increase of baseline and reflexly augmented levels of human vagal-cardiac activity induced by scopolamine. Circulation 71: 797–804, 1985.
48. De Ferrari GM, Mantica M, Vanoli E, Hull SS Jr, Schwartz PJ: Scopolamine increases vagal tone and vagal reflexes in patients after myocardial infarction. J Am Coll Cardiol 22: 1327–1334, 1993.
49. Verrier RL, Lown B: Sympathetic-parasympathetic interactions and ventricular electrical stability. In Schwartz PJ, Brown AM, Malliani A, Zanchetti A (eds): Neural Mechanisms in Cardiac Arrhythmias. New York, Raven Press, 1978, pp 75–85.
50. Verrier RL: Neurochemical approaches to the prevention of ventricular fibrillation. Fed Proc 45:2191–2196, 1986.
51. Stramba-Badiale M, Vanoli E, De Ferrari GM, Cerati D, Foreman RD, Schwartz PJ: Sympathetic-parasympathetic interaction and accentuated antagonism in conscious dogs. Am J Physiol 260:H335–H340, 1991.
52. Vanoli E, De Ferrari GM, Stramba-Badiale M, Hull SS Jr, Foreman RD, Schwartz PJ: Vagal stimulation and prevention of sudden death in conscious dogs with a healed myocardial infarction. Circ Res 68:1471–1481, 1991.
53. Schwartz PJ, Vanoli E: Cardiac arrhythmias elicited by interaction between acute myocardial ischemia and sympathetic hyperactivity: A new experimental model for the study of antiarrhythmic drugs. J Cardiovasc Pharmacol 3:1251–1259, 1981.
54. Schwartz PJ, Vanoli E, Zaza A, Zuanetti G: The effect of antiarrhythmic drugs on life-threatening arrhythmias induced by the interaction between acute myocardial ischemia and sympathetic hyperactivity. Am Heart J 109:937–948, 1985.
55. Schwartz PJ, Priori SG, Vanoli E, Zaza A, Zuanetti G: Efficacy of diltiazem in two experimental feline models of sudden cardiac death. J Am Coll Cardiol 8:661–668, 1986.
56. Priori SG, Zuanetti G, Schwartz PJ: Ventricular fibrillation induced by the interaction between acute myocardial ischemia and sympathetic hyperactivity: Effect of nifedipine. Am Heart J 116:37–45, 1988.
57. De Ferrari GM, Salvati P, Grossoni M, Ukmar G, Vaga L, Patrono C, Schwartz PJ: Pharmacologic modulation of the autonomic nervous system in the prevention of sudden cardiac death. A study with propranolol, methacholine and oxotremorine in conscious dogs with a healed myocardial infarction. J Am Coll Cardiol 22:283–290, 1993.
58. De Ferrari GM, Vanoli E, Stramba-Badiale M, Hull SS Jr, Foreman RD, Schwartz PJ: Vagal reflexes and survival during acute myocardial ischemia in conscious dogs with healed myocardial infarction. Am J Physiol 261:H63–H69, 1991.
59. Kunze DL: Reflex discharge patterns of cardiac vagal efferent fibres. J Physiol 222: 1–15, 1972.
60. Minisi AJ, Thames MD: Effect of chronic myocardial infarction on vagal cardiopulmonary baroreflex. Circ Res 65:396–405, 1989.
61. Bigger JT Jr, La Rovere MT, Steinman RC, et al: Comparison of baroreflex sensitivity and heart period variability after myocardial infarction. J Am Coll Cardiol 14:1511–1518, 1989.
62. Pomeranz M, Macaulay RJB, Caudill MA, et al: Assessment of autonomic function in humans by heart rate spectral analysis. Am J Physiol 248:H151–H153, 1985.

7

Critical Mass Hypothesis in the Initiation and Sustenance of Ventricular Fibrillation

FRANCIS X. WITKOWSKI
PATRICIA A. PENKOSKE
KATHERINE M. KAVANAGH

This chapter provides an overview of the knowledge gathered from animal models of sudden cardiac death (SCD) regarding the hypothesis that a critical mass of ventricular tissue is necessary for the initiation and sustenance of ventricular fibrillation (VF), and its implications for ventricular defibrillation.

SCD kills approximately 400,000 people each year in North America alone. While coronary artery disease is the principal etiological factor, the majority of these deaths occur suddenly due to rhythms that ultimately degenerate to VF.[1] The only currently successful therapy for VF is electrical defibrillation. The development and application of clinically useful implantable cardioverter-defibrillators has been accelerated by the magnitude of the clinical problem, the catastrophic implications of therapeutic failure, the generic nature of electrical therapy, and frustration in finding pharmacological means of decreasing mortality.[2] The Cardiac Arrhythmia Suppression Trial results[3] have dramatically emphasized the potential hazards of antiarrhythmic therapy and how treatment of a known adverse prognostic factor may worsen rather than improve outcome. The clinical documentation of the dramatic efficacy of the implantable cardioverter-defibrillator has largely been based on historical control groups or projected sudden death rates based on number of appropriate shocks,[4-6] with controlled clinical trials under way to evaluate the effect of implantable cardioverter-defibrillator treatment on survival.[7]

CRITICAL MASS FOR VENTRICULAR FIBRILLATION

Ventricular and atrial fibrillation are inducible in all hearts but are sustained only in heart tissue masses beyond a certain minimal size. Furthermore, the induction and maintenance of these rhythm disturbances are intimately dependent on intrinsic myocardial properties such as conduction velocity, anatomical obstacles to propagation, refractory periods, and their inherent anisotropic inhomogeneities. It has been known for decades that in the heart of large mammal such as a human or a dog, VF rarely converts spontaneously. Wiggers commented in 1940 that in over 400 cases of VF in dogs, only a single spontaneous recovery had been observed.[8] Spontaneous termination of naturally occurring VF in humans is unusual, but rare case reports of self-termination of "paroxysmal VF" have been reported as causes of syncope in patients with chronic third-degree atrioventricular block,[9] as part of the prolonged QT syndrome,[10] and after acute myocardial infarction (MI).[11,12] Electrode catheter stud-

---

Research from the authors' laboratories was supported by grants from the Alberta Heritage Foundation for Medical Research and the Medical Research Council of Canada. It was performed duirng Dr. Witkowski's tenure as a Scholar of the Alberta Heritage Foundation for Medical Research.

ies in humans suggest that maintenance of VF induced by premature electrical stimulation depends on both the mass and the electrophysiological properties of fibrillating myocardium.[13]

The salient features of VF were clearly described over a century ago by MacWilliam[14] and include (1) the complexity of the movement, (2) its persistence, and (3) its rapidity. The description presented by Moe and Abildskov of fibrillating tissue,[15] termed the multiple wavelet theory of fibrillation, has been experimentally confirmed in the atria[16] where the fibrillating activity is essentially limited to two dimensions. Mapping of fibrillating ventricular tissue, with its significant third dimension, has proved more challenging.

VF is an aberration at the level of cellular electrical organization. Direct intracellular recordings of transmembrane alterations in fibrillating ventricular tissue have been significantly hampered by the requirement to use large muscle mass preparation, in which stable impalements are technically challenging. Early intracellular recordings in isolated in vitro guinea pig hearts, in which VF was induced with aconitine applied to the myocardial surface, revealed action potential durations shortened to approximately 70 msec at the beginning of VF from the original 200 msec.[17] Additionally, when two simultaneous intracellular recordings were attempted with insertions approximately 1 mm apart, an element of synchronism of action potentials was found to exist.[17] With increased distances (10 mm) between microelectrodes, less and less synchroism was present,[17] with similar findings reported for in situ dog hearts with electrically induced VF.[18] Mechanically stabilized intracellular microelectrode recordings during VF reveal that individual action potentials, though shortened and irregularly activated, maintain a remarkably normal morphology.[19] Additionally, these intracellular recordings have documented that action potential durations during VF are reduced to the 70–130 msec range, and that the resting membrane potential is depolarized to approximately -60 mV.[19] These observations have been interpreted to favor re-entry as the likely mechanism, with no evidence for pacemaker activity observed.

The perpetuation of the presumed multiple wandering wavelets in VF likely depends on the number of wavelets present, although no detailed ventricular mapping study to date has directly confirmed this hypothesis. Brief refractory periods, slow conduction velocity, and larger tissue mass all would facilitate the occurrence of multiple independent wavelets.[20] Similarly, refractoriness prolongation without alterations in conduction velocity should promote fibrillation termination. Experimental findings have been interpreted to support the need for a critical ventricular mass to maintain VF. Garrey reported that pieces of ventricular muscle with a surface area less than 4 cm^2 shaved from the surface of the fibrillating left ventricle stopped fibrillating immediately.[21] Additionally, he demonstrated that fibrillation spontaneously terminated within 15 seconds in an isolated right ventricular wall cut from a fibrillating dog's heart, whereas the thicker, free left ventricular wall or interventricular septum were capable of fibrillation sustenance. Similar studies have not been duplicated with detailed electrophysiological mapping to address the mechanism for these findings. The effects of chronic hypertrophy, ischemia, ventricular remodeling after MI, or scar would most likely enhance VF persistence.

Fibrillation is rarely seen spatially contained within islands of ventricular tissue but has been described in association with acute myocardial ischemia[22] and in the setting of chronic MI.[23] Presumably, if this fibrillating activity could functionally exit via a mass of tissue of sufficient dimension,[21] then VF would be initiated in the remainder of the ventricular myocardium. That VF can be readily induced through a re-entrant mechanism by a single extra stimulus was theoretically predicted by Winfree[24] and has subsequently been experimentally confirmed using three-dimensional mapping.[25] Accordingly, fibrillation appears to be regenerative in nature. When induced in a local region it has a tendency to initiate a similar disturbance in the remainder of the ventricular myocardium. What the exact dimensions are for the ventricular mass necessary for VF stability and how this mass may be affected by electrical or pharmacological interventions, the presence of scarring, etc. are yet to be determined. The critical mass for VF initiation is therefore a small fraction of the ventricular mass but enlarges considerably when one considers the requisite mass for VF sustenance.

VENTRICULAR DEFIBRILLATION AND THE CRITICAL MASS HYPOTHESIS

Studies addressing VF termination have principally involved pharmacological and electrical modes of defibrillation. The "critical mass hypothesis" for defibrillation[26] is an electrical extension of the original anatomical observations made by Garrey,[21] and extended through electropharmacological means by Zipes et al.[26] According to this theory, a sufficient volume of fibrillating ventricular myocardium must be electrophysiologically altered to render it incapable of sustaining VF. How the defibrillation shock alters the presumed multiple reentrant wavelets of VF is uncertain.[27] Utilizing simultaneously obtained directly coupled cardiac mapping of both the voltage gradient produced by the defibrillation shock as well as the underlying myocardial electrical activity, we have obtained further evidence supporting the critical mass hypothesis for defibrillation.[28] We have demonstrated that there exists a progression from significantly subthreshold shocks to shocks that completely terminate fibrillation. For markedly subthreshold shocks, multiple areas were found to be left fibrillating post shock, and VF resumed post shock initiated from these multiple sites. As one approached the defibrillation threshold, the fibrillating activity in greater volumes of ventricular myocardium was found to be terminated with resultant smaller areas left fibrillating. The locations of these residual fibrillating areas were found to coincide with regions in which the voltage gradient field produced by the shock was lowest. Near defibrillation threshold, if a single site was found to be fibrillating post shock, it could either go on to reinitiate global VF or not, depending on factors that appeared to be randomly distributed. These factors might include the geometry of the prior activation loops, fiber orientation, loading effects presented by the adjacent nonfibrillating ventricular muscle, and shock field direction.

Recent evidence using optically interrogated electrically paced ventricular myocardium suggests that a defibrillation shock excites a new action potential independent of the phase of the ongoing action potential it encounters.[29] This proposed interpretation would explain the observed alterations in repolarization and excitation recovery. Similar studies from arrays of optically interrogated sites during actual VF and defibrillation have not yet been reported but should prove most interesting.

An alternative explanation for the observed postdefibrillation electrophysiological alterations is the "upper limit of vulnerability" hypothesis.[25,30–33] In contrast to the critical mass hypothesis, the upper limit of vulnerability hypothesis of defibrillation suggests that a subthreshold shock eliminates all the areas of fibrillation in the myocardium; however, the shock itself induces a new episode of fibrillation, owing to the intersection of a critical shock strength with a critical degree of ventricular refractoriness. Thus, according to the upper limit of vulnerability hypothesis, a shock must be strong enough to exceed the critical or vulnerable shock strength which results in the reinduction of VF.

Both of these hypotheses, the critical mass and the upper limit of vulnerability, are subject to the difficulties inherent in defining true local activation from extracellular recording electrodes during VF with the consequential challenges at interpretation of what is truly a continuation of preshock activity.[34] The development of improved means of defining local activation during VF from extracellular recording electrodes would significantly improve the ability to elucidate a mechanistic interpretation for defibrillation.

REFERENCES

1. Eisenberg MS, Hallstrom A, Bergner L: Long-term survival after out-of-hospital cardiac arrest. N Engl J Med 306:1340, 1982.
2. Klein LS, Miles WM, Zipes DP: Antitachycardia devices: Realities and promises. J Am Coll Cardiol 18:1349, 1991.
3. The Cardiac Arrhythmia Suppression Trial (CAST) investigators: Preliminary report: Effect of encainide and flecainide on mortality in a randomized trial of arrhythmia

suppression after myocardial infarction. N Engl J Med 321:406, 1989.
4. Mirowski M: The automatic implantable cardioverter-defibrillator: An overview. J Am Coll Cardiol 6:461, 1985.
5. Echt DS, Armstrong K, Schmidt P, et al.: Clinical experience, compliance, and survival in 70 patients with the automatic implantable cardioverter/defibrillator. Circulation 71:289, 1985.
6. Tchou PJ, Kadri N, Anderson J, et al.: Automatic implantable cardioverter defibrillators and survival of patients with left ventricular dysfunction and malignant ventricular arrhythmias. Ann Intern Med 109:529, 1988.
7. Bigger JT: Future studies with the implantable cardioverter defibrillator. PACE 14(II): 883, 1991.
8. Wiggers CJ: The mechanism and nature of ventricular fibrillation. Am Heart J 20:399, 1940.
9. Jensen G, Sigurd B, Sandoe E: Adams-Stokes seizures due to ventricular tachydysrhythmias in patients with heart block: Prevalence and problems in management. Chest 67:43, 1975.
10. Wellens HJJ, Vermenlen A, Durrer D: Ventricular fibrillation occurring on arousal from sleep by auditory stimuli. Circulation 46:661, 1972.
11. Choquette G, Wasserman F, Lisker S, et al: Spontaneous reversion of ventricular fibrillation to normal sinus rhythm in a case of acute myocardial infarction. Am Heart J 51: 455, 1963.
12. Moskowitz RM, Schwartz AB: Spontaneous termination of prolonged ventricular fibrillation after acute myocardial infarction. Arch Intern Med 147:171, 1987.
13. Josephson ME, Spielman SR, Greenspan AM, et al: Mechanism of ventricular fibrillation in man. Am J Cardiol 44:623, 1979.
14. MacWilliam JA: Fibrillar contaction in the heart. J Physiology 8:296, 1887.
15. Moe GK, Abildskov JA: Atrial fibrillation as a self-sustaining arrhythmia independent of focal discharge. Am Heart J 58:59, 1959.
16. Allessie MA, Lammers WJEP, Bonke FIM, et al: Experimental evaluation of Moe's multiple wavelet hypothesis of atrial fibrillation. In Zipes DP, Jalife J (eds): Cardiac Electrophysiology and Arrhythmias. New York, Grune & Stratton, 1985, p 265.
17. Hogancamp CE, Kardesch M, Danforth WH, et al: Transmembrane electrical potentials in ventricular tachycardia and fibrillation. Am Heart J 57:214, 1959.
18. Sano T, Tsuchihasiii H, Shimamoto T: Ventricular fibrillation studied by the microelectrode method. Circ Res 51:41, 1958.
19. Akiyama T: Intracellular recording of in situ ventricular cells during ventricular fibrillation. Am J Physiol 240:H465, 1981.
20. Zipes DP: Electrophysiological mechanisms involved in ventricular fibrillation. Circulation 51, 52(III):120, 1975.
21. Garrey WE: The nature of fibrillary contraction of the heart: Its relation to tissue mass and form. Am J Physiol 33:397, 1914.
22. Waldo AL, Kaiser GA: A study of ventricular arrhythmias associated with acute myocardial infarction in the canine heart. Circulation 47:1222, 1973.
23. Durrer D, Van Dam RTh, Freud GE, et al: Re-entry and ventricular arrhythmias in local ischemia and infarction of the intact dog heart. Proc Kon Ned Akad Wetensch [C] 74:321–334, 1971.
24. Winfree AT: When Time Breaks Down. Princeton, NJ, Princeton University Press, 1987, p 125.
25. Chen P-S, Wolf PD, Dixon EG, et al: Mechanism of ventricular vulnerability to single premature stimuli in open-chest dogs. Circ Res 62:1191, 1988.
26. Zipes DP, Fischer J, King RM, et al: Termination of ventricular fibrillation in dogs by depolarizing a critical amount of myocardium. Am J Cardiol 36:37, 1975.
27. Witkowski FX, Penkoske PA: Refractoriness prolongation by defibrillation shocks. Circulation 82:1064, 1990.
28. Witkowski FX, Penkoske PA, Plonsey R: Mechanism of cardiac defibrillation in open-chest dogs with unipolar DC-coupled simultaneous activation and shock potential recordings. Circulation 82:244, 1990.
29. Dillon SM: Optical recordings in the rabbit heart show that defibrillation strength shocks prolong the duration of depolarization and the refractory period. Circ Res 69: 842, 1991.
30. Chen P-S, Shibata N, Dixon EG, et al: Activation during ventricular defibrillation in open-chest dogs: Evidence of complete cessation and regeneration of ventricular fibrillation after unsuccessful shocks. J Clin Invest 77:810, 1986.
31. Chen P-S, Shibata N, Dixon EG, et al: Comparison of the defibrillation threshold and the upper limit of ventricular vulnerability. Circulation 73:1022, 1986.
32. Shibata N, Chen P-S, Dixon EG, et al: Epicardial activation after unsuccessful defibrillation shocks in dogs. Am J Physiol 255: H902, 1988.
33. Chen PS, Shibata N, Dixon EG, et al: Comparison of activation during ventricular fibrillation and following unsuccessful defibrillation shocks in open-chest dogs. Circ Res 82:244, 1990.
34. Chen PS, Wolf PD, Ideker RE: Mechanism of cardiac defibrillation: A different point of view. Circulation 84(2):913, 1991.

8

Myocardial Activation at the Onset of and During Ventricular Fibrillation

SUSAN M. BLANCHARD
ERIC E. JOHNSON
RAYMOND E. IDEKER

Until recently, the technical problems of recording simultaneously from many electrodes made studies of the onset and maintenance of ventricular fibrillation (VF) difficult. With advances in digital hardware,[1] electrode construction,[2] and identification of activation during VF,[3] it is now possible to use hundreds of electrodes placed directly on and in the ventricles to map activation sequences during the transition from ventricular tachycardia (VT) as well as during VF. In the past decade, the basic mechanisms responsible for the initiation and continuance of VF have been shown to include both re-entrant and nonre-entrant mechanisms. Even with recent improvements in mapping techniques, there are still many unanswered basic questions concerning the exact mechanisms and location of the critical electrophysiological events that are responsible for VF. Cardiac mapping represents an important tool because it can be used to pinpoint the site of origin for a particular fibrillatory event. Once the arrhythmogenic site has been identified, other techniques such as biochemical analysis, identification of receptor levels, and determination of refractory periods can be focused on the area to provide additional information.

MYOCARDIAL ACTIVATION AT THE ONSET OF VENTRICULAR FIBRILLATION

Induction by Ischemia

Janse et al[4] studied the flow of injury current and the patterns of excitation during early ventricular arrhythmias in acute regional myocardial ischemia by simultaneously recording electrograms from 60 extracellular epicardial and intramural sites of the left ventricle of isolated porcine and canine hearts during the first 15 minutes after occlusion and subsequent reperfusion of the left anterior descending artery. Fragmentation of wave fronts occurred during VF, and multiple wandering wavelets were seen following tortuous paths on the epicardial surface. Circus movements were seldom complete and had small diameters (0.5 cm) when they were. These data suggested that two mechanisms were responsible for the arrhythmias in early ischemia: (1) a "focal" mechanism located at the normal side of the ischemic border, possibly induced by injury currents, and (2) re-entry in the ischemic myocardium. However, a definitive assessment of the underlying mechanism could not be made since mapping was limited to only a portion of the ventricles.

Supported in part by National Institutes of Health research grants HL-42760, HL-44066, HL-28429, HL-33637, and HL-41168, and by National Science Foundation Engineering Research Center grant CDR-8622201.

Ideker et al[5] recorded from 27 epicardial electrodes spaced over both ventricles of the canine heart and demonstrated a period of organized epicardial activation during the transition to VF that was induced by a 15-minute occlusion of the proximal circumflex artery followed by reperfusion. The first 1.5–2.5 seconds of the transition from sinus rhythm or VT to VF were analyzed and revealed that ventricular activation occurred in an orderly, rapidly repeating sequence in all hearts. In each case, the cycle of activation broke through to the epicardium near the border of the ischemic-reperfused region and passed across the nonischemic portion of the ventricles to the opposite side of the heart as a single organized wave front. The decreasing time between successive activations indicated that the rate increased during the onset of fibrillation, while the decreasing distance between isochrones indicated that the duration of each cycle increased concurrently, owing to slowing conduction. As the conduction velocity slowed and the rate of activation increased, less time elapsed between the end of one cycle of activation and the start of the next. The duration of each activation cycle soon grew longer than the interval between epicardial breakthroughs for consecutive cycles. When this occurred, the next activation front would break through to the epicardium in the ischemic-reperfused region before the previous activation front had terminated over the right ventricle. The overlap continued to increase during subsequent cycles and resulted in as many as three successive activation fronts being present on the epicardium simultaneously.[6] This is clearly demonstrated in Figure 8–1, which shows that the 13th cycle in the transition from VT to fibrillation began before cycle 12 terminated and ended after cycle 14 began. The overall duration of the 13th cycle over the entire heart was much longer than the time between cycles 12 and 13 or between cycles 13 and 14 at any given electrode site. Even though the body surface electrocardiogram appeared disorganized during this transition period, the experimental results demonstrated that there was actually organization and periodicity in the underlying cardiac activation sequence. The actual mechanism by which activation was initiated during the transition to fibrillation could not be determined because of the limited number of electrodes, the wide spacing between the epicardial electrodes, and the lack of intramyocardial and subendocardial electrodes.

In a series of experiments by Pogwizd and Corr,[7] the electrophysiological mechanisms responsible for malignant ventricular arrhythmias associated with reperfusion of ischemic myocardium were further delineated by using a computerized three-dimensional mapping system to simultaneously record from 232 bipolar sites at eight transmural levels located throughout the feline heart. In six cats, 10 minutes of occlusion of the left anterior descending coronary artery were followed by reperfusion to induce regional ischemia. Total ventricular activation time during sinus rhythm was significantly delayed just before reperfusion. VT occurred within 15 seconds after reperfusion in all six animals and progressed to VF in three. Initial activation occurred at the border of the reperfused zone in the subendocardium in 75% of cases of nonsustained VT and did not involve re-entry. The nonre-entrant nature of the arrhythmia was demonstrated by the lack of continuous activity and the failure to find any association between intervening depolarizations and the time from the end of the sinus beat to the beginning of the VT. The remaining 25% of cases of nonsustained VT were initiated when delayed midmyocardial activation from the preceding sinus beat re-entered the adjacent subendocardium. These re-entrant tachycardias were characterized by a marked prolongation in activation of the preceding sinus beat. This delay was comparable to that produced during early ischemia without reperfusion and resulted in continuous activation which initiated the first beat of the tachycardia in the subendocardium.

VT leading to VF was most commonly initiated in the subendocardium at the border of the reperfused zone by a nonre-entrant mechanism, although intramural re-entry contributed in some cases, and was maintained by both nonre-entrant and re-entrant mechanisms that sometimes occurred in the same beat. Nonre-entrant mechanisms arose from both the subendocardium and subepicardium, led to a very rapid acceleration of the tachycardia during

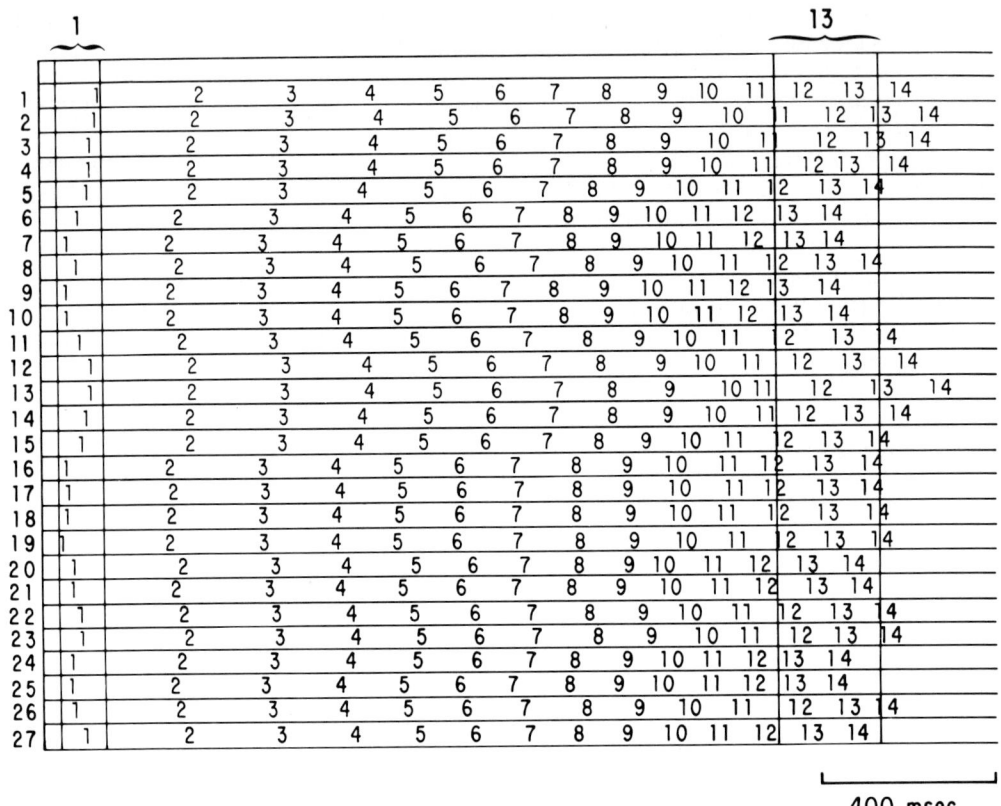

Fig. 8–1. Overlapping cycles during the transition to ventricular fibrillation. Electrodes are numbered along the ordinate; the abscissa represents time. The times at which local activation occurred for each electrode are numbered consecutively. The time between activation fronts at an individual electrode site decreased as time progressed (e.g., the time between cycles 1 and 2 versus the time between cycles 13 and 14 at any electrode) while the time within an individual cycle throughout the heart increased (e.g., the duration of cycle 1 versus the duration of cycle 13 for all electrodes). Thus, activation occurred in repeating, overlapping cycles. (Reprinted by permission of the American Heart Association, from Ideker RE, et al: The transition to ventricular fibrillation induced by reperfusion following acute ischemia in the dog: A period of organized epicardial activation. Circulation 63:1371, 1981.)

the transition from VT to VF, and resulted in enhanced functional block and further conduction delays. During nonre-entrant tachycardia, the total activation time of the transition beats exceeded the coupling interval and resulted in overlapping cycles of activation. The nature of this nonre-entrant excitation remains unexplained but may involve an abnormal form of automaticity or triggered activity.

The mechanisms underlying the development of VF during early myocardial ischemia without reperfusion were also examined by Pogwizd and Corr.[8] In four of 15 animals studied with the previously described mapping system, occlusion of the proximal left anterior descending coronary artery led to VT that degenerated into VF in 1–5 minutes. Intramural re-entry involving multiple activation sites in and around the border region of the ischemic zone was the primary factor in maintaining the VT that led to VF in three of four animals. In the fourth animal the initiating mechanism could not be determined. Nonre-entrant mechanisms that arose in the subendocardium and subepicardium also contributed to the maintenance of VT. However, intramural re-entry with initiation of re-entrant beats occurring in the subendocardium and occasionally the subepicardium was exclusively responsible for the transition from VT to VF. During intramural re-entry, increased functional block and conduction delay as well as very rapid and inhomogeneous recovery of excitability resulted from acceleration of the tachycardia. Thus, the total activation time for a given beat exceeded the coupling interval for that beat.

The mechanism underlying the transition from VT to VF during ischemia differs from the mechanism operating during subsequent reperfusion. After reperfusion, the transition to VF is due to acceleration by non-re-entrant mechanisms that arise in both the subendocardium and subepicardium, whereas nonre-entrant mechanisms were not observed to contribute to acceleration of the tachycardia in cases involving ischemia without reperfusion. Once acceleration of the tachycardia occurred, subsequent development of VF was similar during ischemia and reperfusion.

Induction by Electrical Stimulus

A large electrical stimulus delivered prematurely during the vulnerable period of the cardiac cycle can give rise to VF. This procedure was thought to result in an activation front that propagates away from the site of stimulation in all directions and then blocks unidirectionally when it reaches regions that have not yet recovered excitability.[9] In this theory, re-entry results from the nonuniform dispersion of refractoriness that occurs when one site remains refractory long after an adjacent site has recovered. In these cases, activation continues to propagate through the adjacent regions that are more recovered and later circles back to excite the formerly blocked regions following their recovery. These later activation fronts then propagate back into the tissue that was immediately excited after the premature stimulus, causing re-entry and VF (Fig. 8–2). Although nonuniform dispersion of recovery or refractoriness probably plays a role in the mechanism of the initiation of VF during ischemia, investigators from Duke University[10–12] have demonstrated that it is not a requirement for the electrical stimulation of fibrillation during the vulnerable period. VF can still be induced in some cases of uniformly distributed refractoriness in which refractoriness changes approximately the same amount over a given distance throughout the region.

In a study of 14 dogs by Frazier et al,[10] recordings were made simultaneously from 117 epicardial electrodes in a 30 × 30-mm region of the anterior right ventricle. Uniform, parallel activation fronts were created by giving a train of ten regularly spaced S1 stimuli simultaneously through a row of eight pacing wires on one side of the mapped region. Refractory periods were determined at 24 to 44 different sites after the tenth S1. These periods were found to be similar at all sites, indicating that recovery was dispersed uniformly across the mapped region. The earliest recovery occurred near the row of S1 pacing electrodes (Fig. 8–3). After it was verified that both activation isochrones and isorecovery lines were uniform and parallel, the recovery period was scanned using 25–250-V monophasic S2 shocks that were given prematurely following the tenth S1 through a mesh electrode that spanned one side of the mapped area. This side of the mapped region was adjacent to and at a right angle to the side at which the S1 shock was delivered so that the potential gradient electrical field of the S2 shock, which indicates how rapidly the extracellular potential changes with distance, was perpendicular to the isorecovery lines. The potential gradient is usually estimated in the heart by recording potentials from electrodes spaced known distances apart and then dividing the difference in potential at adjacent electrodes by the distance between them. The potential at a site must always be measured with respect to some reference potential and will differ for different reference potentials; however, the potential difference between two myocardial electrodes will be the same no matter where the reference electrode is placed. The potential gradient at each point is a vector quantity, since the potential at a site can change at different rates in different directions away from the site. Isogradient lines were found to be parallel with highest gradients near the S2 mesh electrode.

Re-entrant activation leading to VF was induced by the S2 shock at some coupling intervals in all animals. Circus re-entry in a leading circle activation pattern was created by the shock (Fig. 8-4). Earliest activation

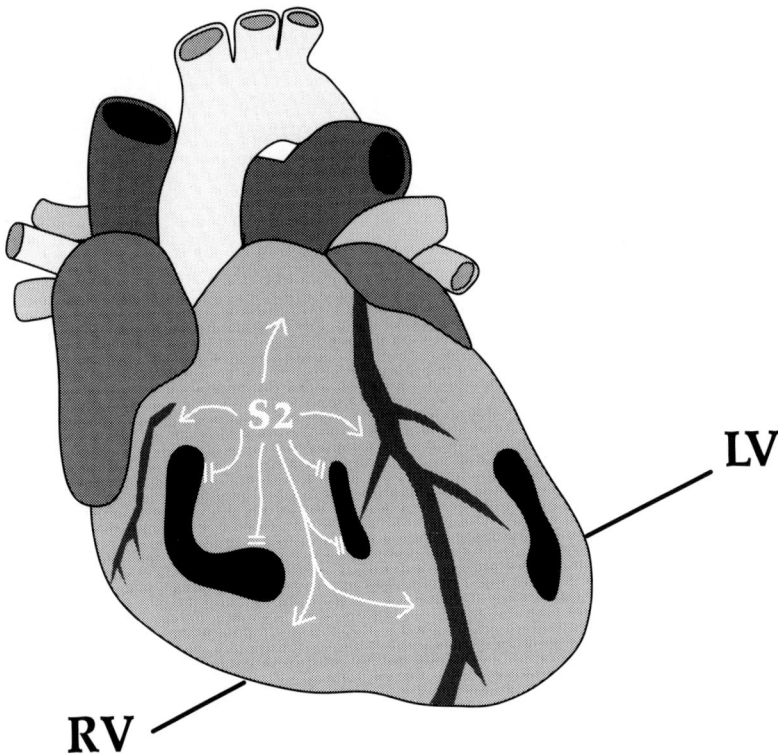

Fig. 8–2. Nonuniform dispersion of refractoriness and re-entry. Refractoriness or recovery is dispersed nonuniformly when it changes at different rates in different places and changes rapidly over a small distance. In this case, one site remains refractory long after an adjacent site has recovered. As shown in the figure, an activation front is thought to propagate away in all directions from the site of stimulation when an electrical stimulus is delivered prematurely during the vulnerable period. The activation front blocks unidirectionally when it reaches regions that have not yet recovered excitability and continues to propagate through adjacent regions that are more recovered. Later, the activation front circles back to excite the blocked regions that have since had time to recover. These later activation fronts may cause re-entry and ventricular fibrillation by propagating into the tissue that was excited soon after the premature stimulus and has had time to recover. (Reprinted by permission of Elsevier Science Publishing Co, Inc, from Johnson EE, Ideker RE: Ventricular fibrillation: Update. In Fisch C, Surawicz B (eds): Cardiac Electrophysiology and Arrhythmias. New York, 1991.)

after the shock occurred at the opposite side of the mapped region from the S2 electrode and at the edge of the directly excited regions, not in the region adjacent to the mesh S2 electrode, where the shock field was the greatest. The "critical point" about which re-entry was created was that point at which critical values of the S2 field strength and the refractoriness intersected. The critical point of the shock potential gradient field averaged approximately 5 V/cm. This was the area at which conduction propagated away from the directly excited border, where potential gradients were weaker, and did not conduct away from the border, where gradients were stronger. Activation circled around this point to form a circus re-entrant pattern. Re-entry was clockwise when the row of S1 electrodes was at the right and the S2 mesh electrode was at the top of the mapped region, and when the S1 electrodes were at the left and the S2 mesh electrode was at the bottom of the mapped region. In the latter case, a spatial shift of 180 degrees in phase occurred. Re-entry was counterclockwise when the row of S1 electrodes were at the right and the S2 electrode was at the bottom, and when the S1 electrodes were at the left and the S2 electrode was at the top of the mapped region

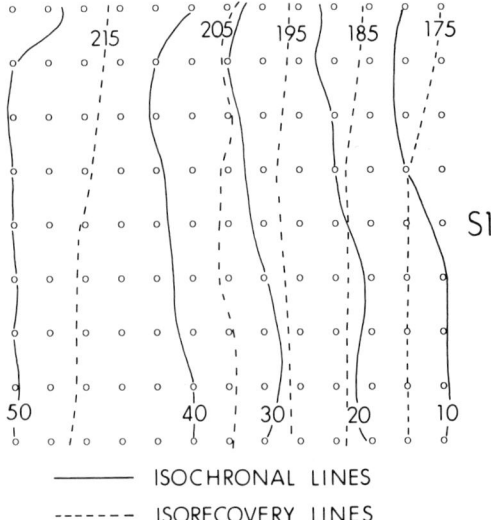

Fig. 8-3. S1 activation and isorecovery patterns. Eight epicardial pacing wires were tied together as a single source (S1) and pulsed at 10 mA. Approximately parallel isochronal lines (solid lines) resulted from this S1 pacing. Conduction velocities between the isochrones were 0.5 to 0.7 m/sec. In this example, recovery periods (dashed lines) were calculated at 32 electrode sites evenly spaced across the array. Refractoriness was essentially homogeneous, as indicated by the similar refractory periods at all electrode sites (166 ± 3 msec). The mean epicardial fiber orientation under this array was 24 ± 5 degrees with respect to the horizontal. (Reprinted by permission of the American Society for Clinical Investigation, Inc, from Frazier et al: Stimulus-induced critical point: Mechanism for electrical initiation of reentry in normal canine myocardium. J Clin Invest 83:1039, 1989.)

(Fig. 8–5), but it was also shifted spatially 180 degrees in phase. The location of the rotor could be moved predictably by changing either the strength or the timing of the S2.

Thus, the initiation and location of reentry were functions of the interaction of refractoriness with the strength of the shock field and not just a function of intrinsic differences in refractoriness throughout the mapped region. Conduction block which led to re-entry and VF was caused by the interaction of a uniformly dispersed change in refractoriness, forming a critical point around which activation fronts rotated. Contrary to predictions based on the nonuniform dispersion of recovery hypothesis, re-entry was not caused by an activation front that conducted away from the S2 electrode in all directions and later blocked in a region where there was a large change in refractoriness. Thus, nonuniform dispersion of refractoriness was not the mechanism for the electrical induction of VF in this study. This does not mean that nonuniform dispersion of refractoriness may not be the mechanism for the VF that occurs naturally in cases of acute ischemia or for VF induced by low-voltage stimuli or by S1 and S2 stimuli given from the same site.

In a study by Chen et al,[11] an array of 40 plunge needles was used for transmural recording after delivery of S1 and S2 stimuli from point sources 1 cm apart in the right ventricular outflow tract of seven dogs. The S2 stimulus was given at the center of the needle array following an S1 stimulus that was given just to the left of the mapped area. Earliest activation following the S2 stimulus occurred at a site between the S1 and S2 stimulation sites and not at the site of S2 stimulation. Activation fronts formed a figure-of-eight re-entrant pattern by spreading toward the S1 site where the tissue was more recovered after circling around both sides of an arc of block near the S2 site. The area around the S2 site was excited last, and if the difference in times between the adjacent early site and the S2 site was large, the front re-entered the tissue toward the S1 site (Fig. 8–6). When two areas with the critical level of potential gradient (one "above" and the other "below" the S2 site) were present, a pair of mirror image rotors was induced and figure-of-eight re-entry was initiated.

The critical point theory predicts that increasing the S2 strength should move the two critical points away from the S2 site and also farther apart, since the critical level of potential gradient will occur at a greater distance from the S2 electrode. This prediction was tested in a third study on seven dogs,[12] in which the S1 stimulus was delivered to the base of either the right or left ventricle and the S2 stimulus was delivered through defibrillation electrodes on the left ventricular apex and right atrium. Two mirror image rotors of re-entry were created on opposite sides of the ventricles, presumably where two critical points existed as a result of the large premature S2 shock.

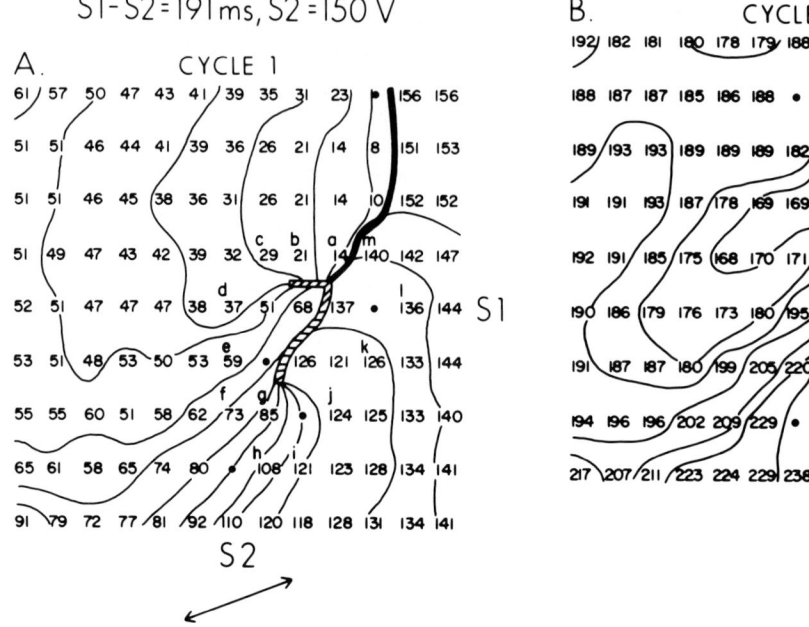

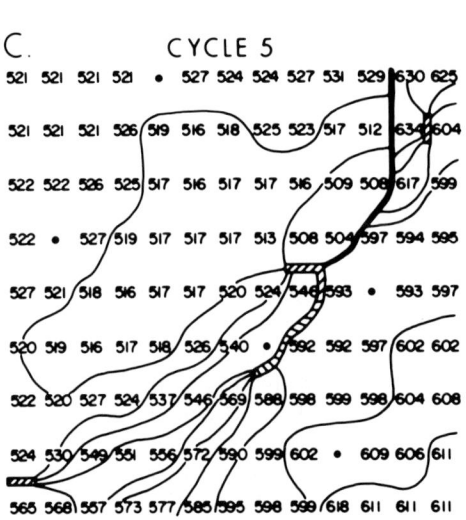

Fig. 8–4. Activation patterns for perpendicular isorefractory and isogradient lines. The patterns of activation following S1 pacing from the right and S2 shock from the bottom are shown in **A** (cycle 1), **B** (cycle 2), and **C** (cycle 5). Activation times, shown in milliseconds, are measured from the start of the 3-msec S2 shock. Solid dots represent sites of inadequate recordings. The solid line represents the transition between successive activation maps and is called a "frame line." It is required because each static isochronal map can show only a single cycle of a continuous dynamic re-entrant circuit. The hatched line represents a zone of conduction block and is called a "block line." Isochrones are at 10-msec intervals. The double-headed arrow for this figure represents the mean epicardial fiber orientation in the area of conduction block, in this case 21 degrees with respect to the horizontal. **A.** The initial activation pattern following the S2 shock at an S1–S2 interval of 191 msec and an S2 strength of 150 V. Earliest postshock activation occurs distant from the S2 site, with no early activation wave fronts conducting away from the region located between the S2 site and the critical point, i.e., the point where the activation front blindly ends at the junction between the frame line and the block line. A counterclockwise re-entrant circuit is formed around the region containing the critical point and the line of block. The potential gradient equals 5.8 V/cm and the preshock interval equals 171 msec at the critical point (critical refractory period = 169 msec). **B.** The second cycle of the re-entrant pattern. No slow conduction occurs at the frame line between the first and second re-entrant cycles. The activation pattern is similar to the first cycle except that the time to complete the circuit is decreased to 122 msec. **C.** The fifty cycle of the re-entrant pattern. The re-entrant pattern is similar to the previous cycles, but the total circuit time has further decreased to 101 msec. (Reprinted by permission of the American Society for Clinical Investigation, Inc, from Frazier et al: Stimulus-induced critical point: Mechanism for electrical initiation of reentry in normal canine myocardium. J Clin Invest *83*:1039, 1989.)

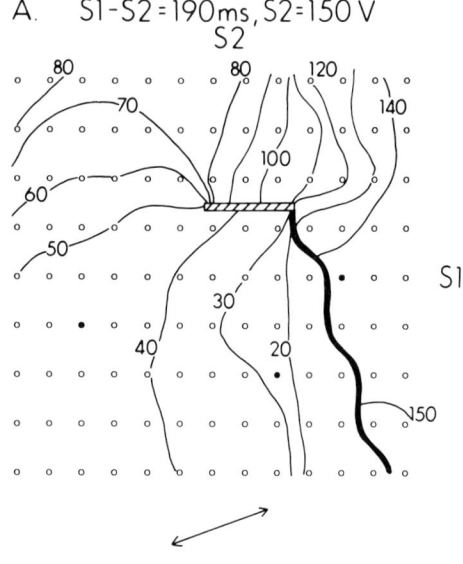

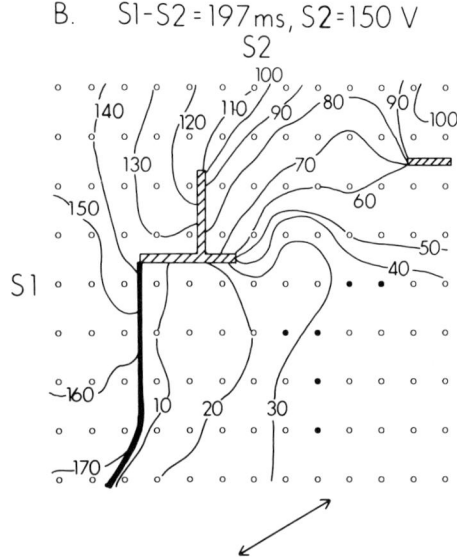

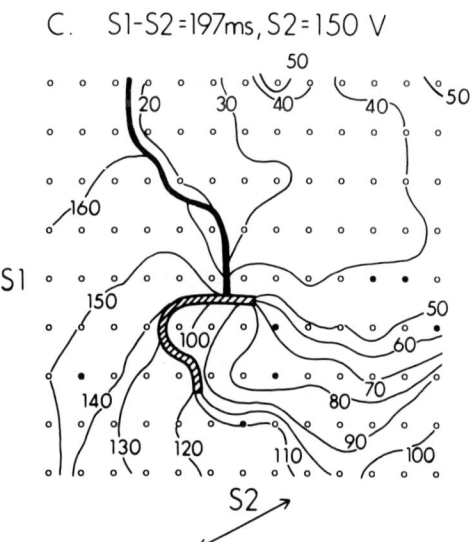

Fig. 8–5. Effect of locations of S1 and S2 on direction of re-entrant circuits. **A.** The first cycle of re-entry following a 150-V S2 at an S1–S2 interval of 190 msec is shown with S2 at the top and S1 toward the septum. Earliest activation occurred distant from the S2 site, with activation wave fronts experiencing slow conduction near the S2 site and conducting in a clockwise manner around a line of block (as compared to the counterclockwise circuit in Figure 8–4A, which resulted from having S2 at the bottom). In addition, the re-entrant circuits in Figures 8–4A and 8–5A differ in phase by approximately 180 degrees, with earliest activation occurring at the top of the array when S2 was at the bottom (Fig. 8–4A) and at the bottom of the array when S2 was at the top (Fig. 8–5A). The potential gradient was 5.4 V/cm and the preshock interval was 172 msec (critical refractory period = 168 msec) at the critical point. In Figure 8–5B and C, as in Figure 8–4A, earliest activation occurred distant from the S2 site with activation fronts forming a re-entrant circuit by conducting around a line of block and through a region of slow conduction near the S2 site. In Figure 8–5B (S2 = 150 V, S1–S2 = 197 msec) with S2 at the top and S1 at the side near the right ventricle, a counterclockwise re-entrant circuit was formed, as in Figure 8–4A (septal S1 with bottom S2). The two re-entrant patterns differ in phase by approximately 180 degrees. The potential gradient was 5.2 V/cm and the preshock interval was 173 msec (critical refractory period = 171 msec) at the critical point. In Figure 8–5C (S2 = 150 V, S1–S2 = 197 msec), with S2 at the bottom and S1 at the side near the right ventricle, a clockwise re-entrant circuit was formed, as in Figure 8–5A (septal S1 with top S2). These two re-entrant patterns also differ in phase by approximately 180 degrees. The potential gradient was 5.9 V/cm and the preshock interval was 169 msec (critical refractory period = 170 msec) at the critical point. (Reprinted by permission of the American Society for Clinical Investigation, Inc, from Frazier et al: Stimulus-induced critical point: Mechanism for electrical initiation of reentry in normal canine myocardium. J Clin Invest 83:1039, 1989.)

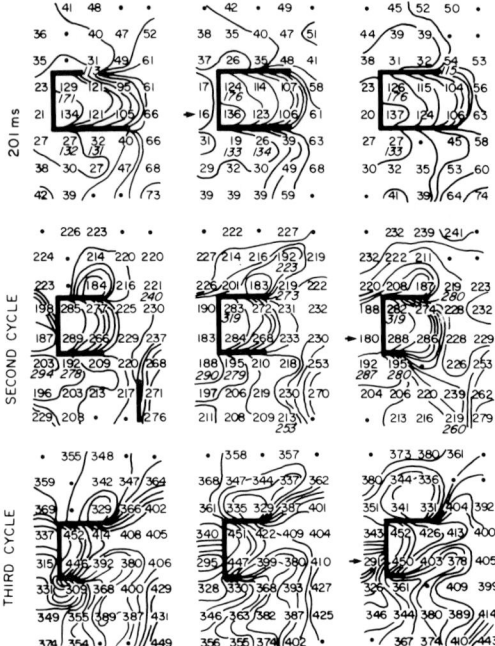

Fig. 8–6. Figure-of-eight re-entry at the onset of ventricular fibrillation. The three maps from left to right in each panel represent the subendocardial, midmyocardial, and subepicardial layers of recording electrodes. The top panel shows activation times for the first cycle following a 5-msec S2 of 50 mA which was given prematurely with a coupling interval of 201 msec and was delivered to the endocardium from a point electrode at the center of the recording array. Activation times for the next two cycles of ventricular fibrillation are shown in the lower two panels. Each number gives the activation time at an electrode site in milliseconds after the S2 stimulus. S1 stimuli were delivered to the endocardium from a point electrode at the left side of the array. Small closed circles represent bad recording electrodes. The heavy black bar in the center of the mapped region represents the frame line. The small arrows indicate the earliest recorded site of activation for each cycle. (Reprinted by permission of the American Heart Association, from Chen et al: Mechanism of ventricular vulnerability to single premature stimuli in open-chest dogs. Circ Res 62:1191, 1988.)

In all three studies, a region directly excited by the S2 field was present, and the border of this directly excited region was dependent on both the strength of the S2 field and the stage of refractoriness of the cells. When the S2 potential gradient was weak (less than approximately 5 V/cm for 3-msec square monophasic waveforms), the border of the directly excited region was in cells that were only mildly refractory. In these cases, an activation front conducted away from this border through the tissue that was not directly excited by the S2 field. When the S2 potential gradient was greater than 5 V/cm, myocardium that was even more refractory was directly excited. In these cases, a zone of temporary unidirectional block was created when activation fronts failed to conduct away from the border of the directly excited region. This block may have resulted from prolongation of refractoriness by the electrical field of the S2 stimulus.[13] The situation in which activation spread away from one portion of the directly excited region but not another after S2 stimulation created an activation front that ended blindly in the tissue and led to re-entry and VF. Whether re-entry was leading-circle or figure-of-eight depended on the location of the S1 and S2 sites and the spatial relationship of the S2 isogradient field to the distribution of refractoriness. The different shape and intersections of the isogradient and isorefractory lines could be used to predict the type of re-entrant pattern.[14,15]

MYOCARDIAL ACTIVATION DURING VENTRICULAR FIBRILLATION

Whether it is initiated by a re-entrant or a nonre-entrant mechanism, VF is thought to be maintained by multiple, disorganized, wandering wavelets that follow constantly changing re-entrant pathways. Several pieces of evidence support the hypothesis that only a small number of wavelets is present during the first minute. Based on cinematographic studies, Wiggers[16] stated that incoordination and asynchronism first involved comparatively large sections of myocardium and that VF could not be adequately described as asynchronous contraction of individual myocardial fibers. Over the first 5 minutes of VF, these large sections progressively decreased in size and increased in number. Garrey[17] dissected the heart into pieces of various sizes and showed that a critical mass of myocardium must be present for VF to persist. The critical mass in dogs is about one fourth of the total ventricular mass. VF is frequently difficult to induce in smaller hearts, such as in frogs, and can be sustained only in larger hearts, such as in humans and dogs.[16] Frequency analysis of VF in humans and dogs has resulted in a power spectrum with a well-defined peak and its higher harmonics, which suggests some degree of organized activation.[18] This evidence, which has been recognized for decades, suggests that VF is sufficiently organized that it could be mapped with closely spaced electrodes if the electrodes do not cause excessive damage to the tissue.[9]

Multiple Wandering Wavelets

Based on the previous work of Garrey[17] and Mines[19] and a series of astute observations, Moe[20] revived the theory of re-entry as a mechanism for fibrillation and developed the well-known multiple wandering wavelet hypothesis. Simultaneous multichannel recordings from a large number of electrodes could not be made from the heart at the time Moe developed his theory, so he and his colleagues tested his hypothesis by developing a mathematical computer model in which the heart was represented as an electrophysiologically inhomogeneous two-dimensional sheet of hexagonal cells.[21] Using this model, they were able to demonstrate multiple wandering wavelets that exhibited self-sustained turbulent activity that resembled fibrillation. The studies using the computer model strengthened the probability that the multiple wavelet hypothesis represented a mechanism for fibrillation in the heart.

In 1964, Sano and Scher[22] were among the first to use cardiac mapping techniques to study fibrillation in vivo. They placed 36 bipolar electrodes on the intact dog atria and induced atrial fibrillation (AF) by giving single electrical shocks. An average of 20 electrograms was successfully recorded at the onset of fibrillation and during recovery. Based on these studies, they proposed that ectopic impulse formation was the initiating mechanism for AF but that re-entry was probably the mechanism responsible for its maintenance.

Allessie et al[23] confirmed Moe's multiple wavelet theory as a basis of AF in a series of in vivo experiments using isolated Langendorff-perfused canine hearts. Two solid egg-shaped multiple electrodes, each containing 480 electrodes, were used to reconstruct excitation of the atria during stable atrial fibrillation. One multiple electrode was placed in the right atrium and the other in the left. During one episode of AF the right atrium would be mapped, with the left atrium mapped during a second episode of fibrillation that would be initiated a couple of minutes later. They demonstrated that multiple wandering wavelets due to intra-atrial re-entry of the leading-circle type provided the basis for the continuity of impulse conduction during fibrillation.[24] Activation patterns in one atrium that appeared to be "foci" of new impulses were interpreted to be endocardial breakthrough sites of impulses coming from the other atrium. They did note that it was possible that the presence of a normal or abnormal pacemaker might sometimes succeed in supporting the continuation of multiple wandering wavelets and might actually be necessary for the perpetuation of AF. If the simultaneous extinction of all activation fronts occurred by chance, then the generation of an impulse either by the sinus node or by some abnormal pacemaker shortly after cancellation of the fibrillatory wavelets would almost certainly restart the arrhythmia. Thus, it is possible that multiple rapidly firing ectopic foci and multiple re-entry may act together in maintaining chronic AF.[23]

Degree of Organization

Some evidence exists that suggests that VF, at least during the 15- to 40-second period that follows an initial tachysystolic stage, is organized. Chen et al[25] used 40 plunge needles anchored 5 mm apart to record from the right ventricles of six dogs after 20 seconds of VF. Three bipolar electrodes with 1 mm between poles were located 1 mm apart on the plunge needle to provide transmural information. They observed coherent activation fronts with dimensions and path lengths of several centimeters. The cycle length averaged 96 ± 16 msec, which was compatible with the frequency of activation of between 600 and 660 per minute that Wiggers[26] had observed and described as stage II VF. The activation fronts during stage II frequently collided with each other or blocked when they approached tissue that remained refractory following a previous activation front. Moe's theory that fibrillation reflected a series of wandering wavelets of activation was consistent with these findings. Additional evidence that organization of VF increases during the first minute has recently been provided by Johnson et al.[27] They mapped VF in pigs with 121 electrodes spaced 0.28 mm apart and found a sharper peak in the power spectra and less conduction block after 1 minute than just after the onset of fibrillation. Some pigs also exhibited a high degree of beat-to-beat repeatability of the activation sequences after 1 minute of fibrillation. Damle et al[28] mapped VF in 13 dogs with myocardial infarctions and 4 without and used vector analysis to show that electrical activation was both spatially (for electrodes 2.5 mm apart) and temporally (from one beat to the next at adjacent electrode sites) organized at the onset of VF and that the degree of organization decreased during the first 5 seconds. On the other hand, Witkowski and Penkoske[29] concluded from phase plane plots and state space diagrams of VF that there was no evidence or recurring spatial patterns during detailed mapping studies of VF.

Frequency Characteristics

During VF, there is frequently a clear dominant frequency with a narrow bandwidth and a peak in the power spectrum at around 9–12 Hz.[18,30] In their study of the power spectrum following the induction of VF in dogs by several different methods, Carlisle et al[31] used fast Fourier transform analysis to determine frequency characteristics and found that the initial frequency of around 12 Hz rapidly fell to 5–6 Hz by 120 seconds. Limb lead recordings were similar for VF induced by ischemia, by reperfusion, or by electrical stimulation in the presence of ischemia. Recordings from the endocardium initially showed a dominant frequency similar to that recorded at the body surface, but there was no significant drop in frequency after 3 minutes from onset. The cause of the fall in frequency in the limb leads after 1–2 minutes of continued fibrillation is unknown. These results are, however, consistent with those presented by Worley et al,[32] in which direct bipolar recordings from the left ventricular endocardium showed that activation rates in the endocardium continued at a rapid rate for many minutes even though activation rates in the myocardium and epicardium were decreasing markedly.

The decrease in the peak frequency associated with VF over time may be of clinical significance since the success rate in the treatment of VF varies inversely with the duration of the time between the onset of VF and the initiation of cardiopulmonary resuscitation and transthoracic defibrillation, i.e., the down time.[33] Dzwonczyk et al[34] used the median frequency of the power spectrum to track the decrease in frequency with the increase in time of fibrillation in pigs. Using the algorithm they developed, they were able to predict the total elapsed time since onset of VF with an average error of −0.86 min. This information may eventually prove useful in the prehospital treatment of ventricular fibrillation.

WHY NOT VENTRICULAR TACHYCARDIA INSTEAD OF VENTRICULAR FIBRILLATION?

Until recently, VT was thought to be caused by re-entry around anatomical blocks in areas of patchy necrosis and scar tissue that resulted from myocardial ischemia and infarction and that were interspersed with small bundles of viable myocardium, while VF was thought to arise from re-entry caused by functional block.[35] Conditions such as slow conduction and variable degrees of conduction block, which are necessary for re-entry to occur, have been demonstrated in ischemic myocardium.[36-40] Although these factors may be responsible for VT in some cases, recent experimental evidence has demonstrated that they are not required for it to occur. Spach and co-workers have shown that re-entry can result from the anisotropy in the safety factor for conduction along and across fibers.[41] Okumura and coworkers[42] have shown in patients that regions of slow conduction during re-entry do not exhibit slow conduction during normal sinus rhythm. These results from several groups suggest that functional block may also be responsible for VT as well as for VF.

Sustained Ventricular Tachycardia from Functional Block

El-Sherif et al looked at isochronal maps of ventricular activation during spontaneous ventricular rhythms and pacing-induced ventricular tachyarrhythmias 1 day[43] and 4 days[44] after myocardial infarctions were produced in canine hearts. In both studies, they used 64 electrograms to record from the entire epicardial surface and from selected endocardial and intramural sites and were able to demonstrate circus movement re-entry in the surviving epicardial tissue overlying the infarction. In the study of 1-day infarcts, spontaneous ventricular rhythms had foci that originated in the surviving subendocardial Purkinje network underlying the infarction and that showed frequent shifts in the pacemaker site. Bursts of rapid ventricular pacing or programmed premature stimulation consistently induced fast ventricular tachyarrhythmias that tended to degenerate into VF. The last

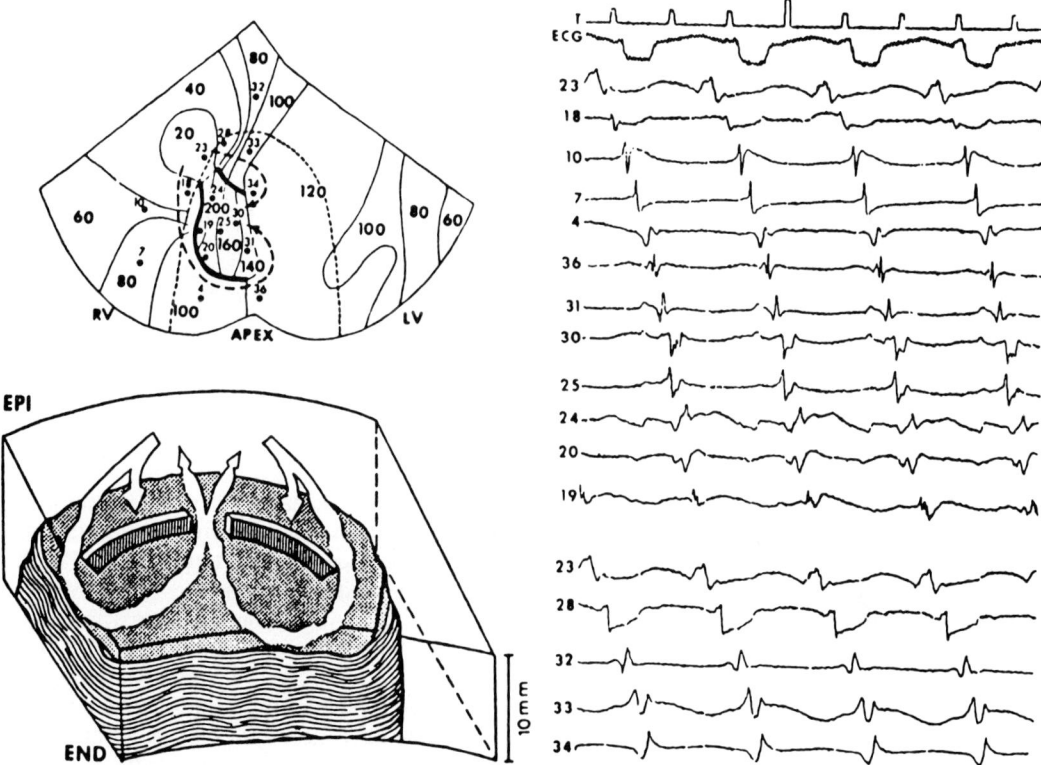

Fig. 8–7. Figure-of-eight model of re-entry. Isochronal activation map during monomorphic re-entrant ventricular tachycardia. Recordings were obtained from a dog 4 days after ligation of the left anterior descending coronary artery. Activation isochrones are drawn at 20-msec intervals. The re-entrant circuit has a characteristic figure-of-eight activation pattern whereby two circulating wave fronts advance in clockwise and counterclockwise directions, respectively, around two zones (arcs) of conduction block (represented by heavy solid lines). The epicardial surface is depicted as if the ventricles were folded out after a cut was made from the crux to the apex. The right panel shows selected simultaneous electrograms recorded along the two arcs of functional conduction block and the common re-entrant wave front and depicts the presence of diastolic bridging between re-entrant beats. A three-dimensional diagrammatic illustration of the ventricular activation pattern during the re-entrant tachycardia is shown at the lower left of the figure. In this experimental model, re-entrant activation occurs in the surviving thin epicardial layer overlying the infarction. RV, right ventricle; LV, left ventricle; EPI, epicardium; END, endocardium; T, time lines at 100-msec intervals. (Reprinted by permission of Futura Publishing Co, Inc, from El-Sherif N: Reentry revisited. PACE *11:* 1358, 1988.)

stimulated beat that initiated re-entry resulted in a continuous arc of functional conduction block and two activation fronts that slowly circled around both ends of the arc of block. The activation fronts rejoined on the distal side of the block before breaking through and reactivating the area proximal to the block. Sustained VT continued owing to the two synchronous circuits that conducted in clockwise and counterclockwise directions in a figure-of-eight re-entry pattern (Fig. 8–7).

Ventricular Fibrillation versus Ventricular Tachycardia

VT is normally induced by electrical stimulation in which a small S2 (<2 mA) is given outside the infarct so that a premature activation front conducts into the infarct, blocks, and leads to re-entry,[45] while VF is normally induced by giving a large S2 (>20 mA) during the vulnerable period. As noted previously, El-Sherif et al[44] used programmed electrical stimulation from electrodes placed outside a 4-day-old nonreperfused infarct to maintain VT in a figure-of-eight re-entry pattern in a thin sheet of viable spared myocardium in the epicardium over the infarct. As seen in the study by Chen et al,[11] VF was initiated by figure-of-eight re-entry near the S2 site when a large S2 stimulus was given in normal myocardium during the vulnerable period, with S1 given at another site.

In a study by Kavanagh et al,[46] ten dogs underwent 30 minutes of partial and 90 minutes of complete left anterior descending coronary artery occlusion followed by reperfusion in order to test the hypothesis that a large S2 stimulus given during the vulnerable period to a site over an infarct may induce VT and not VF. Four days after the infarction was induced, ten S1 stimuli were given to right or left ventricular sites and the vulnerable period was scanned with an S2 stimulus given to the center of the region of epicardial sparing over the infarct. The S2 strength was increased until VT or VF was induced. Sustained VT in a figure-of-eight re-entry pattern was induced repeatedly from 23 S1 sites with a mean S2 of 39 mA, while VF was obtained from ten S1 sites with a mean S2 of 56 mA. The mean difference in the arrhythmia cycle lengths for the initial six cycles was 153 ± 33 msec for VT and 110 ± 8 msec for VF ($p < 0.001$). The mean transmural extent of infarction, determined histologically, was 80% in five dogs with only VT from all S1 sites, 60% in three dogs with VT from some and VF from other S1 sites, and 20% from two dogs with only VF from all S1 sites. Increasing the S2 strength above the lowest strength that initiated VT up to 100 mA yielded only VT, not VF, in animals with large, nearly transmural infarcts. Although the infarct lowered the VF threshold for large S2 stimuli given outside the infarcted region, the infarct had a protective effect for large S2 stimuli given over the center of the infarct during the vulnerable period by causing slower rotational velocity and increased stability of rotors. However, it was probably much easier to initiate the slower rotors during VT in an infarcted heart than it would be to initiate rotors leading to VF in a noninfarcted heart. This study demonstrated that both VT and VF could begin with figure-of-eight re-entry and that both could be induced by giving a large S2 stimulus during the vulnerable period.

SUMMARY AND CONCLUSION

With recent advances in cardiac mapping, both re-entrant and nonre-entrant mechanisms have been shown to play a role in the initiation and maintenance of VF. The mechanism underlying the transition from VT to VF during early ischemia differs from that during reperfusion. The transition to VF after reperfusion is due to acceleration by nonre-entrant mechanisms, whereas acceleration of the tachycardia by a nonre-entrant mechanism was not observed during the transition to VF during ischemia without reperfusion. Once acceleration of the tachycardia occurred, the development of VF during ischemia and reperfusion was similar.

Although the re-entrant mechanism for the initiation of VF by electrical stimulation during the vulnerable period was thought to be due to nonuniform dispersion of refractoriness, it has been shown that VF may be initiated electrically in the presence of uniform dispersion of refractoriness. Conduction block leading to re-entry and VF can be caused by the interaction of a uniformly dispersed change in refractoriness with the strength of a shock field which forms a critical point around which activation fronts rotate. This does not rule out the likelihood that nonuniform dispersion of refractoriness may be the mechanism for naturally occurring VF, such as that caused by acute ischemia, or for VF induced by low-voltage stimuli.

Evidence has been found both experimentally and through computer simulations to suggest that VF is maintained by multiple wandering wavelets. Maintenance of VF also requires a critical mass of available cardiac tissue, for it is difficult to induce and impossible to sustain VF in small hearts, such as in frogs. Results from experiments involving atrial fibrillation indicate that multiple rapidly firing ectopic foci and multiple re-entry may act together to maintain fibrillation. A dominant frequency of 12 Hz occurs during early VF and soon falls to around 5-6 Hz, with rates in the myocardium and epicardium decreasing before those in the endocardium. A relationship between the peak frequency of VF and the time since onset has been found in pigs and may be useful in determining prehospital treatment of VF in humans.

The extent of surviving epicardial tissue overlying an infarct may determine whether a particular heart will develop VT or VF following pacing from the center of the spared region. Animals with a thin layer of spared tissue developed VT, while those with infarcts corresponding to only 20% of the wall thickness developed VF. These results may lead to new methods for predicting which patients are at risk for VF rather than sustained VT.

REFERENCES

1. Smith WM, Wharton JM, Blanchard SM, Wolf PD, Ideker RE: Direct cardiac mapping. In Zipes DP, Jalife J (eds): Cardiac Electrophysiology: From Cell to Bedside. Philadelphia, WB Saunders, 1990, pp 849-858.
2. Mastrototaro JJ, Pilkington TC, Ideker RE, Massoud HZ: Thin-film multielectrode arrays for potential gradient measurements in the heart. In Harris G, Walker C (eds): Proceedings of the 10th Annual Conference of the IEEE Engineering in Medicine and Biology Society. New Orleans, IEEE, 1988, p 90.
3. Cabo C, Wharton JM, Simpson EV, Ideker RE, Smith WM: Use of coherence in activation detection during ventricular fibrillation. In Kim Y, Spelman FA (eds): Proceedings of the 11th Annual Conference of the IEEE Engineering in Medicine and Biology Society. New York, NY, IEEE, 1989, pp 1733-1734.
4. Janse MJ, van Capelle FJL, Morsink H, et al: Flow of "injury" current and patterns of excitation during early ventricular arrhythmias in acute regional myocardial ischemia in isolated porcine and canine hearts: Evidence for two different arrhythmogenic mechanisms. Circ Res 47:151-165, 1980.
5. Ideker RE, Klein GJ, Harrison L, et al: The transition to ventricular fibrillation induced by reperfusion following acute ischemia in the dog: A period of organized epicardial activation. Circulation 63:1371-1379, 1981.
6. Ideker RE, Bardy GH, Worley SJ, German LD, Smith WM: Patterns of activation during ventricular fibrillation. In Josephson ME, Wellens HJJ (eds): Tachycardias: Mechanisms, Diagnosis, Treatment. Philadelphia, Lea and Febiger, 1984, pp 519-536.
7. Pogwizd SM, Corr PB: Electrophysiologic mechanisms underlying arrhythmias due to reperfusion of ischemic myocardium. Circulation 76:404-426, 1987.
8. Pogwizd SM, Corr PB: Mechanisms underlying the development of ventricular fibrillation during early myocardial ischemia. Circ Res 66:672-695, 1990.
9. Moe GK, Harris AS, Wiggers CJ: Analysis of the initiation of fibrillation by electrographic studies. Am J Physiol 134:473-492, 1941.
10. Frazier DW, Wolf PD, Wharton JM, Tang ASL, Smith WM, Ideker RE: Stimulus-induced critical point: Mechanism for electrical initiation of reentry in normal canine myocardium. J Clin Invest 83:1039-1052, 1989.
11. Chen P-S, Wolf PD, Dixon EG, Danieley ND, Frazier DW, Smith WM, Ideker RE: Mechanism of ventricular vulnerability to single premature stimuli in open-chest dogs. Circ Res 62:1191-1209, 1988.
12. Shibata N, Chen P-S, Dixon EG, et al: Influence of shock strength and timing on induction of ventricular arrhythmias in dogs. Am J Physiol 255:H891-H901, 1988.
13. Kao CY, Hoffman BF: Graded and decremental response in heart muscle fibers. Am J Physiol 194:187-196, 1958.
14. Ideker RE, Frazier DW, Krassowska W, et

al: Experimental evidence for autowaves in the heart. In Jalife J (ed): Mathematical Approaches to Cardiac Arrhythmias. Ann NY Acad Sci 591:208–218, 1990.
15. Winfree AT: When Time Breaks Down: The Three-Dimensional Dyanamics of Electrochemical Waves and Cardiac Arrhythmias. Princeton, Princeton University Press, 1987.
16. Wiggers CJ: The mechanism and nature of ventricular defibrillation. Am Heart J 20:399–412, 1940.
17. Garrey WE: The nature of fibrillatory contractions of the heart: Its relation to tissue mass and form. Am J Physiol 33:397–414, 1914.
18. Herbschleb JN, Heethaar RM, Tweel L, Meijler RL: Frequency analysis of the ECG before and during ventricular fibrillation. In Ripley KL, Ostrow HG (eds): Proceedings of Computers in Cardiology. Washington, DC, IEEE Computer Society Press, 1980, pp 365–368.
19. Mines GR: On circulating excitations in heart muscles and their possible relation to tachycardia and fibrillation. Trans R Soc Can 4:43–52, 1914.
20. Moe GK: Cardiac arrhythmias: Introductory remarks to part III. Ann NY Acad Sci 64:540–542, 1956.
21. Moe GK, Rheinboldt WC, Abildskov JA: A computer model of atrial fibrillation. Am Heart J 67:200–220, 1964.
22. Sano T, Scher AM: Multiple recording during electrically induced atrial fibrillation. Circ Res 14:117–125, 1964.
23. Allessie MA, Lammers WJEP, Bonke FIM, Hollen J: Experimental evaluation of Moe's multiple wavelet hypothesis of atrial fibrillation. In Zipes DP, Jalife J (eds): Cardiac Electrophysiology and Arrhythmias. Orlando, Grune & Stratton, 1985, pp 265–275.
24. Allessie MA, Bonke FIM, Schopman FJG: Circus movement in rabbit atrial muscle as a mechanism of tachycardia: III. The "leading circle" concept: A new model of circus movement in cardiac tissue without the involvement of an anatomical obstacle. Circ Res 41:9–18, 1977.
25. Chen P-S, Wolf PD, Melnick SB, Danieley ND, Smith WM, Ideker RE: Comparison of activation during ventricular fibrillation and following unsuccessful defibrillation shocks in open chest dogs. Circ Res 66:1544–1560, 1990.
26. Wiggers CJ: Studies of ventricular fibrillation caused by electric shock: Cinematographic and electrocardiographic observations of the natural process in the dog's heart. Its inhibition by potassium and the revival of coordinated beats by calcium. Am Heart J 5:351–365, 1930.
27. Johnson EE, Idriss SF, Cabo C, Melnick SB, Smith WM, Ideker RE: Evidence that organization increases during the first minute of ventricular fibrillation in pigs mapped with closely spaced electrodes [abstract]. J Am Coll Cardiol 19:90A, 1992.
28. Damle RS, Kanaan NM, Robinson NS, Ge Y-Z, Goldberger JJ, Kadish AH: Spatial and temporal linking of epicardial activation directions during ventricular fibrillation in dogs: Evidence for underlying organization. Circulation 86:1547–1558, 1992.
29. Witkowski FX, Penkoske PA: Activation patterns during ventricular fibrillation. In Jalife J (ed): Mathematical Approaches to Cardiac Arrhythmias. New York, New York Academy of Sciences, 1990, pp 219–231.
30. Carlisle EJF, Allen JD, Bailey A, et al: Fourier analysis of ventricular fibrillation and synchronization of DC countershocks in defibrillation. J Electrocardiol 21:337–343, 1988.
31. Carlisle EJF, Allen JD, Kernohan WG, et al: Fourier analysis of ventricular fibrillation of varied aetiology. Eur Heart J 11:173–181, 1990.
32. Worley SJ, Swain JL, Colavita PG, et al: Development of an endocardial-epicardial gradient of activation rate during electrically induced, sustained ventricular fibrillation in the dog. Am J Cardiol 55:813–820, 1985.
33. Yakaitis RW, Ewy A, Otto CW, et al: Influence of time and therapy on ventricular defibrillation in dogs. Crit Care Med 8:157–163, 1980.
34. Dzwonczyk R, Brown CG, Werman HA: The median frequency of the ECG during ventricular fibrillation: Its use in an algorithm for estimating the duration of cardiac arrest. IEEE Trans Biomed Eng BME-37:640–646, 1990.
35. Michelson EL, Spear JF, Moore EN: Electrophysiologic and anatomic correlates of sustained ventricular tachyarrhythmias in a model of chronic myocardial infarction. Am J Cardiol 45:583–590, 1980.
36. Boineau JP, Cox JL: Slow ventricular activation in acute myocardial infarction: A source of re-entrant premature ventricular contractions. Circulation 48:702–713, 1973.
37. Williams DO, Scherlag BJ, Hope RR, et al: The pathophysiology of malignant ventricular arrhythmias during acute myocardial ischemia. Circulation 50:1163–1172, 1974.
38. Elharrar V, Foster PR, Jirak TL, et al: Alterations in canine myocardial excitability during ischemia. Circ Res 40:98–105, 1977.
39. Lazzara R, El-Sherif N, Hope RR, et al: Ventricular arrhythmias and electrophysiological consequences of myocardial is-

chemia and infarction. Circ Res 42:740–749, 1978.
40. Janse MJ, Kléber AG: Electrophysiological changes and ventricular arrhythmias in the early phase of regional myocardial ischemia. Circ Res 49:1069–1081, 1981.
41. Spach MS, Dolber PC, Heidlage JF: Influence of the passive anisotropic properties on directional differences in propagation following modification of the sodium conductance in human atrial muscle: A model of reentry based on anisotropic discontinuous propagation. Circ Res 62:811–832, 1988.
42. Okumura K, Olshansky B, Henthorn RW, et al: Demonstration of the presence of slow conduction during sustained ventricular tachycardia in man: Use of transient entrainment of the tachycardia. Circulation 75:360–378, 1987.
43. El-Sherif N, Mehra R, Gough WB, Zeiler RH: Ventricular activation patterns of spontaneous and induced ventricular rhythms in canine one-day-old myocardial infarction: Evidence for focal and reentrant mechanisms. Circ Res 51:152–166, 1982.
44. El-Sherif N, Gough WB, Restivo M: Reentrant ventricular arrhythmias in the late myocardial infarction period: 14. Mechanisms of resetting, entrainment, acceleration, or termination of reentrant tachycardia by programmed electrical stimulation. PACE 10:341–371, 1987.
45. Dillon SM, Allessie MA, Ursell PC, Wit AL: Influences of anisotropic tissue structure on reentrant circuits in the epicardial border zone of subacute canine infarcts. Circ Res 63:182–206, 1988.
46. Kavanagh KM, Kabas JS, Rollins DL, et al: High-current stimuli to the spared epicardium of a large infarct induce ventricular tachycardia. Circulation 85:680–698, 1992.

C
Underlying Substrates in Sudden Cardiac Death

9

Sudden Death Late After a Myocardial Infarction: Substrate and Risk Stratification

HEIN J. J. WELLENS

Coronary artery disease is the most common cause of sudden death. Death may occur in the acute phase of ischemia or may happen at a time remote from a previous myocardial infarction (MI). This chapter considers the patient who dies suddenly after having sustained an MI in the past.

SUBSTRATE OF SUDDEN DEATH IN THE LATE PHASE OF MYOCARDIAL INFARCTION

Observations during ambulatory monitoring of patients dying suddenly indicate that in patients known to have had a previous MI, either ventricular tachycardia (VT) deteriorating into ventricular fibrillation (VF) or VF is the most common mode of death.[1-3]

Information from animal experiments,[4,5] programmed electrical stimulation,[6,7] and ventricular activation mapping in the human heart,[8,9] as well as the effects of pharmacological and nonpharmacological interventions,[10-12] suggest re-entry as the most common underlying mechanism of the arrhythmia.

Animal experiments have shown that after an MI, an electrical impulse may travel over a pathway consisting of surviving myocardial muscle cells embedded in fibrotic tissue.[4,5] In 1972 it was demonstrated that in patients who had a sustained VT late after an MI the arrhythmia could be reproducibly initiated by programmed electrical stimulation of the heart.[6] The observation that the arrhythmia could not only be initiated but also terminated by a critically timed premature beat made the authors suggest re-entry as the most likely mechanism of the arrhythmia. Two years later[7] workers from the same institution showed that the ability to re-initiate the clinically documented VT by critically timed premature stimuli during programmed stimulation of the heart was much greater in patients who had had sustained VT late after MI than in patients who had the onset of VT early (in the acute phase) after MI. These observations suggested that a "stable" phase with the development of a well-defined re-entrant pathway was required for perpetuation of the arrhythmia. Subsequently, again using the technique of programmed electrical stimulation of the heart, it was shown that pharmacological interventions could influence the ability to initiate and to modify the rate of the arrhythmia in patients with recurrent VT late after MI.[10]

Of major importance for our understanding of the substrate of life-threatening ventricular arrhythmias has been the ability to map ventricular activation during the arrhythmia.[8] The demonstration of fragmented, repetitive, low-voltage electrical activity in the area of abnormal impulse formation covering most of the interval between two successive tachycardia beats was originally interpreted as indicative of a re-entry circuit with markedly slowed conduction velocity.[8] Thereafter, however, it was shown that the cells incorporated in the circuit may have a normal intracellular ultrastructure and exhibit normal electrical behavior,[13] and that severe loss of lateral intercellular connections (isolation) can lead to very long, spaghetti-like circuits,[14] falsely giving the impression of marked slowing of the conduction velocity in the circuit.

Most of our observations on the substrate for life-threatening ventricular arrhythmias after MI in humans are based on studies done in the catheterization laboratory and operating room. In order to be able to make those observations, the arrhythmia had to be sustained and hemodynamically tolerated. This obviously leads to a bias because studies were made in sustained VT rather than VF.[15] This should be taken into account and may lead to an overestimation of our ability to identify persons prone to die suddenly outside the hospital after a remote MI. It cannot be denied, however, that scar tissue after an MI plays an important role as a possible pathway for life-threatening ventricular arrhythmias.

Other Factors Playing a Role in Sudden Death

As indicated in Figure 9–1, many factors alone or in combination can play a role in the process of sudden arrhythmic death. Three main factors, left ventricular dysfunction, ischemia, and electrical instability, have to be mentioned. Each of these factors has static (size of the scar, chronic stenosis of the coronary artery, ventricular hypertrophy) and dynamic components, such as changes in degree of ischemia, triggers (ventricular premature beats), blood platelet function, influence of the autonomic nervous system, electrolyte levels, time of day, and so forth. Table 9–1 indicates how all these different factors may lead to different arrhythmogenic mechanisms. It also shows that, in addition, our therapeutic measures may induce new arrhythmia mechanisms. One should also realize that different mechanisms may play a role in the initiation and perpetuation of the arrhythmia. Therefore, in the patient with a previous MI, a complex situation is present

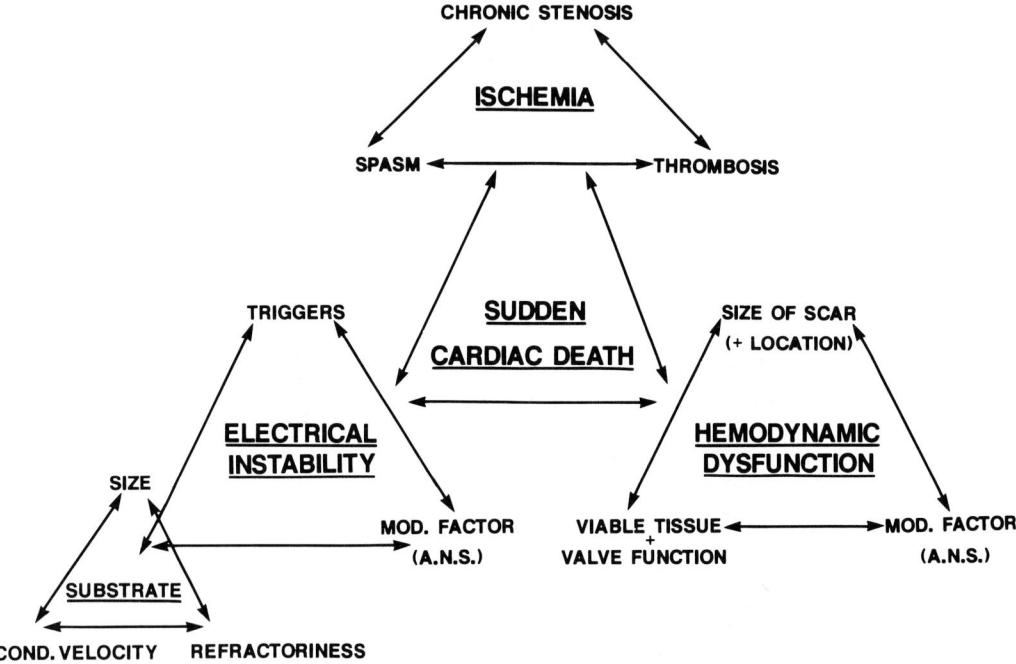

Fig. 9–1. Factors that play a role in sudden death. The basic triangle is formed by hemodynamic dysfunction, ischemia, and electrical instability. Each of these three cornerstones has static and dynamic components. Modulatory (M.O.D.) factors include the autonomic nervous system (A.N.S.), electrolytes, hormones, and drugs.

Table 9–1
Different Mechanisms of Arrhythmias Subsequent to Changes Induced by Myocardial Infarction or Its Treatment

	Re-entry	EAD	DAD	AA
Structural				
Scar	+			
Fibrosis	+			
Dilation	+		+	
Hypertrophy		+	+	
Ischemia	+			+
Functional				
Wall stress ↑			+	
Diastolic pressure ↑			+	
Neuro-control				
Sympathetic		+	+	+
Electrolytes				
K		+		
Mg		+		
Drugs				
Digitalis			+	
Diuretics		+		
Vasodilators	+			+
Inotropes	+			
Antiarrhythmic agents	+	+		

Abbreviations: AA, abnormal automaticity; DAD, delayed after depolarizations; EAD, early after depolarizations.

therapy is decided upon, a programmed electrical stimulation study with intracardiac mapping is performed in an effort to localize the substrate for the arrhythmia. This requires a stable, hemodynamically tolerated, sustained ventricular arrhythmia. Unfortunately, because of that prerequisite a search for the substrate is possible only in a minority of patients with sustained monomorphic VT or VF. If one is able to localize the substrate, surgical excision or destruction of the area by surgical, chemical, or electrical means can cure the patient. Inability to initiate a previously inducible arrhythmia after antiarrhythmic drug therapy with many factors determining the chance of dying suddenly.

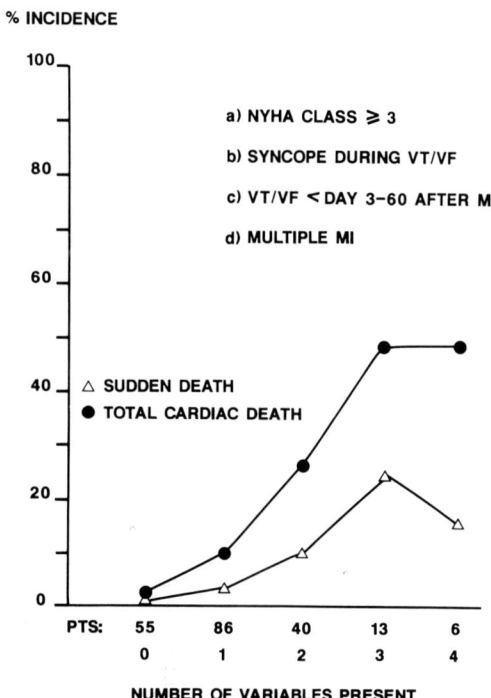

Fig. 9–2. Incidence of total cardiac death and sudden cardiac death in relation to the total score of four clinical variables in 200 patients with sustained monomorphic VT (169 patients) or VF (31 patients) after MI. The four clinical variables, listed in the upper right corner of the figure, were (a) a New York Heart Association class of dyspnea outside the arrhythmia of 3 or more; (b) the presence of circulatory collapse during VT or VF; (c) the occurrence of VT or VF during day 3 to day 60 after MI; and (d) more than one previous MI. Depending on the number of variables present, these are marked differences in sudden and total cardiac death during 2 years of follow-up.

RISK STRATIFICATION

The Patient with Myocardial Infarction and a Spontaneous Episode of Sustained Ventricular Tachycardia or Ventricular Fibrillation

Recently we discussed the risk assessment and prognosis of patients after aborted SCD or suffering from symptomatic ventricular tachyarrhythmias.[16] In a patient with a remote MI suffering from these complications, four clinical questions can help stratify the patient as to prognosis and to select therapy. Figure 9–2 shows that the presence of two or three of these clinical variables identifies a group of patients at high risk of dying suddenly during a 2-year follow-up period. In most of these patients, before apy predicts a reduced chance of spontaneous recurrences of VT.[17–19] Most of these patients, however, and especially those with arrhythmias leading to circulatory collapse, will have to be treated with a defibrillator.

The Survivor of Myocardial Infarction Without Spontaneous Sustained Ventricular Arrhythmias

One would like to be able to stratify MI survivors as to their risk of dying suddenly at the time of discharge from hospital. Much time and money have been spent in the past decade to establish a reliable risk stratification protocol. As shown in Table 9–2, several tests have been suggested for that purpose.[20–34] Some tests, like the signal-averaged electrocardiogram (ECG) or programmed stimulation of the heart, will give information about a possible substrate for VT. Others, like the left ventricular ejection fraction (LVEF), are better predictors of VF.[35] It is important to realize that all these tests, alone or in combination, although they have a high negative predictive value, also have a low positive predictive accuracy. In other words, it is easy to recognize patients at low risk for dying suddenly but difficult to predict accurately which patient will die suddenly. This would not be a serious problem if sudden death could be adequately prevented by a treatment of low cost and no side effects, but unfortunately, no such treatment is currently available. This makes it extremely difficult, if not impossible, to select post-MI patients who have not yet experienced a spontaneous episode of life-threatening ventricular arrhythmia for an expensive prophylactic treatment, such as implantation of a defibrillator. It is rare, even when using combinations of different tests, to come to a positive predictive accuracy of more than 40%. In practical terms, 100 defibrillators have to be implanted to protect the 40 patients who otherwise would die suddenly.

One should also realize that numerically more sudden deaths will occur in the low-risk group than in the high-risk group. This is illustrated in Figure 9–3, which shows the sequence of events in 231 patients less than 75 years old who were admitted to our coronary care unit in 1991 because of an acute MI. Fifteen patients died in the hospital, 12 within 24 hours after admission. Of the 216 patients discharged, 20 were not included in risk stratification because of bundle-branch block (one of those patients died in the 12 months after discharge). In 196 patients the LVEF was determined and a signal-averaged ECG was recorded before discharge. These 196 patients were grouped according to positivity or negativity of the signal-averaged ECG and an LVEF of <40% or ≥40%. "High-risk" patients with both a positive signal-averaged ECG and LVEF below 40% were asked to undergo a programmed electrical stimulation study. That study was considered to be positive if a monomorphic sustained VT could be induced with a cycle length of ≤270 msec. The protocol used right apical ventricular pacing with three basic cycle lengths and a maximum of three extrastimuli. Of the 21 patients eligible for the stimulation study, 9 patients refused and only one of the 12 remaining patients had a positive study. Six patients died during a follow-up of 1 year. Three patients (the ones within brackets in Fig. 9–3) died suddenly. Two of the sudden deaths occurred in the 108 patients with a negative signal-averaged ECG and a reasonable LVEF.

Figure 9–3 clearly shows some of the problems in risk stratifying patients after an acute MI. First, in the 1990s, with current treatment modes, both in-hospital and post-discharge mortality are low if the patient survives the first day after admission. This

Table 9–2
Risk Stratification for Sudden Death After Myocardial Infarction[20–34]

Pump function:	Functional class
	LVEF
	Exercise duration
	Heart rate variability
	Baroreflex sensitivity
Ischemia	Exercise testing (+nuclear)
	Holter
Arrhythmias:	Signal-averaged ECG
	Holter monitoring
	QT interval duration and disparity
	Exercise testing
	PES

Abbreviations: ECG, electrocardiogram; LVEF left ventricular ejection fraction; PES, programmed electrical stimulation.

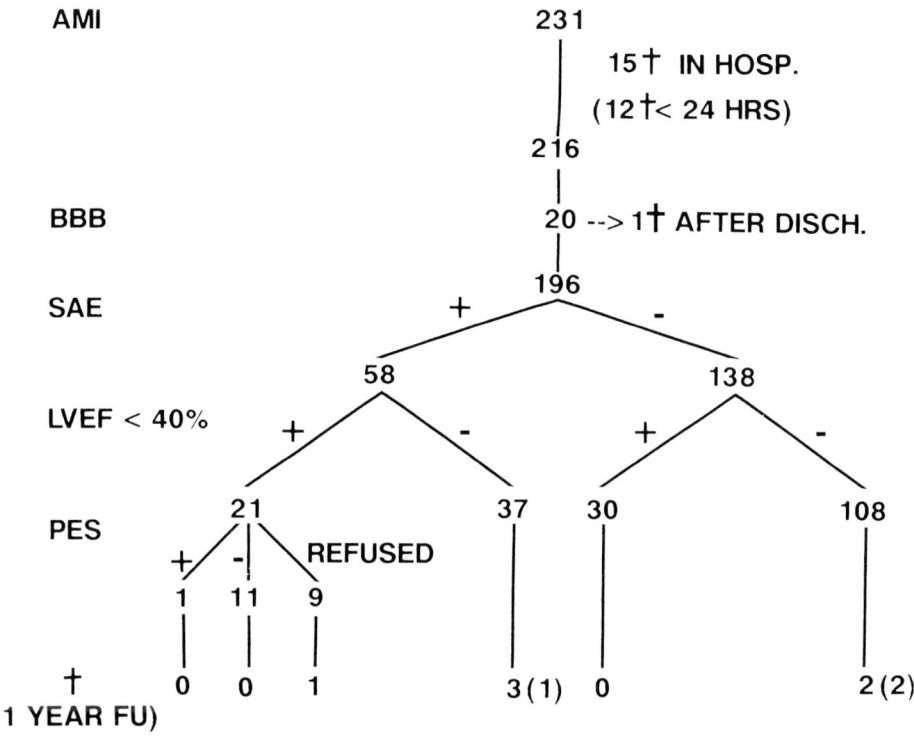

Fig. 9-3. Risk stratification using the signal-averaged electrocardiogram (SAE), left ventricular ejection fraction (LVEF), and programmed electrical stimulation (PES) of the heart in 231 patients less than 75 years old who were admitted to the Maastricht University Hospital in 1991 because of an acute MI, and who had no spontaneous sustained ventricular arrhythmia. Fifteen of the 231 patients died in hospital, 12 within 24 hours after admission. Of the remaining 216 patients, 20 patients were excluded because of bundle-branch block (one died after discharge). That resulted in risk stratification of 196 patients. Patients were stratified according to positivity or negativity of the SAE and an LEVF of <40% or ≥40%. A programmed electrical stimulation study was intended in patients with both a positive SAE and an LVEF <40%. PES was considered to be positive when a sustained monomorphic VT could be induced with an R-R interval of 270 msec or more. Note: (1) Only six patients died during the 1 year of follow-up; of these, three (the ones within brackets) died suddenly; and (2) nine of the 21 patients scheduled for PES refused the investigation.

means that very large series of patients are required to evaluate the effect of therapy in preventing sudden death. Second, a substantial number of patients refuse an invasive procedure like programmed electrical stimulation. Third, because of the large "low-risk" group, the number of sudden deaths may be higher in the "low-risk" group than in the "high-risk" group.

In 1992 Pedretti et al[36] published their approach to 283 patients after acute MI (Fig. 9-4). They used three variables for basic risk stratification—LVEF < 40%, a positive signal-averaged ECG, and the presence of nonsustained VT on 48-hour Holter monitoring. Patients were categorized according to the presence of one variable and two or more of the variables. Patients falling in the second category underwent programmed electrical stimulation with induction of a sustained monomorphic VT of less than 270 beats/min as a positive finding. As shown in Figure 9-4, that approach resulted in the correct prediction of a serious late arrhythmic event in 13 of the 20 high-risk patients. From the article[36] it is not clear how many of the 13 patients died suddenly or were resuscitated from VF.

From the different studies on risk stratification at the time of hospital discharge after acute MI, it is clear that combining different tests might increase positive predictive ac-

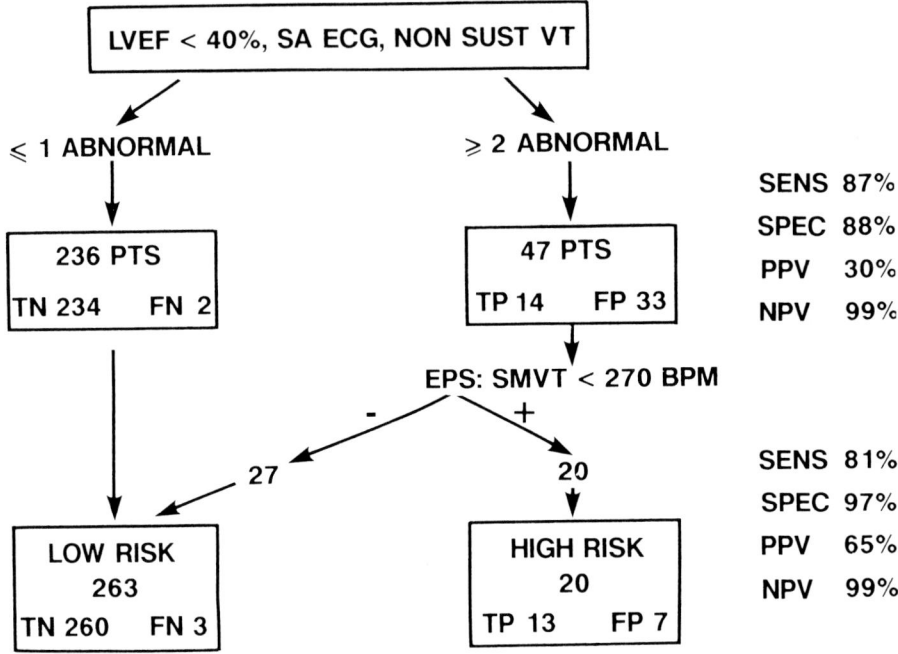

Fig. 9-4. Risk stratification as performed by Pedretti et al[36] in survivors of acute MI without spontaneous sustained ventricular arrhythmias. Patients were initially classified by three parameters: left ventricular ejection fraction (LVEF) <40%, positive signal-averaged electrocardiogram (SA ECG), and the presence of nonsustained VT on 48-hour Holter monitoring. Patients were then divided into two groups. One group had no or only one parameter positive and the other group had two or more parameters positive. The figure shows the sensitivity, specificity, positive predictive value, and negative predictive value of that approach for serious late ventricular arrhythmias by listing the true negatives (TN), false negatives (FN), true positives (TP), and false positives (FP). In addition, in 47 patients an electrophysiological (EPS) study was performed that was considered positive if a sustained VT of less than 270 beats/minute was initiated. As shown, this resulted in a higher positive identification of patients developing a serious late arrhythmic event. (Reproduced with permission from Pedretti R, et al: Am J Cardiol 69:866-872, 1993.[36])

curacy, but that most institutions will be able to identify only a very small number of patients, and at great expense.

LESSONS FROM SUDDEN DEATH OUT OF HOSPITAL

Sudden cardiac death is a common mode of death in patients with coronary artery disease. Most SCDs take place outside the hospital. It would be very helpful to know the characteristics of these patients in order to be able to construct a strategy to reduce that problem.

In Maastricht, a city with 180,000 inhabitants and only one hospital, one office of records, and one ambulance service, all sudden deaths in persons between 20 and 75 years of age have been registered as of January 1, 1991. In about 50% of cases permission for autopsy is obtained. Interim analysis of 300 sudden deaths revealed that in 40% of cases, sudden death was the first manifestation of coronary artery disease. Two thirds of the remaining patients with known coronary artery heart disease had had a documented MI in the past. However, when we examined the hospital data on these patients, we found that only 30% would have been recognized in hospital prior to discharge as high-risk candidates for sudden death! Those observations suggest that our current methods of risk estimation are not able to recognize with sufficient accuracy the majority of patients with coronary heart disease who will die suddenly.

SUMMARY

In the past two decades much new information has become available concerning the occurrence of serious ventricular arrhythmias and sudden death late after an MI. It has become clear that many (static and dynamic) factors play a role in the formation of the substrate and the initiation and perpetuation of these suddenly occurring, life-threatening events. The complexity of the problem makes it difficult to identify the high-risk candidate accurately, especially the patient dying suddenly outside the hospital.

REFERENCES

1. Nicolic G, Bishop RL, Singh JB: Sudden death during Holter monitoring. Circulation 66:218–225, 1982.
2. Kempf FC, Josephson ME: Cardiac arrest recorded on ambulatory electrocardiograms. Am J Cardiol 53:1577–1582, 1984.
3. Bayes de Luna A, Coumel P, Léclercq JF: Ambulatory sudden death: Mechanisms of production of a fatal arrhythmia on the basis of data from 157 cases. Am Heart J 117:151–159, 1989.
4. Friedman PL, Stewart JR, Wit AL: Spontaneous and induced cardiac arrhythmias in subendocardial Purkinje fibers surviving extensive myocardial infarction in dogs. Circ Res 33:612, 1973.
5. El-Sherif N, Scherlag BJ, Lazzara R, Hope RR: Re-entrant ventricular arrhythmias in the late myocardial infarction period: 1. Conduction characteristics in the infarction zone. Circulation 55:686, 1977.
6. Wellens HJJ, Schuilenburg RM, Durrer D: Electrical stimulation of the heart in patients with ventricular tachycardia. Circulation 46:215, 1972.
7. Wellens HJJ, Lie KI, Durrer D: Further observations on ventricular tachycardia as studied by electrical stimulation of the heart: Chronic recurrent ventricular tachycardia and ventricular tachycardia during acute myocardial infarction. Circulation 49:647–653, 1974.
8. Josephson ME, Horowitz LN, Farshidi A, Spear JF, Kastor JA, Moore EN: Recurrent sustained ventricular tachycardia: 2. Endocadial mapping. Circulation 57:440–447, 1978.
9. Josephson ME, Horowitz LN, Spielman SR, et al: Comparison of endocardial catheter mapping with intraoperative mapping of ventricular tachycardia. Circulation 61:395–404, 1980.
10. Wellens HJJ, Bär FW, Lie KI, Düren DR, Dohmen H: Effect of procainamide, propranolol and verapamil on mechanism of recurrent ventricular tachycardia. Am J Cardiol 40:579–585, 1977.
11. Josephson ME, Harken AH, Horowitz LN: Endocardial excision: A new surgical technique for the treatment of recurrent ventricular tachycardia. Circulation 60:1430–1439, 1979.
12. Josephson ME: Treatment of ventricular arrhythmias after myocardial infarction. Circulation 74:653–658, 1986.
13. Gardner PJ, Ursell PC, Fenoglio JJ, Wit AL: Anatomical and electrophysiological bases for electrograms showing fractionated activity. Circulation 66:78–93, 1982.
14. De Bakker JMT, Van Capelle FJV, Janse MJ, et al: Reentry as a cause of ventricular tachycardia in patients with chronic ischemic heart disease: Electrophysiologic and anatomic correlation. Circulation 77:589–601, 1988.
15. Stevenson WG, Linssen GCM, Havenith MG, Brugada P, Wellens HJJ: Late death after myocardial infarction: Mechanisms, etiologies, and implications for prevention of sudden death. In Brugada P, Wellens HJJ (eds): Cardiac Arrhythmias: Where to Go From Here? Mount Kisco, NY, Futura, 1987, pp 377–438.
16. Wellens HJJ, Rodriguez LM, Gorgels APM, Smeets JL: Risk assessment and prognosis of patients after aborted sudden cardiac death or suffering form symptomatic ventricular tachyarrhythmias. In Kapoor AS, Singh BN (eds): Prognosis and Risk Assessment in Cardiovascular Disease. New York, Churchill Livingstone, 1992, pp 403–411.
17. Fisher JD, Cohen HL, Mehra R, Altschuler H, Escher DJW, Furman S: Cardiac pacing and pacemakers: II. Serial electrophysiologic-pharmacologic testing for control of recurrent tachyarrhythmias. Am Heart J 93:658–668, 1977.
18. Mason JW, Winkle RA. Electrode-catheter arrhythmia induction in selection and assess-

ment of antiarrhythmic drug therapy for recurrent ventricular tachycardia. Circulation 58:971–985, 1978.
19. Horowitz LN, Josephson ME, Farshidi A, Spielman SR, Michelson EL, Greenspan AM: Recurrent sustained ventricular tachycardia: 3. Role of the electrophysiologic study in selection of antiarrhythmic regimens. Circulation 58:986–987, 1978.
20. McNamara RF, Carleen E, Moss AJ, the Multicenter Post-Infarction Research Group: Estimating left ventricular ejection fraction after myocardial infarction by various clinical parameters. Am J Cardiol 62:192–196, 1988.
21. Bigger JT Jr, Fleiss JL, Kleiger R, Miller JP, Rolnitzky LM, the Multicenter Post-Infarction Research Group: The relationships among ventricular arrhythmias, left ventricular dysfunction, and mortality in the 2 years after myocardial infarction. Circulation 69:250–258, 1984.
22. Weld FM, Chu K-L, Bigger JT Jr, Rolnitzky LM: Risk stratification with low-level exercise testing 2 weeks after acute myocardial infarction. Circulation 64:306–314, 1981.
23. Lombardi F, Sandrone G, Pernpruner S, et al: Heart rate variability as an index of sympatho-vagal interaction in patients after myocardial infarction. Am J Cardiol 60:1239–1245, 1987.
24. Kleiger RE, Miller JP, Bigger JT Jr, Moss AJ, the Multicenter Post-Infarction Research Group: Decreased heart rate variability and its association with increased mortality after acute myocardial infarction. Am J Cardiol 59:256–262, 1987.
25. La Rovere MT, Specchia G, Mortara A, Schwartz PJ: Baroreflex sensitivity, clinical correlates, and cardiovascular mortality among patients with a first myocardial infarction: A prospective study. Circulation 78:816–824, 1988.
26. Hammermeister KE, DeRouen TA, Dodge HT: Variables predictive of survival in patients with coronary disease: Selection by univariate and multivariate analyses from the clinical, electrocardiographic, exercise, arteriographic, and quantitative angiographic evaluations. Circulation 59:421–430, 1979.
27. Gomes JA, Winters SL, Stewart D, Horowitz SL, Milner M, Barreca P: A new noninvasive index to predict ventricular tachycardia and sudden death in the first year after myocardial infarction: Based on signal averaged electrocardiogram, radionuclide ejection fraction and Holter monitoring. J Am Coll Cardiol 10:349–357, 1987.
28. Kuchar DL, Thorburn CW, Sammel NL: Prediction of serious arrhythmic events after myocardial infarction: Signal-averaged electrocardiogram, Holter monitoring and radionuclide ventriculography. J Am Coll Cardiol 9:531–538, 1987.
29. Moss AJ, Davis HT, DeCamilla J, Bayer LW: Ventricular ectopic beats and their relation to sudden and nonsudden cardiac death after myocardial infarction. Circulation 60:998–1003, 1979.
30. Denniss AR, Richards DA, Cody DV, et al: Prognostic significance of ventricular tachycardia and fibrillation induced at programmed stimulation and delayed potentials detected on the signal-averaged electrocardiograms of survivors of acute myocardial infarction. Circulation 74:731–745, 1986.
31. Richards DA, Cody DV, Denniss AR, Russell PA, Young AA, Uther JB: Ventricular electrical instability: A predictor of death after myocardial infarction. Am J Cardiol 51:75–80, 1983.
32. Cripps TR, Bennett ED, Camm AJ, Ward DE: High gain signal averaged electrocardiogram combined with 24-hour monitoring in patients early after myocardial infarction for bedside prediction of arrhythmic events. Br Heart J 60:181–187, 1988.
33. Farrell TG, Bashir Y, Cripps T, et al: Risk stratification for arrhythmic events in post-infarction patients based on heart rate variability, ambulatory electrocardiographic variables and the signal-averaged electrocardiogram. J Am Coll Cardiol 18:687–697, 1991.
34. Bigger JT, Fleiss JL, Steinman RC, Rolnitzky LM, Kleiger RE, Rottman JN: Frequency domain measures of heart period variability and mortality after myocardial infarction. Circulation 85:164–171, 1992.
35. Rodriguez LM, Smeets J, O'Hara GE, Geelen P, Brugada P, Wellens HJJ: Incidence and timing of recurrences of sudden death and ventricular tachycardia during antiarrhythmic drug treatment in patients with sudden death or ventricular tachycardia after myocardial infarction. Am J Cardiol 69:1403–1406, 1992.
36. Pedretti R, Laporta A, Etro MD, et al: Influence of thrombolysis on signal-averaged electrocardiogram and late arrhythmic events after acute myocardial infarction. Am J Cardiol 69:866–872, 1992.

10

Sudden Death in Patients with Idiopathic Dilated Cardiomyopathy

PATRICK J. TCHOU
STEPHEN G. KEIM
ROBERT KINN

Nonischemic dilated cardiomyopathy is becoming a more common entity in patients with cardiac disease because of the increasing incidence of this entity and the decreasing incidence of coronary artery disease.[1] Overall survival after clinical diagnosis is estimated to be approximately 70% at 1 year and 50% at 2 years.[2-5] The incidence of sudden death varies in different reports but ranges from 28% to 72% of total deaths.[6-9] Most studies have shown that a majority of deaths were sudden in nature and likely to be secondary to tachyarrhythmias. The differing percentages of sudden deaths may be due to differing populations. Patients who have relatively preserved ventricular function may well have a comparatively low short-term risk of death from cardiac pump failure but may nevertheless be at a higher risk for arrhythmic deaths.

ETIOLOGY OF MALIGNANT ARRHYTHMIAS

Several factors may contribute to sudden arrhythmic deaths in patients with nonischemic dilated cardiomyopathy. Sustained ventricular tachyarrhythmias of the monomorphic variety or of the polymorphic variety have been seen in these patients and may be the most common cause of sudden cardiac death in this population. Reports of patients dying suddenly while being monitored generally show that tachyarrhythmia is the most common cause.[10-13] However, bradyarrhythmias may also play a role, especially in patients with very advanced heart failure.[14]

The inciting mechanism for the onset of primary polymorphic ventricular tachycardia (VT) or ventricular fibrillation (VF) in idiopathic dilated cardiomyopathy is unclear. Ischemia is known to cause this type of arrhythmia in both animal models and humans.[15] However, there is no evidence to support that mechanism in patients with nonischemic dilated cardiomyopathy. Although thromboembolic coronary occlusion is certainly possible in this entity, the frequency with which such an event might lead to polymorphic VT is unknown. There is evidence, however, that patients with diseased ventricles may be more sensitive to initiation of polymorphic ventricular tachyarrhythmias during programmed stimulation.[16] Premature beats in diseased ventricles appear to generate more conduction slowing and thus greater dispersion of activation. Such dispersion may form the substrate for the onset of sustained polymorphic VT. Whatever the mechanism whereby polymorphic VT is initiated in patients with nonischemic dilated cardiomyopathy, the occurrence of polymorphic VT is a malignant event. Figure 10-1 shows the electrocardiogram (ECG) tracings of a patient with idiopathic dilated cardiomyopathy who

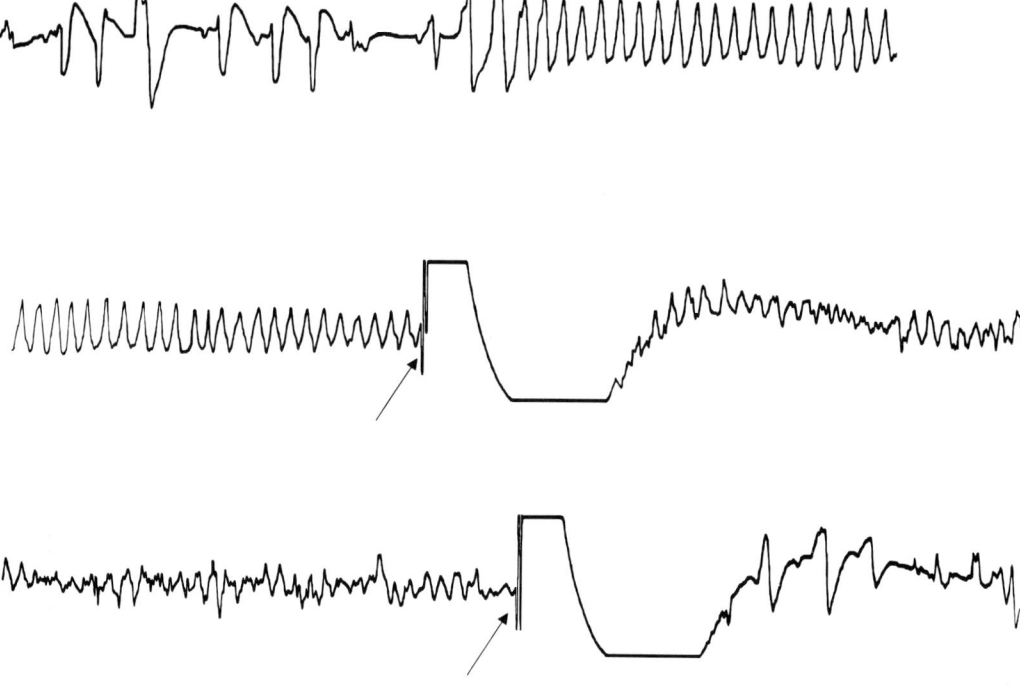

Fig. 10–1. ECG recordings of a spontaneous polymorphic ventricular tachycardia (VT) in a patient with idiopathic dilated cardiomyopathy and normal coronary arteries. The QT interval immediately preceding the onset of VT was not prolonged. The patient had no evidence of ischemia on ECG and no clinical symptoms of angina. The patient lost consciousness during the episode. The implantable defibrillator detected the arrhythmia and responded appropriately. However, it had to deliver two shocks before successfully defibrillating the patient.

spontaneously went into a rapid polymorphic VT. The patient's electrolytes were all in the normal range. The QT interval on the ECG was not prolonged. The patient was not taking antiarrhythmic agents at the time and had no evidence of ischemia, as the coronary arteriograms appeared normal. The tachycardia was terminated by two shocks delivered by an automatic implantable cardioverter-defibrillator. Although the patient was lying in bed, he had lost consciousness prior to receiving the first shock, which indicates the malignant nature of this type of arrhythmia in causing hemodynamic collapse.

Secondary causes of polymorphic VT can readily occur in patients with idiopathic dilated cardiomyopathy. They are frequently treated with diuretics, which can cause electrolyte imbalances such as hypokalemia and hypomagnesemia. These electrolyte abnormalities can cause torsade de pointes, especially in patients who have an underlying susceptibility to developing such arrhythmias with electrolyte disturbances. These patients are at risk for atrial tachyarrhythmias such as atrial fibrillation and flutter. Antiarrhythmic medications used to treat these arrhythmias can also cause polymorphic VT.

Rapid sustained monomorphic VT, while usually not as malignant as the polymorphic variety in causing immediate cardiovascular collapse, can nevertheless be the initiating event in a sudden death episode. Two categories of monomorphic VTs have been described from results of cardiac electrophysiological studies. One mechanism involves re-entry around a relatively large circuit, including the right and left bundle branches, the Purkinje network, and the ventricular muscle.[17] A single re-entrant beat of this sort has been well described and is commonly seen during delivery of ventricular premature stimuli in the right ventricular apex.[18] The ability of this circuit to sustain a re-entrant tachycardia in the dilated, diseased ventricle probably relates to an increase in ventricular activation times consequent on enlargement of the ventricles, and to slowing of conduction within muscle and His-Purkinje tissues as a result of the disease process. These factors would allow the re-entrant circuit to sustain a tachycardia where a normal heart could not. This macro re-entry, also called bundle-branch re-entry, accounts for a significant proportion of sustained monomorphic VTs induced during programmed ventricular stimulation in this patient population. It has been estimated that 40% of patients with dilated cardiomyopathy who have inducible monomorphic VT in the electrophysiology laboratory have macro re-entry as the mechanism of tachycardia.[19] A recent survey of all patients with inducible monomorphic VT at the University of Pittsburgh Medical Center over a 1-year period revealed that 14% had bundle-branch re-entrant VT. In the subgroup of patients with nonischemic dilated cardiomyopathy, 64% had bundle-branch re-entry as the mechanism of inducible sustained VT.

The clinical importance of recognizing this entity as a cause of VT lies in the fact that the re-entrant mechanism can be readily interrupted with catheter ablation techniques.[17,20] Such a treatment would avoid drug therapy, which frequently is not well tolerated by these patients because of their poor ventricular function. At present, radiofrequency catheter ablation of the right bundle branch appears to be the treatment of choice for this tachycardia. An example of this type of tachycardia is illustrated in Figure 10–2. A 55-year-old man with idiopathic dilated cardiomyopathy presented with recurrent episodes of rapid monomorphic VT causing hemodynamic collapse. Multiple electrophysiological studies using standard pacing protocols of up to three premature beats failed to reproduce the clinical arrhythmia. The patient was therefore treated with an implantable defibrillator. However, amiodarone therapy had to be initiated because of frequent clinical recurrence of the tachycardia. Within 2 years, the patient developed intolerance to amiodarone, which had to be discontinued. Approximately 6 months after discontinuation of amiodarone, the patient again began to receive frequent shocks secondary to rapid monomorphic VT. Electrophysiological studies were repeated, and the clinical tachycardia was repeatedly reproduced with the delivery of four premature beats. This tachycardia was demonstrated to be due to bundle-branch re-entry, and the patient underwent radiofrequency ablation of the right bundle. No tachycardia was inducible after the ablation, and the patient has not experienced any further clinical events. This case illustrates the fact that, despite frequently occurring clinical events, reproducing this tachycardia during programmed stimulation can be difficult at times. Because of a high degree of clinical suspicion, an unusually aggressive pacing protocol was employed that allowed reproduction of the clinical tachycardia.

Monomorphic VT not due to bundle-branch re-entry makes up a significant proportion of all inducible monomorphic VTs in this patient population, in the range of 40–60%. A few of these may be due to fascicular re-entry within the left bundle branch system. Most, however, are likely due to smaller re-entrant circuits within the myocardium, although experimental data to support this observation are lacking, and therefore one cannot exclude automatic mechanisms as the cause of these VTs. The potential substrate for re-entry certainly exists in these patients, since there frequently is microscopic scarring in the ventricular muscle that can be quite extensive.

There has been some recent evidence that bradyarrhythmias could be a cause of sudden death in this type of patient. Luu et al[14] noted in a recent report that 62% of patients who had cardiac arrest as inpatients while awaiting cardiac transplantation had bradycardia or electrical mechanical dissociation as the precipitating event of the arrest. However, they also pointed out that this was a rather unstable population that required hospitalization, and therefore, one may not be able to extrapolate the data to patients who do not need continuous hospitalization. Because electrical mechanical dissociation with sinus node arrest is frequently seen in the dying heart, it is not too surprising to observe this phenomenon in a critically ill patient population. Alterna-

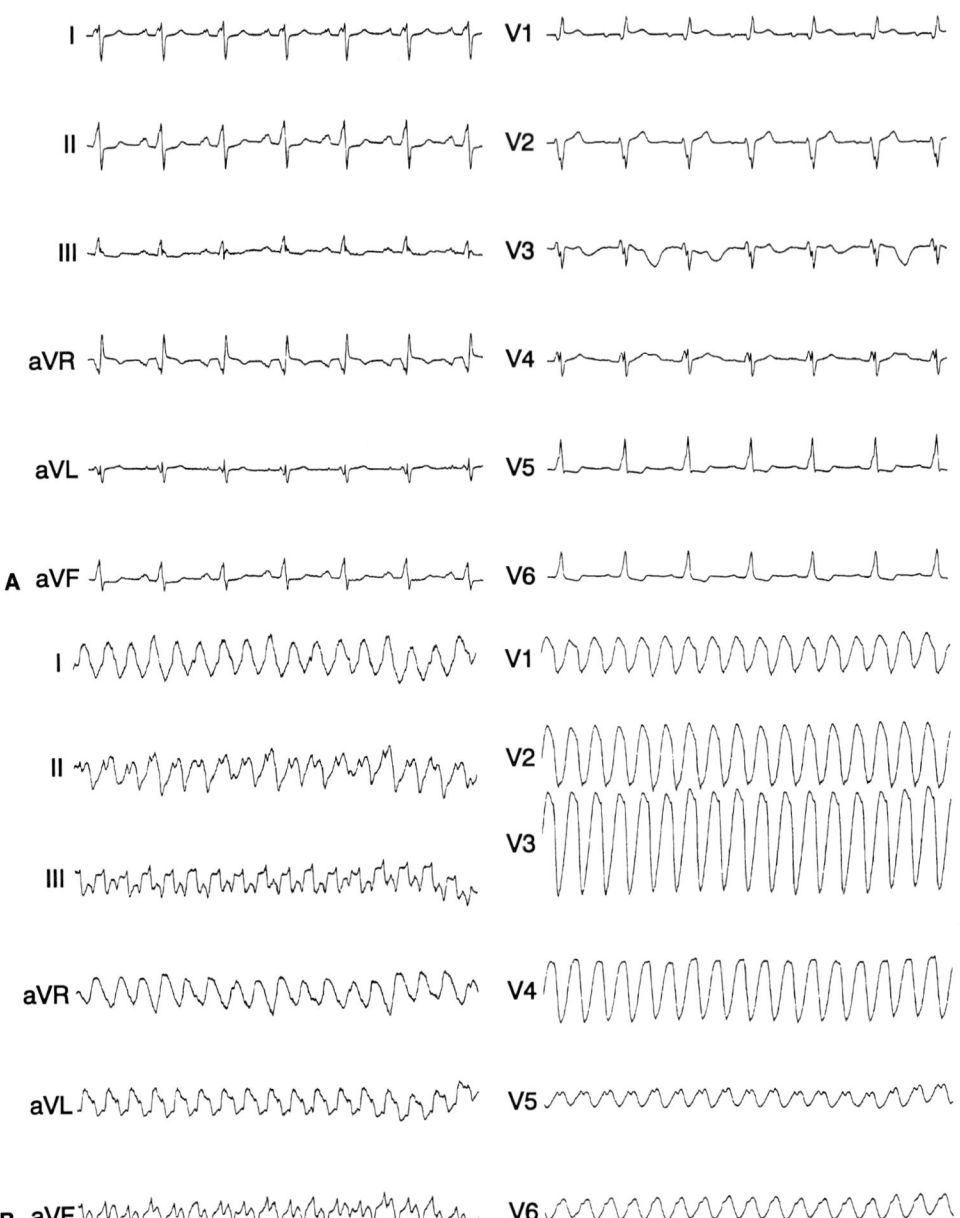

Fig. 10–2. **A.** Twelve-lead ECG during sinus rhythm of a patient with nonischemic dilated cardiomyopathy and recurrent sustained VT. The ECG shows a right bundle-branch block pattern type of conduction defect with a marked right axis deviation. The patient had frequent clinical episodes of VT, which were terminated by shocks from an implanted defibrillator.

B. Bundle-branch re-entrant VT induced during electrophysiological study in the same patient, which reproduced the clinical tachycardia. The QRS morphology has several characteristics common to bundle-branch re-entrant tachycardia. It has a typical left bundle-branch block pattern with a rapid downstroke to the S wave in the anterior precordial leads. This rapid downstroke appears to be characteristic of ventricular activation via the right bundle branch and right-sided Purkinje network. The axis is always left to superior. In some patients, the axis could be in the −90 to −120 degree range. Note that the presence of a right bundle-branch block pattern during sinus rhythm did not exclude conduction down the bundle during tachycardia. See text for discussion.

tively, such observation can also be accounted for by a sudden catastrophic event, such as a massive pulmonary embolism, coronary embolism, exsanguination from rupture of a large artery, or pericardial tamponade from an arterial rupture. Patients in advanced heart failure certainly are at risk for some of those events.

RISK ASSESSMENT

Assessing risk for sudden death in a patient with nonischemic dilated cardiomyopathy is controversial. Several clinical variables have been associated with an increased incidence of sudden death, at least in some reports. These variables include a prior cardiac arrest, left ventricular systolic dysfunction, ambulatory arrhythmias documented on Holter recordings, syncopal events, and the results of programmed electrical stimulation.

Large follow-up studies assessing the recurrence of sudden death in patients who had experienced a cardiac arrest indicate that the recurrence rate is quite high, approximately 30% at 1 year and 45% at 2 years.[21,22] While these studies did not separately analyze the outcome of patients with idiopathic dilated cardiomyopathy, it would be reasonable to suggest that prior cardiac arrest is the strongest risk factor for recurrent sudden death in this population.

Left ventricular (LV) dysfunction in the presence of ventricular arrhythmia has been reported to have a strong association with sudden cardiac death.[6,7,9,23,24] Others, however, have raised doubts about the relationship of ambulatory asymptomatic ventricular arrhythmias to sudden death.[25,26] While depressed LV function appears to be a strong prognosticator of sudden death in this population, most of the reports in the literature suggest that the presence of high-grade ventricular arrhythmia, especially ventricular couplets and runs of VTs, is independently associated with a higher incidence of sudden death.

The use of programmed electrical stimulation to assess the risk of arrhythmic death in patients with idiopathic dilated cardiomyopathy is controversial.[8,27–33] Most studies have found that the absence of inducible arrhythmias does not confer protection from sudden death in this population. The reason for this finding may relate to the changing substrate for malignant ventricular arrhythmias in this population. The varying contribution from electrolyte disturbances, neurohormonal abnormalities, LV filling pressures, stress, dilation, and progressive scarring may all contribute to the substrate for arrhythmias, making predictions based on a test at a single time less useful. However, several studies indicate that the presence of inducible arrhythmias correlates with the later occurrence of clinical sustained arrhythmia[30] and their suppression with drugs or devices is associated with a low incidence of subsequent sudden death.[27,28,32,33] Others, however, were unable to detect a beneficial effect in patients who had drug suppression of inducible ventricular tachyarrhythmias.[31]

Syncope in this patient population may be a particularly poor prognostic sign, even in the absence of documented sustained cardiac arrhythmia. A recent report indicated that patients with idiopathic dilated cardiomyopathy who presented with syncope had a high incidence of sudden death (44% sudden death survival in 4 years) despite the absence of inducible VT during electrophysiological testing.[34] In fact, those patients who appeared to be at the highest risk because of the clinical occurrence of sustained VT not amenable to drug therapy fared quite well, as they were treated with implantable defibrillators (no sudden death mortality).[35] In these reports, it was clear that the absence of inducible ventricular tachyarrhythmias did not confer protection from sudden death in patients who presented with syncope. These patients were at high risk, and the only available therapy that appeared effective would be an implanted device.

THERAPEUTIC CONSIDERATIONS

Some general principles should be kept in mind when considering medical therapy of patients with nonischemic dilated cardiomyopathy. Electrolyte disturbances should be closely monitored during diuretic therapy to prevent arrhythmias that may arise from hypokalemia and depressed serum magnesium levels. Metabolic and renal functions may be depressed due to low cardiac output. The elimination half-lives of many drugs can be prolonged in these patients. The dosages of antiarrhythmic drugs and other drugs that may have an arrhythmic toxic effect should be properly adjusted and monitored to lessen their proarrhythmic potential. Anticoagulation should be considered in all patients in whom ventricular function is sufficiently depressed to increase the risk for thromboembolic events, especially if they have atrial fibrillation. Aside from reducing the risk for stroke and other peripheral embolic complications, such therapy may reduce the risk for embolic myocardial infarction or ischemia, which can be a cause of sudden death in this patient population.

Patients with idiopathic dilated cardiomyopathy who have experienced a sudden death episode not clearly due to a reversible event that can be corrected with a high degree of certainty should undergo electrophysiological testing. If inducible sustained monomorphic tachycardia can be identified, appropriate drug suppression therapy or ablative therapy may be attempted. The response to drug therapy, however, appears to be poor at best, no better than 20%.[28] If a bundle-branch re-entrant tachycardia is identified, right bundle ablation should be effective therapy to prevent recurrence. However, a complete electrophysiological study should be performed after ablation to ensure that other tachycardias are not present but previously obscured by the bundle-branch re-entry. The only therapy for patients with non-bundle-branch re-entrant VT that is not suppressible with antiarrhythmic drugs is an implantable defibrillator. Although there is some risk associated with implantation, these devices appear to offer the best long-term protection against arrhythmic deaths. Patients who have no inducible ventricular tachyarrhythmias after experiencing a cardiac arrest or a sustained episode of VT should be also considered for an implantable defibrillator.

It is much more difficult to make recommendations regarding prophylactic therapy for patients who have not experienced documented, sustained clinical tachycardia. It appears from the data mentioned earlier regarding patients with syncopal events that they should be considered for an implantable device if other causes of syncope such as excessive doses of vasodilator or diuresis cannot be identified as a cause of the syncopal events. An electrophysiological study should be performed to see if sustained monomorphic VT can be induced and whether it would respond to drug therapy or right bundle ablation. Because absence of inducible VT does not necessarily mean that the patient is not at risk, in the absence of an identified correctable or treatable cause, consideration should be given to implanting a cardioverter-defibrillator.

If a patient falls into the higher-risk category based on poor ventricular function and having high-grade ventricular ectopy but has not experienced a clinical syncopal or sustained tachycardic event, any recommendation for prophylactic therapy is even more problematic. There is no evidence that empirical drug therapy with antiarrhythmic medication reduces the risk for malignant tachyarrhythmic events. Patients with an intraventricular conduction defect on an ECG may be at higher risk for bundle-branch re-entrant VT. An electrophysiology study may demonstrate the ability of this patient's heart to sustain bundle-branch re-entry. Under those circumstances, one may recommend "prophylactic" right bundle ablation. It is reasonable to assign a low risk to this procedure. There is no evidence from several reports in the literature that these patients develop third-degree AV block as a result of such ablation.[17,19,20] Right bundle-branch block is not thought to have significant hemodynamic effects on cardiac function. Therefore, the overall risk of such a procedure should be low and may be justified by the potential for preventing a clinical tachycardia. If other types of rapid monomorphic VT could be induced with programmed stimulation, treatment with antiarrhythmic drugs or an implantable device would be more problematic. Antiarrhythmic drug treatment or device implantation probably carries more risk than a right bundle ablation. Therefore, the benefit of such therapy in a patient who had not experienced any clinical event would be more questionable.

SUMMARY

Arrhythmic deaths are a major cause of mortality in patients with idiopathic dilated cardiomyopathy. Patients who have demonstrated sustained clinical ventricular arrhythmias should be treated with modalities that have a high degree of success. Patients presenting with syncope appear to be at high risk for sudden death, especially if specific reversible causes for the syncope cannot be found. They should also be treated with reliable means. Although risk stratification in asymptomatic patients is helpful for prognostication, the benefits of various therapeutic options that are now available may not outweigh the risks of such therapy. Therefore, a clear recommendation cannot be made for these patients. In evaluating any of these patients for VT, the clinician should pay particular attention to the possibility of bundle-branch re-entry as a mechanism. Up to half of these patients who have inducible monomorphic VTs have this mechanism. The ready availability of a low-risk procedure for treating this entity makes it imperative that this entity be properly identified during electrophysiological studies.

REFERENCES

1. Gillum RF: Idiopathic cardiomyopathy in the United States, 1970–1982. Am Heart J *111*:752–755, 1986.
2. Francis GS: Development of arrhythmias in the patient with congestive heart failure: Pathophysiology, prevalence and prognosis. Am J Cardiol *57*:3B–7B, 1986.
3. Unverferth DV, Magorien RD, Moeschberger ML, Baker PB, Fetters JK, Leier CV: Factors influencing the one-year mortality of dilated cardiomyopathy. Am J Cardiol *54*:147–152, 1984.
4. Fuster V, Gersh BJ, Giuliani ER, Tajik AJ, Brandenburg RO, Frye RL: The natural history of idiopathic dilated cardiomyopathy. Am J Cardiol *47*:525–531, 1981.
5. Franciosa JA, Wilen M, Ziesche S, Cohn JN: Survival in men with severe chronic left ventricular failure due to either coronary heart disease or idiopathic dilated cardiomyopathy. Am J Cardiol *51*:831–836, 1983.
6. Meinertz T, Hofmann T, Kasper W, et al: Significance of ventricular arrhythmias in idiopathic dilated cardiomyopathy. Am J Cardiol *53*:902–907, 1984.
7. Hofmann T, Meinertz T, Kasper W, et al: Mode of death in idiopathic dilated cardiomyopathy: A multivariate analysis of prognostic determinants. Am Heart J *116*:1455–1463, 1988.
8. Meinertz T, Treese N, Kasper W, et al: Determinants of prognosis in idiopathic dilated cardiomyopathy as determined by programmed electrical stimulation. Am J Cardiol *56*:337–341, 1985.
9. Chakko CS, Gheorghiade M: Ventricular arrhythmias in severe heart failure: Incidence, significance, and effectiveness of antiarrhythmic therapy. Am Heart J *109*:497–504, 1985.
10. Goldstein S, Friedman L, Hutchinson R, et al, and the Aspirin Myocardial Infarction Study Group: Timing, mechanism and clinical setting of witnessed deaths in postmyocardial infarction patients. J Am Coll Cardiol *3*:1111–1117, 1984.
11. Nicolic G, Bishop RL, Singh JB: Sudden death recorded during Holter monitoring. Circulation *66*:218–225, 1982.
12. Savage HR, Kissane JQ, Becher EL, Maddocks WQ, Murtaugh JT, Dizadji H: Analysis of ambulatory electrocardiograms in 14 patients who experienced sudden death during monitoring. Clin Cardiol *10*:621–632, 1987.
13. Kempf FC, Josephson ME: Cardiac arrest recorded on ambulatory electrocardiogram. Am J Cardiol *53*:1577–1582, 1984.
14. Luu M, Stevenson WG, Stevenson LW, Baron K, Walden J: Diverse mechanisms of unexpected cardiac arrest in advanced heart failure. Circulation *80*:1675–1680, 1989.
15. Tchou P, Atassi K, Jazayeri M, McKinnie J, Avitall B, Akhtar M: Etiology of polymorphic ventricular tachycardia in the absence of prolonged QT. J Am Coll Cardiol *13(2)*:21A, 1989.
16. Avitall B, McKinnie J, Jazayeri M, Akhtar M, Tchou P: Induction of ventricular fibrillation versus monomorphic ventricular tachycardia during programmed stimulation: Role of premature beat conduction delay. Circulation [in press].
17. Tchou P, Jazayeri M, Denker S, Dongas J, Akhtar M: Transcatheter electrical ablation of right bundle branch: A method of treating macro-reentrant ventricular tachycardia due to bundle branch reentry. Circulation *78*:246–257, 1988.
18. Akhtar M, Damato AN, Batsford WP, Ogonkelu JB, Ruskin JN: Demonstration of reentry within the His-Purkinje system in man. Circulation *50*:1150, 1974.
19. Caceres J, Jazayeri M, McKinnie J, et al: Sustained bundle branch reentry as a mechanism of clinical tachycardia. Circulation *79*:256–270, 1989.
20. Cohen TJ, Chien WW, Lurie KG, et al: Ra-

diofrequency catheter ablation for treatment of bundle branch reentrant tachycardia: Results and long-term follow-up. J Am Coll Cardiol 18:1767–1773, 1991.
21. Liberthson RR, Nagel EL, Hirschman JC, Nussenfeld SR: Prehospital ventricular fibrillation: Prognosis and follow-up course. N Engl J Med 291:317–321, 1974.
22. Myerburg RJ, Conde CA, Sung RJ, et al: Clinical, electrophysiologic, and hemodynamic profile of patients resuscitated from prehospital cardiac arrest. Am J Med 60: 568–576, 1980.
23. Fowler MB, Schroeder JS, Stevenson WG, Dracup KA, Fond V: Poor survival of patients with idiopathic cardiomyopathy considered too well for transplantation. Am J Med 83:871–876, 1987.
24. Holmes J, Kubo SH, Cody RJ, Kligfield P: Arrhythmias in ischemic and nonischemic dilated cardiomyopathy: Prediction of mortality by ambulatory electrocardiography. Am J Cardiol 55:146–151, 1985.
25. Packer M: Lack of relation between ventricular arrhythmias and sudden death in patients with chronic heart failure. Circulation 85(suppl I):150–156, 1992.
26. Von Olshausen K, Schafer A, Mehmel HC, Schwarz F, Senges J, Kubler W: Ventricular arrhythmias in idiopathic dilated cardiomyopathy. Br Heart J 51:195–201, 1984.
27. Naccarelli GV, Prystowsky EN, Jackman WM, Heger JJ, Rahilly GT, Zipes DP: Role of electrophysiologic testing in managing patients who have ventricular tachycardia unrelated to coronary artery disease. Am J Cardiol 50:165–171, 1982.
28. Poll DS, Marchlinski FE, Buxton AE, Josephson ME: Usefulness of programmed stimulation in idiopathic dilated cardiomyopathy. Am J Cardiol 58:992–997, 1986.
29. Das SK, Morady F, DiCarlo L, et al: Prognostic usefulness of programmed ventricular stimulation in idiopathic dilated cardiomyopathy without symptomatic ventricular arrhythmias. Am J Cardiol 58:998–1000, 1986.
30. Poll DS, Marchlinski FE, Buxton AE, Doherty JU, Waxman HL, Josephson ME: Sustained ventricular tachycardia in patients with idiopathic dilated cardiomyopathy: Electrophysiologic testing and lack of response to antiarrhythmic drug therapy. Circulation 70:451–456, 1984.
31. Milner PG, Dimarco JP, Lerman BB: Electrophysiological evaluation of sustained ventricular tachyarrhythmias in idiopathic dilated cardiomyopathy. PACE 11:562–568, 1988.
32. Rae AP, Spielman SC, Kutalek SP, Kay HR, Horowitz LN: Electrophysiologic assessment of antiarrhythmic drug efficacy for ventricular tachyarrhythmias associated with dilated cardiomyopathy. Am J Cardiol 59:291–295, 1987.
33. Liem LB, Swerdlow CD: Value of electropharmacologic testing in idiopathic dilated cardiomyopathy and sustained ventricular tachyarrhythmias. Am J Cardiol 62:611–616, 1988.
34. Tchou PJ, Krebs AC, Sra J, et al: Syncope: A warning sign of sudden death in idiopathic dilated cardiomyopathy patients. J Am Coll Cardiol 17:196A, 1991.
35. Tchou PJ, Krebs AC, Axtell K, et al: Implantable defibrillators: Antiarrhythmic therapy of choice in high risk patients with dilated cardiomyopathy. J Am Coll Cardiol 17:351A, 1991.

11

Mechanisms of Sudden Death in Patients with Hypertrophic Cardiomyopathy

KELLEY P. ANDERSON

Although reports of a disorder that might now be classified as hypertrophic cardiomyopathy appeared as early as 1869,[1,2] its recognition as a clinical entity occurred with the descriptions of Brock in 1957[3] and Teare in 1958.[4] Its association with sudden death was established with Teare's series of nine patients, eight of whom had died suddenly.[4] More than 30 years later sudden death in patients with hypertrophic cardiomyopathy remains a major problem because its occurrence is unpredictable and practical methods of preventing it have not been identified. Indeed, the list of potential causes has lengthened during this period of great technological strides in the detection of genetic, metabolic, and electrophysiological abnormalities.

INCIDENCE

Hypertrophic cardiomyopathy is defined by the absence of left ventricular (LV) dilation and the presence of myocardial hypertrophy that is not due to another recognized cause of hypertrophy such as systemic hypertension or aortic stenosis.[5] The breadth of this definition, the lack of pathognomonic sign, and the fact that many patients are asymptomatic confound estimation of its incidence.[6] Codd et al[7] found the age- and sex-adjusted incidence to be 2.5/100,000 person-years based on data obtained in Olmsted County, Minnesota. The 95% confidence interval was 1.4 to 3.7 per 100,000 person-years, and the population prevalence in this study was 19.7/100,000. The prevalence in Iceland was estimated to be 33/100,000.[8] Two studies using echocardiography as a screening tool estimated prevalences of 830/100,000 in the United States[9] and 170/100,000 in Japan.[10] Studies involving primarily patients referred to centers with a special interest in hypertrophic cardiomyopathy have reported mortalities of 2–4% per year.[11–14] Most of the deaths in these studies were sudden, the percentages varying from 50 to 90%. Despite this relatively low incidence, hypertrophic cardiomyopathy retains a high profile because it is a common cause of unexpected sudden cardiac death (SCD) in young persons, especially in those engaged in athletic competition.[15–17]

FUNCTIONAL AND STRUCTURAL ABNORMALITIES

It is generally acknowledged that there may be several mechanisms of sudden death in patients with hypertrophic cardiomyopathy. Hypertrophic cardiomyopathy is remarkable in that it seems to encompass almost every disturbance known to participate in the genesis of fatal arrhythmias. It should be recognized that although the factors presented here are separated for the purpose of exposition, they are highly interrelated and in some cases represent different aspects of the same phenomenon.

Cellular Function

Calcium Ion Regulation

Gwathmey et al[18] observed that relaxation from peak tension was markedly prolonged in myocardial tissue samples from patients with hypertrophic cardiomyopathy. Increasing the external concentration of calcium ion accentuated the difference from the control tissues. In contrast, peak tension was greater in the hypertrophic tissue than in controls despite the fact some of the tissue samples were obtained from three patients with hypertrophic cardiomyopathy and end-stage congestive heart failure. However, when the temperature of the tissue bath was increased from 30° C to 38° C and the stimulation frequency was increased from 20/min to 60/min or greater, the active tension was lower and end-diastolic tension increased. This suggests that systolic and diastolic function would be worsened at rapid heart rates. Intracellular calcium ion concentration was measured with the intracellular bioluminescent indicator aequorin, which emits light when it combines with calcium ions (a "transient") as the muscle twitches. The calcium ion transient recorded from control tissue consisted of a single component that rose rapidly to a peak and declined to the baseline. In trabeculae from patients with hypertrophic cardiomyopathy, the falling phase of the transient was very prolonged and appeared to consist of two components, an initial decline (L_1) followed by a much more gradual decline toward baseline (L_2). When the rate of stimulation was increased, the amplitude of the transient and of the twitch increased in normal and hypertrophic tissue, indicating an increase in intracellular calcium ion concentration. But because of the slower decline of the transient in tissue from patients with hypertrophic cardiomyopathy, there was fusion of transients and twitches that resulted in higher end-diastolic intracellular calcium and tension. These findings suggest that calcium ion movement is disturbed in patients with hypertrophic cardiomyopathy, and that the abnormalities are associated with diastolic dysfunction. The addition of a digitalis glycoside aggravated the decline in active tension and the increment of end-diastolic tension with higher stimulation rates. Verapamil decreased the amplitude of the aequorin signal and the twitch, indicating a reduction in peak intracellular calcium ion concentration and a negative inotropic effect. Verapamil also prevented the rise in end-diastolic tension at higher pacing rates. Gwathmey et al concluded that there is a failure of calcium ion homeostasis in ventricular tissue from patients with hypertrophic cardiomyopathy, and that there is cytosolic calcium ion overload that is in part responsible for abnormalities of diastolic function. The cause of the abnormality in calcium metabolism could not be determined in this study. Of interest, the authors found no difference between tissue obtained from right and left ventricles, which suggests that the changes were diffuse and not solely due to hemodynamic stresses occurring in the LV.

A possible mechanism of increased intracellular calcium ion concentration is suggested by reports of increased density of voltage-sensitive calcium channels in the sarcolemma of myocardial cells in patients with hypertrophic cardiomyopathy.[19,20] A large body of evidence from animal models supports the findings of disturbed calcium ion movement in myocardial hypertrophy.[21-24] Abnormal calcium currents may be responsible for arrhythmias due to triggered automaticity.[25-27] In addition, elevations in intracellular calcium can impede intercellular electrical transmission and slow propagation.[28] It should be noted that the patients from whom tissue was obtained for these studies were undergoing operation for symptomatic disease, so it is not known if calcium regulation is abnormal in other groups of patients with hypertrophic cardiomyopathy.

Other Aspects of Cellular Electrophysiology

Action potential duration (APD) is prolonged in tissue from patients with hypertrophic cardiomyopathy,[18,29] which may be a cause or consequence of abnormal calcium ion regulation. Prolongation of repolarization is thought to be antiarrhythmic.[30] On the other hand, nonuniform distribution of changes in APD has been identified in other forms of hypertrophy[31-33] and could promote re-entry.[34] A number of other abnormalities have been demonstrated in animal models of myocardial hypertrophy, including reduced action potential upstroke velocity,[35] reduced membrane potential,[36,37] abnormal function of sodium-potassium ATPase,[37] and altered passive electrical properties.[38]

Cardiac Morphology

Fibrosis and Myocyte Disarray

The bizarre histological appearance of the myocardium is a hallmark of hypertrophic cardiomyopathy.[4,39-41] There are great variations in the sizes and shapes of the cardiac myocytes.[40] Myocytes and bundles of myocytes are malaligned,[4,39-41] and fibrosis may be extensive.[39-42] These changes may be partly responsible for abnormalities in systolic and diastolic dysfunction in hypertrophic cardiomyopathy.[39,41] However, the electrophysiological effects of the abnormal myocardial architecture may be of even greater significance for the problem of sudden death. All of these changes are likely to result in deviations from uniform anisotropic propagation, which requires the parallel arrangement of myocardial fibers, a normal distribution of gap junctions, and a normal geometry of the extracellular space. Maron and coworkers observed multiple intercalated disks that were markedly convoluted in patients with hypertrophic cardiomyopathy and other forms of hypertrophy.[40,43] Factor et al[41] performed detailed histological studies of the distribution of connective tissue in ventricular septal tissue removed at operation for obstructive hypertrophic cardiomyopathy and from tissue obtained from two patients who died suddenly. The average collagen content of tissue from patients with hypertrophic cardiomyopathy was considerably greater than in hypertrophies resulting from other disorders and in nonhypertrophied hearts. Increases at all levels of the connective tissue matrix were demonstrated. Of particular interest was the finding of extensive pericellular connective tissue that appeared to encase individual myocytes in a "dense weave of connective tissue."[41] The implication of these findings for intercellular electrical coupling is unclear. However, Spach and colleagues[44,45] have extensively investigated the relation between the distribution of connective tissue and myocardial propagation. Their work in human atrial tissue and in atrial and ventricular tissue from animals indicates that the collagenous septa that course between myocytes and muscle bundles create discontinuities in the spread of activation and can decrease the effective conduction velocity to very low values in the direction transverse to fiber orientation.[44,45] They have shown that the presence of extensive collagenous tissue is associated with loss of electrical coupling between myocytes and bundles,[46] and that these alterations can create sufficient nonuniformity of propagation for re-entry to occur.[45,46] Nonuniform activation has been associated with increased fibrous tissue in other forms of human cardiomyopathy,[47] and the electrical activation sequence has been shown to be disturbed in hypertrophic cardiomyopathic hearts,[48,49] but detailed studies relating myocardial structure and electrical activation in hypertrophic cardiomyopathic tissue have not been reported. Obliteration of electrical connections between myocytes by infiltration of fibrous tissue could also affect recovery of excitability. Burgess et al[50] demonstrated that nonuniform activation produces alterations in repolarization that could increase dispersion of repolarization, and Lesh et al showed that a loss of electrotonic activity due to uncoupling of myocytes can "unmask" dispersion of repolarization.[51]

In addition to the changes present at a microscopic level, some patients demonstrate large confluent areas of scar tissue[39,40,52] that could create an anatomical obstacle around which re-entry could occur. This may be the mechanism of the ventricular tachycardia (VT) that occurs in a distinctive group of patients with the triad of midventricular hypertrophy, apical aneurysm, and sustained monomorphic VT.[53-56]

Myocardial Mass

Massive myocardial hypertrophy is sometimes observed in patients with hypertrophic cardiomyopathy who die suddenly. An intriguing question is whether increased LV mass per se predisposes to arrhythmias. Although cardiac hypertrophy in a number of disorders is associated with an increased risk of sudden death,[57] it would be difficult to dissociate the effects of myocardial mass and various other abnormalities in structure and function. Nevertheless, experimental and theoretical work has shown that the mass of normal myocardium is positively related to the ability to induce and sustain fibrillation.[58-62]

Myocardial Perfusion

Myocardial hypertrophy usually is not accompanied by a proportional increase in capillaries, so the distance over which nutrients and metabolites must diffuse is increased.[63] Since diffusion is driven by concentration gradients, the partial pressure of oxygen will be lower and the concentration of potentially toxic metabolites will be higher at cells farther from capillaries. Extramural coronary disease appears to follow the normal age and sex distribution, but intramural coronary arteries are often abnormal in patients of all ages with hypertrophic cardiomyopathy, including infants.[52,64-66] Morphological studies reveal thickening of the arterial walls due to intimal and medial thickening and narrow lumina.[52,64-66] In some cases these abnormalities are associated with fibrosis,[64] and in some cases abnormal vessels appear to supply the sinus node, atrioventricular (AV) node, or His bundle.[65,66]

Evidence for myocardial ischemia in patients with hypertrophic cardiomyopathy without epicardial coronary artery disease includes stress-related angina pectoris,[67-69] ST-segment abnormalities,[67,69,70] thallium-201 imaging defects,[70,71] changes in positron emission tomography,[72] reduced great cardiac vein flow,[67-70] decreased lactate consumption,[67-70] and diastolic dysfunction.[68-70] The capacity to increase myocardial flow in response to demand is clearly limited in patients with hypertrophic cardiomyopathy. In the patients with hypertrophic cardiomyopathy reported by Cannon et al,[68] myocardial flow increased as the heart rate was increased by pacing to 130 beats/min, but average flow actually decreased as the rate was increased to 150 beats/min, in contrast to a group of control patients in whom flow continued to increase with more rapid pacing rates. The failure to increase flow at more rapid pacing rates in the patients with hypertrophic cardiomyopathy was accompanied by complaints of chest pain, metabolic evidence of myocardial ischemia, and elevation of LV end-diastolic pressure. These findings were present in patients with and without obstruction to LV outflow. Myocardial oxygen consumption and coronary blood flow were higher in the patients with obstruction, and lactate production and clinical evidence of ischemia occurred at lower pacing rates in this group.[69] However, myocardial ischemia occurred at lower coronary flow and lower myocardial oxygen consumption in the group without obstruction, suggesting more severely impaired myocardial perfusion.

The precise mechanisms by which myocardial ischemia causes arrhythmias are controversial,[73] but there is no doubt that where a potential for ischemia exists, there is a high likelihood of fatal arrhythmias. Furthermore, degrees of ischemia that might be insignificant in normal myocardium could prove fatal by exacerbating preexisting electrophysiological or hemodynamic abnormalities. One possible common target is the intracellular calcium ion concentration, which tends to rise in response to ischemia,[74,75] an effect that is suspected to be partly responsible for the alterations in contractile function and arrhythmias associated with ischemia.[73-75] The threshold for these effects might be lessened and the time course shortened if calcium ion regulation is already disturbed as described above. Myocardial ischemia is also an important focal point for positive feedback because its effects on systolic and diastolic function[76] will tend to reduce myocardial perfusion further. However, ascertaining the role of ischemia in the process of sudden death is complicated by the fact that it is likely to be part of the final common pathway no matter which factors initiate the process.

Hemodynamic Factors

Left Ventricular Outflow Tract Obstruction

Obstruction to LV outflow is present in about 25% of patients with hypertrophic cardiomyopathy who present for medical evaluation.[39,77] It is another point where positive feedback could occur because obstruction can cause systemic hypotension that, in turn, exacerbates obstruction by reducing LV cavity size and by increasing sympathetic activity.[39,78]

Diastolic Dysfunction

Diastolic dysfunction is present in a large proportion of patients with hypertrophic cardiomyopathy[39,78] and results from a combination of passive (e.g., fibrosis and myocyte disarray) and active abnormalities (e.g., calcium ion movement) and loading conditions.[39] Prolongation of the time required for ventricular filling impairs the ability to maintain cardiac output during tachycardia, while even modest increases in heart rate result in sufficient ischemia to worsen diastolic function.[68,69] This too is a potential focus for positive feedback because reduced diastolic filling can compromise cardiac output and increased diastolic filling pressures can enhance subendocardial ischemia.[68] The reduction in cardiac output could lower myocardial perfusion and increase sympathetic activity and heart rate, which would increase myocardial oxygen requirements, and so on. In addition, high atrial pressures and atrial dilation resulting from reduced ventricular compliance could promote atrial tachyarrhythmias or result in the release of vasodepressor hormones.[79]

Peripheral Vasodilation

Frenneaux et al[80] reported abnormal blood pressure responses during exercise in a group of patients with hypertrophic cardiomyopathy. The authors measured systolic blood pressure during treadmill exercise testing in 129 patients with hypertrophic cardiomyopathy. Four patterns of blood pressure response were observed: (1) A normal response was observed in 48%, with a linear increase in blood pressure to peak exercise and a decline during recovery. (2) The systolic pressure fell continuously from the first minute of exercise in 4% of patients. (3) The systolic blood pressure initially rose but then fell 20–100 mm Hg during exercise in 29% of the group. (4) In 18% of patients a normal blood pressure response occurred during exercise, but during recovery it fell initially and increased later. Invasive hemodynamic studies were performed in 14 patients with and 14 patients without a normal blood pressure response. Systemic vascular resistance decreased in both groups at peak exercise, but the fall was greater in the abnormal group. In a subsequent study these authors detected abnormal forearm vasodilation in response to exercise.[81] A drop in systemic and forearm vascular resistances could result from a number of neural or humoral mechanisms,[82,83] but previous investigations suggest that LV stretch receptors mediate this response. In particular, Mark et al[84] found that forearm vascular resistance decreased during lower extremity exercise in patients with aortic stenosis while it increased in patients with mitral valve stenosis or in patients without valvular disease. Moreover, the drop in forearm resistance vanished after aortic valve replacement. In animal preparations in which the coronary and systemic circulations were isolated, systemic hypotension occurred in response to increased myocardial contractility produced by intracoronary injection of catecholamines, by electrical stimulation of a sympathetic cardiac nerve, and by obstructing the flow of blood from the LV.[85] These findings indicate that the exercise-related fall in blood pressure observed in some patients with hypertrophic cardiomyopathy probably results from a normal reflex mechanism. The cause of the inappropriate activity of the reflex in patients with hypertrophic cardiomyopathy is unknown, but patients with exercise-induced hypotension were younger and had smaller LV end-diastolic dimensions.[80,81] The resulting hypotension could exacerbate LV outflow tract obstruction or cause myocardial ischemia.[80,86] Johnson originally proposed and elegantly explained this mechanism of sudden death in patients with aortic stenosis.[86]

Neurohumoral Function

Sympathetic Activity

Sympathetic activity is likely to play a central role in the pathophysiology of sudden death in patients with hypertrophic cardiomyopathy because of its direct and indirect effects, which can increase heart rate, contractility, LV outflow obstruction, myocardial oxygen consumption, intracellular calcium concentration, and because it may facilitate both re-entrant and automatic arrhythmias,[87,88] It is not clear that sympathetic function is abnormal in patients with hypertrophic cardiomyopathy. Kawai et al[89] found that the average concentrations of norepinephrine and epinephrine in plasma and myocardial biopsy specimens were no higher than those of a control group without cardiomyopathy, although individual patients with hypertrophic cardiomyopathy had high levels. These findings were corroborated by more recent reports.[90,91] Maisel et al[92] found significantly higher plasma norepinephrine concentrations and greater systemic release rates of this catecholamine, but the high mean age of their patients (63 years) may account for concentrations greater than were found in other studies.[91] Brush et al[90] assessed the uptake and release of norepinephrine in the cardiac circulation and found that the percentage of norepinephrine extracted from arterial blood was less in patients with hypertrophic cardiomyopathy, suggesting decreased uptake by cardiac sympathetic nerve endings compared to the control group. However, coronary flow was greater in the patients with hypertrophic cardiomyopathy, so that the rate of uptake (i.e., the amount of norepinephrine per unit of time) was not significantly different between the two groups. Toshima and Koga[91] and Sugishita et al[93] reported increased effects of catecholamine infusions on echocardiographic indices of LV function and concluded that patients with hypertrophic cardiomyopathy have greater sensitivity to catecholamines. However, the smaller cavity sizes present in patients with hypertrophic cardiomyopathy may result in lower wall tension, which could account for greater fractional shortening and larger ejection fractions.[94] Golf et al[95] found that neither β-receptor density, relative amounts of β-receptor subtypes, nor response of adenylate cyclase differed between patients with hypertrophic cardiomyopathy and a group of patients with other forms of cardiac disease. These findings regarding the absence of changes in β-receptor density have been confirmed by others.[19,20] Therefore, although some investigations indicate abnormalities in sympathetic activity in patients with hypertrophic cardiomyopathy, a consistent pattern has not emerged.

Other Neurohumoral Factors

A reflex resulting in inappropriate vasodilation was mentioned earlier. It seems likely that other autonomic and hormonal influences[82,85] participate in the process of sudden death in patients with hypertrophic cardiomyopathy, but definite evidence of abnormalities in these systems is not yet available.

Electrophysiological Findings in the Intact Heart

Sinus Node Dysfunction and Atrioventricular Block

Abnormalities in the sinus node or in the AV conduction system could cause bradyarrhythmias. Morphological abnormalities in these structures have been detected in patients with hypertrophic cardiomyopathy who died suddenly.[65,66] Spontaneous abnormalities of sinus node function or AV block are not commonly recorded on long-term ECG monitoring in patients with hypertrophic cardiomyopathy.[13,96-102] However, abnormalities of sinus node function are often observed at electrophysiological study; 7% of the patients studied by Fananapazir et al[103] had elevated sinus node recovery times and 66% had long sinoatrial conduction times. Abnormalities of AV conduction are also common.[104] Fananapazir et al[103] found that 6% of patients had atrial-His (AH) intervals greater than 120 msec, 4% had refractory periods of the AV node greater than 450 msec, and 6% had Wenckebach cycle lengths greater than 500 msec. Thirty percent had His bundle-ventricular (HV) intervals greater than 55 msec, and in six patients the HV interval increased or infranodal block was observed in response to atrial pacing.

Supraventricular Arrhythmias

The importance of supraventricular arrhythmias has become increasingly apparent because elevated heart rates cause myocardial ischemia and because the ability of the hypertrophied heart to maintain cardiac output during tachycardia is limited. Long-term ambulatory ECG recordings reveal atrial premature complexes in most patients and episodes of supraventricular tachycardia in about 15–30% of patients.[96,97,100,102,105] About 5% of patients with hypertrophic cardiomyopathy referred to medical centers have atrial fibrillation (AF), and about 10% more develop AF during follow-up.[106] A small percentage of patients may have additional conditions that may predispose to supraventricular tachyarrhythmias or rapid ventricular response rates such as accessory AV connections or facile AV nodal conduction.[102-104,107]

Ventricular Arrhythmias

Spontaneous nonsustained ventricular arrhythmias are of interest because they may initiate or be markers of a predisposition to sustained ventricular tachyarrhythmias. Over 80% of patients with hypertrophic cardiomyopathy who undergo ambulatory ECG monitoring have ventricular arrhythmias,[96,98,101,108] although the prevalence is lower in younger patients.[102,109] Nonsustained VT, i.e., three or more consecutive ventricular beats, is present in 8–32% of patients.[96,98,99,101,102,108,110] The etiology of ventricular ectopic activity is not known. The arrhythmias show no particular relation to activity and are as frequent and as complex during sleep.[96] Although exercise testing appears to "provoke" ventricular arrhythmias in some cases, it is generally acknowledged that the arrhythmias that occur at exercise rarely exceed the frequency or grade of arrhythmias that occur spontaneously during the day or night.[96,98,108] ST-segment depression during exercise testing is not associated with arrhythmias.[96] McKenna et al[108] found that the administration of drugs that block β-adrenergic receptors did not significantly affect the prevalence of ventricular arrhythmias during ambulatory ECG monitoring or exercise testing despite substantial reductions in the heart rates at rest and during maximum exercise. Investigators who have produced ischemia in patients with hypertrophic cardiomyopathy by rapid atrial pacing[70,111,112] or catecholamine administration[70,91,93,111] have not noted the emergence of ventricular ectopic activity. These data suggest that the premature ventricular beats and runs of nonsustained VT commonly recorded in patients with hypertrophic cardiomyopathy are not directly caused by myocardial ischemia, sympathetic activity, or acute hemodynamic stresses related to exertion. Ventricular ectopic activity bears no relation to sex, severity of symptoms, presence of obstruction, LV diastolic cavity dimension, or LV end-diastolic pressure.[96,108,109,113] Several studies have reported an association between the presence of nonsustained VT and the degree of ventricular hypertrophy,[96,109,113] but other investigations have not confirmed such an association.[101,108]

Sustained ventricular tachyarrhythmias can be induced with programmed electrical stimulation in a high percentage of patients with hypertrophic cardiomyopathy. Anderson et al[114] induced sustained polymorphic VT or VF in 82% of 17 patients with obstructive hypertrophic cardiomyopathy undergoing myotomy-myectomy; only one had had a previous cardiac arrest. The arrhythmias remained inducible after the initiation of cardiopulmonary bypass, suggesting that the arrhythmias were not related to an immediately reversible effect of outflow tract obstruction. An identical stimulation protocol did not induce a sustained arrhythmia in five patients undergoing operation for severe coronary artery disease without previous myocardial damage, which suggested that the induced arrhythmias were not caused by myocardial ischemia. Geibel et al[115] studied a broader cross section of patients with hypertrophic cardiomyopathy and induced sustained ventricular arrhythmias in 59% of 22 patients, only three of whom had had prior cardiac arrests. Fananapazir et al[103] induced sustained ventricular arrhythmias in 43% of 155 patients; 22 had had previous cardiac arrests. The clinical significance of the induced arrhythmias is hotly debated.[103,115-117] However, it is clear that sustained ventricular tachyarrhythmias can be induced in patients with hypertrophic cardiomyopathy more readily than in other groups of patients,[118] which at least suggests heightened vulnerability to ventricular arrhythmias.

PREDICTORS AND ASSOCIATED FACTORS

Only a few of the large number of potential factors have been associated positively or negatively with sudden death in patients with hypertrophic cardiomyopathy with sufficient consistency to provide some degree of confidence in their contribution. Almost all studies show that sudden death occurs more commonly in patients less than 30 years old.[11-13,119,120] McKenna et al[12] reported an annual mortality of 5.9% in patients less than 15 years old and an annual mortality of 2.5% in adults. In some studies the ages of the sudden death victims were higher than those of the survivors,[97,121] but against the weight of other series, these findings indicate that the risk of sudden death in older patients is not trivial.

A higher risk of sudden death in patients with a family history of hypertrophic cardiomyopathy and sudden death has been repeatedly observed by McKenna and colleagues,[12,97,102,122] but not in some other studies.[11,120] However, the existence of families in which several members have hypertrophic cardiomyopathy and succumb suddenly supports the importance of this factor.[123-125]

A particular form of hypertrophic cardiomyopathy characterized by hypertrophy of the apical portion of the septum, deep negative T waves, and a spadelike shape on the left ventricular angiogram is associated with a low risk of sudden death.[14,120,126-133] This variety of hypertrophic cardiomyopathy, which is common in Japan but rare in Western countries, may have a distinct etiology.[133]

Nonsustained VT identified patients who subsequently died suddenly in early studies of ambulatory monitoring. Defined as three or more consecutive ventricular beats, nonsustained VT was detected by Maron et al[13] in only 19% of the entire group of patients with hypertrophic cardiomyopathy, but in four of six patients who died suddenly or had a cardiac arrest. The annual risk of sudden death in the patients with VT was 8.6%, compared to 1.0% in the patients without VT. Very similar results were published by McKenna et al[97]: five of seven patients who died suddenly had had VT on ECG monitoring, while only 24% of survivors had the finding. The predictive value of nonsustained VT has not been confirmed by more recent studies, in part because treatment was affected by the early results. In a subsequent study of young patients, McKenna et al[102] treated all patients with nonsustained VT with amiodarone, and none died suddenly. Nevertheless, 7 of 53 patients still died suddenly or had a cardiac arrest, and no factors or combination of factors could distinguish this group from the survivors. Spirito et al[134] reported no sudden deaths in a group of patients with hypertrophic cardiomyopathy with characteristics similar to other studies, including a 24% prevalence of nonsustained VT. Nonsustained VT was a poor predictor of cardiac arrest in another recent study.[103]

Most studies found no consistent association between sudden death and sex,[11,13,119,120] New York Heart Association functional class, or symptoms such as dyspnea, angina, dizziness, or syncope,[11,13,119,120] although McKenna et al[12] reported that a history of syncope and severe dyspnea at last follow-up visit occurred more frequently in patients who died suddenly than in survivors. The assessment of hemodynamic variables showed that neither the presence of a gradient to LV outflow nor its magnitude bore a discernible relation to sudden death.[12,97,102,119,120] Victims of sudden death had higher LV end-diastolic pressures in at least two studies,[97,120] but this was not noted by others.[12,102,119] A large LV end-diastolic volume and a small end-systolic volume were found to have independent predictive value in one study.[135] Left ventricular hypertrophy was reported to be greater in patients with hypertrophic cardiomyopathy who died suddenly.[136] In other studies neither ventricular septal nor posterior wall thickness was significantly greater in patients who died suddenly than in survivors, although a trend was sometimes described.[97,102,120] Analysis of findings on the 12-lead ECG, including the presence of AF, QRS duration, left axis deviation, voltage, and QT interval, did not identify patients who died suddenly.[12,119,120] Ambulatory ECG monitoring has been useful because of the detection of nonsustained VT. Also, sudden death victims tend to have more frequent single and paired premature ventricular complexes.[97] However, neither atrial premature complexes nor episodes of supraventricular arrhythmias have been found to be of prognostic value.[97]

EFFECTS OF MEDICAL AND OPERATIVE TREATMENT

No well-controlled trials of preventing sudden death have been published, but some information has been gathered by comparing the treatments administered to victims of sudden death and survivors. Treatment with β-adrenergic-receptor blockers and calcium ion antagonists does not prevent sudden death.[11–13,97,102,119,137] Myotomy-myectomy and mitral valve replacement in patients with hypertrophic cardiomyopathy also do not prevent sudden death[11,12,119]; however, a trend for less sudden death has been noted in some studies.[11–13,138,139]

Antiarrhythmic drugs, which include drugs that block sodium channels or potassium channels or both, have not been used in a uniform fashion, which makes assessment of efficacy very unreliable. In several studies patients died suddenly during treatment with various antiarrhythmic drugs, including quinidine, disopyramide, mexiletine, and procainamide.[13,137,140–142] In addition, proarrhythmic effects have been reported with disopyramide, sotalol, and flecainide.[143–145]

The use of amiodarone in patients with hypertrophic cardiomyopathy is highly controversial. McKenna and colleagues[110,137,146,147] reported administration of amiodarone to patients with hypertrophic cardiomyopathy at high risk for sudden death, including patients with nonsustained VT, supraventricular tachycardia due to the Wolff-Parkinson-White syndrome, AF, recurrent syncope, or a family history of hypertrophic cardiomyopathy and multiple sudden deaths. None of the patients who received amiodarone died suddenly, which was a significant improvement over the sudden death rate in an earlier series of patients treated with other antiarrhythmic drugs.[137] The observations of other investigators have been less encouraging. Fananapazir et al[148] administered amiodarone to 50 patients with hypertrophic cardiomyopathy. Nonsustained VT was eliminated in 19 of 21 patients who received amiodarone. Nevertheless, during a mean follow-up period of 2.2 years eight patients died, seven suddenly, and six of the deaths occurred within the first 5 months of amiodarone treatment, suggesting a proarrhythmic effect.[148,149] None of the patients who died had had nonsustained VT on ECG monitoring after the initiation of amiodarone. Others have reported cardiac arrests despite amiodarone therapy, including one instance in which VF was documented at the onset of collapse.[142,150]

EVIDENCE FOR AND AGAINST THE CONTRIBUTION OF SPECIFIC FACTORS TO SUDDEN DEATH

The inability to demonstrate a relation between a factor or treatment and sudden death does not mean, of course, that the factor does not participate in the pathogenesis of sudden death or that the treatment is not effective, for several reasons: (1) The presence or contribution of a factor may be obscured by a limited ability to detect or measure it. Contractility, for instance, has a well-recognized relationship to arrhythmia vulnerability,[151] but measurements used to estimate it such as ejection fraction and fractional shortening are affected by loading conditions, wall thickness, and the like, which may not be directly related to contractility. (2) The statistical power of the investigation may be inadequate due to small sample sizes, few end points, and large variances in clinical variables, all characteristic of studies of sudden death in hypertrophic cardiomyopathy. Few studies have offered any analysis of statistical power, and usually all factors are analyzed together, as if the statistical power were equal. (3) The contribution of a factor may vary between individuals. If, for instance, obstruction to LV flow had a predominant contribution in some patients while ischemia predominated in others, the lack of obstruction in the "ischemic" group could result in the failure to detect obstruction as an important mechanism of death. (4) The presence or amplitude of a factor may change between the time of measurement and the time of sudden death or cardiac arrest. (5) Interventions may neutralize, mask, or accentuate the contribution of a factor. Finally, it should be emphasized that although none of the therapies mentioned above completely prevents sudden death, none has been subjected to a rigorous clinical trial, so the possibility that any or all of them reduce the risk of sudden death should not be discounted. With the reliability of the available information thus qualified, it is appropriate at this point to review the evidence for or against the contribution of specific factors to the process of sudden death.

Calcium Ion Regulation

There is no direct evidence for involvement of abnormal calcium ion regulation since such measurements are difficult to obtain. The fact that calcium ion antagonists do not prevent sudden death[120,122,152] and the fact that diastolic dysfunction has not been noted to have a major effect[135,140] do not favor a predominant role for this factor. On the other hand, it has been reported that verapamil treatment is associated with fewer sudden deaths than therapy with β-adrenergic-blocking agents.[152]

Prolonged Action Potential Duration

Studies that include direct measurements of APD and its effects on risk of sudden death are not yet available. The QT interval was prolonged in some patients with hypertrophic cardiomyopathy,[140] but no differences have been reported between patients who died suddenly and others.[12,119]

Myocyte Disarray and Fibrosis

Sufficient histological data are generally not available from survivors to make comparisons with autopsy findings in victims of sudden death. However, isolated observations are suggestive. Transmural infarction was identified in a patient who died suddenly,[119] and aneurysm formation has been noted in some patients who presented with VT.[53,153] Extensive fibrosis has been noted in several cases of sudden death,[52,125,153,154] including four victims of sudden death who were members of a single family.[125] Numerous foci of disorganized myocardial cells without abnormal fibrosis were observed in a young patient who died suddenly.[124] In contrast, Maron and Roberts[155] found no correlation between the degree of myocardial disorganization and the mode of death (sudden versus chronic decompensation). On the other hand, muscle disorganization was greater in patients less than 18 years old, and in patients who had more than one relative who died suddenly with hypertrophic cardiomyopathy.

Myocardial Mass

Sudden death victims had greater degrees of myocardial hypertrophy than other patients with hypertrophic cardiomyopathy in a few investigations,[136,140,142] but the differences were not always significant.[140] This trend was particularly noticeable when only patients with minimal symptoms at the time of sudden death were considered.[136] However, the range of myocardial masses observed in sudden death victims overlaps with the normal range,[123] and case reports indicate that increased myocardial mass is absent in some patients with sudden death.[124,125]

Myocardial Ischemia

Prolonged hypotension or excessive tachycardia can produce ischemia and VF in a normal heart. For pertinence as a mechanism of sudden death, ischemia should be present at or before the time of collapse or there should be an unusual propensity for ischemia. Several findings do not favor an exclusive role for ischemia. Exertional angina was not more prevalent in patients who died suddenly than in those who did not.[11,12,119] Of course, ischemia could be present without angina. Verapamil prevents silent perfusion abnormalities,[156] but neither calcium ion antagonists[12,97,120,142,152] nor β-adrenergic-blocking agents[11-13,102,119,140,142,152] have been shown to reduce the risk of sudden death. To the contrary, Koga et al[120] found that ST-segment depression in response to exercise testing was present in several patients who died suddenly during exertion. Fananapazir and Epstein reported five patients from a group of 30 cardiac arrest survivors who showed signs of ischemia (ST-segment depression) in response to atrial pacing and treadmill exercise testing and who had reversible perfusion defects with thallium imaging techniques.[141] The presence of extramural coronary disease seems to confer an unusually high risk of sudden death,[140] although most patients who die suddenly do not have extramural coronary disease. Several case reports indicate an important role for ischemia in precipitating malignant ventricular arrhythmias. Stafford et al[157] reported a 15-year-old boy with asymptomatic hypertrophic cardiomyopathy who had a cardiac arrest while jogging. No abnormalities of sinus node function or AV conduction were noted at electrophysiological study, and no ventricular tachyarrhythmias could be induced. However, ST-segment changes were noted during incremental atrial pacing and after initiation of AF, although the average ventricular response rate was less than 200 beats/min. These changes were accompanied by complaints of chest pain and hypotension, and after 100 seconds VF occurred. Several other cases of tachycardia associated with ischemic ST-segment alterations followed by ventricular tachyarrhythmias have been reported.[107,141,158]

The finding that a high proportion of sudden deaths occur during or shortly after vigorous activity could be cited as favoring an ischemic cause.[13,120,121,140] However, there are so many changes during exertion (sympathetic activity, peripheral vasodilation, etc.) that this observation must be considered somewhat nonspecific.

Operative relief of LV outflow tract obstruction has been shown to reduce myocardial oxygen consumption at rest and during atrial pacing and to increase the heart rate at which angina occurs.[112] This, and other changes such as a reduction in outflow tract obstruction itself, are possible mechanisms for decreasing sudden death after surgery. Despite encouraging trends, however, the impact of myotomy-myectomy or mitral valve replacement on the occurrence of sudden death remains equivocal.[11-13,138,139]

Left Ventricular Outflow Tract Obstruction

A gradient to LV outflow is certainly not required for sudden death to occur, nor are sudden death victims more likely to have a gradient, nor is there a correlation of the magnitude of the gradient and risk of sudden death.[12,97,102,119-121,140] Nevertheless, recordings obtained during syncope and sudden death in patients with aortic stenosis underscores the potential importance of obstruction to LV outflow,[159] and a role for obstruction could account, in part, for the trend in improved survival after operation to relieve obstruction. Moreover, measurements of LV outflow tract obstruction at rest or even with provocative maneuvers may not perfectly reflect the degree of obstruction during all the physiological states to which an individual might be subject.

Diastolic Dysfunction

A number of measurements have been used to assess diastolic function. Several studies have not demonstrated significant differences in LV end-diastolic pressure between patients who died suddenly and those who did not,[12,119,140] but in one study a higher risk of sudden death was associated with an LV end-diastolic pressure greater than 20 mm Hg.[120] Newman et al[135] found that a low peak filling rate, as assessed by LV angiography, predicted sudden death. Chikamori et al[122] also found that poor diastolic function as measured by radionuclide angiography was associated with sudden death, but did not improve predictive accuracy over other factors.

Peripheral Vasodilation

Frenneaux, Counihan, and colleagues[80,81] argued that "hemodynamic instability" resulting from inappropriate peripheral vasodilation initiates sudden death in some patients. In their studies 33% of patients with hypertrophic cardiomyopathy had an abnormal blood pressure response to exercise,[80] and 38% had inappropriate forearm vasodilation in response to exercise.[81] Patients with abnormal hemodynamic responses to exercise were significantly younger and more likely to have a family history of hypertrophic cardiomyopathy and sudden death. Eight of the nine patients with a family history of sudden death had abnormal vascular responses and none had an LV outflow tract gradient or severe myocardial hypertrophy.[81] Two patients evaluated after out-of-hospital VF had abnormal results on forearm plethysmography,[81] and three of the patients with abnormal vascular responses died suddenly but did not have other risk factors for sudden death such as ventricular arrhythmias during ECG monitoring. Although these findings are undoubtedly relevant to the problem of sudden death in patients with hypertrophic cardiomyopathy, the degree of blood pressure inadequacy observed in many of the "abnormal" patients does not seem sufficient to cause severe problems. For instance, the mean systolic blood pressure at peak exercise in the patients with "exercise hypotension" (119 ± 35 mm Hg) was quite close to the mean pressure before exercise (118 ± 26 mm Hg).[80] Therefore, as the authors point out, other factors must be involved.

Neurohumoral Dysfunction

Abnormal sympathetic activity has not been related to sudden death in patients with hypertrophic cardiomyopathy. Moreover, drugs that block β-adrenergic receptors do not prevent sudden death.[11–13,102,119,140,142,152] As noted earlier, however, neurohumoral mechanisms probably mediate inappropriate vasodilation during exertion and other effects that could contribute to sudden death.

Sinus Node Dysfunction

James and Marshall[66] found fibrosis or narrowing of the artery to the sinus node in several victims of sudden death. Asystole has been documented at the time of cardiac arrest.[142] In 30 patients who survived a cardiac arrest and underwent electrophysiological study, Fananapazir et al[141] found prolonged sinoatrial conduction times (> 120 msec) in 47%, and a corrected sinus node recovery time greater than 500 msec in one patient. One patient had documented sinus pauses associated with syncope, and two other patients had sinus bradycardia associated with presyncope. Long periods of asystole due to sinus arrest[98] and sinus arrest after exercise testing have been reported.[160] Sinus pauses and bradycardia could also occur in response to changes in autonomic tone despite normal sinus node function.

Atrioventricular Conduction

James and others reported abnormalities of the AV node and the His-Purkinje system in patients with hypertrophic cardiomyopathy who died suddenly.[65,66] Abnormal AV nodal function was observed in 10% of cardiac arrest survivors, and prolonged His to ventricular conduction times or infranodal block in response to atrial stimulation was noted in 23%.[141] Complete heart block associated with syncope or requiring cardiopulmonary resuscitation and emergency pacing have been reported,[161–163] as has a familial pattern of hypertrophic cardiomyopathy and heart block.[164]

Supraventricular Arrhythmias

There is no consistent relationship between sudden death and the presence of atrial premature beats or episodes of supraventricular tachyarrhythmias detected on ECG monitoring,[97] or the presence of AF.[106,120] Among a group of 30 patients with a history of cardiac arrest, 10% had inducible AF, 10% had inducible re-entrant atrial tachycardia, and one patient had inducible re-entrant tachycardia due to an accessory AV connection.[141] On the other hand, several case reports have shown that spontaneous or induced supraventricular tachyarrhythmias could initiate a sequence of events leading to death.[107,141,157,158,165]

Ventricular Arrhythmias

Recordings obtained within minutes of collapse in patients with hypertrophic cardiomyopathy almost always reveal VF,[140,142] but do ventricular arrhythmias initiate the events leading to collapse? Sustained ventricular arrhythmias were induced in 70% of 30 survivors of cardiac arrest,[141] but ventricular tachyarrhythmias can be induced in many patients with hypertrophic cardiomyopathy who have not had spontaneous ventricular tachyarrhythmias.[103,114,115,166] As noted earlier, the presence of nonsustained VT has been associated with sudden death.[13,97] These spontaneous arrhythmias usually have much longer intervals between beats than is usually required to initiate ventricular arrhythmias with programmed stimulation,[97,110,114,115,141,147,166] but it is conceivable that longer coupling intervals could initiate malignant arrhythmias if the site of impulse formation was critically located. That VT is a mechanism of sudden death is strongly suggested by the recording of spontaneous, sustained polymorphic VT in the absence of preceding tachycardia, hypotension, or evident ischemia.[141]

Miscellaneous Factors and Concomitant Disorders

Mechanisms not necessarily related to hypertrophic cardiomyopathy could obviously cause sudden death, including pulmonary embolism, cerebrovascular accidents,[140] anomalous coronary arteries,[167] and accessory connections.[165]

THE PROCESS OF SUDDEN DEATH

Figure 11–1 summarizes our current understanding of sudden death in patients with hypertrophic cardiomyopathy: A rather long list of abnormalities has been detected in patients with this disorder, but it is not yet known how the "dynamical system" of normal and abnormal processes present in an individual with hypertrophic cardiomyopathy are transformed into a system that is not compatible with life. Sudden death could result from a well-defined discrete event such as a pulmonary embolism that blocks cardiac output, but it may also result from a complex interplay of an array of factors. The number of possible interactions between the known list of abnormalities and normal processes that could produce a fatal outcome is large. In addition, sudden death is often temporarily related to some identifiable "stress" such as physical exertion,[140,168,169] which multiples the number of potentially malignant combinations.

Valuable clues have been obtained from individual cases in which physiological data were recorded during an episode of sudden death or cardiac arrest. Zee-Cheng et al,[107] for instance, described a 24-year-old woman who was resuscitated from out-of-hospital VF. The patient was asymptomatic until shortly before collapse, when she experienced chest pain and shortness of breath. An echocardiogram showed marked ventricular septal hypertrophy. An LV outflow tract gradient of 33 mm Hg at rest was detected at cardiac catheterization, but coronary arteries appeared normal. On electrophysiological study there was no evidence of abnormal sinus node function or of delayed AV conduction, although a discontinuous AV refractory curve was present. A ventricular tachyarrhythmia could not be induced. However, ventricular stimulation initiated an AV junctional tachycardia with a rate of 162 beats/min that accelerated to 222 beats/min (Fig. 11–2). During the tachycardia the blood pressure dropped to 60 mm Hg and marked ST-segment deviation was noted on the ECG. Twenty-one seconds after the onset of tachycardia, VF occurred which was converted by a DC shock. An automatic defibrillator was implanted, but since initiation of diltiazem the patient has had no symptomatic recurrences of tachycardia or discharges from the defibrillator during the subsequent 4 years (R. Ruffy, pers. commun.).

If it is assumed that the events observed in the electrophysiology laboratory were similar to the one that resulted in the initial cardiac arrest, then the changes responsible for the cardiac arrest seem logical and straightforward. Nevertheless, it is difficult to assign causality to any particular phenomenon. Obviously, if the supraventricular tachycardia had not occurred, then the

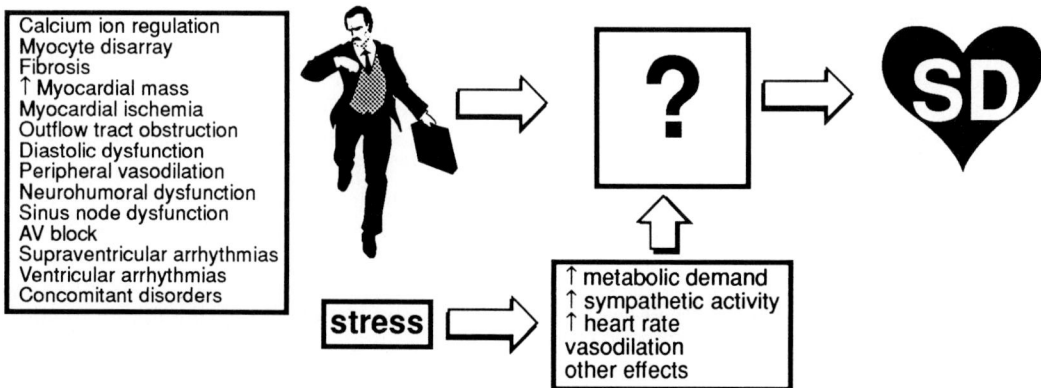

Fig. 11–1. Factors contributing to sudden death (SD) in patients with hypertrophic cardiomyopathy. See text for discussion.

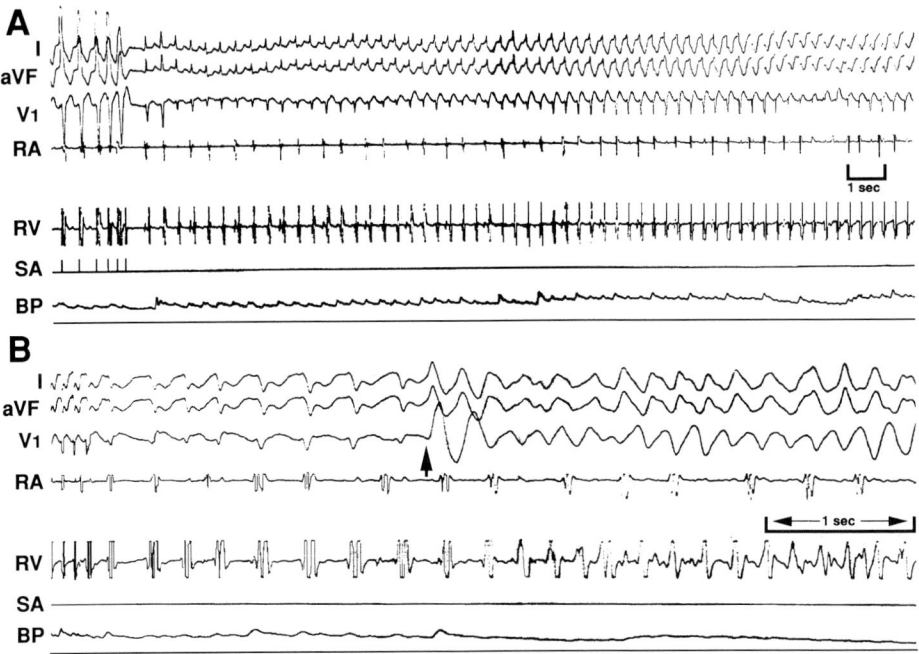

Fig. 11–2. Supraventricular tachycardia followed by ventricular fibrillation in a patient with hypertrophic cardiomyopathy. (Reproduced with permission from Zee-Cheng C-S, et al: J Electrophysiol 2:251–254, 1988.[107]) Body surface ECG leads I, aV_F, and V_1 were recorded with intracardiac electrograms from the high right atrium (RA) and the right ventricle (RV) in addition to a stimulus artifact (SA) and arterial blood pressure (BP) traces. The figure was retouched for clarity. **A.** Three ventricular extrastimuli delivered after a train of eight beats induced a narrow QRS complex tachycardia with a pattern consistent with atrioventricular junctional re-entry with variable atrial capture (retrograde type I AV node block with a 3:2 pattern initially). The rate of tachycardia increased from 162 beats/min to 202 beats/min. ST-segment depression developed in leads I and a V_F, and ST-segment elevation in lead V_1. **B.** Continuation of tracings in **A.** The paper speed was increased after the first few beats of this panel. The arrow indicates the onset of ventricular fibrillation. See text for further discussion.

arrest would not have occurred. On the other hand, this was a very unusual response to a common arrhythmia. Knowledge of the abnormalities commonly present in hypertrophic cardiomyopathy makes it possible to speculate that the several of the factors listed in Figure 11–1 contributed to the process that resulted in VF, but it may not be possible to identify a single "cause" or even a predominant cause. Nor may it be possible to specify linear sequence of causes and effects, since many processes are occurring simultaneously.

Myerburg et al[170,171] have emphasized the importance of the interplay between structural and functional aspects of the cardiovascular system in the pathophysiology of sudden death. Arnsdorf has used a matrical approach to examine the interaction of electrophysiological effects.[172,173] A similar approach can be used to conceptualize the interactions of important elements in hypertrophic cardiomyopathy. The diagrams in Figure 11–3 are similar to those used by Arnsdorf.[172,173] Figure 11–3A shows an arrangement of six physiological entities connected by bars representing possible interactions. The depiction of this dynamical system is limited by the number of elements that are practically shown in a two-dimensional drawing, by the arbitrary choice of the elements selected, and by the arbitrary distinction between overlapping entities. A mathematical representation could include many other elements in addition to a number of subsidiary systems. Figure 11–3B shows how the system might respond to a supraventricular tachycardia in an individual without hypertrophic cardiomyopathy. The perturbation caused by the

Mechanisms of Sudden Death in Patients with Hypertrophic Cardiomyopathy 177

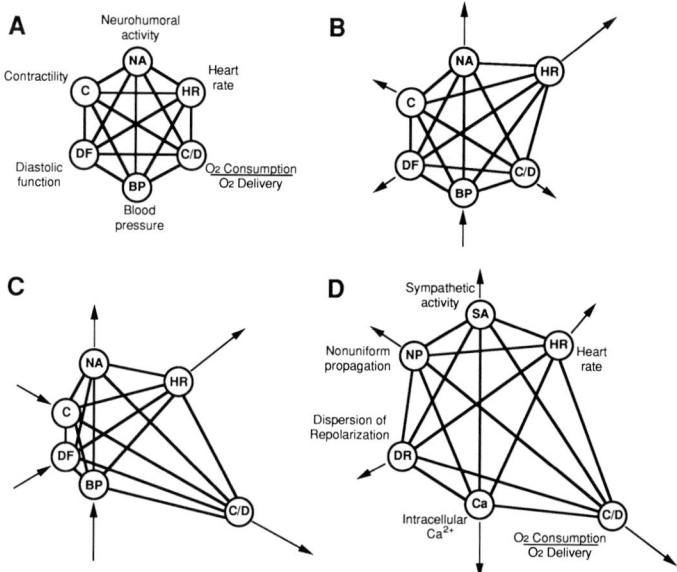

Fig. 11-3. Depiction of a "dynamical system" to represent physiological changes in response to tachycardia. (Adapted with permission from Arnsdorf.[172,173]) The components of the system are shown as circles and the bars between components indicate interactions. **A.** Several hemodynamic components and a neurohumoral component of the dynamical system in its baseline state. **B.** The dynamical system of a normal subject perturbed by supraventricular tachycardia. Arrows pointing away from the center of the system with extension of the interaction bars represent an increase in the value of the component (e.g., increased heart rate), while arrows pointing inward (shortening of bars) indicate a lower value of the component (e.g., blood pressure). **C.** The dynamical system of a patient with hypertrophic cardiomyopathy perturbed by supraventricular tachycardia. **D.** Perturbed dynamical system illustrating possible electrophysiological components. See text for discussion.

sudden increase in heart rate is represented by increasing the distance of the heart rate element (HR) from the center of the system. There is a drop in the blood pressure (BP), an increase in the ratio of myocardial oxygen consumption to delivery (C/D), and enhanced sympathetic activity (NA). Coronary artery vasodilation restores C/D to some extent. Elevated NA increases contractility (C) and improves diastolic function (DF), but it might enhance AV conduction, which further increases HR; all of these effects increase C/D. On the other hand, improved DF will tend to minimize compromised diastolic filling due to tachycardia. This effect plus increased C- and NA-induced peripheral vasoconstriction tends to restore BP, which in turn diminishes C/D. Thus, the tachycardia alters the state of the system depicted in Figure 11-3B, but appropriately functioning control mechanisms prevent excessive deviation from a viable state.

In the person with hypertrophic cardiomyopathy, several compensatory mechanisms may malfunction (Fig. 11-3C). Reduced coronary reserve impairs the ability to restore C/D for the same degree of tachycardia. LV filling is compromised to a greater extent by pre-existing disturbances in DF, and DF will be diminished further by tachycardia and developing ischemia. Increased NA will improve DF somewhat, but at the expense of increased C/D. The reduction in LV filling and increased C mediated by increased NA exacerbate the LV outflow tract gradient, which prevents the needed restoration of BP. Sufficient increases in C/D result in myocardial ischemia, which will impair C and DF further, resulting in greater diminutions of BP, and so on, creating a positive feedback loop. This makes restoration of a viable system impossible without termination of tachycardia. Figure 11-3C represents a possible electrophysiological system. Although ischemia (elevated C/D) is probably sufficient cause for VF, numerous other abnormalities could facilitate arrhythmogenesis with lesser degrees of ischemia. These include nonuniform propagation (NP) and dispersion of repolarization (DR) due to fibrosis or myocyte disarray, and disturbed intracellular calcium ion movement (Ca).

The possibility of sudden death resulting predominantly from hemodynamic influences was demonstrated in a patient with aortic stenosis who was undergoing ambulatory ECG monitoring and simultaneous ear densitographic monitoring, which reflects phasic blood flow.[174] The patient had a history of syncopal episodes associated with angina and ST-segment changes on the ECG. Just before collapse, the patient was in normal sinus rhythm with relatively large external pulse waves (Fig. 11–4A). Progressive ST-segment depression was accompanied by progressive decreases in the amplitude and slope of the external pulse wave. The ECG showed a slight increase in heart rate from about 60 beats/min to 75 beats/min. Finally, the pulse wave became flat with marked sinus bradycardia. The concomitant depression of pulse wave amplitude and the ST segment suggests positive feedback between blood pressure, myocardial perfusion, and contractility, with minor effects on heart rate (Fig. 11–4C), until profound hypotension and myocardial ischemia were presumably present (Fig. 11–4D). In addition to aortic stenosis, the autopsy of this patient revealed abnormalities frequently observed in victims of sudden death with hypertrophic cardiomyopathy: extensive myocardial hypertrophy, fibrosis, and patent coronary arteries. Case reports of syncope during normal sinus rhythm suggest that a similar scenario could be responsible for sudden death in some patients with hypertrophic cardiomyopathy.[175]

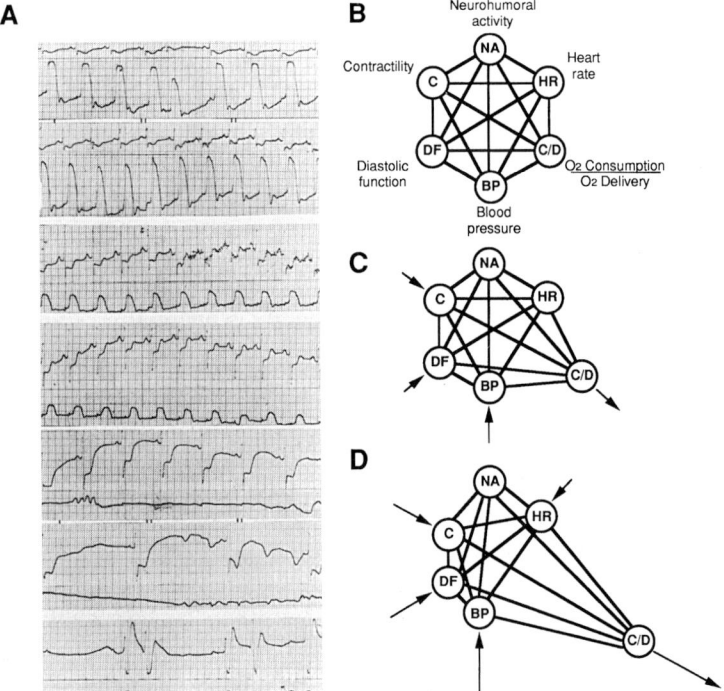

Fig. 11–4. Sudden death in a patient with aortic stenosis. **A.** Sequential tracings of an ECG and ear densitographic pulse waves. (Reproduced with permission from Nikolic G, et al: Am Heart J *104:* 311–312, 1982.[174]) **B.** Baseline state (see Fig. 11–3). **C.** Early phase of the perturbed state, representing development of myocardial ischemia with mild reductions in contractility (C) and diastolic function (DF) and systemic blood pressure (BP). **D.** Depiction of a system with progressive ischemia accompanied by further reductions in C, DF, BP, and now heart rate (HR).

Curiously, sudden death was associated with nonsustained VT in this case report since it had been recorded without significant symptoms by ambulatory monitoring 2 days before death.[174] But in an ironic twist, its detection may have actually contributed to the patient's demise because quinidine sulfate was then added to her previous therapy, which included nitrates, nifedipine, and furosemide. The combined vasodilator effects of these drugs may have prevented the peripheral vasoconstriction needed to maintain myocardial perfusion.[183] Thus, this case is a poignant illustration of how the association between a sign (nonsustained VT) and sudden death can lead to incorrect and potentially harmful conclusions about the mechanism of sudden death and how to prevent it.

TOWARD A THEORY OF SUDDEN DEATH

Unfortunately, it is not yet possible to address other crucial aspects of the problem. For instance, what initiated the supraventricular tachycardia that presumably led to the cardiac arrest reported by Zee-Cheng et al?[107] Perhaps left atrial stretch resulting from an elevation in LV filling pressure provoked an atrial premature beat that initiated the tachycardia; perhaps LV mechanoreceptor stimulation resulted in a reflex withdrawal of sympathetic tone and enhanced vagal tone, which altered the electrophysiological properties of the AV node sufficiently to permit re-entry; or perhaps a salvo of nonsustained ventricular beats initiated the arrhythmia, as suggested by the findings at electrophysiological study. Prediction and prevention of sudden death require an understanding not only of the "triggers" of sudden death but of the precursors of those triggers. In addition to the acquisition of more detailed data, a theory of sudden death is needed to provide a framework for interpreting the data and for making testable predictions. This is of particular importance for a relatively uncommon disorder for which there are no adequate animal models because a well-formulated theory can direct more efficient use of limited resources.

A model of sudden death would have to address several characteristics of the process in patients with hypertrophic cardiomyopathy (not necessarily unique to this disorder). In many cases the victims have no inkling of heart disease and are not merely asymptomatic, but have sufficient functional capacity to engage in athletic competitions. In addition, the time course of sudden death is striking. In their description of 16 witnessed deaths, James and Marshall[66] commented, "In every case it was virtually instantaneous and silent. One child did complain of being tired just before collapsing, and two adult victims tried to speak but were unable, but in all 13 others there was not even an effort to utter a word." Since cerebral function may persist for a few seconds in the absence of flow, the rapidity with which collapse can occur suggests that cerebral blood pressure falls to very low levels within seconds. A theory of sudden death also would have to reconcile the observation that a relatively high percentage of events (about 40%) are associated with vigorous exercise, while most sudden deaths occur during minimal activity or during sleep.[13,102,120,121,140,142]

Another prominent property of sudden death is its erratic occurrence. Cecchi et al[142] studied 33 patients with hypertrophic cardiomyopathy who survived a cardiac arrest. Although patients who can be resuscitated may not represent the entire spectrum of patients who die suddenly, such patients would still be expected to be at very high risk of sudden death. In this sense, the outcome was surprisingly good: only four patients died suddenly and five other patients had another cardiac arrest during a mean follow-up period of 6 years. One could conclude that the treatments were highly effective. However, therapy consisted largely of conventional antiarrhythmic drugs and surgery, which, as noted earlier, have not been definitely associated with improved survival, and no pattern of treatment appeared particularly effective in this study (one patient received amiodarone and none received an implantable defibrillator). Importantly, there was no apparent pattern to the interval between the index cardiac arrest and subsequent cardiac arrest or sudden death. The sudden deaths occurred anywhere between 7 months and 4 years later. The cardiac arrests occurred at 3 weeks and

5, 6, 9, and 40 months after the initial arrest. In another study, five patients had had a cardiac arrest before dying suddenly. In these patients the intervals between cardiac arrest and sudden death were between 3 weeks and 26 months.[140]

Finally, a feature that mocks most proposed mechanisms of sudden death is the inability to reproduce it. In a few instances, a sequence of events that appeared to recreate important features of the process of sudden death has occurred during atrial pacing,[165] after the initiation of supraventricular arrhythmias,[107,157] and during exercise testing.[150,160,176] However, these case reports constitute a tiny percentage of the patients who have undergone rapid pacing,[70,111,112] supraventricular arrhythmia induction attempts,[103,115,141,175] catecholamine infusions,[70,91,93,111] or exercise testing.[14,70,80,96,98,100,108,120,148,177–180]* Moreover, there is little doubt that these maneuvers are producing effects that have been proposed to be important contributors to sudden death, including tachycardia, ischemia, hypotension, and diastolic dysfunction.

These two characteristics, the irregular occurrence of sudden death and the inability to reproduce it, do not favor a classical deterministic process. Take, for instance, a patient in whom a cardiac arrest occurs during vigorous exercise. A deterministic hypothesis might be that cardiac arrest in this individual required a certain degree of myocyte disarray plus reduced myocardial perfusion reserve plus enhanced sympathetic activity plus myocardial ischemia. One would therefore expect to be able to reproduce the cardiac arrest with an exercise test or similar maneuver, but, as noted above, this has rarely been possible. Furthermore, if such a deterministic process were in control, one would anticipate that the risk of death would be highest near the time of the cardiac arrest, since the patient's "substrate" would be closest to its "critical" state. Instead, recurrence of cardiac arrest occurs at irregular intervals after the initial event. The irregular pattern of cardiac arrhythmias has been noted in other contexts. Pritchett and colleagues[181] found that the times of occurrence or paroxysmal supraventricular tachycardia were clinically independent, and that the temporal distribution of occurrences suggested a type of random event called a Poisson process. Thus, the occurrence of sudden death in patients with hypertrophic cardiomyopathy could be the result of a nondeterministic process, which would make prediction of sudden death impossible in individual cases. Alternatively, chaos, a deterministic process, could account for this irregular behavior. Chaotic processes are characterized by extreme sensitivity to initial conditions. This latter feature could explain the inability to reproduce sudden death, since it is never possible to reproduce perfectly the conditions under which sudden death occurred spontaneously, and it could explain how small differences in initial conditions could result in very divergent responses.[182]

PREVENTION OF SUDDEN DEATH

In the absence of proven treatment strategies or a tenable theory of sudden death, there is no firm basis for making management recommendations. Without a technique for reproducing sudden death, or at least the reversible portions of the process, there is no way to test treatments. Instead, one must depend on intuition and past experience, which tend to be heavily biased and notoriously unreliable. The current lack of agreement on the evaluation and management of patients with hypertrophic cardiomyopathy at high risk for sudden death testifies to this unfortunate situation. It would seem logical to hunt for potential contributors to sudden death that could be ameliorated. An electrophysiological study, for example, could be performed to assess the potential for a rapid ventricular rate to advance to supraventricular arrhythmias. A treadmill test could be performed to ascertain the presence of exercise-induced myo-

---

* It is debatable whether ventricular tachyarrhythmia induction with programmed stimulation reproduces the cardiac arrest that precedes sudden death or is an irrelevant finding present in a large proportion of patients with hypertrophic cardiomyopathy. A balanced view would be that this phenomenon measures something about vulnerability to sustained ventricular arrhythmias that could interact at some stage of the process, but it seems unlikely that the stimulation program usually required reproduces an event that occurs often naturally.

cardial ischemia or hypotension. However, many of the possible factors, such as myocyte disorganization or calcium regulation, cannot be practically examined, so there will always be doubts about the relation of clinical observations and tests to the risk of sudden death. Furthermore, it is not yet possible to determine the impact of treatment on the biological matrix. Verapamil, for instance might reduce myocardial ischemia but might also result in a dangerous decrease in systolic function or peripheral vascular resistance.[183]

The therapies that tend to provide the most confidence for prevention of sudden death do nothing to prevent the process itself. Use of the automatic internal defibrillator is based on the premise that terminating a ventricular tachyarrhythmia will prevent death. As the foregoing discussion indicates, this premise is quite questionable. Obviously, defibrillation alone may not prevent death caused by severe bradyarrhythmias or by a supraventricular arrhythmia that is not terminated by the defibrillator as well. The defibrillator may not be effective against arrhythmias due to advanced myocardial ischemia, and it may be helpless against myocardial "stunning" resulting from myocardial ischemia and VF.[184] The experience with the use of internal defibrillators in patients with hypertrophic cardiomyopathy is limited.[185-188] On the other hand, there is no indication that patients with hypertrophic cardiomyopathy do any worse than others treated with this device. Although evidence suggests that increased myocardial mass increases defibrillation thresholds, the literature on automatic internal defibrillators does not indicate that this is a problem in practice. Thus, intuition, experience in other patient populations, and absence of negative experience in patients with hypertrophic cardiomyopathy suggest that automatic defibrillator implantation is an effective method of preventing sudden death. Nevertheless, its apparent effectiveness may in part be due to other aspects of treatment, including concomitant medical therapy and prohibition of vigorous physical activity. Enthusiasm for this device should be tempered by the fact that it may not prevent dangerous events such as syncope during driving, swimming, and the like, by its potential for both somatic and psychological complications,[189] and by its expense. Although cardiac transplantation undoubtedly reduces the risk of sudden death, it is still associated with a relatively high mortality[190] and should therefore be reserved for patients with debilitating symptoms refractory to other therapy.

CONCLUSION

Hypertrophic cardiomyopathy retains a fascination for investigators out of proportion to its incidence because of its diverse clinical expression and multiplicity of pathological processes. The individuals afflicted with it, however, face an uncertain future, and their clinicians cannot confidently manipulate the clinical course. Several hurdles remain in the way of further elucidation of the mechanisms of sudden death. First, there appear to be a large number of paths by which death could occur. Second, it seems unlikely that a single mode of therapy will be sufficient. Third, it is a relatively uncommon disorder so that it will be difficult to mount the clinical trials needed to verify mechanisms and treatment. On the other hand, the pace of progress in the understanding of basic biological processes provides hope of, in the words of Charles Dickens' Mr. Micawber, "an immediate prospect of something turning up!"

REFERENCES

1. Liouville H: Rétrécissement cardiaque sous aortique. Gazette Med Paris 24: 161–163, 1869.
2. Hallopeau M: Rétrécissement ventriculo-aortique. Gazette Med Paris 24:683–684, 1869.
3. Brock R: Functional obstruction of the left ventricle (acquired aortic subvalvular stenosis). Guys Hosp Rep 106:211–212, 1957.
4. Teare D: Asymmetrical hypertrophy of the heart in young adults. Br Heart J 20:1–18, 1958.
5. World Health Organization: Report of the WHO/ISFC Task Force on the Definition and Classification of Cardiomyopathies. Br Heart J 44:672–673, 1980.
6. Maron BJ: Hypertrophic cardiomyopathy: Historical perspective, nomenclature and definition. In Toshima H, Maron BJ (eds):

Cardiomyopathy Update 2: Hypertrophic Cardiomyopathy. Tokyo, University of Tokyo Press, 1988, pp 3–11.
7. Codd MB, Sugrue DD, Gersh BJ, Melton LJ: Epidemiology of idiopathic dilated cardiomyopathy and hypertrophic cardiomyopathy. Circulation 80:564–572, 1989.
8. Bagger JP, Baandrup U, Rasmussen K, Møller M, Vesterlund T: Cardiomyopathy in Western Denmark. Br Heart J 52:327–331, 1984.
9. Savage DD, Castelli WP, Abbott RD, et al: Hypertrophic cardiomyopathy and its markers in the general population: The great masquerader revisited. The Framingham study. J Cardiovasc Ultrasonogr 2:41–47, 1983.
10. Hada Y, Sakamoto T, Amano K, et al: Prevalence of hypertrophic cardiomyopathy in a population of adult Japanese workers as detected by echocardiographic screening. Am J Cardiol 59:183–184, 1987.
11. Shah PM, Adelman AG, Wigle ED, et al: The natural (and unnautral) course of hypertrophic obstructive cardiomyopathy: A multicenter study. Circ Res 34, 35(suppl II):II-179–195, 1973.
12. McKenna WJ, Deanfield J, Faruqui A, England D, Oakley C, Goodwin J: Prognosis in hypertrophic cardiomyopathy: Role of age and clinical, electrocardiographic and hemodynamic features. Am J Cardiol 47:532–538, 1981.
13. Maron BJ, Savage DD, Wolfson JK, Epstein SE: Prognostic significance of 24 hour ambulatory electrocardiographic monitoring in patients with hypertrophic cardiomyopathy: A prospective study. Am J Cardiol 48:252–257, 1981.
14. Koga Y, Itaya K, Toshima H: Prognosis in hypertrophic cardiomyopathy. Am Heart J 108:351–359, 1984.
15. Waller BF: Exercise-related sudden death in young (age <30 years) and old (>30 years) conditioned subjects. Cardiovasc Clin 15:9–73, 1985.
16. Maron BJ, Epstein SE, Roberts WC: Causes of sudden death in competitive athletes. J Am Coll Cardiol 7:204–214, 1986.
17. Burke AP, Farb A, Virmani R, Goodin J, Smialek JE: Sports-related and non-sports-related sudden cardiac death in young adults. Am Heart J 121:568–575, 1991.
18. Gwathmey JK, Warren SE, Briggs GM, et al: Diastolic dysfunction in hypertrophic cardiomyopathy: Effect on active force generation during systole. J Clin Invest 87:1023–1031, 1991.
19. Ferry DR, Kaumann AJ: Relationship between β-adrenoceptors and calcium channels in human ventricular myocardium. Br J Pharmacol 90:447–457, 1987.
20. Wagner JA, Sax FL, Weisman HF, et al: Calcium-antagonist receptors in the atrial tissue of patients with hypertrophic cardiomyopathy. N Engl J Med 230:755–761, 1989.
21. Moore RL, Yelamarty RV, Misawa H, et al: Altered Ca^{2+} dynamics in single cardiac myocytes from renovascular hypertensive rats. Am J Physiol [Cell Physiol] 260:C327–C337, 1991.
22. Schouten VJA, Vliegen HW, Van der-Laarse A, Huysmans HA: Altered calcium handling at normal contractility in hypertrophied rat heart. J Mol Cell Cardiol 22:987–998, 1990.
23. Bing OHL, Brooks WW, Conrad CH, Sen S, Perreault CL, Morgan JP: Intracellular calcium transients in myocardium from spontaneously hypertensive rats during the transition to heart failure. Circ Res 68:1390–1400, 1991.
24. Ito Y, Suko J, Chidsey CA: Intracellular calcium and myocardial contractility: V. Calcium uptake of sarcoplasmic reticulum fractions in hypertrophied and failing rabbit hearts. J Mol Cell Cardiol 6:237:247, 1974.
25. Aronson RS: Afterpotentials and triggered activity in hypertrophied myocardium from rats with renal hypertension. Circ Res 48:720–727, 1981.
26. Marban E, Robinson SW, Wier WG: Mechanisms of arrhythmogenic delayed and early after depolarizations in ferret ventricular muscle. J Clin Invest 78:1185–1192, 1986.
27. Nordin C: Abnormal Ca^{2+} handling and the generation of ventricular arrhythmias in congestive heart failure. Heart Failure 5:143–154, 1989.
28. Spray DC, Burt JM: Structure-activity relations of the cardiac gap junction channel. Am J Physiol 258:C195–C205, 1990.
29. Coltart DJ, Meldrum SJ: Hypertrophic cardiomyopathy: An electrophysiological study. Br Med J 4:217–218, 1970.
30. Hondeghem LM, Snyders DJ: Class III antiarrhythmic agents have a lot of potential but a long way to go: Reduced effectiveness and dangers of reverse use dependence. Circulation 81:686–690, 1990.
31. Keung ECH, Aronson RS: Non-uniform electrophysiological properties and electrotonic interaction in hypertrophied rat myocardium. Circ Res 49:150–158, 1981.
32. Cameron JS, Miller LS, Kimura S, et al: Systemic hypertension induces disparate localized left ventricular action potential lengthening and altered sensitivity to verap-

amil in left ventricular myocardium. J Mol Cell Cardiol 18:169–175, 1986.
33. Kowey PR, Friehling TD, Sewter J, et al: Electrophysiological effects of left ventricular hypertrophy: Effect of calcium and potassium channel blockade. Circulation 83: 2067–2075, 1991.
34. Kuo C, Munakata K, Reddy CP, Surawicz B: Characteristics and possible mechanism of ventricular arrhythmia dependent on the dispersion of action potential durations. Circulation 67:1356–1367, 1983.
35. Tritthart H, Luedcke H, Bayer R, Stierle H, Kaufmann R: Right ventricular hypertrophy in the cat: An electrophysiological and anatomical study. J Moll Cell Cardiol 7:933–942, 1975.
36. Gelband H, Bassett AL: Depressed transmembrane potentials during experimentally induced ventricular failure in cats. Circ Res 32:625–634, 1973.
37. Houser SR, Freeman AR, Jaeger JM, et al: Resting potential changes associated with Na-K pump in failing heart muscle. Am J Physiol 240:H168–H176, 1981.
38. Keung ECH, Keung C-S, Aronson RS: Passive electrical properties of normal and hypertrophied rat myocardium. Am J Physiol 243:H917–H926, 1982.
39. Maron BJ, Bonow RO, Cannon RO III, Leon MB, Epstein SE: Hypertrophic cardiomyopathy: Interrelations of clinical manifestations pathophysiology and therapy. Part I. N Engl J Med 316:780–789, 1987.
40. Maron BJ, Ferrans VJ, Henry WL, et al: Differences in distribution of myocardial abnormalities in patients with obstructive and nonobstructive asymmetric septal hypertrophy (ASH): Light and electron microscopic findings. Circulation 50:436–446, 1974.
41. Factor SM, Butany J, Sole MJ, Wigle ED, Williams WC, Rojkind M: Pathologic fibrosis and matrix connective tissue in the subaortic myocardium of patients with hypertrophic cardiomyopathy. J Am Coll Cardiol 17:1343–1351, 1991.
42. Tanaka M, Fujinara H, Onodera T, Wu D-J, Hamashina Y, Kawai C: Quantitative analysis of myocardial fibrosis in normals, hypertensive hearts and hypertrophic cardiomyopathy. Br Heart J 55:575–581, 1986.
43. Maron BJ, Ferrans VJ: Significance of multiple intercalated discs in hypertrophied myocardium. Am J Pathol 73:81–87, 1973.
44. Spach MS, Miller WT III, Dolber PC, Kootsey JM, Sommer JR, Mosher CE Jr: The functional role of structural complexities in the propagation of depolarization in the atrium of the dog: Cardiac conduction disturbances due to discontinuities of effective axial resistivity. Circ Res 50:175–191, 1982.
45. Spach MS, Dolber PC: The relation between discontinuous propagation in anisotrophic cardiac muscle and the "vulnerable period" of reentry. In Zipes DP, Jaliffe J (eds): Cardiac Electrophysiology and Arrhythmias. Orlando, Fla, Grune & Stratton, 1985, pp 241–252.
46. Spach MS, Dolber PC: Relating extracellular potentials and their derivatives to anisotropic propagation at a microscopic level in human cardiac muscle: Evidence for electrical uncoupling of side-to-side fiber connections with increasing age. Circ Res 58: 356–371, 1986.
47. Anderson KP, Ershler PR, Lux RL, et al: Nonuniform electrical activation in idiopathic dilated cardiomyopathy [abstract]. Circulation 80(suppl II):II-431, 1989.
48. Anderson KP, Stinson EB, Block PJ, et al: Epicardial mapping in patients with hypertrophic cardiomyopathy. J Appl Cardiol 1: 285–307, 1986.
49. van Dam RTh, Roos JP, Durrer D: Electrical activation of the ventricles and interventricular septum in hypertrophic cardiomyopathy. Br Heart J 34:100–112, 1972.
50. Burgess MJ, Steinhaus BM, Spitzer KW, Ershler PR: Nonuniform epicardial activation and repolarization properties of in vivo canine pulmonary conus. Circ Res 62: 233–246, 1988.
51. Lesh MD, Pring M, Spear JF: Cellular uncoupling can unmask dispersion of action potential duration in ventricular myocardium. Circ Res 65:1426–1440, 1989.
52. Yutani C, Imakita M, Ishibashi-Ueda H, et al: Three autopsy cases of progression to left ventricular dilatation in patients with hypertrophic cardiomyopathy. Am Heart J 109:545–553, 1985.
53. Alfonso F, Prenneaux MP, McKenna WJ: Clinical sustained uniform ventricular tachycardia in hypertrophic cardiomyopathy: Association with left ventricular apical aneurysm. Br Heart J 61:178–181, 1989.
54. Macina G, Singh A, Drew TM, Moran RM, Most AS: Asymmetric myocardial hypertrophy, left ventricular aneurysm, mural thrombus and sudden death. Am Heart J 111:175–178, 1986.
55. Miyajima S, Aizawa Y, Suzuki K, et al: Sustained ventricular tachycardia responsive to verapamil in patients with hypertrophic cardiomyopathy: Clinical and electrophysiological assessment of drug efficacy. Jpn Heart J 30:241–249, 1989.
56. Gordon EP, Henderson JA, Rakowski H,

Wigle ED: Midventricular obstruction with apical infarction and aneurysm formation [abstract]. Circulation 70(suppl II):II–145, 1984.
57. Anderson KP: Sudden death, hypertension and hypertrophy. J Cardiovasc Pharmacol 6:S498–S503, 1984.
58. Garry WE: Nature of fibrillary contraction of the heart: Its relation to tissue mass and form. Am J Physiol 22:397–414, 1914.
59. Moe GK, Abildskov JA: Atrial fibrillation as a self-sustaining arrhythmia independent of focal discharge. Am Heart J 58:59–70, 1969.
60. Zipes DP, Fischer J, King RM, Nicoll AB, Jolly WW: Termination of ventricular fibrillation in dogs by depolarizing a critical amount of myocardium. Am J Cardiol 36:37–44, 1975.
61. Winfree AT: Ventricular reentry in three dimensions. In Zipes DP, Jalife J (eds): Cardiac Electrophysiology: From Cell to Bedside. Philadelphia, WB Saunders, 1990, pp 224–234.
62. Damiano RJ Jr, Asano T, Smith PK, Cox JL: Effect of the right ventricular isolation procedure on ventricular vulnerability to fibrillation. J Am Coll Cardiol 15:730–736, 1990.
63. Tomanek RJ: Response of the coronary vasculature to myocardial hypertrophy. J Am Coll Cardiol 15:528–533, 1990.
64. Maron BJ, Wolfson JK, Epstein SE, Roberts WC: Intramural ("small vessel") coronary artery disease in hypertrophic cardiomyopathy. J Am Coll Cardiol 8:545–557, 1986.
65. James TN, Jordan JD, Riddick L, Bargeron LM: Subaortic stenosis and sudden death. J Thorac Cardiovasc Surg 95:247–254, 1988.
66. James TN, Marshall TK: De subitaneis mortibus: XII. Asymmetrical hypertrophy of the heart. Circulation 51:1149–1166, 1975.
67. Pasternac A, Noble J, Streulens Y, Elie R, Henschke C, Bourassa MG: Pathophysiology of chest pain in patients with cardiomyopathies and normal coronary arteries. Circulation 65:778–789, 1982.
68. Cannon RO III, Rosing DR, Maron BJ, et al: Myocardial ischemia in patients with hypertrophic cardiomyopathy: Contribution of inadequate vasodilator reserve and elevated left ventricular filling pressures. Circulation 71:234–243, 1985.
69. Cannon RO III, Schenke WH, Maron BJ, et al: Differences in coronary flow and myocardial metabolism at rest and during pacing between patients with obstructive and patients with nonobstructive hypertrophic cardiomyopathy. J Am Coll Cardiol 10:53–62, 1987.
70. Cannon RO III, Dilsizian V, O'Gara PT, et al: Myocardial metabolic, hemodynamic, and electrocardiographic significance of reversible thallium-201 abnormalities in hypertrophic cardiomyopathy. Circulation 83:1660–1667, 1991.
71. O'Gara PT, Bonow RO, Maron BJ, et al: Myocardial perfusion abnormalities in patients with hypertrophic cardiomyopathy. Circulation 76:1214–1223, 1987.
72. Camici P, Chiriatti G, Lorenzoni R, et al: Coronary vasodilation is impaired in both hypertrophied and nonhypertrophied myocardium of patients with hypertrophic cardiomyopathy: A study with nitrogen-13 ammonia and positron emission tomography. J Am Coll Cardiol 17:879–886, 1991.
73. Janse MJ, Wit AL: Electrophysiologic mechanisms of ventricular arrhythmias resulting from myocardial ischemia and infarction. Physiol Rev 69:1049–1154, 1989.
74. Marban E, Kitakaze M, Koretsune Y, Yue DT, Chacko VP, Pike MM: Quantification of $[Ca^{2+}]_i$ perfused hearts: Critical evaluation of the 5F-BAPTA and nuclear magnetic resonance method as applied to the study of ischemia and reperfusion. Circ Res 66:1255–1267, 1990.
75. Opie LH, Clusin WT: Cellular mechanism for ischemic ventricular arrhythmias. Annu Rev Med 41:231–238, 1990.
76. Braunwald E, Kloner RA: The stunned myocardium: Prolonged, postischemic ventricular dysfunction. Circulation 66:1146–1149, 1982.
77. Wigle ED, Heimbecker RO, Gunton RW: Idiopathic ventricular septal hypertrophy causing muscular subaortic stenosis. Circulation 26:325–340, 1962.
78. Wigle ED, Lenkei SCM, Chrysohou A, Wilson DR: Muscular subaortic stenosis: The effect of peripheral vasodilation. Can Med Assoc J 89:896–899, 1963.
79. Atlas SA, Laragh JH: Atrial natriuretic peptide: A new factor in hormonal control of blood pressure and electrolyte homeostasis. Annu Rev Med 37:397–414, 1986.
80. Frenneaux MP, Counihan PJ, Caforio ALP, Chikamori T, McKenna WJ: Abnormal blood pressure response during exercise in hypertrophic cardiomyopathy. Circulation 82:1995–2002, 1990.
81. Counihan PJ, Frenneaux MP, Webb DJ, McKenna WJ: Abnormal vascular responses to supine exercise in hypertrophic cardiomyopathy. Circulation 84:686–696, 1991.
82. Abboud FM: Pathophysiology of hypoten-

sion and shock. In Hurst JW (ed): The Heart, New York, McGraw-Hill, 1986, pp 370–382.
83. Furchgott RF, Vanhoutte PM: Endothelium-derived relaxing and contracting factors. FASEB J 3:2007–2018, 1989.
84. Mark AL, Kioschos JM, Abboud FM, Heistad DD, Schmid PC: Abnormal vascular responses in patients with aortic stenosis. J Clin Invest 52:1388–1394, 1973.
85. Chevalier PA, Weber KD, Lyons GW, Nicoloff DM, Fox IJ: Haemodynamic changes from stimulation of left ventricular baroreceptors. Am J Physiol 227:719–728, 1974.
86. Johnson AM: Aortic stenosis, sudden death and the left ventricular baroreceptors. Br Heart J 33:1–5, 1971.
87. Wit AL, Cranefield PF: Triggered and automatic activity in the canine coronary sinus. Circ Res 41:435–445, 1977.
88. Waxman MB, Wald RW, Cameron D: Interactions between the autonomic nervous system and tachycardias in man. Cardiol Clin 1:143–185, 1983.
89. Kawai C, Yui Y, Hoshino T, Sasyama S, Matsumori A: Myocardial catecholamines in hypertrophic and dilated (congestive) cardiomyopathy: A biopsy study. J Am Coll Cardiol 2:834–840, 1983.
90. Brush JE Jr, Eisenhofer G, Garty M, et al: Cardiac norepinephrine kinetics in hypertrophic cardiomyopathy. Circulation 79:836–844, 1989.
91. Toshima H, Koga Y: Increased cardiovascular responses to epinephrine and norepinephrine in patients with hypertrophic cardiomyopathy. In Toshima H, Maron B (eds): Cardiomyopathy Update 2: Hypertrophic Cardiomyopathy. Tokyo, University of Tokyo Press, 1988, pp 141–153.
92. Maisel AS, Wright M, Wilner KD, Ziegler MG: Norepinephrine kinetics in hypertrophic cardiomyopathy. In Toshima H, Maron B (eds): Cardiomyopathy Update 2: Hypertrophic Cardiomyopathy. Tokyo, University of Tokyo Press, 1988, pp 129–139.
93. Sugishita Y, Iida K, Yukisada K: Autonomic nervous function in hypertrophic cardiomyopathy. In Toshima H, Maron B (eds): Cardiomyopathy Update 2: Hypertrophic Cardiomyopathy. Tokyo, University of Tokyo Press, 1988, pp 155–167.
94. Pouleur H, Rousseau MF, van Eyll C, Brasseur LA, Charlier AA: Force-velocity-length relations in hypertrophic cardiomyopathy: Evidence of normal or depressed myocardial contractility. Am J Cardiol 52:813–817, 1983.
95. Golf S, Myhre E, Abdelnoor M, Anderson D, Hansson V: Hypertrophic cardiomyopathy characterized by beta-adrenoceptor density, relative amount of beta-adrenoceptor subtypes, and adenylate cyclase activity. Cardiovasc Res 19:693–699, 1985.
96. Savage DD, Seides SF, Maron BJ, Myers DJ, Epstein SE: Prevalence of arrhythmia during 24 hour electrocardiographic monitoring and exercise testing in patients with obstructive and nonobstructive hypertrophic cardiomyopathy. Circulation 59:866–875, 1979.
97. McKenna WJ, England D, Doi YL, Deanfield JE, Oakley CM, Goodwin JF: Arrhythmia in hypertrophic cardiomyopathy: I. Influence on prognosis. Br Heart J 46:168–172, 1981.
98. Canedo MI, Frank MJ, Abdulla AM: Rhythm disturbances in hypertrophic cardiomyopathy: Prevalence, relation to symptoms and management. Am J Cardiol 45:848–855, 1980.
99. Frank MJ, Watkins LO, Prisant LM, Stefadouros MA, Abulla AM: Potentially lethal arrhythmias and their management in hypertrophic cardiomyopathy. Am J Cardiol 53:1608–1613, 1984.
100. Tamari I, Rabinowitz B, Glaziewski V, Motro M, Neufeld HN: Detection of arrhythmia in idiopathic hypertrophic subaortic stenosis by means of continuous electrocardiogram monitoring and ergometry. Cardiovasc Rev Rep 4:1258–1284, 1983.
101. Bjarnason I, Hardarson T, Jonsson S: Cardiac arrhythmias in hypertrophic cardiomyopathy. Br Heart J 48:198–203, 1982.
102. McKenna WJ, Franklin RCG, Nihoyannopoulos P, Robinson KC, Deanfield JE: Arrhythmia and prognosis in infants, children and adolescents with hypertrophic cardiomyopathy. J Am Coll Cardiol 11:147–153, 1988.
103. Fananapazir L, Tracy CM, Leon MB, et al: Electrophysiologic abnormalities in patients with hypertrophic cardiomyopathy. Circulation 80:1259–1268, 1989.
104. Ingham RE, Mason JW, Rossen RM, Goodman DJ, Harrison DC: Electrophysiologic findings in patients with idiopathic hypertrophic subaortic stenosis. Am J Cardiol 41:811–816, 1978.
105. Nienaber CA, Hiller S, Spielmann RP, Geiger M, Kuck K-H: Syncope in hypertrophic cardiomyopathy: Multivariate analysis of prognostic determinants. J Am Coll Cardiol 15:948–955, 1990.
106. Robinson K, Frenneaux MP, Stockins B, Karatasakis G, Poloniecki JD, McKenna

WJ: Atrial fibrillation in hypertrophic cardiomyopathy: A longitudinal study. J Am Coll Cardiol 15:1279–1285, 1990.
107. Zee-Cheng C-S, Quattromani A, Barbey JT, Ruffy R: Aborted sudden death in a young adult with hypertrophic cardiomyopathy and atrioventricular nodal tachycardia. J Electrophysiol 2:251–254, 1988.
108. McKenna WJ, Chetty S, Oakley CM, Goodwin JF: Arrhythmia in hypertrophic cardiomyopathy: exercise and 48 hour ambulatory electrocardiographic assessment with and without beta adrenergic blocking therapy. Am J Cardiol 45:1–5, 1980.
109. Spirito P, Watson RM, Maron BJ: Relation between extent of left ventricular hypertrophy and occurrence of ventricular tachycardia in hypertrophic cardiomyopathy. Am J Cardiol 60:1137–1142, 1987.
110. McKenna WJ, Harris L, Rowland E, Kleinebenne A, Krikler DM, Oakley CM, Goodwin JF: Amiodarone for long-term management of patients with hypertrophic cardiomyopathy. Am J Cardiol 54:802–810, 1984.
111. Udelson JE, Cannon RO III, Bacharach SL, Rumble TF, Bonow RO: β-adrenergic stimulation with isoproterenol enhances left ventricular diastolic performance in hypertrophic cardiomyopathy despite potentiation of myocardial ischemia. Circulation 79:371–382, 1989.
112. Cannon RO III, McIntosh CL, Schenke WH, Maron BJ, Bonow RO, Epstein SE: Effect of surgical reduction of left ventricular outflow obstruction on hemodynamics, coronary flow and myocardial metabolism in hypertrophic cardiomyopathy. Circulation 79:766–775, 1989.
113. Lazzeroni E, Domenicucci S, Finardi A, et al: Severity of arrhythmias and extent of hypertrophy in hypertrophic cardiomyopathy. Am Heart J 118:734–738, 1989.
114. Anderson KP, Stinson EB, Derby GC, Oyer PE, Mason JW: Vulnerability of patients with obstructive hypertrophic cardiomyopathy to ventricular arrhythmia induction in the operating room. Am J Cardiol 49:869–874, 1983.
115. Geibel A, Brugada P, Zehender M, Stevenson W, Waldecker B, Wellens HJJ: Value of programmed stimulation using a standardized ventricular stimulation protocol in hypertrophic cardiomyopathy. Am J Cardiol 60:738–739, 1987.
116. McKenna WJ, Camm AJ: Sudden death in hypertrophic cardiomyopathy. Circulation 80:1489–1492, 1989.
117. Fananapazir L, Epstein SE: VT and sudden death in HCM patients [letter]. Circulation 80:1923, 1989.
118. Cooper MJ, Anderson KP, Mason JW: Invasive electrophysiologic studies. In Zipes DP, Jalife J (eds): Cardiac Electrophysiology: From Cell to Bedside. Philadelphia, WB Saunders, 1990, pp 837–849.
119. Maron BJ, Henry WL, Calrk CE, Redwood DR, Roberts WC, Epstein SE: Asymmetric septal hypertrophy in childhood. Circulation 53:9–19, 1976.
120. Koga Y, Ogata M, Kihara K, Tsubaki K, Toshima H: Sudden death in hypertrophic and dilated cardiomyopathy. Jpn Circ J 53:1546–1556, 1989.
121. Sakurai T, Kawai C: Sudden death in idiopathic cardiomyopathy. Jpn Circ J 47:581–585, 1983.
122. Chikamori T, Dickie S, Poloniecki JD, Myers MJ, Lavender JP, McKenna WJ: Prognostic significance of radionuclide-assessed diastolic function in hypertrophic cardiomyopathy. Am J Cardiol 65:478–482, 1990.
123. Maron BJ, Lipson LC, Roberts WC, Savage DD, Epstein SE: "Malignant" hypertrophic cardiomyopathy: Identification of a subgroup of families with unusually frequent premature death. Am J Cardiol 41:1122–1140, 1978.
124. Maron BJ, Kragel AH, Roberts WC: Sudden death in hypertrophic cardiomyopathy with normal left ventricular mass. Br Heart J 63:308–310, 1990.
125. McKenna WJ, Stewart JT, Nihoyannopoulos P, McGinty F, Davies MJ: Hypertrophic cardiomyopathy without hypertrophy: Two families with myocardial disarray in the absence of increased myocardial mass. Br Heart J 63:287–290, 1990.
126. Sakamoto T, Tei C, Murayama M, Ichiyasu H, Hada Y: Giant T wave inversion as a manifestation of asymmetrical apical hypertrophy (AAH) of the left ventricle: Echocardiographic and ultasono-cardiotomographic study. Jpn Heart J 17:611–629, 1976.
127. Yamaguchi H, Ishimura T, Nishiyama S, et al: Hypertrophic nonobstructive cardiomyopathy with giant negative T waves (apical hypertrophy) ventriculographic and echocardiographic features in 30 patients. Am J Cardiol 44:401–412, 1979.
128. Maron BJ, Bonow RO, Seshagiri TN, Roberts WC, Epstein SE: Hypertrophic cardiomyopathy with ventricular septal hypertrophy localized to the apical region of the left ventricle (apical hypertrophic cardiomyopathy). Am J Cardiol 49:1838–1847, 1982.
129. Louie EK, Maron BJ: Apical hypertrophic cardiomyopathy: Clinical and two-dimensional echocardiographic assessment. Ann Intern Med 106:663–670, 1987.

130. Keren G, Belhassen B, Sherez J, Miller HI, Megidish R, Berenfeld D, Laniado S: Apical hypertrophic cardiomyopathy: Evaluation by noninvasive and invasive techniques in 23 patients. Circulation 71:45–56, 1985.
131. Webb JG, Sasson Z, Rakowski H, Liu P, Wigle ED: Apical hypertrophic cardiomyopathy: Clinical follow-up and diagnostic correlates. J Am Coll Cardiol 15:83–90, 1990.
132. Alfonso F, Nihoyannopoulos P, Stewart J, Dickie S, Lemery R, McKenna WJ: Clinical significance of giant negative T waves in hypertrophic cardiomyopathy. J Am Coll Cardiol 15:965–971, 1990.
133. Koga Y, Nohara M, Miyazaki Y, Toshima H: Two forms of apical hypertrophic cardiomyopathy: Japanese and western forms. In Toshima H, Maron BJ (eds): Cardiomyopathy Update 2: Hypertrophic Cardiomyopathy. Tokyo, University of Tokyo Press, 1988, pp 293–308.
134. Spirito P, Chiarella F, Carratino L, Berissol MZ, Bellotti P, Vecchio C: Clinical course and prognosis of hypertrophic cardiomyopathy in an outpatient population. N Engl J Med 320:749–755, 1989.
135. Newman H, Sugrue D, Oakley CM, Goodwin JF, McKenna JW: Relation of left ventricular function and prognosis in hypertrophic cardiomyopathy: An angiographic study. J Am Coll Cardiol 5:1064–1074, 1985.
136. Spirito P, Maron BJ: Relation between extent of left ventricular hypertrophy and occurrence of sudden cardiac death in hypertrophic cardiomyopathy. J Am Coll Cardiol 15:1521–1526, 1990.
137. McKenna WJ, Oakley CM, Krikler DM, Goodwin JF: Improved survival with amiodarone in patients with hypertrophic cardiomyopathy and ventricular tachycardia. Br Heart J 53:412–416, 1985.
138. Seiler C, Hess OM, Schoenbeck M, Turina J, Jenni R, Turina M, Krayenbuehl H-P: Long-term follow-up of medical versus surgical therapy for hypertrophic cardiomyopathy: A retrospective study. J Am Coll Cardiol 17:634–642, 1991.
139. Morrow AG, Koch JP, Maron BJ, Kent KM, Epstein SE: Left ventricular myotomy and myectomy in patients with obstructive hypertrophic cardiomyopathy and previous cardiac arrest. Am J Cardiol 46:313–316, 1980.
140. Maron BJ, Roberts WC, Epstein SE: Sudden death in hypertrophic cardiomyopathy: A profile of 78 patients. Circulation 65:1388–1394, 1982.
141. Fananapazir L, Epstein SE: Hemodynamic and electrophysiologic evaluation of patients with hypertrophic cardiomyopathy surviving cardiac arrest. Am J Cardiol 67:280–287, 1991.
142. Cecchi F, Maron BJ, Epstein SE: Long-term outcome of patients with hypertrophic cardiomyopathy successfully resuscitated after cardiac arrest. J Am Coll Cardiol 13:1283–1288, 1989.
143. Miyajima S, Aizawa Y, Matsuoka A, Okabe M, Shibata A: Danger of use of disopyramide in patients with hypertrophic obstructive cardiomyopathy. Jpn Heart J 29:115–119, 1988.
144. Kuck KH, Dernedde J, Geiger M, Kunze KP: Inefficacy and adverse effect of sotalol on arrhythmia in hypertrophic cardiomyopathy [abstract]. J Am Coll Cardiol 5:450, 1985.
145. Falk RH: Flecainide-induced ventricular tachycardia and fibrillation in patients treated for atrial fibrillation. Ann Intern Med 111:107–111, 1989.
146. McKenna WJ, Harris L, Perez G, Krikler DM, Oakley CM, Goodwin JF: Arrhythmia in hypertrophic cardiomyopathy: II. Comparison of amiodarone and verapamil in treatment. Br Heart J 46:173–178, 1981.
147. Counihan PJ, McKenna WJ: Low-dose amiodarone for the treatment of arrhythmias in hypertrophic cardiomyopathy. J Clin Pharmacol 29:436–438, 1989.
148. Fananapazir L, Leon MB, Bonow RO, Tracy CM, Cannon RO III, Epstein SE: Sudden death during empiric amiodarone therapy in symptomatic hypertrophic cardiomyopathy. Am J Cardiol 67:169–174, 1991.
149. Fananapazir L, Epstein SE: Value of electrophysiologic studies in hypertrophic cardiomyopathy treated with amiodarone. Am J Cardiol 67:175–182, 1991.
150. Mercereau D, Kubac G, Klinke WP: Failure of amiodarone to prevent ventricular fibrillation (sudden death) in hypertrophic cardiomyopathy. Can J Cardiol 5:77–80, 1989.
151. Multicenter Postinfarction Research Group: Risk stratification and survival after myocardial infarction. N Engl J Med 309:331–336, 1983.
152. Pelliccia F, Cianfrocca C, Romeo F, Reale A: Hypertrophic cardiomyopathy: Long-term effects of propranolol versus verapamil in preventing sudden death in "low risk" patients. Cardiovasc Drug Ther 4:1515–1518, 1990.
153. Warnes CA, Maron BJ, Roberts WC: Massive cardiac ventricular scarring in first-de-

gree relatives with hypertrophic cardiomyopathy. Am J Cardiol 54:1377–1379, 1984.
154. Unverferth DV, Baker PB, Pearce LI, Lautman J, Roberts WC: Regional myocyte hypertrophy and increased interstitial myocardial fibrosis in hypertrophic cardiomyopathy. Am J Cardiol 59:932–936, 1987.
155. Maron BJ, Roberts WC: Quantitative analysis of cardiac muscle cell disorganization in the ventricular septum of patients with hypertrophic cardiomyopathy. Circulation 59:689–706, 1979.
156. Udelson JE, Bonow RO, O'Gara PT, et al: Verapamil prevents silent myocardial perfusion abnormalities during exercise in asymptomatic patients with hypertrophic cardiomyopathy. Circulation 79: 1052–1060, 1989.
157. Stafford WJ, Trohman RG, Bilsker M, Zaman L, Castellanos A, Myerburg RJ: Cardiac arrest in an adolescent with atrial fibrillation and hypertrophic cardiomyopathy. J Am Coll Cardiol 7:701–704, 1986.
158. Nicod P, Polikar R, Peterson KL: Hypertrophic cardiomyopathy and sudden death. N Engl J Med 318:1255–1257, 1988.
159. Schwartz LS, Goldfischer J, Sprague GJ, Schwartz SP: Syncope and sudden death in aortic stenosis. Am J Cardiol 23:647–658, 1969.
160. Joseph S, Balcon R, McDonald I: Syncope in hypertrophic obstructive cardiomyopathy due to asystole. Br Heart J 34:974–976, 1972.
161. Touboul P, Kirkorian G, Atallah G, Cahen P, de Zuloaga C, Moleur P: Atrioventricular block and preexcitation in hypertrophic cardiomyopathy. Am J Cardiol 53:961–963, 1984.
162. Khair GZ, Soni JS, Bamrah VS: Syncope in hypertrophic cardiomyopathy: II. Coexistence of atrioventricular block and Wolff-Parkinson-White syndrome. Am Heart J 110:1083–1086, 1985.
163. Chmielewzski CA, Riley RS, Mahendran A, Most AS: Complete heart block as a cause of syncope in asymmetric septal hypertrophy. Am Heart J 93:91–93, 1977.
164. Louie EK, Maron BJ: Familial spontaneous complete heart block in hypertrophic cardiomyopathy. Br Heart J 55:469–474, 1986.
165. Krikler DM, Davies MJ, Rowland E, Goodwin JF, Evans RC, Shaw DB: Sudden death in hypertrophic cardiomyopathy: associated accessory atrioventricular pathways. Br Heart J 43:245–251, 1980.
166. Kuck KH, Kunze KP, Schluter M, Nienaber CA, Costard A: Programmed electrical stimulation in hypertrophic cardiomyopathy: Results in patients with and without cardiac arrest or syncope. Eur Heart J 9:177–185, 1988.
167. Waller BJ, Bournique VM, Nasser TK, Reeck M: Sudden death in two competitive athletes. Choices Cardiol 5:34–36, 1991.
168. Maron BJ, Roberts WC, Edwards JE, McAllister HA Jr, Foley DD, Epstein SE: Sudden death in patients with hypertrophic cardiomyopathy: Characterization of 26 patients without functional limitation. Am J Cardiol 41:803–810, 1978.
169. Krelhaus W, Kuhn H, Loogen F: Analysis of deaths in the course of hypertrophic obstructive cardiomyopathy. In Kaltenbach M, Loogen F, Olsen JGJ (eds): Cardiomyopathy and Myocardial Biopsy. New York, Springer-Verlag, 1978, pp 300–307.
170. Myerburg RJ, Kessler KM, Bassett AL, Castellanos A: A biological approach to sudden cardiac death: Structure, function and cause. Am J Cardiol 63:1512–1516, 1989.
171. Myerburg RJ, Kessler KM, Interian A Jr, et al: Clinical and experimental pathophysiology of sudden cardiac death. In Zipes DP, Jalife J (eds): Cardiac Electrophysiology: From Cell to Bedside. Philadelphia, WB Saunders, 1990, pp 666–678.
172. Arnsdorf MF: Basic understanding of the electrophysiologic action of antiarrhythmic drugs: Sources, sinks and matrices of information. Med Clin North Am 68:1247–1280, 1984.
173. Arnsdorf MF: Cardiac excitability the electrophysiologic matrix and electrically induced ventricular arrhythmias: Order and reproducibility in seeming electrophysiologic chaos. J Am Coll Cardiol 17:139–142, 1991.
174. Nikolic G, Haffty BG, Bishop RL, Singh JB, Flessas AP, Spodick DH: Sudden death in aortic stenosis monitored by ear densitographic pulse and ECG: Am Heart J 104: 311–312, 1982.
175. Schiavone WA, Maloney JD, Lever HM, Castle LW, Sterba R, Morant V: Electrophysiologic studies of patients with hypertrophic cardiomyopathy presenting with syncope of undetermined etiology. PACE 9:476–481, 1986.
176. Linker NJ, Stewart JT, Griffith MJ, et al: Investigation of the mechanism of syncope in patients with hypertrophic cardiomyopathy [abstract]. J Am Coll Cardiol 15:98A, 1990.
177. Edwards RHT, Kristinsson A, Warrel DA, Goodwin JF: Effects of propranolol on response to exercise in hypertrophic cardiomyopathy. Br Heart J 32:219–225, 1970.

178. Frenneaux MP, Porter A, Caforia AL, et al: Determinants of exercise capacity in hypertrophic cardiomyopathy. J Am Coll Cardiol 13:1521–1526, 1989.
179. Ingham RE, Rossen RM, Goodman DJ, Harrison DC: Treadmill arrhythmias in patients with idiopathic hypertrophic subaortic stenosis. Chest 68:759–674, 1975.
180. Bonow RO, Dilsizian V, Rosing DR, Maron BJ, Bacharach SL, Green MV: Verapamil-induced improvement in left ventricular diastolic filling and increased exercise tolerance in patients with hypertrophic cardiomyopathy: Short- and long-term effects. Circulation 72:853–864, 1985.
181. Pritchett ELC, Smith MS, McCarthy EA, Lee KL: The spontaneous occurrence of paroxysmal supraventricular tachycardia. Circulation 70:1–6, 1984.
182. Glass L, Mackey MC: From Clocks to Chaos. Princeton, NJ, Princeton University Press, 1988, pp 36–56.
183. Epstein SE, Rosing DR: Verapamil: Its potential for causing serious complications in patients with hypertrophic cardiomyopathy. Circulation 64:437–441, 1981.
184. Koretsune Y, Marban E: Cell calcium in the pathophysiology of ventricular fibrillation and in the pathogenesis of postarrhythmic contractile dysfunction. Circulation 80:369–379, 1989.
185. Mirowski M, Reid PR, Mower MM, et al: Termination of malignant ventricular arrhythmia with an implanted automatic defibrillator in human beings. N Engl J Med 303:322–324, 1980.
186. Mirowski M, Reid PR, Watkins L, Weisfeldt ML, Mower MM: Clinical treatment of life-threatening ventricular tachyarrhythmias with the automatic implantable defibrillator. Am Heart J 102:265–270, 1981.
187. Kron J, Oliver RP, Norsted S, Silka MJ: The automatic implantable cardioverter-defibrillator in young patients. J Am Coll Cardiol 16:896–902, 1990.
188. Winkle RA, Mead RH, Ruder MA, et al: Long-term outcome with the automatic implantable cardioverter-defibrillator. J Am Coll Cardiol 13:1353–1361, 1989.
189. Pycha C, Gulledge AD, Hutzler J, Kadri N, Maloney J: Psychological responses to the implantable defibrillator: Preliminary observations. Psychosomatics 27:841–845, 1986.
190. Kriett JM, Kaye MP: The Registry of the International Society for Heart and Lung Transplantation: Eighth Official Report—1991. J Heart Lung Transplant 10:491–498, 1991.

12

Role of Left Ventricular Ejection Fraction

J. THOMAS BIGGER JR.

The identification of increased mortality and morbidity risk in patients with coronary heart disease provides a rational and cost-effective basis for individualizing diagnostic and therapeutic strategies. Risk stratification is used to plan large-scale intervention trials and to guide the use of conventional diagnostic or therapeutic procedures. This chapter reviews information about left ventricular function as a predictor of risk, particularly the risk of sudden cardiac death (SCD). Left ventricular dysfunction possibly is linked to sudden death by being an indicator of a myocardium vulnerable to sustained ventricular tachycardia (VT) or ventricular fibrillation (VF). Some additional transient factor such as ischemia, drug toxicity, electrolyte abnormality, or change in autonomic nervous system activity may be required to provoke the vulnerable myocardium into sustained VT or VF. Conversely, myocardial scarring, the anatomical correlate of left ventricular dysfunction, can substantially amplify the adverse effect of one of these transient factors.

LEFT VENTRICULAR DYSFUNCTION

Infarct Size

In coronary heart disease, infarct size importantly determines left ventricular dysfunction, which in turn is a prime determinant of sudden or arrhythmic death as well as total mortality early and late after myocardial infarction (MI). The fraction of left ventricle that is infarcted has a strong association with hospital death in acute MI.[1] Infarct size is dependent on the amount of myocardium supplied by the occluded or stenotic coronary artery, the extent and timing of spontaneous or therapeutic thrombolysis, the extent and effectiveness of coronary collaterals, and the magnitude of the myocardial oxygen demand. Recent animal and patient studies indicate that the evolution of MI is a dynamic and time-dependent process.[2] In 1971, quantitative estimates of infarction size became possible through the analysis of serial changes in the serum creatine kinase (CK) activity.[3] Refined methods that measure the myocardial band (MB) CK provide more precise quantitation.[4,5]

Studies using these methods showed that infarction size was a major predictor of death during all phases of MI.[5–8] Geltman et al studied 173 patients younger than 66 years of age who survived their first acute MI for at least 24 hours.[5] Overall survival was significantly better after small (infarct size index < 15 units) or moderate-size infarcts (15–30 units) than with large infarcts (>30 units). The mean infarct size index of those who died averaged 46.5 ± 5.8 (SEM) units, compared with 21.1 ± 1.4 units for survivors ($p < 0.001$). Regardless of the infarct location, patients with small infarcts had a better prognosis than those with larger infarcts. Patients with anterior infarcts had a higher mortality than those with inferior

---

Supported in part by NIH grants HL-41552 from the National Heart, Lung, and Blood Institute, Bethesda, MD and RR-00645 from the Research Resources Administration, NIH; and by funds from the Bugher Foundation, the Dover Foundation, and Mrs. Adelaide Segerman, New York, NY.

infarction, but this difference in survival was accounted for by infarct size: anterior infarcts were roughly twice as big as inferior infarcts. Multivariate analysis indicated that infarct size was an independent predictor of death in patients experiencing their first infarct. Also, ventricular premature complexes (VPCs) occurred more frequently in the coronary care unit (CCU) in patients with large infarcts, regardless of infarct location.[5]

Marmor et al studied a sample of 200 patients and found that non-Q-wave infarctions were associated with less myocardial damage than Q-wave infarctions, i.e., 11 vs. 25 CK-MB units.[7] Also, 43% of the non-Q-wave and 8% of the Q-wave infarctions exhibited early recurrence or an extension of the initial infarct, manifested by a second rise in CK-MB activity beginning 48 hours or more after the onset of the primary infarct. In patients with non-Q-wave infarcts that extended, the hospital mortality was 16%, compared to 7% when no extension occurred. Also, in patients with infarct extension, left ventricular ejection fraction (LVEF) decreased from 0.56 ± 0.11 to 0.34 ± 0.10 10 days later ($p < 0.01$). Infarct extension in patients with non-Q-wave infarctions was associated with an increased mortality between hospital discharge and 1 year. Behorin et al studied the independent risk carried by nonfatal reinfarction for subsequent cardiac death in 1234 patients treated with placebo and followed up for 1–4 years after acute MI in the Multicenter Diltiazem Postinfarction Trial.[9] One hundred sixteen patients had at least one nonfatal reinfarction during follow-up, and 14 (12%) subsequently died. Cox regression analyses, using nonfatal reinfarction as a time-dependent predictor variable along with baseline clinical variables, revealed that nonfatal reinfarction carried a significant and independent risk for subsequent cardiac mortality (hazard ratio 3.0, $p = 0.002$) which was greater than that carried by other significant predictor variables (New York Heart Association functional class, pulmonary congestion on chest x-ray, LVEF, and ventricular arrhythmias). The risk of cardiac death associated with nonfatal reinfarction was even higher in patients whose index infarction was their first (hazard ratio 5.4, $p = 0.0006$). Thus, nonfatal reinfarction carries a strong, significant, and independent risk for subsequent cardiac death in patients discharged alive after acute MI.

Clinical Variables During the CCU Phase of Acute Myocardial Infarction That Predict Short- and Long-Term Risk of Death

Many clinical variables that can be assessed in the CCU phase of acute MI predict death during the acute phase of infarction and after discharge from the hospital.[10-15] Most of the CCU predictor variables reflect marked left ventricular dysfunction; among these are shock, low blood pressure, rales, increased heart rate, increased respiratory rate, and pulmonary venous congestion or cardiomegaly on chest x-ray. Prognostic indices derived from these data, such as the Norris and Peel indices,[16,17] can predict short- and long-term outcome, and these findings indicate that extensive myocardial damage at the time of infarction is a permanent liability.

Noninvasive Evaluation of Left Ventricular Function

Radionuclide ventriculography, dye angiography, and echocardiography are three commonly used laboratory techniques for evaluation of ventricular function after MI. Radionuclide methods or dye angiography have been used more commonly in clinical trials and clinical practice, but newer echocardiographic methods are gaining wider acceptance. Echocardiography and angiography lack the precision of MUGA scans, but LVEF is such a potent risk predictor that the difference is of little practical significance.

Radionuclide Methods

In 1975, Schulze et al[18] studied 81 postinfarction patients and found an association between LVEF below 0.40 and mortality events during a 6-month follow-up. Our Multicenter Post-infarction Program (MPIP) determined a radionuclide ejection fraction in 811 of 867 patients during hospitalization for acute MI.[19] About one third of the patients had an LVEF below 0.40 1 week after infarction. One-year cardiac

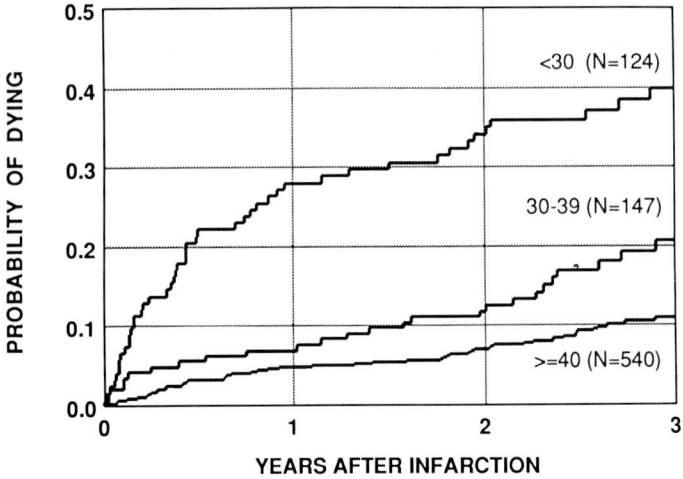

Fig. 12-1. Relationship between left ventricular ejection fraction and all-cause mortality. (From the Multicenter Post-Infarction Program, reference 31.)

mortality increased progressively as the ejection fraction decreased below 0.40 (Fig. 12-1). Cox survival analyses identified an ejection fraction below 0.40 and rales heard in the upper two thirds of the lung fields while the patient was in the CCU as the two most significant independent risk factors. Patients with both of these indicators of left ventricular dysfunction had an eightfold mortality risk compared to patients with neither. In another report from MPIP, Greenberg et al[20] concluded that rales in the CCU provide information about acute phase ventricular dysfunction, possibly ischemia-related reduction in ventricular compliance, whereas the radionuclide ejection fraction obtained a week or so later provides information about residual ventricular performance after the infarct has stabilized. The rales and low ejection fraction findings provide different hemodynamic information at different times during the evolving MI. These interpretations are further substantiated by the observations of Warnowicz et al,[21] who noted a marked disparity between acute phase ventricular dysfunction (pulmonary edema) and recovery phase ventricular performance (normal ejection fraction) in selected patients with acute MI. Dwyer et al[22] found that an ejection fraction below 0.40 and an independent predictor of nonfatal cardiac events (angina, heart failure, arrhythmia, and coronary artery surgery) that prompted rehospitalization during the year following MI, but not of reinfarction in the first year after the index infarction.

The resting radionuclide ejection fraction clearly has prognostic value, and high-risk patients with ejection fractions below 0.40 can be easily identified. A significant percentage of patients with ejection fractions above 0.40 still experience mortality and morbidity, and exercise radionuclide ejection fraction studies may have value in this subgroup. Corbett et al[23] studied ejection fractions on submaximal exercise in 67 post-infarction patients before hospital discharge. The mean ejection fraction in this population was 0.55, and the patients with major cardiac events during 6-month follow-up had a significant reduction in peak exercise ejection fraction (0.44 at rest to 0.37 with exercise), compared to minimal change in patients with minor cardiac events and an increase in patients with no cardiac events (0.66 at rest to 0.76 with exercise). A reduction in the exercise ejection fraction in patients with a normal resting ejection fraction is associated with multivessel coronary disease,[24] explaining the unfavorable outcome for patients with this finding.

Echocardiographic Methods

The echocardiogram may prove useful for evaluating ventricular function to assess risk after MI. Postmortem studies in patients dying within 30 days after acute MI have shown that 72% of the hearts have thinning and dilation of the infarcted area.[25] Furthermore, approximately one third of hearts with transmural infarction had significant expansion of the infarct zone. Infarct expansion may be deleterious to the heart as a result of increased oxygen demands associated with increased wall tension. Two-dimensional echocardiography can demonstrate acute alterations in cardiac topography, including regional myocardial dilation and wall thinning. Eaton et al[26] looked for these changes with serial echocardiography in 28 patients during the first 2 weeks after acute Q-wave MI. Eight patients (29%) showed infarct expansion with disproportionate dilation and transmural thinning in the infarcted zone. The eight patients with regional expansion had a higher 8-week mortality, even though their peak CK levels and Killip classification were similar to those in patients without this finding, suggesting that aneurysm formation has independent prognostic significance.

Several echocardiographic studies report the extent of left ventricular dysfunction complicating an acute MI as a "wall motion index" derived from scores for wall movement and thickening in 11 myocardial segments.[27–29] Gibson et al[28] observed severe wall motion abnormalities remote from the infarct zone in 47% of 75 patients. Wall motion abnormalities were associated with increased mortality ($p < 0.05$), shock ($p < 0.01$), progression to a worse Killip class ($p < 0.001$), reinfarction ($p < 0.01$), and angina ($p < 0.10$). In 66 patients initially classified as Killip Class I or II, the wall motion index predicted subsequent hemodynamic deterioration.

Stamm et al[30] studied the relationship between coronary anatomy (using coronary angiography) and left ventricular wall motion abnormalities detected by two-dimensional echocardiography during acute MI in 30 patients. In single-vessel disease, MI produced a distinctive pattern of asynergy with remote compensatory hyperkinesis in 50% of patients. In contrast, 75% of patients with multivessel coronary disease had remote asynergy. The extent of asynergy during acute MI overestimated the extent of wall motion abnormality present after recovery. The authors concluded that remote asynergy soon after infarction identifies a subset of patients with jeopardized myocardium and is associated with early reinfarction and a poor prognosis.[26] Coronary angiography is indicated when remote asynergy is detected by echocardiography soon after MI. Patients with critical coronary lesions in noninfarct vessels should be considered for revascularization, especially when the resting LVEF is below 0.40.

RELATIONSHIP BETWEEN LEFT VENTRICULAR DYSFUNCTION AND VENTRICULAR ARRHYTHMIAS AFTER MYOCARDIAL INFARCTION

Four large multicenter studies have evaluated the relationships among left ventricu-

Table 12–1
Relationship Between Ventricular Arrhythmias, Left Ventricular Dysfunction, and Mortality After Myocardial Infarction

Study*	Total No. of Pts.	Left Ventricular Ejection Fraction <0.40					Left Ventricular Ejection Fraction ≥0.40				
		VPC <10/hr		VPC ≥10/hr			VPC <10/hr		VPC ≥10/hr		
		N	Mortality Rate	N	Mortality Rate	Relative Risk	N	Mortality Rate	N	Mortality Rate	Relative Risk
MPIP	766	184	17.3%	72	32.2%	1.87	432	6.3%	78	11.7%	1.84
MILIS	533	141	19.1%	40	40.0%	2.09	314	5.1%	38	18.4%	3.61
MDPIT	955	203	15.2%	75	30.2%	1.99	589	7.0%	88	12.6%	1.81
UCSD SCOR	749	84	17.9%	101	26.7%	1.50	357	5.0%	207	14.5%	2.87

Abbreviations: MDPIT, Multicenter Diltiazem Post Infarction Trial; MILIS, Multicenter Investigation of the LImitation of Infarct Size; MPIP, Multicenter Post-infarction Program; UCSD SCOR, University of California San Diego, Special Center of Research in Ischemic Heart Disease; VPCs, ventricular premature complexes.

* Values for MPIP and MDPIT are Kaplan-Meier estimates of mortality rates at 24 months of follow-up; values for MILIS are crude mortality rates after an average follow-up of 18 months. The UCSD SCOR arrhythmia data are partitioned, not by VPC value of 10/hr, but by grade <2 and ≥2 (many patients in the ≥2 group have infrequent VPCs and no repetitive ventricular arrhythmias). The mortality values are crude rates at the end of 12 months of follow-up.

lar dysfunction, ventricular arrhythmias, and mortality in a total of more than 3000 postinfarction patients.[31-35] These studies are summarized in Table 12–1. The overall strength of the association between LVEF and death in the four studies was strong (odds ratio = 3.38). The strength of association was similar among the four studies (range of odds ratios, 2.90–4.46). The overall strength of association between ventricular arrhythmia and death in the four studies also was strong (odds ratio = 3.37). The strength of association was similar among the four studies (range of odds ratios, 2.41–6.60). There was a weak but statistically significant association between left ventricular dysfunction and ventricular arrhythmias after MI. On average, patients with an LVEF below 0.40 were 1.6 times as likely to have ventricular arrhythmias as patients with an LVEF of 0.40 or above (range among the relative risks for the four studies, 1.49–2.08). There was no statistical interaction between ventricular arrhythmias and LVEF with respect to their ability to predict mortality—that is, these two factors each predict risk independent of the other. When both of these important risk factors are present, their relative risks can be multiplied to obtain the combined risk (e.g., 3.38 × 3.37 = 11.39-fold increase in risk). In the MPIP, LVEF predicted deaths occurring in the first 6 months after MI better than ventricular arrhythmias, while the converse was true for deaths occurring after 6 months (Fig. 12–2).[31]

Infarct Size and Prevalence of Inducible Ventricular Tachycardia Early After Acute Myocardial Infarction

In dogs with experimental MI, the probability of having sustained VT as a response to programmed ventricular stimulation is strongly related to infarct size (Fig. 12–3).[36,37] In studies involving more than 100 dogs, infarct size expressed as a percentage of the left ventricular mass was related to the probability of inducing sustained VT, as follows: infarct size < 10%, 5% inducible; infarct size 10–19%, 25% inducible; and infarct size > 20%, 70% inducible.[36,37] Wilber et al[38] showed that dogs with large MIs were not only more likely to have inducible VT, but also they were more likely to have spontaneous VF during a period of myocardial ischemia.

Left Ventricular Dysfunction and Inducible Ventricular Tachycardia

Richards et al[39] studied 165 survivors of MI and found that inducible patients had lower LVEFs, 0.47 ± 0.03, than noninducible patients, 0.58 ± 0.02 ($p < 0.01$). These findings suggest that inducible VT is more likely in patients who have large infarcts. Denniss et al studied 403 patients after acute MI and found a strong relationship between LVEF and the probability of inducing sustained VT.[40] The overall probability of inducing sustained VT was 20%. The probability of inducing sustained VT was 52% in patients with an LVEF below 0.40, vs. 5%

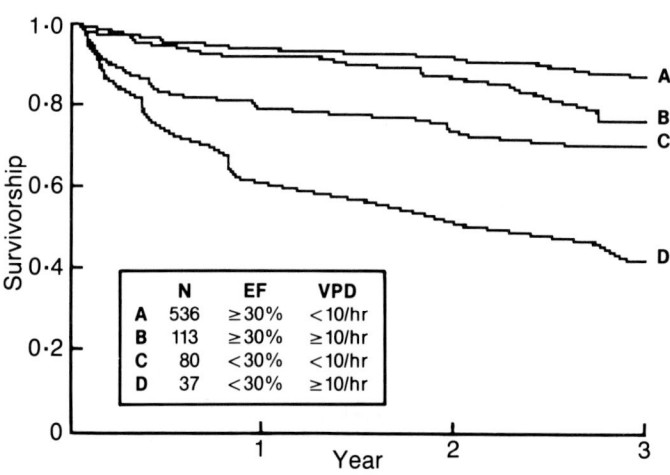

Fig. 12–2. Time course for all-cause mortality in patients classified by left ventricular ejection fraction and ventricular arrhythmias. (From the Multicenter Post-Infarction Program, reference 31).

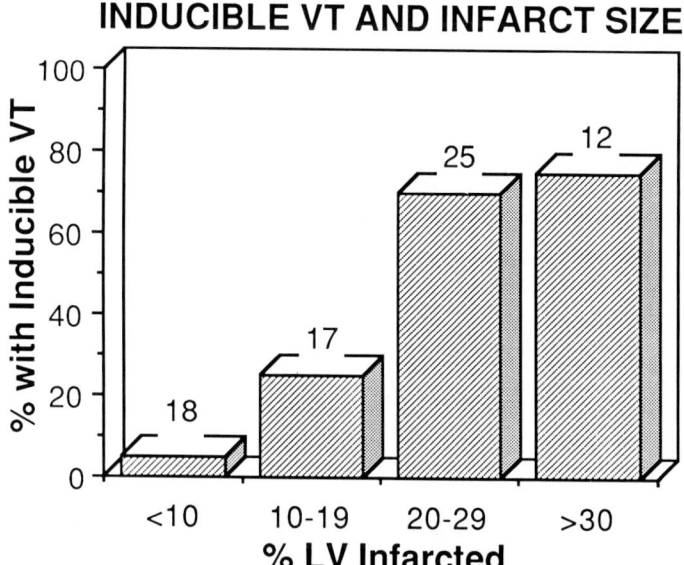

Fig. 12–3. Relationship between size of myocardial infarction and the probability of inducing ventricular tachycardia or fibrillation in an animal model of postinfarction ventricular tachycardia. (From references 36,37.)

in patients with an LVEF of 0.40 or greater. Patients with chronic coronary heart disease and large scars, particularly those with ventricular aneurysms, are more likely to have sustained VT induced by programmed ventricular stimulation. Spielman and colleagues studied 58 patients with previous MI who had at least ten VPCs per hour and LVEFs below 0.50.[41,42] In this group, 50% had inducible sustained VT, a much higher rate than those found in studies of unselected patients. Bourke et al reported the largest experience with postinfarction electrophysiological studies.[43] They studied 1209 patients 6–28 days after acute MI. In a subgroup of 423 patients in whom the ejection fraction was measured and who also underwent programmed ventricular stimulation, they evaluated the combined use of these two tests to predict arrhythmic events (documented spontaneous VT, VF, or witnessed instantaneous death) (Table 12–2). They found that using an ejection fraction of <0.40 alone was sensitive (73%), but the positive predictive value for arrhythmic events was only 6%. Programmed ventricular stimulation on all patients yielded a 10% prevalence of sustained VT and had a positive predictive accuracy of 20% for predicting arrhythmic events in the first year after infarction. Bourke et al then evaluated a policy of performing programmed ventricular stimulation only in patients who have an ejection fraction below 0.40. This policy restricted programmed stimulation to only 30% of the infarct survivors, in 20% of

Table 12–2
Left Ventricular Ejection Fraction and Electrophysiology Studies to Predict Arrhythmic Events in the First Year After Myocardial Infarction (N = 423)

	LVEF <0.40	Positive Electrophysiologic Study	Both Studies Positive
Positive tests (%)	30	10	6
Sensitivity (%)	73	73	64
Positive predictive value (%)	6	20	28
Negative predictive value (%)	99	99	99
Overall predictive accuracy (%)	72	91	97

Source: Bourke JP, et al: J Am Coll Cardiol 18:780–788, 1991.[43] Reproduced by permission.

whom sustained VT could be induced. The positive predictive accuracy of the two tests together was 28%. Although the data in humans are still meager, they suggest that large infarcts are strongly associated with inducible, sustained VT in man just as in dogs. Studies are not available to show whether inducible sustained VT predicts death or spontaneous sustained ventricular arrhythmias independent of LVEF. Such studies are badly needed.

LEFT VENTRICULAR EJECTION FRACTION COMPARED WITH OTHER NONINVASIVE PREDICTORS OF ARRHYTHMIC RISK

Farrell et al studied the predictive value of several tests done early after MI: LVEF, 24-hour Holter electrocardiographic (ECG) recording, heart period variability, and signal-averaged ECG.[44] The study included 416 patients in whom a battery of tests was done, after which patients were followed for 1.7 years to determine survival status and occurrence of nonfatal arrhythmic events. Twenty-four arrhythmic events and 47 cardiac deaths occurred during follow-up. LVEF ranked seventh as a predictor of arrhythmic event (relative risk) and third as a predictor of cardiac death (Table 12–3). LVEF ranked sixth in positive predictive accuracy for arrhythmic events during follow-up (Table 12–4). Combinations of LVEF with other risk predictors were not as strong (relative risk, 5–7) as the relative risk of a positive signal-averaged ECG combined with heart period variability (relative risk, 18.5) for predicting arrhythmic events. This study suggests that LVEF does not predict arrhythmic events as well as cardiac death. It is possible that LVEF would have performed better if a cutpoint of 0.30 or 0.35 had been used.

LEFT VENTRICULAR DYSFUNCTION AND ANTIARRHYTHMIC DRUG ASSESSMENT

Sustained Ventricular Tachycardia or Ventricular Fibrillation

Meissner et al assessed the relation between acute antiarrhythmic drug efficacy and left ventricular function in 201 patients with coronary artery disease and sustained ventricular tachyarrhythmias.[45] In the 201 patients, 560 electrophysiological studies were done to evaluate antiarrhythmic drug therapy. Ejection fraction was dichotomized at 0.30. At least one successful acute antiarrhythmic regimen was found for 47% of patients. Success was significantly more common in the 81 patients with an ejection fraction of 0.30 or higher (64%) than in the 120 with an ejection fraction below 0.30 (36%; $p < 0.001$) (Fig. 12–4). Drug trials

Table 12–3
Relative Risk for Risk Predictors in 416 Patients Studied 7 to 10 Days After Myocardial Infarction

Rank*	Risk Predictor	Number Below Cutpoint	Relative Risk Arrhythmic Events† (95% CI)	Relative Risk Cardiac Mortality (95% CI)
1	R-R variability <20 msec	113	32.4 (7.6–138.2)	6.7 (3.6–12.3)
2	Signal-averaged ECG positive	89	6.5 (2.9–14.9)	2.2 (1.2–4.0)
3	VPCs ≥10/hr	84	5.0 (2.2–11.1)	3.0 (1.7–5.4)
4	Repetitive ventricular arrhythmias	86	4.9 (2.2–10.9)	2.5 (1.4–4.6)
5	Mean R-R interval <750 msec	126	4.9 (2.1–11.5)	3.5 (2.0–6.2)
6	Killip class ≥2	83	2.6 (1.1–6.0)	5.6 (3.2–10.0)
7	LVEF <0.40	110	2.5 (1.1–5.6)	3.7 (2.1–6.5)

Source: Farrell TG, et al: J Am Coll Cardiol 18:687–697, 1991.[44] Reproduced by permission.
* Ranked by relative risk for arrhythmic events.
† Sustained ventricular tachyarrhythmia or arrhythmic death by the CAPS definition.

Table 12-4
Prediction of Arrhythmic Events After Myocardial Infarction Using Noninvasive Risk Measures (N = 416)

Risk Predictor	Below Cutpoint	Positive Predictive Accuracy (%)	Negative Predictive Accuracy (%)
Signal-averaged ECG positive	21.4	17	81
R-R variability <20 msec	27.2	17	77
VPCs ≥10/hr	20.2	16	82
Repetitive ventricular arrhythmias	20.7	15	97
Mean R-R <750 msec	30.3	13	97
LVEF <0.40	26.4	10	75

SOURCE: Farrell TG, et al: J Am Coll Cardiol *18*:687–697, 1991.[44] Reproduced by permission.

were successful (initiation of <15 repetitive ventricular responses) in 32% of patients with an ejection fraction of 0.30 or greater vs. 19% of those with an ejection fraction below 0.30 ($p < 0.001$). A logistic regression analysis with many clinical covariates showed that LVEF was the only factor that was significantly associated with drug success or failure ($p < 0.002$).

Unsustained Ventricular Tachycardia

Pratt et al did a similar study using 24-hour continuous ECG recordings instead of programmed ventricular stimulation to assess antiarrhythmic drug treatment. They evaluated the relationship between LVEF and the likelihood of achieving suppression of ventricular arrhythmias as judged by 24-hour ECG recordings.[46] A total of 246 patients (42% with an ejection fraction below 0.40) had complex ventricular arrhythmias and were treated with one of eight antiarrhythmic drugs. A total of 132 (54%) of the 246 had unsustained VT. For patients with an ejection fraction of 0.30 or higher, 67% had suppression of VT, compared with 36% suppression in patients with an ejection fraction below 0.30 ($p = 0.001$) (see Fig. 12–4). Life-threatening complications of antiarrhythmic therapy occurred most frequently in the 61 patients with an ejection

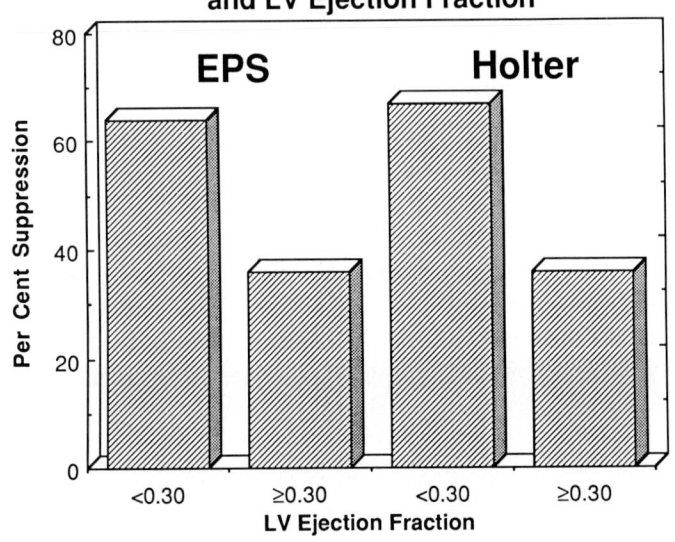

Fig. 12–4. Relationship between left ventricular ejection fraction and the likelihood of suppressing inducible, sustained ventricular tachycardia (EPS, *left*) or spontaneous, unsustained ventricular tachycardia (Holter, *right*). (From references 45,46).

fraction below 0.30, compared to the 185 patients with an ejection fraction of 0.30 or higher (15% vs. 2%; $p = 0.001$).

Asymptomatic Ventricular Arrhythmias After Myocardial Infarction

These results were confirmed in the Cardiac Arrhythmia Pilot Study (CAPS).[47] In CAPS, titration of antiarrhythmic drugs included dose ranging and, if the first drug tried did not work, a second drug was tried. Based on results of treatment with the first drug, there was a clear relationship between successful suppression of ventricular arrhythmias and LVEF. Overall, the percentage suppression for the four active treatments, taken together, were: 58% for an ejection fraction below 0.30, 68% for an ejection fraction of 0.30–0.44, and 76% for an ejection fraction of 0.45 or above. It is notable that placebo treatment had a similar trend with LVEF: there was a lower rate of apparent drug response in the group with an ejection fraction below 0.30. This finding suggests less spontaneous variation in VPC rates in the low ejection fraction group.

IS SUDDEN CARDIAC DEATH A VALID END POINT?

It is not clear that LVEF predicts SCD any better than it predicts all-cause mortality. Assessing mechanisms of death of patients after MI is problematic. If arrhythmic death could be accurately classified, then arrhythmic death would be the most appropriate end point to assess for benefit of treatments aimed at reducing death due to ventricular arrhythmias. Unfortunately, neither SCD nor arrhythmic death has been validated. Classification of deaths as due to myocardial failure has not been validated either.

The Multicenter Postinfarction Program (MPIP) investigators classified deaths, during 1 to 4 years of follow-up, as sudden or nonsudden, and also by mechanism.[48] To assign a mechanism to each death, the classification by Hinkle and Thaler was used.[49] The major categories in this classification are arrhythmic death, death due to circulatory failure, and noncardiac death. Arrhythmic death was defined by Hinkle and Thaler as "abrupt loss of consciousness and disappearance of pulse without prior collapse of the circulation." Circulatory failure was defined as collapse of circulation before disappearance of the pulse. Deaths due to cancer, cerebral emboli, accidents, suicide, and complications of procedures were classified as noncardiac deaths.

Of the 143 deaths in the MPIP, 70% were witnessed and 30% were unwitnessed.[48] Of the 104 cardiac deaths with known onset of symptoms, 43% were sudden (<1 hour). By the Hinkle-Thaler classification, 56% of the deaths were arrhythmic, 20% were due to myocardial failure, and 24% were not cardiac. About two thirds of the arrhythmic deaths were not preceded by disabling heart failure. Even deaths that were preceded by disabling heart failure were abrupt and occurred without prior evidence of circulatory collapse. Of the sudden deaths, 98% were classified as arrhythmic by the Hinkle-Thaler classification; 54% of the nonsudden cardiac deaths were arrhythmic by the Hinkle-Thaler classification. Similar results have been obtained using the CAPS definition,[50] which is similar to the Hinkle-Thaler definition of SCD.

Classification of deaths as sudden or arrhythmic has not been validated. Patients with low LVEFs after acute MI are at least as likely to die "arrhythmic deaths" as deaths due to "myocardial failure" (Table 12–5). There is no difference in the relative risk for arrhythmic death and myocardial failure deaths for patients with LVEFs below 0.30 versus those with LVEFs of 0.30 or above. Similarly, patients with frequent or repetitive VPCs are as likely to die of myocardial failure as of arrhythmias. Newer risk predictors, such as the signal-averaged ECG or R-R variability, have not been evaluated in this way.

Multiple and Competing Risks after Myocardial Infarction

The MPIP investigators found that patients with coronary heart disease usually have multiple functional deficits as they approach death. Many have both arrhythmias and heart failure, and about half have either angina pectoris or recurrent MI in the last few weeks of life. How the three important mechanisms interact pathophysiologically

Table 12-5
Independent Association of Postinfarction Risk Predictors with Arrhythmic Death and Death Due to Myocardial Failure (Hinkle-Thaler classification)*

Risk Predictor	Arrhythmic Deaths ($n = 71$)		Myocardial Failure Deaths ($n = 24$)		Z Score‡
	Relative† Risk	95% CI	Relative Risk	95% CI	
LVEF	1.9	1.5–2.4	1.6	1.0–2.4	0.7
Rales in CCU	2.1	1.2–3.5	3.3	1.4–7.7	−0.9
NYHA functional class	1.7	1.0–2.9	2.6	1.1–6.0	−0.8
VPC frequency	1.4	1.1–1.8	1.3	0.8–2.0	0.4

SOURCE: Marcus FI, et al: Am J Cardiol 61:8–15, 1988.[48] reproduced by permission.
* Cox proportional hazards model with all four risk predictors in the model.
† Ratio of risk for patients with/without the factor, adjusted for the other factors.
‡ Comparison of the relative risk for arrhythmic deaths with the relative risk for heart failure deaths ($Z \geq 1.96$ have a $p < 0.05$).

to lead to death is almost impossible to determine. A single functional mechanism of death is difficult to identify even when a patient dies in an intensive care unit under continuous ECG and hemodynamic observation. Because several pathophysiological factors often contribute to death in coronary heart disease, it was difficult to link baseline indicators—left ventricular dysfunction, arrhythmias, or ischemia—to the mechanism of death. Competing risks can confound functional classifications of death. A postinfarction patient who has frequent and repetitive ventricular arrhythmias on a baseline 24-hour ECG recording may experience a second MI and die a few days later of myocardial failure. If the death is classified as primarily due to heart failure or ischemia, this case represents a lack of validity: arrhythmic risk was detected on baseline examination but the death was not arrhythmic. Had the fatal infarct not occurred, the patient may have died an arrhythmic death at some later point in time, but we can never know. The competing risk concept makes it clear why it is difficult to validate mechanistic classifications of death.

The difficulty in validating sudden death will cloud the interpretation of studies that attempt to show treatment effects on sudden or arrhythmic death. However, collateral information can strengthen the inference that a reduction in sudden death indicates an effect on lethal arrhythmias. For example, the inference would be strengthened if the treatment reduces arrhythmias and known arrhythmogenic factors as well as sudden death.

REFERENCES

1. Miller RR, Olson HG, Vismara LA, Bogren HG, Amsterdam EA, Mason DT: Pump dysfunction after myocardial infarction: Importance of location, extent and pattern of abnormal left ventricular segmental contraction. Am J Cardiol 37:340–344, 1976.
2. Reimer KA, Jennings RB: Myocardial ischemia, hypoxia, and infarction. In Fozzard HM, et al (eds): The Heart and Cardiovascular System: Scientific Foundations. Boston, Martinus Nijhoff, 1986, pp 1133–1201.
3. Shell WE, Kjekshus JK, Sobel BE: Quantitative assessment of the extent of myocardial infarction in the conscious dog by means of analysis of serial changes in serum creatine phosphokinase activity. J Clin Invest 50:2614–2625, 1971.
4. Roberts R, Sobel BE, Parker CW: Radioimmunoassay for creatine kinase isoenzymes. Science 194:855–857, 1976.
5. Geltman EM, Ehsani AA, Campbell MK, Schechtman K, Roberts R, Sobel BE: The influence of location and extent of myocardial infarction on long-term ventricular dysrhythmia and mortality. Circulation 60:805–814, 1979.
6. Roberts R, Henry PD, Sobel BE: An improved basis for enzymatic estimation of infarct size. Circulation 52:743–754, 1975.
7. Marmor A, Sobel BE, Roberts R: Factors

presaging early recurrent myocardial infarction ("extension"). Am J Cardiol 48:603–610, 1981.
8. Roberts R: Non-transmural myocardial infarction. Council Clin Cardiol Newslett 11:1–17, 1985.
9. Benhorin J, Moss AJ, Oakes D: Prognostic significance of nonfatal myocardial reinfarction: Multicenter Diltiazem Postinfarction Trial Research Group. J Am Coll Cardiol 15:253–258, 1990.
10. Rutherford BD, McCann WD, O'Donnovan TPB: The value of monitoring pulmonary artery pressure for early detection of left ventricular failure following myocardial infarction. Circulation 43:655–666, 1971.
11. Ratshin RA, Rackley CE, Russell RO: Hemodynamic evaluation of left ventricular function in shock complicating myocardial infarction. Circulation 45:127–139, 1972.
12. Forrester JS, Diamond GA, Swan HJC: Correlative classification of clinical and hemodynamic function after myocardial infarction. Am J Cardiol 39:137–145, 1977.
13. Weber KT, Janicki JJ, Russell RO, Rackley CE: Identification of high risk subsets of acute myocardial infarction: Derived from the Myocardial Infarction Research Units Cooperative Study Data Bank. Am J Cardiol 41:197–203, 1978.
14. Shell W, Peter T, Mickle D, Forrester JS, Swan HJC: Prognostic implications of reduction of left ventricular filling pressure in early transmural acute myocardial infarction. Am Heart J 102:334–340, 1981.
15. Cohn JN, Franciosa JA, Francis GA, et al: Effects of short term infusion of sodium nitroprusside on mortality rate in acute myocardial infarction complicated by left ventricular failure. N Engl J Med 306:1129–1235, 1982.
16. Norris RM, Brandt PWT, Caughey DE, Deeming LW, Scott PJ: A new coronary prognostic index. Lancet i:274–278, 1969.
17. Peel AAF, Semple T, Wang I, Lancaster WM, Dall JLG: A coronary prognostic index for grading the severity of infarction. Br Heart J 24:745–760, 1962.
18. Schulze RA Jr, Rouleau J, Rigo P, Bowers S, Strauss HW, Pitt B: Ventricular arrhythmias in the late hospital phase of acute myocardial infarction: Relation to left ventricular function detected by gated cardiac blood pool scanning. Circulation 52:1006–1011, 1975.
19. Multicenter Post-infarction Research Group: Risk stratification after myocardial infarction. N Engl J Med 309:331–336, 1983.
20. Greenberg H, McMaster P, Dwyer EM Jr, and the Multicenter Post-infarction Research Group: Left ventricular dysfunction after acute myocardial infarction: Results of a prospective multicenter study. J Am Coll Cardiol 4:867–874, 1984.
21. Warnowicz MA, Parker H, Cheitlin MD: Prognosis of patients with acute pulmonary edema and normal ejection fraction after myocardial infarction. Circulation 67:330–334, 1983.
22. Dwyer EM Jr, McMaster P, Greenberg H, and the Multicenter Post-infarction Research Group: Non-fatal cardiac events and recurrent infarction in the year following acute myocardial infarction. J Am Coll Cardiol 4:695–702, 1984.
23. Corbett JR, Dehmer GJ, Lewis SE, et al: The prognostic value of submaximal exercise testing with radionuclide ventriculography before hospital discharge in patients with recent myocardial infarction. Circulation 64:535–544, 1981.
24. Wasserman AG, Katz RJ, Cleary P, Varma JM, Reba RC, Ross AM: Noninvasive detection of multivessel disease after myocardial infarction by exercise radionuclide ventriculography. Am J Cardiol 50:1242–1247, 1982.
25. Hutchins GM, Bulkley BH: Infarct expansion versus extension: Two different complications of acute myocardial infarction. Am J Cardiol 41:1127–1132, 1978.
26. Eaton LW, Weiss JL, Bulkley BH, Garrison JB, Weisfeldt ML: Regional cardiac dilatation after acute myocardial infarction. N Engl J Med 300:57–62, 1979.
27. Heger JJ, Weyman AE, Wann LS, Rogers EW, Dillon JC, Feigenbaum H: Cross-sectional echocardiographic analysis of the extent of left ventricular asynergy in acute myocardial infarction. Circulation 61:1113–1118, 1980.
28. Gibson RS, Bishop HL, Stamm RB, Crampton RS, Beller GA, Martin RP: Value of early two-dimensional echocardiography in patients with acute myocardial infarction. Am J Cardiol 49:1110–1119, 1982.
29. Nixon JV, Narahara A, Smitherman TC: Estimation of myocardial involvement in patients with acute myocardial infarction by two-dimensional echocardiography. Circulation 62:1248–1255, 1980.
30. Stamm RB, Gibson RS, Bishop HL, Carabello BA, Beller GA, Martin RP: Echocardiographic detection of infarct-localized asynergy and remote asynergy during acute myocardial infarction: Correlation with extent of angiographic coronary disease. Circulation 67:233–244, 1983.
31. Bigger JT Jr, Fleiss JL, Kleiger R, Miller JP, Rolnitzky LM, and the Multicenter Post-infarction Research Group: The relationship

among ventricular arrhythmias, left ventricular dysfunction and mortality in the 2 years after myocardial infarction. Circulation 69: 250–258, 1984.
32. Mukharji J, Rude RE, Poole KE, et al, and the MILIS Study Group: Risk factors for sudden death after acute myocardial infarction: Two-year follow-up. Am J Cardiol 54: 31–36, 1984.
33. Coromilas J, Bigger JT Jr, Kleiger RE, Rolnitzky LM, Fleiss JL, and the MDPIT Research Group: Relations among left ventricular dysfunction, ventricular arrhythmias, and mortality after myocardial infarction. Circulation 80(suppl II):48, 1989.
34. Nicod P, Gilpin E, Dittrich H, Henning H, Ross J Jr: Prognostic significance of complex ventricular arrhythmia for cardiac death during the first year after myocardial infarction. J Electrophysiol 1:93–102, 1987.
35. Ahnve S, Gilpin E, Henning H, Curtis G, Collins D, Ross J Jr: Limitations and advantages of the ejection fraction for defining high risk after acute myocardial infarction. Am J Cardiol 58:872–878, 1986.
36. Gang ES, Bigger JT Jr, Livelli FD Jr: A model of chronic ischemic arrhythmias: The relationships among electrically inducible ventricular tachycardia, ventricular fibrillation threshold and myocardial infarct size. Am J Cardiol 50:469–477, 1982.
37. Coromilas J, Bigger JT Jr, Gang ES, Zimmerman JM: Relationship between infarct size and ventricular arrhythmias. In Zipes DP, Jalife J (eds): Cardiac Electrophysiology and Arrhythmias. New York, Grune & Stratton, 1985, pp 523–530.
38. Wilber DJ, Lynch JJ, Montgomery D, Lucchesi BR: Postinfarction sudden death: Significance of inducible ventricular tachycardia and infarct size in a conscious canine model. Am Heart J 109:8–18, 1985.
39. Richards DA, Cody DV, Denniss AR, Russell PA, Young AA, Uther JB: Ventricular electrical instability: A predictor of death after myocardial infarction. Am J Cardiol 51: 75–80, 1983.
40. Denniss AR, Richards DA, Cody DV, et al: Prognostic significance of ventricular tachycardia and fibrillation induced at programmed stimulation and delayed potentials detected on the signal-averaged electrocardiograms of survivors of acute myocardial infarction. Circulation 74:731–745, 1986.
41. Spielman SR, Yacone LA, Greenspan AM, Webb CR, Horowitz LN: Electrophysiologic testing in high-risk patients with non-sustained ventricular tachycardia and abnormal ventricular function. Circulation 68(suppl III):III-56, 1983.
42. Spielman SR, Greenspan AM, Kay HR, et al: Electrophysiologic testing in patients at high risk of sudden death: Nonsustained ventricular tachycardia and abnormal ventricular function. J Am Coll Cardiol 6:31–40, 1985.
43. Bourke JP, Richards DAB, Ross DL, Wallace EM, McGuire MA, Uther JB: Routine programmed electrical stimulation in survivors of acute myocardial infarction for prediction of spontaneous ventricular tachyarrhythmias during follow-up: Results, optimal stimulation protocol and cost-effective screening. J Am Coll Cardiol 18: 780–788, 1991.
44. Farrell TG, Bashir Y, Cripps T, et al: Risk stratification for arrhythmic events based on heart rate variability, ambulatory electrocardiographic variables and the signal-averaged electrocardiogram. J Am Coll Cardiol 18: 687–697, 1991.
45. Meissner MD, Kay HR, Horowitz LN, Spielman SR, Greenspan AM, Kutalek SP: Relation of acute antiarrhythmic drug efficacy to left ventricular function in coronary artery disease. Am J Cardiol 61:1050–1055, 1988.
46. Pratt CM, Eaton T, Francis M, et al: The inverse relationship between baseline left ventricular ejection fraction and outcome of antiarrhythmic therapy: A dangerous imbalance in the risk-benefit ratio. Am Heart J 118:433–440, 1989.
47. Cardiac Arrhythmia Pilot Study (CAPS) Investigators: Effects of encainide, flecainide, imipramine, and moricizine on ventricular arrhythmias during the year after acute myocardial infarction: The CAPS. Am J Cardiol 61:501–509, 1988.
48. Marcus FI, Cobb LA, Edwards JE, et al, and the Multicenter Post-infarction Research Group: Mechanism of death and prevalence of myocardial ischemic symptoms in the terminal event after acute myocardial infarction. Am J Cardiol 61:8–15, 1988.
49. Hinkle LE, Thaler JT: Clinical classification of cardiac deaths. Circulation 65:457–464, 1982.
50. Greene HL, Richardson DW, Barker AH, et al, and the CAPS Investigators: Classification of deaths after myocardial infarction as arrhythmic or nonarrhythmic (the Cardiac Arrhythmia Pilot Study). Am J Cardiol 63: 1–6, 1989.

13
Sudden Death in Patients with Structural Heart Disease

JOHN P. DiMARCO

Sudden death is most frequently encountered among patients with advanced forms of structural heart disease. Even if the patient had been unaware of any cardiac problem prior to the event, evaluation after resuscitation or during a postmortem examination will usually identify one or more specific cardiac lesions that constitute an anatomical substrate for fatal or life-threatening arrhythmias. However, in both autopsy series[1-3] and previously reported studies on the electrophysiological evaluation of patients resuscitated from out-of-hospital cardiac arrest,[4-6] a small percentage of patients have had no identifiable structural heart disease. Several small series of young patients without heart disease who suffered cardiac arrest have also been reported.[7-9] This chapter highlights several points in the evaluation and management of such patients.

DIFFERENTIAL DIAGNOSIS

A number of different conditions should be considered when a patient without previously identified structural heart disease experiences cardiac arrest. Hypertrophic cardiomyopathy will often be asymptomatic until the appearance of significant and even fatal arrhythmias.[10] However, the diagnosis is usually easily made by echocardiography and may often be suspected on the basis of a standard electrocardiogram (ECG). Previously healthy patients with sickle cell trait may collapse and die suddenly during vigorous exercise, probably due to red cell changes induced by heat and dehydration.[11] These patients may well have normal hearts, and the precise mechanism for death is uncertain. The congenital long QT syndrome may appear as an isolated phenomenon even without a family history of premature sudden death.[12] Coronary artery anomalies may cause sudden death either due to scarring from a prior, unsuspected myocardial infarction or from transient ischemia caused by the abnormal course of the anomalous coronary artery.[13] Occult coronary artery abnormalities from Kawasaki's disease may lead to similar problems. Coronary artery spasm which may or may not be associated with pain may cause ischemia-related arrhythmias that can be fatal.[14,15] Ergonovine testing may confirm the diagnosis if spasm and early arrhythmias can be induced. Arrhythmogenic right ventricular dysplasia may first manifest with arrhythmias. The diagnosis of dysplasia or other form of right ventricular myopathy must be considered if appropriate diagnostic studies are to be undertaken.[16,17] Careful interpretation of the ECG and echocardiogram may be required to detect right ventricular abnormalities. Magnetic resonance imaging or contrast right ventriculography are also useful. Sudden death can occur in the setting of congenital atrioventricular (AV) block, particularly if very slow escape pacemaker rates lead to ventricular arrhythmias.[18] Although sudden death is uncommon in patients with supraventricular tachycardia, occasional patients may achieve extremely rapid ventricular rates in supraventricular tachycardia that may then deteriorate to ventricular fibrillation (VF). The majority of such patients will have Wolff-Parkinson-White syndrome with pre-excited atrial fibrillation, but atrial flutter with 1:1 conduction, rapid AV reciprocating tachycardia, and even AV node re-entry may also rarely manifest in this fashion.[19] Patients with neurocardiogenic syncope often have prolonged periods of asystole. Although rare, bradycardia-dependent polymorphic ventricular arrhythmias have been reported in this syndrome.[4] Drug ingestion or intoxication should also be considered as a possible cause of sudden death.[3] Cocaine and alcohol have been the agents most commonly reported to cause sudden death, but many other drugs of abuse may cause either arrhythmias or respiratory depression. Other commonly used drugs may also rarely prolong ventricular repolarization and lead to polymorphic ventricular tachycardia (VT) and cardiac arrest in susceptible individuals.[20] Subclinical myocarditis has been found at autopsy in up to 10% of young patients who died suddenly,[1] but the results of studies on the use of myocardial biopsy in patients with sustained ventricular tachyarrhythmias have been inconsistent.[21,22]

At least two other poorly understood syndromes have been described as the cause of unexpected sudden death in patients with structurally normal hearts. Pokkuri disease is a syndrome of nocturnal sudden death in young males that has been reported from Japan.[23-25] Paroxysmal ventricular arrhythmias are thought to be the cause of death, and fibrotic changes in the conduction system have been reported in some patients. A somewhat similar syndrome of sudden death has been reported to occur in young male Southeast Asian immigrants to the United States.[26,27] Ventricular fibrillation and polymorphic VT are the arrhythmias that have been documented in these patients in isolated cases.

UNIVERSITY OF VIRGINIA EXPERIENCE

Over a 10-year period, 191 patients with aborted sudden cardiac death and documented VF at the time of resuscitation have undergone electrophysiological studies at the University of Virginia (Fig. 13–1). Patients in whom the cardiac arrest was preceded by an acute MI or was associated with hypotension, shock, or some other obvious noncardiac cause are excluded from this number. Patients who presented with syncope without documented sustained ventricular arrhythmias also were not included. All patients underwent diagnostic cardiac catheterization, two-dimensional echocardiography, and, in selected cases, myocardial biopsy, in addition to the electrophysiological evaluation. Patients with structural heart disease identified by these investigations were then excluded (Fig.

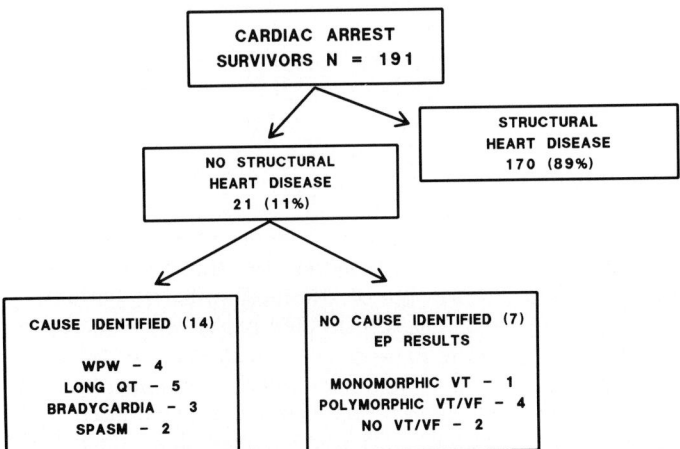

Fig. 13–1. Cardiac arrest without structural heart disease. The chart shows the University of Virginia experience with cardiac arrest survivors who underwent an electrophysiological evaluation. VF, ventricular fibrillation; VT, ventricular tachycardia; WPW, Wolff-Parkinson-White syndrome.

Table 13-1
Characteristics of Patients With Cardiac Arrest and No Structural Heart Disease: University of Virginia, 1981–91

Pt. No.	Age (yr)/Sex	LVEF	No. of Episodes	History of Syncope	Initial EPS	Other Finding	Therapy	Outcome
1	48/M	60%	1	Yes	VF (3 ES)		Quin.	Well
2	65/M	51%	1	No	VT (2 ES)		Amio.	Nonfatal VT
3	59/M	55%	3	Yes	VF (2 ES)		Amio./ICD	Nonfatal VT
4	15/M	70%	2	Yes	No VT		ICD/β-blocker	Recurrent VF after patient discontinued treatment
5	45/F	54%	2	No	No VT		β-blocker	Well
6	32/F	70%	3	Yes	VF (3 ES)		ICD/β-blocker	Nonfatal VT
7	38/M	60%	1	No	VF (2 ES)		Quin.	Well
8	59/M	58%	1	Yes	No VT	Neurocardiac syncope	Pacer/β-blocker	Well
9	49/M	55%	1	Yes	No VT	Neurocardiac syncope	Pacer/β-blocker	Well
10	40/M	60%	1	Yes	No VT	Spasm	Calcium blocker	Well
11	38/F	65%	1	No	No VT	Spasm	Calcium blocker	Well
12	19/F	65%	2	Yes	No VT	Cong. AV block	Pacing	Well
13	65/F	60%	2	Yes	No VT	PAF LQTS	Pacer/β-blocker	Well
14	34/F	60%	4	Yes	No VT	LQTS	β-blocker	Well
15	55/F	67%	2	Yes	No VT	PAF LQTS	β-blocker	Well
16	41/F	55%	1	No	No VT	LQTS	β-blocker	Well
17	19/F	65%	1	No	No VT	LQTS	β-blocker	Well
18	19/F	55%	1	No	AF/SVT	WPW	Ablation	Well
19	17/F	55%	1	Yes	AF/SVT	WPW	Quin./β-blocker	Well
20	42/M	62%	1	No	AF	WPW	Ablation	Well
21	21/M	65%	1	No	AF	WPW	Ablation	Well

Abbreviations: LVEF, left ventricular ejection fraction; EPS, electrophysiologic study; VF, ventricular fibrillation; Quin., quinidine; Amio., amiodarone; VT, ventricular tachycardia; ICD, implantable cardioverter-defibrillator; ES, extrastimuli; Cong., congenital; AV, atrioventricular; PAF, paroxysmal atrial fibrillation; LQTS, long QT syndrome; AF, atrial fibrillation; SVT, supraventricular tachycardia.

13–1). There were 21 patients, or 11.5% of the total group, in whom no structural heart disease or obvious precipitating factor was identified (Table 13–1). Four of these patients (Nos. 18 through 21) were found to have Wolff-Parkinson-White syndrome with rapidly conducting accessory pathways but had cardiac arrest as their initial presentation. Five additional patients had documented fixed or dynamic QT interval prolongation. One patient had well-described congenital AV block but presented at age 19 with syncope and repeated episodes of VF. A detailed discussion of the management of these three conditions as causes of sudden death is found elsewhere in this volume. The remaining 11 patients ranged in age from 15 to 71 years and had experienced between one and ten episodes of cardiac arrest prior to their presentation for electrophysiological study.

Electrophysiological studies were carried out in all patients in the absence of any antiarrhythmic drug therapy. The protocol we routinely use includes single, double, and triple extrastimuli at two drive cycle lengths from two right ventricular sites. Left ventricular stimulation was used in only two patients and was negative in both. Isoproterenol infusions were employed in all patients with a negative response to ventricular stimulation at baseline, but this did not change the results of stimulation in any patient.

The results of electrophysiological testing in the patients were very diverse. Only one patient had sustained monomorphic VT. This patient had a history of sustained, well-tolerated VT and had experienced a cardiac arrest only after treatment with quinidine. Of note, during this same period we also studied 38 other patients with recurrent sustained monomorphic VT and structurally normal hearts. None of these had experienced a cardiac arrest. These observations illustrate the marked difference in prognosis between patients presenting with sustained monomorphic VT and no structural heart disease, and those presenting with cardiac arrest. In four patients VF could be induced with either two or three extrastimuli. Three of these four patients had spontaneous episodes of cardiac arrest during telemetry monitoring, and the spontaneous rhythms documented were also polymorphic VT that degenerated to VF (Fig. 13–2). Neither sustained monomorphic VT nor sustained polymorphic VT or VF could be induced in the remaining 16 patients.

Even though no ventricular arrhythmias could be initiated with programmed ventricular stimulation, other abnormalities were identified in 14 of the 16 other patients. Five patients in the series had long QT intervals. None of these patients, who ranged in age from 19 to 65 had a family history of premature sudden death, family members with long QT intervals, or symptoms during childhood. The two oldest long QT patients experienced cardiac arrest in association with dynamic QT changes only after they had had episodes of paroxysmal atrial fibrillation with very irregular R-R intervals. ECGs recorded earlier in life had shown QT intervals at the upper limit of normal. Four patients had Wolff-Parkinson-White syndrome with accessory pathways capable of rapid conduction during atrial fibrillation. Two of these had had no prior symptoms of arrhythmia, and none of the four had had documentation of pre-excitation prior to cardiac arrest. Bradycardia was identified as a cause of cardiac arrest in three patients. A 19-year-old woman with congenital AV block was totally asymptomatic until she suddenly collapsed and was found to be in VF. Two other patients experienced an episode of syncope followed by cardiac arrest during monitoring while being transported to the hospital. The rhythm strips obtained showed severe sinus slowing terminating in

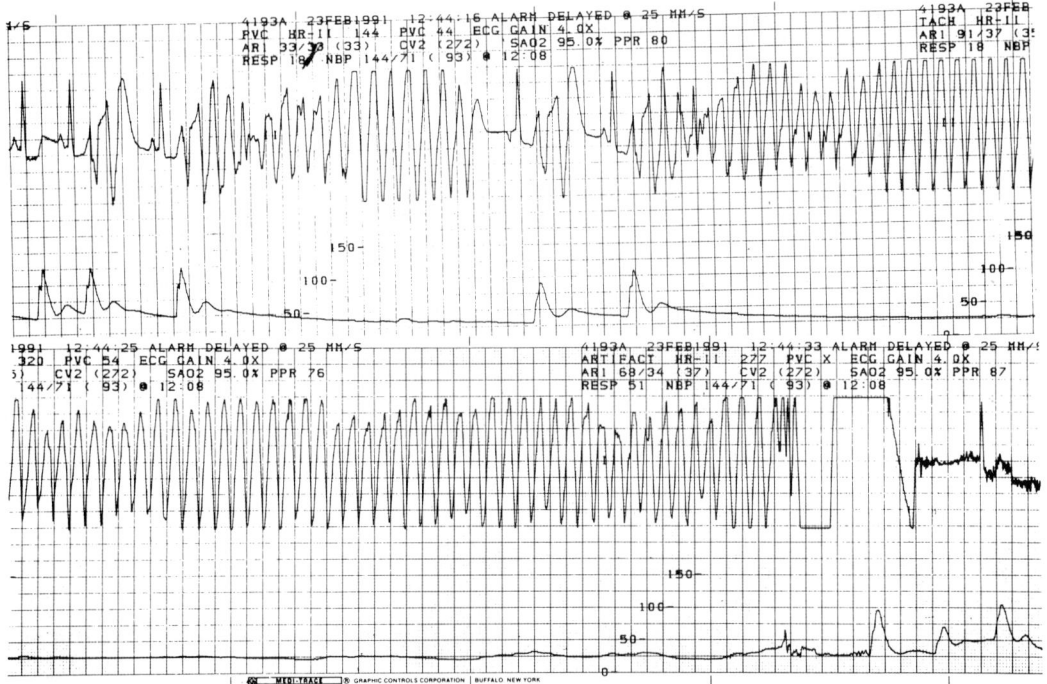

Fig. 13–2. Telemetry recording in patient No. 6. The tracing shows a rapid polymorphic ventricular tachycardia with hypotension that is terminated in the lower recording by a defibrillator discharge. This same polymorphic arrhythmia could be initiated with programmed ventricular stimulation.

a bradycardia-induced polymorphic VT. These two patients were seen prior to the introduction of tilt table testing for the provocation of neurocardiogenic syncope. It would have been of interest to see if their arrhythmias could be reproduced by head-up tilt. Finally, in two patients cardiac arrest occurred after brief periods of chest pain, with associated hyperventilation in one patient. They had normal coronary arteriograms at baseline, but severe focal coronary spasm with pain and nonsustained polymorphic VT in response to ergonovine. Ergonovine testing was negative in the two remaining patients with no inducible arrhythmia.

Therapy in the group was prescribed based on the results of their evaluation. Among the patients with long QT syndrome, Wolff-Parkinson-White syndrome, bradycardia, or spasm-related cardiac arrest, therapy specific for these conditions has been uniformly successful. Two patients with inducible VF have done well on quinidine, but three other patients have had recurrent arrhythmias that have been managed in two with an implantable cardioverter-defibrillator. Two patients have remained asymptomatic on β-blocker therapy only, with one of these having requested explantation of a defibrillator after 4 years without a discharge. This patient later discontinued his β-blocker and had a repeat cardiac arrest.

COMPARISON TO OTHER STUDIES

There have only been a few series of patients with cardiac arrest and no structural heart disease reported. Numerous additional single case reports have also been published and have been reviewed by Viskin and Belhassen.[27] Data from several representative series are summarized in Table 13–2 and may be seen to be similar to those reported here.[7,9,28,29] Not all studies included patients with known Wolff-Parkinson-White syndrome or with the long QT interval syndrome. If one considers only those patients without other causes for cardiac arrest, such as spasm or bradycardia, it becomes clear that the responses to programmed stimulation are variable. Sixteen (50%) of the 32 patients without another cause for cardiac arrest had either polymorphic VT or VF induced. Aggressive stimulation protocols using three or more extrastimuli were usually required. The specificity of VF in response to such a protocol has been questioned.[30] Monomorphic VT, usually considered to be a much more specific and useful finding, was induced in

Table 13–2
Cardiac Arrest in Patients Without Structural Heart Disease—Selected Reports

| Institution | No. of Pts. | Sex (M/F) | Prior Syncope | EP Results | | | Other Findings (n) |
				Monomorphic VT	Polymorphic VT or VF	No VT, No Other Cause	
Tel Aviv[28]	5	3/2	1	—	5	—	—
Miami[9]	9	7/2	NR	2	2	2	WPW (1) LQTS (1) Brady (1)
Minnesota[7]	6	5/1	NR	2	1	2	WPW (1)
Maastricht[29]	6	6/0	4	—	4	2	—
Virginia	21	10/11	12	1	4	2	WPW (4) LQTS (5) Spasm (2) Brady (3)
Total	47	31/16	—	5	16	8	19

Abbreviations: EP, electrophysiologic; VT, ventricular tachycardia; VF, ventricular fibrillation; NR, not reported; WPW, Wolff-Parkinson-White syndrome; LQTS, long QT syndrome; Brady, bradycardia.

only five (16%) patients. No arrhythmia at all was induced in eight (34%) patients. The ability of serial electropharmacological testing to predict future drug efficacy is also not well defined in the literature. Belhassen et al reported an excellent response to Class I antiarrhythmic agents.[28] Results of drug therapy in other series were less favorable. Therefore, unless a specific correctable cause can be identified, therapy has remained largely empirical. Prior to the widespread availability of antiarrhythmic devices, some authors favored empirical therapy with β-adrenergic blockers.[31,32] Recently there has been a tendency to recommend implantable defibrillators to most patients, since the natural history of their disorder is uncertain. However, reported recurrences of cardiac arrest during continued drug therapy have not been common, and the comparative effectiveness of the various approaches proposed remains to be determined.

SUMMARY

Approximately 10% of patients resuscitated from a cardiac arrest unassociated with MI will have no identifiable structural heart disease despite thorough investigation. Some of these patients will have characteristic electrophysiological findings such as long QT intervals, pre-excitation, or bradycardia that predisposed them to VF. In the remaining patients, electrophysiological studies are often inconclusive, and no firm consensus about the optimal management of these patients exists.

REFERENCES

1. Neuspiel DR, Kuller LH: Sudden and unexpected natural death in childhood and adolescence. JAMA 254:1321, 1985.
2. Raymond JR, van den Berg EK Jr, Knapp MJ: Nontraumatic prehospital sudden death in young adults. Arch Intern Med 148:303, 1988.
3. Topaz O, Edwards JE: Pathologic features of sudden death in children, adolescents, and young adults. Chest 87:476, 1985.
4. Hays LJ, Lerman BB, DiMarco JP: Nonventricular arrhythmias as precursors of ventricular fibrillation in patients with out-of-hospital cardiac arrest. Am Heart J 118:53, 1989.
5. Wilber DJ, Garan H, Finkelstein D, et al: Out-of-hospital cardiac arrest: Use of electrophysiologic testing in the prediction of long-term outcome. N Engl J Med 318:19, 1988.
6. Roy D, Waxman HL, Kienzle MG, Buxton AE, Marchlinski FE, Josephson ME: Clinical characteristics and long-term follow-up in 119 survivors of cardiac arrest: Relation to inducibility at electrophysiologic testing. Am J Cardiol 52:969, 1983.
7. Benson DW Jr, Benditt DG, Anderson RW, et al: Cardiac arrest in young, ostensibly healthy patients: Clinical, hemodynamic, and electrophysiologic findings. Am J Cardiol 52:65, 1983.
8. Morady F, Scheinman MM, Hess DS, Chen R, Stanger P: Clinical characteristics and results of electrophysiologic testing in young adults with ventricular tachycardia or ventricular fibrillation. Am Heart J 106:1306, 1983.
9. Topaz O, Perin E, Cox M, Mallon SM, Castellanos A, Myerburg RJ: Young adult survivors of sudden cardiac arrest: Analysis of invasive evaluation of 22 subjects. Am Heart J 118:281, 1989
10. Maron BJ, Fananapazir L: Sudden cardiac death in hypertrophic cardiomyopathy. Circulation 85(suppl I):I-57, 1992.
11. Kark JA, Posey DM, Schumacher HR, Ruehle CJ: Sickle-cell trait as a risk factor for sudden death in physical training. N Engl J Med 317:781, 1987.
12. Moss AJ, Schwartz PJ, Crampton RS, Locati E, Carleen E: The long QT syndrome: A prospective international study. Circulation 71:17, 1985.
13. Garson A Jr: Sudden death in the young. Hosp Pract (Off Ed) 26:51, 1991.
14. Miller DD, Waters DD, Szlachcic J, Théroux P: Clinical characteristics associated with sudden death in patients with variant angina. Circulation 66:588, 1982.
15. Fellows CL, Weaver WD, Greene HL: Cardiac arrest associated with coronary artery spasm. Am J Cardiol 60:1397, 1987.
16. Martini B, Nava A, Thiene G, et al: Ventricular fibrillation without apparent heart disease: Description of six cases. Am Heart J 118:1203, 1989.
17. Thiene G, Nava A, Corrado D, Rossi L, Pennelli N: Right ventricular cardiomyopathy and sudden death in young people. N Engl J Med 318:129, 1988.
18. Dewey RC, Capeless MA, Levy AM: Use of ambulatory electrocardiographic monitoring to identify high-risk patients with congenital

complete heart block. N Engl J Med *316*:835, 1987.
19. Wang Y, Scheinman MM, Chien WW, Cohen TJ, Lesh MD, Griffin JC: Patients with supraventricular tachycardia presenting with aborted sudden death: Incidence, mechanism and long-term follow-up. J Am Coll Cardiol *18*:1711, 1991.
20. Monahan BP, Ferguson CL, Killeavy ES, Lloyd BK, Troy J, Cantilena LR Jr: Torsades de pointes occurring in association with terfenadine use. JAMA *264*:2788, 1990.
21. Hosenpud JD, McAnulty JH, Niles NR: Unexpected myocardial disease in patients with life threatening arrhythmias. Br Heart J *56*:55, 1986.
22. Brooks R, Burgess JH: Idiopathic ventricular tachycardia. A review. Medicine (Baltimore) *67*:271, 1988.
23. Hayashi M, Murata M, Satoh M, et al: Sudden nocturnal death in young males from ventricular flutter. Jpn Heart J *26*:585, 1985.
24. Gotoh K: A histopathological study on the conduction system of the so-called "Pokkuri disease" (sudden unexpected cardiac death of unknown origin in Japan). Jpn Circ J *40*:753, 1976.
25. Kirschner RH, Eckner FAO, Baron RC: The cardiac pathology of sudden, unexplained nocturnal death in Southeast Asian refugees. JAMA *256*:2700, 1986.
26. Otto CM, Tauxe RV, Cobb LA, et al: Ventricular fibrillation causes sudden death in Southeast Asian immigrants. Ann Intern Med *100*:45, 1984.
27. Viskin S, Belhassen B: Idiopathic ventricular fibrillation. Am Heart J *120*:661, 1990.
28. Belhassen B, Shapira I, Shoshani D, Paredes A, Miller H, Laniado S: Idiopathic ventricular fibrillation: Inducibility and beneficial effects of class I antiarrhythmic agents. Circulation *75*:809, 1987.
29. Lemery R, Brugada P, Bella PD, Dugernier T, Wellens HJJ: Ventricular fibrillation in six adults without overt heart disease. J Am Coll Cardiol *13*:911, 1989.
30. Stevenson WG, Brugada P, Waldecker B, Zehender M, Wellens HJJ: Can potentially significant polymorphic ventricular arrhythmias initiated by programmed stimulation be distinguished from those that are nonspecific? Am Heart J *111*:1073, 1986.
31. Brodsky MA, Sato DA, Allen BJ, Chesnie BM, Henry WL: Solitary beta-blocker therapy for idiopathic life-threatening ventricular tachyarrhythmias. Chest *89*:790, 1986.
32. Coumel P, Rosengarten MD, Leclercq J-F, Attuel P: Role of sympathetic nervous system in non-ischaemic ventricular arrhythmias. Br Heart J *47*:137, 1982.

14

Sudden Cardiac Death in the Long QT Syndrome

ARTHUR J. MOSS

The idiopathic long QT syndrome (LQTS) is an infrequently occurring disorder in which affected individuals have delayed repolarization (QT prolongation), usually with bifid T-wave configurations in several leads; relative sinus bradycardia; and a propensity to recurrent syncope and sudden cardiac death.[1,2] This disorder has a strong familial pattern consistent with a genetic mechanism. Autosomal recessive[3] and autosomal dominant[4,5] modes of inheritance were suggested in the first reported LQTS families. Recently, LQTS was linked to a DNA marker (Harvey-*ras*-1) on the short arm of chromosome 11 in a large LQTS pedigree,[6] a finding that confirms the genetic basis for this disorder in this kindred. Several other families with LQTS have shown similar linkage to Harvey-*ras*-1,[7] but this has not been a consistent finding in all families investigated to date, thus raising the issue of genetic heterogeneity. Sporadic cases of LQTS without familial involvement occasionally occur, less than 10% of the reported cases, suggesting that new genetic mutations may be responsible for this disorder in some patients.

HISTORICAL BACKGROUND

In 1957, Jervell and Lange-Nielsen described the first family with LQTS.[3] In this family, three sudden deaths occurred in four deaf children (three girls and one boy). The deaf children had several fainting attacks precipitated by exercise and acute emotions. Three of the deaf children underwent electrocardiography (ECG), and the QT interval was prolonged in each of them. The three children died at the ages of 4, 5, and 9 years. Two other children and the parents were healthy with normal hearing and normal ECGs. This combination of congenital deafness, QT prolongation, recurrent syncope, and death in children of normal parents was interpreted as indicative of an autosomal recessive inheritance. Levine and Woodworth,[8] Fraser et al,[9] and Hashiba[10] reported similar families. Of note, there was a 2:1 ratio of females to males among the first 21 reported cases.

Romano et al in 1963[4] and Ward in 1964[5] described individual families with QT prolongation in one of the parents and several affected children with QT prolongation, recurrent syncope, and sudden death. There was normal hearing in these two families. In 1978, Hashiba[10] described an additional 28 families in Japan with similar clinical findings. The 28 probands consisted of two males and 26 females, and segregation analysis supported an autosomal dominant inheritance.

PHENOTYPIC CONSIDERATIONS

The diagnosis of LQTS is usually based on an abnormally prolonged QT interval. Precise quantification of the QT interval is frequently confounded by the imprecision

Table 14-1
The Heart Rate–Corrected QT Interval (QTc): Suggested Values for Diagnosis of the Long QT Syndrome

	QTc Values* By Age Group and Gender		
	1–15 yr	Adult Males	Adult Females
Normal	<0.44	<0.43	<0.45
Borderline	0.44–0.46	0.43–0.45	0.45–0.47
Prolonged	≥0.47	≥0.46	≥0.48

* The QTc values are calculated by dividing the observed QT interval in seconds by the square root of the RR cycle length in seconds. The QTc unit is in square root of seconds (sec$^{1/2}$), and the values are derived from a normal population of 578 healthy subjects.[11]

in accurately identifying the end of the T wave on the 12-lead ECG. Under normal physiological conditions, the QT interval shortens as the heart rate increases. The traditional criterion for the diagnosis of QT prolongation is a heart rate–corrected QT interval (QTc) greater than 0.44 sec$^{1/2}$, with QTc = QT/RR$^{1/2}$. Recently, Gottlieb et al[11] studied a large normal population and found that the QT interval is influenced by sex and age as well as by heart rate. A suggested categorization of QTc is to use a three-level classification (normal, borderline prolonged, and prolonged) adjusted for age and sex (Table 14-1).

In addition to QTc prolongation, other ECG features of LQTS include unusual T-wave configurations such as double-humped or bifid T waves in several leads and relative sinus bradycardia with resting heart rates frequently less than 50 beats/min in the absence of any medication.

CLINICAL CONSIDERATIONS

In 1979 our research group initiated a prospective long-term study of LQTS families, including first- and second-degree relatives, to better understand the clinical aspects of this disorder. Recently we reported on the clinical course of individuals from 328 families in which one or more members were identified with LQTS (QTc > 0.44 sec$^{1/2}$).

The disorder was largely familial in that 85% of the probands (the first member of a family to be identified with LQTS) had one or more family members with QTc > 0.44 sec$^{1/2}$. Some families were too small to allow proper evaluation of the inheritance pattern. Our best estimate at this time is that approximately 7% of affected probands have the sporadic form of the disorder. The study population (n = 2020) was nearly equally divided between those with QTc > 0.44 sec$^{1/2}$ (n = 1016) and those with QTC ≤ 0.44 sec$^{1/2}$ (n = 1004). There was variable expression among those with QTc > 0.44 sec$^{1/2}$, suggesting that genetic factors other than the length of the QT interval affect the manifestations of this disease process. As in earlier reported studies, females predominated among the probands (69%) and affected family members (60%).

The proband was usually brought to medical attention because of a syncopal episode during childhood or the teenage years. Probands (n = 328) were younger at first contact (21 ± 15 [SD] years), were more likely to be female (69%), and had a higher frequency of pre-enrollment syncope or aborted cardiac arrest (80%), congenital deafness (7%), a resting heart rate less than 60 beats/min (31%), QTc > 0.50 sec$^{1/2}$ (52%), and a history of repetitive ventricular arrhythmias (47%) than other affected (n = 688) family members.

Arrhythmogenic syncope often occurred in association with acute physical, emotional, or auditory arousal. Among those for whom information was available about factors associated with syncopal events prior to enrollment, 47% of the LQTS patients with syncope had one or more events occurring in association with intense emotions (anger or fright), 41% with vigorous physical activity exclusive of swimming, 19% on awakening, 15% while swimming, and 8% on arousal by auditory stimuli such as the ringing of an alarm clock or a telephone, or the sound of thunder. By age 12, 50% of the probands had experienced at least one syncopal episode or death.

The rates of post-enrollment syncope (one or more episodes) and LQTS-related sudden death before age 50 years were 5.3% per year and 0.9% per year, respectively, for probands, and 0.5% per year and 0.2%

per year, respectively, for affected family members.

Cox model analysis identified different risk factors for post-enrollment cardiac events (syncope or LQTS-related sudden death before age 50 years) among probands and family members. For probands, QTc and heart rate were the independent risk factors. For example, a patient with a QTc of $0.60\ \text{sec}^{1/2}$ had a 2.2-fold greater risk of experiencing a cardiac event than a patient with a QTc of $0.45\ \text{sec}^{1/2}$; a patient with a heart rate of 80 beats/min had a 1.7-fold greater risk of experiencing a cardiac event than a patient with a heart rate of 50 beats/min. A patient with both a QTc of $0.60\ \text{sec}^{1/2}$ and a heart rate of 80 beats/min would have 3.7 times (2.2 × 1.7) the risk of experiencing a cardiac event than a patient with a QTc of $0.45\ \text{sec}^{1/2}$ and a heart rate of 50 beats/min. For family members, the risk factors for a post-enrollment cardiac event were a history of a prior cardiac event (hazard ratio 6.7) and female sex (hazard ratio 3.9).

Arrhythmogenesis

LQTS is tightly linked to the Harvey-*ras*-1 gene on chromosome 11 in several reported families,[6,7] and Keating et al[6] have speculated that Harvey-*ras*-1 may be the candidate LQTS gene. This is an intriguing hypothesis, since Harvey-*ras*-1 is known to regulate G proteins, membrane proteins involved in signal transduction between activated receptors and ionic channels.[12] In vitro studies have shown[13-15] that alterations in G protein activity can: (1) alter the delayed potassium rectifier current, a functional change that could prolong action potential duration, augment early afterdepolarizations, and prolong the QT interval on the surface ECG; and (2) reduce the I_f current in pacemaker cells, a functional change that could contribute to sinus bradycardia. Thus, the two major ECG manifestations of LQTS, QT prolongation and relative sinus bradycardia, might be mechanistically linked to a mutation in the Harvey-*ras*-1 gene.

Delayed ventricular repolarization and profound bradycardia are the substrate for the development of polymorphous ventricular tachycardia, torsade de pointes, and ventricular fibrillation—malignant arrhythmias that are responsible for sudden cardiac death in LQTS. Sympathetic stimulation with exercise, excitement, or acute arousal seems to trigger or initiate many of the episodes of torsade de pointes, especially in patients with pre-existing slow heart rates. The exact mechanism by which sympathetic stimulation triggers this arrhythmia is unclear. Sympathetic stimulation may augment the amplitude of early afterdepolarizations, lower the threshold for afterdepolarization firing, or act by a combination of both mechanisms. Altered signal transduction of catecholamine-activated receptors may be an important mechanism in triggering these arrhythmias. The heart rate appears to be a two-edged sword. Profound bradycardia as well as tachycardia can augment afterdepolarizations,[16,17] thus setting the stage for triggered activity.

Evaluation of LQTS Patients

The three hallmarks of LQTS are (1) QTc prolongation, (2) syncopal episodes, and (3) family members with QTc prolongation, syncope, or premature sudden cardiac death. Abrupt-onset syncope, especially that occurring in the setting of acute physical, emotional, or auditory arousal, is almost always due to a transient malignant tachyarrhythmia with cerebral hypoperfusion. These syncopal events clear rapidly when an adequate rhythm is spontaneously re-established, but they indicate a high risk for subsequent sudden cardiac death. Abrupt onset/offset syncope is of concern in all patients with LQTS, but especially in pediatric patients.[18]

Once the clinical diagnosis of LQTS is established in a given patient, ECGs should be obtained on all living first-degree relatives. A family pedigree should be recorded with special attention to syncope and premature sudden cardiac death. Such pedigrees provide valuable insight into the potential virulence of the LQTS disorder in the identified family.

Twenty-four-hour ambulatory (Holter) ECG recordings may be useful in evaluating the arrhythmia potential in a given patient. The Holter recording may reveal periods of profound bradycardia, transient extreme QT prolongation, brief runs of ventricular tachyarrhythmias, or episodes of T-wave alternans, findings indicative of ventricular electrical instability in this disorder.

The exercise test is frequently used to evaluate the variability of the QT interval over a range of heart rates that occur during exercise and recovery. Failure of the QT interval to shorten during the tachycardia associated with exercise is said to be a feature of LQTS, but this has not been my experience. Rather, we have observed exaggerated QT prolongation in the recovery phase after exercise,[19] and this has also been noted by Weintraub et al in children.[18] T-wave alternans and ventricular tachyarrhythmias are rarely observed during exercise testing.

The signal-averaged ECG has been recorded in only a limited number of patients with LQTS. It is unlikely that a signal-averaged ECG will uncover any late potentials in this disorder since there is nothing to support delay or fragmentation of depolarization in LQTS. Fast Fourier transform analysis of the T wave may be useful in uncovering early afterdepolarizations, and this requires further investigation. Electrophysiological testing has been unrewarding, and programmed stimulation does not induce repetitive ventricular arrhythmias in this disorder. Monophasic action potential recordings from the endocardium have identified afterdepolarizations and non-uniform recovery of repolarization in a few LQTS patients.[20]

A recent report by Nador et al[21] describes an echocardiographic abnormality in the ventricular contraction pattern in LQTS, a finding more frequent in symptomatic (syncope/cardiac arrest) than in asymptomatic patients. The unusual contraction pattern consisted of a more rapid early contraction phase and a slower late thickening phase before rapid relaxation. How this altered contraction pattern relates to the electrophysiological abnormality in LQTS is unclear at this time. Confirmation of these interesting observations is required.

THERAPY FOR LQTS

The primary goal of therapy in LQTS is to prevent life-threatening arrhythmogenic syncope and sudden cardiac death. At present, the four modalities of treatment for patients with LQTS are β-blockers,[1] pacemaker,[22] left cervicothoracic sympathetic ganglionectomy,[23] and implantable defibrillators. β-blockers remain the therapy of first choice for symptomatic LQTS patients with a history of syncope or aborted cardiac arrest, and in some asymptomatic LQTS patients who are members of high-risk families. The β-blocker dose should be maximized to ensure adequate competitive blockade of the myocardial β-adrenergic receptors. The effectiveness of this blockade can be ascertained by an attenuated heart rate response to treadmill or bicycle exercise testing.

Many LQTS patients have underlying sinus bradycardia, and β-blocker therapy can sometimes exacerbate the bradycardia and actually increase the propensity for malignant ventricular arrhythmias. Profound bradycardia can further prolong repolarization and provoke pause-dependent afterdepolarizations and triggered arrhythmias of the torsade de pointes type. Eldar et al[24] in 1987 reported favorable results from implanted pacemakers in eight LQTS patients. In 1991, Moss et al reported beneficial results of pacing in 30-high-risk LQTS patients.[22] All 30 patients had experienced syncope and/or aborted cardiac arrest before pacemaker implantation, and almost all patients had failed antiadrenergic therapy. Permanent pacing prevents bradycardia and pauses, and it might contribute to more homogeneous repolarization. Thus, there is a physiological rationale for combing β-blockers and permanent pacemakers in the treatment of high-risk LQTS patients with bradycardia.

In 1969, Moss et al[25] reported the control of recurrent syncope and aborted cardiac arrest with left cervicothoracic sympathetic ganglionectomy in one adult patient with LQTS. This surgical therapy was initiated prior to the availability of β-blockers. Recently, Schwartz et al[23] reported on the worldwide experience of left cardiac sympathetic denervation in 85 patients with LQTS refractory to more conservative measures. Left cardiac sympathetic denervation was associated with a marked reduction in the incidence of tachyarrhythmic syncope in this high-risk group. The efficacy of sympathectomy is related, in part, to the extensiveness of the surgical ganglionectomy.

That is, the surgery should involve removal of the lower half of the left stellate ganglion as well as the first four thoracic ganglia in order to achieve adequate cardiac sympathetic denervation. The surgery can be performed through a left supraclavicular approach and does not require a thoracotomy.

Patients with a malignant clinical course may require triple therapy with β-blockers, pacing, and ganglionectomy. The available therapy does not alter the myocellular substrate responsible for LQTS, and some patients with recurrent cardiac events despite triple therapy require an implantable defibrillator. Presently, I am aware of only six LQTS patients with implantable defibrillators.

EPIDEMIOLOGY

Although LQTS is a distinct clinical entity, it is reasonable to speculate that the length of the QT interval is influenced by a complex interplay of genetic and environmental factors. The prognostic implications of modest QTc prolongation in a healthy population has recently been investigated. Algra et al[26] studied 6693 consecutive patients who had undergone 24-hour ambulatory ECG recordings in Rotterdam. One hundred seventy-six patients died suddenly during 2 year follow-up, and the QTc on the initial 12-lead ECG was evaluated in those who died and in a random sample ($n = 467$) of survivors. In patients without intraventricular conduction defects and cardiac dysfunction, QTc prolongation (>0.44 sec$^{1/2}$) was a risk factor for sudden cardiac death (relative risk 2.3; 95% CI 1.4, 3.9) independent of age, history of myocardial infarction, heart rate, and drug use. In a separate study, Schouten et al[27] found that in an apparently healthy population ($n = 3091$), a QTc > 0.44 sec$^{1/2}$ was associated with a relative mortality risk of 1.6 in subjects without signs of heart disease at baseline examination. These findings suggest a continuum of risk for QTc, similar to the risk associated with blood pressure and cholesterol levels. LQTS may represent a unique hereditary disorder much like essential hypertension and familial hypercholesterolemia.

REFERENCES

1. Moss AJ, Schwartz PJ, Compton RS, et al: The long QT syndrome: Prospective longitudinal study of 328 families. Circulation 84: 1136, 1991.
2. Schwartz PJ, Periti M, Malliani A: The long QT syndrome. Am Heart J 89:378, 1975.
3. Jervell A, Lange-Nielsen F: Congenital deaf mutism, functional heart disease with prolongation of the QT interval, and sudden death. Am Heart J 54:59, 1957.
4. Romano C, Gemme G, Pongiglione R: Aritmie cardiache rare dell'eta pediatrica. Clin Pediatr (Phila) 45:656, 1963.
5. Ward OC: New familial cardiac syndrome in children. J Irish Med Assoc 54:103, 1964.
6. Keating M, Atkinson D, Dunn C, et al: Linkage of a cardiac arrhythmia, the long QT syndrome, and Harvey-ras-1 gene. Science 252: 704, 1991.
7. Keating M, Atkinson D, Dunn C, et al: Linkage of the long-QT syndrome to the Harvey-ras-1 locus on chromosome 11. Hum Genet 49:1335, 1991.
8. Levine SA, Woodworth CR: Congenital deaf-mutism, prolonged Q-T interval, syncopal attacks and sudden death. N Engl J Med 259:412, 1959.
9. Fraser GR, Froggatt P, James TN: Congenital deafness associated with electrocardiographic abnormalities, fainting and sudden deaths. Q J Med 33:361, 1963.
10. Hashiba K: Hereditary QT prolongation syndrome in Japan: Genetic analysis and pathological findings of the conducting system. Jpn Circ J 42:1133, 1978.
11. Gottlieb S, Moss AJ, Hall WJ, et al: Statistical identification of delayed repolarization: Applicability in long QT syndrome (LQTS) population. J Am Coll Cardiol 17:241A, 1991.
12. Holmer SR, Homcy CJ: G Proteins in the heart: A redundant and diverse transmembrane signaling network. Circulation 84: 1891, 1991.
13. Brown AM, Birnbaumer L: Ionic channels and their regulation by G protein subunits. Ann Rev Physiol 52:197, 1990.
14. Yatani A, Okabe K, Polakis P, et al: ras p21 and GAP inhibit coupling of muscarinic receptors to atrial K$^+$ channels. Cell 61:769, 1990.
15. Yatani A, Okabe K, Codina J, et al: Heart rate regulation by G proteins acting on the cardiac pacemaker channel. Science 249: 1163, 1990.
16. Brachmann J, Scherlag BJ, Rosenshtraukh LV et al: Bradycardia-dependent triggered activity: Relevance to drug-induced multi-

form ventricular tachycardia. Circulation 68: 846, 1983.
17. Jackman WM, Friday KJ, Anderson JL, et al: The long QT syndromes: A critical review, new clinical observations and a unifying hypothesis. Prog Cardiovas Dis 31:115, 1988.
18. Weintraub RG, Gow RM, Wilkinson JL: The congenital long QT syndrome in childhood. J Am Coll Cardiol 16:674, 1990.
19. Benhorin J, Hewitt D, Moss AJ: Relationship between repolarization duration and cycle length during exercise testing in normals and long QT syndrome patients. J Am Coll Cardiol 17:60A, 1991.
20. Schechter E, Greeman CC, Lozzara R: Afterdepolarizations as a mechanism for the long QT syndrome. J Am Coll Cardiol. 3: 1556, 1984.
21. Nador F, Beria G, De Ferrari GM, et al: Unsuspected echocardiographic abnormality in the long QT syndrome: Diagnostic, prognostic, and pathogenetic implications. Circulation 84:1530, 1991.
22. Moss AJ, Liu JE, Gottlieb S, et al: Efficacy of permanent pacing in the management of high-risk patients with long QT syndrome. Circulation 84:1524, 1991.
23. Schwartz PJ, Locati EH, Moss AJ: Left cardiac sympathetic denervation in the therapy of congenital long QT syndrome: A worldwide report. Circulation 84:503, 1991.
24. Eldar M, Griffin JC, Abbott JA, et al: Permanent cardiac pacing in patients with the long QT syndrome. J Am Coll Cardiol 10:600, 1987.
25. Moss AJ, McDonald J: Unilateral cervicothoracic sympathetic ganglionectomy for the treatment of long QT interval syndrome. N Engl J Med 285:903, 1970.
26. Algra A, Tijssen JGP, Roelandt JRTC, et al: QTc prolongation measured by standard 12-lead electrocardiography is an independent risk factor for sudden death due to cardiac arrest. Circulation 83:1888, 1991.
27. Schouten EG, Dekker JM, Meppelink P et al: QT interval proplongation predicts cardiovascular mortality in an apparently healthy population. Circulation 84:1516, 1991.

15

Sudden Cardiac Death in the Wolff-Parkinson-White Syndrome

WEE SIONG TEO, GEORGE J. KLEIN, RAYMOND YEE, JAMES LEITCH

Sudden death in the Wolff-Parkinson-White (WPW) syndrome is rare but is particularly devastating because it often occurs in young, otherwise healthy individuals.[1,2] The symptomatic patient can be readily assessed by electrophysiological techniques and offered appropriate pharmacological, ablative, or operative therapy.[3,4] The asymptomatic individual with the WPW pattern poses a greater challenge since potential diagnostic and therapeutic measures must be weighed against a very low risk of sudden death in this group.[5,6] The estimated prevalence of WPW varies from 0.1% to 0.3% of the population[7-9] but is difficult to determine exactly since this would require a tremendous longitudinal study of healthy subjects from birth to advanced age. Sudden death in these individuals is very uncommon, as evidenced by the low incidence of WPW in autopsy series of young individuals with sudden cardiac death.[10-16] The incidence of sudden death in WPW has been suggested to be from 0 to 4%, and the most pessimistic estimate in asymptomatic individuals would be no greater than 1 per 100 patient-years of follow-up.[5,6,17-35]

Work was supported by the Heart and Stroke Foundation of Ontario, Toronto, Canada. Dr. Klein is a Distinguished Research Professor of the Heart and Stroke Foundation of Ontario.

MECHANISM OF SUDDEN DEATH IN WOLFF-PARKINSON-WHITE SYNDROME

Sudden death in the majority of patients with WPW occurs as a result of atrial fibrillation (AF) with a very rapid ventricular response over the accessory pathway, leading to ventricular fibrillation (VF) for hemodynamic reasons.[1,2] AF may occur as a primary arrhythmia but probably occurs more frequently in the course of atrioventricular (AV) reciprocating tachycardia that degenerates to AF (Figs. 15-1 to 15-3). The ventricular response during AF is determined by several factors, the most important of which is the refractory period of the accessory pathway. Other determinants include ventricular refractoriness, AV nodal properties, and dynamic influences such as concealed conduction into the accessory pathway.[36-39] Patients with concomitant heart disease, of course, experience sudden death secondary to the organic disease or to the interplay of arrhythmia in the context of left ventricular dysfunction.[40,41]

PROFILE OF THE PATIENT WITH SUDDEN CARDIAC DEATH

An examination of patients resuscitated from VF who are found to have the WPW pattern provides our best estimate of the characteristics leading to this complica-

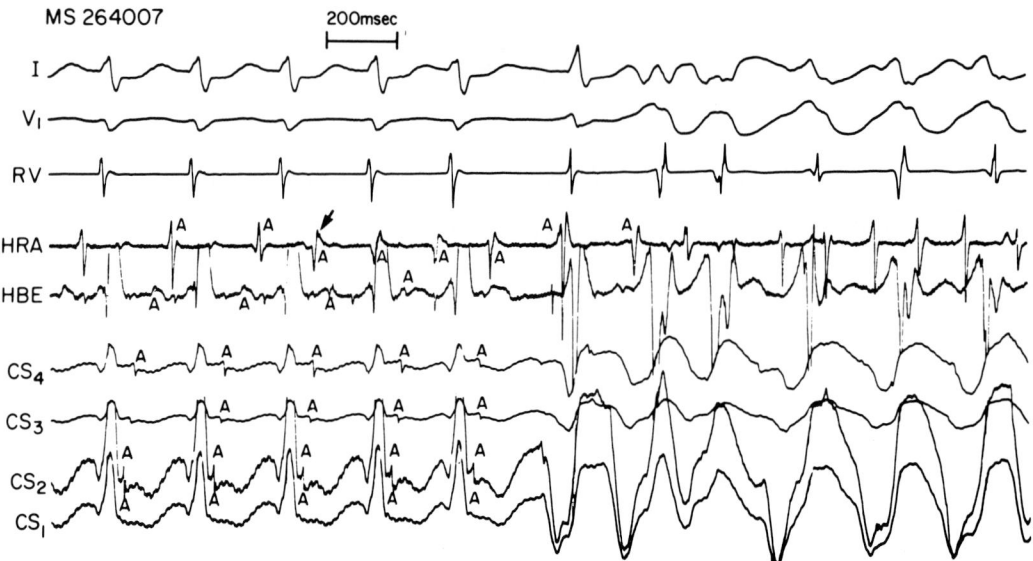

Fig. 15–1. Transition of reciprocating tachycardia to atrial fibrillation. Orthodromic reciprocating tachycardia utilizing a left lateral accessory pathway is observed on the left half of the panel. Earliest retrograde atrial activation occurs at the distal coronary sinus atrial electrogram. At the arrow, an atrial ectopic is observed at the high right atrial electrogram, which heralds the onset of atrial fibrillation. Transition from reciprocating tachycardia is considered to be the most common mechanism for the occurrence of atrial fibrillation in the clinical setting. I and V_1, surface ECG leads; CS_1 to CS_4, coronary sinus electrograms from distal to proximal; HBE, His bundle electrogram; HRA, high right atrial electrogram; RV, right ventricular electrogram.

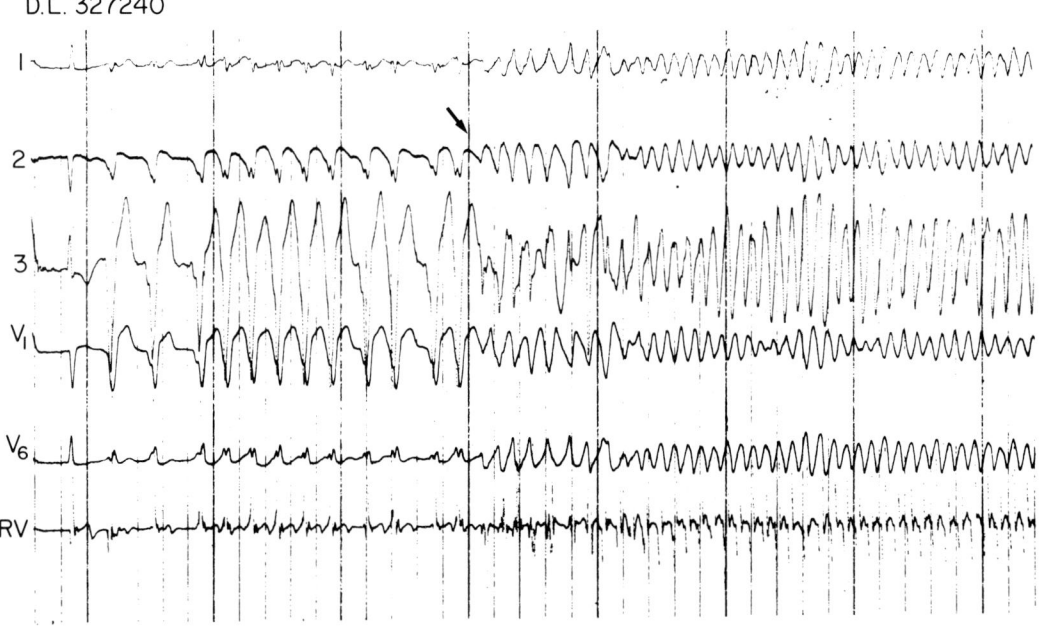

FIG. 15–2. Transition from atrial fibrillation (AF) to ventricular fibrillation (VF). The left side of the panel demonstrates AF with a rapid ventricular response over a posteroseptal accessory pathway. At the arrow, VF began and was accompanied by a clinical cardiac arrest. See legend for Figure 15–1 for abbreviations.

MS 363475

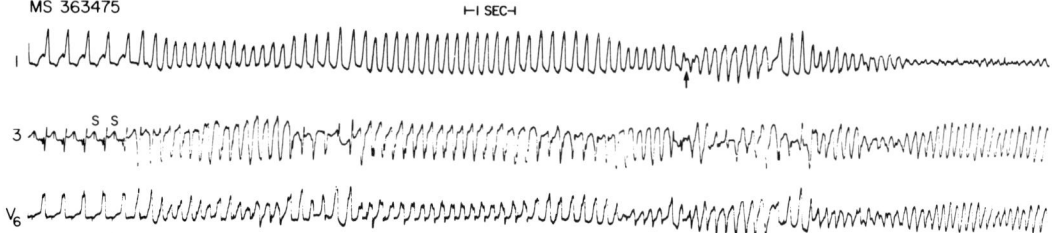

Fig. 15–3. Atrial vulnerability leading to ventricular fibrillation (VF). A single atrial extrastimulus in this patient with an accessory pathway leads immediately to atrial fibrillation (AF) with a rapid ventricular response over the accessory pathway. VF is observed on the right half of the figure and probably begins at the arrow or close to it. Reciprocating tachycardia could never be induced in this patient, who was considered to have had clinical VF secondary to primary AF.

tion.[1,2] Approximately 70% of such patients have had significantly symptomatic arrhythmias, while 20% had relatively minor symptoms and approximately 10% were entirely asymptomatic. When compared with a control group of symptomatic patients without VF, patients with VF have a higher prevalence of both AV re-entrant tachycardia and AF and are more likely to have multiple accessory pathways. The most striking observation in patients with VF is a rapid ventricular response over the accessory pathway during AF (Fig. 15–4). With few exceptions, the shortest R-R (SRR) interval between pre-excited beats is <250 msec (Fig. 15–5). These retrospective data consequently sug-

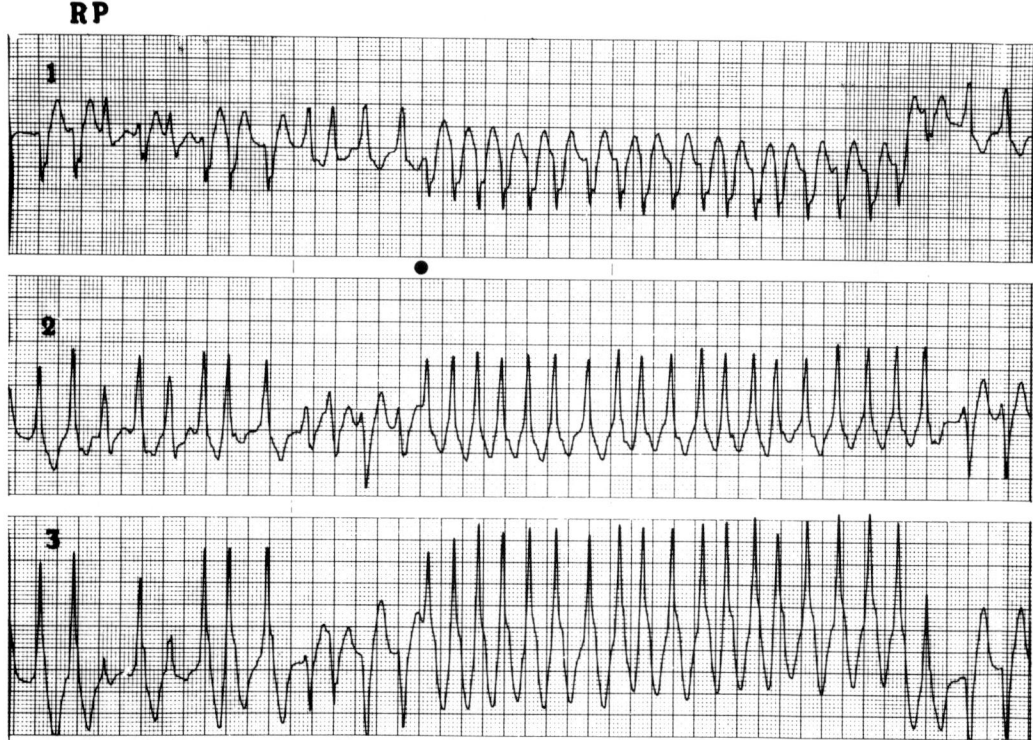

Fig. 15–4. Atrial fibrillation in Wolff-Parkinson-White syndrome. This patient had two accessory pathways, a left lateral and a right anteroseptal pathway. These are discernible as two distinct morphologies on the surface ECG during atrial fibrillation. Both accessory pathways are capable of providing a rapid ventricular response, with the SRR < 200 msec for each pathway.

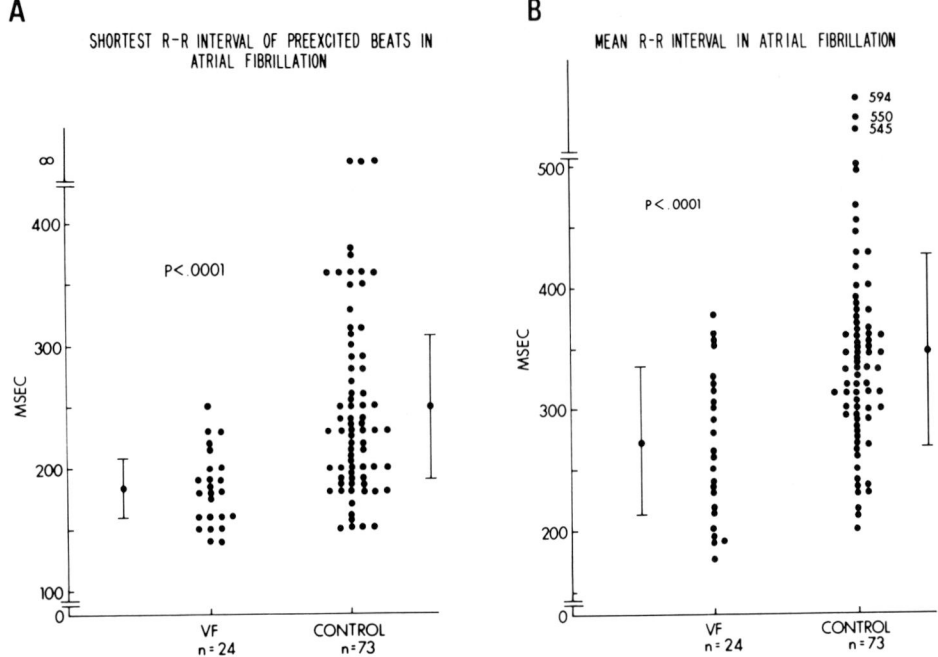

Fig. 15–5. R-R intervals in atrial fibrillation in Wolff-Parkinson-White syndrome associated with sudden death. **A.** The SRR of pre-excited beats is indicated for a population of patients resuscitated from ventricular fibrillation (VF) and a control group studied concurrently for symptoms other than VF. Patients with VF have a shortest R-R < 250 msec, and the majority have an SRR < 200 msec. Many of the control symptomatic patients, however, had similarly rapid rates. **B.** Mean R-R intervals in atrial fibrillation illustrated in similar fashion. (Reproduced with permission from Klein JG, et al: N Engl J Med *301*:1080–1085, 1979.[1])

gest "risk factors" for the development of VF, the most important of which would be a rapid ventricular response over the accessory pathway during AF (SRR ≤ 250 msec). Other risk factors include the presence of symptoms (especially a history of both reciprocating tachycardia and AF) and the presence of multiple accessory pathways.[42] The patient with Ebstein's anomaly[43] or other concomitant organic heart disease is probably also at greater risk for VF than the individual without these problems. Finally, inducibility of AF during standard electrophysiological assessment ("atrial vulnerability") is more frequently observed in patients with a history of AF[44] and may also be a risk factor, although this is less clear.

ASSESSING RISK OF SUDDEN DEATH

Who Should Be Assessed?

Patients with WPW syndrome can be divided into three groups on the basis of clinical presentation for the purposes of this discussion. The three groups are:

1. Presentation with VF or hemodynamically significant AF.
2. Presentation with symptoms other than the above, such as AV re-entrant tachycardia.
3. Asymptomatic patients found to have the WPW pattern as an incidental electrocardiographic abnormality.

There is probably little disagreement that patients presenting with VF or hemodynamically poorly tolerated AF merit full electrophysiological investigation and serious consideration of either catheter ablative or operative therapy. These patients are clearly in a high-risk group. The management of patients with less serious symptoms remains less certain. Electrophysiological assessment with a view to therapy will be done in the patient who desires resolution of symptoms. In other patients with less severe or more infrequent symptoms, the decision may be made to withhold treatment or to provide drug treatment on a trial-and-error basis. Electrophysiological testing in this group of patients would be geared more toward assessing their ventricular response to induced AF and deciding further therapy with that issue in mind. Finally, considerable controversy exists as to the merits of attempting to assess asymptomatic individuals with the WPW pattern.[6,45,46] These individuals have a small but definite risk of experiencing VF as the first manifestation of their disorder. Electrophysiological testing could readily identify those individuals with a rapid ventricular response during induced AF who are presumably at risk for the development of VF. This approach is limited in practice by two facts. Firstly, approximately 20% of asymptomatic individuals will have inducible AF with a rapid ventricular response over the accessory pathway (SRR < 250 msec).[5] Second, the incidence of sudden death as the first manifestation of the WPW syndrome in the asymptomatic individual is very low, and certainly less than 1 per 100 patient-years of follow-up by the most pessimistic estimate.[6] This event rate is far too low to allow even the most sensitive and specific predictor of sudden death to have a good positive predictive value (Fig. 15–6). Electrophysiological assessment in such individuals can reasonably be recommended only for those patients in whom even this small risk is unacceptable (pilots, professional athletes, others). The evolution of catheter ablation as a simple, safe, and effective approach may, in the future, lower the physician's threshold for recommending this therapy in the asymptomatic individual considered to be at risk.

What Investigations?

Electrophysiological testing provides a definitive assessment of the properties of the accessory pathways and evaluation of potential arrhythmias. It serves as the definitive diagnostic test prior to catheter ablative or operative ablative therapy and as a direct measure of the efficacy of antiarrhythmic agents. In some instances, the physician may only wish to assess the anterograde refractory properties of the acces-

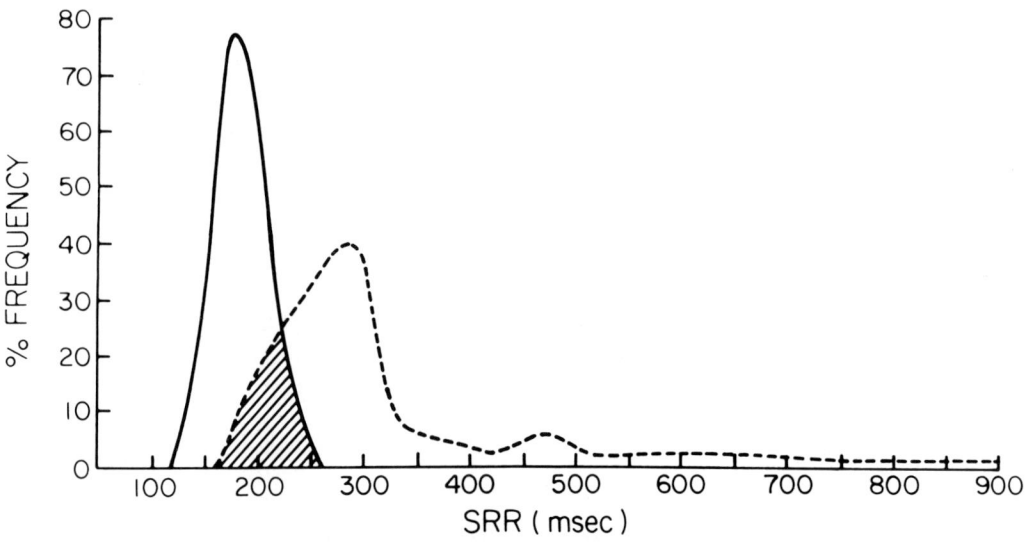

Fig. 15–6. Depiction of shortest R-R intervals during atrial fibrillation in asymptomatic patients with the Wolff-Parkinson-White pattern. The lefthand curve shows the frequency of R-R intervals in a population of patients who had been resuscitated from ventricular fibrillation.[1] The dashed-line curve provides this information for asymptomatic patients with the Wolff-Parkinson-White pattern. There is a large overlap between the frequency distributions of the R-R intervals within these two populations. (Reproduced with permission from Leitch JW, et al: Circulation 82:1718–1723, 1990.[5])

sory pathway either directly or indirectly to obtain a reasonable estimate of the ventricular response in the event of AF. As stated earlier, this is usually an issue in the minimally symptomatic individual in whom the physician wishes to withhold therapy or to provide empirical therapy but with some assurance that the patient is not at risk for a rapid ventricular response in the event of AF. Elective induction of AF by electrophysiological tests is the most definitive way of obtaining this information. The anterograde refractory period of the accessory pathway correlates with the SRR interval during AF but is an imperfect surrogate for this measure.[1,36,37,46–49] Other noninvasive or less invasive methods have been advocated for approximating this information. These are described below.

Electrocardiography

Rest or ambulatory ECGs may reveal an intermittent loss of pre-excitation (Fig. 15–7) that indicates a low margin of safety for anterograde conduction over an accessory pathway.[50] With few exceptions, this is a marker for a slow ventricular response in the event of AF. This is also intuitively attractive, since intermittent pre-excitation is compatible with "precarious" conduction over the accessory pathway. In interpreting loss of pre-excitation, it is important to rule out other factors that can cause apparent normalization of the delta wave.[51] The most important factor is shortening of AV nodal conduction time as a result of sympathetic stimulation or vagolysis, which can result in disappearance of pre-excitation without loss of conduction over the accessory pathway. This is most likely to occur when the delta wave is "subtle" and pre-excitation is minimal to begin with. Loss of pre-excitation is diagnosed most reliably when the delta wave is prominent and normalization is accompanied by a lengthening of the PR interval and repolarization changes. Normalization of the QRS in the absence of loss of conduction over the accessory pathway can also occur with junc-

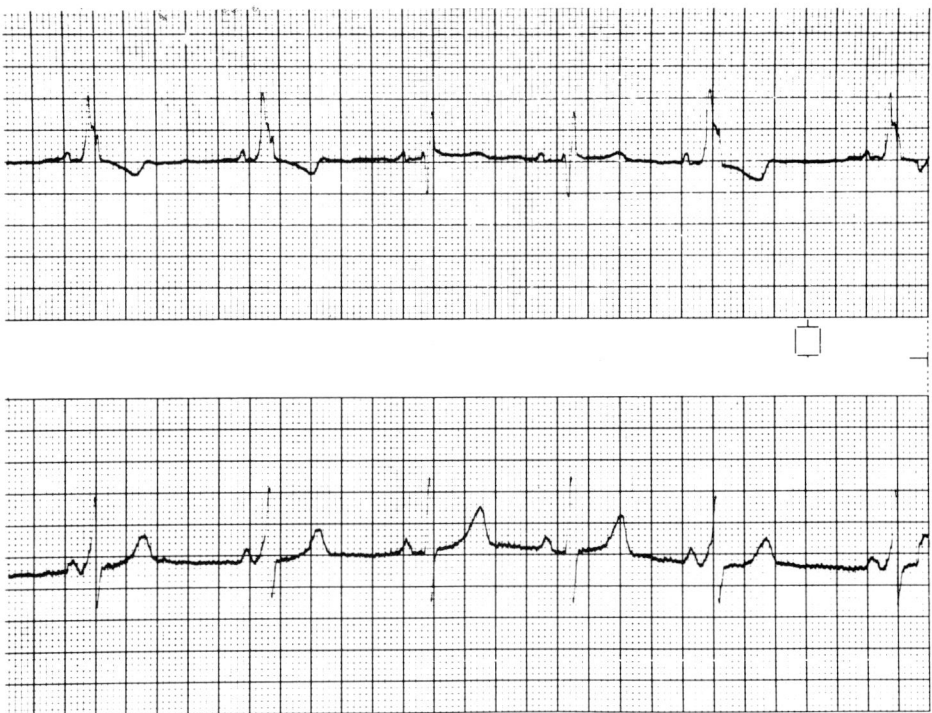

Fig. 15–7. Demonstration of intermittent loss of pre-excitation in a Holter recording. There is abrupt loss of a typical pre-excitation pattern on the third cycle with prolongation of the PR interval and repolarization changes. The pre-excitation pattern returns on the fifth cycle.

tional extrasystoles and immediately after ventricular ectopic beats that may penetrate the accessory pathway retrogradely and prevent anterograde conduction over the pathway in the next cycle. When these other causes of normalization are excluded, intermittent pre-excitation is a reliable predictor of a slow ventricular response in the event of AF.

Treadmill stress testing

Intermittent pre-excitation is an equally reliable finding when observed in the course of an exercise stress test.[51-56] However, the enhancement of AV nodal conduction during exercise testing tends to normalize the QRS as a result of enhancement of AV nodal conduction, making assessment of accessory pathway conduction difficult. To avoid this potential pitfall, loss of pre-excitation with exercise should be diagnosed cautiously and only when the delta wave is rather prominent and its disappearance is abrupt and associated with repolarization changes. Multiple ECG channels should be recorded continuously throughout this test.

Pharmacological Challenge

Wellens observed that the effectiveness of Class I antiarrhythmic drugs in prolonging the refractory period of accessory pathways is proportional to the initial refractory period of the pathway. That is, accessory pathways with short refractory periods were affected less by these agents than those with long refractory periods. He sub-

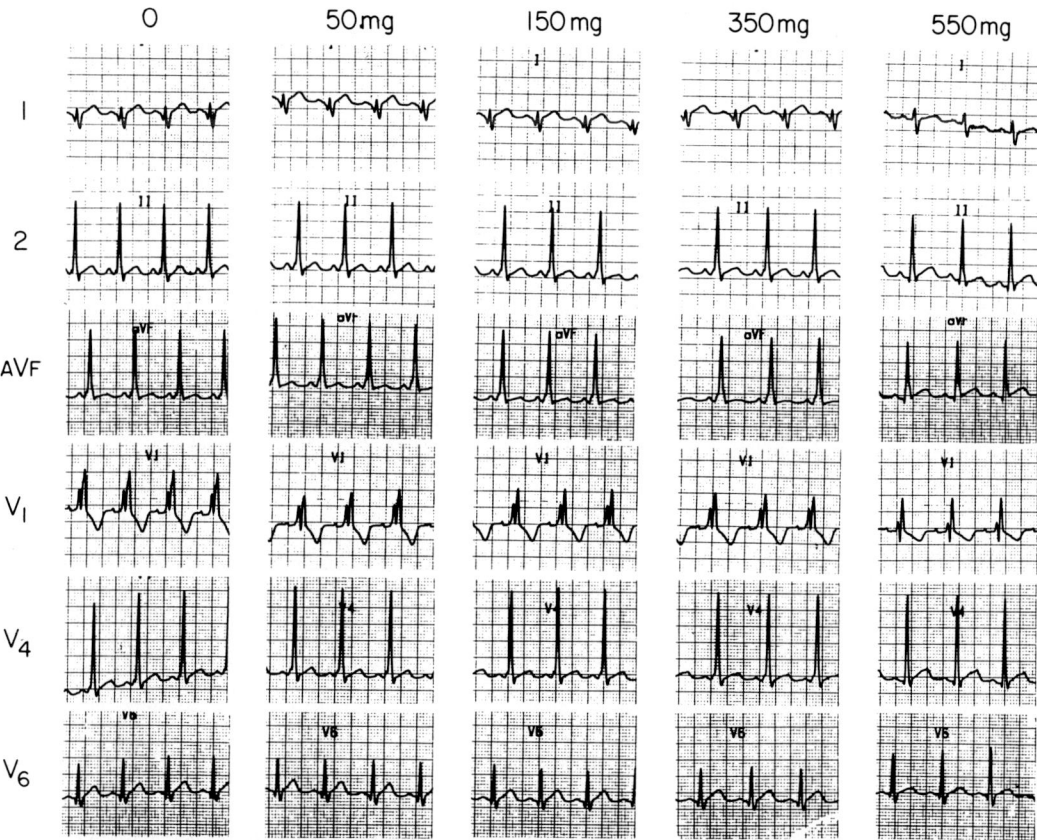

Fig. 15–8. Illustration of a modified procainamide test to assess pre-excitation. A graded infusion of procainamide was given to this patient with manifest pre-excitation. At a cumulative dose of 550 mg, pre-excitation disappears abruptly with prolongation of the PR interval and repolarization changes. This is perhaps most evident in lead 1. (Reproduced with permission, from Boahene KA, et al: Am J Cardiol 65:195–200, 1990.[63]).

sequently proposed that intravenous infusion of ajmaline or procainamide be used to separate patients with long from those with short refractory periods, since these agents will normalize the QRS in patients in whom the ERP is >270 msec and will not normalize it if it is less.[57,58] Other agents, including disopyramide, propafenone, and flecainide, were subsequently reported to yield similar results.[55,59,60] Others have suggested that ajmaline[61] and procainamide[62] are not useful since normalization may frequently occur in patients with short refractory periods, and vice versa. Boahene et al used an incremental infusion regimen of procainamide to assess the value of this test at different dosages (Fig. 15–8).[63] As might be expected, it was concluded that the effect of procainamide on accessory pathway refractoriness was dose dependent. Patients exhibiting loss of pre-excitation after procainamide infusion had both higher baseline refractory periods and a steeper dose-response curve (Fig. 15–9). Procainamide blocked conduction over accessory pathways at the higher infusion rates regardless of initial ERP of the pathway, whereas block of the accessory pathway at lower doses predicted a long ERP. It was found that a cumulative dose of 550 mg of procainamide provided the best balance between sensitivity (60%) and specificity (89%) for identifying patients destined to have SRR >250 msec during AF. This issue remains controversial, but it is clear that any pharmacological test used in this way must have a strictly controlled and standardized infusion regimen.

Esophageal Pacing

The atrium can be paced via the esophagus, and this route has been used for elective induction of AF in patients with WPW syndrome.[64,65] In addition to providing a direct assessment of AF, this technique can also be used to induce AV reciprocating tachycardia if this can be done by atrial stimulation techniques in the given individual.

Use of Isoproterenol in Assessing Risk

Isoproterenol has been shown to shorten the anterograde refractory period of the accessory pathway and increase the ventricu-

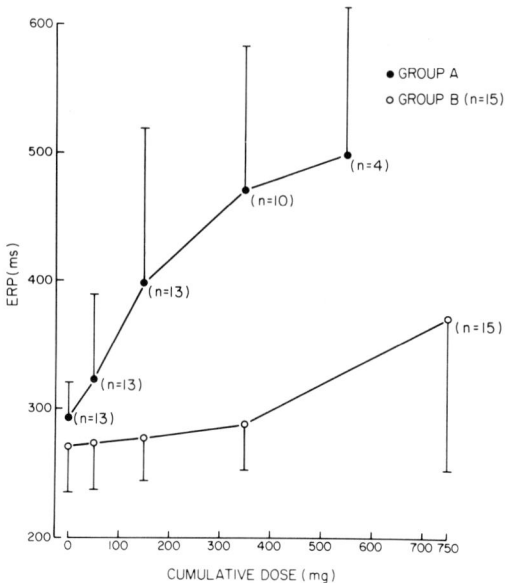

Fig. 15–9. Dose-response relationship of procainamide and loss of pre-excitation. Groups A and B both underwent a modified procainamide infusion test[63] to assess response of the pre-excitation pattern. Pre-excitation disappeared after completion of the protocol in group A patients (solid circles) and pre-excitation persisted in group B patients (open circles). Patients losing pre-excitation (group A) had a longer baseline anterograde effective refractory period of the accessory pathway (ERP) but also had a steeper dose-response curve. The horizontal axis indicates the cumulative dose of procainamide in milligrams.

lar response during AF.[66,67] This raised the issue of the potential role of catecholamine enhancement during electrophysiological assessment of the asymptomatic WPW patient. This strategy is less useful than would be expected, for the following reasons:

1. The data acquired from survivors of VF were obtained under baseline laboratory conditions.[1] Thus, the finding of an SRR < 250 msec only after isoproterenol infusion cannot be interpreted as having predictive value.
2. An SRR < 250 msec is observed in approximately 20% of asymptomatic individuals with the WPW pattern. However, at least 65% of such individuals will have an SRR < 250 msec after isoproterenol.[68] This renders the po-

tential specificity of this observation prohibitively low.

Although an absolute reduction of the SRR to <250 msec by isoproterenol is not helpful, it is possible that the individual at risk for VF has a steeper dose-response curve relating SRR to isoproterenol dose,[68] and this concept may be worthy of further evaluation.

SUMMARY

Sudden death in the individual with Wolff-Parkinson-White syndrome generally occurs as a sequel to AF with a rapid ventricular response over the accessory pathway. The propensity to develop this complication can be accurately assessed by electrophysiological testing. Curative ablative therapy prevents recurrent arrhythmias, including AF.[69] The assessment of asymptomatic individuals by any technique remains controversial, owing to the very low risk of sudden death as the first manifestation of the syndrome in these individuals.

REFERENCES

1. Klein GJ, Bashore TM, Sellers TD, Pritchett EL, Smith WM, Gallagher JJ: Ventricular fibrillation in the Wolff-Parkinson-White syndrome. N Engl J Med 301:1080–1085, 1979.
2. Montoya PT: Ventricular fibrillation in the Wolff-Parkinson-White syndrome [abstract]. Circulation 78(suppl II):II-22, 1988.
3. Gallagher JJ, Pritchett ELC, Sealy WC, Kasell J, Wallace AG: The preexcitation syndrome. Prog Cardiovasc Dis 20:285, 1978.
4. Prystowsky EN, Miles WM, Heger JJ, Zipes DP: Preexcitation syndromes: Mechanisms and management. Med Clin North Am 68:831, 1984.
5. Leitch JW, Klein GJ, Yee R, Murdock C: The prognostic value of electrophysiologic testing in asymptomatic patients with Wolff-Parkinson-White pattern. Circulation 82:1718–1723, 1990.
6. Klein GJ, Prystowsky EN, Yee R, Sharma AD, Laupacis A: Asymptomatic WPW: Should we intervene? Circulation 80:1902–1905, 1989.
7. Hiss RG, Lamb LE: Electrocardiographic findings in 122,043 individuals. Circulation 25:947–961, 1962.
8. Guize L, Soria R, Chaouat JC, Chretien JM, Houe D, Le-Heuzey J: Prevalence and course of Wolff-Parkinson-White syndrome in a population of 138,048 subjects. Ann Med Intern Paris 136:474–478, 1985.
9. Vidaillet HJ, Pressley JC, Henke E, Harrell FE, German LD: Familial occurrence of accessory atrioventricular pathways (preexcitation syndrome). N Engl J Med 317:65–69, 1987.
10. Luke JL, Helpern M: Sudden unexpected death from natural causes in young adults: A review of 275 consecutive autopsied cases. Arch Pathol 85:10–17, 1968.
11. Topaz O, Edwards JE: Pathologic features of sudden death in children, adolescents and young adults. Chest 87:476–482, 1985.
12. Phillips M, Robinowitz N, Higgins JR, Boran KJ, Reed T, Virmani R: Sudden cardiac death in Air Force recruits: A 20 year review. JAMA 256:2696–2699, 1986.
13. Maron BJ, Epstein SE, Roberts WC: Causes of sudden death in competitive athletes. J Am Coll Cardiol 7:204–214, 1986.
14. Raymond JR, Van-den-Berg EK Jr, Knapp MJ: Nontraumatic prehospital sudden death in young adults. Arch Intern Med 148(2):303–308, 1988.
15. Denfield SW, Garson A Jr: Sudden death in children and young adults. Pediatr Clin North Am 37:215–231, 1990.
16. Carrado D, Thiene G, Nava A, Rossi L, Pennelli N: Sudden death in young competitive athletes: Clinicopathologic correlations in 22 cases. Am J Med 89:588–596, 1990.
17. Wolff L: Wolff-Parkinson-White syndrome: Historical and clinical features. Prog Cardiovasc Dis 60:677–690, 1959.
18. Swiderski J, Lees MH, Nadas AS: The Wolff-Parkinson-White syndrome in infancy and childhood. Br Heart J 24:561, 1962.
19. Kaplan MA, Cohen KL: Ventricular fibrillation in the Wolff-Parkinson-White syndrome. Am J Cardiol 24:259–264, 1969.
20. Dreifus LS, Haiat R, Watanabe Y, Arriaga J, Reitman N: A possible mechanism of sudden death in patients with the WPW syndrome. Circulation 43:520–527, 1971.
21. Lim CH, Toh CC, Chia BL: Ventricular fibrillation in type B WPW syndrome. Aust NZ J Med 4:515–517, 1974.
22. Fasth A: Wolff-Parkinson-White syndrome: A fatal case in a girl with no other heart disease. Acta Paediatr Scand 64(1):138–140, 1975.
23. Duvernoy WFC: Sudden death in Wolff-Parkinson-White syndrome. Am J Cardiol 39:472, 1977.

24. Brechenmacher C, Coumel P, Fauchier JP, Cachera JP, James TN: XXII. Intractable paroxysmal tachycardias which proved fatal in type A Wolff-Parkinson-White syndrome. Circulation 55(2):407–417, 1977.
25. Papa LA, Saia JA, Chung EK: Ventricular fibrillation in Wolff-Parkinson-White syndrome, type A. Heart Lung 7:1015–1019, 1978.
26. Cosio FG, Benson DW Jr, Anderson RW, et al: Onset of atrial fibrillation during antidromic tachycardia: Association with sudden cardiac arrest and ventricular fibrillation in a patient with Wolff-Parkinson-White syndrome. Am J Cardiol 50:353–359, 1982.
27. Wiedermann CJ, Becker AE, Hopferwieser T, Muhlberger V, Knapp E: Sudden death in a young competitive athlete with Wolff-Parkinson-White syndrome. Eur Heart J 8:651–655, 1987.
28. Vidaillet HJ, et al: An unusual variant of familial preexcitation. Am J Cardiol 59:371–373, 1987.
20. Gillette PC: Supraventricular arrhythmias in children. J Am Coll Cardiol 5(suppl 6):122B–129B, 1985.
30. Orinius E: Preexcitation: Studies on criteria, prognosis and heredity. Acta Med Scand Suppl 465:5–50, 1966.
31. Berkman NL, Lamb LE: The Wolff-Parkinson-White electrocardiogram: A followup study of 5–28 years. N Engl J Med 278:492, 1968.
32. Flensted-Jensen E: Wolff-Parkinson-White syndrome: A long term followup of 47 cases. Acta Med Scand 186:65–74, 1969.
33. Brembilla-Perrot B, Aliot E, Louis P, et al: (Outcome of 195 patients with Wolff-Parkinson-White syndrome.) Arch Mal Ceur 80(3):271–277, 1987.
34. Proudfit WL, Sterba R: Long-term status and survival in Wolff-Parkinson-White syndrome. Cleve Clin J Med 56:601–606, 1989.
35. Milstein S, Sharma AD, Klein GJ: Electrophysiologic profile of asymptomatic Wolff-Parkinson-White pattern. Am J Cardiol 57:1097–1100, 1980.
36. Castellanos A Jr, Myerburg RJ, Craparo K, Befeer B, Agha AS: Factors regulating ventricular rates during atrial flutter and fibrillation in preexcitation (Wolff-Parkinson-White) syndrome. Br Heart J 35:811–816, 1973.
37. Wellens HJJ, Durrer D: WPW and atrial fibrillation: relation between refractory period of accessory pathway and ventricular rate during atrial fibrillation. Am J Cardiol 34:777–782, 1974.
38. Klein GJ, Yee Y, Sharma AD: Concealed conduction in accessory atrioventricular pathways: An important determinant of the expression of arrhythmias in patients with Wolff-Parkinson-White syndrome. Circulation 70:402–411, 1984.
39. Meijler FL, Van Der Tweel I, Herbschleb JN, Hauer RN, Robles de Medina EO: Role of atrial fibrillation and atrioventricular conduction (Wolff-Parkinson-White syndrome) in sudden death. J Am Coll Cardiol 5(suppl 6):17B–22B, 1985.
40. Krikler DM, Davies MJ, Rowland E, Goodwin JF, Evans RC, Shaw D: Sudden death in hypertrophic cardiomyopathy: Associated accessory atrioventricular pathways. Br Heart J 43(3):245–251, 1980.
41. Prystowsky EN, Fananapazir L, Packer DL, Thompson KA, German LD: Wolff-Parkinson-White syndrome and sudden cardiac death.
42. Teo WS, Klein GJ, Leitch JW, et al: Multiple accessory pathways in the Wolff-Parkinson-White syndrome: A risk factor for ventricular fibrillation. Am J Cardiol [in press].
43. Smith WM, Gallagher JJ, Kerr CR, et al: The electrophysiologic basis and management of symptomatic recurrent tachycardia in patients with Ebstein's anomaly of the tricuspid valve. Am J Cardiol 49:1223–1234, 1982.
44. Rinne C, Klein GJ, Sharma AD, Yee R, Milstein S, Rattes MF: Relation between clinical presentation and induced arrhythmias in the Wolff-Parkinson-White syndrome. Am J Cardiol 60:576–573, 1987.
45. Waldo AL, Akhtar M, Benditt DG, et al: Appropriate electrophysiologic study and treatment of patients with the Wolff-Parkinson-White syndrome. J Am Coll Cardiol 11:1124–1129, 1988.
46. Wellens HJJ, Brugda P, Penn OC: The management of preexcitation syndromes. JAMA 257:2325–2333, 1987.
47. Rowland E, Curry P, Fox K, Kirkler D: Relation between atrioventricular pathways and ventricular response during atrial fibrillation and flutter. Br Heart J 45:83, 1981.
48. Sharma AD, Klein GJ, Yee R, Szabo T, Rinne C: Systematic deviations between the ventricular response to atrial fibrillation and anterograde accessory pathway [abstr]. J Am Coll Cardiol 2(suppl II):78A, 1988.
49. Rakovec P, Cijan A, Kenda MF, Rode P, Jakopin J, Turk J: Failure of the refractory period of the accessory pathway to predict the ventricular rate during atrial fibrillation in Wolff-Parkinson-White syndrome. Int J Cardiol 1:329–330, 1982.
50. Klein GJ, Gulamhussein SS: Intermittent preexcitation in the Wolff-Parkinson-White syndrome. Am J Cardiol 52:292–296, 1983.
51. Klein GJ, Sharma AD, Milstein S: Initial

evaluation of patients with the Wolff-Parkinson-White syndrome. In Benditt DG, Benson DW Jr (eds): Cardiac Preexcitation Syndromes: Origins, Evaluation and Treatment. Boston, Martinus Nijhoff, 1986, pp 305–319.
52. Strasberg B, Ashley WW, Wyndham CRC, et al: Treadmill exercise testing in the Wolff-Parkinson-White syndrome. Am J Cardiol 45:742–748, 1980.
53. Eschar Y, Belhassen B, Laniado S: Comparison of exercise and ajmaline tests with electrophysiologic study in the Wolff-Parkinson-White syndrome. Am J Cardiol 57:782–786, 1986.
54. Levy S, Broustet JP, Clementy J, Vircoulon B, Guern P, Bricaud H: Syndrome de Wolff-Parkinson-White: Correlations entre l'exploration électrophysiologique et l'effet de l'épreuve d'effort sur l'aspect électrocardiographique de préexcitation. (Wolff-Parkinson-White syndrome: Correlation between the results of electrophysiological investigation and exercise tolerance testing on the electrical aspect of preexcitation.) Arch Mal Coeur 72:634–640, 1979.
55. Sharma AD, Yee R, Guiraudon G, Klein GJ: Sensitivity and specificity of invasive and noninvasive testing for risk of sudden death in Wolff-Parkinson-White syndrome. J Am Coll Cardiol 10:373–381, 1987.
56. Daubert C, Ollitrault J, Descaves C, Mabo P, Ritter P, Gouffault J: Failure of the exercise test to predict the anterograde refractory period of the accessory pathway in Wolff-Parkinson-White syndrome. PACE 11:1130–1138, 1988.
57. Wellens HJ, Braat S, Brugada P, Gorgels AP, Bar FW: Use of procainamide in patients with WPW syndrome to disclose a short refractory period of the accessory pathway. Am J Cardiol 50:1087–1089, 1982.
58. Wellens HJJ, Barr FW, Dassen WRM, Brugada P, Vanagt EJ, Farre J: Effect of drugs in the WPW syndrome: Importance of initial length of ERP of the accessory pathway. Am J Cardiol 46:665–669, 1980.
59. Gaita F, Giustetto C, Riccardi R, Mangiardi L, Brusca A: Stress and pharmacologic tests as methods to identify patients with Wolff-Parkinson-White syndrome at risk of sudden death. Am J Cardiol 64:487–490, 1989.
60. Talard P, Cointe R, Bru P, et al: (Wolff-Parkinson-White syndrome: Value of intravenous flecainide for detecting Kent's pathways with short refractory period.) Arch Mal Coeur 83:489–492, 1990.
61. Cavalli A, Maggioni A, Tusa M, Volpi A: Two false negative responses to the ajmaline test in the Wolffe-Parkinson-White syndrome. PACE 8:832–837, 1985.
62. Fananapazir L, Packer DL, German LD, Greer GS, Gallagher JJ, Prystowsky EN: Procainamide infusion test: Inability to identify patients with Wolff-Parkinson-White syndrome who are potentially at risk of sudden death. Circulation 77:1291–1296, 1988.
63. Boahene KA, Klein GJ, Sharma AD, Yee R, Fujimura O: Value of a revised procainamide test in the Wolff-Parkinson-White syndrome. Am J Cardiol 65:195–200, 1990.
64. Gallagher JJ, Smith WM, Kerr CR, et al: Esophageal pacing: A diagnostic and therapeutic tool. Circulation 65:336–341, 1982.
65. Critelli G, Grassi G, Perticone F, Coltorti F, Monda V, Condorelli M: Transesophageal pacing for prognostic evaluation of preexcitation syndrome and assessment of protective therapy. Am J Cardiol 51:513–518, 1983.
66. Wellens HJJ, Brugada P, Roy D, Weiss J, Bar FW: Effect of isoproterenol on the anterograde refractory period of the accessory pathway in patients with the Wolff-Parkinson-White syndrome. Am J Cardiol 50:180–184, 1982.
67. German LD, Gallagher JJ, Broughton A, Guarniere T, Trantham JL: Effects of exercise and isoproterenol during atrial fibrillation in patients with Wolff-Parkinson-White syndrome. Am J Cardiol 61:1203–1206, 1983.
68. Szabo T, Klein GJ, Sharma AD, Yee R, Milstein S: Usefulness of isoproterenol during atrial fibrillation in evaluation of asymptomatic Wolff-Parkinson-White pattern. Am J Cardiol 63:187–192, 1989.
69. Sharma AD, Klein GJ, Guiraudon GM, Milstein S: Atrial fibrillation in patients with Wolff-Parkinson-White syndrome: Incidence after surgical ablation of the accessory pathway. Circulation 72:161–169, 1985.

16
Arrhythmogenic Right Ventricular Dysplasia: Definition and Mechanism of Sudden Death

GUY FONTAINE, FABRICE FONTALIRAN, TORU IWA,
PHILIPPE AOUATE, LISA NADITCH, GILLES LASCAULT,
JOELCI TONET, ROBERT FRANK

Arrhythmogenic right ventricular dysplasia (ARVD) is a clinical entity that is now recognized as a cause of ventricular arrhythmias and sudden cardiac death (SCD) in young people with apparently normal hearts who do not have a coronary heart disease. However, when their arrhythmias are adequately treated, a nearly normal life expectancy can be anticipated.[1]

DEFINITION OF ARVD

Arrhythmogenic right ventricular dysplasia was the name given in 1977 to a new form of cardiomyopathy that showed fatty infiltration of the RV.[2] This condition may be difficult to diagnose clinically or even at postmortem examination except in patients who have extensive dilation of the RV. Until recently, these cases were classified as a variant of Uhl's anomaly, since this entity was somewhat similar.[3] In 1978, we performed studies in two anatomical adult cases[4] that fit the original description made by Uhl in 1952 in a single pediatric patient.

Our cases showed a huge RV mostly devoid of myocardium that was replaced by fibrosis, suggesting apposition of epicardium against endocardium. This led to the striking illustrative images of "paper-thin right ventricle,"[3] "parchment heart,"[5] or "coeur papyracé."[6] Uhl's anomaly is generally recognized in the newborn or the young child since the anomaly is so severe that congestive heart failure results in death in early infancy. Few adult cases of Uhl's anomaly have been reported. Even when the amount of RV damage is not as severe as in the infants, who have nearly total absence of RV myocardium, affected patients experience severe heart failure or sudden death, usually before the age of 40.

In contrast, the patients with RV disease that we studied[2] had only moderate RV dilation. After our initial experience, we appreciated the fatty infiltration of the RV myocardium was a constant feature of the disease. Episodes of life-threatening arrhythmias were the most salient clinical feature. We consider Uhl's anomaly and ARVD two separate clinical entities because of their different clinical and pathological profile.[7] It is possible to make the retrospective diagnosis of ARVD in patients who have been described with RV dilation[8,9] and who have experienced many episodes of ventricular arrhythmia despite a seemingly normal heart.[10]

It is conceivable that ARVD with moderate RV dilation has been largely overlooked as a cause of ventricular arrhythmias and sudden death.

Work was supported in part by grants from Le Centre de Recherche sur les Maladies Cardiovasculaires de l'Association Claude Bernard La Fédération de Cardiologie.

A thorough description of this entity, mainly based on the surgical experience, was reported by our group in 1982.[11] A few years later several groups reported a seemingly similar entity under the name of RV dilated cardiomyopathy[12,13] or ARVD.[14,15] This difference in clinical presentation is probably the result of different patient populations. All of our patients had been referred for surgery after multiple episodes of inadequately controlled ventricular tachycardia (VT).

Recently, our collaboration with a cardiac pathologist led us to review all the biopsy specimens taken during surgery by our group as well as by some others.[16] We concluded that ARVD was frequently the result of a previously healed myocarditis. The main histological pattern was fatty tissue, often associated with a greater amount of fibrous tissue than was seen originally.[17] Two main histological patterns emerged. The first was fatty replacement of subepicardial layers of myocardium with minor amounts of fibrosis and few inflammatory cells. This pattern is consistent with a congenital cause. The other was irregular patchy infiltration with fat, extensive fibrosis and patchy infiltration by lymphocytes in sclerotic areas that could sometimes be found only after a careful examination of the glass slides with high field magnification.

However, if some forms of ARVD are a sequelae of more diffuse myocarditis, their presentation could be similar to some forms of cardiomyopathy in which cardiac arrhythmias originate in the RV.[18,19] In that case it is logical that involvement of the left ventricle would not be uncommon and that the long-term prognosis could be different.

SUDDEN DEATH IN ARVD

The natural history of the disease is not known, and few studies have reported long-term follow-up.[1,20,21] However, there have been some cases of sudden death,[22-24] frequently associated with strenuous exercise or sports.[22,23] Sudden death can be the first manifestation of the disease. We will discuss in more detail the different possible mechanisms of SCD in patients with ARVD, including the data obtained in a series of 67 patients with ARVD studied at the Jean Rostand Hospital in Paris.

PREVALENCE OF SUDDEN DEATH IN PATIENTS WITH ARVD

Blomstrom-Lundqvist et al reported two sudden deaths in a series of 15 patients with a mean follow-up of 8.8 years (range, 1.5–28 years). Both patients who died had had previous syncopal episodes, whereas only two of the 12 survivors had syncope.[20]

Marcus et al reported the follow-up of three series, one from Jean Rostand Hospital and two from the United States. In the 16 patients of the French series studied with a mean follow-up of 8.4 years (range, 3–13 years), no case of sudden arrhythmic death was observed at the time of publication of this paper. In the 12 patients in the American series with a mean follow-up of 5 years (range, 1–9 years), two patients (15%) died suddenly of arrhythmic death.[1,25] Marcus et al reported nine cases of sudden arrhythmic death[1] in a clinical series of 57 cases from the literature (excluding the previous series). In that report, patients were excluded if sudden death was the first manifestation of the disease.

Leclerq reported long-term follow-up of 58 patients. Of these, 39 were followed up for 5 years or more. One patient died suddenly of ventricular fibrillation (VF), and two (5%) died of unknown causes.[26]

Therefore, based on the American and the Swedish series, it could be deduced that SCD in patients with RV dysplasia was observed in about 2% per year despite various forms of pharmacological as well as nonpharmacological treatment.

It is possible that the better outcome observed in the French series demonstrates the benefit of amiodarone. One patient of our series who recently stopped taking the drug died suddenly 1 month later and another patient who discontinued amiodarone was resuscitated after cardiac arrest. These cases will be discussed later.

SUDDEN DEATH AS A RESULT OF ATRIOVENTRICULAR CONDUCTION DISTURBANCES

Atrioventricular (AV) conduction disturbance is a well-recognized cause of SCD in elderly patients.[27] Sudden death due to AV block is rare in young patients who do not have congenital heart block.[28,29] However, during strenuous exercise the increase in venous return could dilate the right atrium and ventricle and stretch the AV conduction system, in which the His bundle is the most fragile structure.[23] Mechanical stretch of the His bundle or the bundle branches could lead to AV block and could also lead to other arrhythmias. However, it is unlikely that AV block led to SCD in most cases. When AV conduction is impaired, different kinds of AV as well as intraventricular conduction disturbances can be observed on the resting electrocardiogram (ECG).[30] Sudden death due to complete AV block implies no resumption of AV conduction for several minutes. This mechanism of sudden death is improbable since loss of consciousness will interrupt effort and subsequently the stress on the AV conduction system. The partial recovery of conduction should prevent a fatal outcome. It also implies the absence of idioventricular escape rhythm, which is uncommon even in elderly patients. Transient or permanent complete AV block is not a common feature of ARVD (Fig. 16–1). Pathological data have been correlated with some forms of AV conduction disturbances, including complete AV block.[31,32] However, even if some morphological and histological patterns have been observed consistent with AV conduction defects, this cannot be considered definite proof of AV conduction disturbance as a cause of sudden death during physical stress in ARVD.

The only clinical information available from the patient who died suddenly and whose heart was described by Osler[33] and later redescribed by Segall in 1950 was that the man died suddenly while climbing a moderately steep hill.[5] The pathology of this heart showed such major alterations involving the four cavities that the cause of death could not be surmised.

Various levels of intraventricular conduction disturbance have been reported by Blomstrom-Lundqvist. Of 21 patients, 33% had complete right bundle-branch block, 29% had incomplete right bundle-branch block, and 29% had nonspecific intraventricular conduction disturbances.[34]

The first case reported by Bharati et al exhibited complete AV block. There was extensive involvement of the AV bundle and the bundle branches. However, this patient also experienced VT.[31] There was also considerable infiltration of mononuclear cells associated with pericarditis. The second case reported by the same author was that of a young patient who died suddenly and in whom various abnormalities were seen in the conduction system.[32] Because myocarditis was suggested by light microscopy, this process may have involved the conduction system.

AV conduction system involvement which may cause complete AV block is a well-known complication of acute myocarditis.[35] However, when the inflammatory process is less pronounced, there is usually only moderate injury to the AV conduction system. This could lead to a delayed conduction in the bundle branches, resulting in incomplete or, less frequently, complete bundle-branch block. However, this phe-

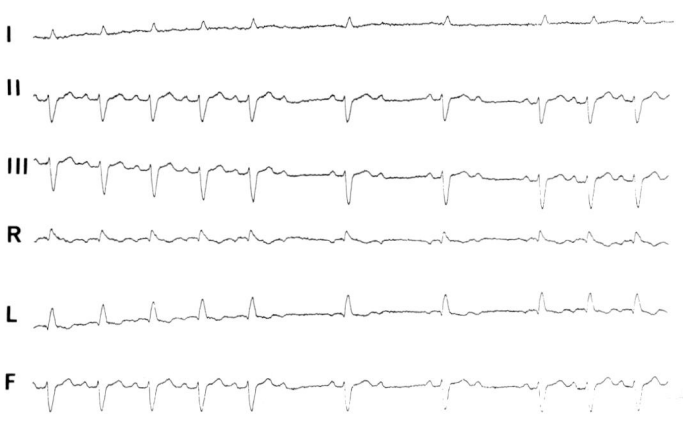

Fig. 16–1. ECG (Leads I, II, III, aVr, aVl, aVf) during a stress test in a patient with arrhythmogenic right ventricular dysplasia who had marked dilatation of the right ventricle. During the test, the heart rate increased up to 80 bpm, followed by 2:1 Mobitz type II block. An electrophysiological study demonstrated a prolonged HV interval. A pacemaker was implanted.

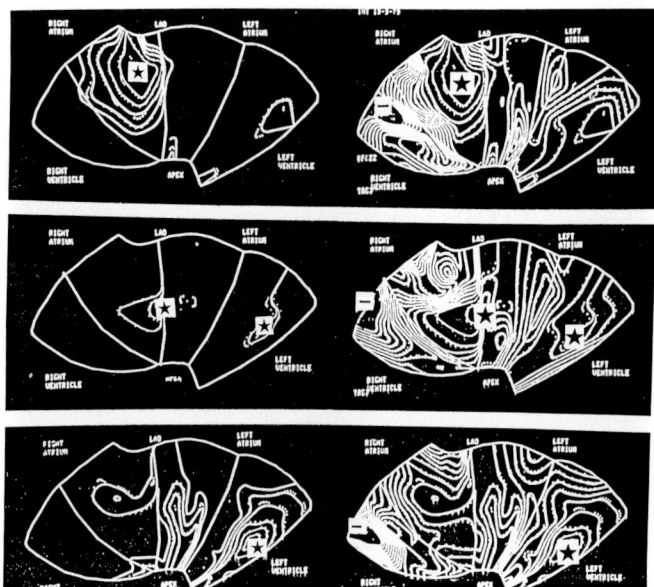

Fig. 16-2. Epicardial maps of three cases of ARVD during sinus rhythm showing initial ventricular activation. These three patients had right ventricular delayed activation on the ECG. Normal activation time of the epicardial exit of the right bundle branch is seen in patient No. 1 (top), simultaneous exit on the epicardium of the right and left ventricle in patient No. 2 (middle), epicardial activation of the right ventricle in patient No. 3 (bottom). Analysis of the completed map showed that all three patients had marked slowing of activation in the free wall of the right ventricle. The most delayed potentials were observed on the posterior diaphragmatic aspect of the right ventricle.

nomenon could increase with time, for two reasons: (1) the aging process of the heart will probably accentuate the degeneration of a structure that has been previously damaged, and (2) the proliferation of fibrosis resulting from myocarditis.

In order to clarify this aspect we correlated the activation epicardial map in sinus rhythm with the surface ECG in seven patients operated on for resistant VT (Fig. 16-2). In most cases it was observed that activation spread over the RV free wall through tightly spaced isochrones. It was therefore concluded that conduction disturbances seen on the ECG in this group of patients was related to parietal block rather than to delay in the right bundle branch.[36]

Therefore, we think that AV conduction disturbances are rarely a cause of sudden death in patients with ARVD/Uhl's anomaly. Ventricular arrhythmias, including VT, have been documented and would seem to be a more frequent cause of death in these patients.

SUDDEN DEATH AS A RESULT OF VENTRICULAR ARRHYTHMIAS

Ventricular fibrillation as the probable mechanism of sudden death in patients with ARVD was first reported by Olsson et al.[24] Ventricular arrhythmias, which are a typical feature of this disease, seem strongly related to the particular histological structure of myocardium. The arrangement of the myocardial tissue and basic concepts of electrophysiology suggest the particular behavior of activation in the zones of abnormal myocardium. The pathophysiology of the arrhythmia was partially deduced from the epicardial maps performed at the time of surgery. One case of typical Uhl's anomaly demonstrated the loop of activation with its two zones of fast and slow conduction suggesting the pathway of a re-entrant phenomenon.[2] The mapping was interesting because, in some places, the remaining myocardium formed a thin layer of tissue that behaved as a two-dimensional structure. A similar organization of fibers is also suggested in some sites on the RV free wall in patients with ARVD.[11,16] In other locations, surviving fibers are embedded in tissue of fat and fibrosis (probably depending on the cause), and in all cases there is a reduction in thickness of individual myocardial fibers (Fig. 16-3). This may help explain delayed potentials and slow conduction in the myocardium.

The thin layers of normal endocardium-myocardium are the result of a pathological

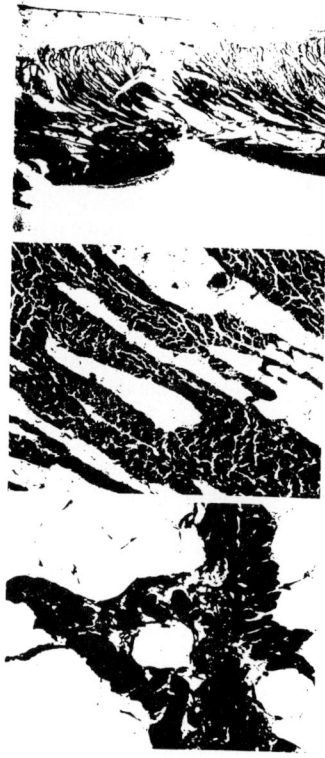

Fig. 16–3. Histology of the patient whose clinical history is presented in the legend of Figure 16–6. **A:** Right ventricular wall showing preservation of endocardium, replacement of myocardial fibers by fatty tissue and normal epicardial fat (original magnification × 10). **B:** Strand of surviving fibers with groups of adipose cells that are the result of replacement of the myocardium by fat. (Original magnification × 100). **C:** Fibrous tissue surrounding cardiomyocytes.

process that has destroyed most of the other layers of mediomural and subepicardial myocardium. Cardiomyocytes have been affected by different forms of degeneration, including fibrosis and transformation to fatty tissue. During this latter process, the cardiomyocytes are replaced by adipose tissue and therefore the total thickness of the wall seems larger than the normal thickness of the RV myocardium. However, this tissue is different histologically from normal fat which is found in the interventricular grooves, since there are myocardial cells embedded in a thin rim of fibrosis.

In patients with ARVD, fatty tissue does not generate a local potential. Only low-amplitude slow waves suggesting far field potentials could be recorded. Therefore, we think that delayed potentials observed on the epicardium, the endocardium, and finally the surface are the result of slow conduction in the surviving strands of fibers.

THE ARRHYTHMOGENIC SUBSTRATE

A large body of evidence suggests that strands of surviving fibers form an arrhythmogenic substrate in ARVD and provide the appropriate conditions necessary to establish a re-entrant pathway. The first condition is slow conduction due to the presence of these strands of myocardium. This can be explained by the cable theory, a classical concept in electrophysiology. According to this theory, the smaller the diameter of fibers, the slower is their conduction velocity. A bridge between this concept of basic electrophysiology and a clinical situation is provided by the permanent form of junctional reciprocating tachycardia (PJRT). In this situation an accessory AV conduction pathway connects atrium and ventricle, as in the Wolff-Parkinson-White syndrome. However, in PJRT this pathway is a thin, serpiginous strand of myocardial fibers located in the left paraseptal posterior aspect of the left ventricle.[37] The anterograde conduction is so slow that no delta wave can be seen on the surface ECG. However, if ablation of the AV conduction is performed at the level of the His bundle, a long P-delta interval can be seen on the surface ECG.[38,39]

In one of the two cases of Uhl's anomaly studied by our group at surgery, it was possible to record the most striking pattern of delayed potentials in a zone of myocardial thinness.[40] This demonstrates that there is at least functional continuity between normal myocardium and the zone of slow conduction. When we are dealing with fibers of small diameter, particular properties may be present.[41,42] For example, conduction from a zone of normal myocardium to a zone of slow conduction does not indicate that conduction in the reverse direction will occur. To elucidate this, we conducted an experiment in a patient with ARVD by delivering stimuli in a zone where delayed potentials had previously been recorded.[43,44] Pacing in these areas demonstrated pacing spikes reactivating the remaining normal myocardium after a long delay. In order to be functional, the strands of fibers should be connected at their two extremities to normal myocardium or should be connected at one point but forming a loop for the activation process.

The second condition is functional: even if the fibers are properly connected, re-entry can occur only if appropriate electrophysiological properties are present to establish and perpetuate the arrhythmia. In order to demonstrate the re-entrant phenomenon we have to find time-dependent properties as well as intraventricular blocks. We demonstrated these characteristics when we studied the electrical behavior of myocardium during premature stimulation, burst pacing, and spontaneous recordings during tachycardia. Both type I and type II block were demonstrated. These data were in agreement with previously reported experimental material by El-Sherif et al.[45,46]

Therefore it is well established that a phenomenon of intraventricular re-entry is a possible mechanism to explain the initiation of major ventricular arrhythmias in ARVD.

An important benefit of our observation of slow conduction and delayed potentials was the initiation of a systematic study that led us to the recording of delayed activity from epicardium to endocardium and finally prompted us to use the signal averaging technique. We are now convinced that this technique is the most simple and sensitive way to identify patients with possible dysplasia (Fig. 16-4).

If an area of myocardium with slow conduction is connected to a subendocardial zone of normal conduction and if the electrophysiological properties for unidirectional block and a re-entry phenomenon are met, the patient could develop extrasystoles, doublets or triplets, or runs of transient or sustained tachycardia and VF. This latter arrhythmia could be the result of the previous arrhythmia (Figs. 16-5 and 16-6) or could occur without arrhythmic precursors. In the case reported by Olsson et al, we do not know if the VF was observed de novo or was the result of deterioration of a previously stable VT.[24] The mechanism by which the arrhythmogenic substrate becomes operative could be explained by the progressive modification of myocardial properties are a result of the aging process or as a result of whatever caused the basic myocardial transformation. This could be modulated by the influence of the autonomic nervous sys-

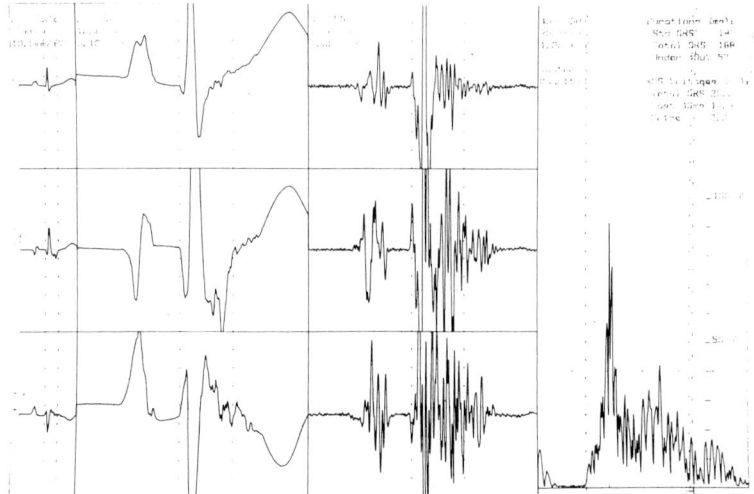

Fig. 16-4. Signal averaged ECG in a patient with ARVD, who had epsilon potentials on the surface tracing in leads Y and Z. The delayed electrical activity is obvious after increasing the amplitude of the ECG signals by a factor of 10. After high amplification and signal processing, the delayed potentials are so long that they are present beyond the limit of the window.

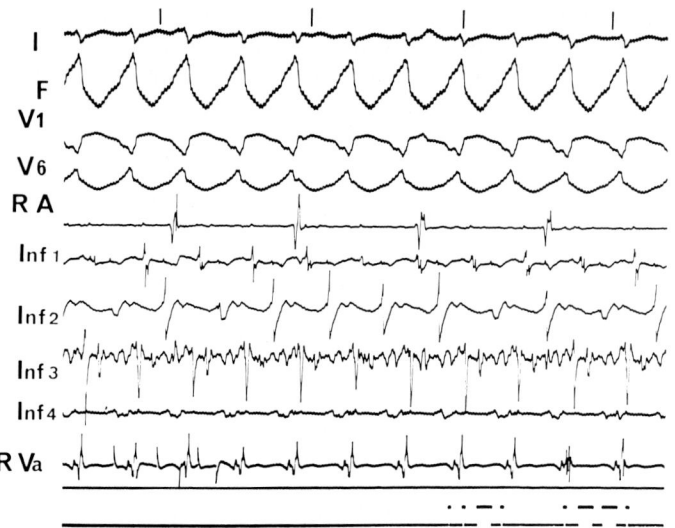

Fig. 16-5. Endocardial recording during ventricular tachycardia of the patient whose signal averaged ECG is shown in Figure 16-4. Note the presence of mid-diastolic potentials in infundibular lead 2, very low potentials in infundibular lead 4, and fragmented potentials of higher amplitude in infundibular lead 3. The pattern is repetitive but shows slight changes of the endocardial signal from beat to beat.

tem, use-dependent properties after extrasystoles, and other factors such as release of catecholamines during physical or psychological stress.[47]

It has been shown that patients with ARVD who have nonsustained runs of VT at rest can develop sustained forms of VT during exercise.[48] We observed patients with ARVD who had premature ventricular complexes (PVCs) at rest. During a stress test, the PVCs tended to increase in number as well as complexity when the heart rate increased during effort. These data suggest that β-blockers could be used as concomitant therapy in patients who have ventricular arrhythmias in ARVD during physical stress and sports.

Sudden death during the recovery phase after effort could be due to the effect of heart rate on PVCs. The increase in heart rate during physical stress may decrease the frequency of premature ventricular contractions. The reversed phenomenon could occur during the recovery phase, increasing

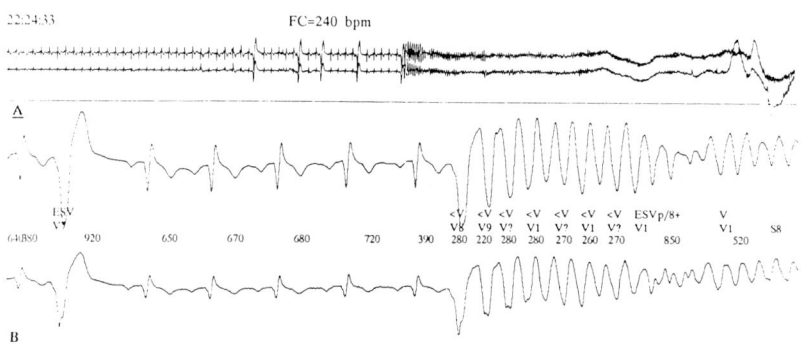

Fig. 16-6. Holter recording of a patient with ARVD who died suddenly during sleep. He had been seen in consultation the day before death because of a period of malaise after drinking a glass of whiskey. Ventricular fibrillation is preceded by isolated single extrasystoles. This patient was scheduled to have an electrophysiological study the next morning. (Reproduced with permission of the publisher from Aouate P, Fontaliran F, Fontaine G, et al: Holter et mort subite. Intérêt dans un cas de dysplasie ventriculaire droite arrythmogène. Arch Mal Coeur 86:363–367, 1993.)

the chances of ventricular arrhythmias. *This is due to the abrupt suppression of the sympathetic tone and a major increase in the vagal tone during the recovery phase after effort. Moreover, there is an abrupt decrease in RV filling that could lead to hypotension by suppression of the pump effect produced by muscular contractions.*

HEMODYNAMIC PHENOMENA

Ventricular arrhythmias could be the result of cardiac failure. We have observed incessant ventricular arrhythmias in a patient with decompensated congestive heart failure. At that time, radiographs showed marked dilation of the RV. The patient was referred for emergency fulguration as a last resort. After the arrhythmia was controlled by amiodarone infusion and multiple applications of programmed stimulation, the heart failure improved in a few days and the jaundice disappeared in 1 week. Eventually, right heart failure was controlled, RV cardiomegaly decreased, and ablation was not necessary. It seemed probable that heart failure increased the stretch of fibers, favoring ventricular arrhythmias, which in turn increased heart failure.

Similarly, one may consider that left heart failure may be caused by sustained or frequent transient VT due to ARVD. These patients may be indistinguishable from patients with idiopathic dilated cardiomyopathy. In such situations, sudden death could be the terminal event of an end-stage progressive ventricular deterioration. Distinguishing between the two diseases is sometimes confused by the pattern of sustained incessant VT.

SUDDEN DEATH AS THE FIRST MANIFESTATION OF ARVD IN YOUNG ATHLETES

Another mechanism of ARVD could be related to the stretch of fibers during exercise. Because of the increase in venous return, enlargement of the RV myocardium as a result of physical stress might be a mechanism of sudden death in competitive athletes. ARVD may have been overlooked as a cause of death during sports. Over a period of 3 years we observed two competitors in the Tour de France who had extrasystoles or sustained VT. These individuals with suspected ARVD had to quit competition or strenuous exercise.

In the United States several cases of sudden death have been reported in basketball players. In some, VT or VF has been documented. The most striking event was reported by Virmani et al from the Institute of Pathology of the Armed Forces of the United States, in Washington, D.C.[23] They reported three cases of sudden death during exercise; two of them in basketball players. The authors were surprised to find almost complete lack of the myocardium of the RV free wall. However, they stressed that the histological pattern was different from the typical aspect of Uhl's anomaly. This paper was published prior to the papers of Marcus et al that alerted the group that their patients had ARVD (Dr. Robinovitz, pers. comm.).

Sugrue et al reported the case of one patient, 21 years old, who had syncope during a football game.[49] The ECG showed VT degenerating into VF and necessitating an external DC shock. The case of a famous American basketball player, Terry Cummings, is similar. He survived several episodes of sudden death during the game. These episodes were finally controlled by amiodarone therapy. The clinical findings were consistent with ARVD (H.C. Palmer, pers. comm.). Virmani et al and Olsson et al noted that their patients were completely asymptomatic before the event, and that sudden death was the first physical manifestation of the disease.[23,24]

Another patient, diagnosed as having adipomatosis cordis, died suddenly while playing. Again, the patient had no cardiac symptoms before death. Gross pathology demonstrated fatty infiltration of the RV. Sudden death occurred in one of his brothers at the age of 17 years, again during effort.[50]

Laurenceau et al reported one case of obvious dysplasia (classified as a partial form of Uhl's anomaly) diagnosed by echocardiography. This patient died suddenly during the recovery phase after playing hockey.[51]

Rakovec et al studied a family in which one daughter died suddenly at the age of 18, during sports. VF was recorded during resuscitation. In addition, a son had repeated syncopal episodes during psychological stress. VF was recorded during one of the episodes.[52]

Leor et al reported two apparently healthy brothers in whom VT was induced by a ball hitting the chest while the patients were playing soccer. In the same family another brother, a father, and a sister had physical signs or symptoms suggesting dysplasia in a family group.[53]

SUDDEN DEATH IN PATIENTS ON DRUG THERAPY

Antiarrhythmia drugs appear to be beneficial in the treatment of ARVD. Our study suggests that patients treated with amiodarone have an excellent prognosis compared to patients treated with other antiarrhythmic drugs or untreated. This was not a randomized or case-controlled study. Nevertheless, it is our impression that amiodarone may prevent major events.[1] A recent anecdotal observation supports the possibly protective effect of this treatment. Antiarrhythmic agents were changed for some reason in two patients who had taken amiodarone for several years. The first patient died suddenly. In the second patient, interruption of treatment led to recurrence of life-threatening VT after a few weeks.

It is possible that arrhythmias in patients with ARVD may be suppressed by amiodarone for several years but that the arrhythmia remains latent and can be initiated with catastrophic consequences if the drug regimen is modified.

CONCLUSION

The spectrum of ARVD is becoming clear. It may manifest as asymptomatic PVCs, transient or sustained VT, or as a cause of sudden unexplained death in young adults, particularly during exercise. Therefore, ARVD patients with documented dangerous ventricular arrhythmias, syncopal or near-syncopal episodes, or a familial history of unexplained SCD should not engage in competitive sports and strenuous exercise. The same restrictions should apply to people in a profession in which sudden loss of consciousness could pose great risk to others. These people include airline pilots, truck drivers, or operators of dangerous equipment.

Signal averaging may be useful to detect possible cases of ARVD in people involved in such activities.[54] When delayed potentials are recorded, this does not mean that the subject will develop ventricular arrhythmias in the future. In order to become dangerous, the arrhythmogenic substrate disclosed by signal averaging should meet the electrophysiological properties to produce re-entry. Holter recording, graded stress testing, and electrophysiological studies should then be performed.

The hearts of young individuals who die suddenly during sports are not being completely examined for ARVD. Autopsies should be performed in all of these cases, as is already done in some countries. When there is no obvious cause of death, analysis of the heart should be performed by an experienced cardiac pathologist.

Patients with ARVD should be managed by electrophysiologists. The effect of drug treatment should be followed by regular Holter recording and exercise testing.

When a drug treatment has been found to be protective, this treatment should not be modified by the patient or physician without first informing the electrophysiologist so that appropriate re-evaluation can be done. The consulting electrophysiologist may advise other forms of treatment, including implantation of an automatic cardioverter-defibrillator, ablation, surgery, or some other treatment.

Finally, a multicenter study of this pathological entity is needed to collect a sufficient number of patients studied over a long period of time to compare the results of different therapeutic strategies. The European Society of Cardiology and the International Society and Federation of Cardiology, which includes the Inter-American, Pan African, European and Asian-Pacific societies of cardiology, have agreed to organize such an international study of arrhythmogenic right ventricular dysplasia/cardiomyopathy.

Note: Since the preparation of this manuscript, new electrocardiographic signs of arrhythmogenic right ventricular dysplasia have been identified on a retrospective study of 50 cases compared to a control group. It was possible to obtain a sensitivity of around 80% for a specificity of 100%. The benefit of a prospective study to identify patients with dysplasia and to demonstrate its prevention of sudden death remains to be determined.[55]

ACKNOWLEDGMENT

We thank Dr. Gilbert Peres for his comments and suggestions concerning the physiology of sports.

REFERENCES

1. Marcus FI, Fontaine G, Frank R, Gallagher JJ, Reiter MJ: Long term follow-up in patients with arrhythmogenic right ventricular disease. Eur Heart J 10(suppl D):68–73, 1989.
2. Fontaine G, Guiraudon G, Frank R, et al: Stimulation studies and epicardial mapping in ventricular tachycardia. Study of Mechanisms and Selection for Surgery. In Kulbertus HE (ed): Reentrant Arrhythmias. Lancaster, MTP, 1977, pp 334–350.
3. Uhl HS: A previously undescribed congenital malformation of the heart: Almost total absence of the myocardium of the right ventricle. Bull Johns Hopkins Hosp 91:197–205, 1952.
4. Vedel J, Frank R, Fontaine G, et al: Tachycardies ventriculaires recidivantes et ventricule droit papyracé de l'adulte. (A propos de deux observations anatomo-cliniques). Arch Mal Coeur 71:973–981, 1978.
5. Segall HN: Parchment Heart (Osler). Am Heart J 40:948–950, 1950.
6. Lepoix J: Le ventricule droit papyrace. Présentation d'un cas personnel. Thèse. Paris, 1958.
7. Fontaine G, Guiraudon G, Frank R, et al: Dysplasie ventriculaire droite arythmogène et maladie de Uhl. Arch Mal Coeur. 75: 361–372, 1982.
8. Miller G, Lowenthal M, Krause S, Rosenbaum P: A saccular outputching of the right ventricle in a child visualized by angiography. Am J Roentgenol 69:69–73, 1953.
9. Tomisawa M, Onouchi Z, Masakutsu G, et al: Right ventricular aneurysm with ventricular premaure beats. Br Heart J 36: 1182–1185, 1974.
10. Froment R, Perrin A, Loire R, Dalloz CL: Ventricule droit papyracé du jeune adulte par dystrophie congénitale. A propos de 2 cas anatomo-cliniques et de 3 cas cliniques. Arch Mal Coeur 61:477–503, 1968.
11. Marcus FI, Fontaine G, Guiraudon G, et al: Right ventricular dysplasia: A report of 24 cases. Circulation 65:384–399, 1982.
12. Thiene G, Nava A, Corrado D, Rossi L, Pennelli N: Right Ventricular Cardiomyopathy and Sudden Death in Young People. N Engl J Med 318:129–133, 1988.
13. Fitchett DH, Sugrue DD, MacArthur CG, Oakley CM: Right ventricular dilated cardiomyopathy. Br Heart J 51:25–30, 1984.
14. Thiene G: Ventricolo destro artimogeno: Displasia, malattia o sindrome? G Ital Cardiol 16:13–15, 1985.
15. Nava A, Scognamiglio R, Thiene G, et al: A polymorphic form of familial arrhythmogenic right ventricular dysplasia. Am J Cardiol 59:1405–1409, 1987.
16. Fontaine G, Fontaliran F, Linares-Cruz E, Chomette G: The arrhythmogenic right ventricle. In Iwa T, Fontaine G (eds): Cardiac Arrhythmias. Recent Progress in Investigation and Management. The Hague, Elsevier Science, 1988, pp 189–202.
17. Fontaine G, Fontaliran E, Lascault G, et al: Dysplasie transmise et dysplasie acquise. Arch Mal Coeur 83:915–920, 1990.
18. Rowland E, McKenna WJ, Sugrue DD, et al: Ventricular tachycardia of left bundle branch block configuration in patients with isolated right ventricular dilatation. Clinical and electrophysiological features. Br Heart J 51:15–25, 1984.
19. Cherrier F, Floquet J, Cuilliere M, Neimann JL: Les dysplasies ventriculaires droites. A propos de 7 observations. Arch Mal Coeur 72:766–733, 1979.
20. Blomstrom-Lundqvist C, Sabel KG, Olsson SB: A long-term follow-up of 15 patients with arrhythmogenic right ventricular dysplasia. Br Heart J 58:477–488, 1987.
21. Higuchi S, Caglar NM, Shimada R, et al: 16-year follow-up of arrhythmogenic right ventricular dysplasia. Am Heart J 108: 1363–1365, 1984.
22. Laurenceau JL, Liehnart JF, Malergue MC, Gilbert M, Dumesnil JG: Données echocardiographiques dans le syndrome du ventricule droit papyracé. Arch Mal Coeur 72:258, 1979.
23. Virmani R, Robinowitz M, Clark MA, McAllister HA: Sudden death and partial absence of the right ventricular myocardium. Arch Pathol Lab Med 106:163–167, 1982.
24. Olsson SB, Edvardsson N, Emanuelsson H, Enestrom S: A case of arrhythmogenic right ventricular dysplasia with ventricular fibrillation. Clin Cardiol 5:591–596, 1982.
25. Reiter MJ, Smith WM, Gallagher JJ: Clinical

spectrum of ventricular tachycardia with left bundle branch morphology. Am J Cardiol 51:113, 1983.
26. Leclercq JF, Coumel PH: Characteristics, prognosis and treatment of the ventricular arrhythmias of right ventricular dysplasia. Eur Heart J 10(suppl D):61–67, 1989.
27. Johansson BW: Adams-Stokes syndrome. Am J Cardiol 8:16, 1966.
28. Ayers CR, Boineau JP, Spach MS: Congenital complete heart block in children. Am Heart J 72:381–389, 1966.
29. Molthan ME, Miller RA, Hastreiter AR, Paul MH: Congenital heart block with fatal Adams-Stokes attacks in childhood. Pediatrics 30:32–41, 1966.
30. Narula OS: Intraventricular conduction defects: Current concepts and clinical significance. In Narula OS (ed): Cardiac Arrhythmias: Electrophysiology, Diagnosis and Management. Philadelphia, Williams & Wilkins, 1979, pp 114.
31. Bharati S, Ciraulo DA, Bilitch M, Rosen KM, Lev M: Inexcitable right ventricle and bilateral bundle branch block in Uhl's disease. Circulation 57:636–644, 1978.
32. Bharati S, Feld AW, Bauernfeind RA, Kattus AA, Lev M: Hypoplasia of the right ventricular myocardium with ventricular tachycardia. Arch Pathol Lab Med 107:249–253, 1983.
33. Osler W: The Principles and Practices of Medicine: Appleton & Co., 1905, pp 1, 820.
34. Blomstrom-Lundqvist C: The Syndrome of Arrythmogenic Right Ventricular Dysplasia. Diagnostic and Prognostic Implications. Goteborg, Medical Thesis, 1987.
35. Sekiguchi M, Hiroe M, Yu ZX, Hasumi M: A serial endomyocardial biopsy study on myocarditis. In Kawai C, Abelmann WH (eds): Pathogenesis of Myocarditis and Cardiomyopathy. Recent Experimental and Clinical Studies. Tokyo, University of Tokyo Press, 1987, pp 213–231.
36. Fontaine G, Frank R, Guiraudon G, et al: The significance of intraventricular conduction defects in arrhythmogenic right ventricular dysplasia. In Levy S, Scheinman MM (eds): Cardiac Arrhythmias. From Diagnosis to Therapy. Mount Kisco, Futura, 1984, pp 233–239.
37. Critelli G, Gallagher JJ, Monda V, Scherillo M, Rossi L: Transvenous catheter ablation of the atrioventricular conduction in permanent junctional reciprocating tachycardia. In Fontaine G, Scheinman MM (eds): Ablation in Cardiac Arrhythmias. Mount Kisco, Futura, 1987, pp 207–221.
38. Critelli G, Scherillo M, Monda V et al: Transvenous catheter ablation of the His bundle in ventricular tachycardia. Am Heart J 111:1106–1113, 1986.
39. Aldakar M, Fontaine G: Invasive and noninvasive approaches for the diagnosis of tachycardias. In Mariani M (ed): Cardiology Up to Date: Diagnosis and Therapy. Bologna, Monduzzi, 1989, pp 3–35.
40. Fontaine G, Frank R, Vedel J, et al: La genèse de certains troubles du rythme ventriculaire. Nouv Presse Med 3:2321, 1974.
41. Cranefield PF: The Conduction of the Cardiac Impulse. The Slow Response and Cardiac Arrhythmias. Mount Kisco, Futura, 1975.
42. de la Fuente D, Sasyniuk BJ, Moe GK:' Conduction through a narrow isthmus in isolated canine atrial tissue. A model of the WPW syndrome. Circulation 44:803, 1971.
43. Fontaine G, Guiraudon G, Frank R: Mechanism of ventricular tachycardia with and without associated chronic myocardial ischaemia: Surgical management based on epicardial mapping. In Narula O (ed): Cardiac Arrhythmias: Electrophysiology, Diagnosis and Management. Philadelphia, Williams & Wilkins, 1979, pp 516–545.
44. Fontaine G, Guiraudon G, Frank R, et al: Surgical management of ventricular tachycardia not related to myocardial ischemia. In Josephson ME, Wellens HJJ (eds): Tachycardias. Mechanisms, Diagnosis and Treatment. Philadelphia, Lea & Febiger, 1984, pp 451–473.
45. El-Sherif N, Mehra R, Gough WB, Zeiler RH: Ventricular activation patterns of spontaneous and induced ventricular rhythms in canine one day old myocardial infarctions. Evidence for focal and reentrant mechanisms. Circ Res 51:152, 1982.
46. El-Sherif N, Hope RR, Scherlag B, Lazzara R: Reentrant ventricular arrhythmias in the late myocardial infarction period. II. Patterns of Initiation and Termination of Reentry. Circulation 55:702, 1977.
47. El-Sherif N: Reentrant ventricular arrhythmias in the late myocardial infarction period. VI. Effect of the autonomic system. Circulation 58:103, 1978.
48. Potenza S, Maison-Blanche P, Cauchemez B, Leclercq JF, Coumel PH: Characteristics of spontaneous ventricular tachycardia onset in arrhythmogenic right ventricular dysplasia (Abstract). Eur Heart J 8:351, 1991.
49. Sugrue DD, Holmes DR, Jr, Gersh BJ: Cardiac histologic findings in patients with life threatening ventricular arrhythmias of unknown origin. J Am Coll Cardiol 4:952–957, 1984.
50. Voigt J, Agdal N: Lipomatous infiltration of

the heart. An uncommon cause of sudden, unexpected death in a young man. Arch Pathol Lab Med 106:497–498, 1982.
51. Laurenceau JL, Dumesnil JG: Right and left ventricular dimensions as determinants of ventricular septal motion. Chest 69:388–393, 1976.
52. Rakovec P, Rossi L, Fontaine G, et al: Familial arrhythmogenic right ventricular disease. Am J Cardiol 58:377–378, 1986.
53. Leor J, Glikson M, Vered Z, Kaplinsky E, Motro M: Ventricular tachycardia after soccer ball blow to the chest: First manifestation of arrhythmogenic right ventricular dysplasia in two brothers. Am J Med 89: 687–688, 1990.
54. Iwa T, Lascault G, Frank R, Tonet J, Fontaine G: Value of the signal averaged electrocardiogram in identifying patients with arrhythmogenic right ventricular dysplasia (Abstract). PACE 14(Part II):749, 1991.
55. Fontaine G, Tsezana R, Lazarus A, et al: Electrocardiographic features of arrhythmogenic right ventricular dysplasia (Abstract). Circulation, in press, 1993.

17

Causes and Implications of Sudden Cardiac Death in Athletes

BARRY J MARON
WILLIAM C. ROBERTS

The highly conditioned, competitive athlete epitomizes the healthiest segment of our society. Nevertheless, both youthful and older athletes may die suddenly, often during athletic activity.[1-4] Such catastrophes are totally unexpected and, while relatively uncommon, have a particularly tragic and devastating impact on the community. In the past few years, the underlying cardiovascular diseases responsible for sudden death in highly trained athletes and youthful asymptomatic individuals became the subject of several reports, and a large measure of clarification has resulted.[1-28] This chapter reviews the published findings and updates our own observations on the causes of sudden cardiac death (SCD) in competitive athletes of various ages and implications for the preparticipation screening of athletic populations.

SUDDEN DEATH IN YOUNG ATHLETES

Definition

For the purposes of this review, which focuses on the highly trained, competitive athlete, we have defined such as individual as one who participates in an organized team or individual sport that requires regular competition against others as a central component, places a high premium on excellence and achievement, and requires vigorous and intense training in a systematic fashion.[29] We also recognize that these definitions are arbitrary and that many individuals may participate in recreational sports in a truly competitive fashion.

Demographics and Mechanisms

Young athletes reported to die suddenly have participated in a variety of sports (most frequently basketball and football) and most are of junior or senior high school age at the time of death[1,2,5]; however, other sudden deaths occur in young athletes who have reached the collegiate or even professional levels of competition. Most athletes who incur sudden death, regardless of their particular underlying disease, have been virtually free of cardiovascular symptoms during their lives; collapse usually (but not always) is associated with exertion, either during training or an actual athletic contest. As a result of these circumstances, death is often attributed (at least in part) to intense physical activity. However, retrospective questioning of survivors may reveal the prior occurrence of transient symptoms (e.g., syncope, chest pain) in a minority of these athletes. Cardiovascular disease is uncommonly suspected during life (in only about 25% of instances). Even if cardiovascular disease is considered in competitive athletes, it is not uncommon for the diagnosis of "athlete's heart"[30,31] to be made rather than structural cardiac disease. The mechanism by which sudden death occurs differs considerably among athletes, depending on the underlying disease responsible.

The vast majority of reported sudden deaths in competitive athletes have been in white men[1-12,20,28]; indeed, of all the sudden deaths reported in young athletes, only about 10% have been in women. It is uncertain whether these findings are due to certain selection biases in reporting or to different relative risks for sudden death.

Previous Investigations

Some previous studies have documented the diseases responsible for sudden death in young competitive athletes while others have been limited to young asymptomatic individuals with active life-styles (who may not have been competitive athletes), or to those in whom death was temporarily related to exercise and sports. In these investigations, deaths related to cerebrovascular accident, heat stroke, or drug abuse[32] were preferentially excluded. It is probably not judicious to assign strict prevalence figures for the relative occurrence of various cardiovascular diseases in studies of sudden death in young athletes because of the patient selection biases and other limitations unavoidably involved in acquiring such data. Indeed, the available published studies not only differ with regard to the methods used to document the diagnoses, but also were derived from a variety of data bases, including populations selected from hospital records, coroner or medical examiner files, referrals based on media reports (Fig. 17-1), or combinations of these.

Even with these considerations in mind, it nevertheless appears that the vast majority of instances of sudden death in young athletes arise from a variety of congenital cardiovascular diseases (Fig. 17-2).[1,2,5-7,10,21,22,25,28] Virtually any cardiovascular disease capable of causing sudden death in young people may do so in young athletes. Among these diseases, hypertrophic cardio-

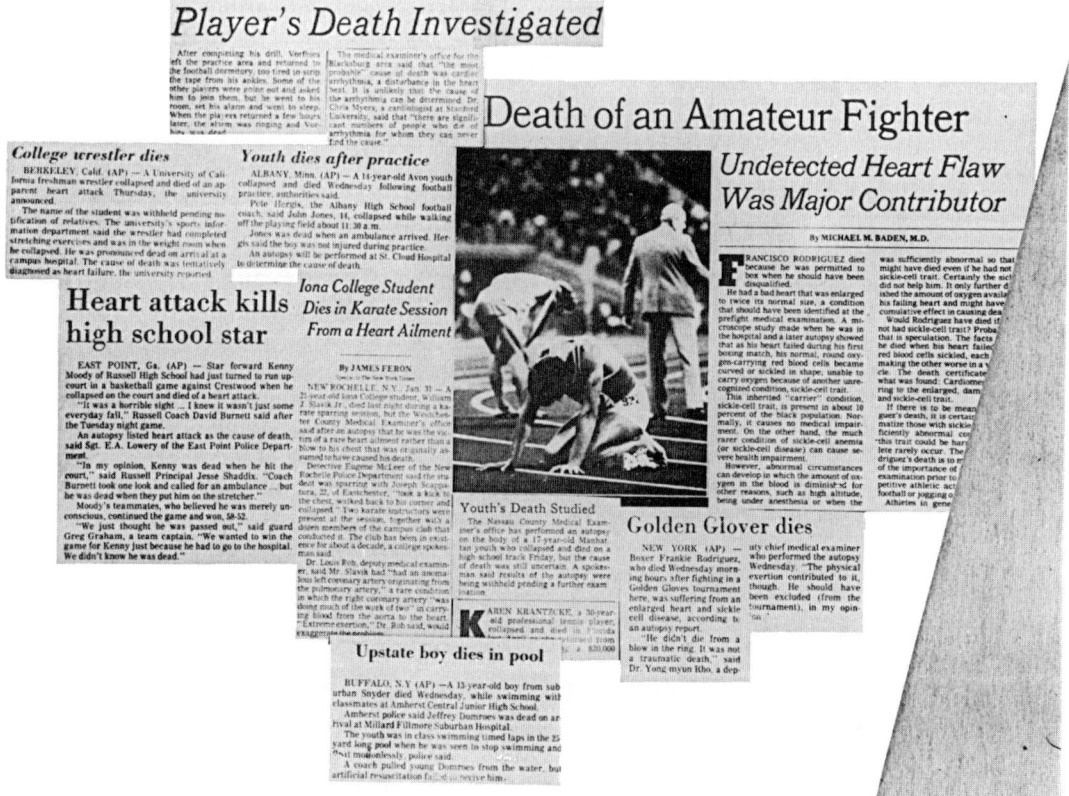

Fig. 17-1. News media reports of sudden death in athletes.

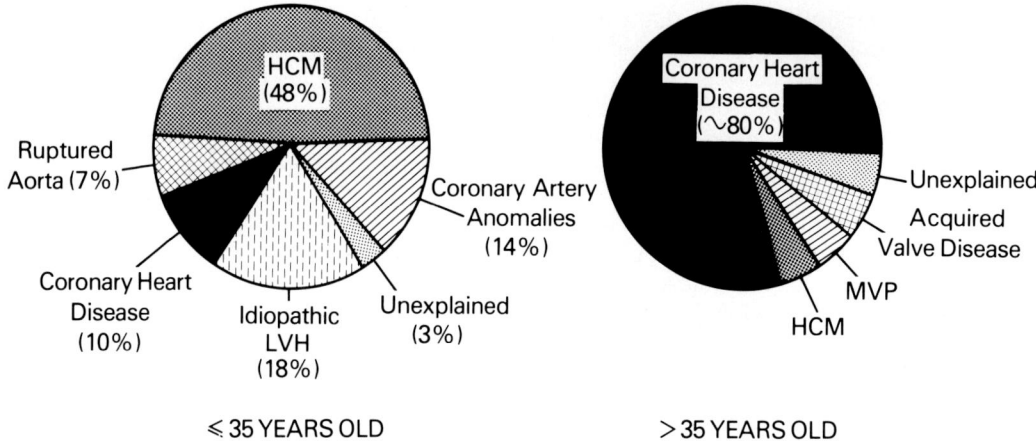

Fig. 17–2. Causes of sudden death in competitive athletes. Estimated prevalences of diseases responsible for death are compared in young (≤35 years old) and older (>35 years old) athletes. Data shown are from Maron et al[1] for young athletes, and collated data from available published studies in older athletes. HCM, hypertrophic cardiomyopathy; LVH, left ventricular hypertrophy; MVP, mitral valve prolapse. (Reproduced by permission of the American College of Cardiology from Maron BJ, et al: Circulation 62:218–229, 1980.[1])

myopathy[1,2,5,10–12,22,25] is probably the most common, although congenital coronary artery anomalies and aortic rupture associated with Marfan syndrome also occur frequently. It should be emphasized that although these diseases may be relatively common in young athletes dying suddenly, each occurs uncommonly in the general population. Two reports have also incriminated sickle cell trait as a predisposing risk factor for SCD with strenuous exertion,[12,33] probably due to sickling induced under the conditions of hypoxia and dehydration.

Based on our own experience and a review of the literature, most published studies suggest that other less common causes of sudden death in competitive athletes include viral myocarditis and rare diseases such as QT-interval prolongation syndromes, RV dysplasia, and mitral valve prolapse.[1,2,11,12,28,34–37] One notable exception to this view is a report from northeastern Italy by Corrado et al[28] that indicated that RV dysplasia was the most common cause of sudden death in athletes. There is no evidence at present that systemic hypertension per se is associated with increased risk for SCD in young athletes, although many older athletes who have died of coronary artery disease may also have had coexisting hypertension.

Most Common Diseases

Hypertrophic Cardiomyopathy

Hypertrophic cardiomyopathy (Fig. 17–3) is a primary disease of cardiac muscle that is usually genetically transmitted[38–41] and is characterized by a hypertrophied but nondilated left ventricle (LV) in the absence of another cardiac or systemic disease that may produce LV hypertrophy.[42] This increase in LV mass usually results in impaired ventricular filling and compliance[38,39]; some patients may also have obstruction to LV outflow produced by systolic anterior motion of the mitral valve.[43]

Competitive athletes dying suddenly of hypertrophic cardiomyopathy in our reported series[1,2] ranged in age from 13 to 30 years (mean, 19 years). Heart weights were 360–630 g, and ventricular septal thickness ranged from 15 to 30 mm (mean, 20 mm). The pattern of LV wall thickening was characteristically asymmetric, with portions of ventricular septum disproportionately thicker than most of the LV free wall.[44,45] In addition, the thickened LV wall (particularly the septum) demonstrated two other characteristic morphological features: bizarre cellular architecture with a markedly disordered arrangement of cardiac muscle cells (Fig. 17–3),[46] and an increased number

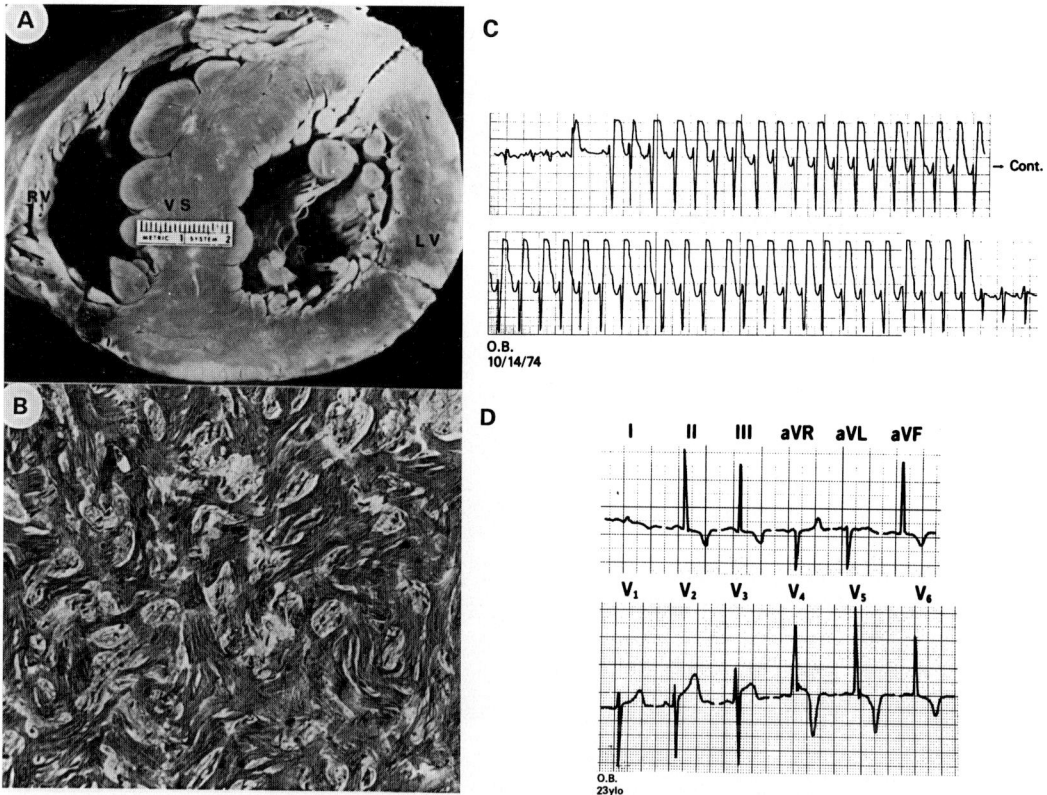

Fig. 17–3. Clinical and morphological features of athletes with hypertrophic cardiomyopathy. **A.** Gross heart specimen showing disproportionate thickening of the ventricular septum (VS) with respect to the left ventricular free wall (LV). RV, right ventricular wall. **B.** Marked disorganization of cardiac muscle cells in the disproportionately thickened ventricular septum. Adjacent hypertrophied cardiac muscle cells are oriented at oblique and perpendicular angles. **C.** ECG showing 4-second period of ventricular tachycardia that occurred in the second minute of recovery after a routine treadmill exercise test, and then terminated spontaneously. **D.** Standard 12-lead ECG showing marked symmetric T-wave inversion (up to 15 mm in depth), as well as evidence of left ventricular hypertrophy. (Reproduced by permission of the American College of Cardiology from Maron BJ, et al: J Am Coll Cardiol 7:204–214, 1986.[2])

of abnormal intramural coronary arteries with thickened walls and apparently narrowed lumina, often associated with fibrosis.[47]

Reports of hospital-based populations with hypertrophic cardiomyopathy have shown the disease to be an important cause of sudden death in the young, usually in patients without prior symptoms (including many in whom sudden death was the first manifestation of disease).[48] Indeed, a clinical profile of 78 patients with hypertrophic cardiomyopathy who died suddenly and had been studied at the National Institutes of Health[49] resembled that of the young competitive athlete with sudden death; 70% of the deaths occurred before 30 years of age, 55% of victims had experienced no functional limitation prior to death, and about 40% had been actively engaged in moderate to severe exertion at or just before death. The fact that a relatively large proportion of these deaths were related to vigorous physical activity suggests an association between participation in sports and risk for SCD in some patients with hypertrophic cardiomyopathy.[50]

Many of the potential mechanisms by which sudden death occurs in athletes with hypertrophic cardiomyopathy are known.[51,52] It is probable that the myocardial structural or functional abnormalities characteristic of this disease[38,39,46,47,52] predispose many susceptible individuals with this disease to a malignant ventricular arrhythmia (which may be primary or possibly preceded by supraventricular tachycardia or bradyarrhythmia). Alternatively, other mechanisms that may be operative include sudden hemodynamic instability in which systemic hypotension is associated with exercise[53] and a reduction in LV volume. On the other hand, it is perhaps remarkable that some competitive athletes with hypertrophic cardiomyopathy (who may or may not die suddenly) are capable of vigorous and prolonged periods of training and may survive with this life-style for many years without being aware of their disease or experiencing significant symptoms.[1,2,54]

Idiopathic Left Ventricular Hypertrophy

Of note, other athletes with SCD and a hypertrophied nondilated LV have been described at autopsy as having "idiopathic left ventricular hypertrophy" (Fig. 17–4).[1,2,5,25] These athletes show relatively symmetric patterns of LV wall thickening, absence of histological evidence of myocardial cell disarray[46] or abnormal intramural coronary arteries,[47] and a family history of hypertrophic cardiomyopathy.[41] Usually such individuals have not been evaluated clinically during life, and hence echocardiographic data are lacking with regard to the distribution of wall thickening[45] and mitral valve motion pattern.[43] Consequently, while it is difficult to categorize such patients definitively as having hypertrophic cardiomyopathy based solely on the available autopsy data, we suspect that many may indeed be part of this broad disease spectrum. For example, it is possible that an asymmetric pattern of LV hypertrophy is present in such patients but obscured by postmortem effects on wall thickness.[55]

Congenital Coronary Artery Anomalies

A variety of congenital malformations of coronary artery anatomy and distribution (unassociated with significant coronary atherosclerosis)[1,2,5,9,25,28,56–65] are not infrequently incriminated as the cause of sudden death in youthful athletes, often exercise-related (Fig. 17–5). Probably the most common of these is anomalous origin of the *left*

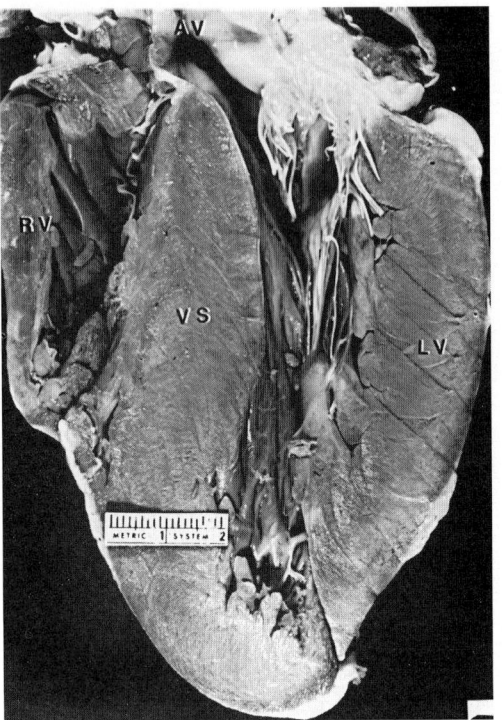

Fig. 17–4. Idiopathic left ventricular hypertrophy in the heart of a 17-year-old soccer player. Note marked concentric (symmetric) thickening of the ventricular septum (VS) and left ventricular (LV) free wall. The heart weighed 465 g. Thickness of the ventricular septum is 23 mm and that of the LV free wall is 20 mm. Histological examination of the LV myocardium and echocardiographic studies in first-degree relatives failed to show evidence supporting the diagnosis of hypertrophic cardiomyopathy. AV, aortic valve; RV, right ventricle. (Reproduced by permission of the American Heart Association from Maron BJ, et al: Circulation 62:218–229, 1980.[1])

main coronary artery from the *right* (anterior) sinus of Valsalva. Cheitlin et al[59] were the first to emphasize that the origin of both the left and the right coronary arteries from the right sinus, with passage of the left main coronary artery between the aorta and pulmonary trunk, was a malformation with relevance to SCD. Of those patients reported with this malformation, most (about 75%) die before age 20, and virtually all of these deaths have occurred during or shortly after vigorous exertion. It is not clear why some individuals with coronary

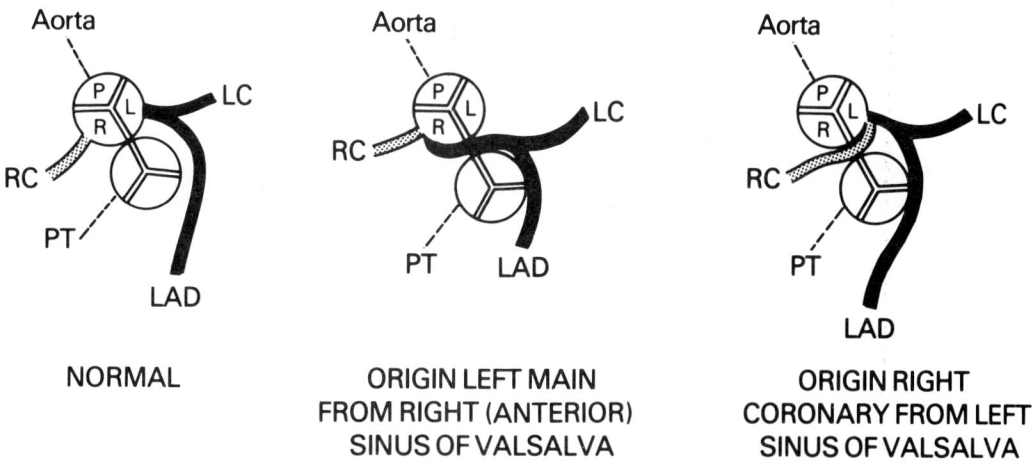

Fig. 17–5. Congenital coronary artery anomalies capable of causing sudden death in young athletes. *Left*, normal anatomy is shown for comparison. *Center*, anomalous origin of the left main coronary artery from the right (anterior) sinus of Valsalva. The left coronary artery may have a separate or common ostium with the right coronary artery, which also arises from the right (R) sinus of Valsalva. Note the acute leftward bend of the left main coronary artery at its origin and its posterior course between the aorta and pulmonary trunk (PT). *Right*, the right coronary (RC) artery arises anomalously from the left (L) coronary sinus in association with the left main coronary artery and shows a similar acute bend at its origin before it courses between the great arteries. LAD, left anterior descending coronary artery; LC, left circumflex coronary artery; P, posterior (noncoronary) cusp.

anomalies survive the course of their natural lives while most die suddenly before age 20, or why some of those who die suddenly can nevertheless tolerate vigorous training and competitive athletics without evidence of myocardial ischemia for prolonged periods of time. Although the correct diagnosis is rarely made during life, a surprising proportion experience prodromal symptoms, most commonly syncope or angina. However, not uncommonly, examples of this anomaly are encountered for the first time at autopsy in patients who had no evidence or symptoms of myocardial ischemia during life. However, in youthful athletes it is possible to identify (or raise a strong suspicion of) this anomaly by means of conventional two-dimensional echocardiography,[58] which can subsequently lead to definitive diagnosis by coronary arteriography.

The mechanism by which this coronary anomaly produces sudden death is not definitively known. However, it has been postulated that the acute takeoff angle of the left main coronary artery from the right sinus results in narrowing of the coronary ostium.[56,57] Presumably, during the basal state or with routine daily activities, the left coronary ostium remains open and oval shaped. With the increased stroke volume and myocardial oxygen requirements associated with exercise, the ascending aorta expands, the takeoff angle of the left coronary artery becomes exaggerated, and the ostium of the left coronary artery is narrowed in a slitlike fashion. This severe compromise of the ostial orifice presumably results in diminished coronary blood flow and myocardial ischemia (particularly in the presence of right coronary artery dominance).[57] It is also possible that as the left main coronary artery courses between the aorta and pulmonary trunk, it may be compressed against the root of the pulmonary trunk (where it is firmly anchored) during exercise when the aortic root and pulmonary trunk dilate. This hypothesis is supported by the observation that sudden exertional death and nonfatal myocardial ischemia have also been described in persons in whom the left main coronary artery originated from the proximal right coronary artery (and then coursed between the great arteries), and therefore could not have an abnormal oblique takeoff from the aortic sinus.

Roberts' group[56,60] and others[65] have emphasized that the "mirror image" coronary anomaly in which the *right* coronary artery arises from the *left* sinus of Valsalva (and courses between the aorta and pulmonary trunk) may also convey risk for sudden death in young individuals. With this lesion an anatomical and pathophysiological situation exists at the right coronary ostium that is analogous to that previously described for the left main coronary ostium when that artery originates from the anterior (right) sinus. Presumably, the mechanism by which myocardial ischemia occurs in these two anatomical variants is similar.

Other unusual variants of coronary arterial anatomy may be rare causes of exercise-related sudden deaths in young conditioned individuals.[1,2,63,66,67] These include hypoplasia of the right coronary and left circumflex arteries (Fig. 17–6), the left anterior descending or right coronary artery emanating from the pulmonary trunk, virtual absence of the left coronary artery,[68] or coronary arterial intussusception causing occlusion of the coronary lumen (Fig. 17–7).[67]

It has also been suggested that major coronary arteries "tunneled" within LV myocardium (myocardial "bridges") constitute a potentially lethal anatomical variant that may cause sudden unexpected death in otherwise healthy young individuals during exertion or stress.[25,69,70] Such coronary arteries (usually the left anterior descending artery) are completely surrounded by myocardium for at least a portion of their course; it has been postulated that in certain susceptible individuals the artery may be subjected to a critical degree of systolic compression and constriction, resulting in myocardial ischemia (even in the absence of hemodynamically significant atherosclerotic disease). However, this hypothetical scenario is less compelling when other issues are considered: (1) most coronary flow occurs during the diastolic phase of the cardiac cycle, and (2) autopsy studies have shown tunneled left anterior descending coronary arteries to occur frequently in about 25% of diseased hearts from patients not dying suddenly.[70] Therefore, at present, convincing evidence that tunneled coronary arteries are responsible for sudden catastrophes in young athletes is lacking.[71]

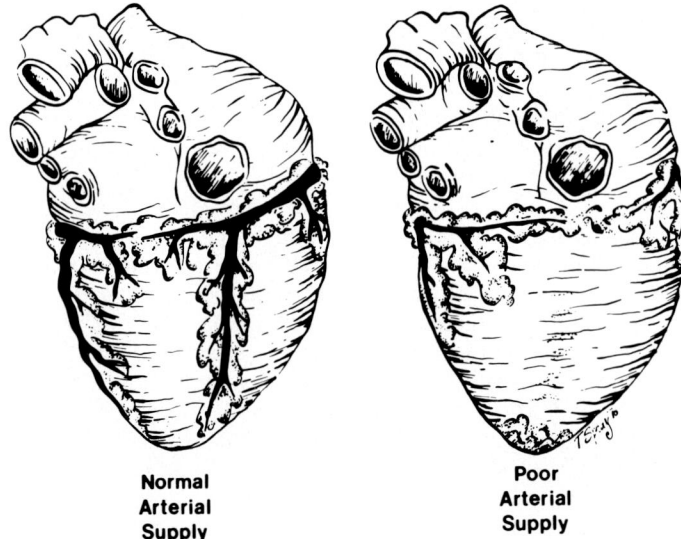

Fig. 17–6. Diagrammatic representation of coronary arterial hypoplasia, a rare congenital coronary abnormality, in a 17-year-old female distance runner who collapsed suddenly and died instantaneously at the end of a race. The coronary arterial distribution to the posterior surface of the heart is greatly diminished in that only two small posterior descending branches to the posterior left ventricular wall arise from the left circumflex coronary artery. Also, the right coronary artery was short and provided only two small branches to the posterior wall of right ventricle and none to posterior wall of left ventricle. (Reproduced by permission of the American Heart Association from Maron BJ, et al: Circulation 62:218–229, 1980.[1])

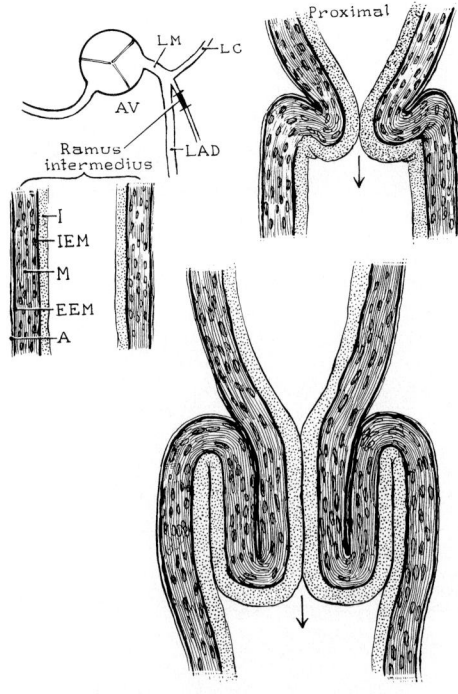

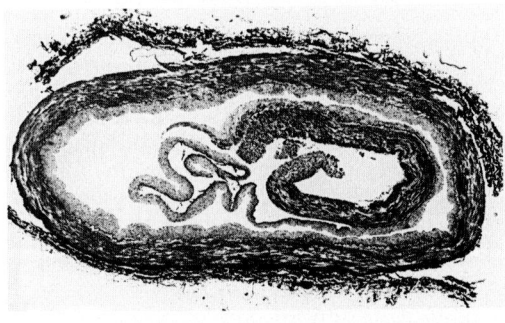

Fig. 17–7. Location and appearance of coronary arterial intussusception in a 19-year-old football player. *Top,* diagrammatic representation. A, adventitia; AV, aortic valve; EEM, external elastic membrane; I, intima; IEM, internal elastic membrane; LAD, left anterior descending coronary artery; LC, left circumflex coronary artery; LM, left main coronary artery; M, media. *Bottom,* photomicrograph of a section containing the intussusception within the ramus intermedius coronary artery. Movat stain, ×34. (Reproduced with permission from Roberts WC, et al: Am J Cardiol 57:179–180, 1986.[67])

Aortic Rupture (Marfan Syndrome)

Young athletes may die suddenly from rupture of the aorta (Fig. 17–8).[1,2] Some such individuals may have the classic physical signs of Marfan syndrome, but others may not. Usually evident at autopsy is disruption of the aortic media with decreased numbers of elastic fibers (i.e., cystic medial necrosis), and it is this abnormality that is responsible for intrinsic weakening of the aortic wall. Certain individuals with Marfan syndrome may participate successfully in strenuous competitive sports for many years without experiencing a catastrophic event, presumably prior to the time aortic dilation becomes marked and the predisposition for dissection/rupture increases critically.

Coronary Heart Disease

Atherosclerotic coronary heart disease is infrequently responsible for sudden death in youthful athletes.[1,2,8,25,28] For example, we have studied three young competitive athletes, ages 24, 26, and 28 years, who had coronary arterial atherosclerosis. At autopsy, two had severe luminal narrowing (>75% reduction in cross-sectional area by atherosclerotic plaque) involving each of the three major extramural coronary arteries. One was a 28-year-old professional football player who had diffuse and severe coronary atherosclerosis and extensive hemorrhage into atherosclerotic plaque, as well as a large healed posterior wall myocardial infarction.[8] On retrospective analysis of his medical history, it was apparent that he had experienced exertional angina on several occasions; however, these symptoms were thought to reflect traumatic injury rather than cardiac disease (Fig. 17–9). In addition, Green et al[72] have reported the case of a 44-year-old marathon runner who collapsed after completing 24 miles of a race and at autopsy proved to have transmural myocardial infarction but no identifiable extramural coronary artery disease.

Less Common Diseases

Myocarditis

Myocarditis (usually of viral origin) has traditionally been considered an important cause of sudden unexplained death in young individuals.[24,25,27,73,74] Although myocarditis may certainly occur in this context (with either no or relatively innocent prodromal symptoms), its frequency as a cause of sud-

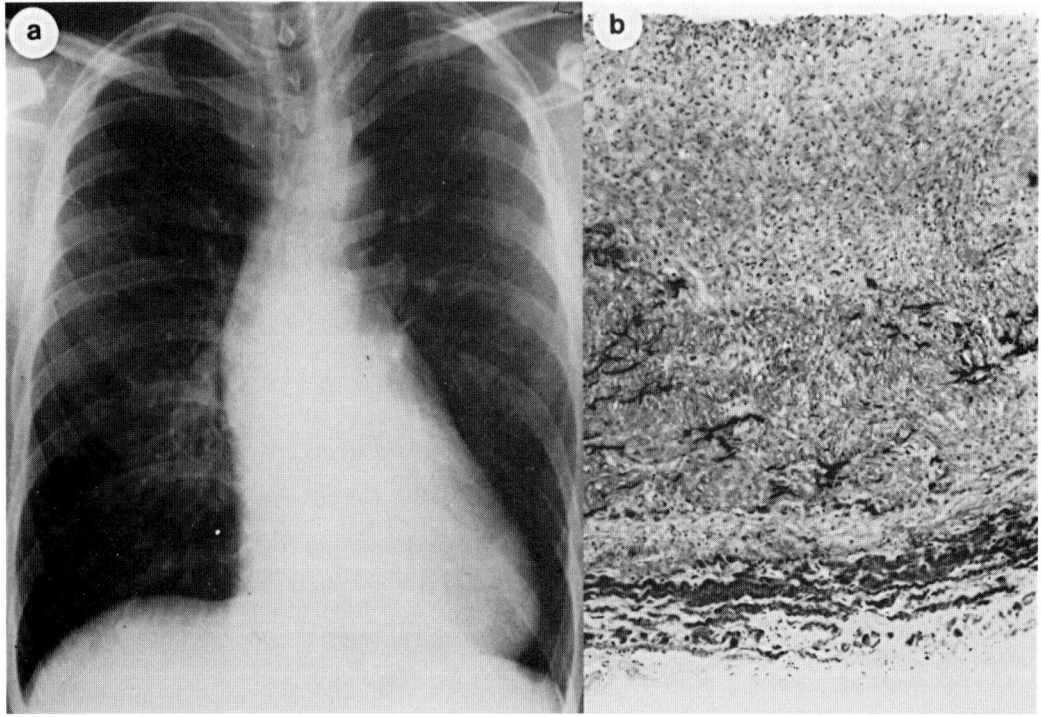

Fig. 17–8. Marfan syndrome. **a.** Posteroanterior chest radiograph obtained from an 18-year-old male collegiate swimmer who died 2 months later of a ruptured aorta during a training session. Prominent dilation of the ascending aorta is apparent. In this patient, the correct diagnosis was made during life and the athlete was apprised of (but ignored) the risks of continued competition. **b.** Histological section of ascending aorta from another athlete who died of a ruptured aorta. Note the markedly diminished number of darkly stained elastic fibers in the aortic media. Intima is toward the top and adventitia is toward the bottom. Elastic van Gieson stain, ×80. (Reproduced by permission of the American Heart Association from Maron BJ, et al: Circulation 62:218–229, 1980.[1])

den death in the young may have been exaggerated because of overinterpretation of the histological findings at autopsy. Indeed, a major limitation in the autopsy diagnosis of myocarditis has been the lack of standardized histological criteria.[75] Of note, myocarditis has been documented in very few true competitive athletes who have died suddenly; Jokl[73] reported the case of a 25-year-old runner who died after a 12-mile road race and proved to have myocarditis that was unsuspected clinically.

Mitral Valve Prolapse

Despite its relative frequency in the general population (probably about 5%),[76] mitral valve prolapse does not appear to be an important cause of sudden death in competitive athletes. To date, fewer than 100 individuals with mitral valve prolapse have been reported with sudden death (average age about 35 years).[28,34,37,50,76–79] Such deaths are uncommonly related to physical exertion or sporting activity, and to date very few have occurred in true competitive athletes.[34,50,79] However, in one autopsy series[79] of children and young adults who died suddenly, mitral valve prolapse and myocarditis were reportedly more common than hypertrophic cardiomyopathy and congenital coronary anomalies; these prevalence figures may well have been influenced by bias in patient selection. In our original series of 29 athletes studied at autopsy,[1] only one had mitral valve morphology consistent with "floppy" mitral valve; however, this patient also had increased LV thickness, a finding that is not consistent with the mitral valve prolapse syndrome.

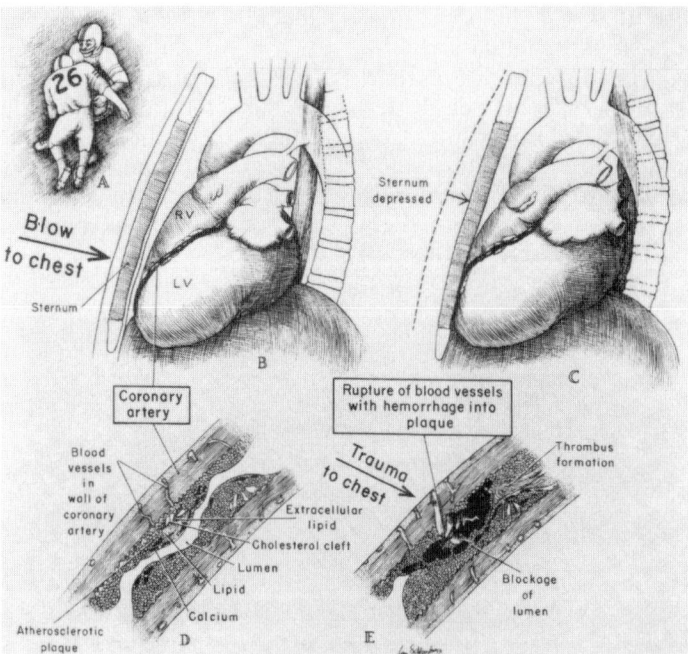

Fig. 17-9. Probable mechanism of hemorrhages into atherosclerotic plaques in the coronary arteries of a 28-year-old professional football player. Tackling and blocking almost surely caused contact of the anterior surface of the heart with the underlying sternum. When the coronary arteries are normal or near-normal, the arteries absorb these blows without consequence, since they are freely pliable. When these arteries are heavily atherosclerotic (as in the present patient) their pliability is lost; subsequent contact of the surface of the heart with the underlying sternum logically might result in "cracking" of the atherosclerotic plaques, allowing hemorrhage into them as shown here. (Reproduced with permission from Roberts WC, et al: Am Heart J *102*:1061-1063, 1981.[8])

Aortic Valvular Stenosis

Aortic stenosis is another congenital cardiac malformation that was previously considered a common cause of sudden death in children and young asymptomatic adults, based on data from hospital-based populations.[22] However, in reported series, aortic stenosis rarely appears to be an explanation for sudden death in young competitive athletes. This is probably due to the fact that aortic stenosis is likely to be identified early in life by virtue of the characteristically loud heart murmur, thereby leading to disqualification of the patient from competitive athletics.

Sarcoidosis

Sarcoid heart disease may cause sudden unexpected death in previously asymptomatic individuals. Roberts et al[11,80] reported that about 25% of patients with sarcoid granulomatous infiltration of the heart died suddenly (average age at death, 36 years), usually associated with exertion and often as the initial clinical manifestation of sarcoidosis. Other individuals with sarcoidosis may experience arrhythmias or complete heart block prior to death. We evaluated a 25-year-old professional basketball player with recurrent clinically overt ventricular tachyarrhythmias who died suddenly and in whom sarcoid infiltration of the heart was demonstrated at autopsy.

Cardiac Conduction System Abnormalities

Some authors[6,7,21,28] have suggested that occult abnormalities of the cardiac conduction system (in the absence of other structural cardiac abnormalities) may be responsible for sudden death in athletes. Thiene et al[6] described three young athletes with a variety of atrioventricular conduction system abnormalities that the authors suggested were responsible for lethal arrhythmias, including one with accessory atrioventricular pathways. James et al[7] described morphological abnormalities of the small intramural artery to the sinoatrial node that consisted of thickened vessel walls and a narrowed lumen, which they incriminated as the cause of the degeneration, scarring, and hemorrhage present in the surrounding conducting tissue. We have also identified morphologically similar alterations of intramural arteries (to either the sinoatrial or atrioventricular nodes) in a small number of the young athletes dying with hypertrophic cardiomyopathy or idiopathic LV hypertrophy (Fig. 17–10).[1,2]

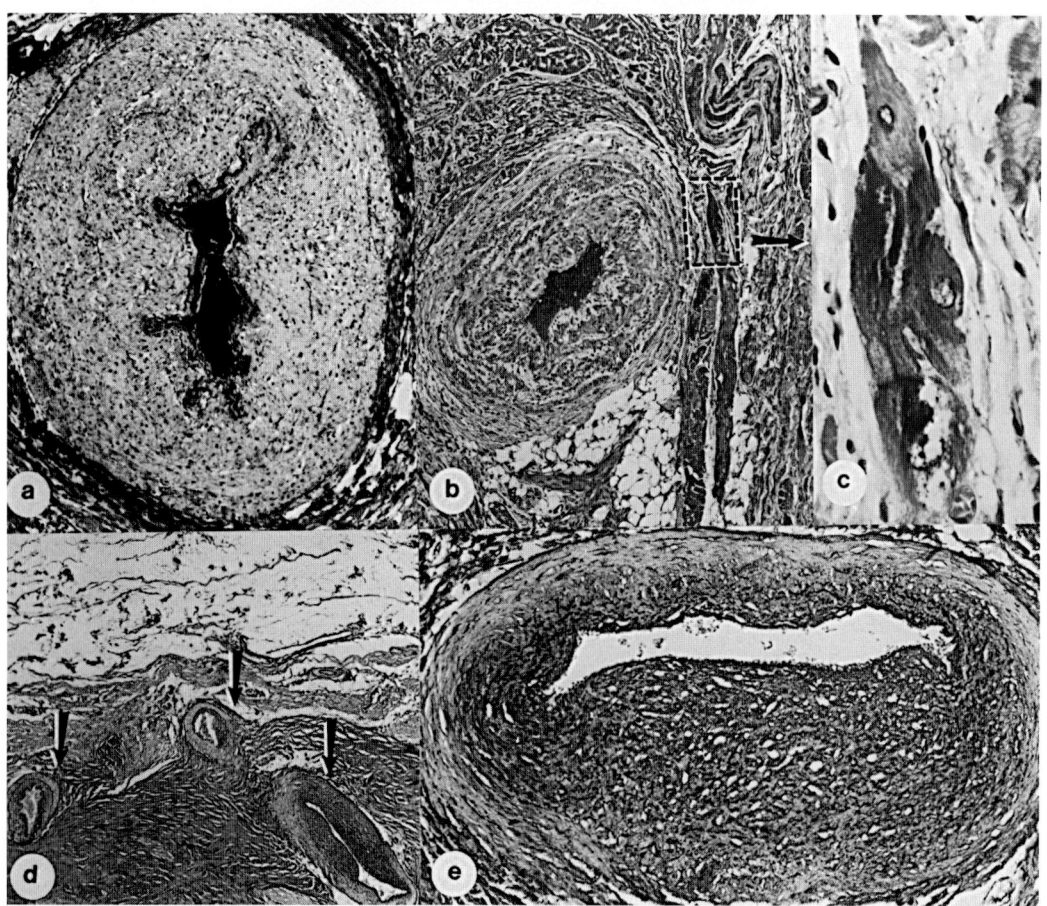

Fig. 17–10. Conduction system disease. Small arteries in the conducting tissue of two athletes who died suddenly. **a–c:** Artery to the sinoatrial node of a 24-year-old basketball player with hypertrophic cardiomyopathy. **d** and **e:** Artery to the AV node of a 17-year-old basketball player with idiopathic concentric left ventricular hypertrophy. **a.** Sinoatrial node artery has markedly narrowed lumen due to extreme thickening of the arterial wall (hematoxylin-eosin, ×95). **b.** Same artery as in **a**, but at a different level and lower magnification (×55), showing calcium deposits in adjacent myocardial fibers (outlined by broken line). **c.** Higher magnification view of a portion of AV nodal tissue that penetrates the central fibrous body (hematoxylin-eosin, ×40). **d.** Three distinctly abnormal small arteries are evident (arrows) (elastic van Gieson, ×40). **e.** High-magnification view (×130) of one of the vessels shown in **d**, but at a different level. The lumen is markedly narrowed due to thickening of the arterial wall. (Reproduced by permission of the American Heart Association from Maron BJ, et al: Circulation 62:218–229, 1980.[1])

Right Ventricular Cardiomyopathy (Dysplasia)

Right ventricular cardiomyopathy is an unusual cardiac disease that is often associated with important ventricular or supraventricular arrhythmias[10,28,81] and has been cited as a cause of sudden death in the young.[10,25,28,36] When recurrent, intractable arrhythmias dominate the clinical picture, the disease is frequently referred to as arrhythmogenic RV dysplasia. Thiene et al[10,28] have stressed that this disease may be more common than was previously thought, and that it is an important cause of SCD in athletes. Indeed, in a study of 22 young competitive athletes who died suddenly in northern Italy,[28] these authors found RV cardiomyopathy to be the most common cause of death; furthermore, in this particular series hypertrophic cardiomyopathy was not identified in any of the athletes. The explanation for such major differences in the prevalence of cardiac diseases responsible for sudden death in athletes reported in the series from Italy[28] and others[1,2,5] is not entirely clear but is undoubtedly related to patient selection.

Right ventricular cardiomyopathy is characterized morphologically by partial or total absence of RV myocardium, which is replaced by fibrous or adipose tissue (Fig. 17–11). In some patients, complete absence of myocardial tissue results in a paper-thin appearance of the RV and the virtual apposition of endocardium and epicardium. This disease process may be segmental or, alternatively, may involve the RV diffusely. In other patients RV wall thickness may be virtually normal.

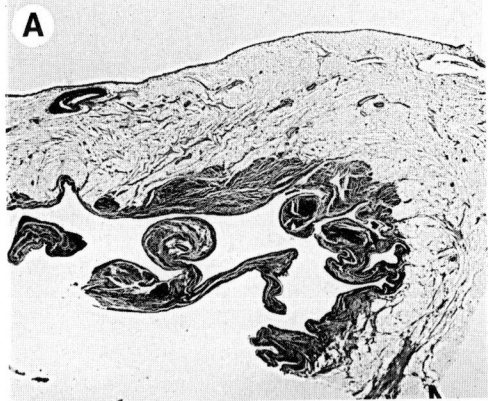

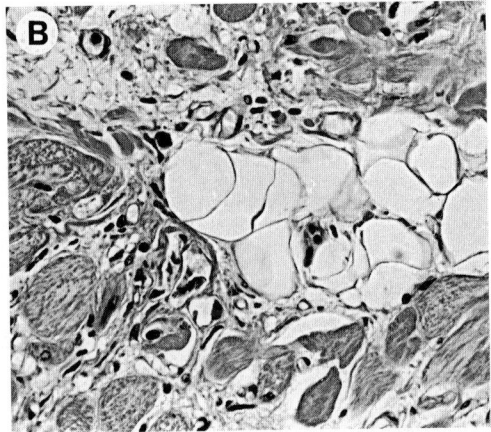

Fig. 17–11. Right ventricular cardiomyopathy (dysplasia) of the lipomatous type. **A.** Low power view of anterior right ventricular wall showing massive lipomatous infiltration (azan, ×5). **B.** High power view of right ventricular myocardium showing myocardial degeneration and lipomatous infiltration (hematoxylin-eosin, ×300). (Reproduced by permission of the *New England Journal of Medicine* from Thiene G, et al: N Engl J Med *318*:129–133, 1988.[10])

Normal Hearts

Occasionally, athletes or other individuals dying suddenly demonstrate no evidence of structural cardiovascular disease, even after careful gross and microscopic examination of the heart.[1,2,4,25,74,79,82] In such instances it may not always be possible to be absolutely certain whether noncardiac factors (such as drug abuse)[32] were responsible for or contributed to the catastrophe, or whether careful inspection of the specialized conducting system and associated vasculature with serial sections would have revealed clinically relevant abnormalities.

While one can only speculate on the potential causes of such deaths, it is possible that some result either from a primary arrhythmia or from rare diseases in which structural abnormalities of the heart and conducting system are characteristically lacking at autopsy, such as QT-interval prolongation syndromes[35] or, conceivably, exercise-induced coronary spasm.[83]

Sudden Death in Soldiers

Although not truly competitive athletes, young military personnel may engage in a rigorous life-style that is similar in many respects to that of athletes. For this reason, it is worth summarizing the data available on the causes of SCD in military recruits. Studies of populations of young soldiers from the United States,[82] Israel,[84] and England[85] report sudden deaths (unrelated to trauma or other noncardiac factors) that are usually due to either myocarditis or congenital cardiac malformations (most commonly hypertrophic cardiomyopathy or coronary artery anomalies). Therefore, myocarditis appears to be a common cause of SCD in this particular population of active young individuals.

CAUSES OF SUDDEN DEATH IN OLDER ATHLETES

Increasing numbers of middle-aged or older individuals are now participating in organized competitive sports and in vigorous physical conditioning programs. However, superior physical fitness in this age group (or any other age group) does not guarantee protection against exercise-related cardiovascular death. As is the case with young competitive athletes, older athletes may harbor occult cardiac disease and die suddenly and unexpectedly while participating in athletic activities. Nevertheless, the incidence of such catastrophes (and therefore the risk) is quite low in light of the large number of older individuals participating in sporting activities.[15,18,19]

Unlike the situation in youthful athletes, the cause of sudden death in older conditioned athletes usually is not a congenital malformation of the heart but, in the vast majority of instances, coronary heart disease (Fig. 17–12). The remaining deaths in older athletes appear to be due to a variety of noncoronary causes, such as hypertro-

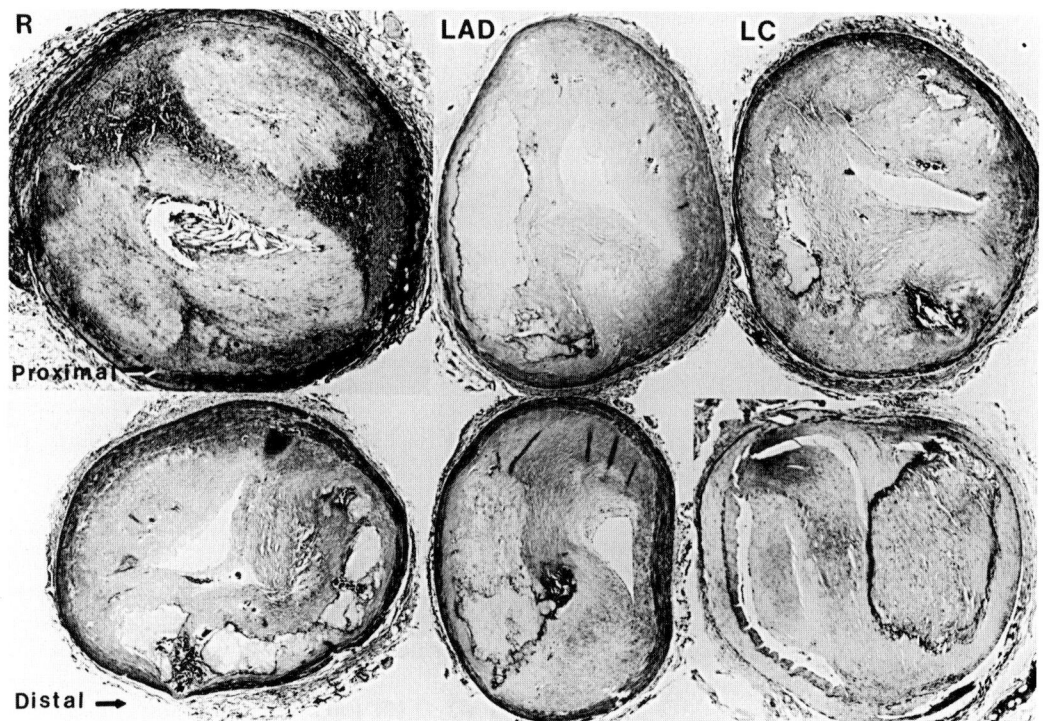

Fig. 17–12. Sections of coronary arteries from a 49-year-old man who ran an average of about 170 km/wk and successfully completed six marathons and seven 80-km races, but who died suddenly of coronary heart disease. The right (R), left anterior descending (LAD), and left circumflex (LC) coronary arteries are shown at the sites of maximal narrowing by atherosclerosis, both in the proximal (*top*) and distal (*bottom*) halves of the respective arteries. (Reproduced by permission of the American College of Cardiology from Maron BJ, et al: J Am Coll Cardiol 7:204–214, 1986.[2]).

phic cardiomyopathy, mitral valve prolapse, or acquired valvular heart disease.[4,14,16] Occasionally the cause of death is not established definitively at autopsy.[4]

To date, almost 150 older trained athletes who have died suddenly of coronary heart disease have been described in several autopsy-based investigations.[3,4,11–13,15–20,23,26,86] These individuals compose a heterogeneous athletic population that includes runners training for competitive long-distance races, joggers, and participants in sports such as rugby and squash. Most of the deaths have occurred during or just after physical activity. In contrast to the young competitive athletes with congenital heart disease, over one half of the older athletes with coronary heart disease had experienced prodromal cardiovascular symptoms, had knowledge of underlying cardiac disease, or had specific documentation of prior myocardial infarction. Although few studies provide detailed or quantitative morphological descriptions of the severity and distribution of arterial narrowing, the available data suggest that most athletes dying of coronary heart disease have significant atherosclerotic narrowing (>75% of the cross sectional luminal area) of two or three major extramural coronary arteries (Fig. 17–12 and 17–13); involvement limited to one major extramural artery has been described in only about 25% of athletes. Also, myocardial scarring is described in about 60% of reported cases in which these data are provided.

PREPARTICIPATION SCREENING IN YOUNG COMPETITIVE ATHLETES

Definition of the causes of sudden death in a young athletic population (as defined earlier) predictably raises the issues of detection and prevention. Prepartication screening is predicated on the generally held belief that individuals with certain underlying cardiovascular diseases are at an enhanced risk for SCD if actively engaged in strenuous and systematic athletic training and competition.[29] Even though the individual occurrences of sudden death in athletes are infrequent and result from a variety of causes, these events command a great deal of public and private attention and raise inevitable questions regarding whether they can be prevented through early detection and ultimately by therapeutic intervention.

Small Populations

Screening young athletes for cardiovascular disease can be undertaken most effec-

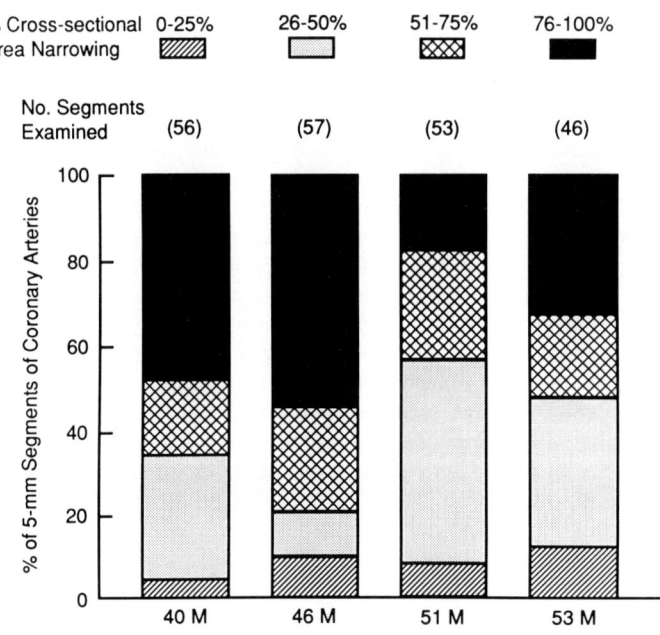

Fig. 17–13. Quantitative assessment of the distribution and extent of coronary atherosclerosis in four trained runners. Data depicted are the percent of 5-mm coronary arterial segments narrowed to various degrees by atherosclerotic plaque.

tively when the number of subjects evaluated is small and the professional fees and costs of the tests can be borne by the athlete's family, school, or a third party. Under these circumstances, a noninvasive evaluation oriented to the cardiovascular diseases known to cause sudden death in athletes would be most appropriate and include at least an informed personal and family history and physical examination, 12-lead electrocardiogram (ECG), and echocardiography.

Athletes with the physical signs of Marfan syndrome are diagnosed or suspected on physical examination; on the other hand, most athletes with hypertrophic cardiomyopathy have the nonobstructive form of the disease and therefore will not have a prominent heart murmur and are unlikely to be identified by physical examination alone. Virtually all patients with hypertrophic cardiomyopathy would, however, be identified by echocardiography,[45] as would patients with Marfan syndrome (by virtue of visualization of the dilated aorta) and often those with anomalous origin of the left or right coronary arteries.[58] Additional invasive or noninvasive testing (e.g., cardiac catheterization and angiography, blood lipid studies) might be indicated, depending on the results of the initial screening tests or on the symptoms or pertinent history reported by the athlete.

Large Populations

The issues surrounding mass screening are complex. Several inherent problems interfere with establishing a successful and economically feasible screening program for identifying relatively rare cardiovascular disease in large populations of asymptomatic athletes.[87,88]

It has been estimated that over 25 million children and young adults participate in organized competitive athletic activities annually in the United States at the youth, interscholastic, and intercollegiate levels. A periodic individualized and comprehensive medical examination for each participant in organized sports is well beyond the capabilities of the current medical care system. This is particularly true since each athlete would essentially require a noninvasive cardiologic workup, including echocardiography.

The expense of such an evaluation could easily exceed $500–$1,000 per athlete. These are prohibitive costs in light of the large numbers of athletes potentially involved in community-based screening. Indeed, all but the least expensive screening efforts would be beyond the financial resources of most institutions.

Another critical problem intrinsic to mass screening is the infrequency with which the cardiovascular diseases responsible for sudden death occur in youthful populations. For example, diseases such as hypertrophic cardiomyopathy and Marfan syndrome are relatively rare, likely occurring in 0.2% or less of young athletes. Hence, it is probably necessary to screen about 1000 athletes to encounter one or two with such cardiovascular diseases.

With these considerations in mind, designing a practical, cost-efficient approach for the mass screening of large populations of young athletes for the detection of cardiovascular diseases known to SCD represents a particularly challenging task. It is perhaps not surprising that such programs have been undertaken only sporadically. Our experience with the screening of intercollegiate athletes at the University of Maryland[87] and Howard University[88] has underlined several relevant issues in this regard. The study of 501 University of Maryland athletes was structured so that the initial clinical screening included the personal and family history, physical examination, and 12-lead ECG (Fig. 17-14). A major impetus for utilization of the ECG (other than its relatively low cost and easy application) was the fact that 90–95% of patients with hypertrophic cardiomyopathy, including those at risk for sudden death, show ECG abnormalities.[89] Also, this study was designed to avoid the routine use of echocardiography as a primary screening test owing to the aforementioned considerations—substantial expense and certain practical and technical problems encountered in its routine application to large athletic populations. About 20% of the athletes tested in our protocol had positive findings on one or more of the initial three tests and were referred for further cardiologic evaluation. The vast majority of the latter athletes ultimately showed no definitive evidence of cardiovascular disease. In three athletes with relatively mild ventricu-

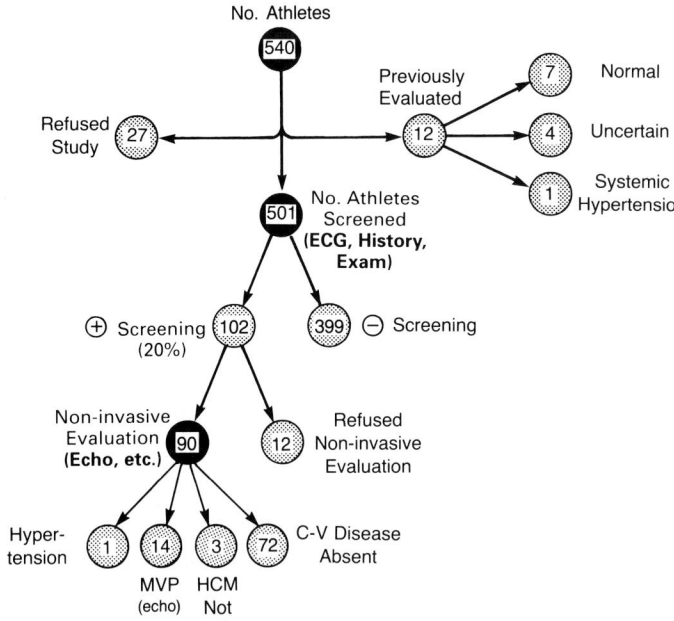

Fig. 17–14. Preparticipation screening of a cohort of 501 intercollegiate competitive athletes at the University of Maryland (College Park). Initial screening included 12-head ECG and personal and family history. Second-tier screening included echocardiography in athletes with a positive study on the initial evaluation. C-V, cardiovascular; HCM, hypertrophic cardiomyopathy; MVP, mitral valve prolapse. (Reproduced by permission of the American College of Cardiology from Maron BJ, et al: J Am Coll Cardiol 10:1214–1222, 1987.[87])

lar septal hypertrophy (thickness of 14–15 mm) it was not possible to be absolutely certain whether the wall thickening was pathological and a manifestation of hypertrophic cardiomyopathy,[38,39,45] or physiological in origin and secondary only to athletic conditioning (i.e., "athlete's heart").[30,31] Therefore, this screening effort identified no athletes with definitive evidence of hypertrophic cardiomyopathy, Marfan syndrome, or other cardiovascular diseases that convey an important potential risk for sudden death or disease progression during athletic training and competition.

In a subsequent study, echocardiography was used as the primary screening test in over 250, predominantly black athletes at Howard University.[88] Definitive evidence of important cardiovascular diseases also proved to be uncommon in this population, despite the routine use of echocardiography. Of note, a substantial minority of athletes surveyed showed borderline LV wall thicknesses of 13–14 mm, which frequently made the morphological distinction between athlete's heart and mild anatomical expressions of nonobstructive hypertrophic cardiomyopathy difficult.[30] The lack of identification of definitive cases of hypertrophic cardiomyopathy or other congenital cardiovascular diseases in this relatively small athletic population again calls attention to the infrequent occurrence of such diseases in the general population.

Despite the practical and philosophical limitations to large population screening, the identification of potentially lethal cardiovascular diseases in young individuals participating in competitive athletics remains a justifiable goal. Although the precise mechanism by which this objective can be most effectively achieved is presently unresolved, an informed personal and family history, physical examination, and perhaps 12-lead ECG would appear to constitute the most realistic and cost-effective primary screening evaluation in large athletic populations. More extensive testing (including echocardiography) could then be pursued in those athletes with evidence of cardiac abnormalities on the primary evaluation.

SUMMARY

A number of necropsy-based studies have shown a variety of cardiovascular diseases to be responsible for sudden unexpected cardiac death in competitive athletes. In young athletes (under 35 years), congenital cardiovascular malformations predominate, and hypertrophic cardiomyopathy appears to be the disease most commonly responsible for these catastrophes. Marfan syndrome and congenital coronary artery anomalies also occur commonly. Several other diseases that appear to be relatively rare but potential causes of sudden death in young athletes are viral myocarditis, right ventricular (RV) dysplasia, QT-interval prolongation syndromes, and aortic valvular stenosis. Mitral valve prolapse, although a relatively common clinical entity, is a rare cause of sudden death in athletes. In older athletes (over 35), acquired coronary heart disease is clearly the most common cause of death.

Sudden collapse in competitive athletes occurs in association with a wide variety of sports and is often exercise-related; the mechanisms responsible for sudden death vary with respect to the responsible underlying disease state.

REFERENCES

1. Maron BJ, Roberts WC, McAllister HA, Rosing DR, Epstein SE: Sudden death in young athletes. Circulation 62:218–229, 1980.
2. Maron BJ, Epstein SE, Roberts WC: Causes of sudden death in the competitive athlete. J Am Coll Cardiol 7:204–214, 1986.
3. Thompson PD, Stern MP, Williams P, Duncan K, Haskell WL, Wood PD: Death during jogging or running: A study of 18 cases. JAMA 242:1265–1267, 1979.
4. Virmani R, Robinowitz M, McAllister HA: Nontraumatic death in joggers: A series of 30 patients at autopsy. Am J Med 72:874–881, 1982.
5. Tsung SH, Huang TY, Chang MH: Sudden death in young athletes. Arch Pathol Lab Med 106:168–170, 1982.
6. Thiene G, Pennelli N, Rossi L: Cardiac conduction system abnormalities as a possible cause of sudden death in young athletes. Hum Pathol 14:706–709, 1983.
7. James TN, Froggatt P, Marshall TK: Sudden death in young athletes. Ann Intern Med 67:1013–1021, 1967.
8. Roberts WC, Maron BJ: Sudden death while playing professional football. Am Heart J 102:1061–1063, 1981.
9. Jokl E, McClellan JT, Ross GD: Congenital anomaly of left coronary artery in a young athlete. JAMA 182:572–573, 1962.
10. Thiene G, Nava A, Corrado D, Rossi L, Pennelli N: Right ventricular cardiomyopathy and sudden death in young people. N Engl J Med 318:129–133, 1988.
11. Virmani R, Roberts WC: Sudden cardiac death. Hum Pathol 18:485–492, 1987.
12. Virmani R, Robinowitz M: Cardiac pathology and sports medicine. Hum Pathol 18:493–501, 1987.
13. Noakes TD, Opie LH, Rose AG, Kleynhans PHT: Autopsy-proved coronary atherosclerosis in marathon runners. N Engl J Med 301: 86–89, 1979.
14. Noakes TD, Rose AG, Opie LH: Hypertrophic cardiomyopathy associated with sudden death during marathon racing. Br Heart J 41:624–627, 1979.
15. Northcote RJ, Ballantyne D: Sudden cardiac death in sport. Br Med J 287:1357–1379, 1983.
16. Northcote RJ, Flannigan C, Ballantyne D: Sudden death and vigorous exercise: A study of 60 deaths associated with squash. Br Heart J 55:198–203, 1986.
17. Northcote RJ, Evans ADB, Ballantyne D: Sudden death in squash players. Lancet 21:148–151, 1984.
18. Maron BJ, Epstein SE, Roberts WC: Hypertrophic cardiomyopathy: A common cause of sudden death in the young competitive athlete. Eur Heart J (Suppl F) 4:135–144, 1983.
19. Thompson PD, Funk EJ, Carleton RA, Sturner WQ: Incidence of death during jogging in Rhode Island from 1975 through 1980. JAMA 247:2535–2538, 1982.
20. Waller BF, Roberts WC: Sudden death while running in conditioned runners aged 40 years or over. Am J Cardiol 45:1292–1300, 1980.
21. Bharti S, Lev M: Congenital abnormalities of the conduction system in sudden death in young adults. J Am Coll Cardiol 8:1096–1104, 1986.
22. Lambert EC, Menon VA, Wagner HR, Vlad P: Sudden unexpected death from cardiovascular diseases in children: A cooperative international study. Am J Cardiol 34:89–96, 1974.
23. Jackson RT, Beaglehole R, Sharpe N: Sudden death in runners. NZ Med J 96:289–292, 1983.
24. Neuspiel DR, Kuller LH: Sudden and unexpected natural death in childhood and adolescence. JAMA 254:1321–1325, 1985.
25. Burke AP, Farb A, Virmani R, Goodin J, Smialek JE: Sports-related and non-sports-related sudden cardiac death in young adults. Am Heart J 121:568–575, 1991.
26. Opie LH: Sudden death and sport. Lancet i:263–266, 1975.
27. Noren GJ, Staley NA, Brandt CM, Kaplan

EL: Occurrence of myocarditis in sudden death in children. J Forensic Sci 22:188–196, 1977.
28. Corrado D, Thiene G, Nava A, Rossi L, Pennelli N: Sudden death in young competitive athletes: Clinicopathologic correlations in 22 cases. Am J Med 898:588–596, 1990.
29. Maron BJ, Epstein SE, Mitchell JE: 16th Bethesda Conference: Cardiovascular abnormalities in the athlete. Recommendations regarding eligibility for competition. Introduction. J Am Coll Cardiol 6:1189–1190, 1985.
30. Maron BJ: Structural features of the athlete heart as defined by echocardiography. J Am Coll Cardiol 7:190–203, 1986.
31. Rost R: The athlete's heart. Eur Heart J 3(suppl A):193–198, 1982.
32. Isner JM, Estes NAM III, Thompson PD, et al: Acute cardiac events temporally related to cocaine abuse. N Engl J Med 315:1438–1443, 1986.
33. Kark JA, Posey DM, Schumacher HR, Ruehle CJ: Sickle-cell as a risk factor for sudden death in physical training. N Engl J Med 317:781–787, 1987.
34. Dollar AL, Roberts WC: Morphologic comparison of patients with mitral valve prolapse who died suddenly with patients who died from severe valvular dysfunction or other conditions. J Am Coll Cardiol 17:921–931, 1991.
35. Schwartz PJ, Periti M, Malliani A: The long Q-T syndrome. Am Heart J 89:378–390, 1975.
36. Virmani R, Robinowitz M, Clark MA, McAllister HA: Sudden death and partial absence of the right ventricular myocardium. Arch Pathol Lab Med 106:163–167, 1982.
37. Jeresaty RM: Sudden death in the mitral valve prolapse click syndrome. Am J Cardiol 37:317–319, 1976.
38. Maron BJ, Bonow RO, Cannon RO, Leon MB, Epstein SE: Hypertrophic cardiomyopathy: Interrelation of clinical manifestations, pathophysiology, and therapy. N Engl J Med 316:780–789, 844–852, 1987.
39. Wigle ED, Sasson Z, Henderson MA, Ruddy TD, Fulop J, Rakowski H, Williams WG: Hypertrophic cardiomyopathy: The importance of the site and extent of hypertrophy. A review. Prog Cardiovasc Dis 28:1–83, 1985.
40. Geisterfer-Lowrance AA, Kass S, Tanigawa G, et al: A molecular basis for familial hypertrophic cardiomyopathy: A beta cardiac myosin heavy chain gene missense mutation. Cell 62:999–1006, 1990.
41. Maron BJ, Nichols PF, Pickle LW, Wesley YE, Mulvihill JJ: Patterns of inheritance in hypertrophic cardiomyopathy: Assessment by M-mode and two-dimensional echocardiography. Am J Cardiol 53:1087–1094, 1984.
42. Maron BJ, Epstein SE: Hypertrophic cardiomyopathy: A discussion of nomenclature. Am J Cardiol 43:1242–1244, 1979.
43. Spirito P, Maron BJ: Patterns of systolic anterior motion of the mitral valve in hypertrophic cardiomyopathy: Assessment by two-dimensional echocardiography. Am J Cardiol 54:1039–1046, 1984.
44. Roberts CS, Roberts WC: Morphologic features. In Zipes DP, Rowlands DJ (eds): Progress in Cardiology 2/2. Philadelphia, Lea & Febiger, 1989, pp 3–22.
45. Maron BJ, Gottdiener JS, Epstein SE: Patterns and significance of the distribution of left ventricular hypertrophy in hypertrophic cardiomyopathy: A wide-angle, two dimensional echocardiographic study of 125 patients. Am J Cardiol 48:418–428, 1981.
46. Maron BJ, Anan TJ, Roberts WC: Quantitative analysis of the distribution of cardiac muscle cell disorganization in the left ventricular wall of patients with hypertrophic cardiomyopathy. Circulation 63:882–894, 1981.
47. Maron BJ, Wolfson JK, Epstein SE, Roberts WC: Intramural ("small vessel") coronary artery disease in hypertrophic cardiomyopathy. J Am Coll Cardiol 8:545–557, 1986.
48. Maron BJ, Roberts WC, Edwards JE, McAllister HA Jr, Foley DD, Epstein SE: Sudden death in patients with hypertrophic cardiomyopathy: Characterization of 26 patients without functional limitation. Am J Cardiol 41:803–810, 1978.
49. Maron BJ, Roberts WC, Epstein SE: Sudden death in hypertrophic cardiomyopathy: A profile of 78 patients. Circulation 65:1118–1194, 1982.
50. Maron BJ, Gaffney FA, Jeresaty RM, McKenna WJ, Miller WW: Task Force III: Hypertrophic cardiomyopathy, other myopericardial diseases and mitral valve prolapse. Bethesda Conference #16: Cardiovascular Abnormalities in the Athlete. Recommendations Regarding Eligibility for Competition. J Am Coll Cardiol 6:1215–1217, 1985.
51. Fananapazir L, Tracy CM, Leon MB, et al: Electrophysiologic abnormalities in patients with hypertrophic cardiomyopathy: A consecutive analysis in 155 patients. Circulation 80:1259–1268, 1989.
52. Maron BJ, Fananapazir L: Sudden cardiac death in hypertrophic cardiomyopathy. Circulation 85(suppl I):I-57–I-63, 1992.
53. Frenneaux MP, Counihan PJ, Caforio ALP, Chikamori T, McKenna WJ: Abnormal blood pressure response during exercise in

hypertrophic cardiomyopathy. Circulation 82:1995–2002, 1991.
54. Maron BJ, Klues HG: Surviving competitive athletics with hypertrophic cardiomyopathy [abstract]. Circulation 82(suppl III):III-293, 1990.
55. Maron BJ, Henry WL, Roberts WC, Epstein SE: Comparison of echocardiographic and necropsy measurements of ventricular wall thicknesses in patients with and without disproportionate septal thickening. Circulation 55:341–345, 1977.
56. Roberts WC: Congenital coronary arterial anomalies unassociated with major anomalies of the heart or great vessels. In Roberts WC (ed): Adult Congenital Heart Disease. Philadelphia, FA Davis, 1987, pp 583–629.
57. Kragel AH, Roberts WC: Anomalous origin of either the right or left main coronary artery from the aorta with subsequent coursing between aorta and pulmonary trunk: Analysis of 32 necropsy cases. Am J Cardiol 62:771–777, 1988.
58. Maron BJ, Leon MB, Swain JA, Cannon RO, Pelliccia A: Prospective identification by two-dimensional echocardiography of anomalous origin of the left main coronary artery from the right sinus of Valsalva. Am J Cardiol 68:140–142, 1991.
59. Cheitlin MD, DeCastro CM, McAllister HA: Sudden death as a complication of anomalous left coronary origin from the anterior sinus of Valsalva. Circulation 50:780–787, 1974.
60. Roberts WC, Siegel RJ, Zipes DP: Origin of the right coronary artery from the left sinus of Valsalva and its functional consequences: Analysis of 10 necropsy patients. Am J Cardiol 49:863–868, 1982.
61. Liberthson RR, Dinsmore RE, Bharati A, et al: Aberrant coronary artery origin from the aorta. Circulation 50:774–779, 1974.
62. Mahowald JM, Blieden LC, Coe JI, Edwards JE: Ectopic origin of a coronary artery from the aorta: Sudden death in 3 of 23 patients. Chest 89:668–672, 1986.
63. McClellan JT, Jokl E: Congenital anomalies of coronary arteries as cause of sudden death associated with physical exertion. In: Medicine and Sports. Vol 5: Exercise and Cardiac Death. Basel, S Karger, 1971, pp 91–98.
64. Roberts WC, Kragel AH: Anomalous origin of either the right or left main coronary artery from the aorta with subsequent coursing of the anomalistically arising artery between aorta and pulmonary trunk. Am J Cardiol 62:1263–1267, 1988.
65. Taylor AJ, Rogan KM, Virmani R: Sudden cardiac death associated with isolated congenital coronary artery anomalies. J Am Coll Cardiol 20:640–647, 1992.
66. Menke DM, Waller BF, Pless JE: Hypoplastic coronary arteries and high take-off position of the right coronary ostium: A fatal combination of congenital coronary artery anomalies in an amateur athlete. Chest 88:299–301, 1985.
67. Roberts WC, Silver MA, Sapala JC: Intussusception of a coronary artery associated with sudden death in a college football player. Am J Cardiol 57:179–180, 1986.
68. Choi JH, Kornblum RN: Pete Maravich's incredible heart. J Forensic Sci 35:981–986, 1990.
69. Faruqui AMA, Maloy WC, Felner JM, Schlant RC, Logan WD, Symbas P: Symptomatic myocardial bridging of coronary artery. Am J Cardiol 41:1305–1310, 1978.
70. Morales AR, Romanelli R, Boucek RJ: The mural left anterior descending coronary artery, strenuous exercise and sudden death. Circulation 62:230–237, 1980.
71. Roberts WC, Dicicco BS, Waller BF, et al: Origin of the left main from the right coronary artery or from the right aortic sinus with intramyocardial tunneling to the left side of the heart via the ventricular septum: The case against clinical significance of myocardial bridge or coronary tunnel. Am Heart J 104:303–305, 1982.
72. Green LH, Cohen SI, Kurland G: Fatal myocardial infarction in marathon racing. Ann Intern Med 84:704–706, 1976.
73. Jokl E: Sudden death after exercise due to myocarditis. In: Medicine and Sport. Vol 5: Exercise and Cardiac Death. Basel, S Karger 1971, pp 99–101.
74. Benson DW Jr, Benditt DG, Anderson RW, et al: Cardiac arrest in young, ostensibly healthy patients: Clinical, hemodynamic, and electrophysiologic findings. Am J Cardiol 52:65–69, 1983.
75. Aretz HT, Billingham ME, Edwards WD, et al: Myocarditis: A histopathologic definition and classification. Am J Cardiovasc Pathol 1:3–14, 1986.
76. Jeresaty RM: Mitral Valve Prolapse. New York, Raven, 1979.
77. Pocock WA, Bosman CK, Chesler E, Barlow RB, Edwards JE: Sudden death in primary mitral valve prolapse. Am Heart J 107:378–382, 1984.
78. Chesler E, King RA, Edwards JE: The myxomatous mitral valve and sudden death. Circulation 67:632–639, 1983.
79. Topaz O, Edwards JE: Pathologic features of sudden death in children, adolescents, and young adults. Chest 87:476–482, 1985.
80. Roberts WC, McAllister HA, Ferrans VJ: Sarcoidosis of the heart: A clinicopathologic study of 35 necropsy patients (group I) and

review of 78 previously described necropsy patients (group II). Am J Med 63:86–108, 1977.
81. Marcus FI, Fontaine GH, Guiraudon G, et al: Right ventricular dysplasia: A report of 24 adult cases. Circulation 65:384–398, 1992.
82. Phillips M, Robinowitz M, Higgins JR, Boran KJ, Reed T, Virmani R: Sudden cardiac death in Air Force recruits: A 20 year review. JAMA 256:2696–2999, 1986.
83. Maseri A, L'Abbate A, Baroldi G, et al: Coronary vasospasm as a possible cause of myocardial infarction: A conclusion derived from the study of "preinfarction" angina. N Engl J Med 299:1271–1277, 1978.
84. Kramer MR, Drory Y, Lev B: Sudden death in young Israeli soldiers: Analysis of 83 cases. Isr J Med Sci 25:620–624, 1989.
85. Lynch P: Soldiers, sports, and sudden death. Lancet i:1235–1237, 1980.
86. Sadaniantz A, Clayton MA, Sturner WQ, Thompson PD: Sudden death immediately after a record-setting athletic performance. Am J Cardiol 63:375, 1989.
87. Maron BJ, Bodison S, Wesley Y, Tucker E, Green KJ: Results of screening a large population of intercollegiate athletes for cardiovascular disease. J Am Coll Cardiol 10:1214–1222, 1987.
88. Lewis JF, Maron BJ, Diggs JA, Spencer JE, Mehrotra PP, Curry CL: Preparticipation echocardiographic screening for cardiovascular disease in a large predominantly black population of collegiate athletes. Am J Cardiol 64:1029–1033, 1989.
89. Maron BJ, Wolfson JK, Ciró E, Spirito P: Relation of electrocardiographic abnormalities and patterns of left ventricular hypertrophy identified by 2-dimensional echocardiography in patients with hypertrophic cardiomyopathy. Am J Cardiol 51:189–194, 1983.

18

Sudden Death in Children

ARNOLD L. FENRICH, JR.
SUSAN W. DENFIELD
ARTHUR GARSON, JR.

Sudden death is a topic that receives much attention in adults but relatively little in children other than the sudden infant death syndrome. Sudden death in children has been linked to a number of cardiovascular causes, including hypertrophic cardiomyopathy, myocarditis, coronary artery anomalies, Wolff-Parkinson-White syndrome, long QT syndrome, and a history of corrective surgery for congenital heart defects such as tetralogy of Fallot or transposition of the great arteries.

In our review of sudden death in children, we will use the following criteria: (1) age 1 year or older at the time of death, (2) occurrence of a sudden event resulting in loss of consciousness until death, (3) death occurring within 24 hours of the sudden event, (4) child participating in usual activities until the event, (5) child not hospitalized when the event occurred.

The incidence of sudden cardiac death (SCD) in adults in the United States is 350,000–450,000 per year.[1–3] SCD accounts for 15–20% of all deaths in adults.[4] The incidence of sudden nontraumatic death in children ranges from 0.6 to 4.6 per 100,000 per year,[5–9] and sudden death accounts for 2.3–7.6% of the total deaths.[6,8,9] Extrapolating from these numbers to a city of 1,000,000 people (with about one third of them children) suggests that 2 to 9 children per year will die suddenly.

This chapter will focus on sudden death in children and young adults. It will evaluate the causes of SCD in apparently healthy children, in young athletes, and in children with known heart disease, followed by other causes of sudden death in children.

SUDDEN CARDIAC DEATH IN APPARENTLY HEALTHY CHILDREN

There are relatively few studies examining sudden death in the pediatric population. Table 18–1 presents the compiled data from five reports on sudden death in apparently healthy children.[6–10] Infection, the leading cause of sudden death, will be discussed later. A cardiovascular etiology is the second most common cause of sudden death. Of the cardiovascular causes, myo-

Table 18–1
Sudden Death in Apparently Healthy Children*

Diagnosis	No. (%)
Infection	106 (32)
Cardiac	100 (31)
Cerebral hemorrhage	37 (11)
Unknown	53 (16)
Other	32 (10)
Total	328 (100)

* Studies reviewed for this table include reports of apparently healthy children only (Driscoll and Edwards,[6] Neuspiel and Kuller,[7] Molander,[8] Keeling and Knowles,[9] and Drory et al[10]).

Table 18–2
Cardiac Causes of Sudden Death in Apparently Healthy Children*

Diagnosis	No.
Myocarditis	32
Hypertrophic cardiomyopathy	21
Conduction system abnormality	11
Myocardial fibrosis	7
Coronary artery anomaly	4
Other	25
Total	100

* Studies reviewed for this table are the same as for Table 18–1.

carditis, hypertrophic cardiomyopathy, conduction system abnormality/primary arrhythmia, myocardial fibrosis, and coronary artery anomaly (Table 18–2) accounted for the highest incidence. Of interest is the large number with an unknown cause of sudden death. A great many who fall into the unknown category may have an abnormality of the conduction system.[11] In many autopsies, a complete examination of the conduction system is not performed.

A profile of some of the more common causes of sudden cardiac death in apparently healthy children follows. Hypertrophic cardiomyopathy and coronary artery anomalies will be discussed later.

Myocarditis

Acute myocarditis is demonstrated on biopsy by lymphocytic infiltration of the myocardium associated with focal necrosis. The prevalence of myocarditis is unknown and the autopsy incidence varies with the definition, etiology, and population studied. In a study from the Armed Forces Institute of Pathology reported shortly after World War II, 3.5% of autopsy specimens had myocarditis.[12] In a study by Noren et al,[13] 17% (15/90) of the children who died suddenly and unexpectedly had myocarditis, although eight of these deaths occurred within the first year of life. In the same study there was a 4% prevalence of myocarditis in children who suffered traumatic deaths. Others report that 5–10% of children dying suddenly were found to have active myocarditis at autopsy.[14,15] Sudden death occurs both at rest and during exercise in children with myocarditis.[16,17] The mechanism of sudden death is probably secondary to inflammation of the conduction system,[13] which may result in atrioventricular (AV) block and ventricular arrhythmias. Ventricular arrhythmias seem to occur in those with more severely compromised ventricular function.[18]

The antemortem diagnosis of myocarditis may be difficult if there are no signs or symptoms of myocardial involvement. Children may be asymptomatic or have only a mild "viral syndrome" and yet die suddenly.

Studies in laboratory animals with myocarditis have shown a significant increase in mortality with strenuous activity.[19] If myocarditis is diagnosed, restriction from athletic participation is recommended for about 6 months. Athletic participation depends on the ventricular function as assessed by echocardiography as well as the absence of clinically significant arrhythmias.[20]

Primary Arrhythmias

Arrhythmias due to primary disorders of automaticity, conduction, and repolarization may occur in children with structurally normal hearts and may be associated with sudden death. Of these disorders the long QT syndrome, Wolff-Parkinson-White syndrome, and congenital atrioventricular block are the most commonly associated with sudden death in children.

Symptoms do not appear to correlate well with a specific type of arrhythmia. Symptoms may include palpitations, weakness, diaphoresis, chest pain, presyncope, and syncope.

Children complaining of fast heartbeats or palpitations generally fall into one of two categories, sinus tachycardia or pathologic tachycardias, usually of supraventricular origin (Table 18–3). Children with sinus tachycardia frequently feel their heart pounding during stressful events or immediately after exercising, with return to normal rate in seconds to minutes with rest. Supraventricular tachycardia tends to start and stop abruptly and may occur any time of the

Table 18-3
Palpitations

	Sinus Tachycardia	Pathologic
When	After exercise	Any time
How often	Once	Many times
How long	Seconds	3-20 min
Where felt	Heart	Neck
Looks like	Red	Pale, sweaty
How stops	Rest	Swallow, gag, etc.

day, lasting from several minutes to hours (usually not seconds). Rapid pulsations may be felt in the neck or seen by a parent. Children sometimes discover how to stop the tachycardia by swallowing, gagging, or using some other vagal maneuver.

Syncope is the most common symptom of serious rhythm disturbances.[21] Typical vasodepressor syncope (the simple faint) occurs in 12-15% of adolescents. Vasodepressor syncope is benign and usually occurs in relation to pain or emotional stress in a hot, crowded environment with the subject upright. Signs and symptoms include nausea, diaphoresis, and a "loud rushing" in the ears, followed by a gradual loss of consciousness. Because the process is gradual, injury usually does not occur. Seizures are uncommon but may occur due to cerebral hypoperfusion if the subject is held upright after fainting.

Of special concern is syncope that does not have a vasodepressor stimulus (Table 18-4). Nonvasodepressor syncope usually has no prodrome; as a result, injury may occur with loss of consciousness. Seizures may occur secondary to cessation of cardiac output. Because nonvasodepressor syncope may occur in conditions that have familial patterns, a family history of sudden death should be sought. Also, inquiry should be made as to a family history of syncope, seizures, and even unexplained accidental death. Nonvasodepressor syncope deserves a thorough evaluation, including electrocardiography (ECG), 24-hour ambulatory recording, treadmill stress ECG, and echocardiography. If the episode was severe and the workup negative, an invasive electrophysiological study should be considered.

The long QT syndrome (LQTS) occurs in an autosomal dominant form, the Jervell and Lange-Nielsen syndrome,[22] and an autosomal recessive form, the Romano-Ward syndrome.[23] Schwartz et al[24] have proposed a group of major and minor criteria for the diagnosis of LQTS. The major criteria are (1) a QTc interval greater than 0.44 seconds, (2) family members with LQTS, and (3) syncope related to noise or anger. The minor criteria consist of (1) congenital deafness, (2) bradycardia, (3) large and bizarre notched T waves, and (4) T-wave alternans. Schwartz requires two major criteria or one major and two minor criteria for the diagnosis of LQTS. In children, one major and one minor criterion may suffice.

There is also an association of a prolonged QTc interval with AV block. Esscher[25] found that 59 (22%) of 273 patients with congenital complete AV block had a prolonged QTc interval. Fifty (85%) of these 59 subjects had symptoms of syn-

Table 18-4
Syncope

	Vasodepressor	Nonvasodepressor
Circumstance	Hot, crowded, hungry, emotion, standing	During exercise, anger, no provocation
Prodrome	Yes	No
Injury	Unusual	Common
Duration	<1 min	Longer
Seizure	Rare	More common
Recurrent	Few with same stimulus	Common

cope. In a recent review of 287 children by the Pediatric Electrophysiology Society, 4% of children with LQTS had AV block, but in the majority it was 2:1 block. The abnormal AV conduction is most likely secondary to abnormal repolarization and a long effective refractory period.[26] In all children with advanced or complete AV block, it is necessary to examine the QTc interval closely. If the QTc interval is prolonged, these infants generally require both β-blocker treatment and a pacemaker.[26,27]

Children with LQTS can present with cardiac arrest or sudden death. In a recent study by Weintraub et al,[27] 19 of 23 children with LQTS presented with symptoms. Of the 19 children with symptoms, 13 (69%) presented with syncope, five (26%) presented with aborted sudden death, and one (5%) was a near-drowning. Thus, it has been recommended that children with the diagnosis of LQTS begin β-blocker treatment whether or not they are symptomatic. If symptoms continue despite β-blocker therapy, an additional antiarrhythmic agent that does not prolong the QTc interval could be added. If the syncopal episodes are secondary to bradycardia with associated ventricular arrhythmias, then a pacemaker should be implanted.[28] Should symptoms persist, a left stellate sympathectomy may be considered. An implantable cardioverter-defibrillator should be considered if recurrent symptoms are present despite maximal therapy.

The two major conditions associated with syncope in LQTS are physical stress and emotional stress. It is recommended that those with LQTS avoid competitive athletics.[28]

The Wolff-Parkinson-White syndrome in children may be subtle; it is documented by ECG when (1) the PR interval is less than 100–120 msec during sinus rhythm; (2) the QRS complex duration exceeds 80–120 msec, with a delta wave in some leads; and (3) there are secondary ST- and T-wave changes. Other helpful evidence that favors the diagnosis of Wolff-Parkinson-White syndrome includes an absent Q wave in the left chest leads or left axis deviation in the frontal plane.[29]

In children there are two dangerous arrhythmias of the Wolff-Parkinson-White syndrome: a rapid reciprocating tachycardia over the accessory pathway and a rapid ventricular response to atrial fibrillation or flutter. Either may cause syncope, and atrial flutter or fibrillation may precipitate ventricular fibrillation and sudden death. It has been shown that in patients with Wolff-Parkinson-White syndrome and documented ventricular fibrillation, the shortest pre-excited R-R interval during induced atrial fibrillation was less than or equal to 250 msec.[30]

In adults with Wolff-Parkinson-White syndrome the risk of sudden death is less than 1%. In children the data are sparse, making it difficult to predict the sudden death risk. The appropriate recommendations in children with Wolff-Parkinson-White syndrome are a current source of debate. With the availability of radiofrequency catheter ablation, we consider catheterization and ablation for children with Wolff-Parkinson-White syndrome who have repetitive symptoms (frequent tachycardia, palpitations or syncope). Those with a short refractory period are individualized; consideration is given to competitive sports.

The incidence of sudden death in congenital complete AV block is 2–3%.[31] Sudden death from this cause is largely avoidable with pacemaker implantation. The indications for pacemaker implantation in children are as defined in the American College of Cardiology/American Heart Association Task Force report.[32]

Mitral Valve Prolapse

Mitral valve prolapse (MVP) has been reported to occur in 1% of males and 6% of females.[33] Despite the frequency of MVP, sudden death is rare, especially in patients less than 20 years of age.[33] The demonstration of MVP as the only autopsy finding in some cases has resulted in the association of sudden death and MVP. In many autopsies a complete examination of the conduction system is not routinely performed, which prevents excluding a conduction system abnormality as a mechanism of sudden death. In fact, there is an increased incidence of dual AV node pathways in subjects with MVP,[34] and a prolonged QTc interval has been related to arrhythmias and sudden death in MVP.[35]

Sudden death in adults with MVP has been related to complex ventricular arrhythmias.[36] In adults, ventricular arrhythmias are more common in patients with MVP and hemodynamically significant mitral regurgitation than in those with MVP alone.[37] This has not been observed in children.[38] In a study by Topaz et al,[39] 12 (24%) of 50 subjects aged 13–30 years who died suddenly had MVP as the only diagnosis at autopsy. Ventricular arrhythmias were present in six, and a family history of sudden death was present in three. The degree of MVP was considered mild in two and moderate to severe in ten. On the other hand, a study by Nishimura et al[40] evaluated the long-term prognosis of 237 subjects aged 10–69 years with echocardiographically documented MVP. The youngest patient who died suddenly was 31 years old, and the overall mortality was not significantly different from that of age- and sex-matched controls. These studies suggest that in subjects with MVP, those who may be at risk of sudden death have ventricular arrhythmias, a family history of sudden death, or significant mitral valve disease.

Children with MVP and complex ventricular arrhythmias should undergo complete evaluation to exclude other causes of ventricular arrhythmias. Invasive electrophysiological study may be indicated, and treatment for ventricular arrhythmias may be necessary. Restriction from competitive sports has been recommended in those with symptoms or those with uncontrolled complex ventricular arrhythmias.

SUDDEN CARDIAC DEATH IN YOUNG ATHLETES

According to Epstein and Maron,[41] an estimated 5 in 100,000 young athletes have a condition that renders them vulnerable to sudden death, and of those at risk, 10% will die suddenly. There are only a few studies evaluating sudden death in young athletes. Table 18–5 lists two major studies as well as the compiled data from ten other studies and case reports.[39,42–52] The most frequent diagnoses include hypertrophic cardiomyopathy, coronary artery anomalies, coronary artery disease, and myocarditis. Arrhythmogenic right ventricular dysplasia (ARVD) was responsible for 27% of the sudden deaths in a study by Corrado et al.[43] Their study population was composed of young athletes in northern Italy. ARVD will be discussed later.

Table 18–5
Sudden Death in Young Athletes

Diagnosis	Maron et al[42] No. (%)	Corrado et al[43] No. (%)	Others[39,44–52] No.
Hypertrophic cardiomyopathy	14 (48)	0	21
Coronary artery anomaly	4 (14)	2 (9)	15
Coronary artery disease	3 (10)	4 (18)	12
Left ventricular hypertrophy	4 (14)	0	10
Myocarditis	0	0	8
Mitral valve prolapse	1 (3)	2 (9)	6
Conduction system abnormality	0	3 (14)	3
ARVD*	0	6 (27)	1
Marfan syndrome	2 (7)	0	0
Unknown	1 (3)	5 (23)	6
Other	0	0	8
Total	29	22	90

*ARVD, arrhythmogenic right ventricular dysplasia.

Hypertrophic Cardiomyopathy

Hypertrophic cardiomyopathy is a major cause of sudden death in children and is the most common cause of sudden death in young athletes.[42] Hypertrophic cardiomyopathy is characterized by a hypertrophied but nondilated left ventricle in the absence of systemic disease or left-sided obstruction capable of producing left ventricular hypertrophy.[53] There is bizarre cellular architecture with a markedly disordered arrangement of cardiac muscle cells. There are two proposed mechanisms of sudden death—malignant ventricular arrhythmias and hemodynamic compromise.[54-56] The thickened ventricle may impede filling, especially during vigorous activity, which increases outflow tract obstruction and results in decreased coronary artery filling and ischemia.

There is a strong correlation between hypertrophic cardiomyopathy and sudden death. Adults with hypertrophic cardiomyopathy have an incidence of sudden death of 2-3% per year. The finding of nonsustained ventricular tachycardia during Holter monitoring in adults appears to provide a marker of increased risk for sudden death.[57,58] In children with hypertrophic cardiomyopathy the annual mortality is approximately 6%,[57,59,60] but there is a problem identifying the child who is at increased risk for sudden death. Possible predictive factors for sudden death include a family history of sudden death,[60] ventricular tachycardia,[61] and a young age at onset of symptoms.[59,60]

The diagnosis of hypertrophic cardiomyopathy can be difficult, as the physical findings are variable and may be altered by the hemodynamic state. Negligible obstruction to outflow does not eliminate the risk of sudden death.[57,58,62,63]

The ECG is abnormal in most, which may be helpful in screening but is not diagnostic.[57,64] Common abnormalities include left ventricular hypertrophy, ST- and T-wave changes, left atrial enlargement, abnormal Q waves, and diminished or absent R waves in the lateral precordial leads.

Inheritance is autosomal dominant with a high degree of penetrance.[55,65] In approximately 60% of cases of hypertrophic cardiomyopathy there is a first-degree relative with clinical or echocardiographic evidence of the disorder. When hypertrophic cardiomyopathy is suspected from a family history or physical examination, the diagnosis is confirmed by echocardiography.[66]

Children and young adults with hypertrophic cardiomyopathy should be restricted from competitive sports but may participate in low-intensity sports.[20] If treatment for ventricular arrhythmias is indicated, children with hypertrophic cardiomyopathy are frequently treated with β-blockers or verapamil; however, sudden death is not always prevented with these antiarrhythmic agents. Data from adults with hypertrophic cardiomyopathy suggesting that amiodarone may prevent sudden death are inconclusive. McKenna et al[67] used amiodarone to treat 53 young adults with hypertrophic cardiomyopathy and found no cases of sudden death at a mean follow-up of 18 months. Fananapazir et al recently found a high early incidence of sudden death after initiating amiodarone therapy.[68,69] The majority of these patients had ventricular arrhythmias; however, some had supraventricular tachycardia and atrial fibrillation-flutter. Placement of an implantable cardioverter-defibrillator in addition to medical treatment should be considered in children with hypertrophic cardiomyopathy who have been resuscitated from a sudden death episode.

Coronary Artery Abnormalities

The congenital anomaly of the coronary arterial system most often reported in association with sudden death is anomalous origin of the left coronary artery from the right (anterior) sinus of Valsalva.[70,71] Although the anomaly itself is rare, it has been a reported cause of sudden death, especially during exercise. Proposed mechanisms for sudden death in anomalous left coronary artery include squeezing of the left coronary artery between the aorta and pulmonary artery during exercise[72] and sudden kinking of the left coronary artery.[73] The most likely mechanism is the acute takeoff angle of the left coronary artery from the right sinus, resulting in narrowing of the coronary ostium.[70] The increased stroke volume during exercise probably causes dilation of the ascending aorta, which results in a more acute takeoff angle. Other coronary artery anomalies associated with sudden death include the right coronary artery originating from the left sinus of Valsalva, a single coronary artery,[74] and a myocardial bridge (tunneled coronary artery).[75]

In general, the physical examination is normal in children with coronary artery anomalies. Symptoms may include those encountered with myocardial ischemia, such as angina and syncope with exertion.[76] More often, however, sudden death is the presenting symptom. Any child who presents with syncope during exercise should be evaluated for a possible coronary artery anomaly.

In nonatherosclerotic acquired coronary artery lesions, such as Kawasaki disease, myocardial infarction is a well-recognized complication.[77] Although sudden death has been reported in Kawasaki disease,[5,78] it is uncommon.

Atherosclerotic coronary artery disease is an extremely rare cause of sudden death in children and young adults. Advanced atherosclerotic heart disease may occur in some children with diabetes mellitus and in children with familial hyperlipidemias (especially type II hypercholesterolemia).

Rupture of the Aorta

Rupture of the aorta, although rare, is a cause of sudden death, especially in young athletes.[42,79] Children with Marfan syndrome represent a high-risk group for aortic rupture. The overall incidence of Marfan syndrome is 5–8 per 100,000.[80] Genetic transmission is autosomal dominant with variable expression.

According to Pyritz and McKusick,[81] two of four major findings are required for the diagnosis of Marfan syndrome. The findings include (1) a positive family history, (2) ectopia lentis, (3) aortic root dilation, and (4) severe kyphoscoliosis or anterior thorax deformities.

Echocardiography is necessary to evaluate the degree of aortic dilation before deciding on sports participation. If the aortic root measurements are normal, strenuous and dynamic activities may be performed, but not static or isometric exercise.[82]

SUDDEN DEATH IN CHILDREN WITH KNOWN HEART DISEASE

In children and young adults who die suddenly, the underlying cardiac diagnosis of

Table 18-6
Sudden Death in Children with Known Heart Disease

Study/Diagnosis	No. (%)
Garson and McNamara[83]	
Palliated CHD	17
PVOD	15
Postoperative TOF	11
Unoperated TOF	7
Dilated Cardiomyopathy	5
Postoperative CAVC	5
LQTS	5
Other	36
Total	101
Lambert et al[84]	
PVOD	41 (18)
Aortic Stenosis	38 (17)
Cyanotic CHD with PS/PA	32 (14)
HCM	17 (8)
Dilated Cardiomyopathy	12 (5)
EFE	12 (5)
Other	74
Total	226

Abbreviations: CHD, congenital heart disease; PVOD, pulmonary vascular obstructive disease; TOF, tetralogy of Fallot; HCM, hypertrophic cardiomyopathy; CAVC, complete atrioventricular canal; PS/PA, pulmonary stenosis or pulmonary atresia; EFE, endocardial fibroelastosis.

those followed in a cardiology clinic or institution differs considerably from those who are apparently healthy. Table 18-6 shows the diagnoses from two large studies in children followed by pediatric cardiologists;[83,84] virtually all had heart disease. From the diagnoses in the two studies, some of the differences may be accounted for by the time frames of the studies as well as by institutional differences. Our study[83] included the records of all patients seen in the Section of Pediatric Cardiology at Texas Children's Hospital between 1958 and 1983. The study by Lambert et al[84] was an international cooperative study from cardiac institutions that was conducted prior to 1973, and the majority of patients did not undergo surgery. Hypertrophic cardiomyopathy and LQTS appear in these studies as well, but were discussed earlier.

The activity at the time of sudden death was known for many of the children (Table

Table 18-7
Activity at Time of Sudden
Death in Children with
Known Heart Disease

Garson[83]	
Sports	22%
Not active	50%
Asleep	28%
Lambert[84]	
Sports	10%
Active	22%
Asleep or not active	58%

18-7). The majority were at rest (not exercising or asleep) at the time of death.

Aortic Stenosis

Aortic valve stenosis occurs in 3-6% of children with congenital heart disease. Excluding infants with critical aortic stenosis, who become symptomatic in the neonatal period, most children are asymptomatic and grow and develop normally. Sudden death is estimated to occur in approximately 1% of children with aortic stenosis per year.[85] Those who appear to be at the highest risk have severe stenosis.[86] These children may manifest left ventricular hypertrophy with strain on ECG and symptoms of syncope, dyspnea, or chest pain. A proposed mechanism of sudden death is decreased cardiac output leading to coronary insufficiency and myocardial ischemia, which results in a terminal arrhythmia.[87]

Aortic valve replacement does not eliminate the risk of sudden death but has been shown to decrease the risk.[86] Ventricular arrhythmias, abnormal hemodynamics, and sudden death appear to be interrelated after valve replacement. Olshausen et al[88] showed that ventricular couplets and ventricular tachycardia were related to postoperative ejection fraction less than 55%, and that sudden death was related to ventricular arrhythmias. Konishi et al[89] found that all patients who died suddenly after aortic valve replacement had frequent or multiform premature ventricular contractions on routine ECG.

Aortic valve stenosis has been associated with sudden death with exercise. The fact that aortic stenosis is not one of the more common causes of sudden death in recent studies may be due to one of several reasons. Most children who die suddenly have severe disease,[90,91] and it is unlikely that a child with severe stenosis would go undetected. In addition, improved identification of patients at risk, appropriate sports restrictions, endocarditis prophylaxis, and timely surgical intervention may have effected a decreased incidence of sudden death.

A normal ECG does not preclude moderate to severe obstruction. Conversely, ECG evidence of left ventricular hypertrophy with ST-segment depression and T-wave inversion generally indicates significant stenosis and should prompt further evaluation and exercise limitations if those limitations were not previously implemented.

Pulmonary Vascular Obstructive Disease

Pulmonary vascular obstructive disease, whether primary or secondary, accounted for a large percentage of the sudden deaths in children with known heart disease. The mechanism of sudden death may be hemodynamic or due to a bradyarrhythmia or tachyarrhythmia.[92] Ventricular arrhythmias, however, are rare in these children.[93-95] We have observed ambulatory ECG recordings on two patients with Eisenmenger syndrome who died during monitoring. In both cases progressive sinus bradycardia and asystole were present.

Tetralogy of Fallot

Children with tetralogy of Fallot appear prominently in studies on sudden death.[83,84] In unoperated cases the mechanism is most likely secondary to acute hypoxic episodes or "Tet spells,"[84] and primary arrhythmic sudden death is rare. Palliative procedures such as shunts do not eliminate the risk of sudden death.

The risk of sudden death after repair of tetralogy of Fallot has been recognized for more than a decade and the cause has been the subject of much speculation. The incidence of sudden death is reported to be as high as 4.6% in children over 10 years of age, or approximately 0.5% per year.[96-103] Most of these children probably die suddenly from ventricular arrhythmias, although an occasional patient may die from sudden AV block or atrial flutter.

Results of a 15-center collaborative study showed that both spontaneous premature ventricular contractions and inducible ventricular tachycardia were significantly related to several factors: older age at repair, longer follow-up interval, symptoms of syncope or presyncope, and right ventricular systolic hypertension (>60 mm Hg).[104] The presence of ventricular arrhythmias and abnormal hemodynamics in the patient who has undergone surgical repair of tetralogy of Fallot has been shown to be statistically related to sudden death. We[105] reviewed 39 studies on 4627 patients after repair of tetralogy of Fallot. Of 57 patients who died suddenly, 80% had the combination of ventricular arrhythmias on Holter and abnormal hemodynamics, whereas only 8% of those who were alive had this combination. Ventricular arrhythmias and abnormal hemodynamics each were statistically related to sudden death as well; however, both were also found in patients who did not die suddenly. This information stresses the importance of evaluating postoperative hemodynamics, especially in the presence of ventricular arrhythmias.

It has been proposed that repair of tetralogy of Fallot in infancy may be associated with a low incidence of ventricular ectopy and sudden death. Walsh et al[106] evaluated 184 patients who underwent tetralogy of Fallot repair between 1 day and 18 months of age (mean age, 7 months). The mean follow-up interval was 5 years. Only two (1.1%) of the 184 patients had ventricular ectopy on any tracing. Of 41 patients who underwent Holter monitoring, 12 had occasional uniform premature ventricular contractions and one had ventricular couplets. No patient received antiarrhythmic medications. There were three late deaths, all reported to be unrelated to arrhythmia. Although these results are encouraging, longer-term follow-up studies (i.e., until after puberty) are necessary.

Treatment criteria remain controversial at present. We reserve antiarrhythmic treatment for children with complex ventricular arrhythmias associated with poor hemodynamics. This group constitutes a subset more prone to sudden death. Consideration should be given to improving hemodynamics if they are abnormal (right ventricular systolic pressure >60 mm Hg, right ventricular end-diastolic pressure >8 mm Hg, poor right ventricular function or perhaps extreme right ventricular dilation as a result of pulmonary regurgitation), especially if medical treatment fails.

In children the electrophysiology study has proved neither as specific nor as sensitive for predicting risk of arrhythmic deaths as it is in adults with coronary artery disease.[104] The major reason for performing electrophysiological testing in the postoperative tetralogy of Fallot patient is to exclude other causes of syncope (i.e., atrial flutter, AV block). If ventricular tachycardia is inducible, repeat electrophysiological study is performed with the patient on antiarrhythmic therapy to determine if the drug effectively eliminates the inducibility of ventricular tachycardia.

Transposition of the Great Arteries (Post Mustard/Senning Procedure)

Studies have shown that only 13% of patients who have undergone the Mustard/Senning procedure for correction of transposition of the great arteries are in sinus rhythm 13 years after surgery.[107,108] Most have bradyarrhythmias secondary to sick sinus syndrome; however, 10–15% have tachyarrhythmias. Atrial flutter is the predominant tachyarrhythmia, but ventricular arrhythmias have been demonstrated as well.[109–111] The presence of atrial flutter appears to be the major risk factor for sudden death in these patients.[107,112] The incidence of late sudden death is reported to be between 2% and 5%.[107,112,113] Sudden death is four times more common when effective suppression of atrial flutter is not achieved.[114] These findings suggest that atrial flutter should be treated aggressively. It is likely that with aging, the incidence of atrial flutter will increase and these patients will be at higher risk than those who have undergone repair of tetralogy of Fallot.

Most centers are now performing the arterial switch operation for repair of transposition of the great arteries. Studies have shown that the incidence of important arrhythmias after the arterial switch operation is low during a 1- to 3-year follow-up period.[115,116] Additional studies will be necessary to determine the incidence of late sudden death in these children. If important arrhythmias are uncommon and coronary artery disease is not premature, occurrence of sudden death following the arterial switch operation is likely to be low.

Arrhythmogenic Right Ventricular Dysplasia

The diagnosis of arrhythmogenic right ventricular dysplasia (ARVD) is made when the following criteria are met: (1) there is a left bundle-branch block ventricular tachycardia, (2) the right ventricle is large, dilated, and poorly functioning, with dyskinetic areas primarily in the right ventricular outflow tract, diaphragmatic surface, and septum, and (3) there is right ventricular conduction delay on the ECG. The pathology of ARVD involves replacement of right ventricular myocardium by fibrosis or adipose tissue. The subepicardial layer appears as a plexiform structure with partially degenerated myocardial fibers that may be the site of slowing necessary for re-entrant ventricular arrhythmias.

The incidence of ARVD is unknown. Among children and young adults with exercise-related ventricular tachycardia, ARVD is a common diagnosis.[117,118] Restriction from competitive sports is recommended if ARVD is diagnosed. ARVD is, however, an uncommon diagnosis in children and a rare cause of sudden death. We have seen one infant with idiopathic ventricular tachycardia in whom the diagnosis of ARVD was made at autopsy after sudden death at 8 years of age.

The diagnosis can be difficult in children as ARVD most often presents in a mild form with subtle trabeculation in, or dilation of, the right ventricular outflow tract. More severe forms occur in adulthood. Because even the most sensitive noninvasive techniques in children may miss the subtle dilation, cardiac catheterization is usually necessary to make the diagnosis.

Idiopathic Dilated Cardiomyopathy

In adults with idiopathic dilated cardiomyopathy, the annual mortality is greater than 20%,[119] and sudden death accounts for approximately one half of the total deaths.[120,121] The outcome is worse in patients with extremely poor left ventricular function.[122,123] Some have reported that the presence of ventricular arrhythmias increases the mortality and the risk of sudden death,[124,125] although others have failed to confirm this relationship.[126,127]

In children with idiopathic dilated cardiomyopathy it appears that the incidence of sudden death is quite low as compared to that in adults.[128] Persistent cardiomegaly and the development of significant arrhythmias have been suggested as risk factors of poor outcome,[129] although no strong correlation has been identified. Even using electrophysiological testing, the presence or absence of inducible ventricular tachycardia does not predict outcome.[130]

Ebstein's Malformation

In a natural history study of patients with unoperated Ebstein's malformation over 1 year of age who died, the incidence of sudden death was 20%.[131] It is not known if these patients had Wolff-Parkinson-White syndrome or ventricular arrhythmias. Despite improved cardiac functional status after repair, the incidence of sudden death remains high. Oh et al[132] reported that five (10%) of 52 patients after surgical repair of Ebstein's malformation died suddenly during a mean follow-up of 33 months. Four of the five had perioperative ventricular tachycardia or fibrillation. As a result, these investigators recommend prophylactic antiarrhythmic treatment for the first 3 months after surgery in all patients who have undergone repair of Ebstein's malformation.

NONCARDIAC SUDDEN DEATH IN CHILDREN

The noncardiac causes of sudden death in children are listed in Table 18–8. Infec-

Table 18–8
Noncardiac Causes of Sudden Death

Abdominal hemorrhage
Cerebral hemorrhage
Infection
Pulmonary abnormality
Seizure disorder
Toxic substance use

tion, not including myocarditis, was responsible for 32% of the sudden deaths in the compiled data from apparently healthy children (see Table 18–1). Respiratory infection, sepsis, and meningitis are most commonly implicated. Children who are in the 1- to 5-year-old group accounted for more than one half of the sudden deaths secondary to an infectious etiology.[7–9] In many instances a severe infection is preceded by mild symptoms, which stresses the importance of observing for early signs of acute deterioration.

Hemorrhage, excluding aortic rupture, was the cause in 11% of the sudden deaths in Table 18–1. Cerebral hemorrhage, predominantly due to arteriovenous malformations and aneurysms, is responsible for the majority of sudden deaths secondary to hemorrhage. Prodromata, usually headache, are a frequent occurrence in children prior to intracranial hemorrhage.[7] Sudden death has also been reported with gastrointestinal hemorrhage and ruptured ectopic pregnancy.[9,10]

Ingestion of toxic substances can be a significant cause of sudden death.[133] Some drugs that have been ingested and implicated in sudden death include tricyclic antidepressants, heroin, cocaine, phenobarbital, methyl alcohol, isopropyl alcohol, and haloperidol.

Chronic illnesses such as asthma (reactive airway disease) and seizure disorders play an important role in sudden death in children.[7,9] Undertreatment in children with asthma[134,135] and subtherapeutic anticonvulsant levels in children with a seizure disorder[136–138] have been associated with sudden death. The majority of those who die suddenly are adolescents,[7,9] a group in which compliance with a medical regimen is likely to be low.

PREVENTION

There are several factors important for the prevention of sudden death in the pediatric population. The goal is to identify children who are at risk so that the appropriate intervention and treatment may be implemented.

Many children who die suddenly have a history of premonitory symptoms, which may include syncope, presyncope, dyspnea, chest pain on exertion, or palpitations. Premonitory symptoms were reported in 25–56% of apparently healthy children,[6,10] 25–50% of young athletes,[42,43] and 40–50% of children with known heart disease[14,83] who died suddenly. Also warranting further evaluation are children with a family history of syncope, arrhythmias, Marfan syndrome, hypertrophic cardiomyopathy, and sudden or unexplained death. A family history of seizures or accidental death (e.g., the pilot in a plane crash) may be masking a history consistent with arrhythmias and sudden death.

The subset of children who may be at increased risk of sudden death during sports includes those with moderate to severe aortic stenosis, hypertrophic cardiomyopathy, Marfan syndrome, LQTS, Wolff-Parkinson-White syndrome, and some postoperative congenital heart disease patients. Restriction of activity in these children should decrease the risk. Screening for these abnormalities, for example with ECG, has been evaluated, but the data are not conclusive.

Arrhythmia suppression may decrease the incidence of sudden death in patients who have undergone operation for congenital heart disease. Arrhythmia suppression is especially important if poor hemodynamics are present. Although not proven, suppression of arrhythmias in hypertrophic cardiomyopathy and other cardiomyopathies may lower the incidence of sudden death. Radiofrequency ablation is now available for patients with Wolff-Parkinson-White syndrome and should be considered for those who are at risk.

Surgery in infants for repair of tetralogy of Fallot, double-outlet right ventricle, and other congenital heart defects appears to decrease the incidence of arrhythmias in the short term. Improved surgical repairs for defects, such as the arterial switch operation for transposition of the great arteries, should help decrease the incidence of sudden death. Also, reoperation to improve hemodynamics may be of benefit if arrhythmias are refractory to medical treatment.

Pacemaker implantation in children with congenital or acquired heart block or sick sinus syndrome should prevent sudden death. Also, pacemaker placement when indicated in patients with LQTS may decrease the risk of sudden death.

The implantable cardioverter-defibrillator can be an important adjunct to therapy in children.[139–141] This may be especially true with the development of smaller devices and the use of tiered therapy.

Because myocarditis has emerged as an important factor in all reported series, the development of blood tests should be extremely helpful. Until such tests are available, it may be that restriction from competitive sports should be recommended for 1–2 weeks after severe systemic viral infections.

SUMMARY

Sudden death in children has been associated with a number of cardiovascular diseases, including hypertrophic cardiomyopathy, myocarditis, coronary artery anomalies, Wolff-Parkinson-White syndrome, LQTS, and a history of corrective surgery for congenital heart defects such as tetralogy of Fallot and transposition of the great arteries. Despite the low incidence of sudden death in the pediatric population, many of these deaths are potentially preventable. The aim of identifying those children at risk is to prevent sudden death with the appropriate intervention and treatment.

REFERENCES

1. DiMarco JP, Haines DE: Sudden cardiac death. Curr Probl Cardiol 186–232, April, 1990.
2. Akhtar M: Sudden cardiac death: Management of high-risk patients. Ann Intern Med 114:499–512, 1991.
3. Singh BN: When is drug therapy warranted to prevent sudden cardiac death? Drugs 41(suppl 2):24–46, 1991.
4. Lown B: Cardiovascular collapse and sudden death. In Braunwald E (ed): Heart Disease: A Textbook of Cardiovascular Medicine. Philadelphia, WB Saunders, 1984, p 774.
5. Niimura I, Takatoshi M: Sudden cardiac death in childhood. Jpn Circ J 53:1571–1780, 1989.
6. Driscoll DJ, Edwards WD: Sudden unexpected death in children and adolescents. J Am Coll Cardiol 5:118B–121B, 1985.
7. Neuspiel DR, Kuller LH: Sudden and unexpected natural death in childhood and adolescence. JAMA 254:1321–1325, 1985.
8. Molander N: Sudden natural death in later childhood and adolescence. Arch Dis Child 57:572–576, 1982.
9. Keeling JW, Knowles SAS: Sudden death in childhood and adolescence. J Pathol 159:221–224, 1989.
10. Drory Y, Turetz Y, Hiss Y, et al: Sudden unexpected death in persons < 40 years of age. Am J Cardiol 68:1388–1392, 1991.
11. Bharati S, Lev M: Congenital abnormalities of the conduction system in sudden death in young adults. J Am Coll Cardiol 8:1096–1104, 1986.
12. Gore I, Saphir O: Myocarditis: A classification of 1,402 cases. Am Heart J 38:827–830, 1947.
13. Noren GR, Staley NA, Bandt CH, et al: Occurrence of myocarditis in sudden death in children. J Forensic Sci 22:188–196, 1977.
14. Harris P, Alexson C, Lewis E, Manning J: Sudden unexpected cardiac death in adolescence. In: Proceedings of the Second World Congress of Pediatric Cardiology. New York, Springer-Verlag, 1985, pp 1183–1185.
15. Vetter VL: Sudden death in children and adolescents. In Morganroth J, Horowitz LN (eds): Sudden Cardiac Death. New York, Grune & Stratton, 1985, pp 33–46.
16. Kramer MR, Drori V, Lev B: Sudden death in young soldiers: High incidence of syncope prior to death. Chest 93:345–347, 1988.
17. Noren GR, Staley NA, Kaplan EL: Nonrheumatic inflammatory diseases. In Adams FH, Emmanouillides GC, Riemenschneider TA (eds): Moss' Heart Disease in Infants, Children, and Adolescents, 4th ed. Baltimore, Williams & Wilkins, 1989, pp 730–746.
18. Hayakawa M, Inoh T, Yakata Y, et al: Long term follow-up study of acute and idiopathic myocarditis. Jpn Circ J 47:1304, 1983.
19. Gatmaitan BG, Chason JL, Lerner AM: Augmentation of the virulence of murine coxsackie virus B-3 myocardiopathy by exercise. J Exp Med 131:1121, 1970.
20. Mitchell JH, Maron BJ, Epstein SE: 16th Bethesda Conference: Cardiovascular abnormalities in the athlete. Recommendations regarding eligibility for competition. J Am Coll Cardiol 6:1186–1232, 1984.
21. Suryard RD, Wengor N: Long QT syndrome. Primary Cardiol 15:13–16, 1989.

22. Jervell A, Lange-Nielsen F: Congenital deaf-mutism, functional heart disease with prolongation of Q-T interval and sudden death. Am Heart J 54:59, 1957.
23. Ward OC: A new familial cardiac syndrome in children. J Ind Med Assoc 54:103, 1964.
24. Schwartz PJ, Locati E, Prioi SG, Zaza A: The idiopathic long QT syndrome. In Zipes DP, Jalife J (eds): Cardiac Electrophysiology: From Cell to Bedside. Philadelphia, WB Saunders, 1990, pp 589–605.
25. Esscher E: Congenital complete heart block in adolescence and adult life: A follow-up study. Eur Heart J 2:281–288, 1981.
26. Scott WA, Dick M: Two:one atrioventricular block in infants with congenital long QT syndrome. Am J Cardiol 60:1409–1410, 1987.
27. Weintraub RG, Gow RM, Wilkinson JL: The congenital long QT syndromes in childhood. J Am Coll Cardiol 16:674–680, 1990.
28. Schwartz PJ, Zaza A, Locati E, Moss AJ: Stress and sudden death: The case of the long QT syndrome. Circulation 83(suppl II):II-71–80, 1991.
29. Perry JC, Giuffre RM, Garson A: Clues to the electrocardiographic diagnosis of subtle Wolff-Parkinson-White syndrome in children. J Pediatr 117:871–875, 1990.
30. Klein GJ, Bashore TM, Sellers TD, Pritchett EL, Smith WM, Gallagher JJ: Ventricular fibrillation in the Wolff-Parkinson-White syndrome. N Engl J Med 301:1980–1985, 1979.
31. Michaelsson M, Engle MA: Congenital complete heart block: an international study of the natural history. In Engle MA (ed): Pediatric Cardiology. Philadelphia, FA Davis, 1972, p 85.
32. Dreifus LS, Fisch C, Griffin JC, et al: Guidelines for implantation of cardiac pacemakers and antiarrhythmia devices. J Am Coll Cardiol 18:1–13, 1991.
33. Jeresaty RM: Mitral valve prolapse: Definition and implications in athletes. J Am Coll Cardiol 7:231–236, 1986.
34. Ware JA, Magro SA, Luck JC, et al: Conduction system abnormalities in symptomatic mitral valve prolapse: An electrophysiologic analysis of 60 patients. Am J Cardiol 53:1075–1078, 1984.
35. Puddu PE, Pasternac A, Tubau JF, Krol R, Farley L, deChamplain J: QT interval prolongation and increased plasma catecholamine levels in patients with mitral valve prolapse. Am Heart J 105:422–428, 1983.
36. Chesler E, King RA, Edwards JE: The myxomatous mitral valve and sudden death. Circulation 67:632, 1983.
37. Kligfield P, Hochreiter C, Kramer H, et al: Complex arrhythmias in mitral regurgitation with and without mitral valve prolapse: Contrast to arrhythmias in mitral valve prolapse without mitral regurgitation. Am J Cardiol 55:1545–1549, 1985.
38. Kavey RW, Blackman MS, Sondheimer HM, Byrum CJ: Ventricular arrhythmias and mitral valve prolapse in childhood. J Pediatr 105:885–890, 1984.
39. Topaz O, Edwards JE: Pathologic features of sudden death in children, adolescents, and young adults. Chest 87:476–482, 1985.
40. Nishimura RA, McGoon MD, Shub C, et al: Echocardiography documented mitral valve prolapse: Long term follow-up of 238 patients. N Engl J Med 313:1305, 1985.
41. Epstein SE, Maron BJ: Sudden death and the competitive athlete: Perspectives on preparticipation screening studies. J Am Coll Cardiol 7:220–230, 1986.
42. Maron BJ, Epstein SE, Roberts WC: Causes of sudden death in competitive athletes. J Am Coll Cardiol 7:204–214, 1986.
43. Corrado D, Thiene G, Nawa A, Rossi L, Pennelli N: Sudden death in young competitive athletes: Clinicopathologic correlations in 22 cases. Am J Med 89:588–596, 1990.
44. James TN, Froggatt P, Marshall TK: Sudden death in young athletes. Ann Intern Med 67:1013–1021, 1967.
45. Burke AP, Farb A, Virmani R, Goodin J, Smialek JE: Sports-related and nonsports-related sudden cardiac death in young adults. Am Heart J 121:568–575, 1991.
46. Phillips M, Robinowitz M, Higgins JR, Boran KJ, Reed T, Virmani R: Sudden cardiac death in Air Force recruits. JAMA 256:2696–2699, 1986.
47. Kramer MR, Drory Y, Lev B: Sudden death in young Israeli soldiers. Isr J Med Sci 25:620–624, 1989.
48. Kennedy HL, Whitlock JA: Sports related sudden death in young persons [abstract]. J Am Coll Cardiol 3:622, 1984.
49. Waller BF, Newhouse P, Pless J, Foster L, Wills E: Exercise-related sudden death in 27 conditioned subjects aged <30 and >30 years: Coronary artery abnormalities are the culprit [abstract]. J Am Coll Cardiol 3:621, 1984.
50. Thomas RJ, Cantwell JD: Sudden death during basketball games. Phys Sports Med 18:75–78, 1990.
51. James TN, Jordan JD, Riddick L, Bargeron LM: Subaortic stenosis and sudden death. J Thorac Cardiovasc Surg 95:247–254, 1988.
52. Tsung SH, Haung TY, Chang HH: Sudden death in young athletes. Arch Pathol Lab Med 106:168–170, 1982.

53. Maron BJ, Bonow RO, Cannon RO, Leon MB, Epstein SE: Hypertrophic cardiomyopathy: Interrelations of clinical manifestations, pathophysiology, and therapy. N Engl J Med 316:780–789, 1987.
54. McKenna WJ, Franklin RCG, Nihoyannopoulos P, Robinson KC, Deanfield JE: Arrhythmias and prognosis in infants, children and adolescents with hypertrophic cardiomyopathy. J Am Coll Cardiol 11:147–153, 1988.
55. Maron BJ: Hypertrophic cardiomyopathy: The leading edge. Cardiology 2:1–12, 1988.
56. Nicod P, Poliker R, Peterson KL: Hypertrophic cardiomyopathy and sudden death. N Engl J Med 318:1255–1256, 1988.
57. McKenna WJ, Deanfield JE, Faruqui A, et al: Prognosis in hypertrophic cardiomyopathy: Role of age and clinical, electrocardiographic and hemodynamic factors. Am J Cardiol 47:532–538, 1981.
58. Newman H, Sugrue D, Oakley CM, Goodwin JF, McKenna WJ: The relation of left ventricular function and prognosis in hypertrophic cardiomyopathy: An angiographic study. J Am Coll Cardiol 5:1064–1074, 1985.
59. Maron BJ, Roberts WC, Epstein SE: Sudden death in hypertrophic cardiomyopathy: A profile of 78 patients. Circulation 67:1288–1294, 1982.
60. McKenna WJ, Deanfield JE: Hypertrophic cardiomyopathy: An important cause of sudden death. Arch Dis Child 59:971–975, 1984.
61. Maron BJ, Savage DD, Wolfson JK, Epstein SE: Prognostic significance of 24 hour ambulatory electrocardiographic monitoring in patients with hypertrophic cardiomyopathy: A prospective study. Am J Cardiol 48:252–257, 1981.
62. Maron BJ, Henry WL, Clark CE, et al: Asymmetric septal hypertrophy in childhood. Circulation 53:9, 1976.
63. Maron BJ, Roberts WC, Edwards JE, et al: Sudden death in patients with hypertrophic cardiomyopathy: Characterization of 26 patients without functional limitation. Am J Cardiol 41:803, 1978.
64. Savage DD, Seides SF, Clark CE, et al: Electrocardiographic findings in patients with obstructive and nonobstructive hypertrophic cardiomyopathy. Circulation 58:402, 1978.
65. Malone R, Covitz W, Lovett EJ: Hypertrophic cardiomyopathy in childhood. J Med Assoc Ga 74:172–175, 1985.
66. St. John Sutton MG, Lie JT, Tajik AJ, Giuliani ER, Danielson GK, Frye RL: Hypertrophic obstructive cardiomyopathy. Heart Failure 152–178, 1985.
67. McKenna W, et al: Amiodarone for long-term management of patients with hypertrophic cardiomyopathy. Am J Cardiol 54:802–810, 1984.
68. Fananapazir L, Epstein SE: Value of electrophysiologic studies in hypertrophic cardiomyopathy treated with amiodarone. Am J Cardiol 67:175–182, 1991.
69. Fananapazir L, Leon MB, Bonow RO, et al: Sudden death during empiric amiodarone therapy in symptomatic hypertrophic cardiomyopathy. Am J Cardiol 67:169–174, 1991.
70. Cheitlin MD, DeCastro CM, McAllister HA: Sudden death as a complication of anomalous left coronary artery origin from the anterior sinus of Valsalva. Circulation 50:780–787, 1974.
71. Maron BJ, Roberts WC, McAllister HA, et al: Sudden death in young athletes. Circulation 62:218, 1980.
72. Benson PA, Lack AR: Anomalous aortic origin of the left coronary artery. Arch Pathol Lab Med 86:214–216, 1968.
73. Jokl E, McClellan JT, Ross GD: Congenital anomaly of left coronary artery in a young athlete. JAMA 182:572–573, 1962.
74. VanCamp SP, Choi JH: Exercise and sudden death. Phys Sports Med 16:49–52, 1988.
75. Morales AR, Romanelli R, Boucek RJ: The mural left anterior descending coronary artery, strenuous exercise and sudden death. Circulation 62:230–237, 1980.
76. Braden DS, Strong WB: Preparticipation screening for sudden cardiac death in high school and college athletes. Phys Sports Med 16:128–140, 1988.
77. Celermajer DS, Sholler GF, Howman-Giles R, Celermajer JM: Myocardial infarction in childhood: Clinical analysis of 17 cases and medium term follow-up of survivors. Br Heart J 65:332–336, 1991.
78. Kohr RM: Progressive asymptomatic coronary artery disease as a late fatal sequela of Kawasaki disease. J Pediatr 108:256, 1986.
79. Cantwell JD: Marfan's syndrome: Detection and management. Phys Sports Med 14:51–55, 1986.
80. Pierpont MEM, Moller JH: Cardiac manifestations of systemic disease. In Adams FH, Emmanouillides GC, Riemenschneider TA (eds): Moss' Heart Disease in Infants, Children and Adolescents, 4th ed. Baltimore, Williams & Wilkins, 1989, pp 792–796.
81. Pyeritz RE, McKusick VA: The Marfan syndrome: Diagnosis and management. N Engl J Med 300:772–777, 1979.
82. McCaffrey FM, Braden DS, Strong WB:

Sudden cardiac death in young athletes. Am J Dis Child 145:177–183, 1991.
83. Garson A, McNamara DG: Sudden death in a pediatric cardiology population. 1958–1983: Relation to prior arrhythmias. J Am Coll Cardiol 5:134B–137B, 1985.
84. Lambert EC, Menon VA, Wagner HR, Vlad P: Sudden unexpected death from cardiovascular disease in children. Am J Cardiol 34:89–96, 1974.
85. Campbell M: The natural history of congenital aortic stenosis. Br Heart J 30:514, 1968.
86. Stewart JR, Paton BC, Blount GS, et al: Congenital aortic stenosis ten to 22 years after valvulotomy. Arch 113:1248, 1978.
87. Schwartz LS, Goldfischer J, Sprague GJ, et al: Syncope and sudden death in aortic stenosis. Am J Cardiol 23:647, 1969.
88. Olshausen K, et al: Ventricular arrhythmias before and later after aortic valve replacement. Am J Cardiol 54:142–146, 1984.
89. Konishi V, Matsuda K, Nishiwaki N, et al: Ventricular arrhythmias late after aortic and/or mitral valve replacement. Jpn Circ J 49:576–583, 1985.
90. Glew RH, Varghese PJ, Krovete LJ, Dorst JP, Rowe RD: Sudden death in congenital aortic stenosis: A review of eight cases with an evaluation of premonitory clinical features. Am Heart J 78:615–625, 1969.
91. Peckman GB, Keith JD, Evan JR: Congenital aortic stenosis: Some observations on the natural history and clinical assessment. Can Med Assoc J 91:639–643, 1964.
92. Graham TP Jr: The Eisenmenger reaction and its management. In Roberts WC (ed): Congenital Heart Disease in Adults. Philadelphia, FA Davis, 1979, p 531.
93. Clarkson RM, Frye RL, DuShane JW, et al: Prognosis for patients with ventricular septal defect and severe pulmonary vascular obstructive disease. Circulation 38:129, 1968.
94. Young D, Mark H: Fate of the patient with Eisenmenger syndrome. Am J Cardiol 28:658, 1971.
95. Brammell HL, Vogel JHK, Pryor R, et al: The Eisenmenger's syndrome: A clinical and physiological appraisal. Am J Cardiol 28:679, 1971.
96. Deanfield JE, McKenna WJ, Hallidie-Smith KA: Detection of late arrhythmia and conduction disturbance after correction of tetralogy of Fallot. Br Heart J 44:248–253, 1980.
97. Fuster V, McGoon DC, Kennedy MA, Ritter DG, Kirklin JW: Long-term evaluation (12–22 years) of open heart surgery for tetralogy of Fallot. Am J Cardiol 46:635–642, 1980.
98. Katz NM, Blackstone EH, Kirklin JW, Pacifico AD, Bargeron LM: Late survival and symptoms after repair of tetralogy of Fallot. Circulation 65:403–410, 1982.
99. Garson A, Porter CJ, Gillette PC, McNamara DG: Induction of ventricular tachycardia during electrophysiologic study after repair of tetralogy of Fallot. J Am Coll Cardiol 6:1493–1502, 1983.
100. Wolff GS, Rowland TW, Ellison RC: Surgically induced right bundle branch block with left anterior hemiblock: An ominous sign in postoperative tetralogy of Fallot. Circulation 46:587–594, 1972.
101. Wessel HU, Bastanier CK, Paul MH, Berry TW, Cole RB, Muster AJ: Prognostic significance of arrhythmias in tetralogy of Fallot after intracardiac repair. Am Cardiol 46:843–848, 1982.
102. Kavey RW, Blackman MS, Sondheimer HM: Incidence and severity of chronic ventricular arrhythmias after repair of tetralogy of Fallot. Am Heart J 103:342–350, 1982.
103. Deanfield JE, Ho S, Anderson RH, McKenna WJ, Allwork SP, Hallidie-Smith KA: Late sudden death after repair of tetralogy of Fallot: A clinicopathologic study. Circulation 67:626–631, 1983.
104. Chandar JS, et al: Ventricular arrhythmias in postoperative tetralogy of Fallot. Am J Cardiol 65:655–661, 1990.
105. Garson A: Ventricular arrhythmias after repair of congenital heart disease: Who needs treatment? Cardiol Young 1(3):177–181, 1991.
106. Walsh EP, Rockenmacher S, Keane JF, et al: Late results in patients with tetralogy of Fallot repaired during infancy. Circulation 77:1062–1067, 1988.
107. Hayes CJ, Gersony WM: Arrhythmias after the Mustard operation for transposition of the great arteries: A long-term study. J Am Coll Cardiol 7:133, 1986.
108. Duster MC, Bink-Boelkens MTE, Lampler D, et al: Long-term follow-up of dysrhythmias following the Mustard procedure. Am Heart J 109:1323, 1985.
109. Saalouke MG, Rios J, Perry LW, et al: Electrophysiologic studies after Mustard's operation for d-transposition of the great vessels. Am J Cardiol 41:1104–1109, 1978.
110. Beerman LB, Neches WH, Fricker FJ, et al: Arrhythmias in transposition of the great arteries after the Mustard operation. Am J Cardiol 51:1530–1534, 1983.
111. Marchal C, Paul T, Garson A: Inducible ventricular tachycardia after Mustard operation for transposition of the great arteries [abstract]. In: Proceedings of the Third World Congress of Pediatric Cardiology, 1989, p 176.

112. Flinn CJ, Wolff GS, Dick M, et al: Cardiac rhythm after the Mustard operation for complete transposition of the great arteries. N Engl J Med 310:1635–1638, 1984.
113. Southall DP, Keeton BR, Leanage R, et al: Cardiac rhythm and conduction before and after Mustard's operation for complete transposition of the great arteries. Br Heart J 43:21–30, 1980.
114. Garson A Jr, Bink-Boelkens M, Hesslein PS, et al: Atrial flutter in the young: A collaborative study of 380 cases. J Am Coll Cardiol 6:871, 1985.
115. Martin RP, Radley-Smith R, Yacoub MH: Arrhythmias before and after anatomic correction of transposition of the great arteries. J Am Coll Cardiol 10:200–204, 1987.
116. Vetter VL, Tanner CS: Electrophysiologic consequences of the arterial switch repair of d-transposition of the great arteries. J Am Coll Cardiol 12:229–237, 1988.
117. Bricker JT, Traweek MS, Smith RT, Moak JP, Vargo TA, Garson A: Exercise related ventricular tachycardia in children. Am Heart J 112:186–188, 1986.
118. Soloman S, et al: Exercise induced ventricular tachycardia and arrhythmias with right ventricular dysplasia: Electrophysiologic and therapeutic considerations. Texas Heart Inst J 10:351–357, 1983.
119. Franciosa JA, Wilen M, Ziesche S, et al: Survival in men with severe chronic left ventricular failure due to either coronary heart disease or idiopathic dilated cardiomyopathy. Am J Cardiol 51:831–836, 1983.
120. Anderson KP, Freedman RA, Mason JW: Sudden death in idiopathic dilated cardiomyopathy. Ann Intern Med 107:104–106, 1987.
121. Olshausen K, Stienen V, Schwarz F, Kubler W, Meyer J: Long-term prognostic significance of ventricular arrhythmias in idiopathic dilated cardiomyopathy. Am J Cardiol 61:146–151, 1988.
122. Johnson RA, Palacios I: Dilated cardiomyopathies in the adult. N Engl J Med 307:1051–1058, 1982.
123. Fuster J, Gersh BJ, Giuliani ER, et al: The natural history of idiopathic dilated cardiomyopathy. Am J Cardiol 47:525–531, 1981.
124. Unverferth OV, Magorien RD, Moeschberger ML, et al: Factors influencing the one-year mortality of dilated cardiomyopathy. Am J Cardiol 54:147–152, 1984.
125. Meinertz T, Hofmann T, Kasper W, et al: Significance of ventricular arrhythmias in idiopathic dilated cardiomyopathy. Am J Cardiol 53:902–907, 1984.
126. Huang SK, Messer JV, Denes P: Significance of ventricular tachycardia in idiopathic dilated cardiomyopathy: Observations in 35 patients. Am J Cardiol 51:507–512, 1983.
127. Costanza-Nordin MR, O'Connell JB, Engelmeier RS, et al: Dilated cardiomyopathy: Functional status; hemodynamics, arrhythmias, and prognosis. Cathet Cardiovasc Diagn 11:445–453, 1985.
128. Friedman RA, Moak JP, Garson A: Idiopathic dilated cardiomyopathy in children: Arrhythmias and clinical implications. J Am Coll Cardiol 18:152–156, 1991.
129. Griffin ML, Hernandez A, Martin TC, et al: Dilated cardiomyopathy in infants and children. J Am Coll Cardiol 11:139–144, 1988.
130. Guarnieri E, et al: Failure of electrophysiologic testing to predict death in congestive cardiomyopathy. Circulation 72(suppl III):159, 1985.
131. Watson H: Natural history of Ebstein's anomaly of tricuspid valve in childhood and adolescence: An international cooperative study of 505 cases. Br Heart J 36:417, 1974.
132. Oh JK, Holmes DR, Hayes DL, et al: Cardiac arrhythmias in patients with surgical repair of Ebstein's anomaly. J Am Coll Cardiol 6:1351–1357, 1985.
133. Raymond JR, van den Berg EK, Knapp MJ: Nontraumatic prehospital sudden death in young adults. Arch Intern Med 148:303–308, 1988.
134. Carswell F: Asthma in New Zealand. N Engl J Med 315:1029, 1986.
135. Greaves IA: Death from asthma. Med J Aust 2:535–536, 1980.
136. Lund A, Gorman H: The role of antiepileptics in sudden death in epilepsy. Acta Neurol Scand 72:444–446, 1985.
137. Terrance CF, Wisotzkey HM, Perper JA: Unexpected unexplained death in epileptic patients. Neurology 25:594–598, 1975.
138. Jay GW, Leetsma JE: Sudden death in epilepsy. Acta Neurol Scand 63(suppl 82):1–66, 1981.
139. Silka MJ, Kron J, Walance CG, Cutler JE, McAnulty JH: Assessment and follow-up of pediatric survivors of sudden cardiac death. Circulation 82:341–349, 1982.
140. Kral MA, Spotnitz HM, Hordof A, et al: Automatic implantable cardioverter defibrillator implantation for malignant ventricular arrhythmias associated with congenital heart disease. Am J Cardiol 63:118–119, 1989.
141. Kron J, Oliver RP, Norsted S, Silka MJ: The automatic implantable cardioverter-defibrillator in young patients. J Am Coll Cardiol 16:896–902, 1990.

19

Role of Specialized Conduction System Abnormalities in Sudden Cardiac Death

SAROJA BHARATI
MAURICE LEV

When death occurs suddenly and unexpectedly, especially in young, healthy people with no prior history of arrhythmias, it is a tragic and emotional experience, not only for the family and friends but also for the pathologist or medical examiner who is unable to determine the cause of death. Although sudden death in young, healthy people is not rare, research in this subject lags far behind research in other areas of cardiology. This may be due to the fact that when death occurs suddenly and unexpectedly and the medical examiner or pathologist is unable to determine its cause, one then thinks in terms of an arrhythmic event that might have triggered the sudden death. If a study of the conduction system is made, we believe that all parts of the conduction system from the sinoatrial (SA) node and its approaches, the atrial preferential pathways, the atrioventricular (AV) node and its approaches, the AV bundle, and the bundle branches up to the periphery should be examined by serial section. In a sense the entire heart should be studied in a semiquantitative fashion to give a meaningful interpretation of the findings, if any.[1] A semiquantitative estimation of the entire heart including the conduction system is an exhaustive task that requires time and expertise to understand the findings. Furthermore, the findings may shed some light for future research in this field.

METHOD OF STUDY OF THE CONDUCTION SYSTEM

The entire conduction system including the SA node and its approaches, the AV node and its approaches, the AV bundle (the penetrating, branching, and bifurcating portions), and the bundle branches up to the peripheral Purkinje fibers are constantly changing their course from beginning to end. The conduction system, therefore, is not a straight line at any point. Thus a method must be developed that will enable the pathologist to follow its entire course. It is therefore mandatory to study this system in its entirety by serial section examination. A complete serial section examination is beyond human capability. However, a semiquantitative analysis can be accomplished by retaining every 10th or 20th serial section for examination. Any other method of study of the conduction system in cases of sudden death would have little value.

METHOD OF OBTAINING BLOCKS

The block containing the SA node and its approaches is made as follows. A cut is made along the proximal margin of the right atrium through the right lateral wall of the superior vena cava. The next cut passes through the original cut made to open the heart, and then passes through the right atrial appendage over the hump of the appendage for a distance of about one-half inch into the posterior wall. The final cut to form the block extends from the end of the previous cut along the superior wall of the right atrium and along the apical aspect of the posterior crest to meet the first cut.

To fashion the blocks containing the approaches to the AV node, the AV node, the AV bundle, and bundle branches, we proceed as follows. A cut is made just posterior to the moderator band and the right anterolateral papillary muscle at an angle of almost 45 degrees to the septal band of the crista supraventricularis and passing below the crux. A second cut is made in the upper aspect of the atrial septum from the roof of the aorta to the center of the fossa ovalis. A third cut is made at right angles to the first cut along a line proximal to the insertion of the eustachian valve so that the coronary sinus region is in the block as well as the crux. A fourth cut is made at a right angle to the first cut through the lower part of the arch of the crista, with the operator making sure that the base of the aorta and most of the pars membranacea are in the block. This block is now subdivided by cuts through the pars membranacea, proximal to the tricuspid valve, and through the muscle of Lancisi.

The blocks are then serially sectioned, and every 10th or 20th section is retained and alternatively stained with hematoxylin-eosin and Weigert–van Geison stains. In this manner, a total of approximately 1000 to 1500 sections are examined and compared with the normal conduction system of a similar age group.[2,3]

We have now studied more than 125 hearts of patients, mostly young and healthy, who died suddenly and unexpectedly. We have also studied the conduction systems of people who died suddenly and unexpectedly with or without a history of documented arrhythmias, and in familial cases. We have studied the conduction system in athletes or athletically trained individuals with and without a history of arrhythmias. When death occurs suddenly and unexpectedly, especially in the young, we usually think of hypertrophic cardiomyopathy, coronary artery anomalies, and Marfan disease, which may remain silent, without any symptoms or warnings. In our examination of the conduction system in sudden death, we have found varying types of congenital and acquired pathological changes affecting the SA node and its approaches, the atrial preferential pathways, the approaches to the AV node, the AV node, the AV bundle and bundle branches, and the surrounding structures.[4] The surrounding structures include the tricuspid, mitral, and aortic valves, the central fibrous body, the membranous septum, and the summit of the ventricular septum, including the left and the right sides. Others who have studied the conduction system in cases of sudden death have reported similar kinds of changes in most instances.[5–12] In this chapter we discuss the changes that might have caused an arrhythmic event during an altered physiological state. For a detailed discussion we refer the reader to a previous publication.[4]

SINOATRIAL NODE AND ITS APPROACHES

The History

A 22-year-old college football player collapsed suddenly and was thought to be in a seizure while relaxing in a bar. He was found to have a carotid pulse of 56 beats/min, and initial monitoring showed sinus bradycardia with wide QRS complexes. He could not be resuscitated.[4] He had a vague history of a heart murmur in high school, but the patient had been medically cleared to play football. The history also suggested a junctional tachycardia in the distant past that disappeared after exercise.

Pathology

The patient was found to have diplomyelia (double spinal cord). The heart weighed 380 g. The right atrium and right ventricle were hypertrophied and enlarged.

Findings in the Conduction System

The SA node was divided into two segments, with a distinct blood supply to each component and atrial myocardium interven-

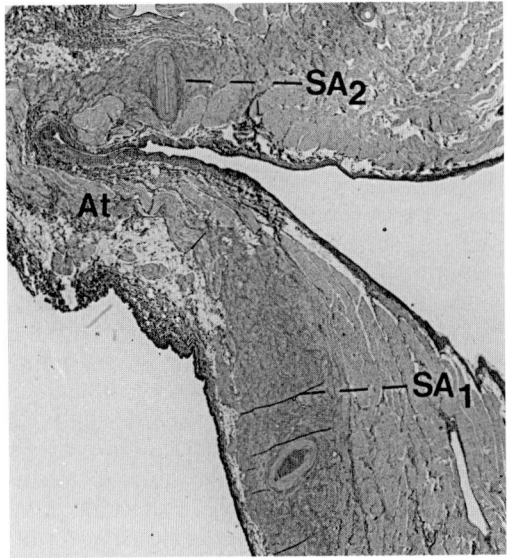

Fig. 19–1. Double sinoatrial node (Weigert–van Geison, ×12). SA_1, first SA node; SA_2, second SA node; At, atrial muscle between the two nodes. Note that the two SA nodes are supplied by separate SA nodal arteries within the substance of each node.

ing between the two nodes (Figs. 19–1 through 19–3). Fibrosis and degeneration of the nerves and epicarditis in the approaches to the SA node were observed (Fig. 19–4).

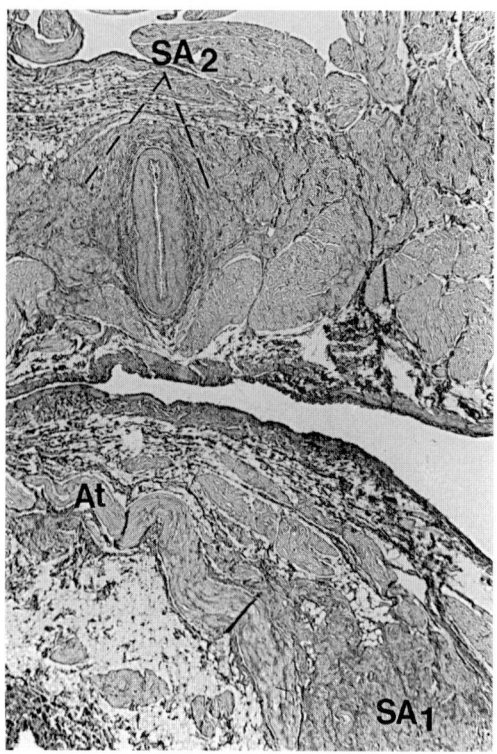

Fig. 19–3. The second SA node (Weigert–van Geison, ×30). SA_2, second SA node; SA_1, first SA node; At, atrial muscle. (Reproduced with permission from Bharati S, Lev M: The cardiac conduction system in unexplained sudden death. Mt. Kisco, NY, Futura, 1990.)

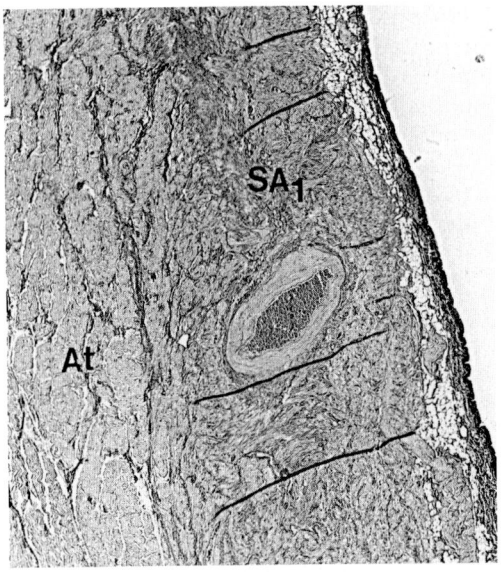

Fig. 19–2. The first SA node (Weigert–van Geison, ×30). SA_1, first SA node; At, atrial muscle.

The AV node was partially separated from its approaches owing to fatty metamorphosis, and the AV nodal artery was narrowed. The node was situated adjacent to the aorta and showed mild to moderate fibrosis. The membranous part of the ventricular septum was considerably shortened and thickened. The penetrating portion of the AV bundle was situated close to the aortic valve and was fibrotic. The right and left bundle branches showed moderate fibrosis.

The presence of a double SA node with a distinct coronary artery supply to each node separately and atrial myocardium in between the two nodes suggests that impulse formation and propagation from the two nodes might have occurred simultaneously, both of which might have formed a substrate for an arrhythmic event. The physiological mechanism of two SA nodes is unknown.

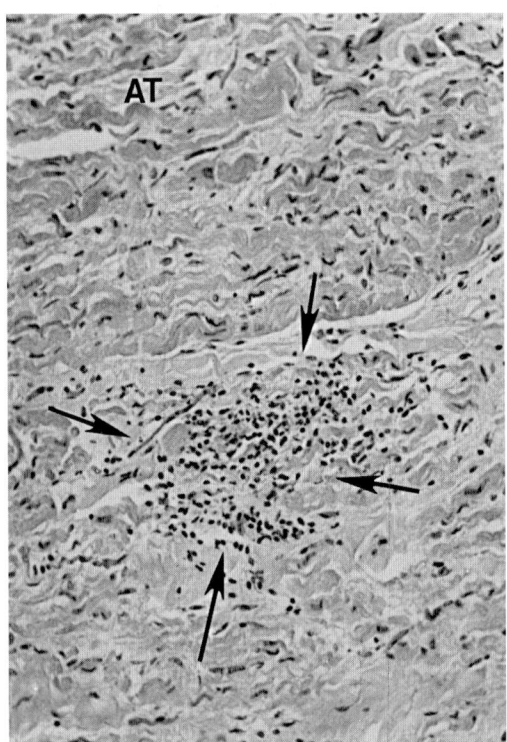

Fig. 19-4. Epicarditis in the approaches to the SA node (hematoxylin-eosin, ×225). AT, atrial myocardium close to the SA node. Arrows point to the accumulation of mononuclear cells.

The double spinal cord is of interest. This case demonstrates that in addition to the abnormal formation of the SA node and the abnormal location of the AV node and AV bundle, there were acquired pathological changes in and around the conduction system that might have contributed to the fatal outcome.

In other cases of sudden death, pathological findings in the SA node and its approaches included marked fibrosis or fatty metamorphosis of the SA node and its approaches, thrombosis of the SA nodal artery and hemorrhage into the SA node and its approaches as a result of blunt trauma, and frequent infiltration of mononuclear cells in and around the node, affecting its function. Although significant pathological findings may be seen in the SA node and its approaches, it is emphasized that there were other findings in and around other parts of the conduction system in many cases.[4,13-15]

THE ATRIOVENTRICULAR NODE

The AV node in many of the cases we studied was situated either within the central fibrous body or within the atrial septum, with tenuous connections to the surrounding atrial myocardium. In some cases the AV node was hypoplastic or situated on the left side, within the tricuspid or the mitral valve anulus, or close to the base of the aorta. The node was sometimes divided into two components, one on the left and one on the right side. Uncommonly, an anterior node was present, situated in the parietal wall close to the septum, or nodelike cells from the mitral valve anulus or atrial muscle were trapped within the central fibrous body and joined the AV node. In some cases it was difficult to differentiate between the AV nodal cells and bundle cells.[4,16] Rarely, an isolated tumor of the AV node had caused sudden death.[17]

History

A 34-year-old trained bicyclist died suddenly while bicycling through town as part of a pre-race exhibition.[4] The paramedics found him to be in coarse ventricular fibrillation (VF) that degenerated into fine VF just before death. He had been bicycling from the age of 12 and throughout adulthood had actively participated in bicycling competition.

Pathology

The heart weighed 510 g. The epicardium on the anterior wall of the right ventricle was markedly thickened. The right atrium and both ventricles were hypertrophied and enlarged. The tricuspid orifice was enlarged, and the valve showed a distinctly increased hemodynamic change.

Findings in the Conduction System

The AV node was within the tricuspid valve anulus (Fig. 19-5) with little communication with the approaches to the node. The AV bundle was on the left side and the ventricular myocardium showed focal areas of fibrosis.

During an altered physiological state, the hemodynamic effects of the tricuspid valve may have affected the AV node, which was

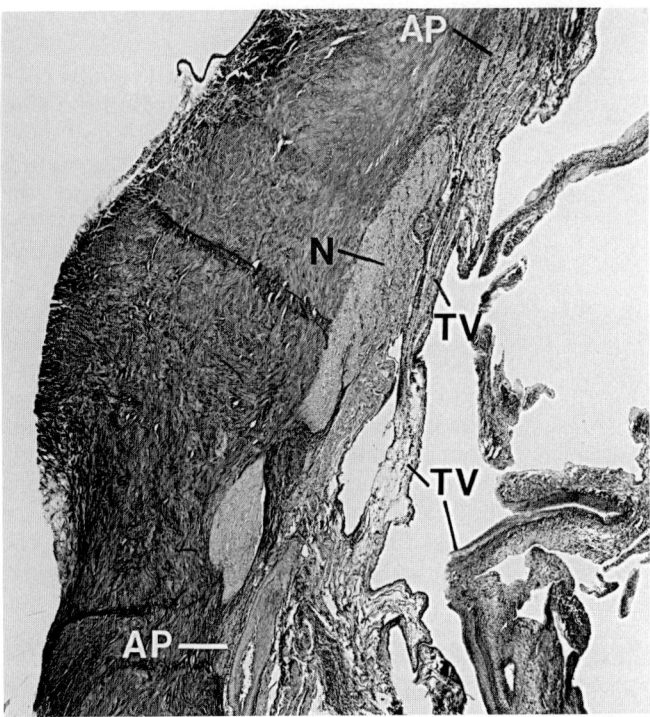

Fig. 19–5. AV node within the tricuspid valve anulus (Weigert–van Geison, ×17). N, AV node; AP, approaches to the AV node; TV, tricuspid valve. Note that the AV node is almost isolated from its approaches. (Reproduced with permission from Bharati S, Lev M: The cardiac conduction system in unexplained sudden death. Mt. Kisco, NY, Futura, 1990.)

located in an abnormal position with few connections to the approaches to the node. In addition there was a left-sided bundle. Also, there were patchy fibrotic scar areas in the ventricular myocardium that might have formed a source for an arrhythmic event. Scars (focal fibrotic areas) in the left ventricle ordinarily are not present in a trained athlete. We were thus confronted with an abnormally located AV node and bundle that were obviously congenital anomalies. In addition, there were focal fibrotic scars in the ventricular myocardium of an acquired nature. Similar observations have been made in other athletes.[4,18,19]

THE ATRIOVENTRICULAR BUNDLE (PENETRATING, BRANCHING, AND BIFURCATING PORTIONS)

In the material we studied, the AV bundle exhibited many variations in size, shape, and location, similar to what we found in the AV node in cases of sudden death. Often there was marked fragmentation of the bundle. The AV bundle frequently was located on the left ventricular side of the ventricular septum, superficial to the subendocardium of the left ventricle, but sometimes the AV bundle was on the right ventricular side. Occasionally the branching bundle, the bifurcating bundle, and the beginning of the left and right bundle branches were present in the pars membranacea and not in the summit of the ventricular septum. The penetrating or branching bundle was occasionally seen in the tricuspid valve anulus. Marked right or left ventricular septal hypertrophy compressed the bundle to a great extent, causing fibrofatty degeneration of the bundle. Atrio-Hisian connections from the right or left atrial side were found in some cases. Rarely, the bundle encircled a piece of the infundibular ventricular septal myocardium on its summit. In many cases there were acquired changes in the bundle in the form of fat, fibrosis, hemorrhage, and infiltration of mononuclear cells.[4,20,21]

History

A 25-year-old man collapsed while playing basketball and was found to be in VF. Despite immediate resuscitative attempts, he died.

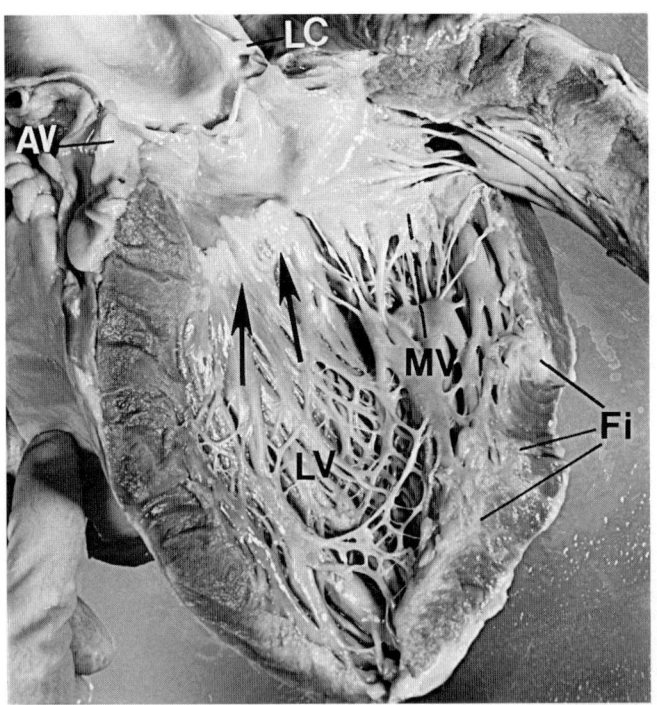

Fig. 19-6. Left ventricular outflow tract demonstrating marked fibroelastic endocardial thickening (arrows) beneath the aortic valve, extending from the anterior part of the ventricular septum up to the aortic-mitral anulus. Note hypertrophy and enlargement of the left ventricle. LV, left ventricle; MV, mitral valve; AV, aortic valve; LC, high origin of the left coronary ostium; Fi, fibrosis in the left ventricular wall.

Pathology

The heart was enlarged, weighing 725 g. All the chambers were hypertrophied and enlarged. The tricuspid valve was somewhat redundant and thickened. The mitral valve revealed distinct thickening and nodularity at the line of closure. The summit of the ventricular septum showed irregular thickening or fibrosis extending from the anterior part of the ventricular septum to the aortic mitral anulus (Fig. 19-6). In addition, there were several scars in the ventricular walls (Fig. 19-6).

Findings in the Conduction System

Epicarditis was noted in the approaches to the SA node, with thickening of the arterioles (Fig. 19-7). The approaches to the AV node revealed marked fatty metamorphosis. The node was entrapped within the central fibrous body and showed arteriolar thickening. The penetrating bundle showed marked fibrosis with lobulation and loop formation (Fig. 19-8). There was marked falling out of cells of the left bundle branch and atrophy of the remaining cells (Fig. 19-9). The bifurcating bundle revealed marked fatty metamorphosis and degenera-

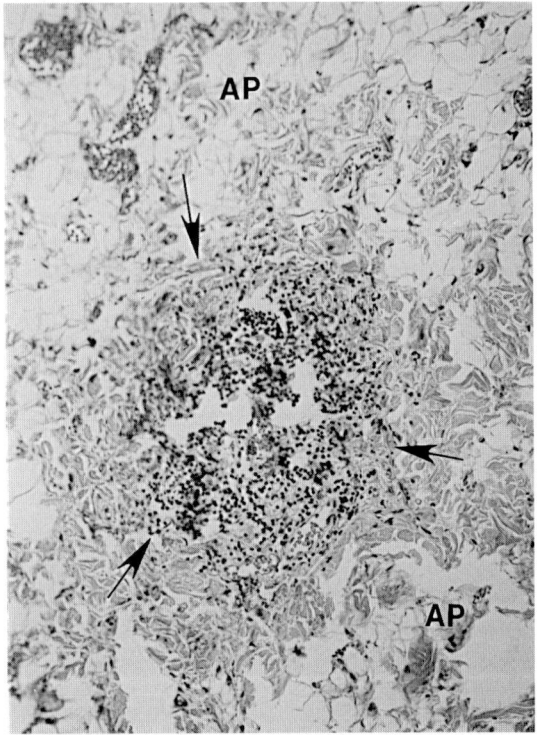

Fig. 19-7. Accumulation of mononuclear cells (arrows) in the approaches to the SA node (hematoxylin-eosin, ×180). AP, approaches to the SA node.

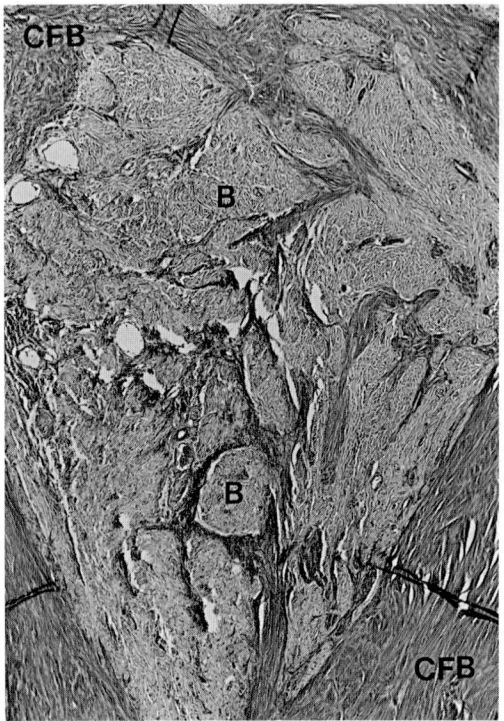

Fig. 19–8. AV bundle, penetrating portion, showing marked fibrosis with lobulation and loop formation (Weigert–van Geison, ×45). B, AV bundle; CFB, central fibrous body.

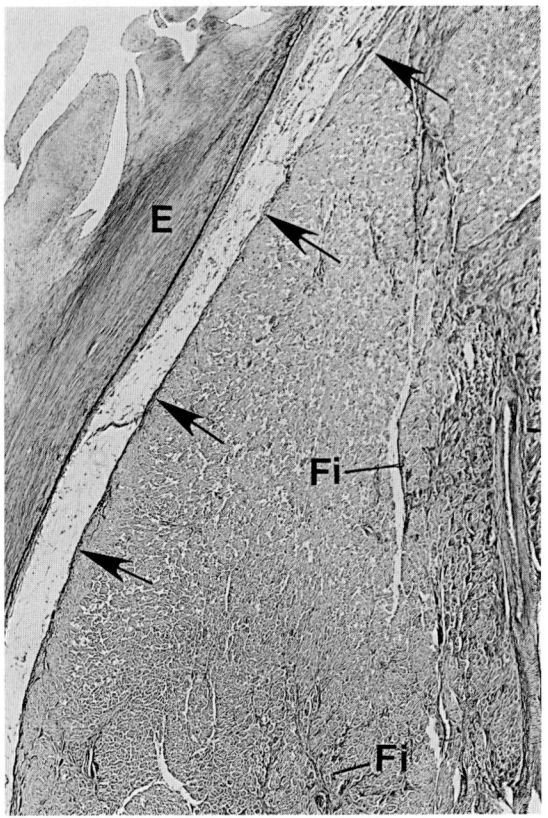

Fig. 19–9. Left bundle branch showing falling out of cells. Note thickening of the endocardium and fibrosis of the ventricular septum. The endocardial thickening corresponds to the endocardial thickening seen in the gross heart specimen (Weigert–van Geison, ×30). E, endocardium; V, ventricular septum; Fi, fibrosis. Arrows point to where left bundle branch should have been.

tion, and the right bundle branch showed moderate fibrosis (Fig. 19–10). The ventricular septum revealed large areas of scar formation (Fig. 19–11).

In this young athlete, the heart was tremendously hypertrophied and enlarged, with distinct fibroelastic scars at the summit of the ventricular septum proceeding to the aortic-mitral anulus. This set of cardiac findings may be considered an atypical form of hypertrophic cardiomyopathy. The thickening of the ventricular septum was not appreciably greater than that of the parietal wall. The marked fibrosis and lobulation of the AV bundle with loop formation, the marked fibrosis on both sides of the bifurcation with fatty metamorphosis, and the falling out of cells of the left bundle branch, as well as entrapment of the AV node within the central fibrous body, may constitute an anatomical substrate for an arrhythmic event and sudden death.

Although this case demonstrated significant findings in the AV bundle, there were additional findings in the form of epicarditis, entrapment of the AV node within the central fibrous body, and scar formation in the ventricular septum. Again some of the findings in the conduction system may be considered congenital and others acquired in nature.

The three cases in athletes just reviewed demonstrate that there are significant pathological findings in the heart to a varying degree with hypertrophy and enlargement of the heart. This observation raises the following questions: (1) Is the hypertrophied and enlarged heart related to athletic training alone? (2) Are the scars related to ath-

Role of Specialized Conduction System Abnormalities in Sudden Cardiac Death 281

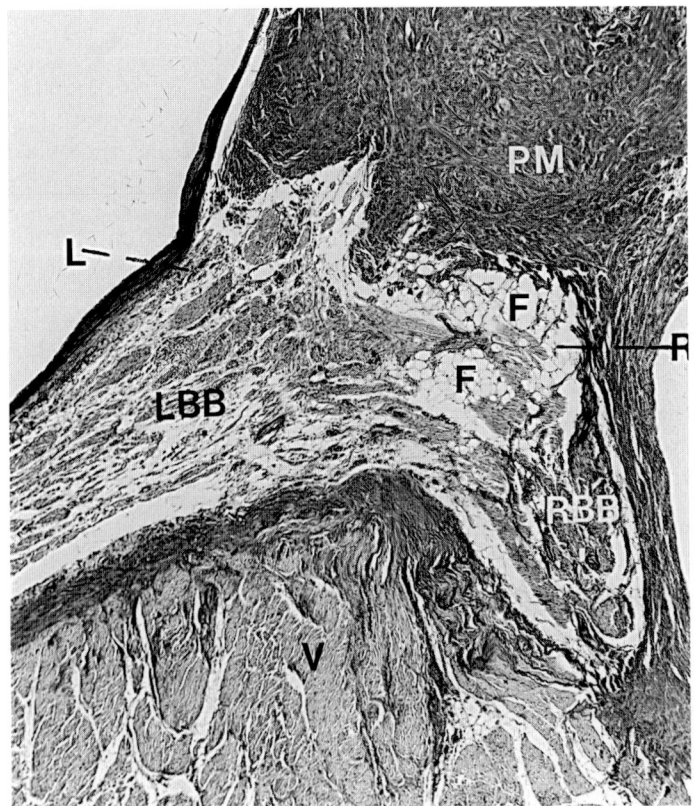

Fig. 19–10. Bifurcating bundle showing fibrosis in the center, falling out of cells of the left and right bundle branch with fatty metamorphosis on the right side (Weigert–van Geison, ×45). V, ventricular septum; L, left side of bifurcating bundle; R, right side of bifurcating bundle; RBB, right bundle branch; LBB, left bundle branch; PM, pars membranacea; F, fat. (Figures 19–8 through 19–10 reproduced with permission from Bharati S, Lev M: The cardiac conduction system in unexplained sudden death. Mt. Kisco, NY, Futura, 1990).

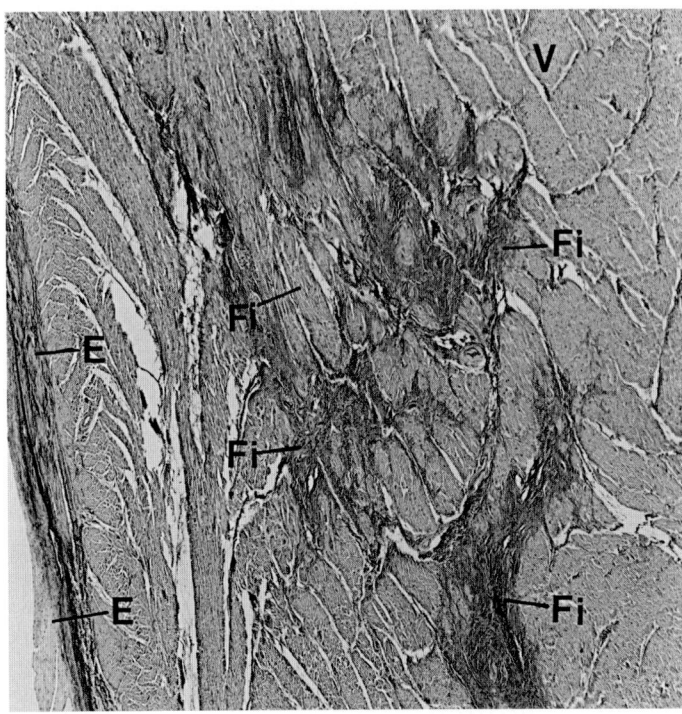

Fig. 19–11. Focal fibrotic scar areas in left ventricle (Weigert–van Geison, ×22.5). V, ventricular myocardium; Fi, fibrosis; E, endocardial thickenings.

letic training? Despite the significant changes in the heart, including the conduction system, presumably some unknown factors protected the athletes and permitted them to perform exceptional physical activity for a long period of time. During an altered physiological state, however, this might have made them vulnerable to an arrhythmic event.

SUDDEN DEATH IN PRE-EXCITATION

When death occurs suddenly in cases of pre-excitation, one may find anomalous AV connections on the right or left side. In a patient who died suddenly with known pre-excitation, we found an anterior AV node in the parietal wall close to the septum that had connections with the infundibular myocardium of the right ventricle.[22]

History

A 26-year-old man was diagnosed as having pre-excitation syndrome with a history of paroxysmal tachycardia of 7 years' duration. He died suddenly at home. The electrocardiogram (ECG) was typical for pre-excitation, suggesting a right free wall anteroseptal anomalous pathway. Two years prior to death, cardiac catheterization had revealed congestive cardiomyopathy with mild mitral regurgitation and moderate pulmonary hypertension.

Pathology

The heart was hypertrophied and enlarged and weighed 640 g. There was diffuse fibroelastosis of the left ventricle.

Findings in the Conduction System

There were copious Mahaim fibers from the AV node to the ventricular septum. The penetrating portion of the AV bundle was markedly septated, with loop formation and copious Mahaim fibers. The branching portion of the AV bundle was septated, with fatty metamorphosis and fibrosis in the region of its bifurcation. There was moderate fibrosis of the right bundle branch. Marked endocardial fibroelastosis was noted in the left ventricle.

Findings in the Right Atrium

There was an accessory anterior AV node situated in the anterior part of the right side of the atrial septum close to the roof. The node made connections with the surrounding atrial myocardium, which joined the infundibular myocardium of the right ventricle where the infundibular septum met the free wall of this chamber (Figs. 19–12 and 19–13).

The paroxysmal supraventricular tachycardia that had been diagnosed during life was probably due to re-entry in the peculiar formation of the anomalous pathway. It is important to realize that an anterior AV node may be present in the anterosuperior parietal wall of the right atrium, close to the ventricular septum, which in turn may be connected to the infundibular right ventricular myocardium close to the membranous septum. This anatomical arrangement may produce Wolff-Parkinson-White syndrome or some other type of AV nodal re-entrant tachycardia. This type of unconventional accessory pathway may be responsible not only for supraventricular tachycardia but also for sudden death. In addition to the anomalous pathway, we found septation and loop formation of the AV bundle as well as copious Mahaim fibers passing from the AV node and bundle to the ventricular septum, which might have contributed to the final outcome. The hypertrophy and enlargement of the heart are most likely the result of recurrent paroxysmal supraventricular tachycardia which the patient had for several years. This is what we call an arrhythmic cardiomyopathy. The cardiomyopathy in turn may initiate an arrhythmic event, creating a vicious cycle of arrhythmic episodes.

SUDDEN DEATH FOLLOWING ABLATIVE PROCEDURES

Radiofrequency catheter ablation is the method of choice today in the management of intractable AV nodal re-entrant tachycardia and tachyarrhythmias associated with Wolff-Parkinson-White syndrome. However, until recently, DC electrical shock was used with reasonable success when arrhythmias could not be controlled pharma-

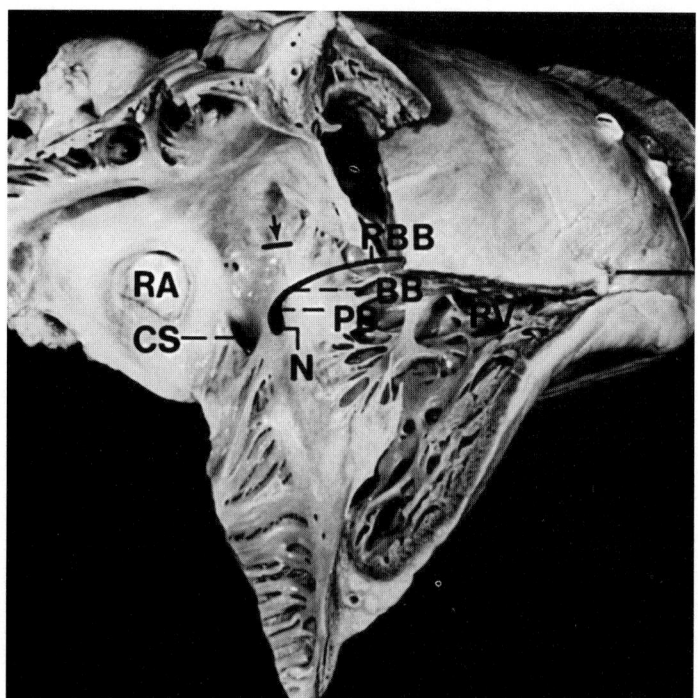

Fig. 19–12. Right atrial and right ventricular view showing the location of the conduction system and the bypass tract (arrow). X indicates the location of the anterior AV node. RA, right atrium; RV, right ventricle; CS, coronary sinus; N, AV node; PB, penetrating portion of AV bundle; PV, branching portion of the AV bundle; RB, right bundle branch.

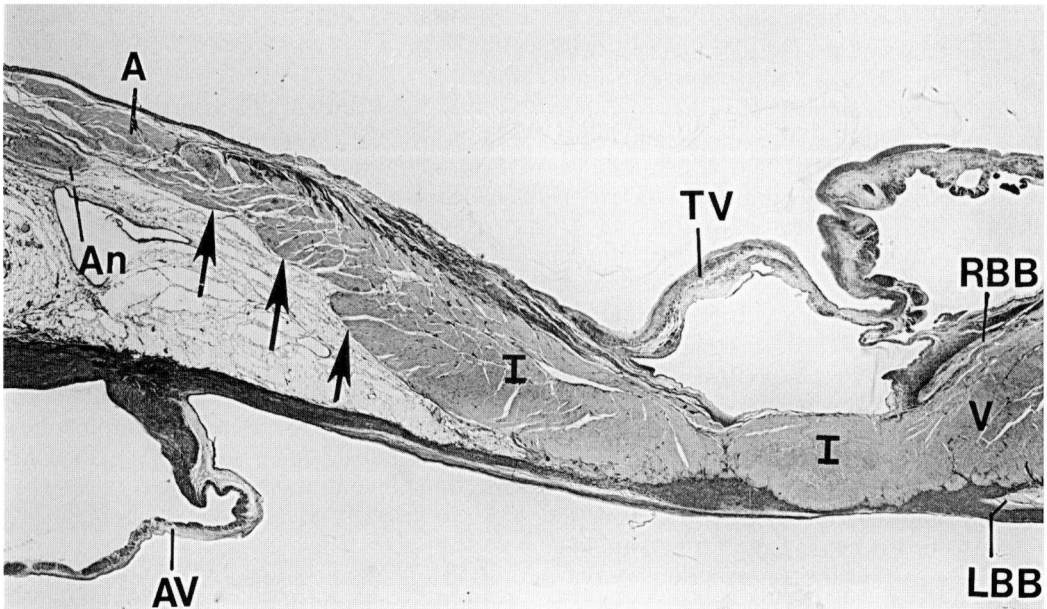

Fig. 19–13. Bypass tract or accessory pathway in the anterior portion of the atrial septum and in the bulbar septum (Weigert–van Geison, ×17). Arrows point to the region of interdigitation of atrial and infundibular myocardial fibers. A, atrial myocardium; An, anterior AV node; AV, aortic valve; I, infundibular musculature; LBB, left bundle branch; RBB, right bundle branch; TV, tricuspid valve; V, ventricular musculature at summit of the ventricular septum. (Figures 19–12 and 19–13 reproduced with permission from Bharati S, et al: Am J Cardiol 48:47–58, 1981.[22])

cologically. Although sudden death may uncommonly occur following ablative procedures performed for intractable supraventricular arrhythmias, there are very few studies of the conduction system in the human in which this had been reported.

History

A 59-year-old woman had recurrent atrial fibrillation refractory to medical management. AV junctional ablation with 500 J (two shocks) was performed and produced complete AV block.[23] A permanent pacemaker was inserted. On physical examination 6 weeks later the woman was doing well. She died suddenly in VF.

Pathology

The heart was somewhat enlarged, weighing 434 g. The pacemaker was in good position and was functioning.

Findings in the Conduction System

There was marked fatty metamorphosis in the SA node and its approaches, the atrial preferential pathways, and the approaches to the AV node. In addition, neuritis was noted in these areas. The AV node showed marked fibroelastosis with moderate infiltration of mononuclear cells, and the node had tenuous connections with the surrounding atrial myocardium. The AV bundle revealed marked fibrosis and fatty metamorphosis with moderate infiltration of mononuclear cells and loop formation. An atrio-Hisian connection was present from the left atrial aspect which joined the AV bundle (Fig. 19–14). The beginning of the right and left bundle branches showed considerable fibrosis. There was marked fibrosis of the summit of the ventricular septum with chronic inflammation.

The chronic inflammatory findings of the summit of the ventricular septum and the marked fibrosis could have formed an anatomical substrate for an arrhythmic event. Likewise, the marked fatty metamorphosis in the atria and the loop formation of the bundle might have formed an anatomical substrate for a re-entry mechanism. The atrio-Hisian fibers could have formed an anatomical substrate for an arrhythmic event.

We have studied four more human hearts

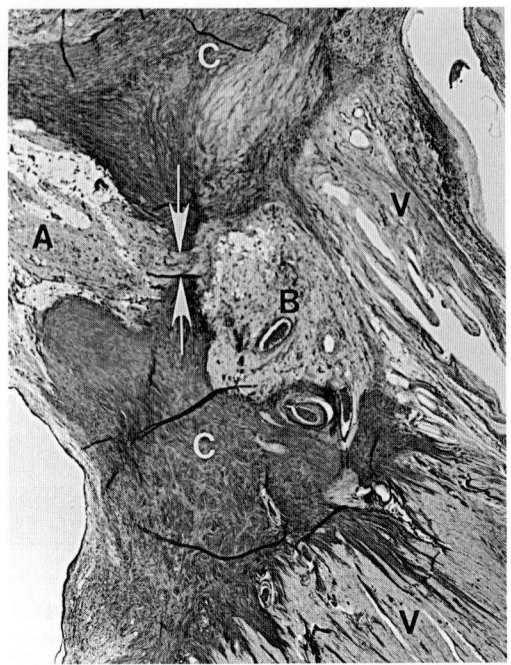

Fig. 19–14. Atrio-Hisian connection (arrows) (Weigert–van Gieson, ×17). A, atrial septum; V, ventricular septal musculature; C, central fibrous body; B, His bundle. (Reproduced with permission from Bharati S, et al: Chest 88: 883–889, 1985.[23])

following ablative procedures,[24] three of them with DC current shock and one with laser ablation, and all showed moderate to marked pathological changes in the surrounding area. In two, marked changes in the form of fibrosis and chronic inflammatory phenomena were found in the summit of the ventricular septum. We believe the chronic inflammatory changes in the adjacent structures, especially in the ventricular septum on the right side, may create a milieu for re-entry, or abnormal automaticity of an impulse, and may cause a fatal arrhythmic event at a later date.

SUDDEN DEATH FOLLOWING OPERATION FOR CONGENITAL HEART DISEASE

Sudden death may occur postoperatively, especially following total surgical correction of tetralogy of Fallot or following the Mustard or Senning operation for complete transposition of the great arteries.[25,26] Sudden death may also occur following surgical correction of atrial septal defect of the secundum or primum types.[25,27] We examined 12 such hearts from patients who died months to years after total surgical correction. Some patients were in normal sinus rhythm and totally asymptomatic at the time of death. Others had a history of arrhythmias but nevertheless were asymptomatic, and were living a relatively normal life clinically.

History

A 17-year-old man diagnosed as having tetralogy of Fallot with pulmonary atresia underwent total surgical correction. A Hancock heterograft valve was placed from the right ventricle to the pulmonary trunk. The ECG revealed premature ventricular contractions. The patient was found dead in bed 6 years after the total surgical correction. Of interest, 24-hour Holter monitoring had revealed not only frequent premature ventricular contractions but also a brief episode of supraventricular tachycardia.

Pathology

The heart was hypertrophied and enlarged and weighed 579 g. All the chambers were hypertrophied and enlarged.

Findings in the Conduction System

The approaches to the SA node and AV node revealed mononuclear cell infiltration, fibrosis, fatty infiltration, and calcification (Fig. 19–15). There was considerable edema of the AV node, and the bundle showed moderate lobulation. Fibrosis and marked fatty metamorphosis of the left-sided branching bundle were noted (Fig. 19–16). The left and right bundle branches revealed fibrosis and fatty metamorphosis. The sum-

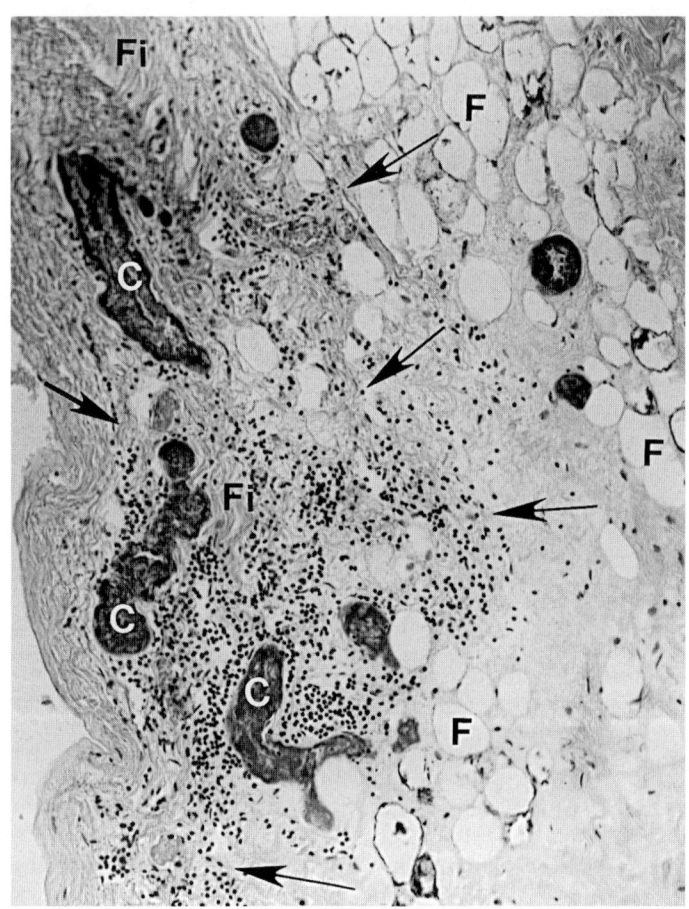

Fig. 19–15. Marked fibrosis, fatty metamorphosis, calcification, and mononuclear cell infiltration (arrows) in the approaches to the SA node. F, fat; Fi, fibrosis; C, calcification.

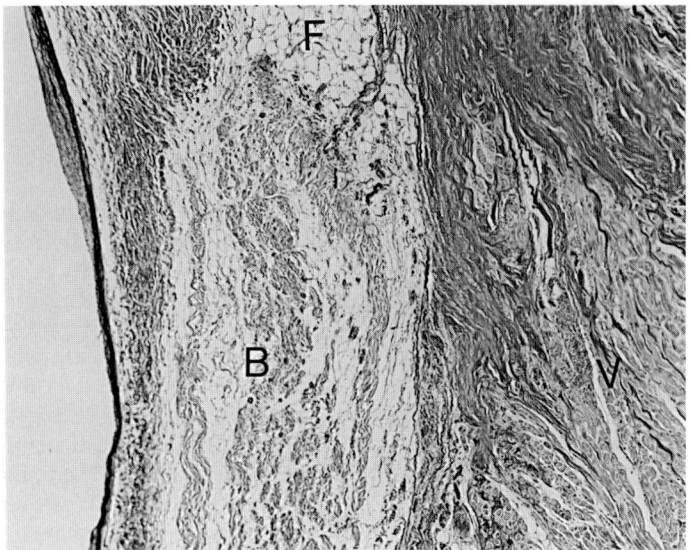

Fig. 19–16. Fatty metamorphosis and falling out of cells of the branching bundle, which is situated on the left ventricular side. V, ventricular septum; F, fatty metamorphosis; B, branching bundle.

mit of the ventricular septum showed immense fibrosis and arteriolo- and arteriosclerosis.

The ubiquitous finding of fatty metamorphosis, fibrosis, and calcification of the approaches to the SA and AV nodes, the fibrosis of the bundle and bundle branches, and fibrosis in other parts of the conduction system and the summit of the ventricular septum could have formed a nidus for a re-entry or other mechanism that might have triggered an arrhythmic event and sudden death. In all the postoperative congenital hearts that we examined, in addition to fat, fibrosis, and calcium in the operated area and the region close to it, there were chronic inflammatory cells and giant cells to a varying degree, regardless of the time when the surgical correction was undertaken. This raises the question of whether these changes represent rejection of the foreign body material used in the operative procedures. The chronic inflammatory cells per se may be responsible for arrhythmias, which may or may not result in a fatal outcome. The causes and effects of fibroelastosis of the chambers in postoperative hearts are unknown.[28]

CONDUCTION SYSTEM FINDINGS IN KNOWN DISEASES WITH SUDDEN DEATH

In addition to changes in the region of the SA node and its approaches, the AV node, and the AV bundle, other disease entities may affect the conduction system and other areas of the heart to a varying degree.[4] Examples of other known diseases that may remain silent clinically or produce asymptomatic or symptomatic arrhythmias include Uhl's anomaly,[29,30] mitral valve prolapse,[31] sarcoidosis of the heart,[32] amyloidosis, Keans-Sayre syndrome,[33] Kawasaki disease,[34] myotonia dystrophica,[35] and other neuromuscular disorders. Although one part of the conduction system in the majority of the cases showed significant pathological change or a congenital anomaly, there were always associated pathological changes in other areas of the conduction system as well. However, there are exceptions to this rule. Mesothelioma of the AV node, which is benign in nature, may infiltrate the AV node and its approaches.[17] This may produce symptoms, or the patient may remain asymptomatic or may have AV block. Sudden death may be the first manifestation of the mesothelioma. This probably is the only condition in which the pathology is quite localized to one area of the conduction system while other parts of the conduction system remain relatively normal. In all other cases with or without a history of familial occurrence, there was involvement of the conduction system in a somewhat diffuse fashion.[36,37] In many cases, the nerves in the approaches to the

SA and AV nodes showed chronic inflammatory cell infiltration and/or fibrosis.

In addition to the above, the following deserve discussion:

Myocarditis

Sudden death can occur in the acute, chronic, or subacute stages of myocarditis. The following information is gleaned from our material. Myocarditis occurred at varying ages and to a varying degree. Whether there was extensive involvement of the heart or selective involvement of the conduction system, clinically the individuals were either totally asymptomatic or had minor complaints such as cold, sore throat, and malaise. Thus there was no correlation between the patient's symptoms in life and the cardiac pathology found at autopsy. We also found an increased tendency for myocarditis to occur in patients who had undergone operation for congenital heart disease or who had a history of chronic arrhythmias. This observation raises the question of whether these individuals are vulnerable to myocarditis, which may be related to the immune system.

QT-Interval Prolongation

We studied the conduction system in five patients with Romano-Ward syndrome and one with the Jervell and Lange-Nielsen syndrome to determine the cause of the prolonged QT interval.[38] The patients included a set of twins. In addition, a prolonged QT interval was found in several members of the family of a sixth patient who died suddenly. Of interest, four of them went into cardiac arrest and two had syncopal episodes. The heart was hypertrophied and enlarged in all, and in four there was fibroelastosis of the left ventricle, possibly related to the fainting spells brought on by the QT prolongation. Pathologically there was marked fatty infiltration in the approaches to the AV node. The AV node was in part situated in the central fibrous body, and often the bundle was segmented with loop formation. Fibrosis of the bundle and the bundle branches was noted. In all cases the ventricular myocardium exhibited chronic inflammatory changes consistent with myocarditis. The varying amount of pathological changes in the ventricular septum may be responsible for abnormal repolarization in this entity. Although there were inflammatory changes in the nerves, they were not extensive. In some cases QT prolongation may be related to linkage between a gene that causes the long QT syndrome and DNA markers on chromosome 11.[39]

Sudden Infant Death Syndrome

There are various theories regarding the cause of sudden unexpected death in infants. We studied 15 such hearts and eight in a control group.[40] The AV node was situated in part within the central fibrous body in some, and the branching bundle was located on the left ventricular side immediately beneath the endocardium in eight of 15. Only two of the eight hearts in the control group showed this finding. We therefore hypothesize that a left-sided AV bundle that is situated quite superficially in the subendocardial region may be vulnerable to arrhythmia during the transition from the relative predominance of the right ventricle at term to the relative predominance of the left ventricle between 2 and 4 months of age. The increase in left ventricular pressure may influence the AV bundle, which is in a superficial subendocardial region in some infants. This may be responsible for an arrhythmia and sudden death. The functional significance of an AV node located partly within the central fibrous body is unknown. We are tempted to speculate a re-entry and/or an abnormal automaticity from an abnormally located AV node. Quite frequently the AV node, the bundle, and the left bundle branch demonstrated fibrosis and neuritis.

Summit of the Ventricular Septum

The summit of the ventricular septum frequently showed an increased amount of fibrosis on the left or right side.[4] The amount of fibrosis was definitively more than one finds normally. The fibrosis extended to a considerable extent into the septum and was frequently associated with arteriolosclerosis. The epicardial coronary arteries were widely patent in almost all cases, especially in the young. The AV nodal artery and its branches, however, exhibited considerable narrowing and thickening in many cases.

SUMMARY

Both congenital and acquired changes may contribute to sudden death in young, healthy subjects by affecting parts of the conduction system and the surrounding myocardium. In the majority of cases we studied there were no symptoms, and some of the individuals were able to perform exceptional physical activity. This raises the issue of the nature and function of diseased tissue. A congenitally malformed structure may remain silent for a long time and might be protected by an unknown factor. During an altered physiological or metabolic state, however, the anatomical abnormalities are probably susceptible to altered function, which may create an arrhythmic event that could degenerate into ventricular tachycardia, fibrillation, and sudden death.

The changes seen in athletically trained individuals were similar to what we found in cases of sudden death in young nonathletes. On the other hand, in individuals with known diseases or a history of arrhythmias and familial sudden death, the pathological changes in the heart and conduction system were more extensive than in young individuals without such a history. We therefore urge the development of better noninvasive techniques to study the normal and abnormal conduction system and the surrounding myocardium. Anatomical changes are seen in all cases of sudden death in young, healthy people, and in most cases the hearts are hypertrophied and enlarged. Unless the clinician is keenly aware of these facts and makes every effort to look for these changes in the living, one may never be able to unravel the enigma associated with sudden death in the young and healthy.

REFERENCES

1. Lev M, Bharati S: Lesions of the conduction system and their functional significance. In Sommers SC (ed): Pathology Annual 1974. New York, Appleton-Century-Crofts, 1974, vol 9, pp 157–208.
2. Lev M: Aging changes in the human sinoatrial node. J Gerontol 9:1–9, 1954.
3. Erickson EE, Lev M: Aging changes in the human atrioventricular node, bundle, and bundle branches. J Gerontol 7:1–12, 1952.
4. Bharati S, Lev M: The Cardiac Conduction System in Unexplained Sudden Death. Mt. Kisco, NY, Futura, 1990.
5. Gotoh K: A histopathological study on the conduction system of the so-called "Pokkuri disease" (sudden unexpected cardiac death of unknown origin in Japan). Jpn Circ J 40: 753–768, 1976.
6. Davies MJ: Pathologic view of sudden cardiac death. Br Heart J 45:88–96, 1981.
7. Rossi L, Thiene G: Recent advances in clinicohistopathologic correlates of sudden cardiac death. Am Heart J 102:478–484, 1981.
8. Rossi L: The pathologic basis of cardiac arrhythmias. Cardiol Clin 1:13–37, 1983.
9. Thiene G, Pennelli N, Rossi L: Cardiac conduction system abnormalities as a possible cause of sudden death in young athletes. Hum Pathol 14:704–709, 1983.
10. Okada R, Kawai S: Histopathology of the conduction system in sudden cardiac death. Jpn Circ J 47:573–580, 1983.
11. James TN: Normal variations and pathologic changes in structure of the cardiac conduction system and their functional significance. J Am Coll Cardiol 5:71B–78B, 1985.
12. James TN, Vikert AM: The fourth USA/USSR symposium on sudden cardiac death. J Am Coll Cardiol 18:1A–109A, 1986.
13. Bharati S, Chervony A, Gruhn J, Rosen KM, Lev M: Atrial arrhythmias related to trauma to sinoatrial node. Chest 61:331–335, 1972.
14. Bharati S, Nordenberg A, Bauernfiend R, et al: The anatomic substrate for the sick sinus syndrome in adolescence. Am J Cardiol 46: 163–172, 1980.
15. Kaplan BM, Langendorf R, Lev M, Pick A: Tachycardia-bradycardia syndrome (so-called "sick sinus syndrome"): Pathology, mechanisms and treatment. Am J Cardiol 31: 497–508, 1973.
16. Bharati S, Bauernfiend R, Scheinman M, et al: Congenital abnormalities of the conduction system in two patients with recurrent tachyarrhythmias. Circulation 59:593–606, 1979.
17. Bharati S, Bicoff JP, Fridman JL, Lev M, Rosen KM: Sudden death caused by benign tumor of the atrioventricular node. Arch Intern Med 136:224–228, 1976.
18. Bharati S, Dreifus LS, Chopskie E, Lev M: Conduction system in a trained jogger with sudden death. Chest 93:348–351, 1988.
19. Brookfield L, Bharati S, Denes P, Halstead RD, Lev M: Familial sudden death: Report of a case and review of the literature. Chest 94:989–993, 1988.
20. Bharati S, Bauernfiend R, Miller LB, Strasberg B, Lev M: Sudden death in three teen-

agers: Conduction system studies. J Am Coll Cardiol *1:*879–886, 1983.
21. Bharati S, Lev M: Congenital abnormalities of the conduction system in sudden death in young adults. J Am Coll Cardiol *8:* 1096–1104, 1986.
22. Bharati S, Strasberg B, Bilitch M, et al: Anatomic substrate for preexcitation in idiopathic myocardial hypertrophy with fibroelastosis of the left ventricle. Am J Cardiol *48:*47–58, 1981.
23. Bharati S, Scheinman MM, Morady F, Hess DS, Lev M: Sudden death after catheter-induced atrioventricular junctional ablation in the human. Chest *88:*883–889, 1985.
24. Bharati S, Moskowitz WB, Scheinman M, Estes NAM III, Lev M: Junctional tachycardias: Anatomic substrate and its significance in ablative procedures. J Am Coll Cardiol *18:*179–186, 1991.
25. Bharati S, Lev M: Conduction system in cases of sudden death in congenital heart disease many years after surgical correction. Chest *90:*861–868, 1986.
26. Bharati S, Molthan ME, Veasy LG, Lev M: Conduction system in two cases of sudden death two years after the Mustard procedure. J Thorac Cardiovasc Surg *77:*101–108, 1979.
27. Bharati S, Lev M: Conduction system in sudden unexpected death a considerable time after repair of atrial septal defect. Chest *94:*142–148, 1988.
28. Bharati S, Lev M: Sequelae of atriotomy and ventriculotomy of the endocardium, conduction system and coronary arteries. Am J Cardiol *50:*580–587, 1982.
29. Bharati S, Feld A, Bauernfiend R, Kattus A Jr, Lev M: A case of hypoplasia of the right ventricular myocardium with ventricular tachycardia. Arch Pathol Lab Med *107:* 249–253, 1983.
30. Bharati S, Ciraulo DA, Bilitch M, Rosen KM, Lev M: Inexcitable right ventricle and bilateral bundle branch block in Uhl's disease. Circulation *57:*636–644, 1978.
31. Bharati S, Granston AS, Liebson PR, Loeb HS, Rosen KM, Lev M: The conduction system in mitral valve prolapse syndrome with sudden death. Am Heart J *101:*667–670, 1981.
32. Bharati S, Lev M, Denes P, et al: Infiltrative cardiomyopathy with conduction disease and ventricular dysrhythmia: Electrophysiological and pathological correlations. Am J Cardiol *45:*163–172, 1980.
33. Gallastegui J, Hariman RJ, Handler B, Lev M, Bharati S: Cardiac involvement in the Kearns-Sayre syndrome. Am J Cardiol *60:* 385–388, 1987.
34. Bharati S, Engle MA, Fatica NS, et al: The heart and conduction system in acute Kawasaki disease: Report of fraternal cases—One lethal, one relapsing. Am Heart J *120:* 359–365, 1990.
35. Bharati S, Bump T, Bauernfiend R, Lev M: Dystrophia myotonia: Correlative electrocardiographic, electrophysiologic and conduction system study. Chest *86:*444–450, 1984.
36. Gault JH, Cantwell J, Lev M, Braunwald E: Fatal familial cardiac arrhythmias: Histologic observation in the cardiac conduction system. Am J Cardiol *29:*548–553, 1972.
37. Husson GS, Blackman MS, Rogers MC, Bharati S, Lev M: Familial congenital bundle branch system disease. Am J Cardiol *32:* 365–369, 1973.
38. Bharati S, Dreifus L, Bucheleres G, et al: The conduction system in cases with prolonged Q-T interval. J Am Coll Cardiol *6:* 1110–1119, 1985.
39. Keating M: Linkage analysis and long QT syndrome: Using genetics to study cardiovascular disease. Circulation *85:*1973–1986, 1992.
40. Bharati S, Krongrad E, Lev M: Study of the conduction system in a population of patients with SIDS. Pediatr Cardiol *6:*29–40, 1985.

D
Role of Triggers in Sudden Cardiac Death

20

Role of Acute Myocardial Ischemia in the Pathogenesis of Sudden Cardiac Death

CHARANJIT S. RIHAL
BERNARD J. GERSH

Since the 1920s, physicians have recognized that patients with "Heberden's angina" are at risk not only for myocardial infarction (MI) but also for sudden unexpected death and that ventricular ectopic beats are a poor prognostic marker in this regard.[1] Prodromal symptoms attributable to coronary artery disease (CAD), such as chest pain and dyspnea, are common in sudden cardiac death (SCD), and in one study they were found in 62% of survivors of SCD.[2]

Of the many manifestations of CAD, SCD represents a particular challenge because logistical constraints radically limit the potential to institute acute therapy. A complete understanding of the pathogenesis of SCD, especially in the context of CAD, is requisite to the effective primary and secondary prevention of SCD. Although a link between CAD and SCD is well established, several unanswered questions remain. How important is myocardial ischemia in the pathogenesis of SCD, how frequently is it the primary inciting factor in SCD, and to what extent does ischemia interact with a fixed substrate in the pathogenesis of SCD? This chapter explores the epidemiological and pathological links between SCD and CAD, discusses the circadian rhythms of cardiovascular diseases, reviews the role of acute and chronic ischemia in the pathogenesis of SCD through examination of several clinical models, and examines the evidence that anti-ischemic treatment modifies SCD event rates.

Definitions of SCD vary, but ideally, the definition should characterize the time from symptom onset, whether the cardiac arrest was witnessed, unexpectedness, and cause.[3] Such a definition would effectively distinguish between the majority of true sudden arrhythmic deaths (whether related to ischemia or not) and those related to congestive heart failure or the mechanical complications of acute MI. As such, witnessed death within 1 hour of onset of symptoms has been advocated as the most useful single operational definition.[4] This definition has been used in numerous epidemiological, pathological, and clinical studies of SCD.

EPIDEMIOLOGICAL EVIDENCE LINKING SUDDEN CARDIAC DEATH AND CORONARY ARTERY DISEASE

Multiple epidemiological studies have demonstrated a link between CAD and SCD. In the Framingham study, more than 50% of coronary *mortality* was related to SCD.[5] CAD and cardiac failure were the two most important risk factors for subsequent SCD (Table 20–1). In men without prior CAD, risk factors for SCD were very similar to those for coronary events in general (Table 20–2).[6] Moreover, no single

Copyright © 1993 Mayo Foundation.

Table 20-1
Risk of Sudden Death by Coronary Heart Disease and Cardiac Failure in 5209 Subjects Aged 35–94 Years: 30-Year Follow-up in the Framingham Study

Cardiovascular Status	Men Biennial Age-Adjusted Rates/1000	Women Biennial Age-Adjusted Rates/1000
No CHD or CHF	3.6	1.5
Previous CHD, no CHF	25.1	4.6
No CHD, previous CHF	24.7	6.1
Previous CHD and CHF	34.2	13.9

SOURCE: Kannel WB, Plehn JF, Cupples LA: Cardiac failure and sudden death in the Framingham study. Am Heart J 115:869, 1988. Reproduced by permission of Mosby–Year Book.
Abbreviations: CHD, coronary heart disease; CHF, congestive heart failure.

characteristic differentiated patients dying of SCD from those dying of MI. In other words, these risk factors were not specific for SCD but only for CAD.[7] In men with known CAD, the only independent risk factors for SCD were the electrocardiographic (ECG) abnormalities of left ventricular (LV) hypertrophy and intraventricular conduction delay,[8,9] presumably in part a reflection of LV dysfunction secondary to ischemic damage.

Further population-based studies have demonstrated that the age-adjusted death rate from ischemic heart disease has decreased by approximately 40% since the early 1960s[10,11] and that this has been paralleled by a similar decrease in out-of-hospital cardiac arrest rates.[12] The 44% decrease in the incidence of out-of-hospital cardiac arrest that occurred in the Worcester Heart Attack Study between 1975 (265/100,000) and 1984 (148/100,000)[13] has been confirmed by numerous other studies.[12,14–18]

On the basis of the epidemiological data, it is apparent that a population at risk for SCD exists and can be identified. In essence, the population at risk is large and consists of patients with risk factors for CAD as well as patients with established CAD. The highest-risk subgroup consists of

Table 20-2
Predictors of Sudden Death by Sex and CHD Status: Framingham Study, 30-Year Follow-up in 5209 Subjects Aged 35–94 Years*

Variable	Men		Women	
	No CHD	Previous CHD	No CHD	Previous CHD
Age (yr)	<0.001	NS	<0.001	<0.01
SBP	NS	NS	NS	NS
Cholesterol	<0.01	NS	NS	NS
Cigarette smoking	<0.01	NS	NS	NS
Glucose intolerance	NS	NS	NS	<0.05
ECG LVH	<0.001	<0.001	NS	NS
Previous CHF	<0.05	<0.01	NS	NS
Previous VA	NS	<0.05	<0.001	NS

SOURCE: Kannel WB, Plehn JF, Cupples LA: Cardiac failure and sudden death in the Framingham study. Am Heart J 115:869, 1988. Modified by permission of Mosby–Year Book.
Abbreviations: CHD, coronary heart disease; CHF, congestive heart failure; LVH, left ventricular hypertrophy; NS, not significant; SBP, systolic blood pressure; VA, ventricular arrhythmia.
* Numbers indicate P value.

patients with cardiac failure secondary to MI. It is also apparent that longitudinal trends in the incidence of SCD closely parallel those of MI. These data strongly suggest a common pathogenetic link between SCD and other acute coronary syndromes and suggest that interventions for CAD may have a substantial impact on SCD.

Circadian Variations in SCD

Not only have longitudinal trends in SCD paralleled those of MI, but circadian variations in the occurrence of SCD and other cardiovascular events are also remarkably similar (Fig. 20–1). A significant diurnal variation in SCD, with a peak incidence at 7 A.M. to 11 A.M., was observed in a study of the death certificates of 2203 patients who sustained out-of-hospital cardiac arrests in Massachusetts in 1983.[19] This diurnal variation was supported by data from the Framingham study that demonstrated a peak incidence of SCD between 7 A.M. and 9 A.M. and a decreased incidence between 9 A.M. and 1 P.M. (the risk of SCD was 70% higher during the peak period).[20]

Analogous circadian rhythms have been demonstrated in other cardiovascular processes, for example nonfatal MI, by the Multicenter Investigation of the Limitation of Infarct Size (MILIS)[21] and Intravenous Streptokinase in Acute Myocardial Infarction (ISAM) studies.[22] Similar diurnal variations have been observed for myocardial ischemia[23,24] as assessed by ST-segment depression on ambulatory ECG[25–28] (even when adjusted for varying sleep time, activity, and heart rate[25]) and for stroke.[29,30]

A number of different physiological processes may underlie the observed diurnal variations, including morning peaks in catecholamine release,[31,32] heart rate, blood pressure,[32,33] and levels of plasma cortisol.[31,34]

Although ischemia is tightly coupled to heart rate in patients with CAD,[35] the ischemic threshold is clearly variable[24] because similar levels of tachycardia are more likely to induce ischemia in the morning.[25] Also, the exercise threshold for ischemia is shorter in the morning in patients with CAD.[36] Such findings may reflect greater morning coronary vascular tone.[36,37]

Not only are there hemodynamic changes

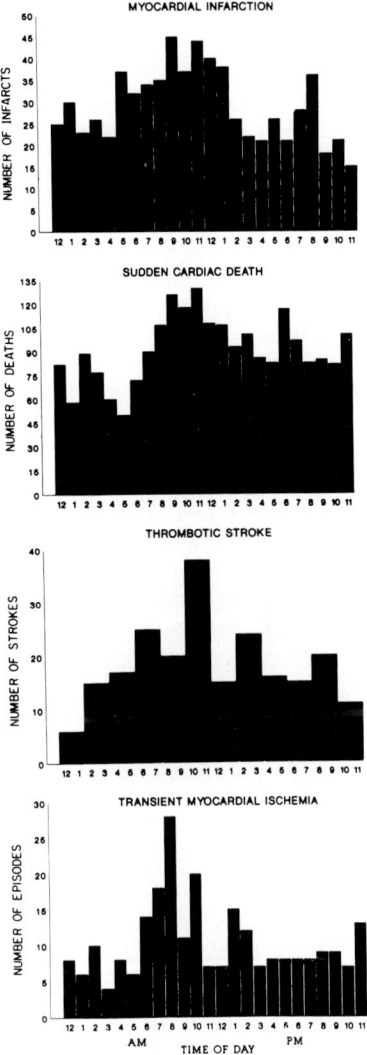

Fig. 20–1. Bar graphs of time of day of onset of myocardial infarction, sudden cardiac death, stroke, and transient myocardial ischemia in four different groups of patients. Number of events is shown on the y-axis and hour of day on the x-axis. Each disorder exhibits a prominent increase in frequency of onset from 6:00 A.M. to noon. (Reproduced by permission of the American Heart Association from Muller JE, et al: Circulation 79:733, 1989.[32])

throughout the course of the day that exert a significant impact on the coronary circulation, but the platelet-clotting system also exhibits important intrinsic physiological diurnal variations.[38–41] In view of the important role that has been suggested for plaque rupture and intracoronary platelet deposition in SCD, such diurnal variations may provide further clues to the links between ischemia in chronic CAD and the triggers of the acute coronary syndromes, including SCD. Major diurnal fluctuations in the intrinsic fibrinolytic system have also been observed (Fig. 20–2).[42–44] Native tissue plasminogen activator activity is lowest in the morning and correlates inversely with plasminogen activator inhibitor activity in patients with CAD and in normal subjects.[43,45]

What physiological processes trigger ischemic sudden death in patients with CAD? Mechanisms that might precipitate ischemia and act as a trigger for arrhythmias in previously asymptomatic patients include abnormal coronary vasomotor responses,[46–50] exercise,[51–53] smoking,[54–58] and mental stress.[59–62] Among patients with LV dysfunction, enhanced cardiac sympathetic activation may contribute importantly in the genesis of malignant ventricular arrhythmias.[63] The role of specific electrophysiological triggers is beyond the scope of this chapter.

ANATOMICAL EXTENT OF CAD IN SCD

Angiographic Series

In general, the clinical and angiographic features of patients suffering SCD are similar to those of patients with unstable angina or MI.[64] The similarity suggests a common pathogenesis.[65–67] Various angiographic and pathological studies have conclusively demonstrated a high prevalence of severe CAD in both survivors and nonsurvivors of SCD.[12,68–71] For example, among 761 patients dying suddenly (1-hour definition) in the Coronary Artery Surgery Study (CASS), 51% had three-vessel disease and 28% had two-vessel disease.[65] It is noteworthy that the majority of these patients had evidence of either LV dysfunction or viable myocardial segments subserved by arteries

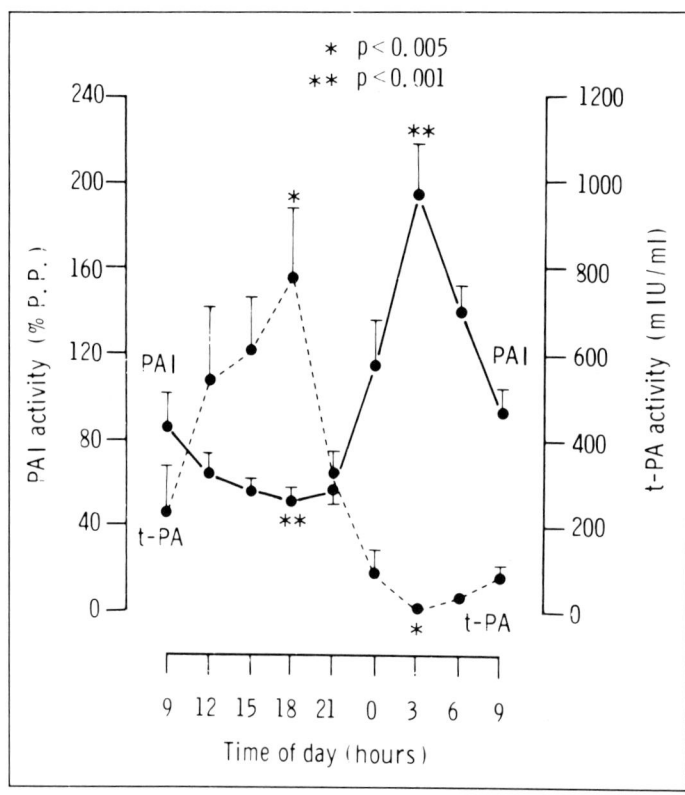

Fig. 20–2. Observed plasma activities of tissue plasminogen activator (t-PA) (dashed curve) and plasminogen activator inhibitor (PAI) (continuous curve) over 24 hours (mean ± SE). Asterisks indicate significant difference ($p < 0.005$ for t-PA; $p < 0.001$ for PAI) between peak and nadir values. (Reproduced by permission of Cahners Publishing Co, a division of Reed Publishing USA, from Andreotti F, et al: Am J Cardiol 62:635, 1988.[43])

with hemodynamically significant stenoses (or both). This suggests the possibility of an interaction between myocardial ischemia and ventricular dysfunction (or scar) in the pathogenesis of SCD (see below). Patients dying of nonsudden but other cardiac causes had similar angiographic and hemodynamic features. Similar results have been reported in other angiographic series of SCD survivors.[68,69,72]

Pathological Series

From a pathological standpoint, an early study from Seattle of 87 cases of SCD occurring within 12 hours of symptoms (the majority were witnessed deaths occurring within 10 minutes of symptom onset) reported a 26% prevalence of recent or healing MI and a 21% prevalence of old MI.[70] Intracoronary thrombus was found only in 10% of the cases, but 59% had at least one coronary occlusion and 39% had at least one 90% stenosis. No major clinical or pathological differences were found between those dying of ventricular fibrillation ($n = 34$) when compared with those dying of asystole ($n = 26$) or when compared with 64 patients successfully resuscitated from ventricular fibrillation (VF).[70] In another autopsy study of 70 patients who died suddenly within 6 hours of onset of symptoms, stenoses of more than 75% diameter were noted in up to 30% of coronary artery segments, and actual intracoronary thrombus was present in 18.6%.[71] CAD has also been demonstrated to be the most important pathological finding in well-conditioned middle-aged subjects suffering SCD.[73]

Role of Acute Arterial Injury

Coronary thrombosis has not been a universal finding in pathological series of SCD. However, Davies[74] pointed out that although the prevalence of intracoronary thrombi varied from 4 to 74% in published series,[70] this range likely reflected methodological differences, interobserver variability, and the fact that many autopsies performed on victims of sudden death were of a forensic, not scientific, nature.

To further elucidate the role of acute arterial injury and platelet deposition in SCD associated with CAD, 100 subjects dying of ischemic heart disease within 6 hours of symptom onset were compared to 78 control subjects who died of noncardiac causes.[75] With the use of rigorous pathological methodology, 74 cases were found to have an intraluminal thrombus and 21 others to have intraintimal thrombi (with plaque fissuring in 19) (Fig. 20–3). Only five subjects in this series did not have an acute arterial lesion. In contrast, only 10.2% of controls had an acute arterial lesion on pathological examination. Although this study may have included some subjects admitted to the hospital with unstable angina or acute MI, subgroup analysis of patients dying within 1 hour (better conforming to strict epidemiological and clinical definitions of SCD) did demonstrate an acute arterial injury in 43 (72.8%) of 59 such patients.

Similarly, platelet aggregates in small *intramyocardial* arteries were found in 27 (30%) of 90 patients dying suddenly of is-

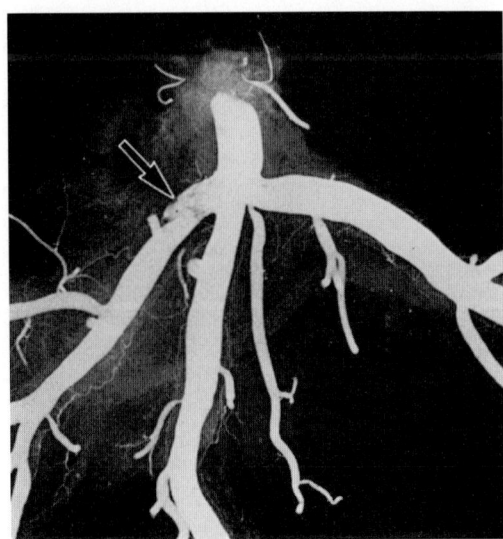

Fig. 20–3. Postmortem angiogram of an extremely fit 44-year-old man with no previous history of angina. During a game of squash he suddenly felt unwell with chest pain and died 30 minutes later. The left anterior descending artery divided into two major branches immediately after its origin. One branch showed an intraluminal filling defect (arrow) associated with an irregular intimal outline. Histology confirmed a fissure of a plaque with overlying thrombus. The remainder of the coronary artery tree was normal on angiography and histology. (Reproduced by permission of the *British Heart Journal* from Davies MJ, et al: Br Heart J 53:363, 1985.[87])

chemic heart disease. In such cases, the proximal major epicardial vessel frequently had evidence of plaque fissuring and mural thrombosis.[76] The prevalence of acute arterial injury in patients dying of SCD or unstable angina was similar, but it was less than in patients dying of acute MI.[67]

The data mentioned above strongly implicate acute arterial injury, platelet deposition, and embolism of platelet aggregates in the pathogenesis of SCD. Furthermore, these data are consistent with epidemiological links between SCD, CAD, and other acute coronary syndromes.

Importance of Coronary Collateralization

A number of convergent lines of clinical investigation suggest an important role for coronary collateral circulation in "protecting" patients with CAD from SCD. It has been demonstrated in *healthy* men ($n = 894$; mean follow-up, 12.7 years) screened by exercise testing that the initial coronary event was MI or SCD in 73% of those with normal results on the exercise test. However, in 80% of the 61 subjects whose test results were abnormal, angina pectoris was the initial manifestation of CAD.[77]

Because coronary collaterals develop in response to chronic, hemodynamically significant CAD[78] and exert a protective effect on regional LV function during coronary occlusion,[79] Epstein et al[80] hypothesized that sudden occlusion of a minimally stenosed coronary artery (putatively precipitated by plaque rupture and superimposed thrombosis) usually results in SCD or acute MI. Conversely, occlusion of a chronic, severe stenosis may be asymptomatic or produce acceleration of angina (Fig. 20–4).

That sudden occlusion of previously minimally stenosed coronary arteries does indeed occur and can result in serious clinical events has been confirmed by retrospective analyses of coronary angiograms that were obtained prior to MI.[81,82] Furthermore, these data are congruent with observations that non-flow-limiting residual coronary stenoses are present in a minority of patients after thrombolytic therapy for acute MI.[83]

The postulated role of occlusion of previously minimally stenosed coronary arteries in the pathogenesis of SCD is consistent with the identified epidemiological risk factors for SCD and may explain why physiological exercise testing cannot specifically identify a subgroup at risk for SCD. However, these concepts are at variance with the angiographic and pathological data cited

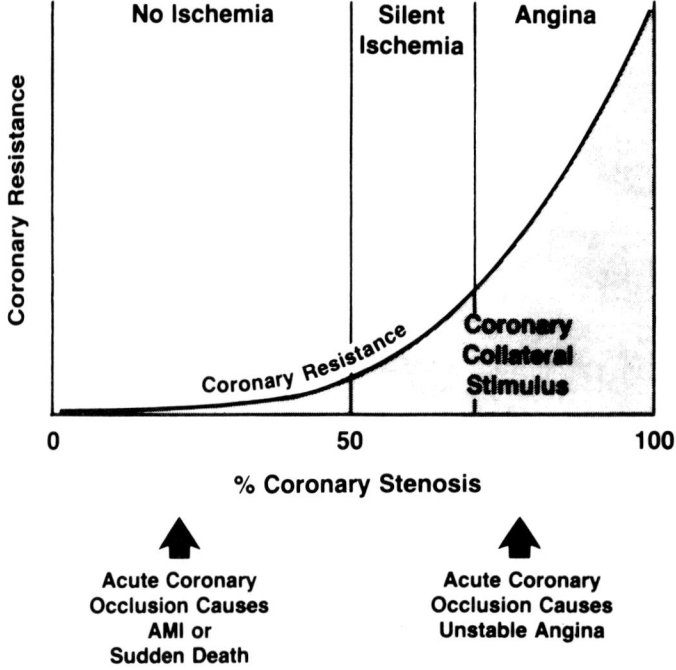

Fig. 20–4. Postulated relationship among severity of stenosis, coronary resistance, development of collaterals, and myocardial ischemia. AMI, acute myocardial infarction. (Reproduced by permission of the *New England Journal of Medicine* from Epstein SE, et al: N Engl J Med *321:* 320, 1989.[80])

above that demonstrate a high prevalence of severe coronary stenoses in patients succumbing to SCD.[84] Further basic and clinical research is required to fully define the pathological mechanisms in SCD.

Unifying Pathological Paradigm

On the basis of the above data, it is apparent that there is an identifiable population of patients at risk for SCD and that these patients are similar to those at risk for other acute coronary events. The frequency with which severe CAD and LV dysfunction are observed at autopsy in these patients confirms the primacy of CAD and congestive heart failure as risk factors for SCD and points to an interaction between ischemia and LV dysfunction in SCD.

In the presence of an as yet unidentified hemodynamic or rheologic trigger(s), plaque fissuring or rupture (or both) occurs and exposes the coronary circulation to highly thrombogenic substances.[85,86] Coronary thrombosis supervenes and in many cases (perhaps especially in patients without the protective shield of arterial collaterals) leads to SCD or acute MI.[87,88] Although these mechanisms may explain many cases of sudden death in patients with CAD, it should be emphasized that in many other patients, SCD undoubtedly is the result of an electrical trigger, such as premature ventricular contractions, that interacts with a fixed electrophysiological substrate. A discussion of such mechanisms is beyond the scope of this chapter and is covered elsewhere.

SCD ASSOCIATED WITH ACUTE MYOCARDIAL INFARCTION

Although the emphasis of this chapter is not on SCD associated with acute MI, the strongest documented link between severe myocardial ischemia and life-threatening ventricular arrhythmias is in this subgroup; for this reason, some discussion is appropriate. It is recognized that VF is not an infrequent complication of acute MI[89] and that it tends to occur with larger infarcts,[90,91] but not exclusively.[92] Of note, conduction delays are more common in MIs complicated by VF.[93] This is consistent with the epidemiological data cited earlier and may reflect infarct size.

Sudden death, most often due to VF, is most common in the 6-month period after MI and is independently predicted by ejection fraction,[94,95] extent of CAD,[96] premature ventricular beats,[94,95,97] late potentials,[98] myocardial ischemia on exercise testing,[99] and decreased heart rate variability.[100,101] In the Multicenter Post-Infarction Prognosis (MPIP) study of 867 patients, symptoms of myocardial ischemia were strongly associated with SCD during the 2-year follow-up period: 107 witnessed SCDs (1-hour definition) occurred, with preceding ischemic symptoms in 60%.[102]

Cellular Mechanisms

Janse and Kléber[103] and Fozzard and Makielski[104] have reviewed the cellular electrophysiological changes that occur during experimental coronary artery ligation. Accumulation of extracellular potassium, increased resting membrane potential, decreased amplitude, upstroke velocity, and duration of the action potential, and dispersion of refractoriness may contribute to electrical instability. Local excitability and conduction velocity increase initially and then decrease. Circus-movement depolarization wave fronts (circulating excitation) around areas of conduction block have been demonstrated 2–10 minutes after ligation of the coronary artery.[103]

It is possible that "reperfusion arrhythmias" may be relevant to SCD in some patients.[105] Manning and Hearse[106] reviewed the mechanisms involved in arrhythmogenesis during reperfusion after coronary artery occlusion and suggested that the heterogeneity in patterns of electrophysiological recovery, including that of refractoriness, may create an unstable electrophysiological milieu capable of sustaining ventricular arrhythmias. Such mechanisms may be important in subsets of patients with variant angina or spontaneous reperfusion after sudden coronary occlusion.

In summary, experimental and, by extrapolation, clinical occlusion of the coronary artery are associated with major electrophysiological abnormalities at the cellular and tissue level that predispose to the initiation and maintenance of re-entrant arrhythmias and ultimately to VF. VF is common during early MI in the presence of acute severe ischemia, and late sudden deaths are frequently preceded by ischemic symptoms. LV dysfunction is a significant factor in *both* situations.[107] Arrhythmogenesis in these subjects is complex and multifactorial.

CLINICAL ARRHYTHMIAS UNDERLYING SCD AND THE ROLE OF ISCHEMIA

Electrocardiographic Studies in Patients with SCD

In the Seattle experience, VF was the most common arrhythmia at the time of resuscitation. VF occurred in 75% of cases, asystole in 20%, and electromechanical dissociation in 5%.[108,109] Ventricular tachycardia (VT) was infrequent and was found in approximately 1% of cases.[110] The high frequency of VF may reflect deterioration from VT (see below), because even in this optimal setting advanced cardiac life support (ACLS) response times averaged 6 minutes. In the Miami experience, based on 352 patients, the initial rhythms recorded were VF in 62% and bradyarrhythmias or asystole in 31%.

Insight into the arrhythmic mechanisms of sudden death and the role of ischemia has been garnered through analyses of ambulatory ECG tracings recorded at the time of SCD (Fig. 20-5).[111-117] Bayés de Luna et al[118] compiled data from ten published series (157 cases) and pointed out that VT degenerating to VF accounted for 62% of the cases, VF without preceding VT for 8%, torsades de pointes for 13%, and bradyarrhythmias for 17%. In five series, ST-segment shifts were noted in only 12.6% of cases prior to the terminal arrhythmia.[118] In

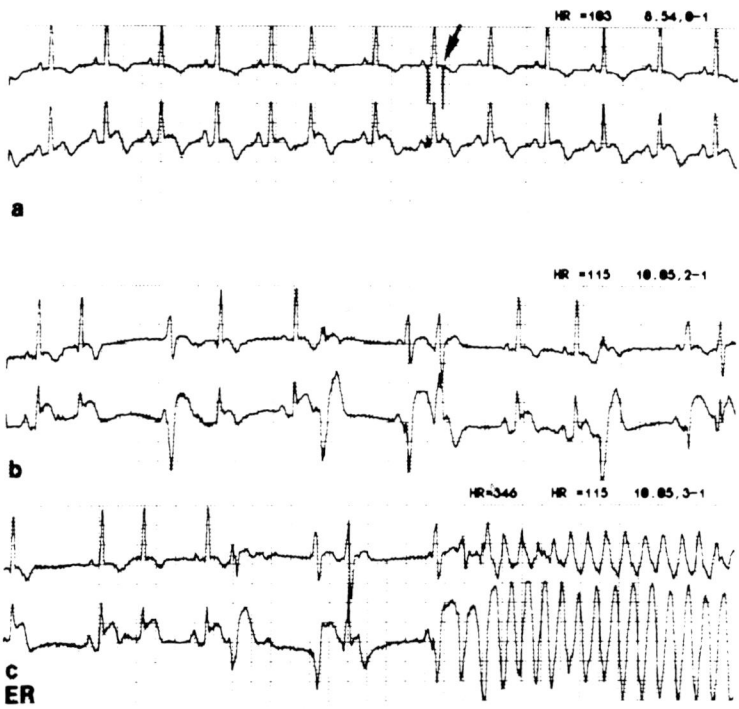

Fig. 20-5. Two-channel Holter electrocardiogram. **a.** Baseline ECG at start of recording period; arrow indicates the two markers for definition of ST segment. **b.** and **c.** Continuous ECG preceding ventricular fibrillation. Marked ST-segment changes (clearly visible in only one lead) are accompanied by complex ventricular arrhythmias. (Reproduced by permission of Cahners Publishing Co, a division of Reed Publishing USA, from Hohnloser SH, et al: Silent myocardial ischemia as a predisposing factor for ventricular fibrillation. Am J Cardiol 61:461, 1988.)

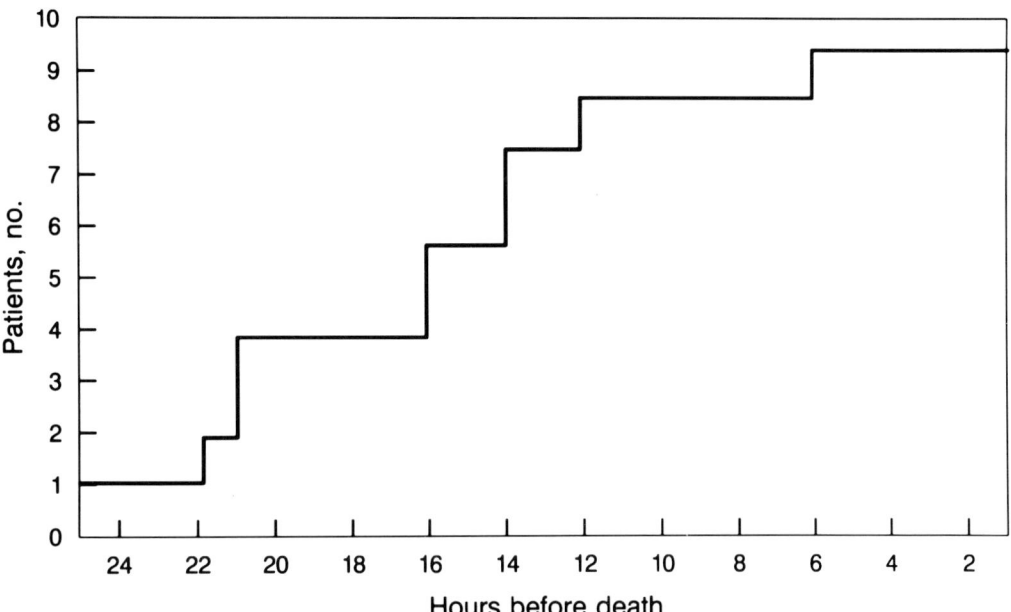

Fig. 20-6. Linear trend analysis of number of patients with ST-segment changes during 24-hour period preceding death ($n = 14$). (Modified with permission from Savage HR, et al: Clin Cardiol *10:* 621, 1987.[119])

one series, in which attention was directed to ischemic changes, the frequency and degree of ST-segment shifts and VT increased during the final 6 hours of life (Fig. 20-6).[119] Ambulatory ECG data obtained more recently demonstrated ST shifts in 34% of cases prior to SCD and suggested that preceding myocardial ischemia may be more common than was previously appreciated.[120]

Although the relatively low incidence of ST-segment shifts prior to terminal events militates against ischemia as a harbinger of SCD in the *majority* of patients, myocardial ischemia may still play an important role in a substantial absolute *number* of patients simply because of the large population of patients with CAD. Ambulatory ECG studies have suggested that, as a conservative estimate, ischemia is present prior to SCD in 10-15% of patients[121] and, in fact, may be present in up to 50%.[120] It is important to note that such studies may underestimate the true incidence of ischemia in ambulatory patients prior to SCD, for a number of reasons: patients wearing ECG monitors are a selected group and may not be representative of the entire population at risk for SCD, and the sensitivity of ambulatory monitoring for myocardial ischemia may be compromised by the usual practice of recording from only one or two leads and by the fact that ST-segment shifts are generally not the initial manifestation of myocardial ischemia.[122]

Clinical Observations in Patients with CAD

Although correlations between SCD and acute MI provide useful mechanistic information, it should be emphasized that SCD generally is not the consequence of acute MI. Acute MI has been diagnosed in as few as 17% of SCD victims,[123] but the reported prevalence of MI in SCD ranges from 17 to 68%.[70]

The hypothesis that sudden death, usually due to VF, may result from profound myocardial ischemia is supported by clinical experience (Fig. 20-7). Asymptomatic (silent) ischemia due to epicardial coronary artery spasm was clearly associated with life-threatening ventricular tachyarrhythmias among five survivors of out-of-hospital cardiac arrest. Only four of the five had had

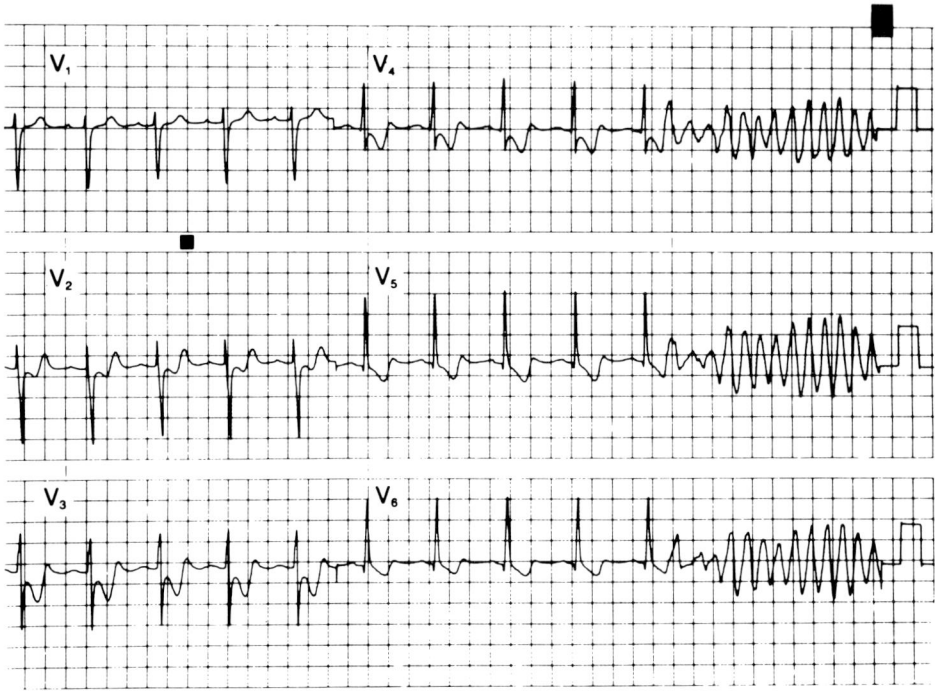

Fig. 20–7. Postexercise 12-lead ECG in a 59-year-old woman with no prior cardiac history who experienced SCD, successful resuscitation, and a negative invasive electrophysiological evaluation. Exercise testing was strongly positive, and VF was initiated by two PVCs during the recovery phase. Coronary angiography disclosed a 60% LAD lesion and occlusion of the first diagonal branch; wall motion was normal. After coronary artery bypass operation, results of exercise study were normal and no cardiac events occurred during 15 months of follow-up on no medications. This case illustrates the interaction between ischemia and electrophysiological triggers in the genesis of SCD. V_1–V_6, precordial ECG leads. (Reproduced by permission of the American Medical Association from Hong RA, et al: Life-threatening ventricular tachycardia and fibrillation induced by painless myocardial ischemia during exercise testing. JAMA 257:1937, 1987.)

an otherwise inducible arrhythmia at electrophysiological study.[124] In an analysis of 17 survivors of exercise-related SCD, Ciampricotti and colleagues[125] pointed out that in all patients, SCD was associated with acute coronary artery occlusion, unstable angina, or asymptomatic ST-segment depression. Exercise-induced painless myocardial ischemia has been demonstrated in survivors of VF, albeit in a minority of them,[126–128] and "silent" ischemia on exercise testing predicted subsequent SCD among CASS registry patients with three-vessel CAD (Fig. 20–8).[129]

True variant angina (defined as chest pain associated with ST-segment elevation, relieved promptly by nitrates, and without evidence of MI) is a useful clinical model of paroxysmal, severe myocardial ischemia.

Ventricular arrhythmias have been closely linked to ischemia in patients with true variant angina: approximately 45% of subjects had serious rhythm disturbances during ischemic episodes. On follow-up, SCD occurred in 42% of patients with arrhythmias during ischemic episodes but in only 6% of those without ischemia-induced arrhythmias.[130] These data have been corroborated in a study of 26 patients with variant angina, in whom VT and complex ectopy occurred only during ST-segment elevation and were more common during symptomatic than during asymptomatic episodes. Most arrhythmias occurred during the resolution (and presumably the "reperfusion") phase of ST-segment elevation.[131] Two studies of patients with Prinzmetal's angina documented that ventricular arrhythmias devel-

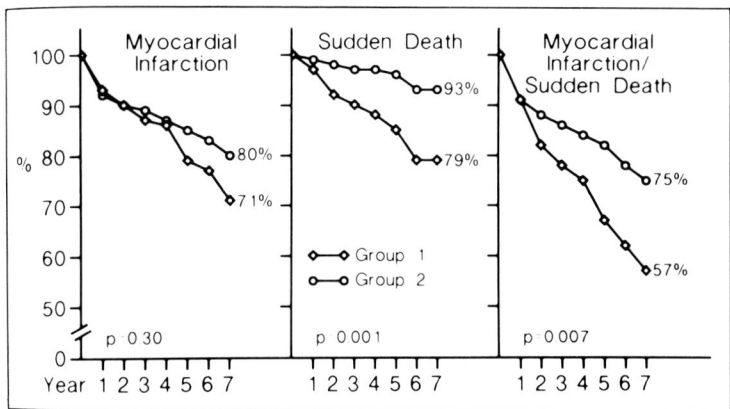

Fig. 20–8. Cumulative 7-year probability of remaining free of myocardial infarction *(left)*, sudden death *(center)*, and the combined end points *(right)* among group 1 and group 2 patients with three-vessel coronary artery disease. Sudden death and combined end points were more frequent among group 1 patients. Group 1, painless ST-segment depression on exercise testing ($n = 424$); group 2, symptomatic ST-segment depression ($n = 456$). (Reproduced by permission of Cahners Publishing Co, a division of Reed Publishing USA, from Weiner DA, et al: Am J Cardiol 62:1155, 1988.[129])

oped in approximately 50% of patients and were likely to be associated with a symptomatic episode of ischemia, longer duration of ischemia, and more extensive ST-segment shifts.[132,133]

That the severity of myocardial ischemia is important in provoking ventricular arrhythmias is further supported by two ambulatory ECG studies of patients with chronic stable angina pectoris. Patients with ectopy during ischemia had greater ST-segment depression, a greater number of ischemic episodes, and longer duration of ischemia.[134,135] Arrhythmias tended to occur more often during the resolution phase of ST-segment elevation and were more frequently associated with R-on-T phenomena.[134] Patients with ectopy had a greater proportion of symptomatic ischemic episodes, and arrhythmias were more likely to occur during symptomatic attacks of ischemia as opposed to "silent" ischemia.[135] In one study, early arrhythmias were of greater frequency, duration, and malignancy than those occurring during resolution.[135] These data point in one direction: The greater the severity of ischemia, the greater is the likelihood of ventricular arrhythmias.

However, it should be emphasized that this association is *not* present in the majority of patients with CAD.[136,137] In three studies of patients ($n = 189$) with chronic stable angina pectoris, ST-segment depression was associated with ventricular ectopy in only 31.[27,134,135]

In the randomized Cardiac Arrhythmia Suppression Trial (CAST) of 1498 patients,[138,139] the use of flecainide or encainide after MI was associated with lower survival when compared to those taking placebo. Of note, there were no differences between these groups in the incidence of *nonfatal* arrhythmic end points or in the incidence of recurrent MI, angina, or bypass operation.[138] These observations suggest that an interaction between ischemia, myocardial scar, and proarrhythmia may exist and may explain the excess mortality among patients treated with antiarrhythmia agents.[140,141] Further basic and clinical investigations are necessary to identify the mechanisms involved.

Other investigators[121,142] have argued against a role for ischemia and have presented evidence to support the pivotal importance of the arrhythmic substrate in patients with CAD. A greater proportion of patients with ventricular arrhythmias had evidence of an arrhythmic substrate (positive programmed stimulation or signal-averaged ECG) when compared to patients with stable angina pectoris but no arrhythmias. Silent ischemia was equally prevalent in both groups.[142] Thus, the authors concluded that in their patient population ischemia did not play a critical role in the pathogenesis of either VT or VF. Instead, electrophysiological triggers, such as the "short-long" sequence, were thought to be more important in the spontaneous initiation of these events[142] and are discussed elsewhere. The same investigators have also identified the presence of late potentials and an ejection fraction below 40% as the most important predictors of late VT or VF after acute MI.[98,143]

Implications of Electrophysiological Studies

Programmed electrical stimulation has not only drawn attention to the importance of a structural substrate in the genesis of malignant ventricular arrhythmias, it has also produced a persuasive argument for a role for other factors, including ischemia, in arrhythmogenesis. Approximately one third of SCD survivors were found to be noninducible at electrophysiological study.[72,144–148] Failure to induce sustained ventricular arrhythmias despite aggressive programmed stimulation implies that the requisite electrophysiological substrate is either transitory or modifiable by such variable external factors as ischemia, autonomic tone, antiarrhythmia drugs, and electrolyte imbalances. In this regard, survivors of SCD who are noninducible more frequently have myocardium subserved by arteries with complicated lesions (irregular or with intraluminal filling defects) or by only collateral vessels (Fig. 20-9).[149] In one study, complex coronary artery lesions were found in 50% of SCD survivors who were noninducible at electrophysiological study but in only 19% of those with inducible ventricular arrhythmias.[150]

In summary, the fact that SCD may occur during angina or exercise in patients with obstructive CAD[151] and that noninducible SCD survivors with obstructive CAD or spasm have an excellent prognosis when treated for the underlying CAD[151,152] supports the hypothesis that in many patients with CAD, the presence of ischemia is a crucial and integral harbinger of the final, fatal arrhythmic event.

Are there important structural differences in the myocardium between subjects who are or are not inducible? SCD survivors with CAD have higher inducibility rates than those without CAD (69% vs. 40%) at electrophysiological study.[146] In the subgroup of SCD survivors with CAD, those who were inducible had a higher prevalence of prior MI, congestive heart failure, low ejection fraction, and akinetic or dyskinetic LV segments.[145,152] Noninducible SCD survivors had a greater number of noninfarcted LV subserved by coronary arteries with lesions of 70% or more in diameter. Also, clinical and ECG features suggestive of acute ischemia at the onset of VF were more common in this group.[152]

The relationship between inducibility at electrophysiological study and myocardial ischemia was determined by direct measurement of arterial–coronary sinus lactate differences in 19 survivors of SCD who had at least one 70% or greater stenosis of the left coronary arterial system. Preceding ischemia (i.e., net myocardial lactate production) was present in 8 of 15 patients with inducible VT; 5 of 6 of these patients were noninducible in the *absence* of ischemia on repeat testing.[153] Programmed ventricular stimulation during variant angina due to angiographically confirmed coronary vasospasm was successful in inducing sustained VT, whereas stimulation during the basal state was not.[154]

In regard to the assessment of long-term prognosis in survivors of SCD, it is known that electrophysiological evaluation (invasive or noninvasive) alone incompletely characterizes prognosis, and other sequelae of CAD must be taken into account.[72,155,156] In one study, reversible defects on thallium-201 scintigraphy had a positive predictive value of 63% and a negative predictive value of 82% for recurrence of ventricular arrhythmias, which is almost as accurate as electrophysiological study (positive predictive value, 83%; negative predictive value, 86%).[157] Similarly, in patients with CAD, prior MI has been demonstrated to be the most important predictor of recurrent SCD and noninducibility to be of lesser value.[146] The data presented above strongly implicate acute myocardial ischemia in the genesis of VF in patients with CAD.

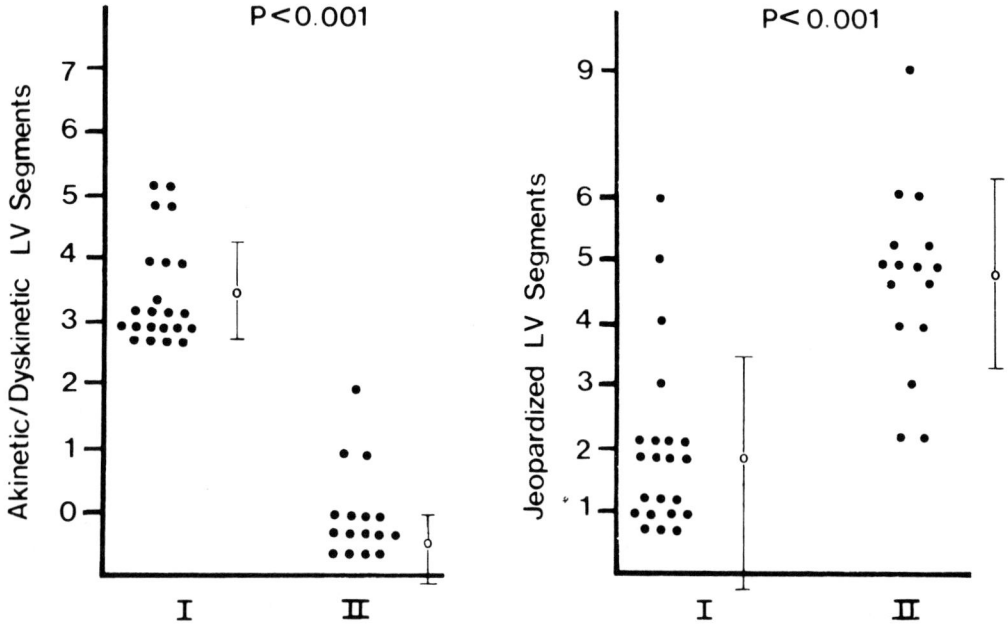

Fig. 20–9. Distribution of akinetic or dyskinetic left ventricular (LV) segments *(left)* and jeopardized LV segments *(right)* for inducible (group I) and noninducible (group II) sudden death survivors. (Reproduced by permission of Mosby-Year Book from Kehoe R, et al: Am Heart J *116:*355, 1988.[152])

Differences Between Patients with Ventricular Fibrillation and Patients with Ventricular Tachycardia

The possibility that the underlying electrophysiological substrate differs between patients presenting with VT and those presenting with VF is supported by direct evidence.[158,159] With the use of signal-averaged ECG and endocardial catheter mapping, Vaitkus and colleagues[147] examined the underlying electrophysiological substrate in 133 patients with angiographically documented CAD, 85 of whom presented with hemodynamically stable sustained monomorphic VT and 48 of whom were resuscitated from a witnessed SCD. Significant differences were found: a greater proportion of patients with sustained monomorphic VT had structural heart damage (previous MI or LV aneurysm), inducible arrhythmias (85% vs. 68%), and abnormalities of endocardial activation (53% vs. 40%) or on the signal-averaged ECG (87% vs. 63%).[147] These data strongly implicate a fixed substrate secondary to previous myocardial damage and reentrant circuits in the pathogenesis of sustained monomorphic VT. On the other hand, in patients with CAD, SCD due to VF may represent a heterogeneous group of cardiac rhythm abnormalities that reflect the interaction between fixed substrate and other transitory factors such as acute myocardial ischemia. Polymorphic VT (without underlying QT prolongation) may also be associated with myocardial ischemia[160,161] and may respond to revascularization.[160] It is noteworthy that approximately one third of SCD survivors are noninducible at electrophysiological study, a finding that is remarkably consistent across different studies.[72,144–148] It is in these patients that factors other than fixed electrophysiological substrate may be implicated.

Similar results demonstrating a greater prevalence of late potentials,[162] inducible ventricular arrhythmias,[148,162] and structural abnormalities[163] among patients with sustained monomorphic VT as compared to those with VF have been reported in the literature. In addition, patients presenting with SCD may have an electrophysiological propensity to lethal arrhythmias because induced ventricular arrhythmias tend to be polymorphic, have shorter cycle lengths, and frequently degenerate into VF.[147,163] In comparison, patients presenting with hemodynamically stable sustained monomorphic VT tend to have the same arrhythmia at electrophysiological study.[147] Although VF is the most commonly observed initial rhythm during resuscitation from SCD, ambulatory ECG studies of SCD have demonstrated that VF is usually preceded by VT.[118]

SCD AND CAD: RESULTS OF THERAPEUTIC STRATEGIES

Medical Therapy

Prospective randomized controlled trials of β-blocker therapy after acute MI have consistently demonstrated a decrease in total mortality[164–166]—related primarily to a decrease in SCD—that is present in the first few months after MI[165,167] and is sustained on long-term follow-up.[164,166] In a meta-analysis of 16 trials (involving more than 18,000 patients) of long-term β-blockade after MI, the risk of death was decreased from approximately 10% to 8% (pooled relative risk was 0.77).[168] Approximately half of all deaths that occurred during follow-up were classified as sudden. Also, a highly significant decrease in the odds ratio of SCD (approximately 30%) was observed, but the decrease in odds ratio of nonsudden deaths was 12% (Fig. 20–10). The greatest decrease in mortality was observed in trials using β-blockers without intrinsic sympathomimetic activity,[168] although this distinction was not absolute.[169] Heterogeneity in study designs is inherent and must be borne in mind in the interpretation of pooled data; however, its effects in this analysis were minimized by comparing only treated with control subjects in the same trial.[168] An important clinical question is whether the primary mechanism of protection is through an antiarrhythmic effect, an anti-ischemic effect, or a combined effect. Thus, it is noteworthy that similar effects have generally not been demonstrated for another class of anti-ischemic agents, the calcium channel blockers.[170–172] Anecdotally, calcium channel blockers have been tried among survivors of cardiac arrest with ventricular arrhythmias documented to be associated with coronary spasm.[124]

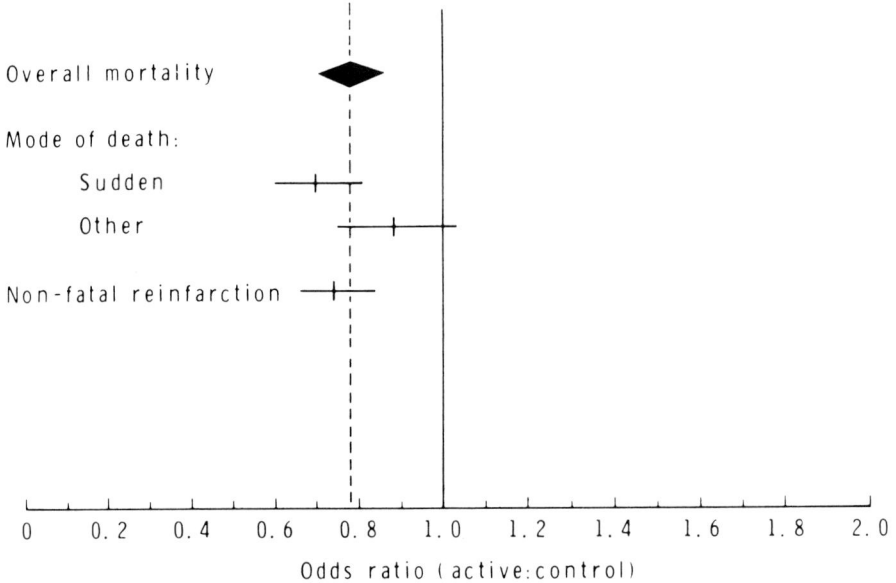

Fig. 20–10. Sudden death, other death, and nonfatal reinfarction in long-term β-blocker trials that reported these end points separately: odds ratios (active:control) with approximate 95% confidence ranges. (Reproduced by permission of WB Saunders from Yusuf S, et al: Prog Cardiovasc Dis 27: 335, 1985.[168])

Because β-blockers have complex actions in CAD, it is possible that the beneficial properties of these agents are due to more than simply an anti-ischemic action. Although sympathetic attenuation and β-receptor blockade decrease myocardial oxygen demand,[173] β-blockers also increase the threshold for VF in ischemic myocardium[174] and have demonstrable benefit in subsets of MI patients who have survived an episode of VF.[164,175] β-Blockers eliminate the circadian morning peaks in MI[21,22,176] and asymptomatic ST-segment depression,[26] and they decrease the incidence of ventricular arrhythmias 6 weeks after MI.[177] These effects are not observed with calcium channel blockers.[26]

It has been postulated that the primary beneficial effect of β-blocker therapy may be to protect vulnerable atherosclerotic plaques from rupture and subsequent thrombosis by attenuating catecholamine surges.[178,179] Thus, the mechanism of benefit of β-blocker therapy in the prophylaxis of SCD after MI is likely multifactorial, with anti-ischemic and other mechanisms playing important roles. Equally important is the fact that such benefits have not been duplicated with pure antiarrhythmic agents after MI in randomized, controlled clinical trials.[138,180] The salutary effects of aspirin and possibly sulfinpyrazone in reducing vascular (many likely sudden) deaths after MI are consistent with the above pathophysiological paradigm.[181–184]

Surgical Therapy

Myocardial revascularization is a frequently used treatment in many patients at risk for SCD[72,146] and may have major clinical electrophysiological consequences.[185–187] In patients with CAD, the major impact of coronary artery bypass surgery (CABG) has been on sudden death rates, as opposed to the prevention of MI or deaths from congestive heart failure.[188–190] In the CASS registry, the proportion of patients suffering SCD (1-hour definition) was significantly decreased over a mean follow-up period of 4.6 years.[190] These differences were most pronounced for higher-risk subsets such as those with three-vessel CAD and a history of congestive heart failure. In this subgroup, 91% of

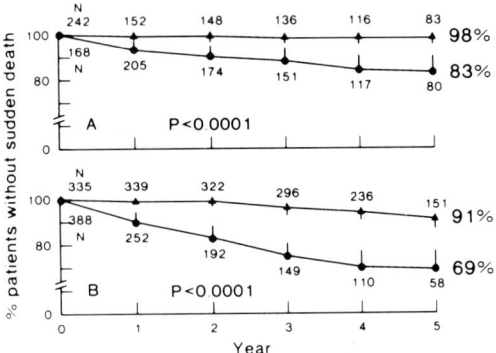

Fig. 20–11. Percent of patients without sudden cardiac death in surgically treated group (triangles) compared with that in medically treated group (circles) in the Coronary Artery Surgery Study (CASS). All patients had a history of congestive heart failure. **A,** Patients with two-vessel disease. **B,** Patients with three-vessel disease. The actual number of patients are given for each survival curve. (Reproduced by permission of the American Heart Association from Holmes DR Jr, et al: Circulation 73:1254, 1986.[190])

patients were free of SCD at 5 years when treated surgically, versus 69% of medically treated patients (Fig. 20–11).[190] Again, these data reinforce the importance of the interaction between ischemia and LV dysfunction in patients susceptible to SCD.

What is the effect of revascularization in survivors of SCD? Although there are few data, two nonrandomized trials imply a benefit of surgical revascularization among survivors of SCD.[191,192] Nevertheless, it should be emphasized that among survivors of out-of-hospital cardiac arrest, particularly those with LV dysfunction, CABG alone is usually not effective therapy.[72,193] Similarly, surgical reperfusion during acute MI has been demonstrated to be associated with lower late SCD rates over 10 years of follow-up,[194,195] and CABG with aortic valve replacement has been shown to reduce late SCD when concomitant CAD was present.[196]

The importance of anti-ischemic therapies in conjunction with automatic implantable cardioverter-defibrillator (AICD) implantation was highlighted in a report of 218 patients.[197] To identify baseline variables associated with first appropriate AICD discharge and long-term survival, Levine and

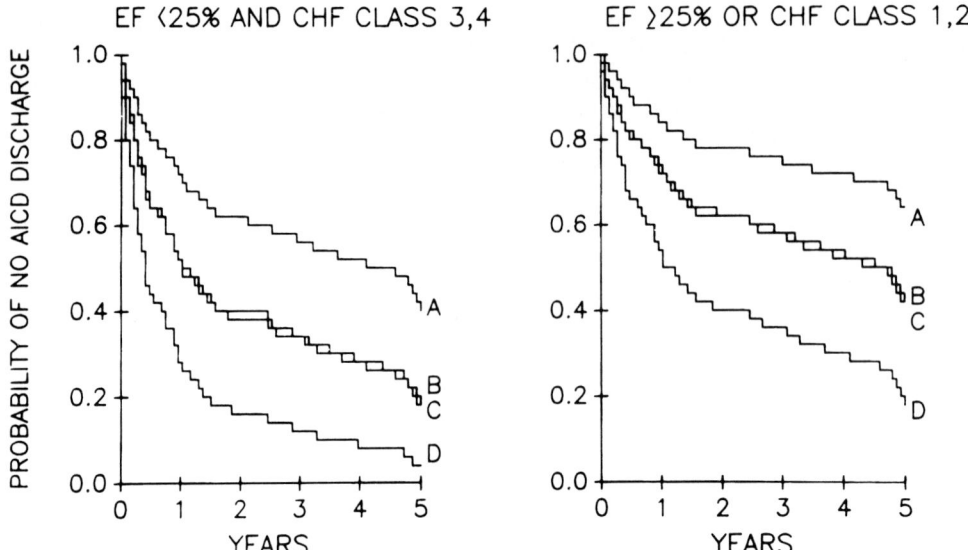

Fig. 20–12. Effect of degree of myocardial dysfunction, use of β-blockers, and coronary artery bypass graft (CABG) on expected cumulative probability of remaining without an automatic implantable cardioverter-defibrillator (AICD) discharge over 5 years (Cox hazards function). Each of the two groups shows effects of the use of β-blockers and CABG: A, β-blockers and CABG; B, β-blockers, no CABG; C, CABG, no β-blockers; D, no β-blockers, no CABG. EF, ejection fraction; CHF, congestive heart failure. (Reproduced by permission of the American Heart Association from Levine JH, et al: Circulation 84:558, 1991.[197])

colleagues[197] performed multivariable analysis controlled for several clinical, electrophysiological, angiographic, surgical, and medical covariates. Severe LV dysfunction was associated with both earlier AICD discharge and shortened survival after first discharge. The use of β-blocking medications and CABG were associated with later AICD discharge. In addition, coronary revascularization was associated with better survival after AICD discharge (Fig. 20–12). The use of antiarrhythmia agents did not correlate with time to first AICD discharge.[197]

SUMMARY AND CONCLUSIONS

Many potentially lethal ventricular arrhythmias, whether spontaneous or induced, and the rates of SCD on long-term follow-up are related to myocardial ischemia. Extensive epidemiological, pathological, and clinical evidence has linked SCD to CAD. A number of population-based cohort studies have demonstrated that patients at risk for SCD share many features with those at risk for other complications of CAD, and that CAD is itself the most important risk factor for subsequent SCD. Further epidemiological evidence demonstrating important circadian variations in various cardiovascular diseases, including sudden death, has suggested that vulnerability to SCD and the triggering of SCD are complex multifactorial processes. Pathological examination has confirmed the presence of severe CAD in a large number of victims of SCD. Close examination of coronary arteries in these patients has led to an appreciation of the role of plaque rupture with superimposed coronary thrombosis in the immediate pathogenesis of SCD.

Fatal and nonfatal ventricular arrhythmias have been associated with myocardial ischemia in clinical and experimental models of myocardial ischemia and are related to the severity of ischemia. Nonetheless, the presence of ST-segment shifts prior to SCD is an infrequent finding, and arrhythmias occur during ischemic episodes in only a minority of patients. Similarly, only in a minority of SCD survivors is ischemia demonstrable on exercise testing.

Invasive electrophysiological testing provides valuable clues to arrhythmic mechanisms in patients resuscitated from SCD and confirms the importance of a well-developed electrophysiological substrate in the genesis of SCD in many patients. Arrhythmias such as sustained monomorphic VT reflect an underlying electrophysiological substrate capable of sustaining re-entrant circuits. As a corollary, VF and polymorphic VT may represent primary manifestations of myocardial ischemia, especially in patients with CAD who are noninducible at electrophysiological study. However, the distinction is not absolute because VT, too, may be more easily manifest (either spontaneously or by programmed stimulation) in the presence of ischemia.

Thus, clinical SCD due to VF may result from ischemia, deterioration of re-entrant arrhythmias, or (in many patients) both. As a conservative estimate, 10–15% of SCDs may be due primarily to myocardial ischemia (leading to VF without preceding sustained monomorphic VT).[121] The one third of patients with SCD who are noninducible at electrophysiological study may represent a population in whom ischemia is particularly important either as a trigger of SCD or to facilitate the induction of re-entrant arrhythmias through modulation of the underlying electrophysiological substrate. In the remaining 45–60% of patients with SCD who have inducible sustained monomorphic VT, electrophysiological triggers such as ventricular ectopic beats may in and of themselves serve to initiate poorly tolerated sustained monomorphic VT, VT that degenerates to VF, or poorly tolerated polymorphic VT. The hemodynamic and electrophysiological responses to sustained monomorphic VT in patients with CAD are undoubtedly further modulated by the presence of LV dysfunction and myocardial ischemia. SCD represents a complex, heterogeneous group of entities with numerous, interacting initiating precursors.

That treatment primarily for CAD can influence SCD rates is confirmed by large randomized controlled trials of medical and surgical therapies in CAD and lends further credence to the hypothesis that ischemia is intimately related to the development of SCD.

Thus, not only is SCD linked to CAD, but acute ischemia is crucial to the development of SCD in many patients, and interventions designed to reduce the frequency and severity of ischemia have important salutary effects on rates of SCD. It is equally clear that a fixed arrhythmic substrate is present in many patients with CAD. In many such patients, the induction of a malignant arrhythmia requires a "trigger," such as ventricular ectopy or myocardial ischemia. What is unclear is in what proportion of patients with SCD is the interaction between ischemia and scar tissue the primary pathophysiological mechanism and in what proportion is ischemia the primary, if not the sole, mechanism.

Further delineation or categorization of the patient subsets is needed because such information could exert a major impact on our ability to tailor therapy to individual patients.

REFERENCES

1. Porter WB: The probably grave significance of premature beats occurring in angina pectoris induced by effort. Am J Med Sci 216:509, 1948.
2. Goldstein S, Medendorp SV, Landis JR, et al: Analysis of cardiac symptoms preceding cardiac arrest. Am J Cardiol 58:1195, 1986.
3. Kuller LH: Sudden death; Definition and epidemiologic considerations. Prog Cardiovasc Dis 23:1, 1980.
4. Goldstein S: The necessity of a uniform definition of sudden coronary death: Witnessed death within 1 hour of the onset of acute symptoms. Am Heart J 103:156, 1982.
5. Kannel WB, Schatzkin A: Sudden death: Lessons from subsets in population studies. J Am Coll Cardiol 5:141B, 1985.
6. Kannel WB, Doyle JT, McNamara PM, Quickenton P, Gordon T: Precursors of sudden coronary death: Factors related to the incidence of sudden death. Circulation 51:606, 1975.
7. Doyle JT, Kannel WB, McNamara PM, Quickenton P, Gordon T: Factors related to suddenness of death from coronary disease: Combined Albany-Framingham studies. Am J Cardiol 37:1073, 1976.
8. Schatzkin A, Cupples LA, Heeren T,

Morelock S, Kannel WB: Sudden death in the Framingham Heart Study: Differences in incidence and risk factors by sex and coronary disease status. Am J Epidemiol *120:* 888, 1984.

9. Kannel WB, Thomas HE Jr: Sudden coronary death: the Framingham study. Ann NY Acad Sci *382:*3, 1982.
10. Sytkowski PA, Kannel WB, D'Agostino RB: Changes in risk factors and the decline in mortality from cardiovascular disease: The Framingham Heart Study. N Engl J Med *322:*1635, 1990.
11. Goldberg RJ: Declining out-of-hospital sudden coronary death rates: Additional pieces of the epidemiologic puzzle. Circulation *79:* 1369, 1989.
12. Gillum RF: Sudden coronary death in the United States: 1980–1985. Circulation *79:* 756, 1989.
13. Goldberg RJ, Gore JM, Alpert JS, Dalen JE: Incidence and case fatality rates of acute myocardial infarction (1975–1984): The Worcester Heart Attack Study. Am Heart J *115:*761, 1988.
14. Gillum RF, Folsom A, Luepker RV, et al: Sudden death and acute myocardial infarction in a metropolitan area, 1970–1980: the Minnesota Heart Survey. N Engl J Med *309:*1353, 1983.
15. Elveback LR, Connolly DC, Melton LJ III: Coronary heart disease in residents of Rochester, Minnesota: VII. Incidence, 1950 through 1982. Mayo Clin Proc *61:*896, 1986.
16. Kuller LH, Perper JA, Dai WS, Rutan G, Traven N: Sudden death and the decline in coronary heart disease mortality. J Chronic Dis *39:*1001, 1986.
17. Beaglehole R, Bonita R, Jackson R, Stewart A, Sharpe N, Fraser GE: Trends in coronary heart disease event rates in New Zealand. Am J Epidemiol *120:*225, 1984.
18. Pell S, Fayerweather WE: Trends in the incidence of myocardial infarction and in associated mortality and morbidity in a large employed population, 1957–1983. N Engl J Med *312:*1005, 1985.
19. Muller JE, Ludmer PL, Willich SN, et al: Circadian variation in the frequency of sudden cardiac death. Circulation *75:*131, 1987.
20. Willich SN, Levy D, Rocco MB, Tofler GH, Stone PH, Muller JE: Circadian variation in the incidence of sudden cardiac death in the Framingham Heart Study population. Am J Cardiol *60:*801, 1987.
21. Muller JE, Stone PH, Turi ZG, et al: Circadian variation in the frequency of onset of acute myocardial infarction. N Engl J Med *313:*1315, 1985.
22. Willich SN, Linderer T, Weg-Scheider K, Schröder R, Steglitz K: Increased risk of myocardial infarction in the morning [abstract]. J Am Coll Cardiol *11:*28A, 1988.
23. Deanfield JE, Shea M, Ribiero P, et al: Transient ST-segment depression as a marker of myocardial ischemia during daily life. Am J Cardiol, *54:*1195, 1984.
24. Panza JA, Quyyumi AA, Diodati JG, Callahan TS, Bonow RO, Epstein SE: Long-term variation in myocardial ischemia during daily life in patients with stable coronary artery disease: Its relation to changes in the ischemic threshold. J Am Coll Cardiol *19:*500, 1992.
25. Rocco MB, Barry J, Campbell S, et al: Circadian variation of transient myocardial ischemia in patients with coronary artery disease. Circulation *75:*395, 1987.
26. Mulcahy D, Keegan J, Cunningham D, et al: Circadian variation of total ischaemic burden and its alteration with anti-anginal agents. Lancet *iii:*755, 1988.
27. Hausmann D, Nikutta P, Trappe H-J, Daniel WG, Wenzlaff P, Lichtlen PR: Incidence of ventricular arrhythmias during transient myocardial ischemia in patients with stable coronary artery disease. J Am Coll Cardiol *16:*49, 1990.
28. Nademanee K, Intarachot V, Josephson MA, Singh BN: Circadian variation in occurrence of transient overt and silent myocardial ischemia in chronic stable angina and comparison with Prinzmetal angina in men. Am J Cardiol *60:*494, 1987.
29. Tsementzis SA, Gill JS, Hitchcock ER, Gill SK, Beevers DG: Diurnal variation of and activity during the onset of stroke. Neurosurgery *17:*901, 1985.
30. Robertson T, Marler J, Muller J, et al: Circadian variation in the frequency of onset of stroke. J Am Coll Cardiol *7(suppl A):* 40A, 1986.
31. Rocco MB, Nabel EG, Selwyn AP: Circadian rhythms and coronary artery disease. Am J Cardiol *59(7):*13C, 1987.
32. Muller JE, Tofler GH, Stone PH: Circadian variation and triggers of onset of acute cardiovascular disease. Circulation *79:*733, 1989.
33. Miller-Craig MW, Bishop CN, Raftery EB: Circadian variation of blood-pressure. Lancet *i:*795, 1978.
34. Weitzman ED, Fukushima D, Nogeire C, Roffwarg H, Gallagher TF, Hellman L: Twenty-four hour pattern of the episodic secretion of cortisol in normal subjects. J Clin Endocrinol Metab *33:*14, 1971.
35. Lambert CR, Coy K, Imperi G, Pepine CJ: Influence of beta-adrenergic blockade de-

fined by time series analysis on circadian variation of heart rate and ambulatory myocardial ischemia. Am J Cardiol 64:835, 1989.
36. Quyyumi AA, Panza JA, Diodati JG, Lakatos E, Epstein SE: Circadian variation in ischemic threshold: A mechanism underlying the circadian variation in ischemic events. Circulation 86:22, 1992.
37. Fujita M, Franklin D: Diurnal changes in coronary blood flow in conscious dogs. Circulation 76:488, 1987.
38. Tofler GH, Brezinski D, Schafer AI, et al: Concurrent morning increase in platelet aggregability and the risk of myocardial infarction and sudden cardiac death. N Engl J Med 316:1514, 1987.
39. Brezinski DA, Tofler GH, Muller JE, et al: Morning increase in platelet aggregability: Association with assumption of the upright posture. Circulation 78:35, 1988.
40. Ehrly AM, Jung G: Circadian rhythm of human blood viscosity. Biorheology 10: 577, 1973.
41. Willich SF, Sintonen SP, Bhatia SS, et al: Morning increase of platelet aggregability in patients with coronary artery disease [abstract]. J Am Coll Cardiol 11:204A, 1988.
42. Ogawa H, Yasue H, Oshima S: Circadian variation of plasma fibrinopeptide A levels in patients with variant angina [abstract]. Circulation 78(suppl II):II-331, 1988.
43. Andreotti F, Davies GJ, Hackett DR, et al: Major circadian fluctuations in fibrinolytic factors and possible relevance to time of onset of myocardial infarction, sudden cardiac death and stroke. Am J Cardiol 62:635, 1988.
44. Rosing DR, Brakman P, Redwood DR, et al: Blood fibrinolytic activity in man: Diurnal variation and the response to varying intensities of exercise. Circ Res 27:171, 1970.
45. Angleton P, Chandler WL, Schmer G: Diurnal variation of tissue-type plasminogen activator and its rapid inhibitor (PAI-1). Circulation 79:101, 1989.
46. Ginsburg R, Bristow MR, Davis K, Dibiase A, Billingham ME: Quantitative pharmacologic responses of normal and atherosclerotic isolated human epicardial coronary arteries. Circulation 69:430, 1984.
47. Furchgott RF, Zawadzki JV: The obligatory role of endothelial cells in the relaxation of arterial smooth muscle by acetylcholine. Nature 288:373, 1980.
48. Gage JE, Hess OM, Murakami T, Ritter M, Grimm J, Krayenbuehl HP: Vasoconstriction of stenotic coronary arteries during dynamic exercise in patients with classic angina pectoris: Reversibility by nitroglycerin. Circulation 73:865, 1986.
49. Brown BG, Lee AB, Bolson EL, Dodge HT: Reflex constriction of significant coronary stenosis as a mechanism contributing to ischemic left ventricular dysfunction during isometric exercise. Circulation 70: 18, 1984.
50. Mudge GH Jr, Grossman W, Mills RM Jr, Lesch M, Braunwald E: Reflex increase in coronary vascular resistance in patients with ischemic heart disease. N Engl J Med 295:1333, 1976.
51. Siscovick DS, Weiss NS, Fletcher RH, Lasky T: The incidence of primary cardiac arrest during vigorous exercise. N Engl J Med 311:874, 1984.
52. Cobb LA, Weaver WD: Exercise: A risk for sudden death in patients with coronary heart disease. J Am Coll Cardiol 7:215, 1986.
53. Schwartz PJ, Billman GE, Stone HL: Autonomic mechanisms in ventricular fibrillation induced by myocardial ischemia during exercise in dogs with healed myocardial infarction: An experimental preparation for sudden cardiac death. Circulation 69:790, 1984.
54. Nicod P, Rehr R, Winniford MD, Campbell WB, Firth BG, Hillis LD: Acute systemic and coronary hemodynamic and serologic responses to cigarette smoking in long-term smokers with atherosclerotic coronary artery disease. J Am Coll Cardiol 4:964, 1984.
55. Deanfield JE, Shea MJ, Wilson RA, Horlock P, deLandsheere CM, Selwyn AP: Direct effects of smoking on the heart: Silent ischemic disturbances of coronary flow. Am J Cardiol 57:1005, 1986.
56. Barry J, Selwyn AP, Nabel EG, et al: Frequency of ST-segment depression produced by mental stress in stable angina pectoris from coronary artery disease. Am J Cardiol 61:989, 1988.
57. Daly LE, Hickey N, Graham IM, Mulcahy R: Predictors of sudden death up to 18 years after a first attack of unstable angina or myocardial infarction. Br Heart J 58:567, 1987.
58. Hallstrom AP, Cobb LA, Ray R: Smoking as a risk factor for recurrence of sudden cardiac arrest. N Engl J Med 314:271, 1986.
59. Rozanski A, Bairey CN, Krantz DS, et al: Mental stress and the induction of silent myocardial ischemia in patients with coronary artery disease. N Engl J Med 318: 1005, 1988.
60. Deanfield JE, Shea M, Kensett M, et al: Silent myocardial ischaemia due to mental stress. Lancet ii:1001, 1984.

61. Verrier RL, Hagestad EL, Lown B: Delayed myocardial ischemia induced by anger. Circulation 75:249, 1986.
62. Frank C, Smith S: Stress and the heart: Biobehavioral aspects of sudden cardiac death. Psychosomatics 31:255, 1990.
63. Meredith IT, Broughton A, Jennings GL, Esler MD: Evidence of a selective increase in cardiac sympathetic activity in patients with sustained ventricular arrhythmias. N Engl J Med 325:618, 1991.
64. DeWood MA, Leimgruber PP, Shields JP, Kunkel RM, Hensley GR, Reisig AH Jr: Thrombosis in acute myocardial infarction and sudden death: Angiographic aspects. Cardiovasc Clin 18(1):195, 1987.
65. Holmes DR Jr, Davis K, Gersh BJ, Mock MB, Pettinger MB, and participants in the Coronary Artery Surgery Study (CASS): Risk factor profiles of patients with sudden cardiac death and death from other cardiac causes: A report from the Coronary Artery Surgery Study (CASS). J Am Coll Cardiol 13:524, 1989.
66. Ciampricotti R, El Gamal M, Relik T, et al: Clinical characteristics and coronary angiographic findings of patients with unstable angina, acute myocardial infarction, and survivors of sudden ischemic death occurring during and after sport. Am Heart J 120:1267, 1990.
67. Kragel AH, Gertz SD, Roberts WC: Morphologic comparison of frequency and types of acute lesions in the major epicardial coronary arteries in unstable angina pectoris, sudden coronary death and acute myocardial infarction. J Am Coll Cardiol 18:801, 1991.
68. Weaver WD, Lorch GS, Alvarez HA, Cobb LA: Angiographic findings and prognostic indicators in patients resuscitated from sudden cardiac death. Circulation 54:895, 1976.
69. Tresch DD, Grove JR, Siegal R, Keelan MH, Brooks HL: Survivors of prehospitalization sudden death: Characteristic clinical and angiographic features. Arch Intern Med 141:1154, 1981.
70. Reichenbach DD, Moss NS, Meyer E: Pathology of the heart in sudden cardiac death. Am J Cardiol 39:865, 1977.
71. Warnes CA, Roberts WC: Sudden coronary death: Relation of amount and distribution of coronary narrowing at necropsy to previous symptoms of myocardial ischemia, left ventricular scarring and heart weight. Am J Cardiol 54:65, 1984.
72. Wilber DJ, Garan H, Finkelstein D, et al: Out-of-hospital cardiac arrest: Use of electrophysiologic testing in the prediction of long-term outcome. N Engl J Med 318:19, 1988.
73. Waller BF: Sudden death in middle-aged conditioned subjects: Coronary artherosclerosis is the culprit. Mayo Clin Proc 62:634, 1987.
74. Davies MJ: Pathological view of sudden cardiac death. Br Heart J 45:88, 1981.
75. Davies MJ, Thomas A: Thrombosis and acute coronary-artery lesions in sudden cardiac ischemic death. N Engl J Med 310:1137, 1984.
76. Davies MJ, Thomas AC, Knapman PA, Hangartner JR: Intramyocardial platelet aggregation in patients with unstable angina suffering sudden ischemic cardiac death. Circulation 73:418, 1986.
77. McHenry PL, O'Donnell J, Morris SN, Jordan JJ: The abnormal exercise electrocardiogram in apparently healthy men: A predictor of angina pectoris as an initial coronary event during long-term follow-up. Circulation 70:547, 1984.
78. Fulton WFM: Arterial anastomoses in the coronary circulation: I. Anatomical features in normal and diseased hearts demonstrated by stereoarteriography. Scott Med J 8:420, 1963.
79. Rentrop KP, Thornton JC, Feit F: Determinants and protective potential of coronary arterial collaterals as assessed by an angioplasty model. Am J Cardiol 61:677, 1988.
80. Epstein SE, Quyyumi AA, Bonow RO: Sudden cardiac death without warning: Possible mechanisms and implications for screening asymptomatic populations. N Engl J Med 321:320, 1989.
81. Ambrose JA, Tannenbaum MA, Alexopoulous D, et al: Angiographic progression of coronary artery disease and the development of myocardial infarction. J Am Coll Cardiol 12:56, 1988.
82. Little WC, Constantinescu M, Applegate RJ, et al: Can coronary angiography predict the site of a subsequent myocardial infarction in patients with mild-to-moderate coronary artery disease? Circulation 78:1157, 1988.
83. Topol EJ, Califf RM, George BS, et al, and the Thrombolysis and Angioplasty in Myocardial Infarction Study Group: A randomized trial of immediate versus delayed elective angioplasty after intravenous tissue plasminogen activator in acute myocardial infarction. N Engl J Med 317:581, 1987.
84. Barbour DJ, Warnes CA, Roberts WC: Cardiac findings associated with sudden death secondary to atherosclerotic coronary artery disease: Comparison of patients with and those without previous angina pectoris and/or healed myocardial infarction. Circulation 75(suppl II):II-9, 1987.

85. Kragel AH, Reddy SG, Wittes JT, Roberts WC: Morphometric analysis of the composition of atherosclerotic plaques in the four major epicardial coronary arteries in acute myocardial infarction and in sudden coronary death. Circulation 80:1747, 1989.
86. Stone PH: Triggers of transient myocardial ischemia: Circadian variation and relation to plaque rupture and coronary thrombosis in stable coronary artery disease. Am J Cardiol 66:32G, 1990.
87. Davies MJ, Thomas AC: Plaque fissuring: The cause of acute myocardial infarction, sudden ischaemic death, and crescendo angina. Br Heart J 53:363, 1985.
88. Falk E: Morphologic features of unstable atherothrombotic plaques underlying acute coronary syndromes. Am J Cardiol 63:114E, 1989.
89. Volpi A, Maggioni A, Franzosi MG, Pampallona S, Mauri F, Tognoni G: In-hospital prognosis of patients with acute myocardial infarction complicated by primary ventricular fibrillation. N Engl J Med 317:257, 1987.
90. Bloor CM, Ehsani A, White FC, Sobel BE: Ventricular fibrillation threshold in acute myocardial infarction and its relation to myocardial infarct size. Cardiovasc Res 9:468, 1975.
91. Roberts R, Husain A, Ambos HD, et al: Relation between infarct size and ventricular arrhythmia. Br Heart J 37:1169, 1975.
92. Hwang S, Stevenson WG, Wiener I: Hearts too good to die: Ventricular fibrillation due to small infarctions or ischemia. Am Heart J 121:938, 1991.
93. Mogensen L, Orinius E, Schenk-Gustafsson K: Electrocardiographic features at onset of ventricular fibrillation in acute myocardial infarction: Relation to intraventricular conduction defects, configuration of initiating QRS complex, preceding heart rate and initiating coupling interval. Eur Heart J 4:86, 1983.
94. Multicenter Postinfarction Research Group: Risk stratification and survival after myocardial infarction. N Engl J Med 309:331, 1983.
95. Bigger JT Jr, Fleiss JL, Kleiger R, Miller JP, Rolnitzky LM, and the Multicenter Post-Infarction Research Group: The relationships among ventricular arrhythmias, left ventricular dysfunction, and mortality in the 2 years after myocardial infarction. Circulation 69:250, 1984.
96. Sanz G, Castañer A, Betriu A, et al: Determinants of prognosis in survivors of myocardial infarction: A prospective clinical angiographic study. N Engl J Med 306:1065, 1982.
97. Mukharji J, Rude RE, Poole WK, et al, and the MILIS Study Group: Risk factors for sudden death after acute myocardial infarction: Two-year follow-up. Am J Cardiol 54:31, 1984.
98. Gomes JA, Winters SL, Ergin A, et al: Clinical and electrophysiologic determinants, treatment and survival of patients with sustained malignant ventricular tachyarrhythmias occurring late after myocardial infarction. J Am Coll Cardiol 17:320, 1991.
99. Théroux P, Waters DD, Halphen C, Debaisieux J-C, Mizgala HF: Prognostic value of exercise testing soon after myocardial infarction. N Engl J Med 301:341, 1979.
100. Billman GE, Schwartz PJ, Stone HL: Baroreceptor reflex control of heart rate: A predictor of sudden cardiac death. Circulation 66:874, 1982.
101. Kleiger RE, Miller JP, Bigger JT Jr, Moss AJ, and the Multicenter Post-Infarction Research Group: Decreased heart rate variability and its association with increased mortality after acute myocardial infarction. Am J Cardiol 59:256, 1987.
102. Marcus FI, Cobb LA, Edwards JE, et al, and the Multicenter Post Infarction Research Group: Mechanism of death and prevalence of myocardial ischemic symptoms in the terminal event after acute myocardial infarction. Am J Cardiol 61:8, 1988.
103. Janse MJ, Kléber AG: Electrophysiological changes and ventricular arrhythmias in the early phase of regional myocardial ischemia. Circ Res 49:1069, 1981.
104. Fozzard HA, Makielski JC: The electrophysiology of acute myocardial ischemia. Annu Rev Med 36:275, 1985.
105. Balke CW, Kaplinsky E, Michelson EL, Naito M, Dreifus LS: Reperfusion ventricular tachyarrhythmias: Correlation with antecedent coronary artery occlusion tachyarrhythmias and duration of myocardial ischemia. Am Heart J 101:449, 1981.
106. Manning AS, Hearse DJ: Reperfusion-induced arrhythmias: Mechanisms and prevention. J Mol Cell Cardiol 16:497, 1984.
107. Gottlieb SH, Ouyang P, Gottlieb SO: Death after acute myocardial infarction: Interrelation between left ventricular dysfunction, arrhythmias and ischemia. Am J Cardiol 61:7B, 1988.
108. Weaver WD, Cobb LA, Hallstrom AP, et al: Considerations for improving survival from out-of-hospital cardiac arrest. Ann Emerg Med 15:1181, 1986.
109. Greene, HL: Sudden arrthythmic cardiac death: Mechanisms, resuscitation and classification. The Seattle Perspective. Am J Cardiol 65:4B, 1990.

110. Weaver WD, Hill D, Fahrenbruch CE, Copass MK, Martin JS, Cobb LA, Hallstrom AP: Use of the automatic external defibrillator in the management of out-of-hospital cardiac arrest. N Engl J Med 319:661, 1988.
111. Kempf FC, Josephson ME: Cardiac arrest recorded on ambulatory electrocardiograms. Am J Cardiol 53:1577, 1984.
112. Lewis BH, Antman EM, Graboys TB: Detailed analysis of 24 hour ambulatory electrocardiographic recordings during ventricular fibrillation or torsade de pointes. J Am Coll Cardiol 2:426, 1983.
113. Milner PG, Platia EV, Reid PR, Griffith LSC: Ambulatory electrocardiographic recordings at the time of fatal cardiac arrest. Am J Cardiol 56:588, 1985.
114. Nikolic G, Bishop RL, Singh JB: Sudden death recorded during holter monitoring. Circulation 66:218, 1982.
115. Panidis IP, Morganroth J: Sudden death in hospitalized patients: Cardiac rhythm disturbances detected by ambulatory electrocardiographic monitoring. J Am Coll Cardiol 2:798, 1983.
116. Pratt CM, Francis MJ, Luck JC, et al: Analysis of ambulatory electrocardiograms in 15 patients during spontaneous ventricular fibrillation with special reference to preceding arrhythmic events. J Am Coll Cardiol 2:789, 1983.
117. Roelandt J, Klootwijk P, Lubsen J, Janse MJ: Sudden death during longterm ambulatory monitoring. Eur Heart J 5:7, 1984.
118. Bayés de Luna A, Coumel P, Leclercq JF: Ambulatory sudden cardiac death: Mechanisms of production of fatal arrhythmia on the basis of data from 157 cases. Am Heart J 117:151, 1989.
119. Savage HR, Kissane JQ, Becher EL, Maddocks WQ, Murtaugh JT, Dizadji H: Analysis of ambulatory electrocardiograms in 14 patients who experienced sudden cardiac death during monitoring. Clin Cardiol 10:621, 1987.
120. Pepine CJ, Morganroth J, McDonald JT, Gottlieb SO: Sudden death during ambulatory electrocardiographic monitoring. Am J Cardiol 68:785, 1991.
121. Meissner MD, Akhtar M, Lehmann MH: Nonischemic sudden tachyarrhythmic death in atherosclerotic heart disease. Circulation 84:905, 1991.
122. Nesto RW, Kowalchuk GJ: The ischemic cascade: Temporal sequence of hemodynamic, electrocardiographic and symptomatic expression of ischemia. Am J Cardiol 57:23C, 1987.
123. Baum RS, Alvarez H III, Cobb LA: Survival after resuscitation from out-of-hospital ventricular fibrillation. Circulation 50:1231, 1974.
124. Myerburg RJ, Kessler KM, Mallon SM, et al: Life-threatening ventricular arrhythmias in patients with silent myocardial ischemia due to coronary artery spasm. N Engl J Med 326:1451, 1992.
125. Ciampricotti R, Taverne R, El Gamel M: Clinical and angiographic observations on resuscitated victims of exercise-related sudden ischemic death. Am J Cardiol 68:47, 1991.
126. Weaver WD, Cobb LA, Hallstrom AP: Characteristics of survivors of exertion- and nonexertion-related cardiac arrest: Value of subsequent exercise testing. Am J Cardiol 50:671, 1982.
127. Sharma B, Asinger R, Francis GS, Hodges M, Wyeth RP: Demonstration of exercise-induced painless myocardial ischemia in survivors of out-of-hospital ventricular fibrillation. Am J Cardiol 59:740, 1987.
128. Amsterdam EA: Relation of silent myocardial ischemia to ventricular arrhythmias and sudden death. Am J Cardiol 62:24I, 1988.
129. Weiner DA, Ryan TJ, McCabe CH, et al: Risk of developing an acute myocardial infarction or sudden coronary death in patients with exercise-induced silent myocardial ischemia: A Report from the Coronary Artery Surgery Study (CASS) Registry. Am J Cardiol 63:1155, 1988.
130. Miller DD, Waters DD, Szlachcic J, Théroux P: Clinical characteristics associated with sudden death in patients with variant angina. Circulation 66:588, 1982.
131. Araki H, Koiwaya Y, Nakagaki O, Nakamura M: Diurnal distribution of ST-segment elevation and related arrhythmias in patients with variant angina: A study by ambulatory ECG monitoring. Circulation 67:995, 1983.
132. Previtali M, Klersy C, Salerno JA, et al: Ventricular tachyarrhythmias in Prinzmetal's variant angina: Clinical significance and relation to the degree and time course of S-T segment elevation. Am J Cardiol 52:19, 1983.
133. Biagini A, Emdin M, Michelassi C, et al: The contribution of ventricular tachyarrhythmias to the genesis of cardiac pain during transient myocardial ischaemia in patients with variant angina. Eur Heart J 9:484, 1988.
134. Carboni GP, Lahiri A, Cashman PMM, Raftery EB: Mechanisms of arrhythmias accompanying ST-segment depression on ambulatory monitoring in stable angina pectoris. Am J Cardiol 60:1246, 1987.

135. Turitto G, Zanchi E, Maddaluna A, Pellegrini A, Risa AL, Prati PL: Prevalence, time course and malignancy of ventricular arrhythmia during spontaneous ischemic ST-segment depression. Am J Cardiol 64: 900, 1989.
136. Mulcahy D, Keegan J, Crean P, et al: Silent myocardial ischaemia in chronic stable angina: A study of its frequency and characteristics in 150 patients. Br Heart J 60:417, 1988.
137. Stern S, Banai S, Keren A, Tzivoni D: Ventricular ectopic activity during myocardial ischemic episodes in ambulatory patients. Am J Cardiol 65:412, 1990.
138. Echt DS, Liebson PR, Mitchell LB, et al, and the CAST investigators: Mortality and morbidity in patients receiving encainide, flecainide, or placebo: The Cardiac Arrhythmia Suppression Trial. N Engl J Med 324:781, 1991.
139. Cardiac Arrhythmia Suppression Trial (CAST) investigators: Preliminary report: Effect of encainide and flecainide on mortality in a randomized trial of arrhythmia suppression after myocardial infarction. N Engl J Med 321:406, 1989.
140. Nattel S, Pedersen DH, Zipes DP: Alterations in regional myocardial distribution and arrhythmogenic effects of aprindine produced by coronary artery occlusion in the dog. Cardiovasc Res 15:80, 1981.
141. Brugada J, Boersma L, Kirchhof C, et al: Double-wave reentry as a mechanism of acceleration of ventricular tachycardia. Circulation 81:1622, 1990.
142. Gomes JA, Alexopoulos D, Winters SL, Deshmukh P, Fuster V, Suh K: The role of silent ischemia, the arrhythmic substrate and the short-long sequence in the genesis of sudden cardiac death. J Am Coll Cardiol 14:1618, 1989.
143. Trusz-Gluza M, Giec L, Dąbrowski A, et al: Proarrhythmic response to antiarrhythmic drug as a risk factor for sudden cardiac death in patients with ischemic heart disease. PACE 14:1947, 1991.
144. Eldar M, Sauve MJ, Scheinman MM: Electrophysiologic testing and follow-up of patients with aborted sudden death. J Am Coll Cardiol 10:291, 1987.
145. Roy D, Waxman HL, Kienzle MG, Buxton AE, Marchlinski FE, Josephson ME: Clinical characteristics and long-term follow-up in 119 survivors of cardiac arrest: Relation to inducibility at electrophysiologic testing. Am J Cardiol 52:969, 1983.
146. McLaran CJ, Gersh BJ, Sugrue DD, et al: Out-of-hospital cardiac arrest in patients without clinically significant coronary artery disease: Comparison of clinical, electrophysiological, and survival characteristics with those in similar patients who have clinically significant coronary artery disease. Br Heart J 58:583, 1987.
147. Vaitkus PT, Kindwall KE, Marchlinski FE, Miller JM, Buxton AE, Josephson ME: Differences in electrophysiological substrate in patients with coronary artery disease and cardiac arrest or ventricular tachycardia: Insights from endocardial mapping and signal-averaged electrocardiography. Circulation 84:672, 1991.
148. Dolack GL, Callahan DB, Bardy GH, Greene HL: Signal-averaged electrocardiographic late potentials in resuscitated survivors of out-of-hospital ventricular fibrillation. Am J Cardiol 65:1102, 1990.
149. Stevenson WG, Wiener I, Yeatman L, Wohlgelernter D, Weiss JN: Complicated artherosclerotic lesions: A potential cause of ischemic ventricular arrhythmias in cardiac arrest survivors who do not have inducible ventricular tachycardia? Am Heart J 116:1, 1988.
150. Lo Y-SA, Cutler JE, Wright A, Kron J, Blake K, Swerdlow CD: Long-segment coronary ulcerations in survivors of sudden cardiac death. Am Heart J 116:1444, 1988.
151. Morady F, DiCarlo L, Winston S, Davis JC, Scheinman MM: Clinical features and prognosis of patients with out-of-hospital cardiac arrest and a normal electrophysiologic study. J Am Coll Cardiol 4:39, 1984.
152. Kehoe R, Tommaso C, Zheutlin T, et al: Factors determining programmed stimulation responses and long-term arrhythmic outcome in survivors of ventricular fibrillation with ischemic heart disease. Am Heart J 116:355, 1988.
153. Morady F, DiCarlo LA Jr, Krol RB, et al: Role of myocardial ischemia during programmed stimulation in survivors of cardiac arrest with coronary artery disease. J Am Coll Cardiol 9:1004, 1987.
154. Lemery R, Gersh BJ: Programmed ventricular stimulation during variant angina: Report of a case. PACE 12:1878, 1989.
155. Ritchie JL, Hallstrom AP, Troubaugh GB, Caldwell JH, Cobb LA: Out-of-hospital sudden coronary death: Rest and exercise radionuclide left ventricular function in survivors. Am J Cardiol 55:645, 1985.
156. Lampert S, Lown B, Graboys TB, Podrid PJ, Blatt CM: Determinants of survival in patients with malignant ventricular arrhythmia associated with coronary artery disease. Am J Cardiol 61:791, 1988.
157. Jordaens L, Hollanders G, De Schrijver A, Simons M, De Backer G, Clement DL: In-

cidence and prognostic significance of asymptomatic ischaemia in patients with sustained ventricular arrhythmias. Eur Heart J *9(suppl N):*128, 1988.
158. Lindsay BD, Ambos HD, Schechtman KB, Arthur RM, Cain ME: Noninvasive detection of patients with ischemic and nonischemic heart disease prone to ventricular fibrillation. J Am Coll Cardiol *16:*1656, 1990.
159. Stevenson WG, Brugada P, Waldecker B, Zehender M, Wellens HJJ: Clinical, angiographic, and electrophysiologic findings in patients with aborted sudden death as compared with patients with sustained ventricular tachycardia after myocardial infarction. Circulation *71:*1146, 1985.
160. Tchou P, Atassi K, Jazayeri M, McKinnie J, Avitall B, Akhtar M: Etiology of polymorphic ventricular tachycardia in the absence of prolonged QT [abstract]. J Am Coll Cardiol *13:*21A, 1989.
161. Zilcher H, Glogar D, Kaindl F: Torsades de pointes: Occurrence in myocardial ischaemia as a separate entity. Multiform ventricular tachycardia or not? Eur Heart J *1:*63, 1980.
162. Freedman RA, Gillis AM, Keren A, Soderholm-Difatte V, Mason JW: Signal-averaged electrocardiographic late potentials in patients with ventricular fibrillation or ventricular tachycardia: Correlation with clinical arrhythmia and electrophysiologic study. Am J Cardiol *55:*1350, 1985.
163. Adhar GC, Larson LW, Bardy GH, Greene HL: Sustained ventricular arrhythmias: Differences between survivors of cardiac arrest and patients with recurrent sustained ventricular tachycardia. J Am Coll Cardiol *12:*159, 1988.
164. β-Blocker Heart Attack Trial Research Group: A randomized trial of propranolol in patients with acute myocardial infarction: I. Mortality results. JAMA *247:*1707, 1982.
165. Herlitz J, Elmfeldt D, Holmberg S, et al: Göteborg Metoprolol Trial: Mortality and causes of death. Am J Cardiol *53:*9D, 1984.
166. Pedersen TR, for the Norwegian Multicenter Study Group: Six-year follow-up of the Norwegian Multicenter Study on Timolol After Acute Myocardial Infarction. N Engl J Med *313:*1055, 1985.
167. The Norwegian Multicenter Study Group: Timolol-induced reduction in mortality and reinfarction in patients surviving acute myocardial infarction. N Engl J Med *304:* 801, 1981.
168. Yusuf S, Peto R, Lewis J, Collins R, Sleight P: Beta blockade during and after myocardial infarction: An overview of the randomized trials. Prog Cardiovasc Dis *27:*335, 1985.
169. Boissel J-P, Leizorovicz A, Picolet H, Peyrieux J-C: Secondary prevention after high-risk acute myocardial infarction with low-dose acebutolol. Am J Cardiol *66:*251, 1990.
170. Held PH, Yusuf S, Furberg CD: Calcium channel blockers in acute myocardial infarction and unstable angina: An overview. Br Med J *299:*1187, 1989.
171. Bigger JT Jr, Coromilas J, Rolnitzky LM, Fleiss JL, Kleiger RE, and the Multicenter Diltiazem Postinfarction Trial Investigators: Effect of diltiazem on cardiac rate and rhythm after myocardial infarction. Am J Cardiol *65:*539, 1990.
172. Roine RO, Kaste M, Kinnunen A, Nikki P, Sarna S, Kajaste S: Nimodipine after resuscitation from out-of-hospital ventricular fibrillation. JAMA *264:*3171, 1990.
173. Frishman WH: Multifactorial actions of beta-adrenergic blocking drugs in ischemic heart disease: Current concepts. Circulation *67(suppl I):*I-11, 1983.
174. Anderson JL, Rodier HE, Green LS: Comparative effects of beta-adrenergic blocking drugs on experimental ventricular fibrillation threshold. Am J Cardiol *51:*1196, 1983.
175. Furberg CD, Hawkins CM, Lichstein E: Effect of propranolol in postinfarction patients with mechanical or electrical complications. Circulation *69:*761, 1984.
176. Peters RW, Muller JE, Golstein S, Byington R, Friedman LM, and the BHAT Study Group: Propranolol and the circadian variation in the frequency of sudden cardiac death: The BHAT experience [abstract]. Circulation *76(suppl 4):*364, 1988.
177. Lichstein E, Morganroth J, Harrist R, Hubble E, for the BHAT Study Group: Effect of propranolol on ventricular arrhythmia: The Beta-Blocker Heart Attack Trial experience. Circulation *67(suppl I):*I-5, 1983.
178. Frishman WH, Lazar EJ: Reduction of mortality, sudden death and non-fatal reinfarction with beta-adrenergic blockers in survivors of acute myocardial infarction: A new hypothesis regarding the cardioprotective action of beta-adrenergic blockade. Am J Cardiol *66:*66G, 1990.
179. Fitzgerald JD: By what means might beta blockers prolong life after acute myocardial infarction? Eur Heart J *8:*945, 1987.
180. Singh BN: Advantages of beta blockers versus antiarrhythmic agents and calcium antagonists in secondary prevention after myocardial infarction. Am J Cardiol *66(9):* 9C, 1990.

181. Anturane Reinfarction Trial Research Group: Sulfinpyrazone in the prevention of sudden death after myocardial infarction. N Engl J Med *302:*250, 1980.
182. ISIS-2 [Second International Study of Infarct Survival] Collaborative Group: Morning peak in the incidence of myocardial infarction: Experience in the ISIS-2 trial. Eur Heart J *13:*594, 1992.
183. Ridker PM, Manson JE, Buring JE, Muller JE, Hennekens CH: Circadian variation of acute myocardial infarction and the effect of low-dose aspirin in a randomized trial of physicians. Circulation *82:*897, 1990.
184. ISIS-2 [Second International Study of Infarct Survival] Collaborative Group: Randomised trial of intravenous streptokinase, oral aspirin, both, or neither among 17,187 cases of suspected acute myocardial infarction: ISIS-2. Lancet *ii:*349, 1988.
185. Kelly P, Ruskin JN, Vlahakes GJ, Buckley MJ, Freeman CS, Garan H: Surgical coronary revascularization in survivors of prehospital cardiac arrest: Its effect on inducible ventricular arrhythmias and long-term survival. J Am Coll Cardiol *15:*267, 1990.
186. Garan H, Ruskin JN, DiMarco JP, et al: Electrophysiologic studies before and after myocardial revascularization in patients with life-threatening ventricular arrhythmias. Am J Cardiol *51:*519, 1983.
187. Kron IL, Lerman BB, Haines DE, Flanagan TL, DiMarco JP: Coronary artery bypass grafting in patients with ventricular fibrillation. Ann Thorac Surg *48:*85, 1989.
188. Vismara LA, Miller RR, Price JE, Karem R, DeMaria AN, Mason DT: Improved longevity due to reduction of sudden death by aortocoronary bypass in coronary atherosclerosis: Prospective evaluation of medical versus surgical therapy in matched patients with multivessel disease. Am J Cardiol *39:*919, 1977.
189. Hammermeister KE, DeRouen TA, Murray JA, Dodge HT: Effect of aortocoronary saphenous vein bypass grafting on death and sudden death: Comparison of nonrandomized medically and surgically treated cohorts with comparable coronary disease and left ventricular function. Am J Cardiol *39:*925, 1977.
190. Holmes DR Jr, Davis KB, Mock MB, et al, and participants in the Coronary Artery Surgery Study: The effect of medical and surgical treatment on subsequent sudden cardiac death in patients with coronary artery disease: A report from the Coronary Artery Surgery Study. Circulation *73:*1254, 1986.
191. Tresch DD, Wetherbee JN, Siegel R, et al: Long-term follow-up of survivors of prehospital sudden cardiac death treated with coronary bypass surgery. Am Heart J *110:*1139, 1985.
192. Every NR, Fahrenbruch CE, Hallstrom AP, Weaver WD, Cobb LA: Coronary surgery reduces mortality in survivors of out-of-hospital cardiac arrest [abstract]. J Am Coll Cardiol *17(suppl A):*209A, 1991.
193. Brooks R, McGovern BA, Garan H, Ruskin JN: Current treatment of patients surviving out-of-hospital cardiac arrest. JAMA *265:*762, 1991.
194. DeWood MA, Notske RN, Berg R Jr, et al: Medical and surgical management of early Q wave myocardial infarction: I. Effects of surgical reperfusion on survival, recurrent myocardial infarction, sudden death and functional class at 10 or more years of follow-up. J Am Coll Cardiol *14:*65, 1989.
195. Koshal A, Beanlands DS, Davies RA, Nair RC, Keon WJ: Urgent surgical reperfusion in acute evolving myocardial infarction: A randomized controlled study. Circulation *78(suppl I):*I-171, 1988.
196. Czer LSC, Gray RJ, Stewart ME, De Robertis M, Chaux A, Matloff JM: Reduction in sudden late death by concomitant revascularization with aortic valve replacement. J Thorac Cardiovasc Surg *95:*390, 1988.
197. Levine JH, Mellits ED, Baumgardner RA, et al: Predictors of first discharge and subsequent survival in patients with automatic implantable cardioverter-defibrillators. Circulation *84:*558, 1991.

21

Acute-on-Chronic Ischemia in the Genesis of Ventricular Arrhythmias

THOMAS G. TROUTON
YOU-HO KIM
HASAN GARAN

Of all sudden cardiac deaths (SCDs), only 20% are believed to be caused by the development of ventricular tachycardia (VT) or ventricular fibrillation (VF) following acute myocardial infarction (MI).[1] This leaves a significant percentage with no evidence of acute infarction precipitating the event. Many patients in this category have chronic coronary artery disease (CAD) with or without myocardial scarring. There is now considerable evidence indicating that acute ischemia superimposed on chronic CAD can trigger serious ventricular arrhythmias, and that the presence of chronic CAD increases the risk of developing such arrhythmias in these patients.

CIRCUMSTANTIAL EVIDENCE FROM HUMAN STUDIES FOR ACUTE-ON-CHRONIC ISCHEMIA AS A FACTOR IN ARRHYTHMIA OCCURRENCE

Over the past 20 years, large prospective studies of patients suffering cardiac arrest secondary to the development of VT or VF have provided several clinical, angiographic, and autopsy data on this patient population.

Although early reports of patients resuscitated from out-of-hospital VF indicated associated acute MI in a high percentage,[2] later studies have demonstrated that VF without acute MI contributes substantially to the numbers of patients suffering sudden death.[3] Large retrospective clinical studies of cardiac arrest victims with CAD give variable estimates of the incidence of acute ischemia heralding SCD, depending on the criteria used to assess ischemia.[4,5] Thus, in a study of 101 patients resuscitated from out-of-hospital cardiac arrest, of whom 52% had a history of prior MI and 50% had a history of angina pectoris, 35% were subsequently shown to have sustained an MI and 32% had ischemia without infarction.[4] In another study of 142 patients, all with CAD, who had been resuscitated from cardiac arrest outside hospital, 44% subsequently satisfied criteria for acute MI, but 34% had electrocardiographic (ECG) changes consistent with ischemia without significant increases in serum cardiac enzymes, and a further 22% had neither significant ECG nor enzyme changes.[5] In a prospective clinical study of survivors of acute MI, symptoms of myocardial ischemia preceded the terminal event in 33 (58%) of a subset of 57 patients with a witnessed arrhythmic death during a 4-year follow-up period.[6] In this study the persistence of angina more than 6 months after acute MI was a significant predictor of subsequent cardiac mortality, suggesting that strategies to prevent ischemia may reduce mortality from sudden as well as nonsudden cardiac deaths within 4 years of acute MI.

Coronary angiography in survivors of

cardiac arrest and in patients with recurrent sustained VT reveals a high prevalence of extensive CAD in this population.[7,8] Both chronic infarction and potentially ischemic areas of myocardium are identifiable. In patients with sustained VT occurring 3–90 days following acute MI, multivessel CAD and anterior MI are independently associated with arrhythmia recurrence.[9]

In general, pathological findings at autopsy in victims of SCD reflect the clinical findings in this patient population and reveal extensive CAD without acute MI in a variable proportion. In three of the larger autopsy studies of patients with SCD and ischemic heart disease, the percentage of those with demonstrable coronary artery thrombosis ranged from 15 to 58%.[10–12] The incidence of recent occlusive thrombus in cases of SCD varies from 4 to 64%, a wide range that reflects, in part, differences in methodology among different pathologists as well as differences in the definition of SCD.[13] From a review of autopsy data, Davies suggests that a luminal stenosis of ≥85% best discriminates those dying suddenly from ischemic heart disease from those dying suddenly from other causes who have coincidental ischemic heart disease.[13]

From a review of 128 autopsies of patients dying with acute MI, Schuster and Bulkley identified 20 patients with severe two- or three-vessel CAD in whom angina associated with transient ECG changes occurred early following acute MI.[14] Of this subgroup, those with ischemia in a noninfarct territory had significantly more deaths due to ventricular arrhythmias than those with ischemia in the territory of the index acute MI. In a subsequent clinical study of 70 patients with early post-MI angina and ECG changes of ischemia, 40 patients died over an average follow-up period of 6 months, and 47% of these died suddenly.[15] The authors hypothesized that postinfarction angina identified a high-risk population that could benefit from surgical intervention.[15]

CLINICAL STUDIES

Several clinical studies have specifically sought evidence of acute ischemia against a background of chronic CAD in patients presenting with life-threatening ventricular arrhythmias.

VT in association with ECG changes indicative of ischemia has been described during exercise treadmill testing in patients with pre-existing ischemic heart disease.[16–19] In one study, patients with exercise-induced ventricular arrhythmias had significantly more extensive CAD and ventricular contraction abnormalities at contrast ventriculography than arrhythmia-free patients with CAD.[17] McHenry et al also showed that patients with three-vessel CAD and abnormal left ventricular (LV) wall motion had a significantly greater incidence of exercise-induced ventricular arrhythmias than those without CAD.[18] These studies support the view that ischemia developing in the setting of an abnormally contracting LV at rest, presumably due to chronic ischemic injury, contributes to the appearance of ventricular arrhythmias. However, the generally low prevalence of exercise-induced ventricular arrhythmias in patients with both conditions and the poor reproducibility suggest that some other humoral or metabolic factors may be required for arrhythmia development during exercise. Experimental data support this suggestion.[20]

More compelling indirect evidence of a role for ischemia in exercise-induced arrhythmias comes from the response to coronary bypass surgery. Weiner et al demonstrated in 80 patients that exercise-induced ventricular arrhythmias were more frequently associated with segmental wall motion abnormalities and myocardial ischemia.[21] Reversal of ischemia following bypass surgery in 22 patients lessened or abolished exercise-induced arrhythmias. Patients with persistent exercise-induced ventricular arrhythmias either had residual ischemia on a postoperative exercise test or had segmental wall motion abnormalities.[21]

Exercise scintigraphy using thallium-201 has been used by some groups to improve the detection of ischemia during exercise. Of 21 long-term survivors of out-of-hospital VF who subsequently underwent myocardial imaging and radionuclide angiography in eight patients (none of whom had sustained an MI at the time of the cardiac arrest) defects were demonstrated both at rest and after exercise in association with exercise-induced ECG changes indicative of ischemia.[22] However, in a more recent study of 38 patients with clinically documented VT or VF, 33 of whom had angiographically proven CAD, only two had reversible defects on exercise scintigraphy to suggest myocardial ischemia.[23] Although 84% of the group had one or more persistent scintigraphic defects suggesting the presence of large areas of irreversibly scarred tissue, only 8% experienced angina with exercise and 29% had exercise-induced ECG changes consistent with ischemia.[23]

DIRECT EVIDENCE FOR MYOCARDIAL ISCHEMIA MEDIATING CLINICAL VENTRICULAR ARRHYTHMIAS

Programmed electrical stimulation has been used to reproduce clinical arrhythmias, enabling identification of mechanism, stratification of risk of recurrence, and definition of end points to guide drug suppression therapy in patients with serious ventricular arrhythmias.[24-26] Direct evidence for the occurrence of ischemia prior to the onset of ventricular arrhythmias has been sought using programmed electrical stimulation to induce VT and measuring myocardial arteriovenous lactate differences as a metabolic indicator of myocardial ischemia.[27] Myocardial lactate production, reflecting myocardial ischemia, was observed during programmed electrical stimulation in eight of 15 cardiac arrest survivors, all of whom had CAD affecting at least one branch of the left coronary artery and seven of whom had abnormal LV contraction. In each case lactate production preceded the induction of VT by 30-60 seconds.[27] In a comparison of patients with and without lactate production during programmed stimulation, there was no significant difference with regard to frequency of a positive stress thallium test or a history of angina. Significant differences occurred in the degree of stenosis of the left anterior descending (LAD) coronary artery, and a history of physical activity at the time of cardiac arrest.[27] Although this study does not demonstrate that ischemia is a necessary requirement for the occurrence of VT, it suggests that myocardial ischemia may contribute to the induction of VT in cardiac arrest survivors with CAD and abnormal LV function.

There is now a large body of evidence demonstrating that coronary artery bypass graft (CABG) surgery reduces the incidence of SCD in patients with critical CAD.[28-30] In the Coronary Artery Surgery Study, of 13,476 patients prospectively assigned to either CABG surgery or medical therapy, a significantly smaller percentage of surgically treated patients died suddenly over a mean follow-up period of 4.6 years (1.6% vs. 4.9%).[30] In addition, the risk of recurrence of cardiac arrest is reduced in cardiac arrest survivors who have undergone CABG.[31,32] In a population of 85 cardiac arrest survivors who underwent CABG, the relative risk of recurrent cardiac arrest was 0.48.[32] Garan et al[33] and Kelly et al[34] used programmed electrical stimulation to examine the effect of CABG surgery on inducible ventricular arrhythmias in patients with life-threatening ventricular arrhythmias and in cardiac arrest survivors. In both studies coronary revascularization abolished inducible ventricular arrhythmias in a substantial proportion. When the inducible arrhythmia was VF, a high percentage of the patients manifested no inducible arrhythmias on programmed electrical stimulation. By contrast, only a small percentage of the patients in whom programmed stimulation induced sustained monomorphic VT had their inducible arrhythmia suppressed by coronary revascularization. In both studies, approximately 50% of patients had sustained a temporally remote MI and approximately 80% had regional segmental wall motion abnormalities.

In an attempt to test the effect of exercise-induced ischemia on the inducibility of ventricular arrhythmias, Thomas et al repeated programmed electrical stimulation in ten patients with no inducible VT or VF at baseline, while the patients were undergoing vigorous supine bicycle exercise.[35] All patients had CAD, a history of remote MI, and prior sustained ventricular arrhythmias with hemodynamic collapse. Despite documented exercise-induced acute myocardial ischemia in nine of the ten patients, programmed electrical stimulation during exercise induced VT in only one patient. In one other patient VT was induced during the recovery period following exercise. A similarly low yield of inducible sustained ventricular arrhythmias was found by Davis et al using a similar protocol of two extrastimuli during programmed ventricular stimulation at the time of rapid atrial pacing to induce ischemia in a group of patients presenting with ventricular arrhythmias during chest pain or exertion.[36] It could be argued that a more aggressive protocol using three extrastimuli during peak cardiac work, although practically not feasible, would have increased the rate of inducibility of ventricular arrhythmias in these studies.

ANIMAL MODELS OF ACUTE-ON-CHRONIC CARDIAC ISCHEMIA

Several animal models of acute superimposed on chronic myocardial ischemia have been developed to investigate the arrhythmogenic potential of this substrate. All involve prior open-chest coronary artery ligation to create anterior wall infarctions of various sizes, followed by reversible occlusion of the circumflex coronary artery from 4 days to 8 weeks later, either again at open-chest surgery or using a transcatheter approach.[37] Although differing in technique and in the sizes of chronic infarction and transient ischemia achieved, these models seem to consistently show an increased incidence of spontaneous VF during later reversible coronary artery occlusion and a higher rate of inducible ventricular arrhythmias during subsequent ischemia than in comparable animals with prior infarction but no superimposed ischemia. However, significant differences exist between the models. While Wilber et al demonstrated that electrically induced VT in a previously infarcted canine heart model predicted spontaneous VF during a later ischemic episode,[38] Garan et al found that programmed electrical stimulation predicted spontaneous ventricular arrhythmias during coronary occlusion in only 21% of postinfarction dogs.[39] In the latter model the LAD coronary artery is occluded distal to the first diagonal branch along with ligation of multiple epicardial branches of the circumflex and posterior descending coronary arteries supplying the apical area. The infarct produced by this technique is confluent and transmural, unlike the former model, although smaller.[40]

In a conscious canine model of SCD, acute occlusion of the left circumflex artery caused spontaneous VF arising in the posterior left ventricle in 97% of dogs when the collateral blood supply was restricted because of prior anterior wall infarction with residual critical stenosis of the LAD coronary artery.[41] This same occlusion in dogs with LAD stenosis but no prior MI resulted in only a 20% incidence of VF. The presence of anterior wall infarction thus increased the frequency of VF when a different area of myocardium was rendered ischemic. The authors interpreted these results as indicating that a "critical mass" of infarcted LV is required to sustain VF triggered by ectopic activity in the area of acute ischemia.[41]

Programmed electrical stimulation has been used to initiate ventricular arrhythmias in both open-chest[42,43] and closed-chest[44] canine models following coronary artery occlusion. The inducibility of ventricular arrhythmias by programmed stimulation and the subsequent survival rate in dogs with acute ischemia in the circumflex artery territory 4–6 days following LAD coronary artery occlusion depend on the size of the anterior wall MI.[38,39] Dogs with larger infarction, as assessed by postmortem tissue staining, had more easily inducible ventricular arrhythmias and worse survival.[38]

Myerburg et al (1982) observed that the incidence of spontaneous ventricular arrhythmias differed between three groups of open-chest cats with healed MI, acute ischemia, and acute ischemia superimposed on healed MI.[45] Spontaneous ventricular arrhythmias occurred in 31% of 61 cats with a 2–4-month-old healed MI, in 42% of 38 cats with acute coronary occlusion, and in 62% of 24 cats in which 90–120 minutes of acute ischemia was superimposed on a 2–4 month-old healed MI.[45] When the hearts were removed and perfused in vitro, programmed stimulation induced sustained ventricular arrhythmias significantly more frequently in the group of cats in which 90–120 minutes of acute ischemia was superimposed on a healed MI than in the other groups.[45]

Kabell et al observed abnormal spontaneous local electrical activity in the form of fractionation and conduction delay in anterior wall electrograms occurring simultaneously with a significant reduction in coronary blood flow through the anterior LV wall in dogs with a 4-day-old anterior wall infarct during circumflex artery occlusion.[46] Spontaneous VT/VF occurred in 4 of 15 dogs in this study. Although the reduction in coronary blood flow to the anterior wall was significant, it was of a much lesser degree than would be expected to produce ventricular arrhythmias in a normal heart. This group concluded that arrhythmogenesis was due to a greater sensitivity of the electrophysiologically abnormal peri-infarction tissue to reversible ischemia.[46]

Other observations also suggest that the mechanism of VT in chronic infarction may differ from the mechanisms responsible for VT or VF when acute ischemia is superimposed on previous infarction. In a canine model of 2-week-old transmural infarction, spontaneous arrhythmias did not correlate with infarct size but did correlate with a reversible decrease in myocardial blood flow to the infarct border zone and peri-infarction zone in the LV wall during reversible circumflex artery occlusion.[39] In contrast, the frequency of electrically induced arrhythmias correlated with infarct size, suggesting a difference in the underlying mechanisms between induced and spontaneous arrhythmias in this model.[39]

CELLULAR ELECTROPHYSIOLOGICAL ABNORMALITIES DURING ACUTE-ON-CHRONIC ISCHEMIA

Intracellular microelectrode techniques have been used to examine cellular electrophysiological changes in in vitro heart preparations since the early 1970s.[47] In subendocardial Purkinje fibers surviving 24 hours after MI, various phenomena, including repetitive depolarizations that are both spontaneous and inducible by programmed stimulation, prolonged action potential durations, and areas of entrance and exit block are observed.[47]

In their series of experiments using cats with healed, acute, and acute-on-healed MI, Myerburg et al have used these techniques to measure transmembrane action potentials from normal and infarcted subendocardium of the excised and superfused hearts.[45] Measurement of transmembrane action potential characteristics revealed that hearts with acute-on-chronic ischemia had the greatest degree of dispersion of action potential duration and ventricular refractoriness during programmed stimulation in comparison with hearts with chronic MI alone or acute ischemia alone.[45] Measurements of transmembrane potentials in hearts with acute-on-chronic ischemia revealed an abnormally prolonged repolarization phase in acutely ischemic cells overlying the healed MI, in contrast to findings in acutely ischemic cells in normal areas of myocardium, in which the action potential duration was shortened. The reason for such an alteration in action potential under these circumstances is not clear. The investigators concluded that healing of surviving cells after acute MI leaves residual long-term electrophysiological abnormalities at a cellular level that predispose to electrical instability during further acute ischemia.[45] Further data from the same group show differential responsiveness of surviving cells overlying a healed MI to the antiarrhythmic agent procainamide, suggesting that an alteration in membrane function persists.[48]

In the in vitro coronary-perfused feline heart preparation with a 2–4-month-old healed MI, differences were again demonstrated in the transmembrane action potential between endocardial cells in normal and infarct zones.[49] There were no significant differences in measured action potential variables and refractory periods between cells in the normal and infarcted zones before acute ischemia. When coronary perfusion was discontinued ("ischemia"), resting potential, action potential amplitude, and action potential duration were reduced and the refractory period was shortened progressively in cells in the normal zone. However, the action potential changes were less prominent and the refractory period was unchanged in the infarct zone. As a result there were significant differences in the resting membrane potential, action potential amplitude, action potential duration, and ventricular refractory period between cells in the normal and infarcted zones at 10 minutes of ischemia. The differences became larger as the ischemic period was prolonged. In addition, spontaneous rapid ventricular activity was observed during the last 20–30 minutes of ischemia in four of eight preparations with healed MI but not in normal hearts.[49]

Thus, cellular electrophysiological characteristics demonstrate heterogeneity during acute ischemia superimposed on healed MI. This dispersion of refractoriness and repolarization is related to the development of arrhythmias in the same animal model during acute ischemia in normal hearts and may be an important mechanism of arrhythmia in both circumstances.[50]

MECHANISMS OF VENTRICULAR ARRHYTHMIAS IN ACUTE-ON-CHRONIC ISCHEMIA

The mechanism of ventricular arrhythmias in acute-on-chronic ischemia is not clear. The mechanism of VT originating in chronic MI has been demonstrated to be re-entry, both in canine models of acute MI[42,43,51] and in humans.[52–56] Whether the VT occurring in acute-on-chronic ischemia also has a re-entrant mechanism remains to be established. In animal models of acute-on-chronic ischemia, abnormal local electrical activity has been recorded both at the site of the prior healed MI[46] and in the remote territory of acute ischemia.[41] Both canine models had 4-day-old anterior LV infarctions with superimposed circumflex territory ischemia, although the model of Kabell and colleagues was anesthetized and open chest, while the model of Patterson and colleagues was conscious and closed chest. In more recent work in the conscious canine model, Patterson et al have demonstrated fractionation and delay of normally conducted beats recorded within 5 minutes of acute left circumflex coronary artery ischemia along with local conduction block.[57] In cases where spontaneous VT occurred, the arrhythmia was accompanied by continuous diastolic electrical activity on the epicardial surface of the circumflex coronary artery territory. Similar changes of a lesser degree were also recorded from the midmyocardium. During a second, delayed phase of ventricular arrhythmia, further increases in latency of midmyocardial activation were observed in the circumflex territory. The site of earliest electrical activation for this second phase of arrhythmia was consistently observed in the midmyocardium.[57] These findings were interpreted as showing localized epicardial re-entry within the acutely ischemic zone, followed by midmyocardial re-entry during the second phase.

Animal studies suggest that the degree of acute collateral ischemia in a chronically infarcted zone of myocardium determines whether the subsequent ventricular arrhythmia is VT or VF.[58] In a canine model, superimposed ischemia increased the likelihood of induction of VT with lesser grades of coronary flow reduction compared with that necessary to allow spontaneous VF, suggesting that the underlying pathophysiology may differ between the two arrhythmias.[58] In the canine model of chronic transmural MI studied by Garan et al, a similar disparity was observed between induced and spontaneous arrhythmias. Induced VT correlated with the size of the 2-week-old infarct, while spontaneous VF during superimposed acute reversible ischemia correlated with a reduction in myocardial blood flow to the infarct border and peri-infarction border zone, suggesting different underlying mechanisms for these arrhythmias.[39] At a cellular level, increased dispersion of refractoriness and repolarization has been observed and may provide a pathophysiological basis for re-entry.[49,50] Some evidence in support of re-entry occurring in humans during the acute ischemia of percutaneous transluminal coronary angioplasty has recently been obtained using a body surface mapping technique. In 25 patients without prior infarction, including five with double-vessel CAD, changes in regional myocardial conduction velocity have been inferred during acute ischemia.[59] This modulation of the arrhythmia substrate by transient ischemia, achieving circumstances favorable for re-entry, was not observed in patients with adequate collateral blood supply to the transiently ischemic territory.[59] Whether such observations also pertain in patients with chronic MI remains to be demonstrated.

Autonomic mechanisms may have an important effect on arrhythmogenesis in acute-on-chronic ischemia. In the conscious canine model of sudden death, left stellectomy reduced the rate of spontaneous VF within 1 hour of acute circumflex ischemia following prior anterior infarction.[20,60] This occurred without measurable electrophysiological changes prior to ischemia and without changes in regional myocardial norepinephrine content.[60] In addition, initial experience with β-adrenergic-receptor antagonists in this model suggests a beneficial effect on spontaneous arrhythmia development.[57]

SUMMARY

Although it has been difficult to demonstrate directly in clinical studies, there is now considerable circumstantial evidence that acute ischemia superimposed on chronic CAD or MI enhances the arrhythmogenic potential both clinically and in animal models. It is likely that a large proportion of SCDs have this combination of acute-on-chronic ischemia. Animal models have been developed which show that the tendency to spontaneous occurrence of ventricular arrhythmias is determined in part by the size of healed infarcted myocardium and the extent of collateral ischemia, possibly modulated by autonomic influences. Recent work using the existing models suggests a beneficial antiarrhythmic effect of β-adrenergic-blocking agents in these circumstances.[57,61-63] However, the mechanisms underlying clinical VT and VF during acute-on-chronic myocardial ischemia remain uncertain, and the information that has been obtained from animal models regarding arrhythmia mechanisms, site of origin, the influence of autonomic factors, and the effects of drugs is yet to be confirmed in clinical studies.

REFERENCES

1. Hurwitz JL, Josephson ME: Sudden cardiac death in patients with chronic coronary heart disease. Circulation 85(suppl I):I-43–I-49, 1992.
2. Adgey AAJ, Nelson PG, Scott ME, et al: Management of ventricular fibrillation outside hospital. Lancet i:1169–1171, 1969.
3. Baum RS, Alvarez H, Cobb LA: Survival after resuscitation from out-of-hospital ventricular fibrillation. Circulation 50:1231–1235, 1974.
4. Liberthson RR, Nagel EL, Hirschman JC, Nussenfeld SR: Prehospital ventricular defibrillation: Prognosis and follow-up course. N Engl J Med 291:317–321, 1974.
5. Goldstein S, Landis R, Leighton R, et al: Characteristics of the resuscitated out-of-hospital cardiac arrest victim with coronary heart disease. Circulation 64:977–984, 1981.
6. Marcus FI, Cobb LA, Edwards JE, et al: Mechanism of death and prevalence of myocardial ischemic symptoms in the terminal event after acute myocardial infarction. Am J Cardiol 61:8–15, 1988.
7. Weaver WD, Lorch GS, Alvarez HA, Cobb LA: Angiographic findings and prognostic indicators in patients resuscitated from sudden cardiac death. Circulation 54:895–900, 1976.
8. Adhar GC, Larson LW, Bardy GH, Greene HL: Sustained ventricular arrhythmias: Differences between survivors of cardiac arrest and patients with recurrent sustained ventricular tachycardia. J Am Coll Cardiol 12:159–165, 1988.
9. Kleiman RB, Miller JM, Buxton AE, Josephson ME, Marchlinski FE: Prognosis following sustained ventricular tachycardia occurring early after myocardial infarction. Am J Cardiol 62:528–533, 1988.
10. Kuller LH, Cooper M, Perper J, Fisher R: Myocardial infarction and sudden death in an urban community. Bull NY Acad Med 49:532–543, 1973.
11. Titus JL, Oxman HA, Connolly DC, Nobrega FT: Sudden unexpected death as the initial manifestation of coronary heart disease: Clinical and pathological observations. Singapore Med J 14:291–293, 1973.
12. Liberthson RR, Nagel EL, Hirschman JC, Nussenfeld SR, Blackbourne BD, Davis JH: Pathophysiologic observations in prehospital ventricular fibrillation and sudden cardiac death. Circulation 49:790–798, 1974.
13. Davies MJ: Pathological view of sudden cardiac death. Br Heart J 45:88–96, 1981.
14. Schuster EH, Bulkley BH: Ischemia at a distance after acute myocardial infarction: A cause of early postinfarction angina. Circulation 62:509–515, 1980.
15. Schuster EH, Bulkley BH: Early post-infarction angina: Ischemia at a distance and ischemia in the infarct zone. N Engl J Med 305:1101–1105, 1981.
16. Gooch AS, McConnell: Analysis of transient arrhythmias and conduction disturbances occurring during submaximal treadmill exercise testing. Prog Cardiovasc Dis 13:293–307, 1970.

17. Goldschlager N, Cake D, Cohn K: Exercise-induced ventricular arrhythmias in patients with coronary artery disease. Am J Cardiol *31*:434–440, 1973.
18. McHenry PL, Morris SN, Kavalier M, Jordan JW: Comparative study of exercise-induced ventricular arrhythmias in normal subjects and patients with documented coronary artery disease. Am J Cardiol *37*: 609–616, 1976.
19. Mokotoff DM, Quinones MA, Miller RR: Exercise-induced ventricular tachycardia. Chest *77*:10–16, 1980.
20. Schwartz PJ, Billman GE, Stone HL: Autonomic mechanisms in ventricular fibrillation induced by myocardial ischemia during exercise in dogs with healed myocardial infarction. Circulation *69*:790–800, 1984.
21. Weiner DA, Levine SR, Klein MD, Ryan TJ: Ventricular arrhythmias during exercise testing: Mechanism, response to coronary bypass surgery and prognostic significance. Am J Cardiol *53*:1553–1557, 1984.
22. Ritchie JL, Hamilton GW, Trobaugh GB, Weaver WD, Williams DL, Cobb LA: Myocardial imaging and radionuclide angiography in survivors of sudden cardiac death due to ventricular fibrillation: Preliminary report. Am J Cardiol *39*:852–857, 1977.
23. Sellers TD, Beller GA, Gibson RS, Watson DD, DiMarco JP: Prevalence of ischemia by quantitative thallium-201 scintigraphy in patients with ventricular tachycardia or fibrillation inducible by programmed stimulation. Am J Cardiol *59*:828–832, 1987.
24. Ruskin JN, DiMarco JP, Garan H: Out-of-hospital cardiac arrest: Electrophysiologic observations and selection of long-term antiarrhythmic therapy. N Engl J Med *303*: 607–613, 1980.
25. Wilber DJ, Garan H, Finkelstein D, et al: Out-of-hospital cardiac arrest: Use of electrophysiologic testing in the prediction of long-term outcome. N Engl J Med *318*: 19–24, 1988.
26. Ruskin JN: Role of invasive electrophysiology testing in the evaluation and treatment of patients at high risk for sudden cardiac death. Circulation *85(suppl I)*:I-152–I-159, 1992.
27. Morady F, DiCarlo LA, Krol RB, et al: Role of myocardial ischemia during programmed stimulation in survivors of cardiac arrest with coronary artery disease. J Am Coll Cardiol *9*:1004–1012, 1987.
28. Vismara LA, Miller RR, Price JE, Karem R, DeMaria AN, Mason DT: Improved longevity due to reduction of sudden death by aortocoronary bypass in coronary atherosclerosis. Am J Cardiol *39*:919–924, 1977.
29. Hammermeister KE, DeRouen TA, Murray JA, Dodge HT: Effect of aortocoronary saphenous vein bypass grafting on death and sudden death. Am J Cardiol *39*:925–934, 1977.
30. Holmes DR, Davis KB, Mock MB, et al: The effect of medical and surgical treatment on subsequent sudden cardiac death in patients with coronary artery disease: A report from the Coronary Artery Surgery Study. Circulation *73*:1254–1263, 1986.
31. Tresch DD, Wetherbee JN, Siegel R, et al: Long-term follow-up of survivors of prehospital sudden cardiac death treated with coronary bypass surgery. Am Heart J *110*: 1139–1145, 1985.
32. Every NR, Fahrenbruch CE, Hallstrom AP, Weaver WD, Cobb LA: Influence of coronary bypass surgery on subsequent outcome of patients resuscitated from out of hospital cardiac arrest. J Am Coll Cardiol *19*: 1435–1439, 1992.
33. Garan H, Ruskin JN, DiMarco JP, et al: Electrophysiologic studies before and after myocardial revascularization in patients with life-threatening ventricular arrhythmias. Am J Cardiol *51*:519–524, 1983.
34. Kelly P, Ruskin JN, Vlahakes GJ, Buckley MJ, Freeman CS, Garan H: Surgical coronary revascularization in survivors of prehospital cardiac arrest: Its effect on inducible ventricular arrhythmias and long-term survival. J Am Coll Cardiol *15*:267–273, 1990.
35. Thomas GS, Garan H, Davis MJE, et al: Exercise electrophysiology testing: The effect of exercise on the induction of ventricular arrhythmias by programmed ventricular stimulation. PACE *13*:17–22, 1990.
36. Davis MJE, Boucher CA, Garan H, Ruskin JN: Programmed ventricular stimulation during myocardial ischemia induced by rapid atrial pacing. J Am Coll Cardiol *9*:107A, 1987.
37. Wit AL, Janse MJ: Experimental models of ventricular tachycardia and fibrillation caused by ischemia and infarction. Circulation *85(suppl I)*:I-32–I-42, 1992.
38. Wilber DJ, Lynch JJ, Montgomery D, Lucchesi BR: Postinfarction sudden death: Significance of inducible ventricular tachycardia and infarct size in a conscious canine model. Am Heart J *109*:8–18, 1985.
39. Garan H, McComb JM, Ruskin JN: Spontaneous and electrically induced ventricular arrhythmias during acute ischemia superimposed on 2 week old canine myocardial infarction. J Am Coll Cardiol *11*:603–611, 1988.
40. Garan H, Ruskin JN, McGovern B, Grant

40. ...G: Serial analysis of electrically induced ventricular arrhythmias in a canine model of myocardial infarction. J Am Coll Cardiol 5: 1095–1106, 1985.
41. Patterson E, Holland K, Eller BT, Lucchesi BR: Ventricular fibrillation resulting from ischemia at a site remote from previous myocardial infarction. Am J Cardiol 50: 1414–1423, 1982.
42. El-Sherif N, Scherlag BJ, Lazzara R, Hope RR: Re-entrant ventricular arrhythmias in the late myocardial infarction period: 1. Conduction characteristics in the infarct zone. Circulation 55:686–701, 1977.
43. El-Sherif N, Hope RR, Scherlag BJ, Lazzara R: Re-entrant ventricular arrhythmias in the late myocardial infarction period: 2. Patterns of initiation and termination of re-entry. Circulation 55:702–719, 1977.
44. Karagueuzian HS, Fenoglio JJ, Weiss MB, Wit AL: Protracted ventricular tachycardia induced by premature stimulation of the canine heart after coronary artery occlusion and reperfusion. Circ Res 44:833–846, 1979.
45. Myerburg RJ, Epstein K, Gaide MS, et al: Electrophysiologic consequences of experimental acute ischemia superimposed on healed myocardial infarction in cats. Am J Cardiol 49:323–330, 1982.
46. Kabell G, Brachmann J, Scherlag BJ, Harrison L, Lazzara R: Mechanisms of ventricular arrhythmias in multivessel coronary disease: The effects of collateral zone ischemia. Am Heart J 108:447–454, 1984.
47. Friedman PL, Stewart JR, Wit AL: Spontaneous and induced cardiac arrhythmias in subendocardial Purkinje fibers surviving extensive myocardial infarction in dogs. Circulation 33:612–626, 1973.
48. Myerburg RJ, Bassett AL, Epstein K, et al: Electrophysiological effects of procainamide in acute and healed experimental ischemic injury of cat myocardium. Circ Res 50:386–393, 1982.
49. Kimura S, Bassett AL, Cameron JS, Huikuri H, Kozlovskis PL, Myerburg RJ: Cellular electrophysiological changes during ischemia in isolated, coronary-perfused cat ventricle with healed myocardial infarction. Circulation 78:401–406, 1988.
50. Kimura S, Bassett AL, Kohya T, Kozlovskis PL, Myerburg RJ: Simultaneous recording of action potentials from endocardium and epicardium during ischemia in the isolated cat ventricle: Relation of temporal electrophysiologic heterogeneities to arrhythmias. Circulation 74:401–409, 1986.
51. Mehra R, Zeiler RH, Gough WB, El-Sherif N: Reentrant ventricular arrhythmias in the late myocardial infarction period: 9. Electrophysiologic-anatomic correlation of reentrant circuits. Circulation 67:11–24, 1983.
52. Josephson ME, Horowitz LN, Farshidi A, Kastor JA: Recurrent sustained ventricular tachycardia: 1. Mechanisms. Circulation 57: 431–440, 1978.
53. Josephson ME, Horowitz LN, Farshidi A, Spear JA, Kastor JA, Moore EN: Recurrent sustained ventricular tachycardia: 2. Endocardial mapping. Circulation 57:440–447, 1978.
54. Josephson ME, Horowitz LN, Farshidi A: Continuous local electrical activity: A mechanism of recurrent ventricular tachycardia. Circulation 57:660–665, 1978.
55. Horowitz LN, Josephson ME, Harken AH: Epicardial and endocardial activation during sustained ventricular tachycardia in man. Circulation 60:1227–1238, 1980.
56. deBakker JMT, van Capelle FJL, Janse MJ, et al: Reentry as a cause of ventricular tachycardia in patients with chronic ischemic heart disease: Electrophysiologic and anatomic correlation. Circulation 77:589–606, 1988.
57. Patterson E, Lucchesi BR: Electrophysiologic and antiarrhythmic actions of nadolol: Acute ischemia in the presence of previous myocardial infarction. Am Heart J 116: 1223–1232, 1988.
58. Furukawa T, Moroe K, Mayrovitz HN, Sampsell R, Furukawa N, Myerburg RJ: Arrhythmogenic effects of graded coronary blood flow reductions superimposed on prior myocardial infarction in dogs. Circulation 84:368–377, 1991.
59. Spekhorst H, Sippens Groenewegen A, David GK, Janse MJ, Dunning AJ: Body surface mapping during percutaneous transluminal coronary angioplasty. Circulation 81:840–849, 1990.
60. Nelson SD, Lynch JJ, Sanders D, Montgomery DG, Lucchesi BR: Electrophysiologic actions and antifibrillatory efficacy of subacute left stellectomy in a conscious, postinfarction model of ischemic ventricular fibrillation. Int J Cardiol 22:365–376, 1989.
61. Chi L, Mu D, Driscoll EM, Lucchesi BR: Antiarrhythmic and electrophysiologic actions of CK-3579 and sematilide in a conscious canine model of sudden coronary death. J Cardiovasc Pharmacol 16:312–324, 1990.
62. Chi L, Mu D, Lucchesi BR: Electrophysiology and antiarrhythmic actions of E-4031 in the experimental animal model of sudden coronary death. J Cardiovasc Pharmacol 17: 285–295, 1991.
63. Patterson E, Lynch JJ, Lucchesi BR: The antiarrhythmic and antifibrillatory actions of the beta-adrenergic receptor antagonist, d,l-sotalol. J Pharmacol Exp Ther 230:519–526, 1984.

22
Electrolyte Abnormalities as Triggers for Lethal Ventricular Arrhythmias

LEONARD S. GETTES

In order to clearly establish a causal relationship between a specific electrolyte abnormality and a lethal arrhythmia, it is important to demonstrate electrophysiological changes in single fibers and in intact hearts of experimental animals that are known or suspected to be arrhythmogenic and to demonstrate an unequivocal relationship between the electrolyte abnormality and lethal or potentially lethal arrhythmias in a reasonably homogeneous population of patients. It is also important to be able to reverse or to prevent a potentially arrhythmogenic electrophysiological change or a potentially lethal arrhythmia by correcting the electrolyte abnormality. Frequently it is difficult to determine whether the electrolyte abnormality contributes to the trigger or to the substrate for the arrhythmia, for in many situations, the electrophysiological changes that are induced by the abnormality may contribute to both. In addition, establishing in man a causal rather than a coincidental relationship between a specific electrolyte abnormality and potentially lethal arrhythmias is often difficult because of the presence of concurrent electrolyte abnormalities, drugs, or disease states known to have arrhythmic potential. Finally, the ability to reverse or prevent an arrhythmia by administration of a specific ion may reflect a specific antiarrhythmic effect unrelated to the cause of the arrhythmia. Even with these qualifications, there is general agreement that alterations in extracellular potassium induce electrophysiological changes that are arrhythmogenic and cause potentially lethal ventricular arrhythmias. It is widely believed that alterations in extracellular magnesium may be arrhythmogenic, and it is known that changes in intracellular calcium cause electrophysiological changes that contribute to the development and maintenance of arrhythmias. There are associations of certain disease states to the above ionic changes and to the appearance of potentially lethal arrhythmias, and there is evidence that the administration of potassium and magnesium salts may reverse or prevent potentially lethal arrhythmias even in the absence of documented abnormalities in the extracellular concentration of these ions.

In this chapter I will briefly review the electrophysiological changes induced by the various ions, which may be arrhythmogenic, and attempt to identify which of these changes are more likely to serve as triggers and which are more likely to contribute to the arrhythmogenic substrate. In addition, the experimental and clinical data suggesting an association between the ionic abnormality and potentially lethal arrhythmias will be presented. Particular attention will be focused on specific situations and/or disease states in which the association of an electrolyte change with lethal arrhythmias is more likely to occur. Three recent journal

---

Work was supported by National Heart, Lung and Blood Institute grants P01 HL 27430 and R37 HL 38885.

CHANGES IN EXTRACELLULAR POTASSIUM

Changes in extracellular potassium affect many components of the action potential, including the resting potential; the upstroke, shape, amplitude, and duration of the plateau; and the shape and duration of the phase of rapid repolarization and spontaneous diastolic depolarization.[4,5] The major potentially arrhythmogenic change induced by an increase in extracellular potassium is a decrease in the maximal rate of rise of the action potential upstroke that occurs secondary to a decrease in the resting membrane potential (Fig. 22–1). The increase in extracellular potassium from 4.8 to 12 mM shown in Figure 22–1 causes a 22-mV depolarization of the resting membrane—e.g., from −81 to −64 mV. As shown in Figure 22–2, a decrease in resting membrane potential of this magnitude is associated with a decrease in the maximum rate of rise of the action potential upstroke ($\dot{V}_{max}$) of approximately 50%,[6] and this decrease will result in conduction slowing. It is this decrease in conduction velocity that causes the diffuse widening of the P wave and QRS complex on the body surface electrocardiogram (ECG) in the setting of systemic hyperkalemia (see Fig. 22–1).[7,8] The decrease in resting membrane potential induced by increasing the extracellular potassium will also lengthen the time course of the recovery of the maximum rate of rise of the action potential upstroke following a preceding depolarization (Fig. 22–3).[6] This will result in postrepolarization or time-dependent refractoriness. As shown in Figure

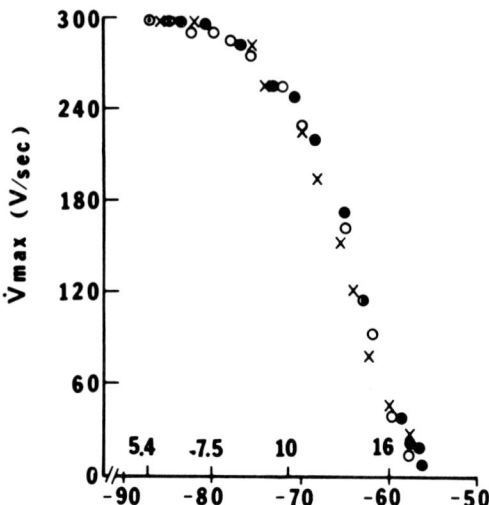

Fig. 22–2. Changes in resting membrane potential (mV, x-axis) and maximum rate of rise of the action potential upstroke ($\dot{V}_{max}$, y-axis) as extracellular potassium is changed from 5.4 mM to more than 16 mM (upper horizontal axis) in superfused guinea pig papillary muscles. Note that between a resting membrane potential of −90 mV and approximately −75 mV, $\dot{V}_{max}$ does not change significantly. A 50% reduction in $\dot{V}_{max}$ occurs when the resting potential is depolarized to approximately −65 mV. $\dot{V}_{max}$ is difficult to obtain when resting potential is less than −55 mV.

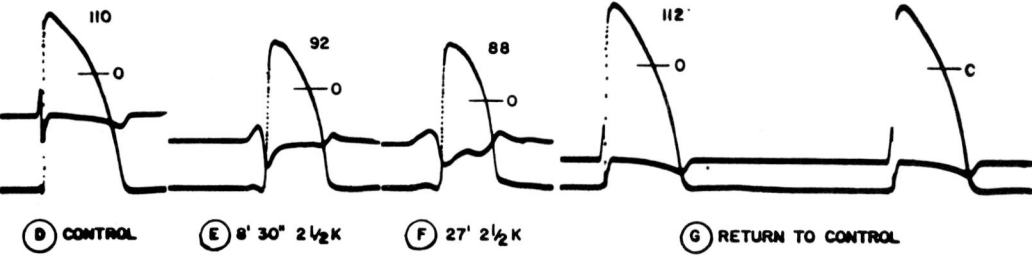

Fig. 22–1. Changes in ventricular action potential and simultaneously recorded electrograms from the epicardial surface of the ventricle in the isolated perfused rabbit heart as extracellular potassium is changed from 4.8 mM (control) to 12 mM (2½ K) and then back to control. Note the diffuse widening of the QRS complex in the electrogram which occurs as K$^+$ is raised. (Reproduced with permission from Gettes LS, et al: Am J Physiol 203:1135–1140, 1962.[4])

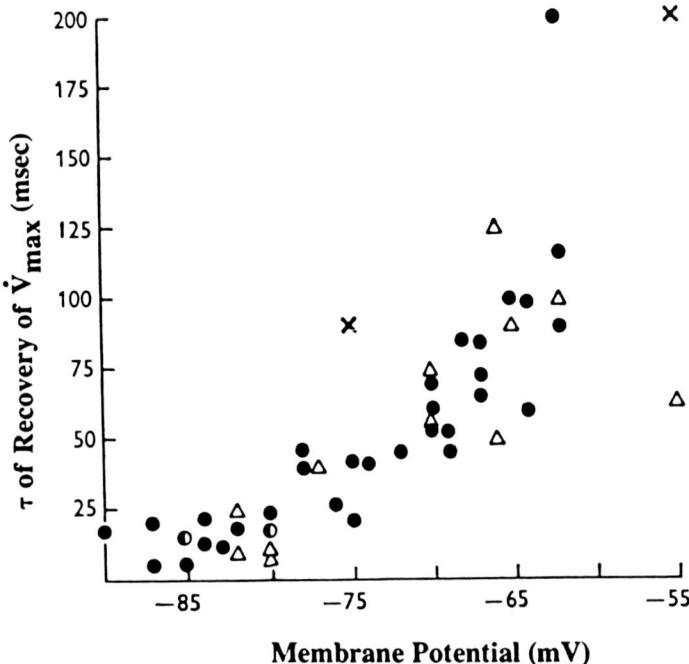

Fig. 22-3. Time course of the recovery of $\dot{V}_{max}$ of the action potential upstroke following the preceding depolarization in superfused guinea pig papillary muscles (solid circles), sheep trabeculae (half-filled circles), pig trabeculae (crosses), and sheep and calf Purkinje fibers (triangles). Note that as the membrane is depolarized from -90 to -55 mV by increasing extracellular potassium, the recovery time constant becomes progressively prolonged. (Reproduced with permission from Gettes LS, et al: J Physiol 240: 703-724, 1974.[6])

22-1, increasing the extracellular potassium also decreases the amplitude of the action potential and the voltage of the plateau, shortens the plateau duration, accelerates the phase of rapid repolarization, and suppresses automaticity. However, it is the slowing of conduction that is most responsible for the induction of ventricular re-entry or of the ventricular inexcitability that characterizes the lethal consequences of systemic hyperpotassemia. These electrophysiological changes contribute more to the substrate for re-entrant arrhythmias than to the trigger. When extracellular potassium is increased rapidly, as may occur in an attempt to reverse systemic hypopotassemia, or when hemolyzed blood is administered, cardiac arrest due to sinus node suppression and/or atrioventricular block as well as ventricular fibrillation (VF) due to re-entry may occur.[9] The terminal cardiovascular event associated with a variety of cardiac and noncardiac diseases, such as chronic renal insufficiency, is most likely due to a terminal increase in extracellular potassium occurring as a result of systemic acidosis and hypoxemia.

An increase in serum potassium has been shown to cause an increase in the diastolic threshold of excitability both in experimental animals and in man.[10,11] Some have reported that in experimental animals, an initial transient decrease in the excitability threshold may precede the increase.[12] The increase in the threshold of excitability decreased in man[10,11] at K^+ levels in excess of 7.0 mM and in the past was regarded as a possible cause of pacemaker failure. An effect of changes in extracellular potassium on defibrillation thresholds should also be regarded as a distinct possibility.

During acute myocardial ischemia, extracellular potassium in the ischemic zone increases (Fig. 22-4).[13] This increase is inhomogeneous (Fig. 22-5)[14-17] and is associated with inhomogeneous slowing of conduction and inhomogeneous changes in refractoriness.[16] These inhomogeneities in conduction and refractoriness are major factors contributing to the substrate for ventricular re-entrant arrhythmias. Indeed, infusion of potassium directly into a coronary artery can by itself cause VF and enhance the vulnerability of the ventricles to applied stimuli.[18] The changes in regional extracellular potassium associated with acute ischemia cause differences in the resting membrane potential of cells in the normal zone and cells in the ischemic zone, while the inhomogeneities within the ischemic

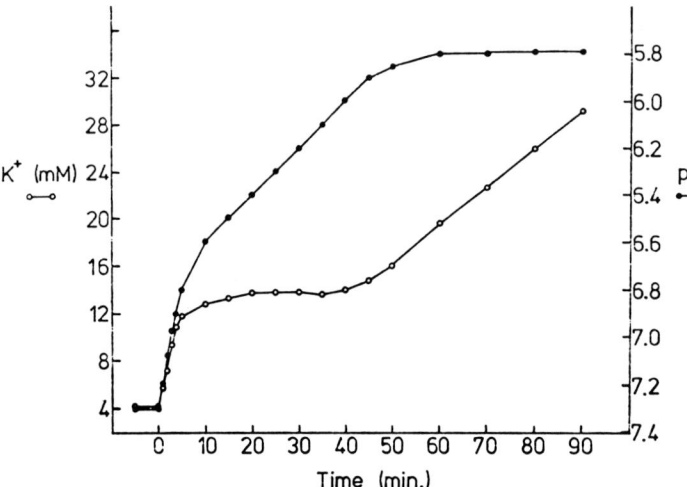

Fig. 22-4. Changes in extracellular myocardial potassium (open symbols) and pH (solid symbols) following occlusion of the left anterior descending coronary artery at time 0 in the in situ anesthetized pig. (Reproduced with permission from Gevers W: J Mol Cell Cardiol 9:867–874, 1979.[94])

zone itself result in inhomogeneous changes in resting potential within this zone. These differences in resting membrane potential lead to the development of injury currents that cause the TQ- and ST-segment changes on the body surface ECG characteristic of acute ischemia.[19] These injury currents are also capable of inducing or enhancing spontaneous diastolic depolarization and of bringing subthreshold afterdepolarizations to the threshold for a propagated response. By so doing, the injury currents provide one mechanism for the premature beats that initiate ventricular tachycardia (VT) and fibrillation.[20] Thus, in acute ischemia, the inhomogeneous changes in extracellular potassium create both the substrate and the trigger for re-entrant arrhythmias. The spontaneous activity induced by the injury current may also create sustained arrhythmias owing to enhanced automaticity or trigger activity.

A decrease in extracellular potassium is a well-recognized cause of lethal and potentially lethal arrhythmias.[21,22] Such a decrease hyperpolarizes the resting membrane and causes an increase in pacemaker activity in Purkinje cells (Fig. 22–6). This enhanced pacemaker activity is clearly a trigger for ventricular arrhythmias. Decreasing the extracellular potassium also shortens plateau duration in ventricular fibers, prolongs the phase of rapid repolarization,[4,5] and may increase the dispersion of the recovery of excitability.[23] It is these changes in repolarization that lead to the characteristic changes in the ST-segment, T and U waves on the body surface ECG that occur in the setting of systemic hypopotassemia, and that contribute to a substrate capable of supporting re-entrant activity.[24,25] Many of the electrophysiological effects of a decrease in extracellular potassium on pacemaker activity and repolarization are identical to those induced by the digitalis glycosides and by the β-sympathetic agonists. It is not surprising, therefore, that the combination of these factors would be associated with an increased incidence of cardiac arrhythmias. Thus, a decrease in extracellular potassium may provide the trigger and contribute to the substrate for re-entrant and nonre-entrant arrhythmias.

In the isolated heart, perfusion with solutions low in potassium causes VT and VF.[4,26] In the experimental animal, the induction of hypopotassemia by diuretics or dialysis results in ventricular ectopy.[27] In man, there are multiple well-documented episodes of supraventricular and ventricular arrhythmias occurring in hypopotassemic patients who do not have obvious underlying heart disease and who are not receiving digitalis therapy (Fig. 22–7).[22,28,29] Clearly, in patients receiving digitalis, hypopotassemia increases the likelihood of supraventricular and ventricular tachyarrhythmias as a consequence of both enhanced automaticity and re-entry. In these situations, the combination of low potassium levels and digitalis contributes both to the trigger and

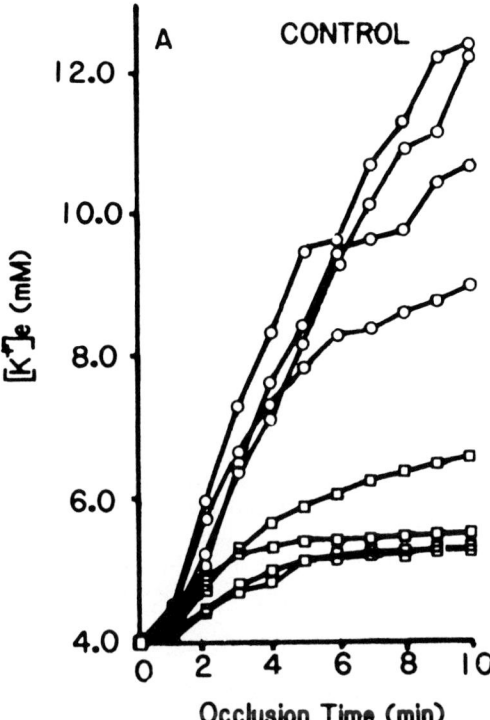

Fig. 22-5. Changes in myocardial extracellular potassium recorded simultaneously by eight K$^+$-sensitive electrodes placed within the ischemic zone following occlusion of the left anterior descending coronary artery at time 0 in the in situ anesthetized pig. The four electrodes rising to the highest levels were closely spaced within the center of the ischemic zone. The remaining four electrodes were closely spaced in the lateral margin of the ischemic area. Note the inhomogeneity of the potassium changes within each zone as well as between the zones. (Reproduced with permission from Coronel R, et al: Circulation 77: 1125–1138, 1988.[16])

to the substrate responsible for the arrhythmia.

There are several discrete clinical situations in which lethal ventricular arrhythmias have been shown to be related to and possibly caused by hypopotassemia. Several studies have documented that the ventricular arrhythmias occurring in hypertensive patients receiving diuretics, particularly thiazide and loop diuretics, correlate with the degree of hypopotassemia and become more frequent as the duration of therapy and the dose of diuretic therapy increases.[30,31] Indeed, there has been spec-ulation that the increased risk of death in hypertensive patients receiving thiazide diuretics, such as reported in the Multiple Risk Factor Intervention Trial (MRFIT),[32] was the result of hypopotassemia and possibly hypomagnesemia. It has been shown that the increase in ectopy associated with the development of hypopotassemia following the onset of thiazide therapy in hypertensive patients is worsened by exercise,[31] suggesting a synergism between the hypopotassemia and the increase in β-sympathetic effect induced by both static and dynamic exercise. It has recently been pointed out[22] that not all studies have been able to link hypopotassemia with arrhythmias.[33,34] However, in most studies failing to show such an association, the duration of thiazide therapy was brief, usually no more than 4 weeks.

A relationship between lethal ventricular arrhythmias occurring in the setting of acute myocardial infarction (MI) and hypopotassemia has been established as the result of studies in close to 10,000 patients.[35-41] These studies have shown that the incidence of VT and VF is greater in patients whose serum potassium level is less than 3.5 mM than in those with normal serum potassium levels (potassium > 3.5 mM). These studies have also shown that the risk of arrhythmia increases as the degree of hypopotassemia becomes more pronounced (Fig. 22-8). This occurs whether or not the patient was receiving diuretic agents prior to the infarction. There have also been reports suggesting an association between out-of-hospital sudden cardiac death (SCD) and hypopotassemia.[42,43] However, in these studies, there is usually no knowledge of the serum potassium level prior to the event. In addition, it is known that serum potassium falls after resuscitation.[44] This is due in part to the β-adrenergic stimulation, which leads to a shift of potassium into the cell.[44-46] The interactions between β-sympathetic stimulation and hypopotassemia may also contribute to the observations made in patients with acute MIs. Not only will the electrophysiological effects of the β-adrenergic stimulation be synergistic with those of hypopotassemia, but the β-adrenergic stimulation associated with acute ischemia might in itself be one cause of hypopotassemia.

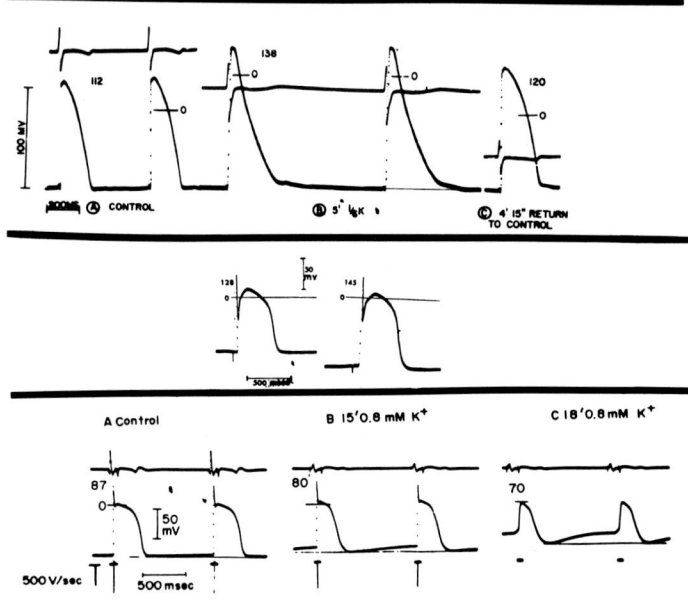

Fig. 22–6. Effect of lowering extracellular potassium from 4.8 mM (control) to 0.8 mM (⅙ K^+) on the ventricular action potential and epicardial electrogram in the isolated perfused rabbit heart *(top)*, and on right bundle-branch action potentials from the perfused pig moderator band *(middle* and *bottom)*. The differentiated upstroke is shown below the action potentials in the bottom panel. (Reproduced with permission from Gettes et al.[4,5])

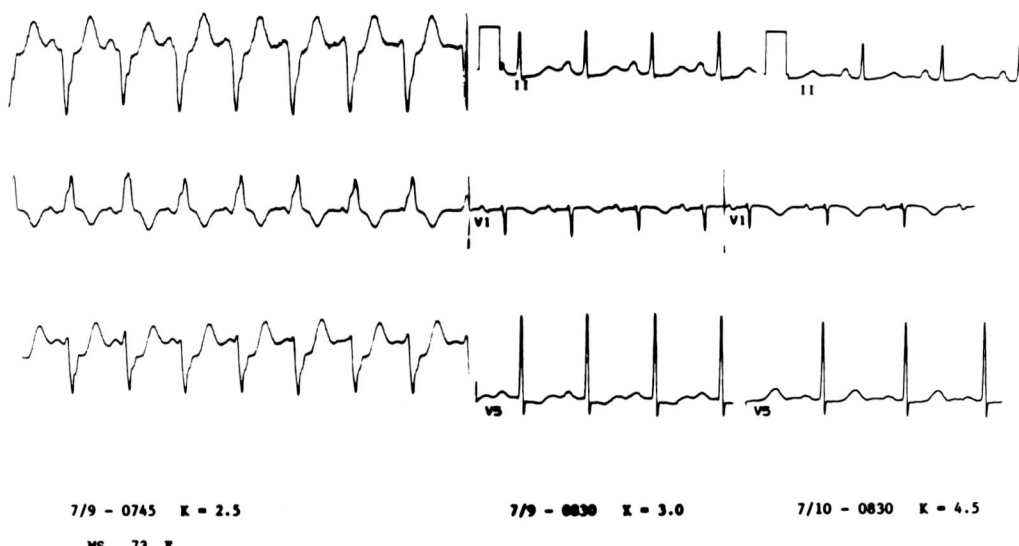

Fig. 22–7. Electrocardiographic leads II *(top)*, V_1 *(middle)*, and V_5 *(bottom)* recorded from a 73-year-old woman receiving thiazide diuretics. At 0745, when K^+ is 2.5 mM *(left)*, the ECG shows ventricular tachycardia with AV dissociation. At 0830, when K^+ is 3.0 mM following intravenous KCl administration *(center)*, the rhythm is sinus and there are ST-, T-, and U-wave changes of hypokalemia. At 0830 the next day, when potassium is 4.5 mM *(right)*, the ECG manifestations of hypokalemia have largely resolved. (Reproduced with permission from Gettes LS: Circulation 85(suppl I):I-70–I-76, 1992.[29])

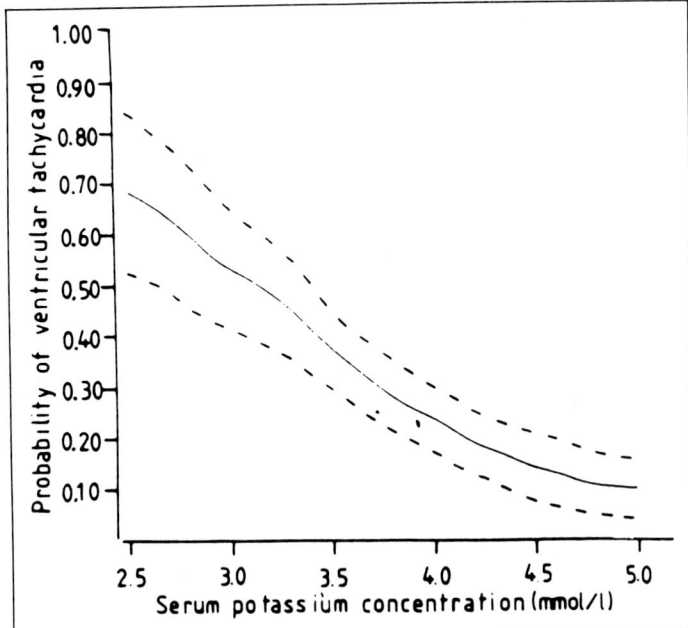

Fig. 22-8. Relationship between serum potassium concentration and probability of ventricular tachycardia in patients with acute myocardial infarction. (Reproduced with permission from Nordrehaug JE, et al: Circulation 71: 645-649, 1985.[37])

There are several other clinical settings in which lethal cardiac arrhythmias are believed to be due, at least in part, to hypopotassemia. These include the arrhythmias associated with acute starvation due to anorexia nervosa, bulimia, or excessive dieting,[47] and the arrhythmias occurring in patients with heart failure,[48,49] particularly those receiving thiazide and loop diuretics. The arrhythmias occurring during acute alcoholic toxicity and withdrawal and the arrhythmias occurring following surgery, particularly cardiac surgery, may also be due, at least in part, to hypopotassemia.

It is believed that in many of the situations in which hypopotassemia is present, hypomagnesemia or magnesium depletion in the absence of hypomagnesemia may contribute to the genesis of the associated arrhythmias. However, the studies on which these conclusions are based are often difficult to interpret because of the hypopotassemia, which by itself could cause the arrhythmia, and because the serum magnesium level may be normal. Moreover, other known arrhythmogenic factors may also be present.[50] A decrease in extracellular magnesium by itself has little effect on the electrophysiological properties of single cells or fibers and no consistent effect on the ECG of experimental animals or man.[50-52] When extracellular calcium is decreased, the concomitant lowering of magnesium will exaggerate the lengthening of the action potential plateau,[51] and there are isolated case reports linking ST-segment and U-wave changes on the body surface ECG to hypomagnesemia.[53] However, frequently the patients reported are suffering from other metabolic problems, have significant underlying cardiac disease, and may be receiving cardioactive drugs. Thus, it is exceedingly difficult to establish a causal relationship between the reported ECG changes and the hypomagnesemia. A causal relationship was suggested in a case report of an alcoholic patient who was receiving thiazide diuretics but who was reported to have a normal serum potassium concentration and a serum magnesium concentration of 0.8 mM. In this patient, T-wave alternans, prolongation of the QT interval, and associated episodes of VT and VF occurred. The ECG abnormalities and the arrhythmias were reversed by administration of magnesium salts.[54]

Several observations have resulted in increasing enthusiasm for the concept that abnormalities in extracellular and intracellular magnesium may contribute significantly to the genesis of lethal cardiac arrhythmias, particularly in patients with hypertension[55,56] or heart failure who have received thiazide and loop diuretic drugs[48,49]; in patients experiencing acute alcohol intoxication or withdrawal[54]; and possibly in patients with acute ischemia.[57,58] The evidence supporting a causal role for hypomagnesemia and arrhythmias is as follows: (1) There are isolated occurrences of ventricular tachycardia, particularly of the torsade de pointes variety, occurring in the absence of abnormalities other than hypomagnesemia.[59,60] These arrhythmias frequently respond to intravenous magnesium therapy. In this situation, one would speculate that hypomagnesemia caused the early afterdepolarizations that are believed to cause this particular arrhythmia. (2) Hypokalemia in patients receiving long-term diuretic therapy and the associated ventricular arrhythmias often require magnesium as well as potassium replacement before either the hypopotassemia or the arrhythmias are reversed.[61] (3) The arrhythmias appearing in hypertensive patients treated with thiazide and loop diuretics correlate not only with the degree of hypopotassemia but also with the serum magnesium concentration, and best of all with the product of the change in the magnesium and potassium extracellular concentrations.[55,56] (4) The known ability of therapy with magnesium salts to treat supraventricular and ventricular tachyarrhythmias occurring in the absence as well as in the presence of digitalis[62-64] and to suppress torsade de pointes induced by type I antiarrhythmic drugs.[65] (5) A possible relationship between hypomagnesemia and arrhythmias in the setting of acute MI[57,58] and reports that prophylactic therapy with magnesium salts lessens the incidence of ventricular arrhythmias and death in the first 24 hours following an infarction.[66-71]

Shechter et al[70] have stressed that the reduction in mortality associated with a 48-hour infusion of magnesium sulfate initiated in the early stages of acute MI may reflect effects on infarct size,[72] decreased platelet aggregation,[73] and coronary vascular tone,[74] rather than a direct electrophysiological effect. However, an increase in extracellular magnesium blocks the L-type calcium channel,[75] shifts the curve relating the maximum rate of rise of the action potential upstroke to the resting potential in the hyperpolarizing direction along the voltage axis,[76] and restores excitability in potassium-depressed fibers.[77] It has been reported that administration of magnesium salts prevents the ECG changes induced by hyperpotassemia in man and attenuates the action potential changes and the depression of conduction velocity that occur in single fibers exposed to an increase in extracellular potassium.[78] An increase in extracellular magnesium also prevents the early afterdepolarizations induced by cesium and quinidine,[79,80] providing a possible explanation for the demonstrated effectiveness of treatment with magnesium salts for torsade de pointes[65] mentioned above. In his review, Shine[81] suggested that the effects of magnesium could best be understood by postulating an interaction of magnesium with other ions, particularly calcium and potassium, and with the ionic channels in the sarcolemmal membrane. Such a construct helps to explain the clinical observations in which the effect of alterations in serum magnesium are manifest primarily in patients with other metabolic and/or ionic disturbances. The take-home message from the existing information is that even though a clear relationship between abnormalities in intracellular and extracellular magnesium and ventricular arrhythmias has not been established, hypomagnesemia should be considered in situations in which hypopotassemia is present and in which ventricular arrhythmias occur, and the use of magnesium salts should be considered to treat refractory ventricular arrhythmias, particularly torsade de pointes and digitalis-induced arrhythmias. The analysis by Teo et al[71] of 1301 patients with acute MI studied in randomized trials suggests that the administration of magnesium salts early in the course of an acute MI may result in a significant reduction in serious ventricular arrhythmias and in mortality. Thus, magnesium therapy should also be considered in this group of patients.

While the ability to prevent or reverse arrhythmias with magnesium may be considered circumstantial evidence suggesting a role of magnesium depletion in the genesis of these arrhythmias, it must be kept in mind that the ability to treat an arrhythmia with an electrolyte solution does not necessarily indicate that the arrhythmia was caused by a deficiency in that electrolyte. As indicated above, increasing extracellular magnesium induces electrophysiological changes that may be antiarrhythmic, regardless of the cause of the arrhythmia. Similarly, the administration of potassium salts has clinically relevant antiarrhythmic effects even in the absence of hypopotassemia or digitalis excess.[82] Moreover, the administration of EDTA to lower ionized calcium has been used successfully to treat arrhythmias induced by digitalis.[83] Thus, the ability of potassium or magnesium salts to affect the frequency of an arrhythmia in any clinical setting should not be taken as proof that the arrhythmias were caused by hypomagnesemia or hypopotassemia.

Although changes in extracellular sodium and calcium cause electrophysiological alterations, as those in the action potential upstroke and shifts in excitability that may be considered arrhythmogenic, the extracellular concentration of these ions necessary to produce these changes are not encountered clinically. Changes in the intracellular concentration of these ions are also associated with electrophysiological alterations that may be arrhythmogenic, and these may occur in the clinical setting. An increase in intracellular calcium causes oscillatory afterpotentials in single cells and fibers. These changes may lead to single or multiple triggered responses.[84] The oscillatory afterpotentials induced by the dihydropyridine calcium ionophore, Bay K-8644,[85] by digitalis glycosides,[86] by catecholamines, and by reperfusion following a period of acute ischemia[87] are each believed to be caused by an increase in intracellular calcium. Some of the ventricular arrhythmias induced by the digitalis glycosides, some exercise-induced ventricular tachyarrhythmias, and some of the ventricular arrhythmias associated with myocardial reperfusion have been attributed to the triggered activity induced by these oscillatory action potentials.[86-88] In these situations, the increase in intracellular calcium serves as the trigger for the arrhythmia.

An increase in intracellular calcium also promotes cellular uncoupling[89-91] and may contribute to the conduction slowing that occurs in the setting of acute ischemia when

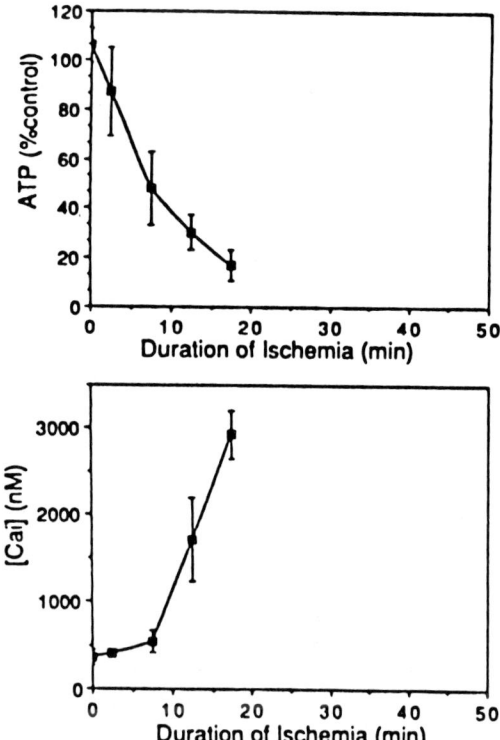

Fig. 22-9. Changes in intracellular ATP and intracellular calcium concentration during global no-flow ischemia in isolated perfused rat hearts as determined by NMR spectroscopy following loading with 5-BAPTA. (Reproduced with permission from Steenbergen C, et al: Circ Res 66: 135-146, 1990.[93])

intracellular calcium rises (Fig. 22-9).[92,93] Thus, the change in intracellular calcium contributes both to the trigger and to the substrate for arrhythmias. Decreases in intracellular and extracellular pH also occur in acute ischemia.[94,95] These changes, together with the increase in intracellular calcium and the changes in extracellular potassium, contribute to cellular uncoupling[90,91] and to the decrease in the maximum rise of the action potential upstroke.[96] Both effects—cellular uncoupling and the decreased maximum rate of rise of the action potential upstroke—will contribute to the slowing of conduction (Fig. 22-10). These changes thereby contribute to the substrate for re-entrant arrhythmias occurring in the setting of acute ischemia when an increase in extracellular K^+, a decrease in both extracellular and intracellular pH, and an in-

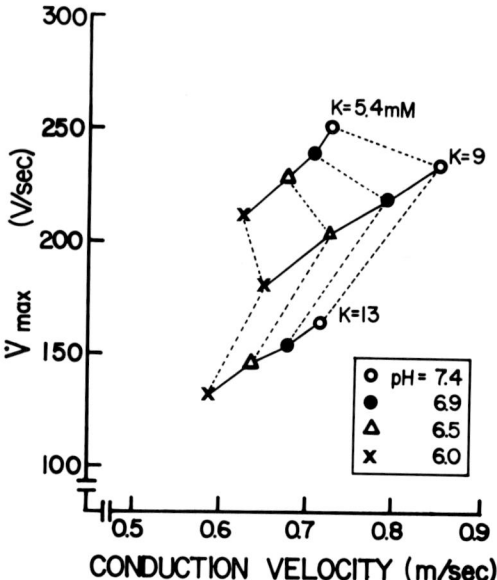

Fig. 22–10. Changes in $\dot{V}_{max}$ of the action potential upstroke and longitudinal conduction velocity in the isolated superfused guinea pig papillary muscle as pH is progressively lowered at the three levels of extracellular potassium shown. At each potassium level, acidosis causes a progressive decrease in $\dot{V}_{max}$ and conduction velocity. (Reproduced with permission from Kagiyama Y, et al: Circ Res 51:614–623, 1982.[96])

crease in intracellular calcium occur simultaneously.

An increase in intracellular sodium would be expected to decrease the sodium inward current and $\dot{V}_{max}$ of the action potential upstroke, thereby leading to slowing of conduction. This ionic change would also contribute to the substrate capable of supporting re-entry. In addition, an increase in intracellular sodium may stimulate an increase in intracellular calcium via the sodium-calcium exchange mechanism.[97] Such an increase in intracellular sodium would be expected in situations in which the sodium/potassium pump is depressed, as may occur during the later stages of acute ischemia. Indeed, an increase in intracellular sodium has been demonstrated under these circumstances.[98,99] Intracellular sodium also increases when the stimulation frequency is suddenly increased.[100] This effect may contribute to the rate-dependent changes in conduction that occur in acute isch-emia[101,102] and thereby contribute to the arrhythmogenic substrate.

SUMMARY

Changes in the extracellular and intracellular ionic milieu induced by a variety of mechanisms are clearly capable of causing electrophysiological changes in single cells and fibers and in intact hearts that may be considered arrhythmogenic. These changes contribute both to the arrhythmogenic trigger and to the arrhythmogenic substrate. It is also clear that in certain groups of patients, particularly those with hypertension and congestive heart failure who have been treated with thiazide and loop diuretics, the presence of ventricular arrhythmias should trigger a search for underlying electrolyte abnormalities, particularly hypopotassemia and/or hypomagnesemia. The arrhythmias occurring in the setting of acute ischemia can be attributed in large part to ionic events, particularly an inhomogeneous increase in extracellular potassium, a decrease in extracellular and intracellular pH, a rise in intracellular calcium, and possibly a rise in intracellular sodium, that occur when coronary flow is acutely interrupted. There is also circumstantial evidence suggesting that hypopotassemia and hypomagnesemia may contribute to the pathogenesis of these arrhythmias. There is solid electrophysiological evidence for considering both an increase and a decrease in extracellular potassium as crucial and often causal in the genesis of lethal cardiac arrhythmias. However, the precise role of changes in extracellular and intracellular magnesium in the genesis of such arrhythmias remains to be defined. The available data, while intriguing and suggestive of an association, are not adequate to permit an unbiased and objective statement of causality. Finally, there is no question that the administration of potassium and magnesium salts may be used to treat specific types of lethal cardiac arrhythmias even when the arrhythmia is unrelated to a primary abnormality in either ion.

The availability of sophisticated methods to determine intracellular ionic changes in a variety of situations, coupled with the ability to determine the effect of such ionic changes on the characteristics of ionic channels and currents in the sarcolemma and at the gap junction, should result in a more definitive understanding of the electrolytic and metabolic abnormalities that underlie lethal ventricular arrhythmias in man.

REFERENCES

1. Hollenberg NK, Hollifield JW (eds): A Symposium: Potassium/Magnesium Depletion: Is Your Patient at Risk of Sudden Death? Am J Med 82(suppl 3a), 1987.
2. Lauler D (ed): A Symposium: Magnesium Deficiency: Pathogenesis, Prevalence, and Strategies for Repletion. Am J Cardiol 63(14), 1989.
3. Packer M (ed): A Symposium: Hormone-Electrolyte Interactions in Congestive Heart Failure. Am J Cardiol 65(10), 1990.
4. Gettes LS, Surawicz B, Shiue J: Effect of high K, low K, and quinidine on QRS duration and ventricular action potential. Am J Physiol 203:1135–1140, 1962.
5. Gettes LS, Surawicz B: Effects of low and high concentrations of potassium on the simultaneously recorded Purkinje and ventricular action potentials of the perfused pig moderator band. Circ Res 23:717–729, 1968.
6. Gettes LS, Reuter H: Slow recovery from inactivation of inward currents in mammalian myocardial fibres. J Physiol 240:703–724, 1974.
7. Surawicz B: Arrhythmias and electrolyte disturbances. Bull NY Acad Sci 43:1160–1180, 1967.
8. Fisch C: Relation of electrolyte disturbances to cardiac arrhythmias. Circulation 47:408–418, 1973.
9. Surawicz B, Gettes LS: Two mechanisms of cardiac arrest produced by potassium. Circ Res 12:415–421, 1963.
10. Surawicz B, Chlebus H, Reeves JT, Gettes LS: Increase of ventricular excitability threshold by hyperpotassemia. JAMA 191:1049–1054, 1965.
11. Gettes LS, Shabetai R, Downs TA, Surawicz B: Effect of changes in potassium and calcium concentrations on diastolic threshold and strength-interval relationships of the human heart. Ann NY Acad Sci 167:693–705, 1969.
12. Han J, de Jalon PG, Moe GK: Adrenergic effects on ventricular vulnerability. Circ Res 14:516–524, 1947.
13. Harris AS, Bisteni A, Russel RA, Brigham JC, Firestone JE: Excitatory factors in ventricular tachycardia resulting from myocardial ischemia: Potassium a major excitant. Science 119:200–203, 1954.
14. Hill JL, Gettes LS: Effect of acute coronary artery occlusion on local myocardial extracellular K^+ activity in swine. Circulation 61:768–778, 1980.
15. Fleet WF, Johnson TA, Graebner CA, Engle CL, Gettes LS: Effects of verapamil on ischemia-induced changes in extracellular K^+, pH, and local activation in the pig. Circulation 73:837–846, 1986.
16. Coronel R, Fiolet JWT, Wilms-Schopman FJG, et al: Distribution of extracellular potassium and its relation to electrophysiologic changes during acute myocardial ischemia in the isolated perfused porcine heart. Circulation 77:1125–1138, 1988.
17. Johnson TA, Engle CL, Boyd LM, Koch GG, Gwinn M, Gettes LS: Magnitude and time course of extracellular potassium inhomogeneities during acute ischemia in pigs: Effect of verapamil. Circulation 83:622–634, 1991.
18. Logic J: Enhancement of the vulnerability of the ventricle to fibrillation (VF) by regional hyperkalaemia. Cardiovasc Res 7:501–507, 1973.
19. Holland RP, Brooks H: TQ-ST segment mapping: Critical review and analysis of current concepts. Am J Cardiol 40:110, 1977.
20. Janse MJ, van Capelle FJL, Morsink H, et al: Flow of "injury" current patterns of excitation during early ventricular arrhythmias in acute regional myocardial ischemia in isolated porcine and canine hearts: Evidence for two different arrhythmogenic mechanisms. Circ Res 47:151–165, 1980.
21. Helfant R: Hypokalemia and arrhythmias. Am J Med 80:13–22, 1986.
22. Podrid P: Potassium and ventricular arrhythmias. Am J Cardiol 65:33E–44E, 1990.
23. Suarwicz B: Electrophysiologic substrate of torsade de pointes: Dispersion of repolarization or early afterdepolarizations? J Am Coll Cardiol 14:172–184, 1989.
24. Surawicz B, Braun HA, Crum WB, Kemp RL, Wagner S, Bellet S: Quantitative analysis of the electrocardiographic pattern of hypopotassemia. Circulation 16:750–763, 1957.
25. Weaver WF, Burchell HB: Serum potassium and the electrocardiogram in hypokalemia. Circulation 21:505–521, 1960.
26. Gettes LS, Surawicz B, Kim KH: Role of myocardial K^+ and Ca^+ in initiation and inhibition of ventricular fibrillation. Am J Physiol 211:699, 1966.
27. Kunin AS, Surawicz B, Sims EA: Decrease

in serum potassium concentrations and appearance of cardiac arrhythmias during infusion of potassium with glucose in potassium-depleted patients. N Engl J Med 266: 228–233, 1962.
28. Davidson S, Surawicz B: Ectopic beats and atrioventricular conduction disturbances in patients with hypopotassemia. Arch Intern Med 120:280–285, 1967.
29. Gettes LS: Electrolyte abnormalities underlying lethal ventricular arrhythmias. Circulation 85(suppl I):I-70–I-76, 1992.
30. Hollifield JW, Slaton PB: Thiazide diuretics, hypokalemia and cardiac arrhythmias. Acta Med Scand (Suppl) 647:67–73, 1981.
31. Hollifield JW: Thiazide treatment of hypertension: Effects of thiazide diuretics on serum potassium, magnesium and ventricular ectopy. Am J Med 80(4A):8–12, 1986.
32. Multiple Risk Factor Intervention Trial: Multiple Risk Factor Intervention Trial Research Group. JAMA 248:1465–1477, 1982.
33. Papademetriou V, Fletcher R, Khatri IM, Freis ED: Diuretic induced hypokalemia in uncomplicated systemic hypertension: Effect of plasma potassium correction on cardiac arrhythmias. Am J Cardiol 52:1017–1022, 1983.
34. Lumme JAJ, Jounela AJ: Cardiac arrhythmias in hypertensive outpatients on various diuretics: Correlation between incidence and serum potassium and magnesium levels. Ann Clin Res 18:186–190, 1986.
35. Dyckner T, Helmers C, Wester PO: Cardiac dysrhythmias in patients with acute myocardial infarction. Acta Med Scand 216:127–132, 1984.
36. Kafka H, Langevin L, Armstrong W: Serum magnesium and potassium in acute myocardial infarction. Arch Intern Med 147:465–469, 1987.
37. Nordrehaug JE, Johannessen KA, von der Lippe G: Serum potassium concentrations as a risk factor of ventricular arrhythmias early in acute myocardial infarction. Circulation 71:645–649, 1985.
38. Nordrehaug JE, Von der Lippe G: Hypokalemia and ventricular fibrillation in acute myocardial infarction. Br Heart J 50:525–529, 1983.
39. Hulting J: In hospital ventricular fibrillation and its relation to serum potassium. Acta Med Scand (Suppl) 647:109–116, 1981.
40. Johansson BW, Dziamski R: Malignant arrhythmias in acute myocardial infarction: Relationship to serum potassium and effect of selective and nonselective beta blockade. Drugs 28(suppl)1:77–85, 1984.
41. Solomon R: Ventricular arrhythmias in patients with myocardial infarction and ischemia: The role of serum potassium. Drugs 31:112–120, 1986.
42. Thompson RG, Cobb LA: Hypokalemia after resuscitation from out of hospital ventricular fibrillation. JAMA 248:2860–2863, 1982.
43. Salerno DM, Asinger RW, Elsperger J, Ruiz E, Hodges M: Frequency of hypokalemia after successfully resuscitated out of hospital cardiac arrest compared with that in transmural acute myocardial infarction. Am J Cardiol 59:84–88, 1987.
44. Salerno DM, Elsperger J, Helseth D, Murakami M, Chepuri V: Serum potassium, calcium and magnesium after resuscitation from ventricular fibrillation: A canine study. J Am Coll Cardiol 10:178–185, 1987.
45. Struthers AD, Reid JL, Whitesmith R, Rodger JC: Effect of intravenous adrenaline on electrocardiogram, blood pressure and serum potassium. Br Heart J 49:90–93, 1983.
46. Brown MJ, Brown DL, Murphy MB: Hypokalemia from beta-2 receptor stimulation by circulating catecholamines. N Engl J Med 307:1414–1419, 1983.
47. Rajs J, Rajs E, Lundman T: Unexpected death in patients suffering from eating disorders. Acta Psychiatr Scand 74:587–596, 1986.
48. Packer M, Gottlieb S, Kessler P: Hormone-electrolyte interactions in the pathogenesis of lethal cardiac arrhythmias in patients with congestive heart failure: Basis of a new physiologic approach to control of arrhythmia. Am J Med 80:23–27, 1986.
49. Packer M: Potential role of potassium as a determinant of morbidity and mortality in patients with systemic hypertension and congestive heart failure. Am J Cardiol 65(suppl):45E–51E, 1990.
50. Surawicz B: Is hypomagnesemia or magnesium deficiency arrhythmogenic? J Am Coll Cardiol 14:1093–1096, 1989.
51. Surawicz B, Lepeschkin E, Herrlich HC: Low and high magnesium concentrations at various calcium levels: Effect on the monophasic action potential, electrocardiogram and contractility of isolated rabbit hearts. Circ Res 9:811–818, 1961.
52. Roden DM, Iansmith DH: Effects of low potassium or magnesium concentrations on isolated cardiac tissue. Am J Med 82:18–23, 1987.
53. Seeling MS: Electrocardiographic patterns of magnesium depletion appearing in alcoholic heart disease. Ann NY Acad Sci 162:906–917, 1969.
54. Reddy CVR, Kiok J, Khan R, El-Sherif:

Repolarization alternans associated with alcoholism and hypomagnesemia. Am J Cardiol 53:390–391, 1984.
55. Hollifield JW: Thiazide treatment of systemic hypertension: Effects on serum magnesium and ventricular ectopic activity. Am J Cardiol 63:22G–25G, 1989.
56. Hollifield JW: Magnesium depletion, diuretics and arrhythmias. Am J Med 82(suppl 3a):30–37, 1987.
57. Sjogren A, Edvinsson L, Fallgren B: Magnesium deficiency in coronary artery disease and cardiac arrhythmias. J Intern Med 226:213–222, 1989.
58. Solomon R: Ventricular arrhythmias in patients with myocardial infarction and ischemia: Relationship to serum potassium and magnesium. Drugs 28:66–76, 1984.
59. Chadda K, Lichstein E, Gupta P: Hypomagnesemia and refractory cardiac arrhythmia in a nondigitalized patient. Am J Cardiol 31:98–100, 1973.
60. Loeb H, Pietras R, Gunnar R, Tobin J: Paroxysmal ventricular fibrillation in two patients with hypomagnesemia: Treatment by transvenous pacing. Circulation 38: 210–215, 1968.
61. Whang R, Flink E, Dyckner T, Wester P, Aikawa J, Ryan M: Magnesium depletion as a cause of refractory potassium repletion. Arch Intern Med 145:1686–1689, 1985.
62. Iseri LT, Chung P, Tobis J: Magnesium therapy for intractable ventricular tachyarrhythmias in normomagnesemic patients. West J Med 138:823–828, 1983.
63. Iseri LT, Freed J, Bures A: Magnesium deficiency and cardiac disorders. Am J Med 58:837–846, 1975.
64. Zwerling H: Does exogenous magnesium suppress myocardial irritability and tachyarrhythmias in the nondigitalized patient? Am Heart J 113:1046–1053, 1987.
65. Tzivoni D, Keren A, Cohen A, et al: Magnesium therapy for torsades de pointes. Am J Cardiol 53:528–530, 1984.
66. Abraham A, Rosenmann D, Kramer M, et al: Magnesium in the prevention of lethal arrhythmias in acute myocardial infarction. Arch Intern Med 147:753–755, 1987.
67. Rasmussen H, Norregard P, Lindeneg, McNair P, Backer V, Balslev S: Intravenous magnesium in acute myocardial infarction. Lancet i:234–236, 1986.
68. Rasmussen H, Suenson M, McNair P, Norregard P, Balslev S: Magnesium infusion reduces the incidence of arrhythmias in acute myocardial infarction: A double-blind placebo-controlled study. Clin Cardiol 10:351–356, 1987.
69. Smith LF, Heagerty AM, Bing RF, Barnett DB: Intravenous infusion of magnesium sulphate after acute myocardial infarction: Effects on arrhythmias and mortality. Int J Cardiol 12:175–180, 1986.
70. Shechter M, Hod H, Marks N, Behar S, Kaplinsky E, Rabinowitz B: Beneficial effect of magnesium sulfate in acute myocardial infarction. Am J Cardiol 66:271–274, 1990.
71. Teo KK, Yusuf S, Collins R, Held PH, Peto R: Effects of intravenous magnesium in suspected acute myocardial infarction: Overview of randomised trials. Br Med J 303:1499–1503, 1991.
72. Morton BC, Nair RC, Smith FM, McKibbon TG, Poznanski WJ: Magnesium therapy in acute myocardial infarction: A double-blind study. Magnesium 3:346–352, 1984.
73. Adams JH, Mitchell JRA: The effect of agents which modify platelet behavior and of magnesium ions on thrombus formation in vivo. Thromb Haemost 42:603–610, 1979.
74. Turplaty PDMV, Altura BM: Magnesium deficiency produces spasms of coronary arteries: Relationship to etiology of sudden death ischemic heart disease. Science 208: 198–200, 1980.
75. Lansman J, Hess P, Tsien R: Blockade of current through single calcium channels by Cd^{2+}, Mg^{2+}, and Ca^{2+}. J Gen Physiol 88: 321–347, 1986.
76. Kiyosue T, Arita M: Magnesium restores high K-induced inactivation of the fast Na channel in guinea pig ventricular muscle. Pflugers Arch 395:78–80, 1982.
77. Watanabe T, Dreifus L: Electrophysiological effects of magnesium and its interactions with potassium. Cardiovas Res 6: 79–88, 1972.
78. Kraft LF, Katholi RE, Woods WT, James TN: Attenuation by magnesium of the electrophysiologic effects of hyperkalemia on human and canine heart cells. Am J Cardiol 45:1189–1195, 1980.
79. Kaseda S, Gilmour RF, Zipes DP: Depressant effect of magnesium on early afterdepolarizations and triggered activity induced by cesium, quinidine, and 4-aminopyridine in canine cardiac Purkinje fibers. Am Heart J 118:458–466, 1989.
80. Nattel S, Quantz, MA: Pharmacological response of quinidine induced early afterdepolarizations in canine cardiac Purkinje fibers: Insights into underlying ionic mechanisms. Cardiovasc Res 22:808–817, 1988.
81. Shine KI: Myocardial effects of magnesium: Am J Physiol 6:H413–H423, 1979.

82. Surawicz B: Role of electrolytes in etiology and management of cardiac arrhythmias. Prog Cardiovasc Dis 8:364–386, 1966.
83. Surawicz B, MacDonald MG, Kaljot V, Bettinger JD: Treatment of cardiac arrhythmias with salts of ethylenediamine tetraacetic acid (EDTA). Am Heart J 58:493–503, 1959.
84. Wit AL, Rosen MR: Afterdepolarizations and triggered activity. In Fozzard HA, Haber E, Jennins RB, Katz AM, Morgan HE (eds): The Heart and Cardiovascular System: Scientific Foundations. New York, Raven, 1986, pp 1449–1490.
85. January CT, Riddle JM, Salata JJ: A model for early afterdepolarizations: Induction with the Ca^{2+} channel agonist Bay K 8644. Circ Res 62:563–571, 1988.
86. Kass RS, Lederer WJ, Tsien RW, Weingart R: Role of calcium ions in transient inward currents and aftercontractions induced by strophanthidin in cardiac Purkinje fibers. J Physiol 281:187–208, 1978.
87. Hawashi H, Ponnambalam C, McDonald TF: Arrhythmic activity in reoxygenated guinea pig papillary muscles in ventricular cells. Circulation 61:124–133, 1987.
88. Woelfel AK, Foster JR, McAllister RG, Simpson RJ, Gettes LS: Efficacy of verapamil in exercise-induced ventricular tachycardia. Am J Cardiol 56:292–297, 1985.
89. Maurer P, Weingart R: Cell pairs isolated from adult guinea pig and rat hearts: Effects of $Ca^{2+}i$ on nexal membrane resistance. Pflugers Arch 409:394–402, 1987.
90. Pressler ML: Effects of pCai and pHi on cell-to cell coupling. Experientia 43:1084–1091, 1987.
91. Noma A, Tsuboi N: Dependence of junctional conductance on proton, calcium and magnesium ions in cardiac paired cells of guinea-pig. J Physiol (London) 382:193–211, 1987.
92. Steenbergen C, Murphy E, Levy L, London RE: Elevation in cytosolic free calcium concentration early in myocardial ischemia in perfused rat heart. Circ Res 60:700–707, 1987.
93. Steenbergen C, Murphy E, Watts JA, London RE: Correlation between cytosolic free calcium, contracture, ATP, and irreversible ischemic injury in perfused rat heart. Circ Res 66:135–146, 1990.
94. Gevers W: Generation of protons by metabolic processes in heart cells. J Moll Cell Cardiol 9:867–874, 1979.
95. Gettes LS, Cascio WE: Effect of acute ischemia on cardiac electrophysiology. In Fozzard H (ed): The Heart and Cardiovascular System: Scientific Foundations, 2nd ed. New York, Raven, 1987, pp 2021–2054.
96. Kagiyama Y, Hill JL, Gettes LS: Interaction of acidosis and increased extracellular potassium on action potential characteristics and conduction in guinea pig ventricular muscle. Circ Res 51:614–623, 1982.
97. Reuter H, Seitz N: The dependence of calcium efflux from cardiac muscle on temperature and external ion composition. J Physiol 195:451–470, 1968.
98. Tani M, Neely JR: Role of intracellular Na^+ in Ca^{2+} overload and depressed recovery of ventricular function of reperfused ischemic rat hearts: Possible involvement of H^+-Na^+ and Na^+-Ca^{2+} exchange. Circ Res 65:1045–1056, 1989.
99. Pike MM, Kitakase M, Marban E: Increase in intracellular free sodium concentration during ischemia revealed by 23Na NMR in perfused ferret hearts [abstract]. Circulation 78:II-151–II-151, 1988.
100. Cohen CJ, Fozzard HA, Sheu SS: Increase in intracellular sodium ion activity during stimulation in mammalian cardiac muscle. Circ Res 50:651–662, 1982.
101. Hope RR, Williams DO, El-Sherif N, Lazzara R, Scherlag BJ: The efficacy of antiarrhythmic agents during acute myocardial ischemia and the role of heart rate. Circulation 50:507–514, 1974.
102. Hiramatsu Y, Buchanan JW Jr, Knisley SB, Koch GG, Kropp S, Gettes LS: Influence of rate-dependent cellular uncoupling on conduction change during stimulated ischemia in guinea pig papillary muscles: Effect of verapamil. Circ Res 65:95–102, 1989.

23

Autonomic Innervation of the Heart and Ventricular Arrhythmias

DOUGLAS P. ZIPES

The mechanisms by which the autonomic nervous system promotes, precipitates, or prevents the development of cardiac arrhythmias are incompletely understood. This review will focus on selected recent observations concerning the effects of myocardial ischemia and myocardial infarction (MI) on autonomic innervation, and how some of these changes can modulate the development of cardiac arrhythmias.[1,2]

FUNCTIONAL PATHWAYS OF SYMPATHETIC AND VAGAL INNERVATION IN CANINE VENTRICLE

Recent functional studies of intracardiac neural pathways indicate that afferent and efferent vagal fibers cross the atrioventricular (AV) groove in the superficial subepicardium and then penetrate the myocardium, at which point they are probably located in the subendocardium.[3-8] Vagal efferent fibers crossing the AV groove are probably postganglionic axons with the ganglion cells located in the atria.[9] In contrast, afferent and efferent sympathetic fibers appear to be located in the superficial subepicardium throughout most of their course (Fig. 23-1).[4,10-12]

Pericardium—An Autonomic Link

Substances in the pericardial fluid, whether normally secreted or present due to disease, can modulate autonomic neural transmission to the heart[13-15] because vagal and sympathetic nerves are located so superficially in the subepicardium, at least during part of their intraventricular course. For example, the pericardium normally synthesizes prostaglandins, and under certain circumstances, such as increased myocardial work and oxygen consumption, a substantial release of pericardial prostaglandin occurs. Pericardial prostaglandins produce an antisympathetic action that may constitute a physiological negative feedback control mechanism regulating efferent sympathetic stimulation of the heart (Fig. 23-2). Thus, when efferent sympathetic input to the heart is heightened or plasma catecholamines are increased, the pericardium could produce prostaglandin I_2 and other prostaglandins, which would bathe the cardiac sympathetic nerves and limit efferent sympathetic input to the heart and further release of catecholamines. Finally, because pericardial prostaglandins do not affect cardiac responses to vagal stimulation, they may act to suppress arrhythmia development in various situations, including acute myocardial ischemia (Fig. 23-3).[15]

Supported in part by the Herman C. Krannert Fund; by grants HL-42370 and HL 07182 from the National Heart, Lung, and Blood Institute of the National Institutes of Health, U.S. Public Health Service; and by the American Heart Association, Indiana Affiliate, Inc.

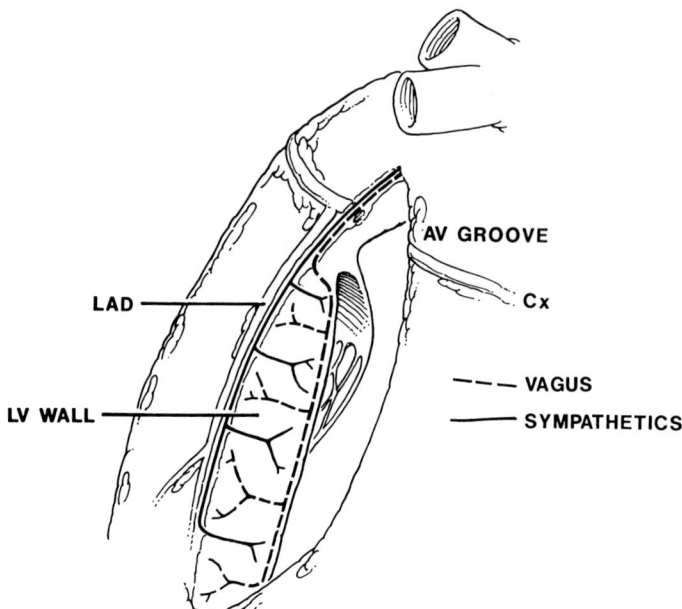

Fig. 23–1. Sagittal view of the left ventricular wall showing pathways of vagal and sympathetic afferent and efferent nerves. Postganglionic sympathetic axons are located superficially in the periadventia of coronary arteries, while (probable) postganglionic vagal axons cross the AV groove in the subepicardium but are then located in the subendocardium. Cx, circumflex coronary artery; LAD, left anterior descending coronary artery; LV, left ventricular.

ISCHEMIA- OR INFARCTION-PRODUCED AFFERENT DENERVATION

Ischemia or infarction, in addition to stimulating mechanosensitive and chemosensitive sensory nerve endings in the ischemic myocardium,[16–18] also impairs neurotransmission.[19] Axons, either because they become ischemic or infarcted or because they lie in an ischemic myocardial milieu that impairs their function, can lose normal function. Initial loss of vagal and sympathetic neural responsiveness after acute myocardial ischemia is probably due to functional derangement of nerve action rather than to structural changes. Nerve fibers serving the apex but traveling through an ischemic segment located more basally develop impaired function. Because the denervated myocardium responds normally to infused norepinephrine, postjunctional target cell dysfunction is not likely. The interaction between ischemically damaged myocardium and altered neural innervation could result in cardiac arrhythmias.

Several minutes after creation of transmural myocardial ischemia, the sympathetic reflex elicited from the epicardium of the ischemic area or apical to it becomes interrupted or attenuated when the myocardial blood flow in the epicardium decreases to approximately 40% or less of the control value.[20] In contrast, nontransmural ischemia does not attenuate the epicardial sympathetic reflex but does attenuate the vagal vasodepressor response, as would be expected from the functional pathways described previously (see Fig. 23–1). Because afferent sympathetic fibers appear to mediate cardiac pain sensation, it is possible that some patients with silent ischemia[21] or infarction have a form of "autodenervation." Ischemia could interrupt afferent neurotransmission, with elimination of pain perception. Recovery of neurotransmission would occur with reperfusion, so that another episode of ischemia, perhaps localized differently (e.g., sparing the epicardium), might then produce pain in the same patient.

ISCHEMIA- OR INFARCTION-PRODUCED EFFERENT DENERVATION

Myocardial ischemia or infarction also alters efferent sympathetic and vagal presynaptic function, probably by affecting neural transmission over axons located within the zone of ischemia or infarction, and can produce efferent sympathetic and vagal de-

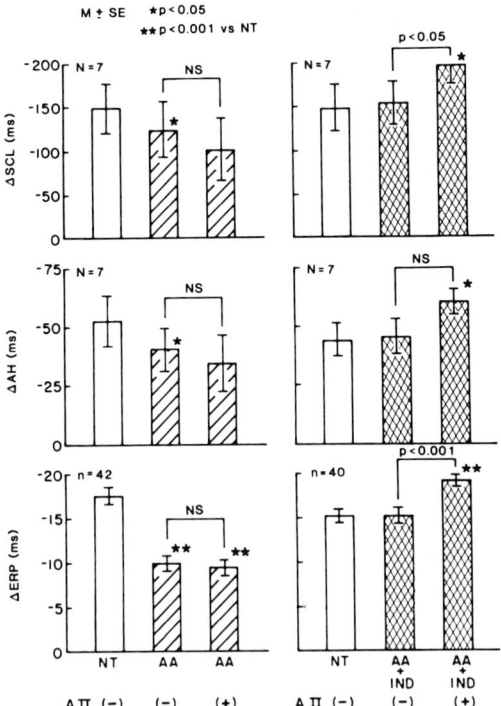

Fig. 23-2. Effects of stimulation of prostaglandin release into the pericardial fluid on changes in cardiac electrophysiological variables elicited by bilateral ansae subclaviae stimulation. *Left panels:* Efferent sympathetic-induced shortening of spontaneous sinus cycle length (ΔSCL), AH interval (ΔAH), and ventricular effective refractory period (ΔERP) determined during controlled superfusion with normal Tyrode's solution (NT) and during subsequent superfusion with arachidonic acid (3 μg/mL, AA) with and without intra-aortic infusion of angiotensin II (30 ng/kg/min, AII). *Right panels:* Data obtained from another 7 dogs that received AA plus indomethacin (1 μg/mL, IND). N, number of test dogs; n, number of ventricular test sites. Reproduced with permission from Miyazaki T, et al: Circ Res 66:163-175, 1990.[14])

nervation at noninfarcted sites apical to that zone (Fig. 23-4).[22,23] Myocardium within the ischemic area also can become denervated.[24] As predicted from the schematic in Figure 23-1, a subendocardial infarction that spares the epicardium interrupts vagal innervation but not sympathetic transmission,[23,25] and may be arrhythmogenic.[26] The noninfarcted myocardial rim overlying a subendocardial infarction also has a transiently depressed response to sympathetic nerve stimulation, possibly owing to local factors released by the adjacent infarct.[27] Initial sympathetic and vagal denervation are due to functional changes in neural activity with measurable decreases in transmitter concentration or enzyme activity lagging behind and following the onset of actual tissue damage as the infarction develops and progresses over time.[28] Myocardial injury that is either functional and transient, or anatomical and permanent, can impair autonomic neural transmission.

PRECONDITIONING ISCHEMIA

The cardiac response to ischemia or infarction is also influenced by the "myocardial history." Four 5-minute episodes of coronary occlusion and reperfusion preserves the efferent sympathetic response during the first hour of the subsequent sustained ischemia and preserves the efferent vagal response for at least 3 hours without an increase in collateral blood flow to the ischemic myocardium.[29] Preconditioning ischemia is not produced by transient exposure of the myocardium to a combination of the ischemic metabolites K^+, H^+, and adenosine.[30] Elevation of these substances during ischemia may be responsible for early denervation.[31]

DENERVATION SUPERSENSITIVITY, ARRHYTHMOGENESIS, AND REINNERVATION

Tissue deprived of its nerve supply responds in an exaggerated fashion to certain agents, a phenomenon called "denervation supersensitivity."[32] Sympathetic supersensitivity, manifested by an exaggerated shortening of refractoriness during both norepinephrine and isoproterenol infusions with an upward and leftward shift in the dose-response curves, occurs in denervated regions of the left ventricle.[33] The mechanism responsible for this type of supersensitivity is not clear. However, the fact that isoproterenol also produces a supersensitive response suggests a postjunctional mechanism.[33,34]

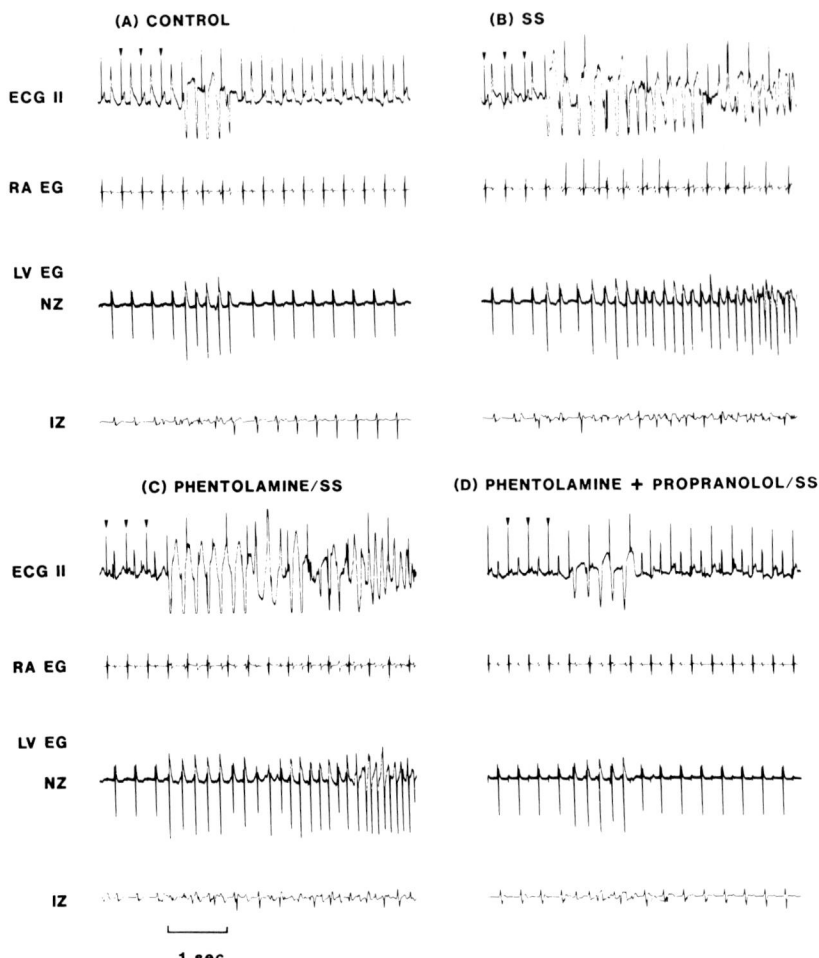

Fig. 23–3. Tracings from a dog showing the effect of stimulation of bilateral ansae subclaviae (SS) on reperfusion-induced ventricular fibrillation and reversal by epicardial superfusion with arachidonic acid solution. Simultaneous recordings of lead II electrocardiogram (ECG II), mean arterial blood pressure (BP), and local bipolar electrograms of the left ventricular normal (NZ) and ischemic (IZ) zones immediately after reperfusion are shown. Arrows in the ECG II indicate the stimuli from right atrial pacing. AA, epicardial superfusion with Tyrode's solution containing arachidonic acid (3 μg/mL); AA ± IND, epicardial superfusion with arachidonic acid (3 μg/mL). (Reproduced with permission from Miyazaki T, et al: Circulation 82:1008–1019, 1990.[15])

Denervation supersensitivity elicits inhomogeneous autonomic and electrophysiological changes and makes the heart more vulnerable to electrical induction of ventricular arrhythmias.[35] Propranolol significantly attenuates this vulnerability. It is tempting to speculate that β-adrenoceptor blockade may reduce the incidence of sudden cardiac death after MI,[36] in part by attenuating the effects of denervation supersensitivity on dispersion of refractoriness, conduction changes, or other electrophysiological properties. In a canine model of postganglionic efferent denervation produced by transmural infarction, reinnervation occurs in 8–17 weeks.[37]

Regional sympathetic denervation and supersensitivity could also modulate drug actions and cause the drugs to affect the myocardium heterogeneously.[38] Such changes could provide another proarrhythmic mechanism.

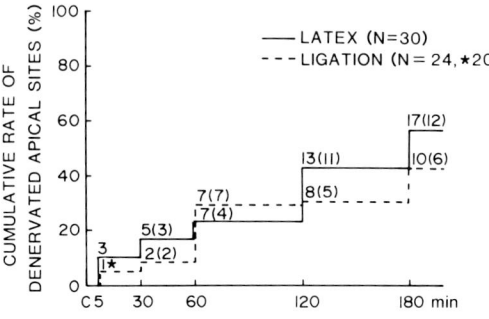
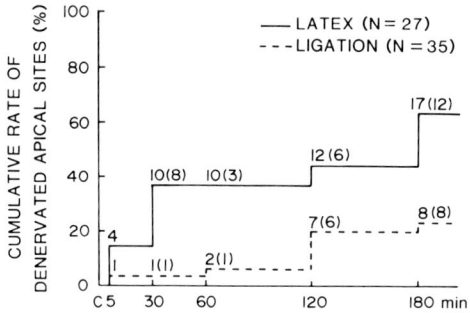

Fig. 23–4. Sympathetic and vagal denervation plots. *Left:* Cumulative percentage of sympathetically denervated apical sites divided by number of total apical test sites (N) is shown on ordinate as function of time. Solid line, data from dogs with latex coronary injection; dotted line, data from dogs with coronary ligation; figures without parentheses, cumulative number of denervated test sites (total number of sites that had shown shortening of effective refractory period ≤2 msec at least once by that moment of determination); figures in parentheses, number of test sites that showed shortening of effective refractory period ≤2 msec at that moment of determination. Presentation in this fashion is necessary because some sites showed variation in response around the cutoff value. For example, 120–180 minutes after latex injection, four new sites (17 minus 13) became denervated, while only 12 of the 17 sites actually still exhibited shortening of effective refractory period ≤2 msec at 180 minutes. The remaining five sites that had shown shortening of effective refractory period ≤2 msec at least once by 120 minutes now exhibited refractory period shortening >2 msec at 180 minutes after infarction. Cumulative rate of denervated sites did not differ between dogs receiving latex injection and coronary artery ligation ($p = 0.41$). C, Control before coronary occlusion. *Data from one dog that developed ventricular fibrillation were not included 5 minutes after ligation. *Right:* Plot showing cumulative percentage of vagally denervated apical sites is shown as in left panel and was greater in dogs receiving latex injection than in dogs with ligation of coronary arteries ($p < 0.002$). (Reproduced with permission from Inoue H, et al: Circ Res 62:1111–1120, 1988.[23])

EFFECTS OF SYMPATHETIC STIMULATION ON ISCHEMIA/INFARCTION

While ischemia/infarction modulates autonomic innervation, sympathetic stimulation in turn modulates ischemia/infarction. It causes an increase in ischemia-related ventricular arrhythmias, particularly reperfusion ventricular fibrillation.[15] Perhaps related to this finding is the fact that sympathetic stimulation increases the extracellular accumulation of potassium during ischemia. Interestingly, infused norepinephrine has an opposite effect.[39] The ATP-sensitive potassium channel opener pinacidil reduces the extent of sympathetic denervation during ischemia, while the potassium channel blocker glibenclamide increases it.[40] It is likely that the extent and site of extracellular K^+ accumulation importantly affect neural innervation and the development of ventricular tachyarrhythmias. Sympathetic stimulation can also alter refractoriness of the myocardium and facilitate the development of ventricular tachycardia (VT).[41]

SYMPATHETIC SCINTIGRAPHY

We investigated whether ^{123}I-labeled metaiodobenzylguanidine (MIBG), a guanethidine analogue taken up by sympathetic nerve terminals,[42] could provide a scintigraphic image that would detect apical sympathetic denervation and possible reinnervation.[37] Dogs underwent MIBG imaging at various times after phenol application or transmural MI. The results of MIBG scintigraphy were then correlated with electrophysiological responses obtained during ansae subclaviae stimulation and norepinephrine infusion to establish the presence of neural denervation, reinnervation, and supersensitivity. Thallium images were obtained concurrently to outline areas of normal blood flow and cell viability. Apical defects on the MIBG scan, which were associated with either normal perfusion by thallium or a thallium defect that was smaller than the MIBG defect, were found consistently in dogs that had apical sympathetic denervation. For all images, the results of MIBG scintigraphy correlated accurately with the presence of denervation and reinnervation established by neuroelectrophysiological testing. Supersensitivity in response to norepinephrine infusion persisted after denervation despite scintigraphic and electrophysiological evidence of reinnervation.[37]

Human Studies

Studies with MIBG scintigraphy in humans have shown abnormalities in MIBG uptake after MI similar to those seen in canine studies. We found evidence of sympathetic denervation in 10 of 12 patients with spontaneous ventricular tachyarrhythmias after MI (Fig. 23–5). Sympathetic denervation was also detected in 2 of 7 postinfarction patients without ventricular arrhythmias.[43] This study[43] provides evidence that regional sympathetic denervation occurs in humans after MI and can be detected noninvasively by comparing MIBG and ^{201}Tl images. These observations have been confirmed recently.[44]

If these denervated areas exhibiting denervation supersensitivity became exposed to circulating norepinephrine, ventricular tachyarrhythmias might result. Recently, Meredith et al[45] demonstrated an almost fivefold increase in cardiac norepinephrine spillover in patients with reduced left ventricular function who had been resuscitated from life-threatening ventricular tachyarrhythmias. The increase in cardiac norepinephrine spillover was probably a result of the reduced left ventricular ejection fraction these patients had. This study[45] provides evidence that areas of denervation supersensitivity could be exposed to excessive concentrations of norepinephrine.

EFFERENT SYMPATHETIC DENERVATION UNRELATED TO CORONARY ARTERY DISEASE

While we have shown unequivocally in the studies cited earlier that myocardial ischemia and infarction produce sympathetic and vagal denervation, it is possible that any pathological process affecting the myocardium that results in cell dropout, remodeling, and fibrosis can cause similar changes. We[46,47] have recently evaluated 16 patients (mean age, 49 ± 19 years) with VT unrelated to coronary artery disease. They had cardiomyopathy ($n = 5$), left ventricular hy-

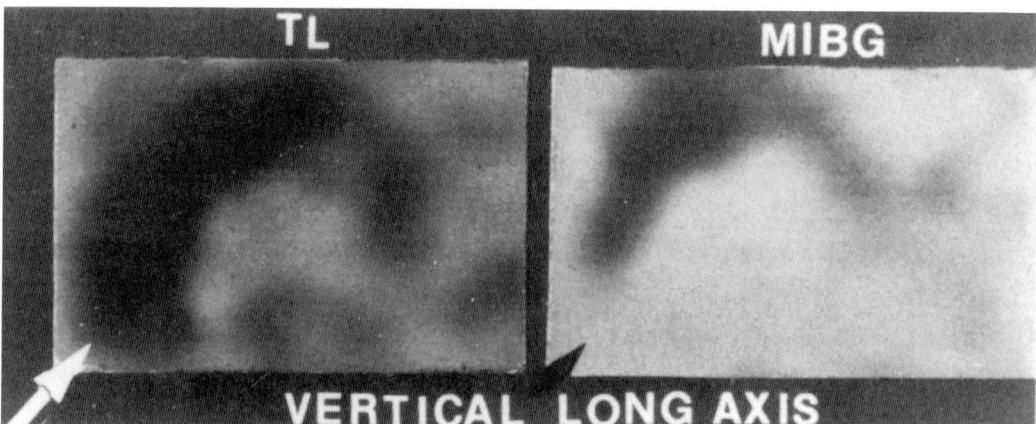

Fig. 23–5. Denervation following myocardial infarction in man. SPECT images of patient with an inferior MI. Note that the apex (arrow) is perfused, as demonstrated by the thallium-201 (TL) images. The metaiodobenzylguanidine (MIBG) images show a defect in the apex (arrow). (Reproduced with permission from Stanton MS, et al: J Am Coll Cardiol 14:1519–1526, 1989.[43])

pertrophy ($n = 1$), or structurally normal hearts ($n = 10$) and presented with monomorphic ($n = 13$) or polymorphic ($n = 3$) VT. We compared their MIBG scans with scans in 12 control patients without VT (mean age, 30 ± 18 years) who had cardiomyopathy ($n = 2$) or structurally normal hearts ($n = 10$). Ten (63%) of 16 patients with VT had regional cardiac sympathetic denervation, compared with 1 (8%) of 12 patients who did not have VT ($p < 0.01$). Of those patients who underwent electrophysiological studies, 8 (57%) of 14 patients with inducible VT had cardiac sympathetic denervation, compared with only 1 (17%) of 6 patients who did not have inducible VT. In the 10 patients with structurally normal hearts and VT, 6 (60%) of 10 patients had regional cardiac sympathetic denervation, compared with none of 10 control patients with structurally normal hearts ($p = 0.01$). Finally, of the 9 patients with structurally normal hearts and inducible VT 5 (55%) of 9 had cardiac sympathetic denervation, while none of 5 patients without inducible VT had sympathetic denervation. From these observations it is clear that patients with VT in the absence of coronary artery disease, including patients with "structurally normal" hearts, have abnormalities of cardiac sympathetic innervation that can be detected by cardiac sympathetic scintigraphy. Regional cardiac sympathetic denervation may play a role in arrhythmogenesis in these patients.

REFERENCES

1. Corr PB, Yamada KA, Witkowski FX: Mechanisms controlling cardiac autonomic function and their relation to arrhythmogenesis. In Fozzard HA, Haber E, Jennings RB, Katz AM, Morgan HE (eds): The Heart and Cardiovascular System. New York, Raven Press, 1986, p 1343.
2. Kulbertus HE, Franck G (eds): Neurocardiology. Mt. Kisco, NY, Futura, 1988, p 3.
3. Kent KM, Epstein SE, Cooper T, Jacobowitz DM: Cholinergic innervation of the canine and human ventricular conducting system. Circulation 50:948-955, 1974.
4. Martins JB, Zipes DP: Epicardial phenol interrupts refractory period responses to sympathetic but not vagal stimulation in canine left ventricular epicardium and endocardium. Circ Res 47:33-40, 1980.
5. Barber MJ, Mueller TM, Davies BG, Zipes DP: Phenol topically applied to left ventricular epicardium interrupts sympathetic but not vagal afferents. Circ Res 55:532-544, 1984.
6. Takahashi N, Barber MJ, Zipes DP: Efferent vagal innervation of the canine left ventricle. Am J Physiol 248 (Heart Circ Physiol 17): H89-H97, 1985.
7. Inoue H, Mahomed Y, Zipes DP: Surgery for Wolff-Parkinson-White syndrome interrupts efferent vagal innervation to the left ventricle and to the atrioventricular node in the canine heart. Cardiovasc Res 22:163-170, 1988.
8. Chilson DA, Peigh P, Mahomed Y, Zipes DP: Encircling endocardial incision interrupts efferent vagal-induced prolongation of endocardial and epicardial refractoriness in the dog. J Am Coll Cardiol 5:290-296, 1985.
9. Blomquist TM, Priola DV, Romero AM: Source of intrinsic innervation of canine ventricles: A functional study. Am J Physiol 252 (Heart Circ Physiol):H638-H644, 1987.
10. Randall WC, Szentivanyi M, Pace JB, Wechsler JS, Kaye MP: Patterns of sympathetic nerve projections onto the canine heart. Circ Res 22:315-323, 1968.
11. Geis WP, Kaye MP: Distribution of sympathetic fibers in the left ventricular epicardial plexus of the dog. Circ Res 23:165-170, 1968.
12. Randall WC, Armour JA: Regional vagosympathetic control of the heart. Am J Physiol 227:444-452, 1974.
13. Miyazaki T, Pride HP, Zipes DP: Modulation of cardiac autonomic neurotransmission by epicardial superfusion: effects of hexamethonium and tetrodotoxin. Circ Res 65:1212-1219, 1989.
14. Miyazaki T, Pride HP, Zipes DP: Prostaglandins in the pericardial fluid modulate neural regulation of cardiac electrophysiologic properties. Circ Res 66:163-175, 1990.
15. Miyazaki T, Zipes DP: Pericardial prostaglandin biosynthesis prevents the increased incidence of reperfusion-induced ventricular fibrillation produced by efferent sympathetic stimulation in dogs. Circulation 82:1008-1019, 1990.
16. Sleight P: A cardiovascular depressor reflex from the epicardium of the left ventricle in the dog. J Physiol (London) 173:321-343, 1964.
17. Malliani A, Schwartz PJ, Zanchetti A: Sympathetic reflex elicited by experimental coronary occlusion. Am J Physiol 217:703-709, 1969.
18. Thames MD, Minisi AJ: Reflex responses to myocardial ischemia and reperfusion: Role

of prostaglandins. Circulation *80:*1878–1885, 1989.
19. Barber MJ, Mueller TM, Davies BG, Gill RM, Zipes DP: Interruption of sympathetic and vagal-mediated afferent responses by transmural myocardial infarction. Circulation *72:*623–631, 1985.
20. Inoue H, Skale BT, Zipes DP: Effects of myocardial ischemia and infarction on cardiac afferent sympathetic and vagal reflexes in the dog. Am J Physiol *255* (Heart Circ Physiol *24*):H26–H35, 1988.
21. Nabil EG, Campbell S, Barry J, Rocco MB, Selwyn AP: Asymptomatic ischemia in patients with coronary artery disease. JAMA *257:*1923–1928, 1987.
22. Barber MJ, Mueller TM, Henry DP, Felten SY, Zipes DP: Transmural myocardial infarction in the dog produces sympathectomy in noninfarcted myocardium. Circulation *67:* 787–796, 1983.
23. Inoue H, Zipes DP: Time course of denervation of efferent sympathetic and vagal nerves after occlusion of the coronary artery in the canine heart. Circ Res *62:*1111–1120, 1988.
24. Martins JB, Kerber RE, Marcus ML, Laughlin DL, Levy DM: Inhibition of adrenergic neurotransmission in ischemic regions of the canine left ventricle. Cardiovasc Res *14:*116–124, 1980.
25. Martins JB, Lewis R, Wenbt B, Lund DD, Schmid PG: Subendocardial infarction produces epicardial parasympathetic denervation in canine left ventricle. Am J Physiol *256* (Heart Circ Physiol *25*):H859–H866, 1989.
26. Herre JM, Wetstein L, Lin YL, Mills AS, Dae M, Thames MD: Effect of transmural versus nontransmural myocardial infarction on inducibility of ventricular arrhythmias during sympathetic stimulation in dogs. J Am Coll Cardiol *11:*414–421, 1988.
27. Hingtgen L, Horn M, Martins JB: Transient depression of refractory period responses to sympathetic nerve stimulation in the epicardial rim overlying subendocardial infarction [abstract]. PACE *12:*639, 1989.
28. Schmid PG, Greif BJ, Lund DD, Roskoski R Jr: Tyrosine hydroxylase and choline acetyltransferase activities in ischemic canine heart. Am J Physiol *243:*H788–H795, 1982.
29. Miyazaki T, Zipes DP: Protection against autonomic denervation following acute myocardial infarction by preconditioning ischemia. Circ Res *64:*437–448, 1989.
30. Rubart M, Zipes DP: Failure of stimulated ischemia to protect against efferent sympathetic denervation during subsequent acute myocardial infarction in dog heart. J Am Coll Cardiol *19:*117A, 1992.
31. Miyazaki T, Zipes DP: Presynaptic modulation of efferent sympathetic and vagal neurotransmission in the canine heart by hypoxia, high K$^+$, low pH and adenosine: Possible relevance to ischemia-induced denervation. Circ Res *66:*289–301, 1990.
32. Cannon WB: A law of denervation. Am J Med *198:* 737–750, 1939.
33. Kammerling JJ, Green FJ, Watanabe AM, Inoue H, Barber MJ, Henry DP, Zipes DP: Denervation supersensitivity of refractoriness in noninfarcted areas apical to transmural myocardial infarction. Circulation *76:* 383–393, 1987.
34. Martins JB: Time course of sympathetic denervation supersensitivity in canine ventricular recovery. Am J Physiol *255* (Heart Circ Physiol *24*):H577–H586, 1988.
35. Inoue H, Zipes DP: Results of sympathetic denervation in the canine heart: Supersensitivity that may be arrhythmogenic. Circulation *75:*877–887, 1987.
36. Frishman WH, Furberg CD, Friedewald WT: Beta-adrenergic blockade for survivors of acute myocardial infarction. N Engl J Med *310:*830–837, 1984.
37. Minardo JD, Tuli MM, Mock BH, Weiner RE, Pride HP, Wellman HN, Zipes DP: Scintigraphic and electrophysiologic evidence of canine myocardial sympathetic denervation and reinnervation produced by myocardial infarction or phenol application. Circulation *78:*1008–1019, 1988.
38. Stanton MS, Zipes DP: Modulation of drug effects by regional sympathetic denervation and supersensitivity. Circulation *84:* 1709–1714, 1991.
39. Warner MR, Kroeker TS, Zipes DP: Effects of sympathetic stimulation on extracellular K$^+$ accumulation during myocardial ischemia. Circulation *84*(suppl II):267, 1991.
40. Itoh M, Pride HP, Zipes DP: ATP-sensitive potassium channel opener protects autonomic denervation after acute coronary occlusion. J Am Coll Cardiol *19:*244A, 1992.
41. Butrous GS, Gough WB, Restivo M, Yang H, El Sherif N: Adrenergic effects on reentrant ventricular rhythms in subacute myocardial infarction. Circulation *86:*247–254, 1992.
42. Sisson JC, Shapiro B, Meyers L, et al: Metaiodobenzylguanidine to map scintigraphically the adrenergic nervous system in man. J Nucl Med *28:*1625–1636, 1987.
43. Stanton MS, Tuli MM, Heger JJ, et al: Regional sympathetic denervation after MI in humans detected noninvasively using I-123 metaiodobenzylguanidine (MIBG). J Am Coll Cardiol *14:*1519–1526, 1989.
44. Wharton JM, Friedman IM, Greenfield RA, Vitullo RN, Strauss HC, Coleman RE:

Quantitative perfusion and sympathetic nerve defect size after myocardial infarction in humans [abstract]. J Am Coll Cardiol *19(suppl A):*264A, 1992.
45. Meredith IT, Broughton A, Jennings GL, Esler MD: Evidence of a selective increase in cardiac sympathetic activity in patients with sustained ventricular arrhythmias. N Engl J Med *325:*618–624, 1991.
46. Zipes DP: Sympathetic stimulation and arrhythmias [editorial]. N Engl J Med *325:* 656–657, 1991.
47. Mitrani R, Klein LS, Miles WM, Burt RW, Wellmar HN, Zipes DP: Regional cardiac sympathetic denervation in patients with ventricular tachycardia in the absence of coronary artery disease. J Am Coll Cardiol, Nov, 1993.

24

Exercise Testing and Its Role in the Management of Patients with Ventricular Arrhythmia

PHILIP J. PODRID

Exercise testing is a well-established and valuable technique for the evaluation of patients with heart disease, as it provides important information about cardiovascular physiology. Although most often applied to patients with coronary artery disease (CAD) for the assessment of myocardial blood flow and oxygen supply, exercise testing produces a number of physiological changes that have a role in arrhythmogenesis. These changes may also alter the action of antiarrhythmic drugs and their effect on the conduction system, the myocardial substrate, and ventricular contractility. Exercise testing is therefore an integral part of the management of patients with any form of arrhythmia, especially those with ventricular arrhythmia.

PHYSIOLOGICAL EFFECTS OF EXERCISE

As a result of exercise, there is withdrawal of vagal tone but, more important, activation of sympathetic nervous system and an increase in circulating catecholamines.[1] These changes in autonomic balance affect mechanical, metabolic, and physiological parameters of myocardial function (Fig. 24–1). As a result of sympathetic stimulation, there is an increase in heart rate, systolic and diastolic blood pressure, and myocardial contractility or inotropy. These changes cause an increase in myocardial oxygen demands. In patients with heart disease who have limited or impaired myocardial oxygen delivery, this increase in demand overwhelms supply, resulting in ischemia and the consequent acidosis and electrolyte shifts, especially the development of extracellular hyperkalemia. These pH and electrolyte abnormalities alter the electrophysiological properties of the membrane, particularly its resting potential, conduction velocity, refractoriness, and automaticity. Changes in these parameters are associated with and affect the basic mechanisms responsible for arrhythmogenesis, namely re-entry, triggered automaticity, and enhanced automaticity.[2]

Sympathetic stimulation can, be a direct inotropic effect, cause mechanical changes, or by increasing blood pressure and afterload can indirectly increase wall stress and tension. Acting in concert with ischemia, these changes may result in regional myocardial dysfunction and contraction abnormalities. These mechanical changes and the increased myocardial stretch are other factors that may be responsible for arrhythmia.

In addition to the metabolic changes that occur in the setting of CAD and ischemia, sympathetic stimulation itself may, even in the absence of CAD, produce regional differences in blood flow and oxygen delivery that may cause localized or regional shifts

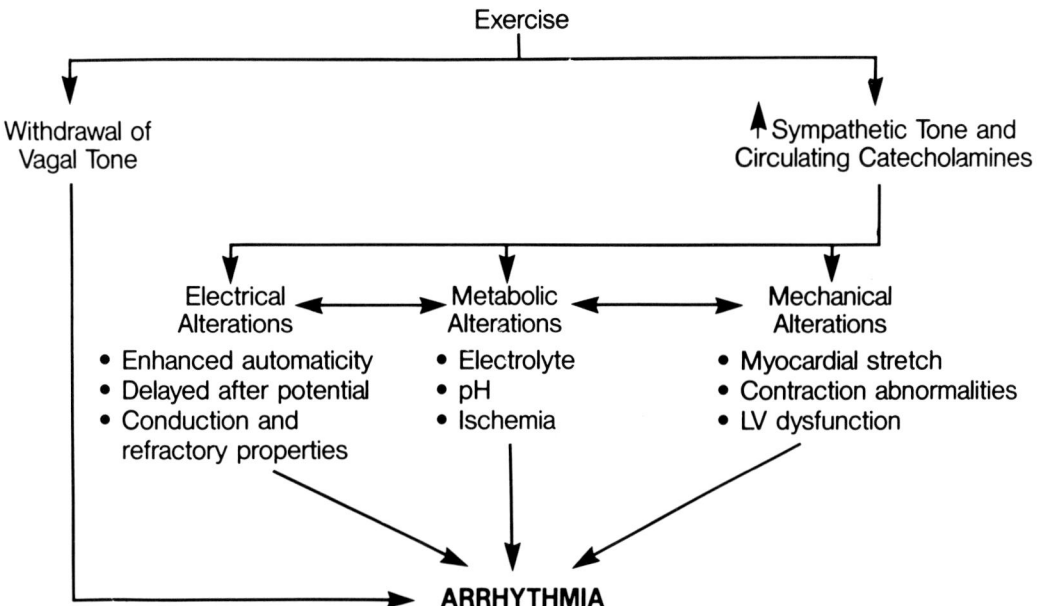

Fig. 24-1. Scheme of physiological changes produced by exercise. The primary effect is activation of the sympathetic nervous system and an increase in circulating catecholamines. This results in electrical, metabolic, and mechanical changes, important in arrhythmogenesis.

in electrolytes and changes in pH. Even in a normal heart there may be regional differences in blood flow due to differences in coronary artery perfusion pressure.[3] During exercise there is the potential for minor or more marked regional abnormality of blood flow and possibly ischemia, even in the normal heart, although this potential is more often realized in the presence of CAD.[4] Differences in pH, electrolytes levels, and oxygen delivery may develop between ischemic and nonischemic tissue as well as between the endocardial and epicardial layers within an ischemic region,[4,5] since a decrease in coronary artery perfusion pressure produces a reduction in blood flow and oxygen supply that is more significant in the endocardial layer than in the epicardium. The regional and local differences in oxygen supply create nonuniformity of extracellular and tissue potassium levels and pH, factors that affect the conduction velocity and refractoriness of the myocardial membrane.[6] The heterogeneity between adjacent areas and nonuniformity between endocardial and epicardial layers produce an appropriate precondition for re-entry, the most important mechanism for arrhythmia.

Lastly, activation of the sympathetic nervous system and an increase in circulating catecholamines can directly augment the very mechanisms responsible for arrhythmogenesis. This effect may be further enhanced by the presence of ischemia and the resultant changes in pH and potassium levels. Catecholamines shorten membrane refractory periods and increase myocardial conduction velocity. However, in the presence of regional ischemia and electrolyte and pH abnormalities, the changes in these electrophysiological parameters may be nonuniform, resulting in further myocardial electrophysiological heterogeneity, an important precondition for re-entry.[2] Sympathetic stimulation also causes an increase in spontaneous automaticity of the membrane by increasing the rate of phase 4 spontaneous depolarization. This enhanced automaticity may be particularly pronounced in diseased myocardial tissue, which already exhibits underlying abnormal automaticity.[7] Finally, sympathetic stimulation increases the influx of calcium ions, thereby increasing the amplitude of delayed afterpotentials, resulting in triggered automaticity.[8]

Exercise testing is therefore important for

the induction of arrhythmia and serves as an adjunct to ambulatory monitoring or electrophysiological testing for evaluating and managing the patient with a history of serious sustained arrhythmia or for stratification of patients with heart disease, in whom the risk of sudden cardiac death (SCD) is increased. It may be of particular importance in patients with a history of a sustained ventricular tachyarrhythmia that cannot be induced in the electrophysiological laboratory, a situation where the normal physiological changes that may be responsible for the arrhythmia cannot be replicated. Exercise testing may also be of use in patients with transient symptoms suggesting arrhythmia in whom other techniques fail to disclose an etiology.

PREVALENCE OF VENTRICULAR ARRHYTHMIA DURING EXERCISE

The type and frequency of ventricular arrhythmia provoked by exercise are related to the presence and extent of underlying heart disease (Table 24–1). Similar to the data from ambulatory monitoring, the occurrence of ventricular arrhythmia is also related to age. Initially the frequency and complexity of ventricular arrhythmia during exercise were not appreciated because of intermittent recording of the rhythm. Continuous monitoring improved the recognition of arrhythmia, especially of repetitive forms, including couplets and runs of nonsustained ventricular tachycardia (VT).[9] In a study of normal subjects, Beard and Owen[10] reported on 1385 exercise tests in which intermittent recording of rhythm was performed. Ventricular premature beats (VPBs) were observed in 110 tests. Master[11] reported an 18.3% overall prevalence in VPBs, which were more frequently documented in patients with heart disease than in normal subjects. This finding was confirmed by Whinnery,[12] who reported VPBs in 5% of normal subjects during exercise but in 50% of those with heart disease.

The reported prevalence of VPBs is higher when the rhythm during exercise is continuously recorded. McHenry and coworkers[13] noted VPBs in 34% of normal subjects during exercise, while 50% of those with heart disease had VPBs. Poblete and coworkers[14] reported a 7% prevalence of VPBs in healthy subjects and a 62% prevalence in those with heart disease. In a study by Jelinek and Lown[15] of 162 normal subjects, 31 (19%) had VPBs during exercise.

Table 24–1
Prevalence of Ventricular Arrhythmia During Exercise

	Percent with Arrhythmia and:			
	Simple VPBs		Repetitive VPBs	
Study	Normal	Heart Disease	Normal	Heart Disease
Beard and Owen[10]	8.0	—	0.3	—
Master[11]	18.0	—	0.3	—
Whinnery[12]	5.0	50.0	0	15.0
McHenry et al[13]	34.0	50.0	6.0	22.0
Poblete et al[14]	7.0	62.0	0	31.0
Cordini et al[23]	—	—	0.1	0.7
Ryan et al[16]	—	55.0	—	20.0
Gooch et al[17]	—	45.0	—	—
Califf et al[20]	14.0	23.0	2.4	8.2
Weiner et al[21]	—	19.0	—	—
Detry et al[24]	—	—	—	0.58*
Jelinek and Lown[15]	19.0	36.0	1.8	3.6

* Ventricular tachycardia or ventricular fibrillation. VPBs = ventricular premature beats.

In contrast, among 100 patients with heart disease, Ryan and coworkers[16] reported exercise-induced VPBs in 55%. Gooch and coworkers[17] reported on 200 patients with heart disease and symptoms suggesting arrhythmia. Arrhythmia occurred in 89 patients (45%) during exercise, while 123 (63%) had VPBs documented on ambulatory monitoring. Although ambulatory monitoring was more helpful for exposing VPBs, in 22 patients (11%) arrhythmia was observed only during exercise testing. The authors concluded that both ambulatory monitoring and exercise testing are important techniques for a complete evaluation of the patient with heart disease, providing complementary information.

Age and sex are important factors associated with the prevalence of VPBs during exercise. In a study by Ekblum and coworkers[18] of 289 normal men and women, the frequency of VPBs with exercise was 35% in men and 14% in women. Among patients less than 30 years old, the prevalence of exercise-induced ventricular arrhythmia was 18%, while 50% of patients more than 50 years of age had ventricular arrhythmia.

Sami and coworkers[19] retrospectively reviewed the data from the Coronary Artery Surgical Study (CASS) involving 1486 patients with CAD documented by cardiac catheterization. VPBs during exercise were observed in only 146 (10%), but there was a relationship between the presence of VPBs and the extent of CAD. Among 245 patients with minimal CAD, only 16 (6.5%) had VPBs, whereas VPBs were documented in 130 (10.5%) of 1241 patients with significant CAD. These authors also observed a relationship between the left ventricular ejection fraction (LVEF) and the presence of VPBs. In the group of patients with minimal CAD, the average LVEF in those with VPBs was 50%, but it was 64% in patients without VPBs ($p < 0.05$). In the group with significant CAD, the occurrence of VPBs was associated with a previous myocardial infarction (MI), a reduced LVEF, and more extensive CAD.

Similar results were reported by Califf and coworkers[20] in a study of 1293 patients, of whom 256 (18%) had VPBs during exercise. The occurrence of VPBs was related to the presence and extent of heart disease, and patients with VPBs had a higher prevalence of significant three-vessel disease and reduced left ventricular function. An association between exercise-induced VPBs and extent of CAD was also reported by Weiner and coworkers.[21] In this study the overall incidence of VPBs was 19% (86 of 446 patients), but 30% of the 120 patients with left main or three-vessel disease had VPBs. As in the other studies the occurrence of arrhythmia with exercise was associated with more extensive CAD, a lower LVEF, more segmental wall motion abnormalities, and a greater amount of ST-segment depression during exercise.

There is also an association between exercise-induced repetitive arrhythmia, particularly runs of nonsustained VT, and the presence and extent of heart disease. In normal subjects, repetitive arrhythmia is infrequently observed during exercise testing. Whinnery[12] and Poblete and coworkers[14] did not observe repetitive arrhythmia in any of their patients who had no heart disease. With continuous monitoring Beard and Owen[10] and Master[11] reported that the prevalence of repetitive arrhythmia in normal subjects was 0.3%. With continuous monitoring Califf and coworkers[20] reported a 2.4% incidence of repetitive arrhythmia, while it was 6% in the study by McHenry and coworkers.[13] In a recent retrospective review of 3351 patients undergoing a routine exercise test, nonsustained VT was observed during exercise in only 50 patients (1.5%).[22]

In contrast, exercise-induced repetitive VPBs, particularly nonsustained VT, are more frequently seen in patients with heart disease. The prevalence ranges from 15% to 31% (Table 24–1). Ryan and coworkers[16] reported that 20% of patients with CAD had repetitive arrhythmia during exercise. Patients with a prior MI had more frequent repetitive arrhythmia than patients who had not had a prior infarction. Although in this study ambulatory monitoring was a more sensitive method for documenting repetitive arrhythmia, observed in 40% of patients, exercise testing was an important adjunctive method. As with single VPBs, there is also a relationship between age and the prevalence of repetitive arrhythmia, as reported by Ekblum and coworkers.[18] In their study of 289 normal subjects, the prevalence of repetitive arrhythmia varied from

1.5% in younger patients (<30 years old) to 5% in older patients (>50 years old).

The occurrence of a serious sustained ventricular tachyarrhythmia during exercise testing is uncommon, even in patients with underlying heart disease. In a report by Yang and coworkers[22] on 3351 patients, sustained VT was provoked during exercise testing in only five (0.2%). Cordini and coworkers[23] reported that 47 (0.8%) of 5750 patients had a sustained VT provoked by exercise. Underlying heart disease was present in 40 of these patients. Detry and coworkers[24] reviewed the data from 7500 consecutive exercise tests and reported that only six patients (0.08%) had an episode of ventricular fibrillation (VF), whereas 40 (0.55%) had VT, which was sustained in 13 (0.17%) and nonsustained in 27 (0.36%). Similar results were reported by Young and coworkers,[25] who retrospectively reviewed 8221 tests performed in 3444 patients with heart disease who did not have a history of a sustained ventricular tachyarrhythmia. During exercise testing there were only four episodes of VF, accounting for 0.05% of tests and 0.12% of patients.

In an attempt to establish differences between patients with and without exercise-induced VT, Rodriguez and coworkers[26] evaluated clinical, angiographic, and electrophysiological characteristics of 112 patients with a history of a sustained ventricular arrhythmia, 13% of whom had VT during exercise. Five of these patients (group A) had CAD and four had VT induced during electrophysiological study. In ten patients (group B) no heart disease was documented and during electrophysiological study eight had VT induced, but four of these patients required isoproterenol. These authors concluded that in contrast to exercise-induced VT in patients with heart disease who have an abnormal substrate, the provocation of this arrhythmia with exercise in those without heart disease is primarily the result of catecholamines. Patients in group A were compared with 27 patients with CAD who had a history of VT but did not have this arrhythmia provoked by exercise testing. On electrophysiological testing, sustained monomorphic VT was induced in 26 patients. There were no clinical, angiographic, or electrophysiological differences between these two groups of patients.

All forms of exercise-induced ventricular arrhythmia are more common in patients who have experienced a clinical episode of a sustained ventricular tachyarrhythmia or SCD. Each of these patients, regardless of the presence or extent of heart disease, has VPBs during exercise testing, and approximately 50–75% has repetitive forms.[27,28] Although ambulatory monitoring is a more sensitive method for exposing repetitive ventricular arrhythmia, especially nonsustained VT, approximately 10% of patients with a history of a serious sustained ventricular tachyarrhythmia will have monomorphic sustained VT exposed only during exercise testing, while no arrhythmia can be documented on ambulatory monitoring,[28] and in some of these patients arrhythmia cannot be induced with electrophysiological testing. A sustained ventricular tachyarrhythmia occurring during exercise is also more frequent in patients with a clinical history of such arrhythmia. In the report by Young and coworkers[25] which included 263 patients with a history of sustained VT or VF who underwent 1377 exercise tests, 24 patients (9.1%) had 32 arrhythmic events (2.3%) requiring emergency therapy. This number included 22 episodes of sustained VT, nine cases of VF, and one bradycardic arrest.

PROGNOSTIC SIGNIFICANCE OF VENTRICULAR ARRHYTHMIA DURING EXERCISE TESTING

Although the majority of data on the prognostic significance of VPBs in patients with heart disease are based on studies utilizing ambulatory monitoring, there are some data about the prognostic important of exercise-induced arrhythmia in patients with heart disease, particularly those with an MI (Table 24-2). In patients with a recent MI, Weld and coworkers[29] reported that the first-year mortality was 12% in patients with VPBs induced by exercise, compared with a 4% incidence of death in those with VPBs at rest but not during exercise. Mortality at the end of the first year was 16% among patients with VPBs occurring both at rest and during exercise. Krone and coworkers[30] performed low-level exercise testing in 667 patients with a recent MI and reported

Table 24-2
Prognostic Significance of Exercise-Induced Ventricular Premature Beats

Study	Population	Follow-Up (yr)	No. of VPBs	Mortality (%) Simple VPBs	Mortality (%) Complex VPBs	Significant?
Califf et al[20]	Normal	3.0	0	0	0	No
Califf et al[20]	CAD	3.0	10	17	25	Yes
Weiner et al[21]	Significant CAD	4.3	11	13	?	No
	Minimal CAD	5.0	2	9	?	No
Udall and Ellestad[32]	CAD (−ST)	1	2	15	29	Yes
	CAD (+ST)	1	10	33	42	Yes
Weld et al[29]	Post MI	1	4	12	?	Yes
Krone et al[30]	Post MI	1	3	7	13	Yes
Henry et al[31]	Post MI	2	8	25	?	Yes
Graboys et al[38]	SCD survivors	2.5	—	2.3	43.6	Yes

Abbreviations: CAD, coronary artery disease; MI, myocardial infarction; SCD, sudden cardiac death; +ST, ST-segment depression; −ST, no ST-segment changes; VPBs, ventricular premature beats.

that the presence of any VPB during exercise increased the first-year mortality from 3% to 7% ($p < 0.05$), whereas exercise-induced couplets increased the mortality threefold, from 4% to 13% ($p < 0.05$). Henry and coworkers[31] retrospectively reviewed the results of exercise testing in 163 patients who had sustained an uncomplicated MI and reported that the occurrence of VPBs during exercise was the only variable associated with an increased risk of sudden death. The incidence was 25% in those with exercise-induced VPBs, compared to 8% in patients without this arrhythmia.

A similar relationship has also been reported in patients with chronic CAD who have not sustained an MI (Table 24-2). Udall and Ellestad[32] reported that among patients with CAD who had no ST-segment depression on exercise testing, the 1-year mortality was 2% when VPBs were absent during exercise testing, 15% in those with simple VPBs, and 29% in patients who had repetitive or complex VPBs with exercise. In contrast, the mortality was higher in patients with CAD and ST-segment depression during exercise testing, regardless of the type of arrhythmia induced. Thus, in these patients without VPBs, the 1-year mortality was 10%, whereas it was 33% in those with simple VPBs and 42% in those with complex VPBs. Califf and coworkers[20] performed exercise testing within 6 weeks of cardiac catheterization in 620 patients with CAD. After a 3-year follow-up, the annual mortality was 25% in patients with repetitive arrhythmia provoked by exercise testing, compared to a 17% yearly mortality in patients with simple VPBs and a 10% mortality in those without exercise-induced arrhythmia. In contrast, there was no cardiac mortality among 673 patients without heart disease, regardless of the presence, type, or frequency of ventricular arrhythmia induced during exercise testing.

Although several studies involving patients with CAD have reported a statistically significant association between the occurrence of VPBs, especially repetitive forms, during exercise testing and an increased risk of SCD, a number of others have failed to confirm this relationship. Weiner and coworkers[21] reported that among 446 patients with CAD treated medically and followed up for an average of 5.3 years, the presence of exercise-induced arrhythmia did not increase cardiac-related mortality. In a CASS reported by Sami and coworkers[19] which included 1486 patients with CAD, VPBs occurring during exercise testing were not associated with cardiac events after a 5-year follow-up. However, these studies did not analyze the relationship between exercise-induced arrhythmia and the presence of ischemia during exercise as determined by ST-segment depression or extent of disease based on coronary angiography.

In conclusion, ventricular arrhythmia provoked by exercise testing may have prognostic importance in patients with a recent infarction or in those with evidence of ischemia during exercise. However, further studies are necessary. Unfortunately, there are no data to indicate that suppression of such an arrhythmia by antiarrhythmic drugs will prevent sudden death and alter mortality.

REPRODUCIBILITY OF EXERCISE-INDUCED ARRHYTHMIA

One of the major problems limiting the use of noninvasive methods is the lack of reproducibility in the occurrence, frequency, and type of VPBs as a result of their random or spontaneous variability. Although spontaneous variability has most often been reported when ambulatory monitoring has been used for documenting arrhythmia, a few studies have reported that random variability of VPBs and lack of reproducibility are also problems with exercise testing. In a study by Sheps and coworkers,[33] 13 patients with documented VPBs during exercise testing underwent a second exercise test approximately 45 minutes after the first. Eight patients had CAD and five were free of underlying heart disease. When the second test was compared to the first, there was a significant reduction in the frequency of recorded VPBs (45 for the first test vs. 16 for the second test, $p < 0.05$). In contrast, Drory and coworkers[34] reported on 76 healthy young men (mean age, 21.5 years) who had arrhythmia with exercise. During a mean of 6.7 years, none of these patients developed heart disease, and with repeat exercise testing arrhythmia was still observed in all.

It has been reported by Faris and coworkers[35] that the reproducibility of exercise-induced VPBs tends to be greater in patients with underlying cardiovascular disease. These authors performed exercise testing in 543 men at baseline and after an average of 2.9 years. The presence of VPBs and their frequency during the exercise testing were reproducible in 55% of subjects aged 25–34 years, in 58% of subjects aged 35–44 years, and in 62% of those aged 45–54 years. However, reproducibility of arrhythmia was greater in patients with underlying cardiovascular disease, and 76% of such patients aged 35–44 years had ventricular arrhythmia during both tests, while 73% of those 45–54 of years had reproducible arrhythmia ($p < 0.05$ when compared to those without heart disease). Handler and Sowton[36] performed an exercise test at the time of discharge and again at 6 weeks in 64 patients who had sustained an acute MI. They reported that ventricular arrhythmia was reproducibly induced by exercise in this cohort.

Age may also be related to the reproducibility of arrhythmia during exercise. In the study by Ekblum and coworkers[18] on 289 normal men and women, reproducibility of exercise-induced arrhythmia was good, for arrhythmias were reproducible in 83% of patients. Reproducibility was greater in patients older than 50 years than in those younger than 50 years.

It has been observed that all forms of VPBs, including repetitive forms, are more frequently induced during exercise testing in patients with a previous history of a sustained ventricular arrhythmia, and that the reproducibility of exercise-induced arrhythmia in this subgroup is good. Saini and coworkers[37] prospectively evaluated 28 patients with complex ventricular arrhythmia, 14 of whom had a clinical history of sustained VT or VF. Arrhythmia was provoked by or increased during exercise in 27 patients. When the test was repeated, 78% had all forms of ventricular arrhythmia reproducibly induced.

USE OF EXERCISE TESTING FOR MANAGEMENT OF PATIENTS WITH VENTRICULAR ARRHYTHMIA

Although the role of exercise tests in identifying patients at risk for sudden death or sustained ventricular arrhythmia is limited, it has an important adjunctive role in managing patients with ventricular arrhythmia, regardless of whether noninvasive ambulatory monitoring or noninvasive electrophysiological testing is used as the primary method for evaluating the patient

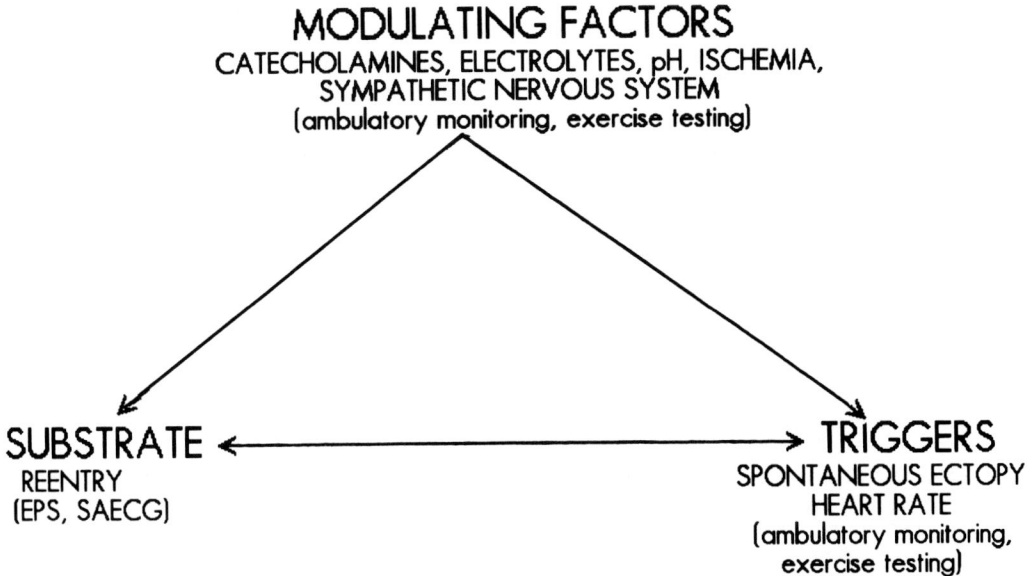

Fig. 24–2. Interrelated factors important in arrhythmia occurrence. The substrate is abnormal and is capable of generating and sustaining arrhythmia. The re-entrant circuit is activated by a number of factors, especially spontaneous arrhythmia. The modulating factors can alter the stability of the substrate and the frequency of the trigger.

and selecting an antiarrhythmic drug. Ambulatory monitoring provides useful information about arrhythmia over an extended period of time, evaluating the frequency and complexity of spontaneously occurring ectopy, which is an important trigger for arrhythmia (Fig. 24–2). Electrophysiological testing evaluates the myocardial substrate and the stability and location of the re-entrant circuit, the usual mechanism for ventricular tachyarrhythmias. However, exercise testing produces important changes within the myocardium that may alter the frequency and type of spontaneous VPBs (the triggers) or the properties and stability of the substrate (the re-entrant circuit). These changes may play a role in the exposure of arrhythmia, but, more important, exercise testing and the resulting physiological effects (electrical, mechanical, and metabolic) have important implications for antiarrhythmic drug therapy. The changes produced by exercise testing, especially an increase in sympathetic tone, an increase in circulating catecholamine levels, and metabolic alterations, particularly of potassium, pH, and oxygen supply, may interact with, negate, or enhance antiarrhythmic drug activity, possibly resulting in arrhythmia recurrence or aggravation.

One group of patients for whom exercise testing is of particular importance as part of a complete evaluation consists of those who have experienced a serious sustained ventricular tachyarrhythmic (VT or VF), as the selection of a drug that is effective under various conditions is critical. Graboys and coworkers[38] reported on 123 patients presenting with a serious ventricular tachyarrhythmia who underwent noninvasive testing for the selection of an effective antiarrhythmic drug. Exercise testing was used as an additional method for evaluating antiarrhythmic drug effect (Fig. 24–3). The continued presence of runs of nonsustained VT during exercise testing, even if absent on monitoring, was associated with a significantly higher annual mortality (43.6%) than in patients in whom such forms were absent during exercise and monitoring as a result of antiarrhythmic drug therapy (annual mortality of 2.3%). An evaluation of antiarrhythmic drug action utilizing either ambulatory monitoring or electrophysiological study is not complete unless an exercise test has been performed, as the latter provides

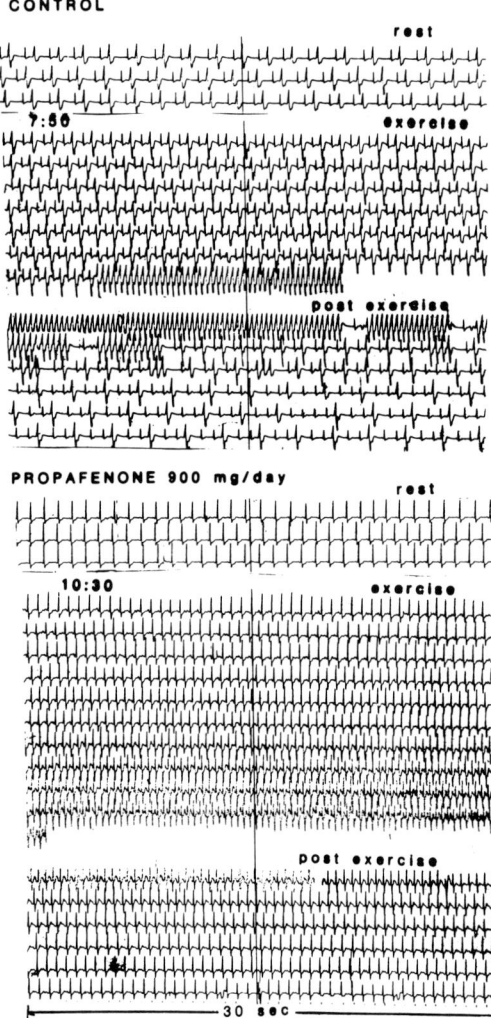

Fig. 24–3. Use of exercise testing as a guide to drug selection. Prior to therapy the rhythm is sinus with ventricular bigeminy. Exercise provokes runs of nonsustained ventricular tachycardia at rates of 220 beats/min. With propafenone therapy, arrhythmia is abolished.

important information about antiarrhythmic drug activity that complements the information derived from the former tests. As indicated, exercise produces important changes in the ventricular myocardium, many of which result from activation of the sympathetic nervous system and an increase in circulating catecholamines, factors that may affect antiarrhythmic drug action. It has been well established that the electrophysiological effects of the antiarrhythmic drugs result in a decrease in myocardial conductivity, prolongation of the membrane refractory period and hence a reduction in excitability, and a decrease in membrane automaticity.[39] In contrast, catecholamines shorten the refractory period, increase membrane excitability, increase membrane conductivity, and augment automaticity, changes that are in direct opposition to those caused by antiarrhythmic drugs (Fig. 24–4).[40] Therefore, catecholamines may interfere with and negate the action of antiarrhythmic drugs by reversing their beneficial effects. In one study, approximately 15% of patients with arrhythmia judged to be controlled based on ambulatory monitoring still had clinically important arrhythmia induced by exercise testing.

A number of studies evaluating the interaction between catecholamines and antiarrhythmic drugs have used electrophysiological techniques to identify a drug effective for preventing the induction of a sustained VT or supraventricular tachycardia.[41–50] In those patients who responded to an antiarrhythmic drug and in whom the clinical arrhythmia was no longer inducible, isoproterenol or epinephrine was infused during antiarrhythmic drug therapy and the electrophysiological test was repeated (Table 24–3). In approximately 50% of patients, the clinical arrhythmia was reinduced during electrophysiological testing when catecholamines were infused, confirming that they negated or reversed antiarrhythmic drug action, resulting in drug inefficacy. During follow-up of patients in whom arrhythmia was reinduced when catecholamines were infused, there was a significant rate of recurrence of the clinical arrhythmia despite the use of an antiarrhythmic drug identified as being effective by electrophysiological techniques. Since exercise testing is a physiological way of activating the sympathetic nervous system and increasing circulating catecholamines, it is a rational and important method for providing a complete evaluation of antiarrhythmic drug action, yielding data that are complementary to those derived from either monitoring or electrophysiological testing. In one study, Van Wijk and coworkers[50] reported on 50 patients with sustained VT or VT that had been treated with flecainide. Exercise testing was performed in 30 patients, and two

Action Potential

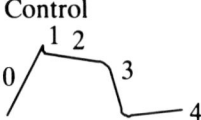

Control

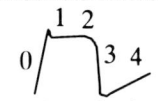

Catecholamines

Phase 0 velocity ↑
Phase 3 refractory period ↓
Phase 4 automaticity ↑

Result: increase in conductivity, excitability and automaticity

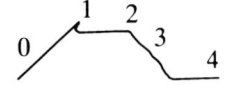

Membrane stabilizing drugs

Phase 0 velocity ↓
Phase 3 refractory period ↑
Phase 4 automaticity ↓

Result: decrease in conductivity, excitability and automaticity

Fig. 24-4. Electrophysiological actions of antiarrhythmic drugs and catecholamines. The effects of catecholamines are in contrast to the depressive actions of the membrane-active agents.

had sustained VT. During follow-up, the clinical arrhythmia recurred in both patients.

In addition to its useful role in evaluating the effect of arrhythmic drugs on arrhythmia, exercise testing is of great importance for exposing potential toxic effects of these agents. As previously indicated, each of the antiarrhythmic drugs reduces membrane conductivity and slows the rate of impulse conduction through the myocardium. The degree of slowing varies among these agents. This reduction of impulse conduction is rate dependent—that is, the depressive effects on conduction are more pronounced at rapid heart rates.[51] This property is known as use or rate dependency. Exercise testing, by causing an increase in heart rate, is an important technique for determining the degree of use dependency and may expose potentially harmful effects of these agents on atrioventricular or ventricular conduction (Fig. 24-5). This may be seen as a rate-related prolongation of PR or QRS intervals, and not infrequently a new right or left bundle-

Table 24-3
Effect of Catecholamine Infusion on Antiarrhythmic Drug Efficacy

Study	No. of Pts.	Arrhythmia	Drug	Reinducible With Catecholamine		Reinducible on Follow-Up
				No.	(%)	No. (%)
Morday[48]	21	VT	Quinidine	10	(48)	NR
Jazayeri[42]	17	VT	Class 1A, 1C	10	(59)	3 (30)
Niazi[45]	16	SVT	Encainide	10	(63)	4 (40)
Brugada[49]	10	SVT	Amiodarone	10	(100)	NR
Helmy[46]	10	SVT	Flecainide	5	(50)	3 (60)
Dubuc[47]	37	SVT	Class 1A, 1C	16	(43)	9 (56)
Akhtar[44]	32	SVT	Encainide	20	(63)	8 (40)
Dongas[43]	8	SVT	Procainamide	5	(63)	NR
Cockrell[41]	21	SVT	Flecainide	11	(52)	7 (64)
Overall	172			97	(56)	34 (47)*

Abbreviations: VT, ventricular tachycardia; SVT, supraventricular tachyarrhythmia; NR, not reported.
* 34/72 patients reported.

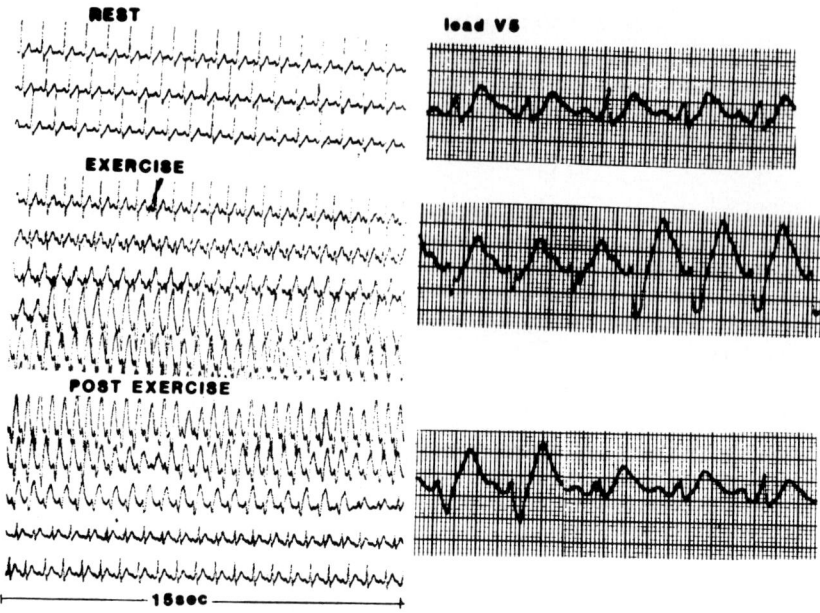

Fig. 24–5. Use of exercise testing to expose conduction abnormalities. Prior to therapy the ECG showed a normal QRS complex at rest and during exercise testing. During therapy with a Class IC antiarrhythmic drug, a rate-related left bundle-branch block occurs during exercise.

branch block will occur during exercise testing. In some cases this rate-dependent slowing of conduction may cause complete blockade of impulse conduction through the atrioventricular node, resulting in complete heart block. The slowing of conduction within the ventricular myocardium may, under certain circumstances, promote arrhythmia aggravation, as the slowing of impulse conduction increases the potential for re-entry and arrhythmia aggravation. Ranger and coworkers[52] exercised 16 patients with arrhythmia treated with flecainide. In these patients there was a significant increase in QRS duration during exercise, from 94 msec to 110 msec ($p < 0.001$) at peak increase, when the mean heart rate had increased by 84 beats/min. Flecainide therapy increased the QRS duration at rest by 12%, while during exercise there was a further increase of QRS duration by 28%. The best predictor of drug-induced QRS interval prolongation with exercise was a change in the QRS width at rest ($p = 0.001$) Importantly, the development of VT with exercise was observed in patients who had the greatest degree of a rate-related increase in QRS duration.

The Class 1A drugs (quinidine, procainamide, and disopyramide) slow impulse conduction and increase the QRS duration only modestly; their effect on the repolarization time is more pronounced. Hence they produce a significant prolongation of the QT interval. In a drug-free state, the increase in heart rate due to exercise decreases the time for membrane repolarization and the QT interval shortens, a result of sympathetic stimulation and increased catecholamine levels. The effect of heart rate on the QT interval may be significantly blunted by antiarrhythmic drugs, and there may be a paradoxical prolongation in repolarization time and the QT interval, a factor that may be responsible for arrhythmogenesis, specifically torsade de pointes. It has been observed that patients with a prolonged QT syndrome (Romano-Ward syndrome or Lange–Jervel Nielson syndrome), who have an abnormally prolonged time for membrane repolarization at baseline, do not have shortening of the QT interval with exercise.[53] These patients may be at greater risk for arrhythmia aggravation (i.e., torsade de pointes) with Class 1A drugs. Vincent and coworkers[54] compared 27 patients with a prolonged QT syndrome (Romano-Ward syndrome) with 27 healthy subjects. With exercise, the QT interval failed to shorten appropriately in patients compared to normal subjects.

It has been suggested that patients with underlying but not clinically obvious abnormalities of repolarization and of QT interval may also be at increased risk for this arrhythmic complication with Class 1A drugs. It has been proposed that failure of the QT interval to shorten appropriately during exercise is a marker for this condition. Kadish and coworkers[55] reported that a paradoxical increase in the QT interval during exercise was observed in patients who experienced arrhythmia aggravation, defined as a polymorphic VT, as a result of drug therapy with Class 1A agents.

It has been reported that aggravation of arrhythmia, which is a frequent and potentially serious complication of antiarrhythmic drugs, may often be exposed by exercise testing (Fig. 24-6). Jordaens and coworkers[56] reported on 11 patients with refractory VT treated with a combination of flecainide and mexiletine. Eight patients responded to the combination, and in these patients arrhythmia became noninducible on electrophysiological testing. However, three of these patients had VT or VF during an exercise test, representing proarrhythmia. Anastasiou Nana and coworkers[57] reported on 55 patients treated with flecainide for complex ventricular arrhythmia. Proarrhythmia was documented in seven patients, five of whom had this complication during exercise testing. In a large series involving mexiletine, encainide, and quinidine, reported by Slater and coworkers,[58] one third of 52 episodes of arrhythmia aggravation occurred during an exercise test, even though ambulatory monitoring demonstrated adequate arrhythmia suppression or the arrhythmia could no longer be induced by electrophysiological testing. Exercise testing may also be useful for exposing potentially serious ventricular arrhythmia in

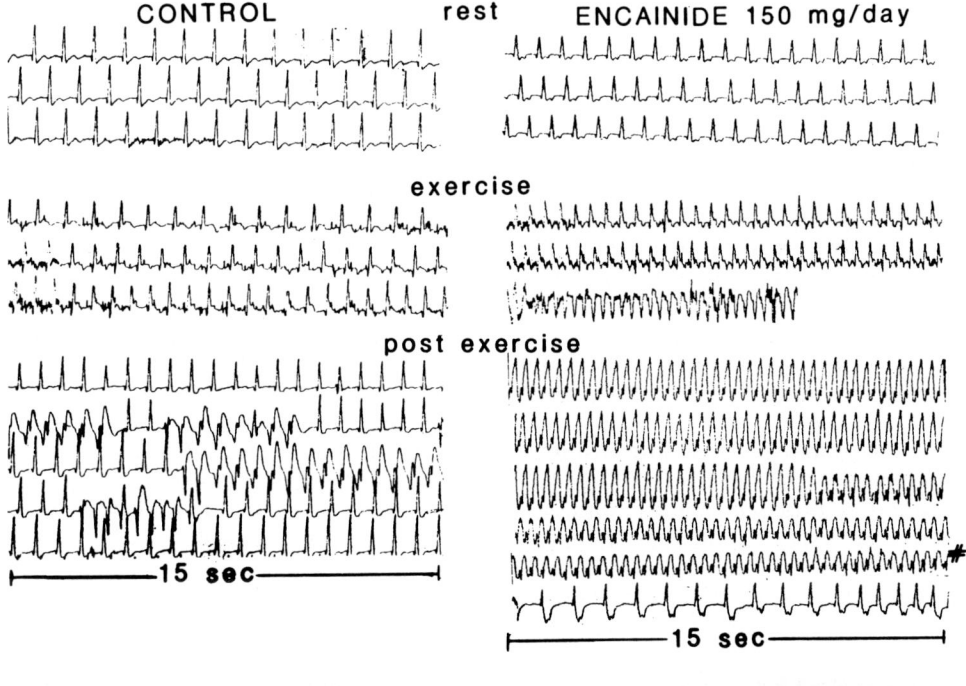

Fig. 24-6. Arrhythmia aggravation exposed by exercise testing. Prior to therapy there were brief episodes of nonsustained ventricular tachycardia. During therapy with encainide, a Class IC antiarrhythmic agent, sustained ventricular tachycardia, resulting in collapse, was provoked. Defibrillation was required.

patients receiving antiarrhythmic drug therapy for suppression of an atrial arrhythmia. Falk[59] reported on 11 patients receiving flecainide therapy for control of ventricular rate during atrial fibrillation, three of whom had VT or VF during exercise.

During exercise there is an increase in sympathetic neural activity and circulating catecholamines, and the occurrence of ischemia and resulting changes in extracellular potassium levels and pH may foster arrhythmia. More important, these changes can affect antiarrhythmic drug action. The development of extracellular hyperkalemia and tissue acidosis resulting from ischemia causes a reduction in resting potential and a slowing of impulse conduction velocity, which may exaggerate the depressive effects on conduction produced by antiarrhythmic drug, possibly resulting in localized intraventricular block. Since the degree of ischemia and the tissue concentration of antiarrhythmic drugs are nonuniform, varying widely from region to region of a diseased myocardium, there is significant regional heterogeneity of electrophysiological properties, an important precondition for re-entry and arrhythmogenesis. Ischemia and acidosis may also alter the tissue binding and hence concentration of these agents, further modifying their electrophysiological actions. In contrast, hypokalemia, which may occur in the absence of ischemia as a result of circulating catecholamines and activation of β_2-mediated insulin secretion,[60] causes a shortening of the refractory period and an increase in membrane excitability, hence negating the prolongation of refractoriness and reduction in excitability produced by antiarrhythmic drugs.

Each of the antiarrhythmic drugs is negatively inotropic and has the potential to depress left ventricular contractility and provoke congestive heart failure.[61] Unfortunately, the LVEF measured while the patient is in a resting state may not demonstrate any significant change resulting from antiarrhythmic drug therapy. Nevertheless, congestive heart failure may occur, and measurement of a resting LVEF is an unreliable method for predicting the patient at risk for this complication. However, it is possible that determination of the LVEF during exercise will be more useful as the effects of ischemia and catecholamines may exacerbate the negative inotropic effect of these agents.[62] In conclusion, exercise testing, in addition to being a helpful tool in the evaluation of antiarrhythmic drug efficacy, is of even greater importance for the evaluation of potential cardiac toxic side effects from these agents.

USE OF EXERCISE TESTING FOR OTHER CONDITIONS

In addition to its important role for evaluating the beneficial or harmful effects of antiarrhythmic drugs, exercise testing has also been useful for the evaluation of other conditions associated with arrhythmia. As indicated earlier, patients with the prolonged QT syndrome do not have the expected shortening of the QT interval during exercise,[54,55] and many will develop serious arrhythmia with exercise, a result of increased sympathetic tone and further autonomic imbalance.[63] It is possible that patients with idiosyncratic reactions to class 1A drugs who develop substantial QT prolongation and the associated increased risk of torsade de pointes even with low serum concentrations of drug have a "forme fruste" of the QT syndrome. Exercise testing may help identify these patients, as the QT interval will not shorten appropriately. Exercise testing has been used to identify patients with the Wolff-Parkinson-White syndrome who are at an increased risk for sudden death.[64] The persistence of pre-excited QRS complexes during exercise testing has a 17% specificity but a 90% sensitivity for identifying patients at risk for sudden death as determined by electrophysiological testing (i.e., shortest R-R interval during atrial fibrillation < 250 msec). The positive predictive value was 40% and the negative predictive value was 88%.

SAFETY OF EXERCISE TESTING

A very important concern about the use of exercise testing in arrhythmia management, particularly in patients with far-advanced heart disease, is its safety. In several surveys involving thousands of patients, mortality due to the precipitation of a serious arrhythmia has been rare, ranging from 0.2% to 0.5%.[65,66] However, in these studies patients had heart disease of different etiologies and severity. Generally, patients with a history of serious ventricular arrhythmia did not undergo exercise testing and were excluded from these reports. Nevertheless, exercise testing appears to be safe in patients with heart disease, and the risk of provoking a serious arrhythmic event is low.

Data on the safety of exercise testing in patients who have a history of ventricular tachyarrhythmia are limited. These patients usually have significant underlying heart disease and impaired left ventricular function. Young and coworkers[25] retrospectively reviewed exercise testing in 263 patients with a history of a serious sustained ventricular tachyarrhythmia, including sustained VT or VF. In this population 1377 exercise tests were performed and a serious arrhythmia complication requiring an intervention (cardioversion, defibrillation, or intravenous drug administration) occurred in 32 tests (2.3%) involving 24 patients (9.1%). There were 22 cases of sustained VT, nine episodes of VF, and one bradycardic arrest. In this population there were no deaths, MIs, or other forms of morbidity as a result of exercise. However, the criteria for a serious arrhythmic event were a sustained tachyarrhythmia or a bradyarrhythmia that caused significant hemodynamic impairment and required emergency intervention. These patients often had episodes of nonsustained VT that did not require immediate therapy. It was also observed in this study that the risk of a sustained tachyarrhythmia during exercise was greater during the administration of an antiarrhythmic drug when compared to testing performed in a baseline state. As part of drug evaluation, 1076 tests were performed and 24 episodes of serious arrhythmia noted, in contrast to only eight events during baseline assessment in a drug-free state. The investigators compared the prevalence of sustained ventricular tachyarrhythmia in these patients with that in a general population of 3444 patients with heart disease who underwent 8221 exercise tests. These patients did not have a history of sustained ventricular arrhythmia, and, as in previous studies, the risk of inducing a life-threatening arrhythmia during exercise testing was extremely small, as there were only four episodes of VF, involving 0.05% of tests and 0.12% of patients. Therefore, it appears that exercise testing in patients with far-advanced heart disease who have a history of sustained ventricular tachyarrhythmia is safe. Although the risk of inducing a serious ventricular tachyarrhythmia during exercise testing was greater in these patients than in patients with heart disease without a clinical history of serious arrhythmia, the majority of events occurred during antiarrhythmic drug use when exercise was performed for an evaluation of efficacy, suggesting that the arrhythmia was a result of aggravation of arrhythmia due to the antiarrhythmic drug. As previously indicated, this is an important use for exercise testing as it helps to identify those patients at risk for this complication. Although serious bradycardic events due to pacemaker failure or conduction problems are rarely seen, such complications are also more likely to occur during drug therapy, and exercise testing is important for exposing the risk for such complications.

SUMMARY

Exercise testing is an established tool for the evaluation of patients with heart disease, being important for diagnosis, management, and prognosis. It is particularly helpful and important for the management of patients with arrhythmia. Although exercise testing has a limited role in establishing a prognosis in patients with arrhythmia, it does have an important role in the evaluation of the beneficial and potentially harmful effects of antiarrhythmic drugs.

REFERENCES

1. Bruce TA, Chapman CP, Baker O, Fisher JN: Role of autonomic and myocardial factors in cardiac control. J Clin Invest 42:721, 1963.
2. Wit AL, Rosen MR: Pathophysiologic mechanisms of cardiac arrhythmias. Am Heart J 106:798, 1983.
3. Marcus ML, Kerber RE, Erhardt JC, Falsetti HL, Davis DM, Abboud FM: Spatial and temporal heterogeneity of left ven-

tricular perfusion in awake dogs. Am Heart J 94:748, 1977.
4. Coggens DL, Flynn AE, Austin RE, et al: Nonuniform loss of regional flow reserve during myocardial ischemia in dogs. Circ Res 67:253, 1990.
5. Kageyama Y, Hill JC, Gettes LS: Interaction of acidosis and increased intracellular potassium on action potential characteristics and conduction in guinea pig ventricular muscle. Clin Res 51:614, 1982.
6. Watanabe I, Johnson TA, Buchanan J, Angle CL, Gettes LS: Effect of graded coronary flow reduction on ionic, electrical and mechanical indices of ischemia in the pig. Circulation 76:1127, 1987.
7. Hauswurth D, Noble D, Tsien RW: Adrenaline mechanism of action of the pacemaker potential in cardiac Purkinje fibers. Science 162:916, 1968.
8. Wit AL, Cranfield PF: Triggered activities in cardiac muscle fibers of the simian mitral valve. Circ Res 38:85, 1976.
9. Antman ES, Graboys TB, Lown B: Comparison of continuous intermittent electrocardiographic monitoring during exercise testing for exposure of cardiac arrhythmias. JAMA 241:2802, 1979.
10. Beard EF, Owen CA: Cardiac arrhythmias during exercise stress testing in healthy men. Aerospace Med 44:286, 1973.
11. Master AM: Cardiac arrhythmias elicited by the two-step exercise test. Am J Cardiol 32:766, 1973.
12. Whinnery JE: Dysrhythmia comparison in apparently healthy males during and after treadmill and accelerated stress test. Am Heart J 105:732, 1983.
13. McHenry PL, Fisch C, Jordan JW: Cardiac arrhythmia observed during maximal exercise testing in clinically normal men. Am J Cardiol 39:311, 1978.
14. Poblete PF, Kennedy HL, Cavalis DG: Detection of ventricular ectopy in patients with coronary heart disease and normal subjects by exercise testing and ambulatory electrocardiography. Chest 74:402, 1978.
15. Jelinek MV, Lown B: Exercise stress testing for exposure of cardiac arrhythmia. Prog Cardiovasc Dis 16:497, 1974.
16. Ryan M, Lown B, Horn H: Comparison of ventricular ectopic activity during 24-hour monitoring and exercise testing in patients with coronary heart disease. N Engl J Med 292:224, 1975.
17. Gooch AS, McConnell D: Analysis of transient arrhythmia and conduction disturbances during submaximal treadmill exercise testing. Prog Cardiovasc Dis 13:293, 1970.
18. Ekblum B, Hartley LH, Day WC: Occurrence and reproducibility of exercise-induced ventricular ectopy in normal subjects. Am J Cardiol 43:35, 1979.
19. Sami M, Chaitman B, Fisher L, Holmes D, Fray D, Alderman E: Significance of exercise-induced ventricular arrhythmia in stable coronary artery disease: A Coronary Artery Surgery Study project. Am J Cardiol 54:118, 1984.
20. Califf RM, McKinnis RA, McNeer F, Harel FE, Leek L, Pryor DB: Prognostic value of ventricular arrhythmias associated with treadmill exercise testing in patients studied with cardiac catheterization for suspected ischemic heart disease. J Am Coll Cardiol 2:1060, 1983.
21. Weiner DA, Levine PR, Klein MD, Ryan TJ: Ventricular arrhythmias during exercise testing: Mechanism, response to coronary bypass surgery, and prognostic significance. Am J Cardiol 53:1553, 1984.
22. Yang JC, Wesley RC, Froelicher VF: Ventricular tachycardia during routine treadmill testing: Risk and prognosis. Arch Intern Med 51:349, 1991.
23. Cordini MA, Sommerfeldt L, Egbil LE: Clinical significance and characteristics of exercise-induced ventricular tachycardia. Cathet Cardiovasc Diag 7:227, 1981.
24. Detry JM, Abouantoun S, Wyms W: Incidence and prognostic implications of severe ventricular arrhythmias during maximal exercise testing. Am J Cardiol 48:35, 1981.
25. Young D, Lampert S, Graboys TB, Lown B: Safety of maximal exercise testing in patients at high risk for ventricular arrhythmia. Circulation 70:184, 1984.
26. Rodriguez LM, Weleffe A, Brugada P, et al: Exercise induced sustained symptomatic ventricular tachycardia: Incidence, clinical, angiographic and electrophysiologic characteristics. Eur Heart J 11:225, 1990.
27. Graboys TB, Lampert S, Lown B: Yield of a ventricular arrhythmia during exercise testing in patients with prior cardiac arrest [abstract]. Circulation 66(suppl II):II-27, 1980.
28. Lown B, Podrid PJ, DeSilva RA, Graboys TB: Sudden cardiac death: Management of the patient at risk. Curr Probl Cardiol 4:1, 1980.
29. Weld FM, Chu KL, Bigger JT, Rolnitzky LM: Risk stratification with low level exercise testing two weeks after myocardial infarction. Circulation 64:306, 1981.
30. Krone RJ, Gillespie JA, Weld FM, Miller JP, Moss AJ, and the Multicenter Postinfarction Research Group: Low-level exercise testing after myocardial infarction: Usefulness in

enhancing clinical risk stratification. Circulation 71:80, 1985.
31. Henry RL, Kennedy GT, Crawford MH: Prognostic value of exercise-induced ventricular ectopy activity for mortality after acute myocardial infarction. Am J Cardiol 59:1251, 1987.
32. Udall JA, Ellestad MJ: Prediction implications of ventricular premature contractions associated with treadmill stress testing. Circulation 56:985, 1977.
33. Sheps DS, Ernst JC, Briese RF, et al: Decreased frequency of exercise-induced ventricular ectopic activity in the second of two consecutive treadmill tests. Circulation 55: 892, 1977.
34. Drory Y, Pines A, Fisman EZ, Kellerman JJ: Persistence of arrhythmia-exercise response in healthy young men. Am J Cardiol 66:1092, 1990.
35. Faris JV, McHenry PC, Jordan JW, Morris SN: Prevalence and reproducibility of exercise-induced ventricular arrhythmias during maximal exercise testing in normal men. Am J Cardiol 37:617, 1976.
36. Handler CE, Sowton E: Stress testing predischarge and six weeks after myocardial infarction to compare submaximal and maximal exercise predischarge and to assess the reproducibility of induced abnormalities. Int J Cardiol 9:173, 1985.
37. Saini V, Graboys T, Towne V, Lown B: Reproducibility of exercise induced ventricular arrhythmia in patients undergoing evaluation for malignant ventricular arrhythmia. Am J Cardiol 63:697, 1989.
38. Graboys TB, Lown B, Podrid PJ, DeSilva R: Long-term survival of patients with malignant ventricular arrhythmia. Am J Cardiol 50:437, 1982.
39. Rosen MR, Wit AL: Electropharmacology of antiarrhythmic drugs. Am Heart J 106: 829, 1983.
40. Wit AL, Hoffman BF, Rosen MR: Electrophysiology and pharmacology of cardiac arrhythmias: IX. Cardiac electrophysiologic effects of beta adrenergic receptor stimulation and blockade. Part A. Am Heart J 90: 521, 1975.
41. Cockrell JL, Scheinman MM, Titus C, et al: Safety and efficacy of oral flecainide therapy in patients with atrioventricular re-entrant tachycardia. Ann Intern Med 114:189, 1991.
42. Jazayeri MR, Wyhe G, Avitall B, McKinna JM, Tchou P, Akhtar M: Isoproterenol reversal of antiarrhythmic effects in patients with inducible sustained ventricular tachyarrhythmias. J Am Coll Cardiol 14:705, 1989.
43. Dongas J, Tchou P, Mahmud R, Lehmann MH, Denker J, Akhtar M: Catecholamine mediated reversal of procainamide induced retrograde block in paroxysmal supraventricular tachycardias: Possible cause of treatment failures [Abstract]. Circulation 72(suppl III):III-126, 1985.
44. Akhtar M, Niazi I, Naccarelli G, et al: Role of adrenergic stimulation by isoproterenol in reversal of effects of encainide in supraventricular tachycardia. Am J Cardiol 62:45L, 1988.
45. Niazi I, Naccarelli G, Dougherty A, Rinkenberger R, Tchou P, Akhtar M: Treatment of atrioventricular nodal re-entrant tachycardia with encainide: Reversal of drug effect with isoproterenol. J Am Coll Cardiol 13:904, 1989.
46. Helmy I, Scheinman MM, Skarkey H, Heler JM, Griffin JC: Isoproterenol reversal of flecainide effects in patients with accessory pathways [Abstract]. Circulation 76(suppl IV):IV-69, 1987.
47. Dubuc M, Kies T, Fromer M, Primeau R, Shenasa M: Reversibility of the electrophysiologic effects of antiarrhythmic drugs by isoproterenol in patients with paroxysmal supraventricular tachycardia (PSVT) [abstract]. Circulation 76(suppl IV):IV-69, 1987.
48. Morday F, Kou WH, Kadish AH, et al: Antagonism of flecainide electrophysiologic effects by epinephrine in patients with ventricular tachycardia. J Am Coll Cardiol 12:388, 1988.
49. Brugada P, Facchini M, Wellens HJJ: Effects of isoproterenol and amiodarone and the role of exercise in initiation of cricus movement tachycardia in the accessory atrioventricular pathway. Am J Cardiol 57: 146, 1986.
50. Van Wijk LM, Crijns HJ, Kingma HJ, et al: Flecainide long-term effects in patients with sustained ventricular tachycardia or ventricular fibrillation. J Cardiovasc Pharmacol 15: 884, 1990.
51. Ranger S, Talajic M, Lemnery R, Roy D, Villemaife C, Nattel, S: Kinetics of use-dependent ventricular conduction slowing by antiarrhythmic drugs in humans. Circulation 83:1987, 1991.
52. Ranger S, Talajic M, Lemery R, Roy D, Nattel S: Amplification of flecainide induced ventricular conduction slowing by exercise: A potentially significant clinical consequence use dependent sodium channel blockade. Circulation 79:1000, 1989.
53. Locati E, Pancaldi A, Pala M, Schwartz PJ: Exercise-induced electrocardiographic changes in patients with the long QT syndrome (LQTS) [abstract]. Circulation 78(suppl II):II-42, 1988.

54. Vincent GM, Jaiswal D, Timothy KW: Effects of exercise on heart rate, QT, QTc and QT/QS2 in the Romano-Ward inherited long QT syndrome. Am J Cardiol 68:498, 1991.
55. Kadish AH, Weisman HF, Veltri EP, Epstein AE, Slepian MJ, Levine JH: Paradoxic effects of exercise on the QT interval in patients with polymorphic ventricular tachycardia receiving type 1A antiarrhythmic agents. Circulation 81:14, 1990.
56. Jordaens LJ, Tavrnier R, Vanmeerhalghi X, Robbins E, Clement DC: Combination of flecainide and mexiletine for the treatment of ventricular tachycardia. PACE 13:1127, 1990.
57. Anastasiou-Nana MI, Anderson JL, Steward JR, et al: Occurrence of exercise-induced and spontaneous wide complex tachycardia during therapy with flecainide for complex ventricular arrhythmia. A possible proarrhythmic effect. Am Heart J 115:1071, 1987.
58. Slater W, Lampert SC, Podrid PJ, Lown B: Clinical predictors of arrhythmia worsening by antiarrhythmic drugs. Am J Cardiol 61: 349, 1988.
59. Falk RH: Flecainide induced ventricular tachycardia and fibrillation in patients treated for atrial fibrillation. Ann Intern Med 111:107, 1989.
60. Brown MJ, Brown DL, Murphy MN: Hypokalemia from beta-2 receptor stimulation by circulating catecholamines. N Engl J Med 307:1414, 1983.
61. Ravid J, Podrid PJ, Lampert S, Lown B: Congestive heart failure induced by antiarrhythmic drugs. J Am Coll Cardiol 14:1326, 1989.
62. Pratt CM, Podrid PJ, Scals A, et al: Effects of ethmozine (morecizine HCL) on ventricular function using echocardiographic, hemodynamic and radionuclide assessments. Am J Cardiol 60:73F, 1987.
63. Schwartz PJ, Periti M, Malliani A: The long QT syndrome. Am Heart J 89:378, 1975.
64. Gaita F, Giustetto C, Riccardi RM, Mangiardi L, Brusca A: Stress and pharmacologic tests as methods to identify patient with Wolff-Parkinson-White syndrome at risk of sudden death. Am J Cardiol 64:487, 1989.
65. Atterhog J, Jonssen B, Samuels MC: Exercise testing: A preoperative study of complication rates. Am Heart J 98:572, 1979.
66. Irving J, Bruce R: External hypertension and post-exertional ventricular fibrillation in stress testing. Am J Cardiol 39:849, 1977.

25

Triggers for Sudden Cardiac Death from the Central Nervous System

RICHARD L. VERRIER
BRUCE D. NEARING
LINDA W. DICKERSON

The fundamental premise that central nervous system (CNS) activity can trigger sudden cardiac death (SCD) requires no debate, as it is soundly embedded in ancient and modern medicine. What is new and exciting is the current depth of understanding of the mechanisms of CNS-induced arrhythmias and the therapeutic insights provided by this information.

Two major concepts have surfaced from extensive investigation of CNS-induced cardiac arrhythmias. The first is that triggering of arrhythmias by the CNS is not only the consequence of intense activation of the autonomic nervous system but is also a function of the specific neural pattern elicited. Thus, the balance in discharge rate through either limb of the autonomic nervous system and the interaction between the two limbs must be considered.[1-6] There is also mounting evidence that release of opioids and neuroactive peptides may play an important role in fine-tuning neurocardiac interactions.[7,8]

The second major theme is that triggering of arrhythmias by CNS activity may depend on several intermediary mechanisms. These include direct effects of neurotransmitters on the myocardium and its specialized conducting system and alterations in myocardial perfusion due to changes in coronary vasomotor tone and/or enhanced platelet aggregability. The processes ultimately engaged thus depend on a complex interplay between the specific neural pattern elicited and the underlying cardiac pathology.

The recent discovery that SCD exhibits a circadian pattern, with a peak in death rates in the early morning, represents a clinical milestone and highlights the importance of neural triggers of life-threatening arrhythmias.[9-15] Specifically, it has been demonstrated that this phenomenon is in large part the consequence of a centrally mediated reciprocal increase in sympathetic activity and a decrease in parasympathetic activity during the early morning hours. This effect occurs prior to waking and assuming the upright posture.[15] Another contributing factor may be increased platelet aggregability, leading to adrenergically mediated thrombosis[16,17] that is exacerbated by arising.[11,12]

This chapter addresses both clinical and experimental studies of brain–heart interactions from the vantage points of several research strategies, including brain stimulation, behavioral stress testing, and sleep state analysis. We conclude by discussing new analytical approaches for the noninvasive assessment of autonomic nervous system activity and cardiac vulnerability that will permit unprecedented exploration of neurocardiac interactions in normal individuals and those at risk for SCD.

Supported by grant HL-33567 from the National Heart, Lung and Blood Institute, National Institutes of Health, Bethesda, Maryland.

CENTRAL NERVOUS SYSTEM STIMULATION STUDIES

Over 70 years ago it was demonstrated that ventricular tachycardia (VT) and other significant arrhythmias could be evoked in normal animals by stimulating certain areas in the hypothalamus.[18] This finding was subsequently confirmed in a variety of species. Hockman and colleagues, using stereotaxic techniques, showed that cerebral stimulation and hypothalamic activation elicited a spectrum of ventricular arrhythmias.[19] These observations are consistent with clinical reports that cerebral vascular disease, and especially intracranial hemorrhage, can produce pronounced cardiac repolarization abnormalities and life-threatening arrhythmias.[20,21]

The posterior hypothalamus is a site of particular importance in CNS-induced arrhythmogenesis. Stimulation of this structure increased tenfold the incidence of ventricular fibrillation (VF) associated with acute coronary artery occlusion.[22] Enhanced vulnerability was due to increased sympathetic activity, because β-adrenergic-receptor blockade but not vagotomy prevented it.[23] Arrhythmias that developed immediately following cessation of diencephalic or hypothalamic stimulation required intact vagi and stellate ganglia.[24,25] The likely basis for the arrhythmogenic effect of vagal activity is that during CNS stimulation, automaticity of cardiac Purkinje fibers is enhanced by adrenergic discharge, and upon cessation of stimulation, the rapid recovery of high vagal tone slows heart rhythm, exposing the increased automaticity of the fibers and leading to ventricular premature beats and tachyarrhythmias. This finding also underscores the complex feedback mechanisms of poststress arrhythmogenic phenomena.[2,26]

Insights into the CNS pathways involved in behaviorally induced arrhythmias have been provided by Skinner and Reed.[27] Cryogenic blockade of the thalamic gating mechanism or its output from the frontal cortex to the brain stem delayed or prevented the occurrence of VF during stress in pigs. Recently, Carpeggiani, Skinner and colleagues showed that cryogenic blockade of the amygdala is also capable of preventing stress-induced VF.[28] Thus, these distinct pathways within the CNS appear to play a critical role in mediating arrhythmogenesis due to intense behavioral arousal. CNS regulation of cardiovascular function has been discussed in detail by Smith and DeVito,[29] Gutterman and colleagues,[30] Jordan,[31] Cechetto and Saper,[32] and LeDoux.[33]

BEHAVIORAL STRESS AND ARRHYTHMIAS

Experimental Studies

Models have been introduced to define the impact of behavioral state on cardiac electrical stability.[2,26,34,35] These models have included both aversive behavioral conditioning paradigms and models eliciting natural emotions, including anger and fear.[2,26,34] Quantification of changes in cardiac electrical stability in the normal as well as ischemic heart was achieved by means of the repetitive extrasystole (RE) threshold technique.[34,36] Aversive conditioning of dogs in a Pavlovian sling with mild chest shock on 3 consecutive days showed that subsequent exposure to the environment without shock reduced the RE threshold by more than 30% (Fig. 25–1).[34,37] The same paradigm elicited a threefold increase in the occurrence of spontaneous VF when occlusion was carried out in the aversive sling compared to the nonaversive cage environment. β-adrenergic blockade with propranolol or the cardioselective drugs tolamolol and metoprolol completely prevented these adverse effects, indicating a primary role of the sympathetic nervous system in stress-induced changes in cardiac vulnerability.[38,39]

An important role of vagal tone in the aversive stress paradigm was also demonstrated. Specifically, when relatively small doses of atropine (0.05 mg/kg) were given to block vagal influences on the heart, vulnerability in the aversive environment was markedly increased.[37] The administration of atropine in the nonstressful cage environment did not alter the RE threshold, suggesting that vagal influences on vulnerability in conscious animals are contingent on the level of adrenergic tone. Furthermore, catecholamines were markedly elevated in the aversive environment but not in the non-

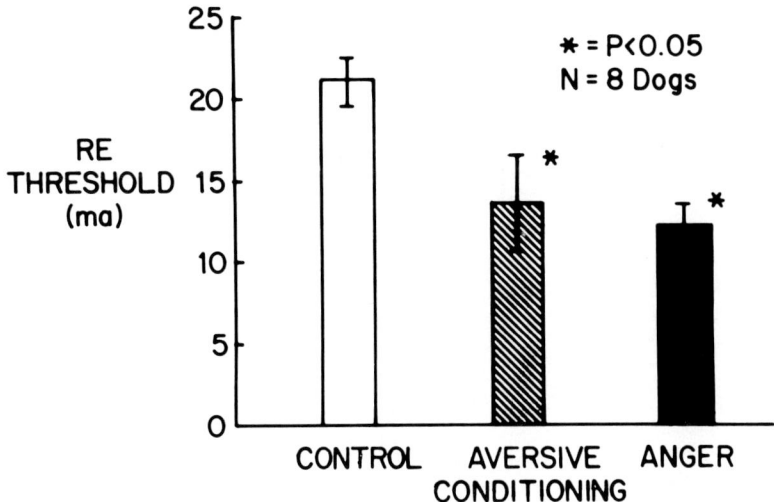

Fig. 25–1. Effects of behavioral stress on the repetitive extrasystole (RE) threshold in normal dogs. Both passive aversive conditioning using a mild electrical shock and induction of an anger-like state by denial of access to food produced significant reductions in the vulnerable period threshold. Heart rate was maintained constant during cardiac electrical testing by ventricular pacing. (Reproduced with permission from Verrier RL, et al: Annu Rev Physiol 46:155–176, 1984.[37])

stressful cage environment.[40] Finally, when β-adrenergic blockade was induced in the aversive environment, atropine failed to alter the RE threshold (Fig. 25–2).[41]

These observations suggest that accentuated antagonism of the profibrillatory effects of enhanced adrenergic activity by muscarinic stimulation operates in the conscious animals affected by behavioral stress[37] as well as in the anesthetized state.[8,42–44] Stramba-Badiale, Vanoli, Schwartz and their coworkers[45,46] have characterized sympathetic–parasympathetic interactions during ischemia and infarction in the conscious state. Even during intense stress there may be sufficient vagal tone to inhibit presynaptically the amount of norepinephrine released at sympathetic nerve endings and to oppose the effects of adrenergic receptor stimulation by muscarinic opposition of second messenger formation (Table 25–1).

Human Studies of Stress

Contemporary clinical investigations have implicated behavioral factors in the genesis of myocardial ischemia and arrhythmias. In a landmark publication, Deanfield, Selwyn, et al[47] reported recurrent episodes of ST-segment depression during daily life

Table 25–1
Sympathetic–Parasympathetic Interactions and Myocardial Electrical Stability

Vagal tone increases myocardial electrical stability and protects against ventricular fibrillation during myocardial ischemia.

Vagally induced reduction in heart rate plays an important role during both myocardial ischemia and reperfusion because it increases diastolic perfusion time and reduces cardiac metabolic demand.

Enhanced vagal activity has an additional antifibrillatory effect owing to antagonism of adrenergic influences.

The bases for sympathetic-parasympathetic interactions are:
- Inhibition of norepinephrine release from nerve endings.
- Attenuation of response to catecholamines at receptor sites.

Beneficial effects of vagal activity may be vitiated if profound bradycardia and hypotension ensue.

Myocardial infarction may alter autonomic influences by damaging neural fibers.

SOURCE: Verrier.[128] Adapted by permission.

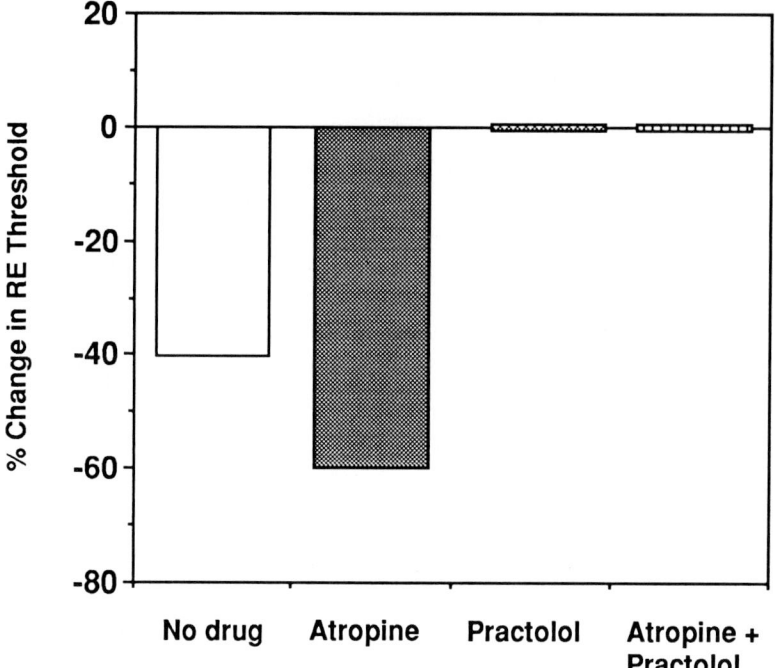

Fig. 25-2. Effect of β-adrenergic blockade with practolol (1 mg/kg IV) on atropine-induced (0.05 mg/kg) changes in the repetitive extrasystole (RE) threshold during aversive conditioning in 6 dogs.[25] In the absence of drug, the aversive environment resulted in a 40% reduction in RE threshold. Following muscarinic receptor blockade, the stress-induced reduction in threshold increased by another 20%. However, when β-receptors were blocked by practolol, atropine no longer exerted an effect on the RE threshold during stress. Thus, the cardioprotective effect of vagal activity during behavioral stress is contingent on the prevailing level of adrenergic stimulation. (Reproduced with permission from Verrier RL, et al.[129])

in patients with stable angina. These abnormalities were induced during ordinary tasks such as conversing, driving a car, or holding a meeting at work and were not correlated with fluctuations in heart rate. The investigators concluded that transient impairment of coronary artery blood flow was the underlying basis for the myocardial ischemia. The group subsequently demonstrated a link between silent ischemia and mental stress[48] when they assessed regional myocardial perfusion and ischemia by measuring the uptake of rubidium-82 with positron tomography after mental arithmetic or physical exercise. During mental arithmetic, 12 (75%) of 16 patients exhibited regional perfusion abnormalities, accompanied in only six by ST-segment depression and in four of these six by angina. Six patients with perfusion abnormalities had neither pain nor electrocardiographic (ECG) changes. Following exercise, all of the patients exhibited abnormal regional myocardial perfusion in the segments that had become ischemic with mental arithmetic. This was associated with ST-segment depression in all and angina in 15 (94%) individuals. The investigators concluded that the interaction between mental activity and myocardial ischemia may operate continuously during everyday life and could be responsible for many transient and symptomless ECG changes in patients with coronary disease.

More recently, Rozanski and associates established a direct link between acute mental stress and myocardial ischemia with a battery of behavioral tests in patients with coronary artery disease (CAD).[49] Their protocol involved comparing the effects of mental arithmetic, the Stroop color-word task, and simulated public speaking and reading with those of exercise. Thirty-nine

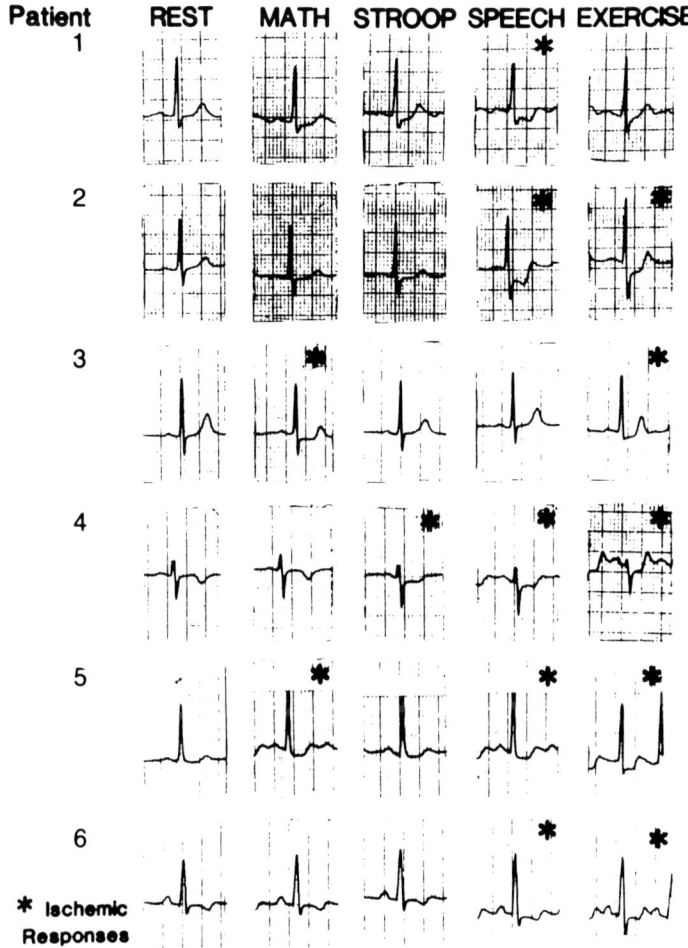

Fig. 25-3. Electrocardiograms obtained during rest, mental tasks, and exercise in the six group I patients with an ischemic ECG response during one or more mental tasks. An ischemic response occurred more frequently during the speaking tasks. The different ECG responses during speech and exercise in patient 1 (2-mm downsloping ST-segment depression vs. none, respectively) occurred despite a slightly higher heart rate during exercise, exemplifying the variable heart rate threshold for ischemia during mental stress and exercise. (Reproduced with permission from Rozanski A, et al: N Engl J Med 318:1005-1012, 1988.[49])

patients with CAD and 12 normal subjects were studied by radionuclide ventriculography. Of the patients with CAD, 23 (59%) exhibited wall motion abnormalities during mental stress and 14 (36%) displayed a decrease in ejection fraction of more than 5%. Ischemia induced by mental stress was symptomatically silent in 19 (83%) of 23 patients with wall motion abnormalities and occurred at lower heart rates than exercise-induced ischemia (Fig. 25-3). Elevations in arterial blood pressure during ischemia induced by mental stress were comparable to those during ischemia induced by exercise. A personally relevant, emotionally arousing speaking task provoked more frequent and greater regional wall motion abnormalities than did less specific cognitive tasks and were of the magnitude of those induced by exercise. This study not only provides a direct link between behavioral stress and ischemia but is an important contribution in the development of standardized clinical behavioral testing.

SLEEP STATES AND STABILITY OF HEART RHYTHM

Autonomic Tone During Sleep

Sleep is associated with dramatic changes in autonomic nervous system activity.[50-52] These changes are particularly evident during rapid eye movement (REM) or active sleep, when the CNS may operate in an "open-loop" mode, independent of feedback control.[51] During non-REM sleep, the system is highly regulated as a result of end-organ feedback and operates in a "closed-loop'' fashion. The apparent transient disruption of homeostatic mechanisms during REM sleep can result both in major surges in cardiac sympathetic activity and in decreases in the baseline vagal tone of sleep. These effects can have an adverse impact on the stability of cardiac rhythm and myocardial perfusion. Surges in sympathetic nervous system activity, particularly during phasic REM sleep, may be responsible for the prevalent but poorly understood phenomenon of nocturnal angina. The significant increase in baroreceptor gain during non-REM sleep is also likely to play an important role in cardiovascular homeostasis in health and disease.[53]

Deep non-REM sleep (slow wave sleep) is associated with marked stability of autonomic regulation.[51] Marked respiratory sinus arrhythmia is present, indicating a high degree of parasympathetic tone. Sympathetic nervous system activity is relatively stable during this stage and its cardiovascular input is reduced. However, during transitions from non-REM to REM sleep, bursts of vagus nerve activity may result in pauses in heart rhythm and frank asystole. Apnea may accentuate the vagal response and result in transient cardiac standstill with the potential for myocardial infarction (MI).[54]

Impact of Sleep States on Myocardial Perfusion and Arrhythmias

Ischemic events and arrhythmias during the nocturnal period[55–58] have been documented in patients with advanced coronary disease[55] or Prinzmetal's variant angina.[56] The REM phase of sleep is especially conducive of ST-segment changes and perfusion abnormalities.[55,56] In fact, 8–10% of ischemic attacks occur during sleep.[59,60] The prevalence of ischemic events associated with nocturnal arousal[14] may be due in part to increased platelet aggregation exacerbated by assumption of the upright posture.[9,12,13] Other factors regulating coronary vascular tone must also be considered.[61–63]

Recent experimental studies have clarified fundamental mechanisms of sleep-induced changes in myocardial perfusion and arrhythmogenesis.[64,67] Both REM sleep and slow wave sleep significantly increase the effective refractory period of the ventricles,[68] an effect independent of alterations in heart rate. The increased excitability of the heart is largely mediated by increases in cardiac vagal tone, since it is abolished by muscarinic blockade with atropine methylnitrate and is not influenced by bilateral stellectomy. Furthermore, even low-intensity electrical scanning of the cardiac cycle induced VF during REM sleep but not during slow wave sleep, suggesting the presence of transient triggers for arrhythmia.

Subsequent investigations revealed that sympathetic activity periodically surges during REM sleep, an action that could destabilize the heart electrophysiologically.[64,65] The heart rate surges occur predominantly during those periods of REM sleep marked by intensely phasic activity.[66] The experiments involved chronically instrumented dogs in which heart rate, arterial blood pressure, coronary arterial blood flow, and electroencephalographic (EEG) data were recorded simultaneously. Coronary stenosis was set to reduce baseline flow by 60%. During REM sleep, there were transient increases in heart rate with concomitant reductions in coronary flow (Fig. 25-4).[65] Because this surge phenomenon is abolished by bilateral stellectomy, it is assumed that increased adrenergic discharge is responsible for the flow deficit.

The increase in adrenergic discharge could lead to a coronary blood flow decrement by at least two mechanisms: (1) stimulation of α-adrenergic receptors on the coronary vascular smooth muscle, and/or (2) a decrease in diastolic coronary perfusion time as a result of the bursts in heart rate. A significant correlation between the magnitude of the increase in heart rate and the decrease in coronary blood flow supports the latter possibility. The link between REM sleep–induced changes in heart rate and coronary insufficiency appears to be consistent with clinical reports of patients with advanced coronary heart disease. In particular, Nowlin and coworkers[55] found in patients with advanced CAD that attacks of nocturnal angina occurred predominantly (32 of 39 episodes in four patients) during REM sleep and were associated with heart rate acceleration (Fig. 25-5).

Triggers for Sudden Cardiac Death from the Central Nervous System 373

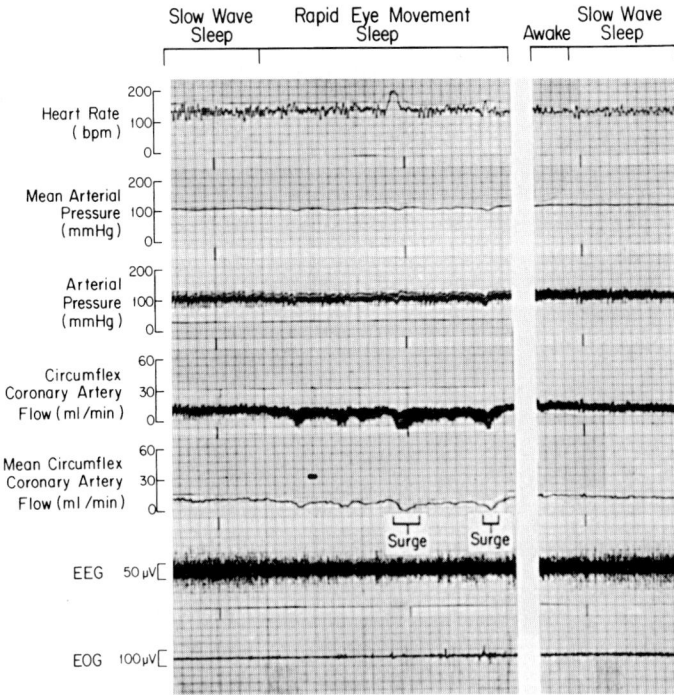

Fig. 25–4. Recordings of effects of sleep stage on heart rate, mean and phasic arterial pressures, and mean and phasic circumflex coronary artery flows in a typical dog during stenosis. Note phasic decreases in coronary flow occurring during heart rate surges while the dog is in rapid eye movement sleep. EEG, electroencephalogram; EOG, electro-oculogram. (Reproduced with permission from Kirby DA, et al: Physiol Behav 45:1, 1989.[65])

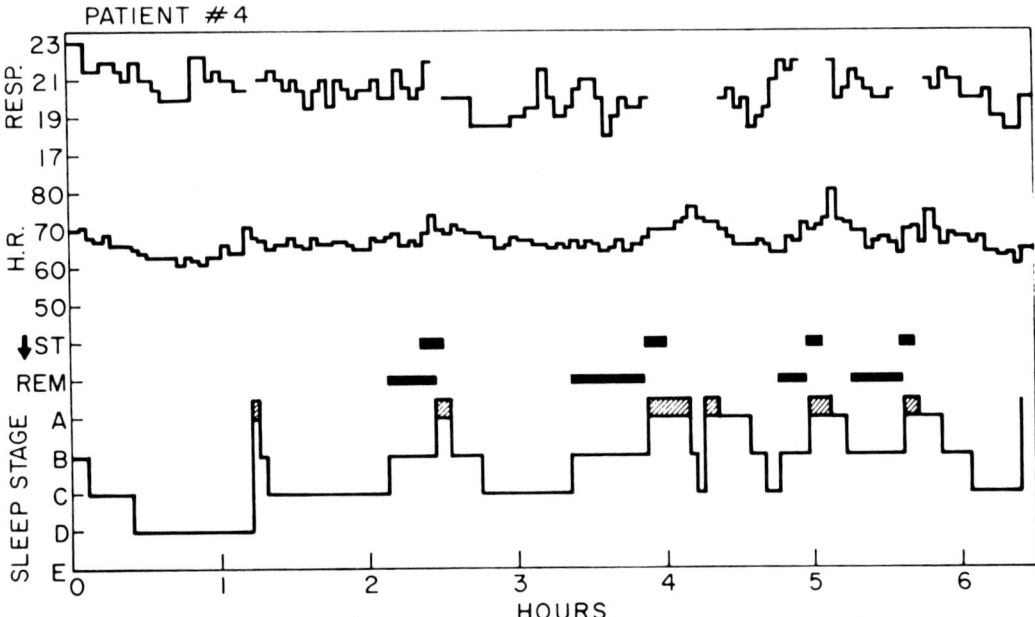

Fig. 25–5. Composite graph of a night of sleep in a patient with nocturnal angina pectoris. Note association between rapid eye movement (REM)–related surges in heart rate and occurrence of ST-segment changes. Resp., respirations; H.R., heart rate; ST, periods of significant ST-segment depression on the electrocardiogram. (Reproduced with permission from Nowlin JB, et al: Ann Intern Med 63:1040, 1965.[55])

Heart Rhythm Pauses and Arrhythmogenesis During Sleep

We recently observed in chronically instrumented dogs prolonged pauses in heart rhythm during transitions from slow wave sleep to periods marked by desynchronized EEG rhythms.[69,70] These pauses persisted from 1 to 8 seconds and were followed by dramatic increases in coronary blood flow averaging 30% and ranging up to 84% (Fig. 25–6).[2] An intense burst of vagal activity appeared to produce the phenomenon, since the pauses developed against a background of marked respiratory sinuses arrhythmia, low heart rate, and varying degrees of heart block with nonconducted P waves. Furthermore, the phenomenon, including the post-pause surge in coronary flow, was emulated by electrical stimulation of the vagus nerve.

These observations carry important implications for diagnosing and treating neurogenically induced ischemia and arrhythmias.[71,72] Nocturnal asystolic events have been reported in both young adults[73] and individuals with obstructive sleep apnea.[54,74] Pauses in heart rhythm could set the stage for triggered activity, as abrupt

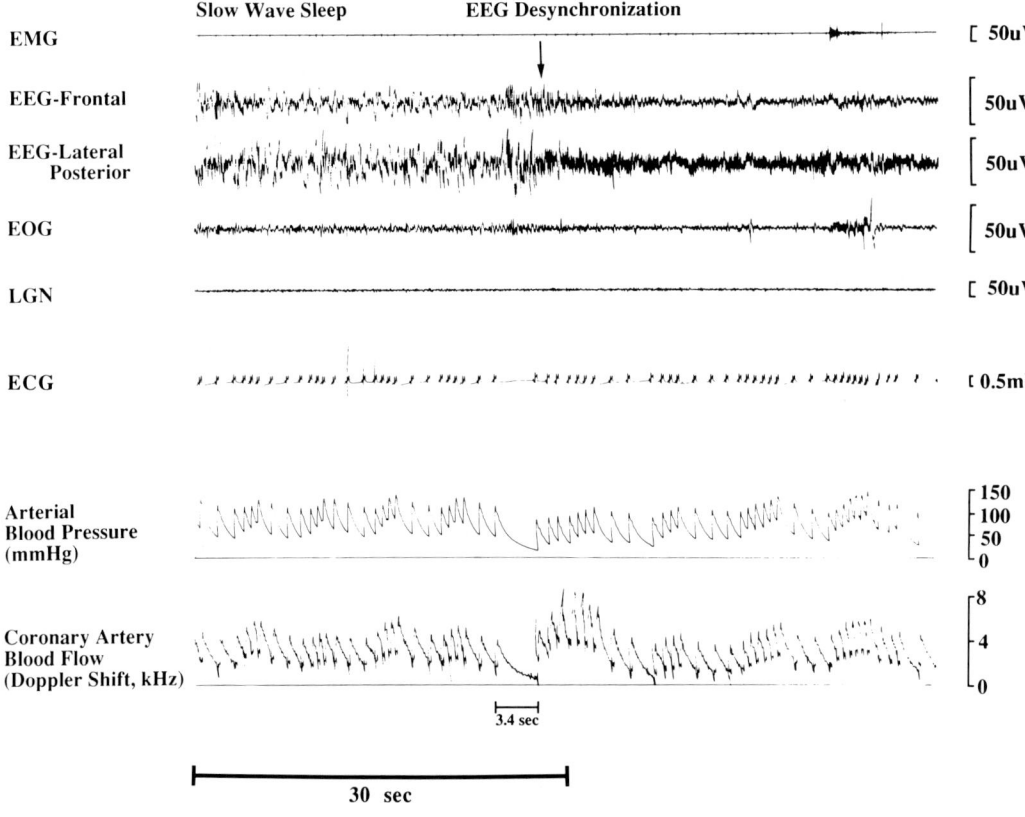

Fig. 25–6. CBF surge during deep SWS interrupted by EEG desynchronization. This response pattern is common and represents a transition to REM sleep. The 3.4-second pause in heart rhythm was followed by a brief increase of 41% in average peak CBF and a decrease of 8% in the HR × SBP product, an indicator of myocardial metabolic demand. EMG, electromyogram; EEG, electroencephalogram; EOG, electro-oculogram; LGN, lateral geniculate nucleus field potential recordings. (Reproduced with permission from Verrier RL, et al.[129])

changes in cycle length are conducive to early and late afterdepolarizations.[75] An intriguing possibility is that in individuals who may be sensitized by proarrhythmic medications, sleep-induced pauses may initiate severe ventricular arrhythmias.

Power Spectrum Analysis of Heart Rate Variability During Sleep

During the past few years, heart rate variability has been analyzed to assess autonomic neural patterning during human sleep.[18,50,76,77] The most commonly employed technique is power spectrum analysis, which identifies interbeat fluctuations by separating the signal into its fundamental frequencies[78] (Cohen in this volume). Accordingly, vagus nerve activity expresses itself as a high-frequency peak (in the 0.4-Hz range in dogs and 0.25-Hz range in humans) coinciding with respiration.[79] Another major peak occurs in a midfrequency bandwidth and represents sympathetic–parasympathetic interactions and baroreceptor responsiveness. A third, low-frequency peak is thought to reflect activity of the renin–angiotensin system and also changes in vasomotor tone associated with thermoregulation.

Zemaityte and coworkers used power spectrum analysis in conjunction with autonomic nervous system blockers such as atropine and propranolol to define autonomic function during sleep in normal human subjects.[77] They found a marked decrease in heart rate and an increase in respiratory sinus arrhythmia during non-REM sleep. The sympathetic input remained relatively constant throughout all stages of sleep except for an initial decrease during drowsy sleep. REM sleep was characterized by irregular fluctuations in autonomic activity on a background of an average increase in heart rate and a decrease in respiratory sinus arrhythmia relative to non-REM sleep. The authors concluded that the periodic structure of the heart rate changes, especially those in respiratory sinus arrhythmia during sleep, is related to the baseline level of autonomic activity during wakefulness. These studies, while informative, should be interpreted with some caution, since both atropine and propranolol cross the blood–brain barrier.

That coronary disease can alter the periodicity of heart rate and blood pressure fluctuations during sleep and dreaming was recognized in the pioneering work of MacWilliams.[80] These early insights have been corroborated and extended in a number of recent studies. Bigger and coworkers compared baroreflex sensitivity and heart period variability after MI during both day and night.[81] They found that baroreflex sensitivity and tonic vagal activity as reflected by heart rate spectral patterns were more greatly reduced in patients with inferior MI than in those with anterior MI. They also observed that baroreceptor sensitivity and the heart period variability were significantly more concordant during the night than during the day. This is consistent with the perception that slow wave sleep has a generally stabilizing effect on heart rhythm and may also enhance the maximal dynamic vagal responsiveness, as indicated by the baroreflex sensitivity test.[82]

Furlan and coworkers[15] raised the intriguing possibility that circadian variations in neural regulation may play a key role in the extensively documented occurrence of early morning cardiovascular mortality.[9,10,11,83] Using spectral analysis, they observed a pronounced and consistent decrease in markers of sympathetic activity and an increase in vagal activity during the night. However, at about 6:00 A.M., patients lying in bed, quietly awake, experienced a progressive rise in spectral indicators of sympathetic activity and a concomitant decrease in markers of vagal tone (Fig. 25–7). The authors proposed that important changes in autonomic function in addition to the putative rise in platelet aggregability[11,13] may contribute to the circadian fluctuations in cardiovascular events, including stroke, MI, and sudden death.[10]

TRACKING NEURALLY INDUCED CARDIAC VULNERABILITY BY ANALYSIS OF T-WAVE ALTERNANS

Renewed interest in this clinically prevalent phenomenon[84–92] has been stimulated by work in several laboratories indicating that computerized analysis of T-wave alternans may provide a quantitative, noninvasive means for assessing susceptibility to

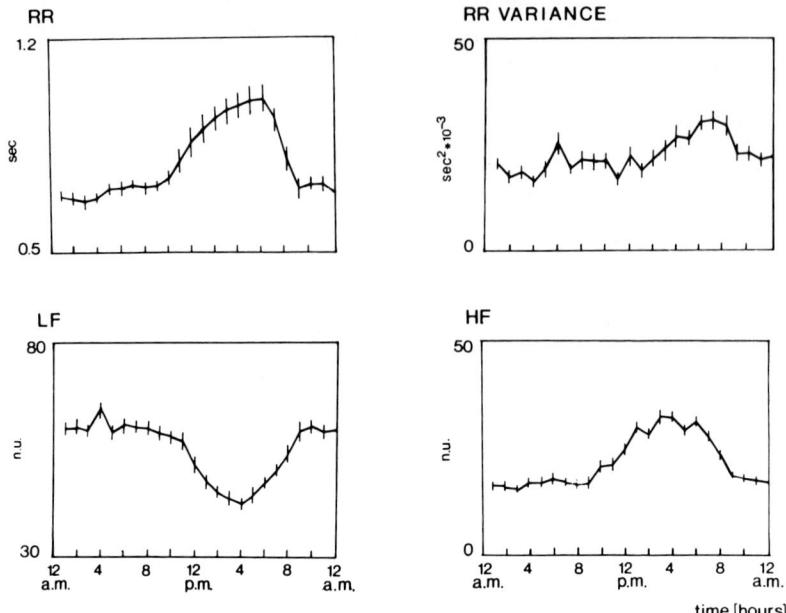

Fig. 25–7. Display of average hourly values of systolic arterial pressure (SAP), its variance, and of low-frequency (LF) and high-frequency (HF) components during 24 hours in a group of 18 ambulatory hospital patients. Note the early morning rise in sympathetic activity, as indicated by the LF component. Concomitantly, there was a progressive decrease in vagus nerve activity, as indicated by the HF component. (Reproduced with permission from Furlan R, et al: Circulation *81*:357, 1990.[15])

VF.[93–97] Adam, Smith and coworkers[93,94] demonstrated a statistically significant correlation between fluctuations in overall T-wave energy and the VF threshold during coronary artery occlusion and hypothermia in dogs. Subsequently a close relationship was shown in humans between the magnitude of T-wave alternans and the inducibility of arrhythmias using programmed electrical stimulation.[97]

Recently we applied the analytical technique of complex demodulation to determine whether the magnitude of T-wave alternans tracks cardiac vulnerability dynamically during both myocardial ischemia and reperfusion.[95] This method was selected because of its adaptability to nonstationary data and because it provides a rapid estimate of physiological events with a time course as brief as 10 seconds.

Left anterior descending (LAD) coronary artery occlusion and reperfusion resulted in marked increases in the magnitude of beat-to-beat alternation in T-wave amplitude (Fig. 25–8). The increase in alternans was manifest within 2–3 minutes of occlusion and progressed until the occlusion was abruptly terminated at 8 minutes (Fig. 25–9). Upon release of the occlusion, there was a rapid increase in alternans that lasted less than 1 minute. A remarkable feature of the alternans pattern was that during reperfusion, the T waves alternated bidirectionally, with waveforms above and below the isoelectric line. It is especially significant that the time course of appearance and disappearance of T-wave alternans during the occlusion/release sequence corresponded precisely with the established time course of the spontaneous emergence of malignant tachyarrhythmias, including VF.[1] The observation that the alternation patterns during occlusion and reperfusion differ is consistent with the well-established concept that differing mechanisms are responsible for ischemia- versus reperfusion-induced arrhythmias.[4,98]

Measuring Sympathetic Nervous System Influences by T-Wave Alternans Analysis

Our studies also demonstrated that the influence of the sympathetic nervous system

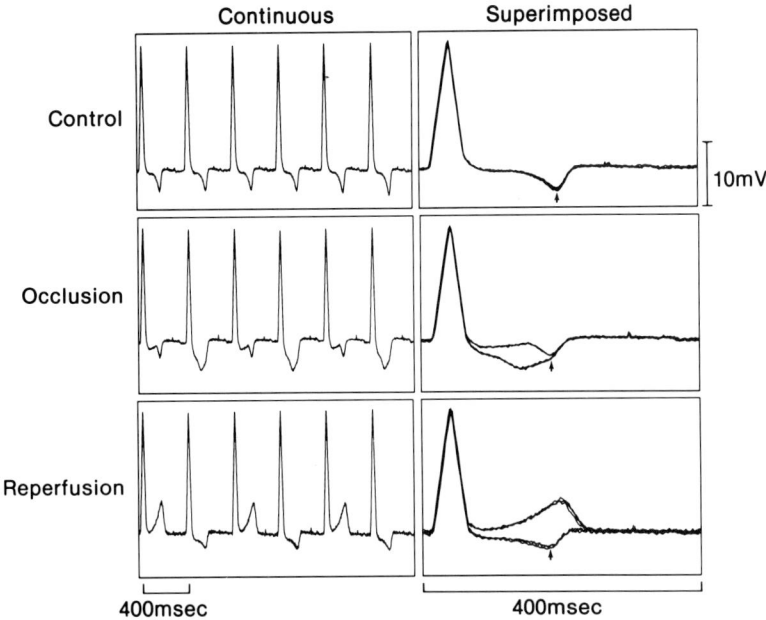

Fig. 25-8. Electrocardiogram recorded within the left ventricle before, during, and after coronary artery occlusion in a single representative animal. Right panels show superimposition of six successive beats. Prior to occlusion (top tracing), the T waves of each succeeding beat are uniform (arrow designates apex of T wave). After 4 minutes of coronary artery occlusion (middle tracing), there is marked alternation of the first half of the T wave, coinciding with the vulnerable period of the cardiac cycle. The second half of the T wave remains uniform. After release of the occlusion (bottom tracing), alternans is bidirectional, with T waves alternately inscribed above and below the isoelectric line. (Reproduced with permission from Nearing BD, et al: Science 252:437, 1991.[95])

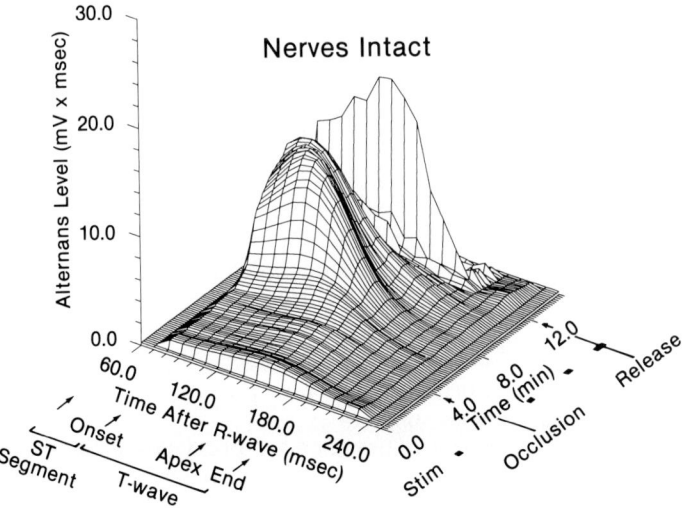

Fig. 25-9. Surface plot display derived by complex demodulation of the T wave of the electrocardiogram before, during, and after coronary artery occlusion in eight dogs with intact cardiac innervation. (Reproduced with permission from Nearing BD, et al: Science 252:437, 1991.[95])

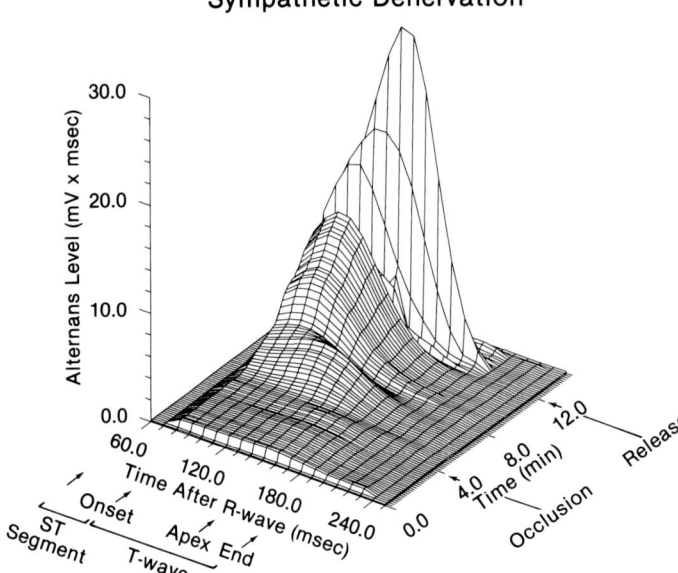

Fig. 25–10. Surface plot display derived by complex demodulation of the T wave of the electrocardiogram before, during, and after coronary artery occlusion after bilateral stellectomy in six dogs. (Reproduced with permission from Nearing BD, et al: Science 252:437, 1991.[95])

on vulnerability in normal and ischemic hearts can be detected with precision. Stellectomy reduced alternans during occlusion with a time course that corresponded to the maximal bursts of neural activity demonstrated in previous studies (Fig. 25–10),[10,87,99] but it did not blunt the reperfusion-induced increase in T-wave alternans. This finding is consistent with the fact that extra-adrenergic factors appear to be decisive during this phase of vulnerability.[4,100,101]

During stellate ganglion stimulation, there was a moderate increase in T-wave alternans before occlusion and a major effect during acute ischemia. These findings are likewise consistent with a number of published reports that indicate that sympathetic activation is highly arrhythmogenic during coronary artery occlusion.[4,87,99] Our recent studies indicate moreover that β-receptor activation appears to be the key factor in sympathetically induced T-wave alternans.[102] Eventually T-wave alternans detection could prove useful in evaluating cardiac electrical stability in patients with the long QT syndrome, wherein major changes in alternans level can be elicited by diverse adrenergic stimuli such as fear and exercise and abolished by antiadrenergic interventions such as β-blockade and stellectomy.[87,88]

Quantifying Parasympathetic Nervous System Influences by T-Wave Alternans Analysis

Vagus nerve stimulation also exerts a significant effect on T-wave alternans in the occlusion–release model.[102] The surge in T-wave alternans that occurs during acute LAD coronary artery occlusion can be markedly suppressed by electrical stimulation of the left vagus nerve. However, vagus nerve excitation did not prevent alternans during reperfusion. These findings concur with reports from several laboratories indicating an important antifibrillatory effect of vagus nerve stimulation during acute myocardial ischemia,[5,103–106] but not during reperfusion, when heart rate was kept constant, as in our study.

The likely basis for these differing effects of vagal stimulation on T-wave alternans during occlusion and reperfusion is that the antifibrillatory influence of this pathway is dependent on accentuated antagonism of adrenergic activity (see Table 25–1). Thus, during coronary occlusion, the profibrillatory surge in sympathetic discharge to the heart is opposed by presynaptic inhibition of the release of catecholamines and by an opposition at the receptor level due to muscarinic stimulation.[8,107] Cyclic nucleotides appear to be responsible for the adrenergic–muscarinic receptor interaction.[8] The failure of vagal stimulation to protect during reperfusion is probably due to the critical role of ischemic by-products rather than to adrenergic factors in reperfusion-induced arrhythmogenesis.[1,105]

Electrophysiological Basis for T-Wave Alternans

It is likely that multiple mechanisms underlie T-wave alternans.[108–110] Therefore, its electrophysiological basis can only be identified in the context of the specific physiological and pathophysiological conditions under which alternans arises. For example, there is strong evidence that T-wave alternans during pericardial tamponade is due to a mechanoelectrical interaction attributable to the swinging action of the heart in the chest.[91] However, in the context of myocardial ischemia and concomitant changes in autonomic tone, the factors are probably far more complex. While it is not possible to discuss all of these mechanisms in detail, we would like to highlight a few concepts that have recurred in the literature.

The first possibility is that alternans represents increased dispersion of repolarization. Smith and Cohen,[111] in their initial article on the subject, proposed that alternation may be due to summation of electrical activity of subpopulations of myocardial cells that generate action potentials only on alternate beats. Our studies also indicate an important link between dispersion of repolarization and alternans, as there is a close temporal correspondence between these two electrophysiological entities.[112]

A second recurring theme is that alternans is due to alteration in action potential morphology of individual cells.[113] Consistent with this suggestion are the observations in a number of laboratories of alternating patterns of action potential morphology.[113–116] Antzelevitch and colleagues have suggested that the appearance and disappearance of the dome portion of the epicardial action potential during simulated ischemia in isolated tissues may account for such alternating T-wave patterns.[114] The activation map studies of Carson and coworkers provide cogent evidence that a change in activation sequence is not the basis for the T-wave alternation phenomenon during myocardial ischemia.[115]

Priori and coworkers have provided evidence that early afterdepolarizations may conduct 2:1 upon reperfusion, and that this pattern may be responsible for the oscillation in T-wave magnitude.[117] This notion is further supported by the work of El-Sherif and coworkers, who reported summation of repolarization activity due to early afterdepolarizatons in animals treated with the inotropic agent anthopleurin A.[118]

Studies by Hashimoto and colleagues[119,120] and ourselves[121] have demonstrated that ionized calcium may represent a final common pathway for ischemia- and reperfusion-induced T-wave alternans. Specifically, it has been shown that calcium channel blockade with either verapamil or diltiazem is capable of preventing alternans during coronary artery occlusion and release–reperfusion. Electrical alternans can be suppressed by this means without concomitant prevention of mechanical alternans. The precise electrophysiological basis whereby ionized calcium can provoke alternans remains to be determined, along with the intracellular compartment from which alternans is elicited.[122]

Finally, the alternation pattern itself provides a compelling suggestion of a prechaotic state, because bifurcative behavior is the hallmark of chaos. Recent studies by Chialvo, Jalife and others indicate that myocardial cells can exhibit chaotic dynamics.[123–126] To establish with certainty that T-wave alternans represents prechaotic behavior requires demonstration of multupling just in advance of fibrillation. Although Ritzenberg and colleagues observed T-wave multupling during infusion of high concentrations of norepinephrine,[127] the progression to lethal arrhythmia remains to be demonstrated. Definitive proof may be elusive because higher order bifurcations represent extremely unstable, transitory states.

SUMMARY

Collectively, the experimental and human studies discussed in this chapter underscore not only the brain's potent influence on the stability of cardiac rhythm but also the astonishing diversity of mechanisms whereby it can exert its arrhythmogenic influence. Notwithstanding this complexity, considerable progress has been made in defining the cardiac receptors involved and the indirect and intermediary hemodynamic factors that predispose to arrhythmias. An important therapeutic corollary is that containment of neurophysiological triggers will require not only intervention at the cardiac adrenergic and muscarinic receptor level, but also at the locus of the coronary circulation and platelets. Finally, recently developed noninvasive methods for spectral analysis of autonomic nervous system activity to the heart and quantification of its influence on cardiac vulnerability by T-wave analysis should prove valuable in the diagnosis and treatment of CNS-triggered arrhythmias.

ACKNOWLEDGMENT

The authors appreciate the editorial contributions of Sandra S. Verrier.

REFERENCES

1. Lown B, Verrier RL: Neural activity and ventricular fibrillation. N Engl J Med 294: 1165–1170, 1976.
2. Verrier RL, Dickerson LW: Autonomic nervous system and coronary blood flow changes related to emotional activation and sleep. Circulation 83(suppl II):II-81, 1991.
3. Schwartz PJ, La Rovere MT, Vanoli E: Autonomic nervous system and sudden cardiac death: Experimental basis and clinical observations for post-myocardial infarction risk stratification. Circulation 85:I-77, 1992.
4. Corr PB, Yamada KA, Witkowski FX: Mechanisms controlling cardiac autonomic function and their relation to arrhythmogenesis. In HA Fozzard, et al (eds): The Heart and Cardiovascular System. New York, Raven, 1986.
5. Zipes DP, Miyazaki T: The autonomic nervous system and the heart: Basis for understanding interactions and effects on arrhythmia development. In DP Zipes, J Jalife (eds): Cardiac Electrophysiology: From Cell to Bedside. Philadelphia, WB Saunders, 1990.
6. Tofler GH, Stone PH, Maclure M, et al: Analysis of possible triggers of acute myocardial infarction (the MILIS study). Am J Cardiol 66:22, 1990.
7. Verrier RL, Carr DB: Stress-specific influences of opioids on cardiac electrical stability. J Cardiovasc Electrophysiol 2(suppl): S124, 1991.
8. Levy MN, Warner MR: Autonomic interactions in cardiac control: Role of neuropeptides. In Zipes DP, Jalife J (eds): Cardiac Electrophysiology: From Cell to Bedside. Philadelphia, WB Saunders, 1990, p 305.
9. Muller JE, Stone PH, Turi ZG, et al: Circadian variation in the frequency of onset of acute myocardial infarction. N Engl J Med 313:1313, 1985.
10. Muller JE, Tofler GH, Stone PH: Circadian variation and triggers of onset of acute cardiovascular disease. Circulation 79:733, 1989.
11. Tofler GH, Brezinski D, Schafer AI, et al: Concurrent morning increase in platelet aggregability and the risk of myocardial infarction and sudden cardiac death. N Engl J Med 316:1514, 1987.
12. Brezinski DA, Tofler GH, Muller JE, et al: Morning increase in platelet aggregability: Association with assumption of the upright posture. Circulation 78:35, 1988.
13. McCall NT, Tofler GH, Schafer AI, Williams GH, Muller JE: The effect of enteric-coated aspirin on the morning increase in platelet activity. Am Heart J 121:382, 1991.
14. Barry J, Campbell S, Yeung AC, et al: Waking and rising at night as a trigger of myocardial ischemia. Am J Cardiol 67: 1067, 1991.
15. Furlan R, Guzzetti S, Crivellar W, et al: Continuous 24-hour assessment of neural regulation of systemic arterial pressure and RR variabilities in ambulant subjects. Circulation 81:537, 1990.
16. Folts JD, Gallagher K, Rowe GG: Blood flow reductions in stenosed canine coronary arteries: Vasospasm or platelet aggregation? Circulation 65:248, 1982.
17. Raeder EA, Verrier RL, Lown B: Influence of the autonomic nervous system on coronary blood flow during partial stenosis. Am Heart J 104:249, 1982.
18. Levy AG: The exciting causes of ventricular fibrillation in animals under chloroform anesthesia. Heart 4:319, 1912.
19. Hockman CH, Mauck HP, Hoff EC: ECG changes resulting from cerebral stimulation: II. A spectrum of ventricular arrhythmias of sympathetic origin. Am Heart J 68: 98, 1966.
20. Cropp GJ, Manning GW: Electrocardiographic changes simulating myocar-

dial ischemia and infarction associated with spontaneous intracranial hemorrhage. Circulation 22:25, 1960.
21. Hugenholtz PG: Electrocardiographic abnormalities in cerebral disorders: Report of six cases and review of the literature. Am Heart J 63:451, 1962.
22. Satinsky J, Kosowsky B, Lown B, et al: Ventricular fibrillation induced by hypothalamic stimulation during coronary occlusion [abstract]. Circulation 44:II-60, 1971.
23. Verrier RL, Calvert A, Lown B, et al: Effect of acute blood pressure elevation on the ventricular fibrillation threshold. Am J Physiol 226:893, 1974.
24. Manning JW, Cotten M de V: Mechanism of cardiac arrhythmias induced by diencephalic stimulation. Am J Physiol 203:1120, 1962.
25. Korteweg GCJ, Boeles TF, Tencate J: Influence of stimulation of some subcortical areas on electrocardiogram. J Neurophysiol 20:100, 1957.
26. Verrier RL, Hagestad EL, Lown B: Delayed myocardial ischemia induced by anger. Circulation 75:249, 1987.
27. Skinner JE, Reed JC: Blockade of frontocortical-brain stem pathway prevents ventricular fibrillation of ischemic heart. Am J Physiol 240:H156, 1981.
28. Carpeggiani C, Landisman C, Montaron M-F, Skinner JE: Cryoblockade in limbic brain (amygdala) prevents or delays ventricular fibrillation after coronary artery occlusion in psychologically stressed pigs. Circ Res 70:600, 1992.
29. Smith OA, DeVito JL: Central neural integration for the control of autonomic responses associated with emotion. Annu Rev Neurosci 7:43, 1984.
30. Gutterman DD, Bonham AC, Arthur JM, et al: Central neural regulation of coronary blood flow. In Buckley JP, Ferrario CM (eds): Brain Peptides and Catecholamines in Cardiovascular Regulation. New York, Raven, 1987, p 125.
31. Jordan D: Autonomic changes in affective behavior. In Loewy AD, Spyer KM (eds): Central Regulation of Autonomic Functions. New York, Oxford University Press, 1990.
32. Cechetto CF, Saper CB: Role of the cerebral cortex in autonomic function. In Loewy AD, Spyer KM (eds): Central Regulation of Autonomic Functions. New York, Oxford University Press, 1990.
33. LeDoux JE: Emotion. In Mountcastle VB, Plum F, Geiger SR (eds): Handbook of Physiology. Vol. 5, part 1. Higher Functions of the Brain. Bethesda, MD, American Physiological Society, 1987.
34. Lown B, Verrier RL, Corbalan R: Psychologic stress and threshold for repetitive ventricular response. Science 182:834, 1973.
35. Skinner JE: Regulation of cardiac vulnerability by the cerebral defense system. J Am Coll Cardiol 5:88B, 1985.
36. Matta RJ, Verrier RL, Lown B: Repetitive extrasystole as an index of vulnerability to ventricular fibrillation. Am J Physiol 230:1469, 1976.
37. Verrier RL, Lown B: Behavioral stress and cardiac arrhythmias. Annu Rev Physiol 46:155–176, 1984.
38. Matta RJ, Lawler JE, Lown B: Ventricular electrical instability in the conscious dog: Effects of psychological stress and beta adrenergic blockade. Am J Cardiol 38:594, 1976.
39. Verrier RL, Lown B: Influence of neural activity on ventricular electrical stability during acute myocardial ischemia and infarction. In Sandoe E, Julian DC, Bell JW (eds): Management of Ventricular Tachycardia: Role of Mexiletine. International Congress Series No. 458. Amsterdam, Excerpta Medica, 1978, p 133.
40. Liang B, Verrier RL, Melman J, et al: Correlation between circulating catecholamine levels and ventricular vulnerability during psychological stress in conscious dogs. Proc Soc Exp Biol Med 161:266, 1979.
41. Verrier RL, Lown B: Vagal tone and ventricular vulnerability during psychological stress [abstract]. Circulation 62:III-176, 1980.
42. Loffelholz K, Muscholl E: Inhibition by parasympathetic nerve stimulation of the release of the adrenergic transmitter. Naunyn Schmiedebergs Arch Pharmacol 267:181, 1970.
43. Revington ML, McCloskey DI: Sympathetic-parasympathetic interactions at the heart, possibly involving neuropeptide Y, in anaesthetized dogs. J Physiol (Lond) 428:359, 1990.
44. Kolman BS, Verrier RL, Lown B: The effect of vagus nerve stimulation upon vulnerability of the canine ventricle: Role of sympathetic-parasympathetic interactions. Circulation 52:578, 1975.
45. Stramba-Badiale M, Vanoli E, DeFerrari GM, et al: Sympathetic-parasympathetic interaction and accentuated antagonism in conscious dogs. Am J Physiol 260:H335–H340, 1991.
46. Vanoli E, De Ferrari GM, Stramba-Badiale M, et al: Vagal stimulation and prevention of sudden death in conscious dogs with a healed myocardial infarction. Circ Res 68:1471, 1991.

47. Deanfield JE, Maseri A, Selwyn AP, et al: Myocardial ischaemia during daily life in patients with stable angina: Its relation to symptoms and heart rate changes. Lancet ii:753–758, 1983.
48. Deanfield JE, Shea M, Kensett M, et al: Silent myocardial ischaemia due to mental stress. Lancet ii:1001–1005, 1984.
49. Rozanski A, Bairey CN, Krantz DS, et al: Mental stress and the induction of silent myocardial ischemia in patients with coronary artery disease. N Engl J Med 318:1005–1012, 1988.
50. Harper RM, Frysinger RC, Zhang J, et al: Cardiac and respiratory interactions maintaining homeostasis during sleep. In Lydic R, Biebuyck JF (eds): Clinical Physiology of Sleep. Bethesda, MD, American Physiological Society, 1988, p 67.
51. Parmeggianni PL, Morrison AR: Alterations in autonomic functions during sleep. In Loewy AD, Spyer KM (eds): Central Regulation of Autonomic Functions. New York, Oxford University Press, 1990.
52. Baust W, Bohnert B: The regulation of heart rate during sleep. Exp Brain Res 7:169, 1969.
53. Smyth HS, Sleight P, Pickering GW: Reflex regulation of arterial pressure during sleep in man. Circ Res 24:109, 1969.
54. Guilleminault C, Connolly SJ, Winkle RA: Cardiac arrhythmia and conduction disturbances during sleep in 400 patients with sleep apnea syndrome. Am J Cardiol 52:490, 1983.
55. Nowlin JB, Troyer WG Jr, Collins WS, et al: The association of nocturnal angina pectoris with dreaming. Ann Intern Med 63:1040, 1965.
56. King MJ, Zir LM, Kaltman AJ, et al: Variant angina associated with angiographically demonstrated coronary artery spasm and REM sleep. Am J Med Sci 265:419, 1973.
57. Murao S, Harumi K, Katayama S, et al: All-night polygraphic studies of nocturnal angina pectoris. Jpn Heart J 13:295, 1972.
58. Quyyumi AA, Wright CA, Mockus LJ, et al: Mechanisms of nocturnal angina pectoris: Importance of increased myocardial oxygen demand in patients with severe coronary artery disease. Lancet i:1207, 1984.
59. Barry J, Selwyn AP, Nabel EG, et al: Frequency of ST-segment depression produced by mental stress in stable angina pectoris from coronary artery disease. Am J Cardiol 61:989, 1988.
60. Campbell S, Barry J, Rebecca GS, et al: Active transient myocardial ischemia during daily life in asymptomatic patients with positive exercise tests and coronary artery disease. Am J Cardiol 57:1010, 1986.
61. Yasue H, Ogawa H, Okumura K: Coronary artery spasm in the genesis of myocardial ischemia. Am J Cardiol 63:29E, 1989.
62. Ludmer PL, Selwyn AP, Shook TL, et al: Paradoxical vasoconstriction induced by acetylcholine in atherosclerotic coronary arteries. N Engl J Med 315:1046, 1986.
63. Maseri A, L'Abbate A, Ballestra AM: Significance of spasm in the pathogenesis of ischemic heart disease. Am J Cardiol 44:788, 1979.
64. Kirby DA, Verrier RL: Differential effects of sleep stage on coronary hemodynamic function. Am J Physiol 256 (Heart Circ Physiol 25):H1378, 1989.
65. Kirby DA, Verrier RL: Differential effects of sleep stage on coronary hemodynamic function during stenosis. Physiol Behav 45:1, 1989.
66. Dickerson LW, Huang AH, Thurnher MM, et al: Relationship between coronary hemodynamic changes and the phasic events of rapid eye movement in sleep in dogs. Sleep, in press, 1993.
67. Verrier RL: Behavioral state and cardiac arrhythmias. In Lydic R, Biebuyck JF (eds): Clinical Physiology of Sleep. Bethesda, MD, American Physiological Society, 1988, p 31.
68. Francis GC, Hagestad EL, Verrier RL: Influence of sleep stage on ventricular refractoriness [abstract]. Physiologist 29:163, 1986.
69. Dickerson LW, Huang AH, Nearing BD, et al: Mechanisms of post-asystole coronary blood flow increase during sleep [abstract]. Soc Neurosci Abst 17:883, 1991.
70. Dickerson LW, Verrier RL: Asystole linked to EEG desynchronization during sleep: Is the initiating event of CNS or cardiovascular origin? [abstract]. Sleep Res 20A:83, 1991.
71. Hung J, Whitford EG, Parsons RW, et al: Association of sleep apnoea with myocardial infarction in men. Lancet 336:261, 1990.
72. De Olazabal JR, Miller MJ, Cook WR, et al: Disordered breathing and hypoxia during sleep in coronary artery disease. Chest 82:548, 1982.
73. Guilleminault CP, Pool P, Motta J, et al: Sinus arrest during REM sleep in young adults. N Engl J Med 311:1006, 1984.
74. Shaw TRD, Corrall RJM, Craib IA: Cardiac and respiratory standstill during sleep. Br Heart J 40:1055, 1978.
75. Rosen MR: The concept of afterdepolarizations. In Rosen MR, Janse MJ, Wit AL

(eds): Cardiac Electrophysiology: A Textbook. Mt. Kisco, NY, Futura, 1990, p 267.
76. Bigger JT, La Rovere MT, Steinman RC, et al: Comparison of baroreflex sensitivity and heart period variability after myocardial infarction. J Am Coll Cardiol *14:*1511, 1989.
77. Zemaityte D, Varoneckas G, Sokolov E: Heart rhythm control during sleep. Psychophysiology *21:*279, 1984.
78. Pagani M, Lombardi F, Guzzetti S, et al: Power spectral analysis of heart rate and arterial pressure variabilities as a marker of sympatho-vagal interaction in man and conscious dog. Circ Res *59:*178, 1986.
79. Akselrod S, Gordon D, Ubel A, et al: Power spectrum analysis of heart rate fluctuation: A quantitative probe of beat-to-beat cardiovascular control. Science *213:* 220, 1981.
80. MacWilliam JA: Blood pressure and heart action in sleep and dreams: Their relation to haemorrhages, angina, and sudden death. Br Med J *22:*1196, 1923.
81. Bigger JT, Kleiger RE, Fleiss JL, et al: Components of heart rate variability measured during healing of acute myocardial infarction. Am J Cardiol *61:*208, 1988.
82. Conway J, Boon N, Jones JV, Sleight P: Involvement of the baroreceptor reflexes in the changes in blood pressure with sleep and mental arousal. Hypertension *5:*746, 1983.
83. Kleiger RE, Miller JP, Bigger JT, et al: Decreased heart rate variability and its association with increased mortality after acute myocardial infarction. Am J Cardiol *59:*256, 1987.
84. Lewis T: Notes upon alternation of the heart. Q J Med *4:*141, 1911.
85. Wellens HJJ: Isolated electrical alternans of the T-wave. Chest *62:*319, 1972.
86. Rozanski JJ, Kleinfeld M: Alternans of the ST segment and T wave: A sign of electrical instability in Prinzmetal's angina. PACE *5:* 359, 1982.
87. Schwartz PJ, Malliani A: Electrical alternation of the T-wave: Clinical and experimental evidence of its relationship with the sympathetic nervous system and with the long Q-T syndrome. Am Heart J *89:*45, 1975.
88. Schwartz PJ: Idiopathic long QT syndrome: Progress and questions. Am Heart J *109:*399, 1985.
89. Belic N, Gardin JM: ECG manifestations of myocardial ischemia. Arch Intern Med *140:*1162, 1980.
90. Raeder EA, Rosenbaum DS, Bhasin R, et al: Alternating morphology of the QRST complex preceding sudden death. N Engl J Med *326:*271, 1992.
91. Goldberger AL, Shabetai R, Bhargava V, et al: Nonlinear dynamics, electrical alternans, and pericardial tamponade. Am Heart J *107:*1297, 1984.
92. Joyal M, Feldman RL, Pepine CJ: ST-segment alternans during percutaneous transluminal coronary angioplasty. Am J Cardiol *54:*915, 1984.
93. Adam DR, Smith JM, Akselrod S, et al: Fluctuations in T-wave morphology and susceptibility to ventricular fibrillation. J Electrocardiol *17:*209, 1984.
94. Smith JM, Clancy EA, Valeri CR, et al: Electrical alternans and cardiac electrical instability. Circulation *77:*110, 1988.
95. Nearing BD, Huang AH, Verrier RL: Dynamic tracking of cardiac vulnerability by complex demodulation of the T wave. Science *252:*437, 1991.
96. Nearing BD, Verrier RL: Personal computer system for tracking cardiac vulnerability by complex demodulation of the T-wave. J Appl Physiol *74:*2606, 1993.
97. Rosenbaum DS, Jackson L, Leigh A, et al: Repolarization alternans: An electrocardiographic marker of arrhythmia vulnerability in man [abstract]. Circulation *84:*II-J, 1991.
98. Janse MJ: Electrical activity immediately following myocardial infarction. In Rosen MR, Janse MJ, Wit AL (eds): Cardiac Electrophysiology: A textbook in Honor of Brian Hoffman. Mt. Kisco, NY, Futura, 1990.
99. Lombardi F, Verrier RL, Lown B: Relationship between sympathetic neural activity, coronary dynamics, and vulnerability to ventricular fibrillation during myocardial ischemia and reperfusion. Am Heart J *105:* 958, 1983.
100. Corbalan R, Verrier RL, Lown B: Differing mechanisms for ventricular vulnerability during coronary artery occlusion and release. Am Heart J *92:*223–230, 1976.
101. Verrier RL, Hagestad EL: Mechanisms involved in reperfusion arrhythmias. Eur Heart J *7(suppl A):*13–22, 1986.
102. Nearing BD, Verrier RL: Evaluation of antifibrillatory interventions by complex demodulation of the T-wave [abstract]. Circulation *84:*II-499, 1991.
103. Kent KM, Smith ER, Redwood DR, et al: Electrical stability of acutely ischemic myocardium: Influences of heart rate and vagal stimulation. Circulation *47:*291, 1973.
104. Kolman BS, Verrier RL, Lown B: The effect of vagus nerve stimulation upon vulnerability of the canine ventricle: Role of sympathetic-parasympathetic interactions. Circulation *52:*578–585, 1975.

105. Verrier RL: Neurogenic aspects of cardiac arrhythmias. In El-Sherif N, Samet P (eds): Cardiac Pacing and Electrophysiology. Philadelphia, WB Saunders, 1991, pp 77.
106. Zuanetti G, De Ferrari GM, Priori SG, et al: Protective effect of vagal stimulation on reperfusion arrhythmias in cats. Circ Res 61:429, 1987.
107. Levy MN, Blattberg B: Effect of vagal stimulation on the overflow of norepinephrine into the coronary sinus during cardiac sympathetic nerve stimulation in the dog. Circ Res 38:81, 1976.
108. Rosenbaum MB, Acunzo RS: Pseudo 2:1 atrioventricular block and T wave alternans in the long QT syndromes. J AM Coll Cardiol 18:1363, 1991.
109. Surawicz B: The pathogenesis and clinical significance of primary T wave abnormalities. In Schlant RC, Hurst JW (eds): Advances in Electrocardiography. New York, Grune & Stratton, 1972, p 377.
110. Sutton PM, Taggart P, Lab M, et al: Alternans of epicardial repolarization as a localized phenomenon in man. Eur Heart J 12:70, 1991.
111. Smith JM, Cohen RJ: Simple finite-element model accounts for wide range of ventricular dysrhythmias. Proc Natl Acad Sci USA 81:233, 1984.
112. Verrier RL, Nearing BD, Huang AH: Method for assessing dispersion of repolarization during acute myocardial ischemia without cardiac electrical testing [abstract]. Circulation 82:III-450, 1990.
113. Kleber AG, Janse MJ, van Capelle FJL, et al: Mechanism and time course of ST and TQ segment changes during acute regional ischemia in the pig heart determined by extracellular and intracellular recordings. Circ Res 42:603, 1978.
114. Antzelevich C, Sicouri S, Litovsky SH, et al: Heterogeneity within the ventricular wall: Electrophysiology and pharmacology of epicardial, endocardial, and M cells. Circ Res 69:1427, 1991.
115. Carson DL, Cardinal R, Savard P, et al: Characterisation of unipolar waveform alternation in acutely ischaemic porcine myocardium. Cardiovasc Res 20:521, 1986.
116. Russell DC, Smith HJ, Oliver MF: Transmembrane potential changes and ventricular fibrillation during repetitive myocardial ischaemia in the dog. Br Heart J 42:88, 1979.
117. Priori SG, Mantica M, Napolitano C, et al: Early afterdepolarizations induced in vivo by reperfusion of ischemic myocardium: A possible mechanism for reperfusion arrhythmias. Circulation 81:1911, 1990.
118. El-Sherif N, Zeiler RH, Craelius W, et al: QTU prolongation and polymorphic ventricular tachyarrhythmias due to bradycardia-dependent early afterdepolarizations: Afterdepolarizations and ventricular arrhythmias. Circ Res 63:286, 1988.
119. Hashimoto H, Suzuki K, Miyake S, et al: Effects of calcium antagonists on the electrical alternans of the ST segment and on associated mechanical alternans during acute coronary occlusion in dogs. Circulation 68:667, 1983.
120. Hashimoto H, Nakashima M: Evidence for a link between mechanical and electrical alternans in acutely ischaemic myocardium of anesthetized dogs. Acta Physiol Scand 141:63, 1991.
121. Nearing BD, Verrier RL: Diltiazem reduces T-wave alternation and vulnerability to fibrillation during both coronary artery occlusion and reperfusion [abstract]. J Am Coll Cardiol 19:346A.
122. Saitoh H, Bailey JC, Surawicz B: Action potential duration alternans in dog Purkinje and ventricular muscle fibers: Further evidence in support of two different mechanisms. Circulation 80:1421, 1989.
123. Chialvo DR, Jalife J: Non-linear dynamics of cardiac excitation and impulse propagation. Nature 330:749, 1987.
124. Chialvo DR, Michaels DC, Jalife J: Supernormal excitability as a mechanism of chaotic dynamics of activation in cardiac Purkinje fibers. Circ Res 66:525, 1990.
125. Smith JM, Kaplan DT, Cohen RJ: The physics of reentry and fibrillation. In Zipes DP, Jalife J (eds): Cardiac Electrophysiology: From Cell to Bedside. Philadelphia, WB Saunders, 1990.
126. Guevara MR, Glass L, Shrier A: Phase locking, period doubling bifurcations, and irregular dynamics. Science 214:1350, 1981.
127. Ritzenberg A, Adam DR, Cohen RJ: Period multupling: evidence for nonlinear behaviour of the canine heart. Nature 307:159, 1984.
128. Verrier RL: Autonomic control of cardiac arrhythmias. In Singh BN, Wellens HJJ, Hiraoka M (eds): Electropharmacologic Control of Cardiac Arrhythmias: To Delay Conduction or to Prolong Refractoriness? Mt. Kisco, NY, Futura [in press].
129. Verrier RL, Dickerson LW: Central nervous system and behavioral factors in vagal control of cardiac arrhythmogenesis. In Levy MN, Schwartz PJ: Vagal Control of the Heart, Mt. Kisco, Futura, in press.

# 26

Role of Electrical Triggers in the Causation of Sudden Cardiac Death

MASOOD AKHTAR
MOHAMMAD R. JAZAYERI
JASBIR S. SRA
ANWER A. DHALA
SANJAY S. DESHPANDE
IMRAN NIAZI

The two main causes of cardiovascular mortality are pump failure and cardiac arrhythmias. In the overall cardiovascular mortality figures, arrhythmic and nonarrhythmic causes account for approximately the same number of deaths. However, in certain subsets of patients, arrhythmic mortality is more common. Some clinical scenarios where this is likely are outlined below.

1. Patients with a prior history of sustained ventricular tachycardia (VT), survivors of ventricular fibrillation (VF), and patients with VT-related syncope have a higher propensity toward arrhythmic death.[1-5]

2. Patients with cardiovascular disease who are in New York Heart Association functional Class I or II seldom die of pump failure.[1] Even though the overall cardiac mortality in this group is low, it is likely to be arrhythmic in nature. Survival into a worse functional class, i.e., Class III and IV, selects patients more prone to pump failure, since advancement to Class III and IV is not likely if cardiac arrest occurs at an earlier stage. Similarly, in patients with a low left ventricular ejection fraction (LVEF) but no history of congestive heart failure or cardiac decompensation, the mode of cardiovascular death is generally arrhythmic.

The arrhythmic and nonarrhythmic forms of cardiac death often present very differently. Arrhythmic deaths in general tend to be instantaneous, and death ensues within minutes after the collapse. Death from pump failure, on the other hand, tends to occur over several hours and days. Occasionally, however, an arrhythmic death may not be instantaneous, and pump-related mortality could be sudden.

Among the arrhythmic causes of cardiovascular mortality, VT and VF are the most common. In fact, when the onset of sudden cardiac death (SCD) is documented during monitoring, VT and VF account for the majority.[6,7] Several factors have been implicated to explain this sudden appearance of a fatal arrhythmic event in an otherwise stable individual. One reason is the abrupt emergence of the so-called electrical triggers. This chapter considers several of these electrical triggers. Because ventricular tachyarrhythmias are the more common precipitating events for SCD, they are addressed first.

VENTRICULAR TACHYCARDIA–VENTRICULAR FIBRILLATION

Even though VF is documented in the majority of SCD victims when the rescue squad arrives, the initial event is often VT, which may be monomorphic or polymorphic.[8,9] Either variety can degenerate into VF after a variable amount of time. Transition to VF from VT may be related to many factors, including a change in myocardial substrate due to hemodynamic deterioration, superimposed myocardial ischemia, or acceleration of the VT rate.[10-12] Additional factors include extensive myocardial fibrosis, hypertrophy, dilation, wall motion abnormalities, and intracavitary pressure alterations.[10,13] Because VT is the initial event, the triggers for VT will be the main subject of this report.

MONOMORPHIC VENTRICULAR TACHYCARDIA

Sustained monomorphic VT can occur in the absence of overt cardiovascular abnormality but is typically seen in patients with structural heart disease.[9] Although acute myocardial changes can produce the same type of arrhythmia, a chronic myocardial substrate is the usual setting. The most extensively studied animal model of VT in association with myocardial scarring is the result of coronary artery occlusion: The resultant fibrosis creates anatomical obstacles that facilitate re-entrant excitation. Propagating impulses, when they encounter areas of block and slow conduction from anisotropy or other factors, can initiate the re-entrant process.[14] If the tissue ahead has recovered excitability, continuation of the process will lead to sustained arrhythmia. A variety of acute triggers such as ischemia, electrolyte abnormalities, and neurohumoral factors (see Chaps. 4, 6, and 20 through 25), can create the environment for VT initiation. There are, however, specific electrophysiological mechanisms that can trigger VT without any of these factors. They are called here electrical triggers.

Role of Premature Beats

Because VT can often be induced in the laboratory with the introduction of premature beats, it is often assumed that clinical episodes have that same basis.[15-17] However, we have analyzed the initiation of spontaneous monomorphic VT with the use of multiple simultaneous surface ECG leads and have reached different conclusions.[18] Observations were made in 25 consecutive patients in whom spontaneous initiation of sustained monomorphic VT was recorded and in whom the same VT was also induced in the laboratory. In only three patients (group A) did the initial beat have a different QRS morphology than subsequent beats, and it is conceivable that a randomly occurring premature ventricular complex initiated re-entry (Fig. 26-1) in a circuit remote from the origin of the premature beat. In the remaining 22 (78%) patients (group B), the first and subsequent QRS complexes of spontaneous VT were identical (Fig. 26-2), suggesting a similar origin for all such complexes. Furthermore, the interval between the first beat (C_1) and the second beat (C_2) was much longer in group A than in group B (see Fig. 26-1 and 26-2), also suggesting different modes for VT initiation in the two groups.

In most cases, therefore, these re-entrant VTs arose without obvious initiating premature beats. Since, in all of the cases in our series, the same VT could also be induced in the laboratory, the underlying mechanism is likely to be re-entrant excitation related to existing re-entrant circuits.[16,18] Although the initiation of VT in group A is in line with conventional thinking, how can one explain the initiation of VT in group B cases without the presence of a prior premature beat?

Repetitive Concealed Re-entry

We propose the following hypothesis to explain these results in group B cases. It is our view that during sinus rhythm or any predominant rhythm, the re-entrant circuits are penetrated. Variable penetration of the circuit with slow, anisotropic, and inhomogeneous conduction creates the appropriate milieu for the start of the re-entrant process. However, several factors may not permit the emergence of these re-entrant impulses, including depolarization of the re-entrant circuit boundaries, keeping the impulse exit areas refractory (Fig. 26-3). Depending on the heart rate, intracavitary pressure, autonomic changes, and possibly other factors, the impulses in the re-entrant circuit may also fail to propagate (Fig. 26-3). This form of concealed and abortive re-entry in all probability is the rule following each spon-

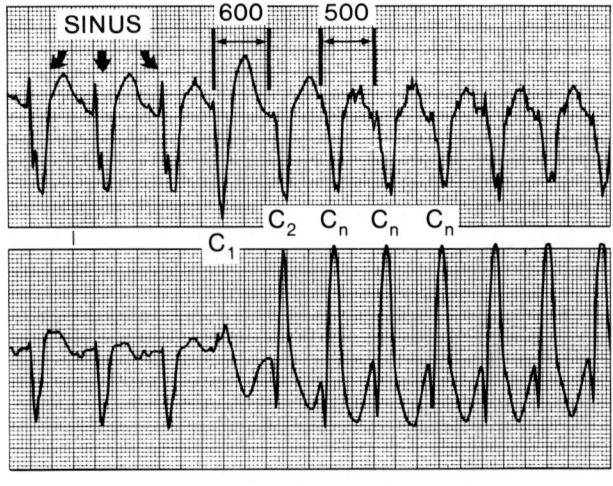

- **First VT complex morphologically distinct from succeeding complexes.**

- **Interval between first and second complexes ($C_1 - C_2$) considerably > VT - CL.**

Fig. 26–1. Spontaneous initiation of sustained monomorphic ventricular tachycardia (MMVT) (group A). Two surface ECG leads are shown (from top to bottom, leads II and V_1). Left bundle-branch block can be appreciated during the first three beats of sinus origin. The fourth complex, labeled C_1, is the first beat of ventricular origin and is followed by MMVT with a cycle length (CL) of 500 msec. Note the distinct difference between the morphology of C_1 and all subsequent beats (labeled C_2, C_n, etc.). Furthermore, the C_1–C_2 interval is 100 msec longer than the CL of VT. PVC, Premature ventricular complex.

taneous beat in patients prone to VT. The existence of such concealed impulses is supported by the observation that, with amplification, one can record continued electrical activity even beyond the completion of ventricular activation on the surface ECG. In fact, it is quite likely that the electrical waveforms recorded on the signal-averaged ECG (abnormal late potentials) represent such abortive concealed re-entrant excitation.[19]

The emergence of the re-entrant impulse at any of the exit points will result in a single QRS that can be interpreted as an isolated premature beat (Fig. 26–3). The continuation of that process will result in two consecutive complexes, nonsustained or sustained VT, all complexes having an identical morphology (Fig. 26–3).

The reason for the change from concealed or abortive process to manifest sustained re-entry could be related to a variety of factors

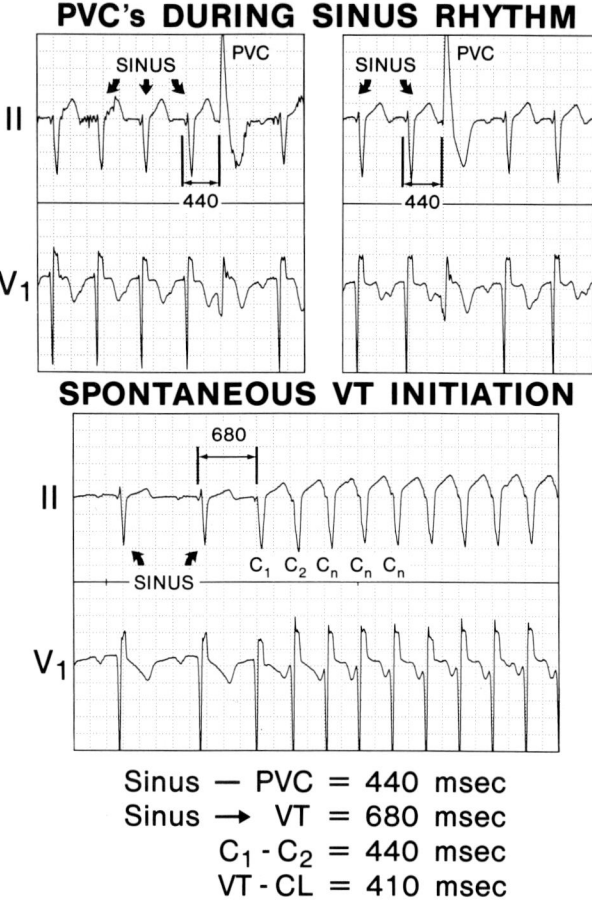

Fig. 26–2. Spontaneous onset of MMVT (group B). The bottom panel shows the spontaneous initiation following two sinus cycles. Note that all complexes of ventricular origin (C_1, C_2, C_n, etc.) have the same QRS morphology. The coupling interval between the last sinus beat and the first of ventricular origin (C_1) is 680 msec, considerably longer than random unifocal PVCs in this patient, shown in the top two panels. It is important to appreciate that these closer coupled PVCs (top panels) did not initiate the VT. Also, there is a relatively small difference in the CL between C_1–C_2 and VT compared to group A (see Fig. 26–1).

and could vary even in the same patient. These reasons include (1) an increased conduction slowing in the circuit, allowing recovery at the area of the previous block during the abortive process, and (2) lesser penetration of the circuit boundaries and exit points during prior sinus or other rhythm, allowing an easier exit for re-entrant impulses. Clearly, changes in heart rate, autonomic tone, and pharmacological and other factors could greatly influence such conduction characteristics of not only the re-entrant circuit but also the circuit boundaries. Interplay of such electrophysiological factors may well be responsible for the emergence of incessant VT in patients with monomorphic VT after antiarrhythmic drugs.[20] It is noteworthy that QRS morphology during such incessant forms of VT is generally similar to the VT seen in patients under treatment. Conceivably, concealed and abortive re-entry, manifest re-entry,

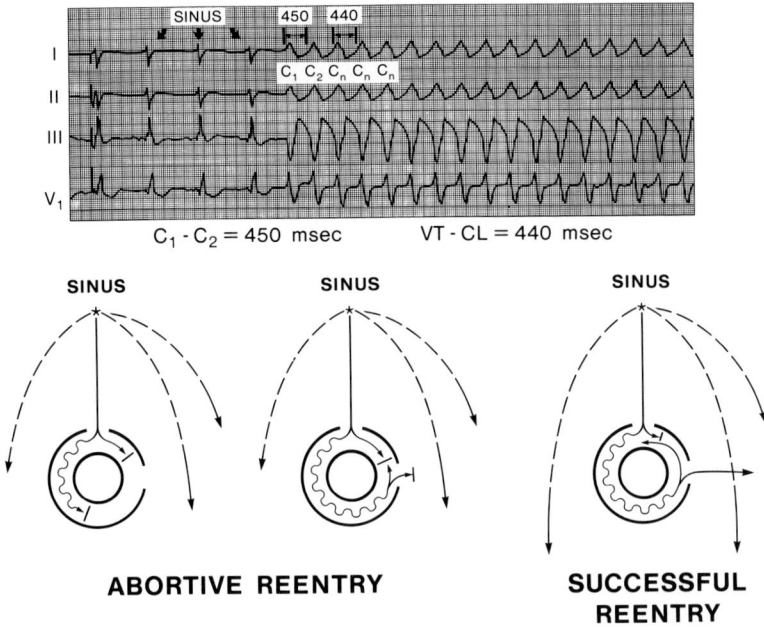

Fig. 26–3. Mechanism of VT initiation in group B. The onset of VT is depicted on the ECG leads in the top panel. The bottom panel provides a simplified visual concept of abortive re-entry in the two left-hand examples. The extreme bottom-left example shows the failure of impulse propagation to the point of exit, while the middle example displays failure at the exit points due to increased refractoriness at the boundary. The right-hand schema shows successful propagation to produce the first complex (C_1). Continuation of the process will depend on the ability of the re-entrant impulse to successfully propagate repeatedly through the re-entrant circuit.

sustained VT, and incessant VT of the same morphology represent different manifestations of the same underlying process.

The following argument supports the concept that random ventricular premature beats seldom start clinical VT.

1. The morphology of the first and subsequent beats of VT is identical, suggesting the same origin (Figs. 26–2 and 26–3). It is illogical to think that the first and subsequent beats with an identical QRS morphology have two different mechanisms, and that the first beat causes the subsequent beats. A better explanation for this observation is that the first and all subsequent beats with identical QRS morphologies have the same origin and mechanism. Such an occurrence is expected if the arrhythmic mechanism is automaticity rather than re-entry. However, in group B cases the mechanism was re-entry, and the sequence at VT initiation can be explained as follows: The first beat represents the first successful emergence of this otherwise concealed re-entry to the adjoining ventricular myocardium, and subsequent beats reflect continuation of the same process.

2. As shown in Figure 26–2, random ventricular premature beats occurring at closer coupling intervals failed to initiate VT in group B cases.

3. Antiarrhythmic drugs that are highly effective in controlling spontaneous ventricular ectopic beats can cause incessant VT with the same QRS morphology as the VT under treatment. This is particularly true of drugs known to prolong conduction such as flecainide and encainide.[21] Suppression of one aspect (ectopy) and worsening of the other (sustained to incessant) suggests the

two respond differently to these drugs. If premature beats were the triggers for sustained VT, the control should lead to VT suppression and not aggravation.

The above description applies to monomorphic VT in association with chronic coronary artery disease, particularly in the background of healed myocardial infarction or any other type of fibrosis. Monomorphic VT is not infrequent in patients with idiopathic dilated cardiomyopathy as well. VT in this substrate may be indistinguishable from VT patients with chronic coronary artery disease. This is indeed the case in 60% of the patients with idiopathic dilated cardiomyopathy who have monomorphic VT. In the remaining 40%, however, a different type of VT is seen.[22,23] The underlying mechanism is bundle-branch re-entry, where both of the bundle branches and the bundle of His form the re-entrant circuit. In this situation as well, ventricular premature beats seldom initiate the clinical VT, and concealed abortive re-entry is common with eventual manifestation as sustained clinical monomorphic VT (Fig. 26–4).

Aside from the above two substrates, there are other clinical scenarios where a sustained form of monomorphic VT is observed. These include hypertrophic cardiomyopathy and valvular heart disease. The amount of data available regarding these substrates is too limited to comment on the mechanism of VT, but it could be similar to the coronary artery disease population if sufficient conduction slowing is created as a result of fibrosis, anisotropy, or other factors.

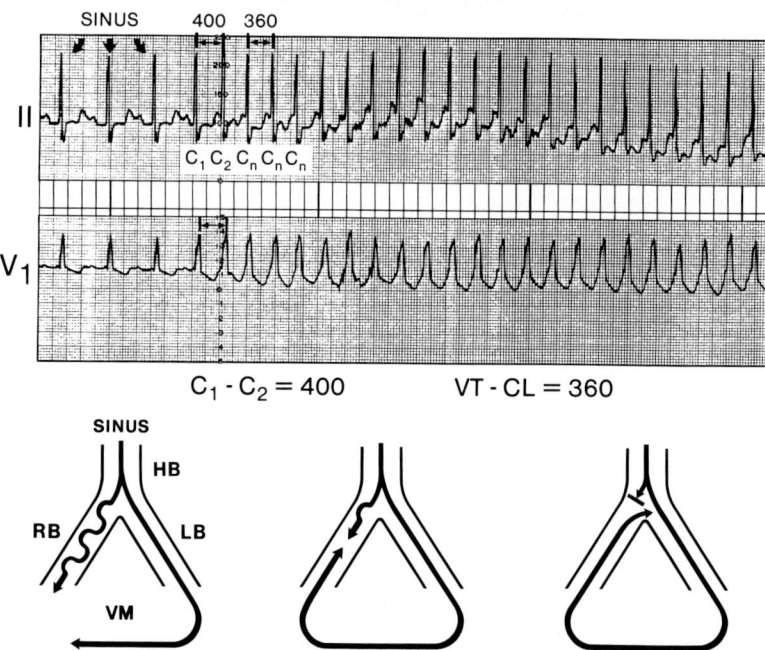

Fig. 26–4. Spontaneous onset of sustained macrore-entrant VT due to bundle-branch re-entry (BBR). The first three beats are of sinus origin, and conduction delay in the right bundle branch (RBB) can be noted. Progressively deeper retrograde penetration of the RB during sinus impulses allows the onset of re-entry without preceding the premature beat. The coupling interval between the sinus beat and the first beat of ventricular origin is 600 msec, too long to initiate BBR on the basis of prematurity alone. A wider QRS during VT is due to lesser His-Purkinje (HP) contribution to ventricular activation, a finding relatively common in patients with BBR as a result of disease in the HP system. The true nature of VT, i.e., bundle-branch re-entry, was documented during electrophysiological evaluation. RB, right bundle; HB, His bundle; LB, left bundle; VM, ventricular myocardium.

POLYMORPHIC VT

Polymorphic VT is generally a highly unstable arrhythmia that usually either spontaneously terminates or degenerates to VF.[6,11,24] Prolonged episodes of polymorphic VT can cause near syncope, syncope, or cardiac arrest. In the clinical setting at least two forms can be identified: (1) polymorphic VT in association with prolonged QT interval (torsade de pointes), and (2) polymorphic VT with a normal QT interval. These are covered in greater detail in Chapter 14, 20, and 21, but some salient aspects relevant to this discussion will be presented.

Polymorphic VT in Association with Prolonged QT Interval

Often referred to as torsade de pointes, this phenomenon is a rapid polymorphic VT that can occur on a congenital basis but can also be seen in an acquired form under certain clinical situations.[9,25] Although it is not entirely certain, the underlying electrophysiological mechanism in both settings may be the emergence of early afterdepolarizations. In the congenital form, adrenergic stimulation seems to trigger the episodes of torsade de pointes. The acquired form of torsade de pointes is seen with electrolyte abnormalities, hypokalemia, hypomagnesemia, antiarrhythmic drugs (i.e., all Class Ia and III antiarrhythmic agents), antidepressants, and several other groups of drugs.

Although seldom initiated by ventricular premature beats, torsade de pointes can be triggered by subsequent pauses. The presence of bradycardia related to sinus node dysfunction or AV block could facilitate the occurrence of torsade de pointes, and the presence of electrolyte abnormalities and the addition of drugs could enhance this possibility. Several clinical scenarios can emerge as a consequence of such interaction.

1. Torsade de pointes can occur at any time, even when there has been no apparent change in medical therapy. As an example, a patient on a stable quinidine dose could develop bradycardia for a variety of reasons, with the emergence of torsade de pointes. Similarly, the addition of other ordinarily innocuous interventions such as diuretics or antihistamines could precipitate torsade de pointes. These aspects should be kept in mind when the trigger for polymorphic VT is not readily apparent.

2. Initial bradycardia could lead to cardiac arrest on the basis of torsade de pointes and not necessarily due to bradycardia. The latter per se is seldom the cause of SCD.

3. The reproduction of torsade de pointes in the laboratory is rarely possible with a conventional stimulation protocol using a series of extrastimuli. A likely method for triggering torsade de pointes in the laboratory should include creation of pauses and adrenergic stimulation such as epinephrine, particularly in the congenital variety.

It is unclear whether the acquired form of the prolonged QT-interval syndrome represents a forme fruste of the congenital counterpart or is a completely different entity. It is conceivable that the acquired type is a more subtle form of the same basic electrophysiological, neurohumoral abnormality that can be unmasked by events that ordinarily result in the prolongation of myocardial recovery. In vulnerable individuals, therefore, the QT prolongation may also be associated with the development of early afterdepolarizations.[25] It should be emphasized that prolongation of the QT interval and development of early afterdepolarization (and hence torsade de pointes) do not necessarily represent a cause-and-effect relationship. This can be appreciated by the fact that amiodarone, a Class III antiarrhythmic drug that invariably prolongs the QT interval (at times to a marked degree), is infrequently associated with torsade de pointes.

The overall prevalence of torsade de pointes–related SCD is not known, but in one communication it was observed in 13% of SCD victims. These observations suggest that torsade de pointes as a trigger for SCD is important. An awareness of this fact alone could help reduce the incidence of arrhythmic death secondary to torsade de pointes, clearly a treatable form of arrhythmia at the present time.

Polymorphic VT in Association with Normal QT Interval

When polymorphic VT is observed in the setting of a normal QT interval, the possibility of underlying acute ischemia must be excluded. The typical clinical picture of ischemia—that is, chest pain, ST- and T-wave changes on the ECG—may not be apparent. Furthermore, when cardiac catheterization is performed, fixed lesions may also not be present, and coronary artery spasm must be entertained as an underlying possibility. This form of VT is highly malignant and is usually lethal if not quickly managed. It is not encountered frequently in clinical practice because out-of-hospital episodes are likely to be fatal. The underlying mechanism is uncertain but could be re-entry in the environment of slow conduction created by acute ischemia. VT cannot be induced in the laboratory in these patients when acute ischemia is not present. Provocation of the ischemia may be necessary to prove the exact nature, particularly in those with no critical lesions in the coronary arteries.[11] When observed in the inpatient setting, immediate cardiac catheterization with or without ergonovine and revascularization should be considered.[24] In the interim, intensive anti-ischemia drug therapy may be necessary to stabilize the patient.

Once torsade de pointes and acute ischemia have been excluded as causes, polymorphic VT is likely to be related to underlying myocardial substrate damaged acutely or harboring hypertrophy or chronic fibrosis.[9] The associated myocardial disease could vary; it might be coronary disease, hypertrophic or dilated cardiomyopathy, and so on. The underlying mechanism is likely to be re-entry initiated either by single or by multiple premature beats, or a manifestation of continuous concealed re-entry. Nonetheless, these arrhythmias can often be induced in the laboratory, suggesting the presence of a myocardial substrate.

SUPRAVENTRICULAR TACHYCARDIA

These arrhythmias, which may arise in the atria or the AV junction, seldom produce cardiac arrest. However, in specific situations SVT might result in a fatal outcome. These are outlined below.

1. *Wolff-Parkinson-White syndrome.* The life-threatening arrhythmia in these patients is atrial flutter–fibrillation. If the refractory period of the accessory pathway is short, ≤250 msec, rapid ventricular response could lead to hemodynamic collapse. Ventricular fibrillation may follow due to rapid consecutive ventricular impulses or secondary to metabolic deterioration of the myocardium. This is one type of electrical cardiovascular mortality encountered in patients with an otherwise structurally normal heart. This topic is discussed in greater detail elsewhere in this book.

2. In patients with *poor cardiovascular status, low LVEF, congestive heart failure, or angina*, rapid ventricular rate in any type of SVT could lead to hemodynamic collapse and precipitate VT/VF. Even though the final event in this situation would be ventricular tachyarrhythmia, the initial trigger is SVT.

BRADYCARDIA AND ASYSTOLE

Although bradycardia in the form of sinus node dysfunction and AV block can produce syncope and cardiac arrest, SCD due to bradycardia per se is not common. When bradycardia/asystole is seen in victims of SCD it is seldom either the precipitating event or the actual cause. This statement can be supported by the following observations: (1) SCD in association with bradycardia/asystole can rarely be salvaged with cardiac pacing.[26] This has been observed during resuscitation efforts where the survival of patients found in bradycardia/asystole is less than 1%, indicating that bradycardia/asystole is the terminal event and not the cause of collapse. (2) Hemodynamic monitoring is seldom available to show that in most of these, hemodynamic collapse precedes the bradycardia/asystole and the latter represents the end result, not the cause of the collapse.

Nonetheless, severe bradycardia/asystole can lead to torsade de pointes and consequently SCD. Therefore, the treatment of severe bradycardia is an important consideration when it is present. Not uncommonly, both bradycardia and VT/VF may need to be addressed in the same patient. The role of bradycardia in SCD is covered in greater detail elsewhere in this book.

REFERENCES

1. Akhtar M, et al: Implantable cardioverter defibrillator therapy for prevention of sud-

1. den cardiac death. In Crawford MH (ed): Cardiac Arrhythmia and Related Syndromes. Cardiol Clin 11:97, 1993.
2. Fogoros RN: The effect of the implantable cardioverter defibrillator on sudden death and on total survival. PACE 16(II):506, 1993.
3. Deshpande S, et al: Is implantable cardioverter defibrillator intervention truly lifesaving in patients receiving such therapy? [abstract]. J Am Coll Cardiol 19(3):208A, 1992.
4. Akhtar M, et al: Implantable cardioverter defibrillator for prevention of sudden cardiac death in patients with ventricular tachycardia and ventricular fibrillation: ICD therapy in sudden cardiac death. PACE 16(II):511, 1993.
5. ESVEM Investigators: Incidence of drug efficacy predictions in the Electrophysiologic Study Versus Electrocardiographic Monitoring Trial (ESVEM) [abstract]. J Am Coll Cardiol 19(3):387A, 1992.
6. Bardy GH, Olson WH: Clinical characteristics of spontaneous-onset sustained ventricular fibrillation in survivors of cardiac arrest. In Zipes DP, Jaliff J (eds): Cardiac Electrophysiology: From Cell to Beside. Philadelphia, WB Saunders, 1990, p 778.
7. deLuna AB, Coumel P, Leclercq JF: Ambulatory sudden cardiac death: Mechanisms of production of fatal arrhythmia on the basis of data from 157 cases. Am Heart J 117:151, 1989.
8. Akhtar M, Garan H, Lehmann H, Troup PJ: Sudden cardiac death: Management of high risk patients. Ann Intern Med 114:499, 1991.
9. Akhtar M: Clinical spectrum of ventricular tachycardia. Circulation 82:1561, 1990.
10. Packer M: Sudden unexpected death in patients with congestive heart failure: A second frontier. Circulation 72:681, 1985.
11. Myerburg RJ, et al: Life-threatening ventricular arrhythmias in patients with silent myocardial ischemia due to coronary artery spasm. N Engl J Med 362(22):1451, 1992.
12. Garan H, McComb JM, Ruskin JN: Spontaneous and electrically induced ventricular arrhythmias during acute ischemia superimposed on 2-week old canine myocardial infarction. J Am Coll Cardiol 11:603, 1988.
13. Messerli FH, et al: Hypertension and sudden death: Increased ventricular ectopic activity in left ventricular hypertrophy. Am J Med 77:18, 1884.
14. Wit AL, et al: Electrophysiologic mapping to determine the mechanism of experimental ventricular tachycardia initiated by premature impulses. Am J Cardiol 49:166, 1982.
15. Myerburg RJ, Kessler KM, Castellanos A: Sudden cardiac death: Structure, function, and time-dependence of risk. Circulation 85: I-2, 1992.
16. Berger MD, et al: Spontaneous compared with induced onset of sustained ventricular tachycardia. Circulation 78:885, 1988.
17. Meissner MD, Akhtar M, Lehmann MH: Nonischemic sudden tachyarrhythmic death in atherosclerotic heart disease. Circulation 84:905, 1991.
18. Niazi I, et al: New insights into initiating mechanisms of clinical ventricular tachycardia [abstract]. Circulation 78(suppl II):II-71, 1988.
19. Borbola J, Ezri MD, Denes P: Correlation between the signal-averaged electrocardiogram and electrophysiologic study findings in patients with coronary artery disease and sustained ventricular tachycardia. Am Heart J 115:816, 1988.
20. Winkle RA, Mason JW, Griffin JC, Ross D: Malignant ventricular tachyarrhythmias associated with use of encainide. Am Heart J 102:857, 1981.
21. The Cardiac Arrhythmia Suppression Trial (CAST) Investigators: Preliminary report: Effect of encainide and flecainide on mortality in a randomized trial of arrhythmia suppression after myocardial infarction. N Engl J Med 321:406, 1989.
22. Caceres J, et al: Sustained bundle branch reentry as a mechanism of clinical tachycardia. Circulation 79:256, 1989.
23. Blanck Z, et al: Bundle branch reentrant ventricular tachycardia: Cumulative experience in 48 patients. J Cardiovasc Electrophysiol [in press].
24. Tchou P, et al: Etiology of QT [abstract]. J Am Coll Cardiol 13:21A, 1989.
25. Jackman WM, et al: The long QT syndromes: A critical review, new clinical observations and a unifying hypothesis. Prog Cardiovasc Dis 31:115, 1988.
26. Luu M et al: Diverse mechanisms of unexpected cardiac arrest in advanced heart failure. Circulation 80:1675, 1989.

27

Pharmacological Triggers of Sudden Death: Lethal Proarrhythmia

RALPH LAZZARA

Proarrhythmia is the induction, facilitation, or exacerbation of arrhythmias. In common usage in relation to pharmacological agents the term implies that the promotion of arrhythmias occurs within ranges of doses and concentrations that are not greatly in excess of those considered usual and therapeutic. Also, the term is most commonly used in relation to a paradoxical effect of agents that are utilized frequently or exclusively for therapeutic actions that are antiarrhythmic. Proarrhythmia can appear as bradyarrhythmias or tachyarrhythmias, benign or malignant. This chapter is primarily concerned with the induction of life-endangering tachyarrhythmias by pharmacological agents.

Myriad agents with diverse actions are implicated in the induction of tachyarrhythmias. Even drugs without significant direct cardiac electrophysiological effects can have very important indirect proarrhythmic actions, such as drug interactions that influence the concentrations of electrophysiologically active agents, changes in concentrations of electrolytes, negative inotropism, changes in blood pressure, changes in coronary flow, influences on endothelial functions and coagulation, and so on. The growing interest in proarrhythmia in the past decade centered on the proarrhythmic actions of those agents with potent electrophysiological actions that warrant their therapeutic use and classification as antiarrhythmic agents.

The recognition that antiarrhythmic agents can paradoxically cause arrhythmias followed soon after the introduction of the prototype antiarrhythmic agent, quinidine, in 1918.[1,2] In the case of cardiac glycosides, recognition of their proarrhythmic actions antedated the appreciation of their value as antiarrhythmic agents. The potential for serious bradyarrhythmia was recognized by Withering,[3] and drug-induced tachyarrhythmias were recognized long before the antiarrhythmic efficacy of cardiac glycosides for various supraventricular arrhythmias was appreciated in the early years of this century.

After a few years of experience with quinidine, sudden death and ventricular tachycardia (VT) and fibrillation (VF) were reported as complications of therapy.[2,4] With the earliest observations of proarrhythmia there was an appreciation that this adverse consequence need not ensue from obvious overdose, but that special conditions might predispose to proarrhythmia. Thus, in the original report of "paroxysmal ventricular fibrillation" attributed to quinidine by Kerr and Bender,[2] the authors stated, "The observations in our case indicate that the unfavorable action of the drug does not always depend on the precise dosage." This concept was emphasized by Selzer and Wray[5] in their report, which concluded that "paroxysmal ventricular fibrillation" (ventricular tachycardia) was the basis for syncope and sudden death due to quinidine.

Kerr and Bender also expressed bemusement at the paradox of proarrhythmia caused by antiarrhythmic agents: "Although this action of bringing fibrillation of the auricles to an end is clearly established, our own case definitely suggests that quinidine may under certain circumstances induce fibrillation. Are these two conclusions necessarily incompatible?"

Although both the term "proarrhythmia" and the concept have come into increasing prominence, these fundamental problems alluded to by Kerr and Bender remain: (1) the ranges of dose and concentration that produce beneficial antiarrhythmic effects and detrimental proarrhythmic effects overlap considerably, and (2) the emergence of proarrhythmia or antiarrhythmia in a patient often is governed by conditions that are inaccessible to analysis by the clinician.

The problem of lethal proarrhythmia was brought into sharp and chilling focus in the Cardiac Arrhythmia Suppression Trial (CAST) in which the antiarrhythmic agents flecainide and encainide induced lethal arrhythmias at a rate exceeding that observed in patients treated with placebo by more than threefold (an excess annual mortality from arrhythmias of approximately 4%).[6] Concomitant with the lethal proarrhythmic action, there was an antiarrhythmic effect in all patients in the form of suppression of ventricular ectopy. Because of the large number of patients and the rigorous placebo control, the CAST study moved the issue of lethal proarrhythmia from the realm of anecdote to the domain of quantitative definition and spotlighted the problem for both the medical and lay communities.

Three mechanisms for drug-induced tachyarrhythmias have received the most attention and support by evidence: (1) the promotion of re-entry, (2) the induction of delayed afterdepolarizations, and (3) the induction of early afterdepolarizations.

The critical dependence of re-entry on slowed conduction and spatially heterogeneous refractoriness has been verified repeatedly.[7] Pharmacotherapy for re-entrant arrhythmias is directed toward terminating propagation in the circuit either by directly reducing excitatory current to a level insufficient to sustain propagation or by prolongation of refractoriness at a site or sites in the circuit sufficiently to exceed the conduction time in the circuit. Consequently, antiarrhythmic agents effective against re-entrant tachyarrhythmias must depress conduction, prolong refractory periods, or accomplish both. Because slowed conduction generally is a prerequisite for the formation of re-entrant circuits, when agents act to slow conduction rather than extinguish it, re-entry is facilitated rather than suppressed. Re-entrant circuits in which the circuit time is only slightly longer than the refractory period at some site might be unstable and tend to terminate spontaneously. An agent that prolongs the circuit time more than the refractory period would make such a circuit more stable and sustain re-entry longer, but at a slower rate. Numerous examples have been observed during electrophysiological testing of nonsustained VTs that are converted to sustained VTs at slower rates by antiarrhythmic agents (Fig. 27-1).

Not only can pre-existing circuits be stabilized at slower rates by antiarrhythmic agents, but circuits can form anew by virtue of both the conduction slowing and the appearance of zones of functional block under the influence of the agents. Potential re-entrant circuits that have circuit times around an anatomical obstacle less than the longest refractory period in the circuit could sustain re-entry if the circuit times were prolonged by an agent that influenced refractoriness to a lesser degree than conduction.

In the case of functional re-entry as originally described in detail by Allessie and co-workers,[8] the circuits form around zones of functional block determined by refractoriness. The fundamental principles regarding re-entry apply as well to functional re-entry. However, in functional re-entry in general the circuit times are determined by, and are nearly equivalent to, the duration of the longest refractory period in the circuits because the impulse proceeds closely on the heels of recovery of excitability.[8] It is the recession of refractoriness that directs the impulse around the circuit. In other words, there is little or no excitable gap. Agents that depress conduction and promote the development of zones of functional block with premature stimulation can generate new functional re-entrant circuits. The formation of functional re-entrant circuits in ventricular myocardium by the actions of flecainide recently was demonstrated by

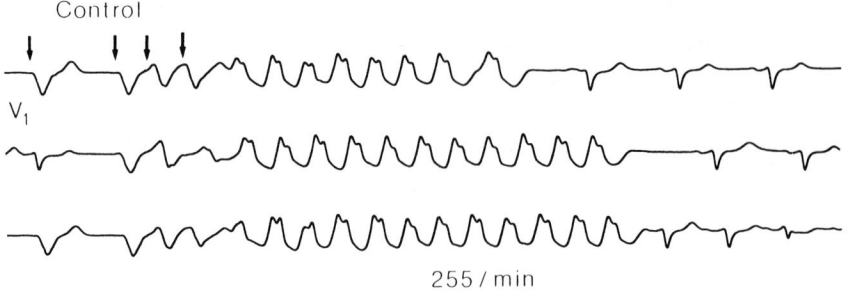
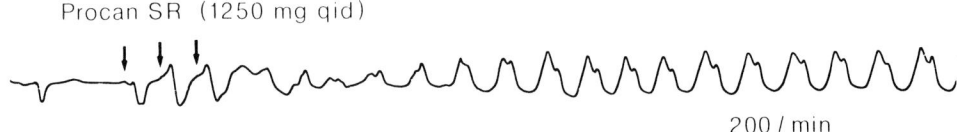

Fig. 27–1. Conversion of nonsustained ventricular tachycardia (VT) to sustained tachycardia by procainamide. In the drug-free state multiple episodes of nonsustained VT at a rate of 255/min were induced by double extrastimuli. After oral administration of Procan SR a sustained tachycardia at a rate of 250/min could be reproduced repeatedly with double extrastimuli.

Brugada and associates[9] by mapping the activation sequence (Fig. 27–2).

With circuits around obstacles, the dimensions are determined by anatomical structures and fixed conduction paths. With functional re-entry the dimensions and configurations of circuits are fluid and labile, depending on refractory periods and conduction velocities, which in turn are variable in space, in time, and with different conditions. The circuit time is the total path length of the circuit divided by the average conduction velocity in the circuit. With greater conduction velocity the dimensions of the circuit must be larger for a given value of the maximum refractory period in the circuit. In an environment of ventricular myocardium with a spatial distribution of a range of refractory periods, a larger functional circuit will traverse a greater range of refractory periods; therefore larger values are obtained. Since the circuit time is determined by the highest value of the refractory periods in the circuit, the larger circuits generally entail longer circuit times and slower rates. Conversely, for any set of refractory periods, if the conduction velocity is slower, the dimensions of the circuits required to sustain re-entry will be smaller. Small regions with relatively shorter refractory periods may not be large enough to accommodate a circuit at higher conduction velocities, but under the influence of an agent that depresses conduction without much altering refractoriness, a small circuit could form within the region with a circuit time equal to the shorter refractory periods of the region. The re-entrant tachycardias could have higher rates than those emanating from larger circuits forming at higher conduction velocities and encompassing longer refractory periods in the absence of the conduction-depressing agent. These considerations are illustrated in Figure 27–3, which illustrates the apparent paradox of a re-entrant tachyarrhythmia of higher rate resulting from an intervention that slows conduction.

It was not appreciated until recently that an agent that slows conduction can speed the rate even in a circuit with an anatomical obstacle. The mechanism for this phenomenon, demonstrated by mapping of the activation sequence in an experimental model, is that of "double-wave re-entry" in which two activation wave fronts circulate around the same barrier, causing two excitations for each complete circuit of one excitation wave.[10] This phenomenon (illustrated in Fig. 27–4) would be more likely in circuits with slow conduction and a large excitable gap. Thus, mechanisms have been de-

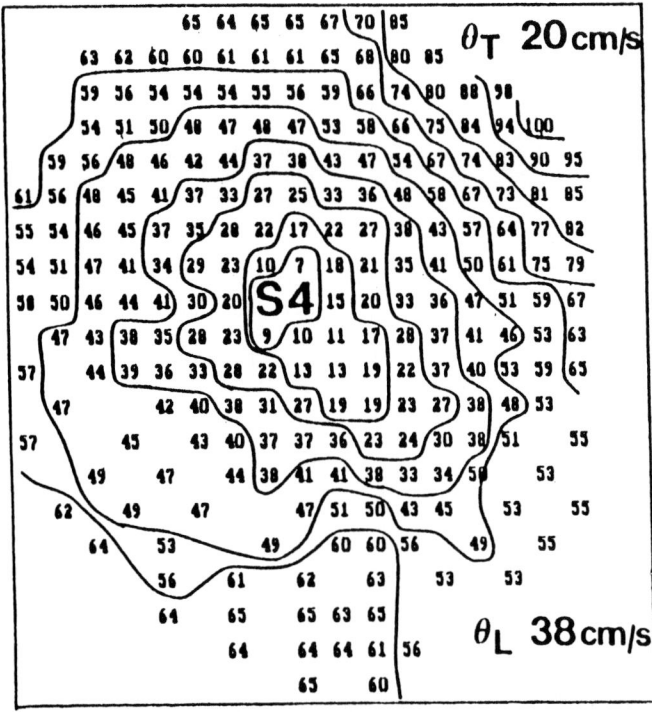

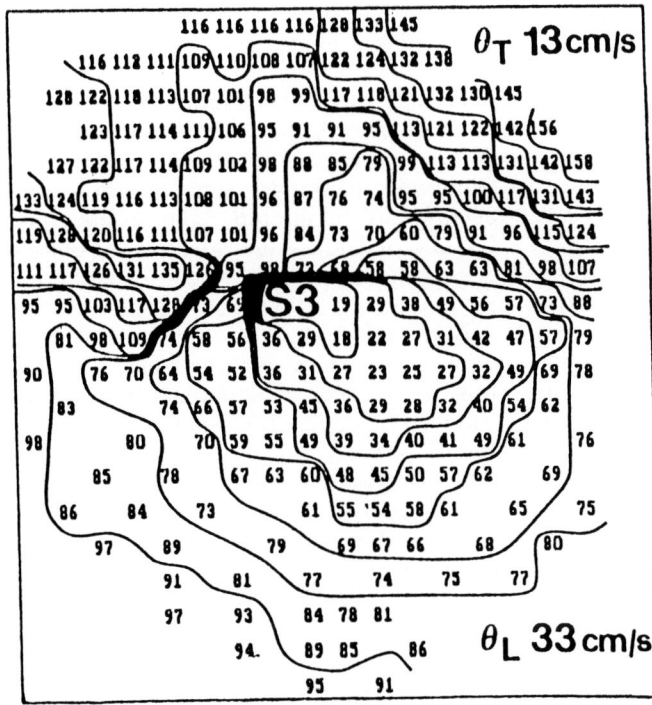

Fig. 27–2. Induction of very slow conduction in zones of block by flecainide in rabbit myocardium in the drug-free state *(left)*. With three extrastimuli the conduction velocity in the transverse direction (ΘT) was 20 cm/sec, that in the longitudinal direction (ΘL) was 38 cm/sec, and there were no zones of functional block. Under the influence of flecainide (1 µg/mL) with two extrastimuli there was greater slowing of conduction, especially in the transverse direction, and the appearance of zones of block (blackened regions). (Reproduced with permission from Brugada J, et al: Circulation 84:1808, 1991, Fig. 7.[9]).

scribed that could account for various observed re-entrant proarrhythmic actions: (1) the conversion of ventricular ectopic beats or nonsustained VT to sustained VT (stabilization of an unstable circuit by conduction slowing, (2) generation of new VT (formation of new circuits by conduction slowing and/or the creation of zones of block), (3)

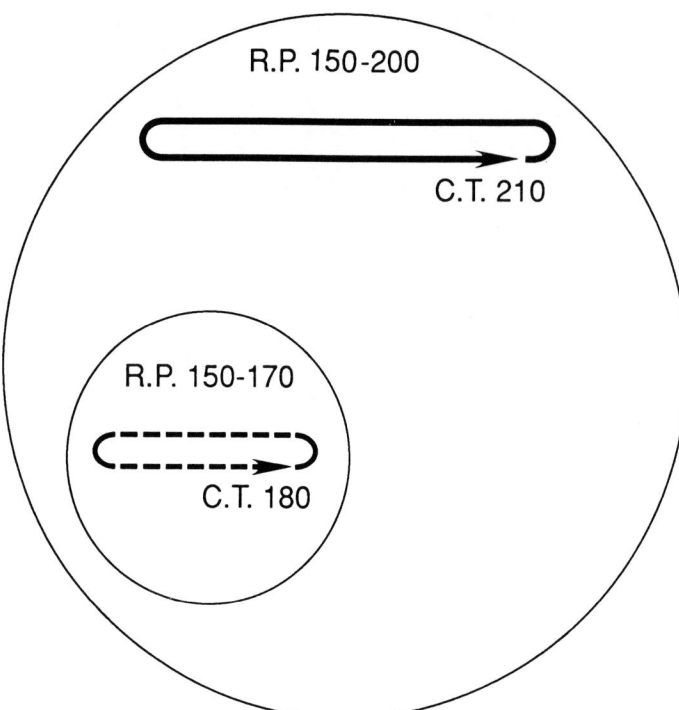

Fig. 27–3. Schematic representation of the formation of a faster re-entrant tachycardia under the influence of an agent that slows conduction. The solid arrow depicts a functioning re-entrant circuit, the smallest circuit that can form with the higher conduction velocities that exist in the drug-free condition. This circuit traverses a relatively large region with a range of refractory periods of 150–200 msec and the circuit time is necessarily longer, 210 msec. When conduction velocity is slowed by sodium channel blockade, a smaller circuit (interrupted arrow) can form in a more circumscribed region (smaller circle), in which the range of refractory periods is 150–170 msec. This circuit can operate with a circuit time of 180 msec, resulting in a more rapid tachycardia.

generation of new VT with faster rates than the pre-existing tachycardia (formation of new functional circuits in regions with lesser refractory periods, or double-wave re-entry).

In the common paroxysmal supraventricular tachycardias due to re-entry—that is, AV nodal re-entrant tachycardia and AV re-entrant tachycardia—the circuits are fixed and proarrhythmia generally takes the form of more frequent, more sustained attacks at slower rates. On the other hand, in the usual VTs occurring in diseased ventricles the potential for multiple circuits in the same or different regions exists, so that drug-induced tachyarrhythmia may take manifold forms.

The situation is further complicated by the influence of disease on the actions and distributions of the antiarrhythmic agents, generally agents that block the sodium channels, i.e., Class I agents in the Vaughan Williams classification.[11] Sodium channel blockade is conditioned by various factors that vary greatly in diseases, such as the magnitude of the resting potential, the local PH, and so forth.[12] With disease of the coronary arteries the distribution of agents may be more heterogeneous.[13] With disease and genetic variations, absorption, binding, distribution, clearance, and metabolism of agents may be altered.[14] These uncertainties complicate the therapeutic uses of these agents and increase the occurrence of proarrhythmia.

Refractoriness, that other critical determinant of re-entry, is targeted for prolongation by a class of antiarrhythmic agents, Class III of Vaughan Williams. That class of agents prolongs refractoriness by delaying repolarization. Refractoriness also can be prolonged by delaying recovery from inactivation of the sodium or calcium channels, a common effect of agents that block those channels.[12] This effect prolongs refractoriness that outlasts repolarization, i.e., post-repolarization refractoriness. This type of refractoriness is characterized by a relatively long refractory period when excitatory current is reduced, action potential upstrokes are slowed and diminished, and conduction is slowed relative to the fully recovered state of the cardiac cells (Fig. 27–5). Ischemically injured cells may mani-

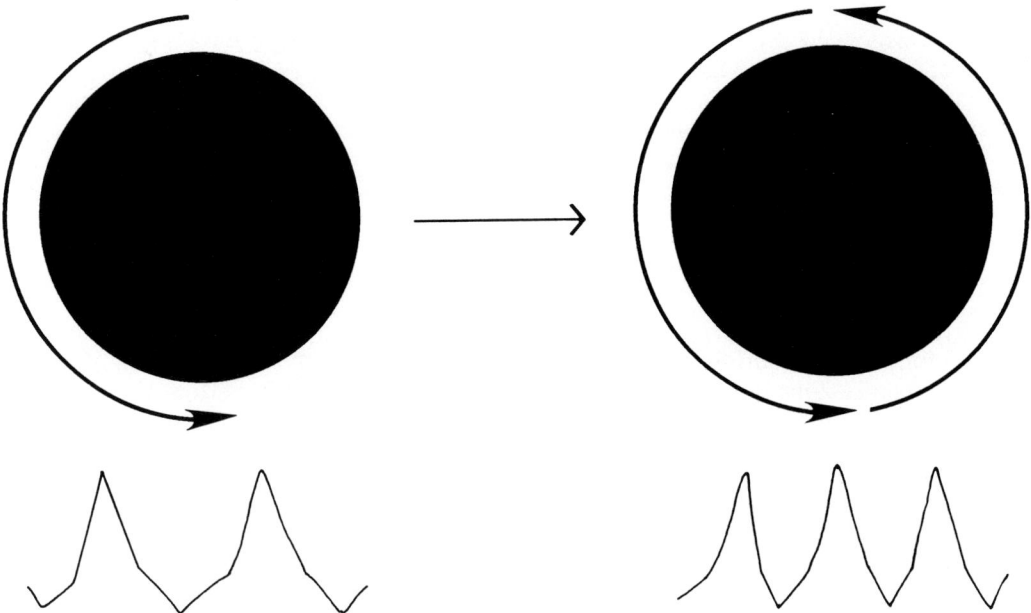

Fig. 27–4. Model for double-wave re-entry. On the left is schematically depicted a wave of re-entrant excitation circling with a large excitable gap around an obstacle. The length of the semicircular arrow represents the refractory wake of the excitation wavefront. Below the circuit are shown two complexes of a ventricular tachycardia emanating from the re-entrant circuit. If an impulse is able to enter the excitatory gap another wave front can be formed, as shown on the right, allowing two wave fronts to simultaneously circle around the barrier. The rate of the tachycardia is approximately doubled.

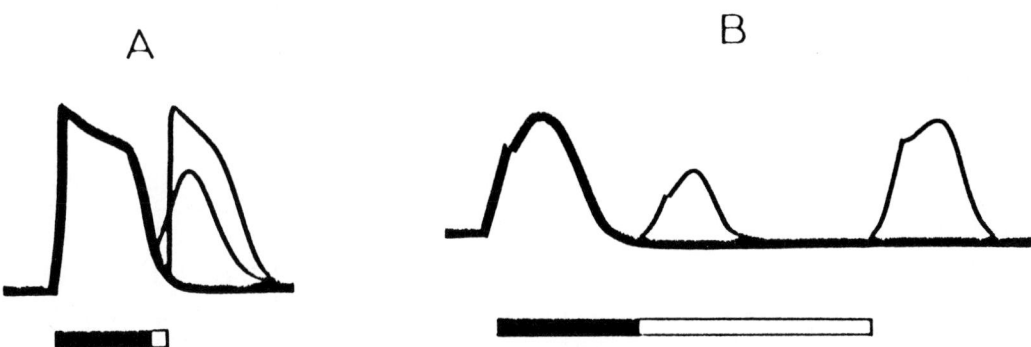

Fig. 27–5. Comparison of refractoriness linked closely to repolarization and refractoriness greatly outlasting repolarization. In *A* a relatively normal myocardial cell can be re-excited with a diminished and slowed upstroke during the terminal phases of repolarization and with a normal upstroke at the termination of repolarization because the recovery from inactivation of the sodium channel is voltage dependent with relatively rapid kinetics. In normal cells of specialized areas, such as the AV node, dependent on calcium current, or in abnormal cells partially depolarized or otherwise altered, the recovery of channels carrying the excitatory current (sodium or calcium) from inactivation is slowed. Re-excitation is not possible until repolarization is complete, and a fully recovered response of the upstroke may not occur until relatively late in diastole. Absolute refractory periods are represented by solid horizontal bars and relative refractory periods (reduced responses with reduced conduction velocity) by open longitudinal bars.

fest postrepolarization refractoriness,[15] which is prolonged by sodium channel blockade, for example with lidocaine.[16] The prolongation by antiarrhythmic agents of the relative refractory period when conduction is relatively slower could promote reentry.

Prolongation of absolute refractoriness of tissues within a re-entrant circuit around an anatomical barrier can only act to suppress re-entry in that circuit. However, prolongation of refractoriness at certain sites of a potential functional re-entrant circuit might spatially expand a zone of functional block, permitting a circuit to form. Moreover, if the prolongation is disparate in normal and diseased myocardium, heterogeneity of refractoriness would be greater. Increased heterogeneity of refractoriness acts to facilitate re-entrant tachycardias as well as fibrillation, a point recognized by Garrey, a pioneering student of re-entrant excitation.[17]

Agents that delay repolarization can cause tachyarrhythmias by a mechanism different from re-entry: the induction of early afterdepolarizations and triggered firing (Fig. 27–6). Early afterdepolarizations and triggered firing emerge under a variety of experimental conditions in which repolarization is retarded.[18] In intact animals induction of these phenomena in ventricular tissues causes an ECG abnormality and polymorphic VT that resemble the long QT syndrome and torsade de pointes.[19] Recordings of monophasic action potentials in intact hearts (Fig. 27–7 and 27–8) have produced evidence highly suggestive of early afterdepolarizations as the triggering mechanism for long QT syndromes and torsade de pointes.[20–27]

Any action that delays repolarization necessarily sets the stage for early afterdepolarization since it tilts the balance among currents toward depolarizing inward currents. Nonetheless, proarrhythmic events related to early afterdepolarizations are an uncommon complication of therapy with Class III agents.[24] It may be that other actions of the same agents, for example sodium channel blockade as in Class IA, may tend to suppress early afterdepolarizations.[19] Perhaps a genetic predisposition related to the prop-

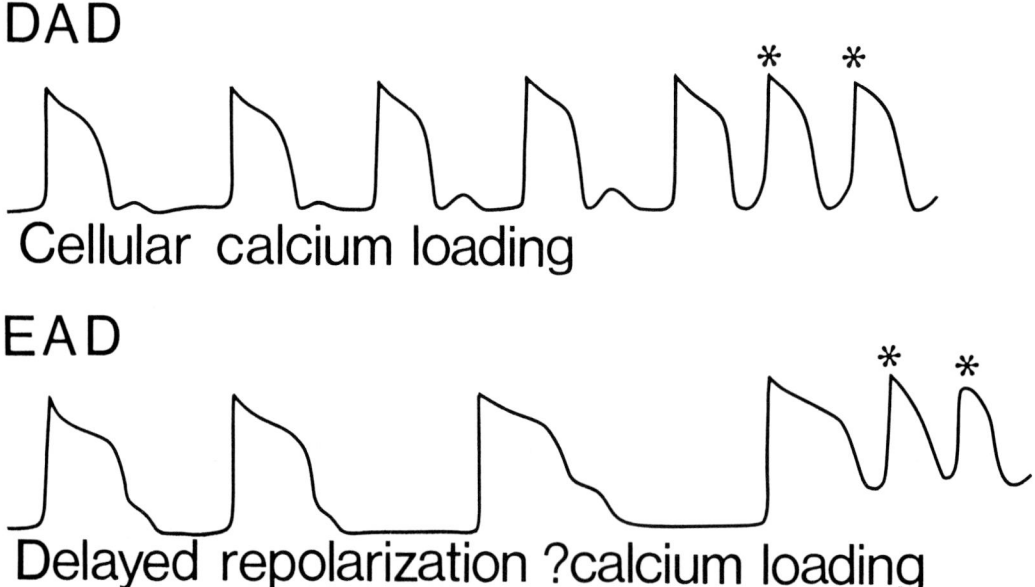

Fig. 27–6. Representation of delayed afterdepolarizations (DAD) and early afterdepolarizations (EAD). DAD, occurring in calcium-loaded cells, show increased amplitude at shorter cycle lengths, whereas EAD, occurring in the setting of delayed repolarization, show increased amplitude at longer cycle lengths. As the amplitudes of DAD and EAD increase, triggered firing (asterisks) can occur. In the case of DAD, triggered beats are usually generated from fully polarized levels of resting potential, whereas in the case of EAD, triggered beats are generated from depolarized levels of diastolic potential and can achieve higher rates. The role of calcium loading in EAD is under investigation.

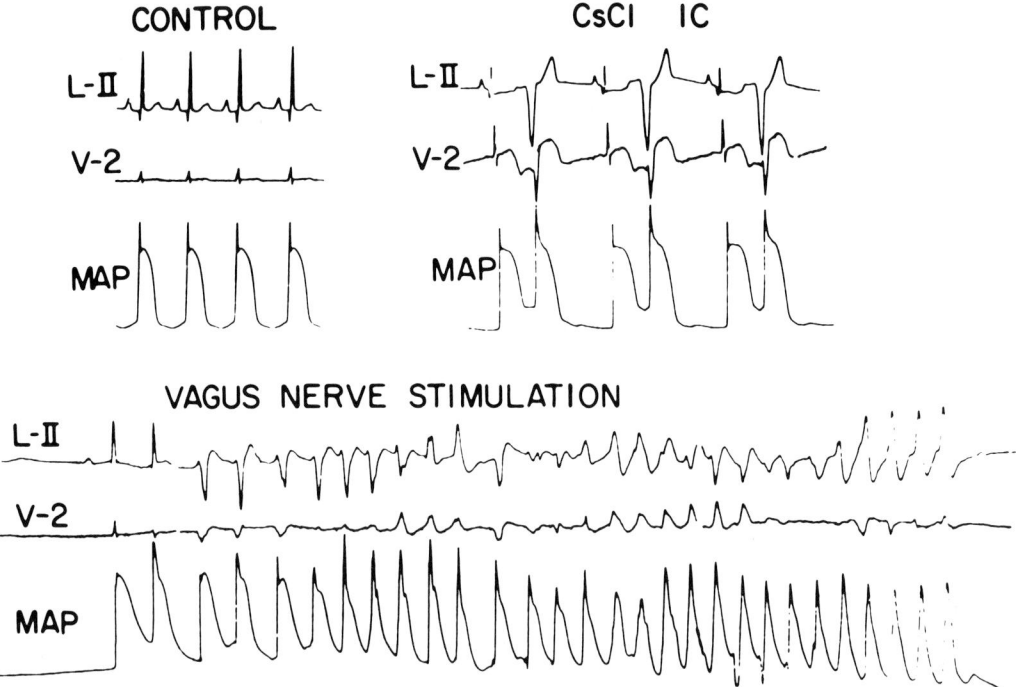

Fig. 27–7. Induction of EAD and polymorphic ventricular tachycardia by intravenous cesium. Cesium chloride (CsCl, 1 mM) was administered by intracoronary (IC) infusion to a closed-chest dog while lead II (L-II) and V_2 and a monophasic action potential (MAP) were recorded. Within 2 minutes after cesium administration (upper right) there were changes in TU waves accompanied by bigeminal PVCs and the appearance of EAD and triggered firing on the MAP. With slowing of the heart rate by vagus nerve stimulation a polymorphic ventricular tachycardia resembling torsades de pointes appeared.

erties of certain ion channels may exist in a subset of the population. Susceptible patients tend to respond with torsade de pointes to multiple agents that prolong the QT interval: there is strong concordance among agents of Class 1A for the induction of torsade de pointes.[24] No reliable identifiers of susceptibility to torsade de pointes have been identified. It is often presumed that QT prolongation may predispose to drug-induced torsade de pointes, but definitive data in support of this presumption are lacking. Certain conditions that in themselves delay repolarization, among them slow heart rates, hypokalemia, hypertrophy, and hypomagnesemia, potentiate this proarrhythmic effect.

Agents that promote the accumulation of calcium in cardiac cells foster the generation of delayed afterdepolarizations (Fig. 27–6) and triggered firing.[18,28] Delayed afterdepolarizations are defined as transient depolarizations of transmembrane potential after repolarization is complete. Delayed afterdepolarizations occur because after excessive accumulation of calcium that sarcoplasmic reticulum tends to spontaneously release calcium. As a result, the normal systolic release of calcium induced by the slow inward current following the action potential upstroke is followed by one or more releases and uptakes following repolarization. Each rise in cytosolic calcium generates an inward (depolarizing) current that can trigger new action potentials. Pharmacological agents that lead to accumulation of cellular calcium promote delayed afterdepolarizations. Induction of this phenomenon by cardiac glycosides has received the most attention,[18] but most positive inotropic agents in therapeutic usage promote cellular calcium accumulation, as do various natural positive

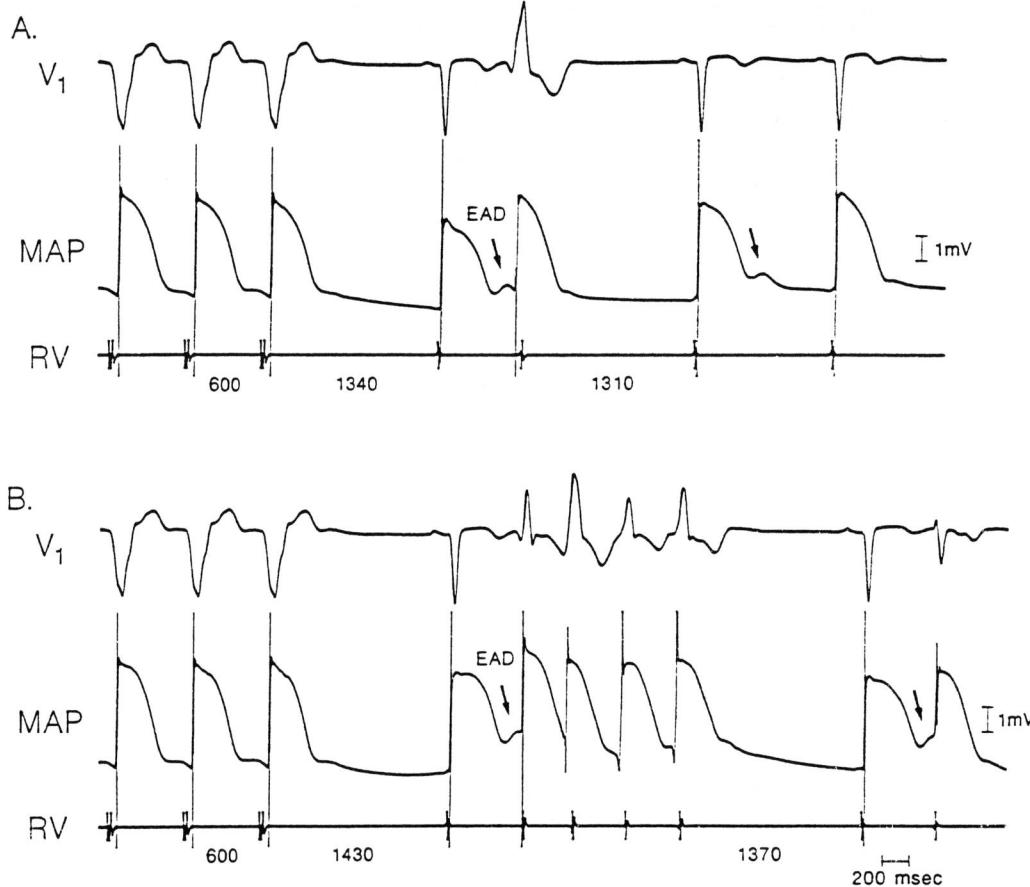

Fig. 27–8. Recordings of EAD in a patient with the pause-dependent long QT syndrome. Tracings from top to bottom are ECG lead V_1, monophasic action potential recording (MAP) from the right ventricular outflow tract, and a bipolar electrogram from the right ventricular apex (RV). Both panels begin with the last three beats of an eight-beat train of RV pacing at a cycle length of 600 msec. **A.** A postpacing pause of 1340 msec is followed by an MAP recording that demonstrates an EAD and a triggered beat associated with a PVC on the ECG. **B.** A longer postpacing pause was followed by a more prominent EAD and a run of apparent triggered firing associated with nonsustained ventricular tachycardia. (Reproduced with permission from Jackman WM, et al: J Cardiovasc Electrophysiol 1: 178, 1990.[28])

inotropic agents, such as the β-adrenergic agonists. The high prevalence of ventricular tachyarrhythmias and excess mortality observed with phosphodiesterase inhibitors and other positive inotropic agents that increase cellular calcium[29–31] may be related to the arrhythmogenic consequences of cellular calcium loading.

While our understanding of the mechanisms of pharmacologically mediated proarrhythmia is increasing, reliable prediction of proarrhythmia in the individual patient remains elusive. Certain groups of patients are known to be at enhanced risk. For example, serious proarrhythmia from agents that block the sodium channel is more likely in patients with structural heart disease who have advanced ventricular dysfunction and have demonstrated pre-existing VT or fibrillation.[32] In light of the previous discussion concerning the formation or facilitation of re-entry, it would seem logical that patients with a fertile milieu for the formation of re-entry circuits—extensive regions of damaged myocardium already able to host reentrant circuits—would be more susceptible to the re-entry-promoting effects of the antiarrhythmic agents. In the case of agents that delay repolarization, promotion of the proarrhythmia by the concomitant action of other factors that delay repolarization, such as slow heart rates and hypokalemia, is well demonstrated. If there is a genuine predisposition to pharmacological induction of torsade de pointes, reliable indicators do not exist.

Some observers have been intrigued by the observation that the tendency to produce torsade de pointes does not appear to be invariably proportional to the intensity of the effect to prolong repolarization, as reflected in prolongation of the QT interval. Prominent discordances have been noted. Amiodarone, an agent very potent in prolonging the QT interval, appears to have less tendency to produce torsade de pointes that many agents with similar or lesser effects on the QT interval.[33–35] It has been postulated that the effects of amiodarone on other currents may counteract the generation of early afterdepolarizations in torsade de pointes.[36] If this explanation is correct, a reasonable strategy for developing agents that could prolong repolarization greatly without generating early afterdepolarizations would be to clarify the crucial currents generating early afterdepolarizations and incorporate blockade of those currents in the actions of the agents developed. On the other hand, the view has been expressed that a strategy to avoid torsade de pointes might be to develop drugs that exhibit use dependence rather than the "reverse use dependence" manifested by currently available agents of Class III, so that prolongation of repolarization would be greater at faster heart rates than at slower rates when early afterdepolarizations occur.[37] It is noteworthy that the effect of amiodarone is more nearly flat across the range of heart rates,[38] whereas other agents coming into clinical use tend to show strong reverse use dependence, i.e., much more prominent effects at slower heart rates than at faster heart rates.

The induction of delayed afterdepolarizations by positive inotropic agents appears to be strongly dependent on concentration and dose because the magnitude of loading of the sarcoplasmic reticulum with calcium appears to be the crucial factor. Since the action of cardiac glycosides, β-adrenergic agonists, and phosphodiesterase inhibitors in common use depends on calcium accumulation, at present there appears to be no way to avoid this complication short of limiting the intensity of the positive inotropic effect. Agents that achieve positive inotropic effect without enhancing cellular calcium uptake presumably would be free of this complication.

The prevalence of possible pharmacological triggers for lethal arrhythmias depends on the population studied. In patients resuscitated from aborted sudden death, about 10% are receiving pharmacotherapy at the time of the cardiac arrest.[39] However, in patients with lethal arrhythmias observed on ambulatory ECG monitoring the prevalence is much higher, as high as 70% in those with tachyarrhythmias fitting the description of torsade de pointes.[40] It is likely that the prevalence observed in patients with aborted sudden death more accurately represents the true prevalence of pharmacological triggers in sudden death since patients undergoing ambulatory ECG monitoring are more likely to be receiving pharmacotherapy. However, there is the possibility that those patients with sudden death induced by pharmacological triggers are more difficult to resuscitate and that a falsely low prevalence is estimated by observing resuscitated survivors.

Evidence is mounting that lethal proarrhythmia is a far from insignificant problem in patients treated with pharmacotherapy, especially with the commonly used, time-honored Class I agents, those that block the sodium channel. In addition to the CAST study, several analyses have suggested that harm exceeds benefit in patients not at high risk from the natural arrhythmia.[41–46] Agents of classes other than Class IC have been implicated, for example quinidine and mexiletine.

Evidence from animal models of ischemic heart disease and late analyses of certain aspects of the results of the CAST study have produced some clues bearing on proarrhythmia in patients with ischemic heart disease. In various animal models with acute ischemia alone or in the setting of chronic coronary occlusion, evidence has been presented that the pre-existence of Class I agents can promote lethal arrhythmias when acute ischemia develops.[47-52] It is thought that in acute ischemia re-entry is the most common basis for arrhythmias.[53,54] It can be inferred that the greater depression of conduction with sodium channel blockers tends to facilitate re-entry in acute ischemia.

Analysis of the mortality in the CAST trial showed findings that could have important implications regarding the mechanism of proarrhythmia. First, contrary to the perception that proarrhythmia should be most frequent early in the course of therapy, the rate of lethal arrhythmia appeared to be uniform throughout the trial.[6] Second, the excess mortality in the treatment limb compared to placebo was greatly concentrated in patients with non-Q-wave MI, in comparison with patients with Q-wave MI.[55] It is recognized that patients with non-Q-wave MI are more vulnerable to acute ischemic events following discharge than patients with Q-wave MI.[56] Finally, the number of new acute ischemic events in the form of angina or new MI in the placebo group exceeded that in the treatment group by almost the exact amount that the sudden deaths or aborted sudden deaths in the treatment group exceeded those in the placebo group.[57] It has been inferred that new ischemic events in the treatment group were lethal, showing as lethal arrhythmias, whereas in the placebo group they manifested as ischemic events. Thus, it appears that in the presence of potent sodium channel blockade such as that achieved by flecainide, the conduction depression that occurs with acute ischemia and leads to re-entry is worsened. This effect might be present with all Class I agents, differing only in intensity, depending on the intensity of blockade of sodium current.

Proarrhythmia remains the challenge of this decade. If pharmacotherapy for the prevention of sudden arrhythmic deaths is to have a major effect on public health, there must be a concerted drive toward greater understanding of the mechanisms in order to derive reliable markers of susceptibility and to develop agents with less risk.

REFERENCES

1. Frey W: Weitere Erfahrungen mit Chinidin bei absoluter Herzunregelmassigkeit. Wien Klin Wochenschr 55:849, 1918.
2. Kerr WG, Bender WL: Paroxysmal ventricular fibrillation with cardiac recovery in a case of auricular fibrillation and complete heart block while under quinidine sulfate therapy. Heart 9:269, 1921.
3. Withering W: An Account of the Foxglove and Some of its Medical Uses: With Practical Remarks on Dropsy and Other Diseases. Printed by M Swinney for GGJ and J Robinson. London, Paternoster-Row, 1785.
4. Viko LE, Marvin HM, White PD: A clinical report on the use of quinidin sulphate. Arch Intern Med 31:345, 1923.
5. Selzer A, Wray HW: Quinidine syncope: Paroxysmal ventricular fibrillation occurring during treatment of chronic atrial arrhythmias. Circulation 30:17, 1964.
6. Cardiac Arrhythmia Suppression Trial (CAST) Investigators: Increased mortality due to encainide or flecainide in a randomized trial of arrhythmia suppression after myocardial infarction. N Engl J Med 321: 406, 1989.
7. Janse MJ: Reentrant arrhythmias. In Fozzard HA, et al (eds): The Heart and Cardiovascular System, 2nd ed. New York, Raven, 1992.
8. Allessie MA, Bonke FIM, Schopman FJG: Circus movement in rabbit atrial muscle as a mechanism for tachycardia: III. The "leading circle" concept. A new model of circus movement in cardiac tissue without the involvement of an anatomic obstacle. Circ Res 41:9, 1977.
9. Brugada J, Boersma L, Kirchhof C, Allessie M: Proarrhythmic effects of flecainide: Experimental evidence for increased susceptibility to reentrant arrhythmias. Circulation 84:1808, 1991.
10. Brugada J, Boersma L, Kirchhof C, et al: Double-wave reentry as a mechanism of ventricular tachycardia acceleration. Circulation 81:1633, 1990.
11. Vaughan Williams EM: Classifications of antiarrhythmic drugs. In Sandoe E, Flensted-Jensen E, Olesen KH (eds): Symposium on Cardiac Arrhythmias. Soderstalje, Sweden, AB Astra, 1970.
12. Snyders DJ, Bennett PB, Hondeghem LM: Mechanisms of drug-channel interaction. In Fozzard HA, et al (eds): The Heart and Cardiovascular System, 2nd ed. New York, Raven, 1992.
13. Nattel S, Pedersen DH, Zipes DP: Alterations in regional myocardial distribution and arrhythmogenic effects of aprindine produced by coronary artery occlusion in the dog. Cardiovasc Res 15:80, 1981.
14. Siddoway L: Initial dosage selection of antiarrhythmic therapy. Am J Cardiol 62:2H, 1988.

15. Lazzara R, El-Sherif N, Hope R, Scherlag BJ: Ventricular arrhythmias and electrophysiological consequences of myocardial ischemia and infarction. Circ Res 42:740, 1978.
16. Lazzara R, Hope RR, El-Sherif N, Scherlag BJ: Effects of lidocaine on hypoxic and ischemic cardiac cells. Am J Cardiol 41:872, 1978.
17. Garrey WE: Auricular fibrillation. Physiol Rev 4:215, 1924.
18. Wit AL, Rosen MR: Afterdepolarizations and triggered activity: Distinction from automaticity as an arrhythmogenic mechanism. In Fozzard HA (ed): The Heart and Cardiovascular System, 2nd ed. New York, Raven, 1992.
19. Brachmann J, Scherlag BJ, Rosenshtraukh LV, Lazzara R: Bradycardia dependent triggered activity: Relevance to drug-induced multiform ventricular tachycardia. Circulation 68:846, 1983.
20. Patterson E, Szabo B, Scherlag BJ, Lazzara R: Early and delayed afterdepolarizations associated with cesium chloride-induced arrhythmias in the dog. J Cardiovasc Pharmacol 15:323, 1990.
21. Levine JH, Spear JF, Guarnieri T: Cesium chloride induced long QT syndrome: Demonstration of afterdepolarizations and triggered activity in vivo. Circulation 72:1092, 1985.
22. Bonatti V, Rolli A, Botti G: Monophasic action potential studies in human subjects with prolonged ventricular repolarization and long QT syndromes. Eur Heart J 6:823, 1985.
23. Bonatti V, Rolli A, Botti G: Recording of monophasic action potentials of the right ventricle in long QT syndromes complicated by severe ventricular arrhythmias. Eur Heart J 4:168, 1983.
24. Jackman WM, Friday KJ, Anderson JL, Aliot EM, Clark M, Lazzara R: The long QT syndromes: A critical review. New clinical observations and a unifying hypothesis. Prog Cardiovasc Dis 31:115, 1988.
25. El-Sherif N, Bekhein SS, Henkin R: Quinidine-induced long QTU interval and torsade de pointes: Role of bradycardia-dependent early afterdepolarizations. J Am Coll Cardiol 14:252, 1989.
26. Jackman WM, Szabo B, Friday KJ, et al: Ventricular tachyarrhythmias related to early afterdepolarizations and triggered firing: Relationship to QT interval prolongation and potential therapeutic role for calcium channel blocking agents. J Cardiovasc Electrophysiol 1:170, 1990.
27. Patterson E, Jackman WM, Scherlag BJ, Lazzara R: The monophasic action potential in clinical cardiology. Clin Cardiol 14:505, 1991.
28. Tsien RW, Kass RS, Weingart R: Cellular and subcellular mechanisms of cardiac pacemaker oscillations. J Exp Biol 81:205, 1979.
29. DiBianco R, Shabetai R, Kostik W, Schlant C, Wright R, for the Milrinone Trial Group: A comparison of oral milrinone, digoxin, and their combination in the treatment of patients with chronic heart failure. N Engl J Med 320:677, 1989.
30. Packer M, Carver JR, Rodeheffer RJ, et al, and the PROMISE Study Investigators: Effect of oral milrinone on mortality in severe chronic heart failure. N Engl J Med 320:677, 1989.
31. Yusuf S: Obtaining reliable information from randomized controlled trials in congestive heart failure and left ventricular function. In Dietz R, Kubler W, Brachman J (eds): Ventricular Arrhythmias and Heart Failure. Berlin, Springer-Verlag, 1990, pp 147–160.
32. Morganroth J: Risk factors for the development of proarrhythmic events. Am J Cardiol 59:32E, 1987.
33. Nguyen PT, Scheinman MM, Seger J: Polymorphous ventricular tachycardia: Clinical characterization, therapy, and the QT interval. Circulation 74:340, 1986.
34. Mattioni TA, Zheutlin TA, Sarmiento JJ, Parker M, Lesch M, Kehoe RF: Amiodarone in patients with previous drug-mediated torsade de pointes. Ann Intern Med 111:575, 1989.
35. Mattioni TA, Zheutlin TA, Dunnington C, Kehoe RF: The proarrhythmic effects of amiodarone. Prog Cardiovasc Dis 31:439, 1989.
36. Lazzara R: Amiodarone and torsades de pointes. Ann Intern Med 111:549, 1989.
37. Hondeghem LM, Snyders DJ: Class III antiarrhythmic agents have a lot of potential but a long way to go: Reduced effectiveness and dangers of reverse use dependence. Circulation 81:686, 1990.
38. Anderson KP, Walker R, Dustman T, et al: Rate-related electrophysiologic effects of long-term administration of amiodarone on canine ventricular myocardium in vivo. Circulation 79:948, 1989.
39. Greene HL: The ventricular fibrillation survivor: When and how to treat. Mod Med 53:64, 1985.
40. de Luna AB, Coumel P, Leclercq JF: Ambulatory sudden cardiac death: Mechanisms of production of fatal arrhythmias on the basis of data from 157 cases. Am Heart J 117:151, 1989.
41. Furberg CD: Effect of antiarrhythmic drugs on mortality after myocardial infarction. Am J Cardiol 52:32C, 1983.

42. IMPACT Research Group: International Mexiletine and Placebo Antiarrhythmic Coronary Trial: I. Report on arrhythmia and other findings. J Am Coll Cardiol 4:1148, 1984.
43. Morganroth J, Goin JE: Quinidine-related mortality in the short-to-medium-term treatment of ventricular arrhythmias: A meta-analysis. Circulation 84:1977, 1991.
44. Coplen SE, Antman EM, Berlin JA, Hewitt P, Chalmers TC: Efficacy and safety of quinidine therapy for maintenance of sinus rhythm after cardioversion: A meta-analysis of randomized control trials. Circulation 82:1106, 1990.
45. Leighton R, Ritter G, Vasu M, Acheson A: Effect of empiric antiarrhythmic therapy in resuscitated out-of-hospital cardiac arrest victims with coronary artery disease. Am J Cardiol 65:1192, 1990.
46. Hine L, Larid N, Hewitt P, Chalmers T: Meta-analysis of empirical long-term antiarrhythmic therapy after myocardial arrest. JAMA 262:3037, 1989.
47. Elharrar V, Gaum WE, Zipes DP: Effect of drugs on conduction delay and incidence of ventricular arrhythmias induced by acute coronary occlusion in dogs. Am J Cardiol 39:544, 1977.
48. Nattel S, Pederson DH, Zipes DP: Alterations in regional myocardial distribution and arrhythmogenic effects of aprinidine produced by coronary artery occlusion in the dog. Cardiovasc Res 15:80, 1981.
49. Geren MG, Kulbertus HE: Effects of various antiarrhythmic agents on conduction delay and incidence of ventricular arrhythmias induced by acute coronary occlusion in the dog. In Sande E, Julian DE, Bell JW (eds): Management of Ventricular Tachycardia: Role of Mexiletine. Amsterdam, Excerpta Medica, 1978.
50. Kou WH, Nelson SD, Lynch JL, Montgomery DG, DiCarlo L, Lucchesi BR: Effect of flecainide acetate on prevention of electrical induction of ventricular tachycardia and occurrence of ischemic ventricular fibrillation during the early postmyocardial infarction period: Evaluation in a conscious canine model of sudden death. J Am Coll Cardiol 9:359, 1987.
51. Lynch JJ, DiCarlo LA, Montgomery DG, Lucchesi BR: Effects of flecainide acetate on ventricular tachyarrhythmia and fibrillation in dogs with recent myocardial infarction. Pharmacology 35:181, 1987.
52. Lederman SN, Wenger TL, Bolster E, Strauss HC: Effects of flecainide on occlusion and reperfusion arrhythmias in dogs. J Cardiovasc Pharmacol 13:541, 1989.
53. Lazzara R, El-Sherif N, Hope RR, Scherlag BJ: Ventricular arrhythmias and electrophysiological consequences of myocardial ischemia and infarction. Circ Res 42:740, 1978.
54. Pogwizd SM, Corr PB: Reentrant and non-reentrant mechanisms contribute to arrhythmogenesis during early myocardial ischemia: Results using three-dimensional mapping. Circ Res 61:352, 1987.
55. Wyse DG: Risk stratification: Does it determine who we should treat or how we should treat? J Cardiovasc Electrophysiol 2:S205, 1991.
56. Zema MJ: Q-wave, S-T segment, and T wave myocardial infarction: Useful clinical distinction. Am J Med 78:391, 1985.
57. Echt DS, Liebson PR, Mitchell LB, et al, and the CAST investigators: Mortality and morbidity in patients receiving encainide, flecainide or placebo. N Engl J Med 324:781, 1991.

28

Mechanisms of Bradyarrhythmic Sudden Death

STEPHEN REMOLE
RONNELL HANSEN
DAVID G. BENDITT

Sudden death due to a primary cardiac bradyarrhythmia is far less common than that due to tachycardia. Nonetheless, given the relatively high prevalence of sudden death in the population, the importance of bradycardic death is, in absolute terms, underappreciated. In this chapter we examine the estimated frequency of bradycardia-related sudden death and provide an overview of some of the mechanisms believed to contribute to this syndrome.

PREVALENCE

The prevalence of bradycardic sudden death varies depending on the manner in which it is defined and the nature of the patient population studied. For example, Myerburg et al[1] reported outcomes for 352 patients with out-of-hospital cardiac arrest in whom rhythm strips were obtained by emergency medical personnel. Bradycardia or asystole was recorded as the initial rhythm in 37% (n = 108) of these patients. However, since bradyarrhythmias can evolve secondarily from preceding tachycardias due to myocardial ischemia, an effort was made to define a subgroup of patients in whom a primary bradycardia or asystole was more likely to have been the primary event. In this regard, there were 37 patients in whom cardiac arrest was witnessed by a bystander and where trained emergency personnel arrived and documented a bradyarrhythmia within 4 minutes of the summons. Thus, the prevalence of a primary bradycardic origin for sudden death could be estimated to be one third of those patients with bradycardia or asystole as their initial rhythm, or 11% of the total population (Fig. 28–1). In a similar analysis, Iseri et al[2] reported an incidence of 25% (33/133 patients) of bradycardic/asystolic arrest using the less strict criterion of attendance at cardiac arrest by emergency personnel within 10 minutes of onset of the episode.

Bayés de Luna et al[3] have provided a meta-analysis of arrhythmias resulting in sudden death fortuitously recorded by ambulatory electrocardiographic (ECG) monitoring. When patients with acute coronary syndromes and those in the terminal stage of any disease were excluded, the incidence of bradycardia causing sudden death was 17% (26/231 patients). More recently, Olshausen et al[4] reported Holter monitoring data from 61 patients, excluding those with acute or recent coronary syndromes, New York Heart Association (NYHA) Class IV congestive heart failure, evident pulmonary embolus, cardiac tamponade, or trauma-induced congestive heart failure. In this

---

Dr. Remole is a recipient of a Grant-in-Aid from the American Heart Association—Minnesota Affiliate. Mr. Hansen is a recipient of a research award from the Howard Hughes Medical Institute.

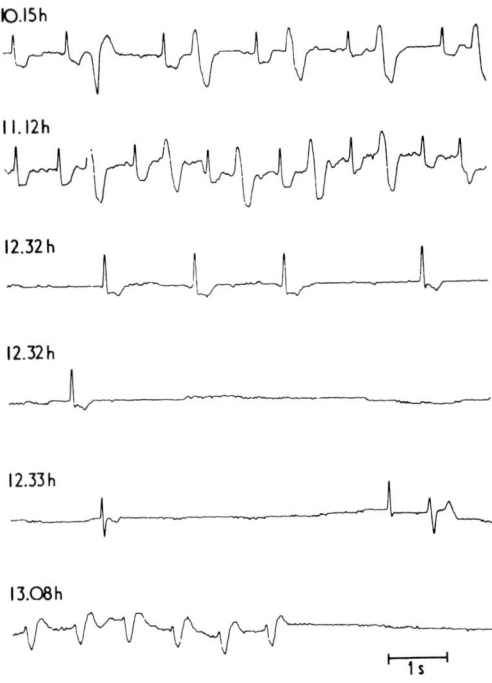

Fig. 28–1. Ambulatory electrocardiographic recording depicting a sudden cardiac arrest episode due to a primary bradyarrhythmia. After preceding periods of ventricular bigeminy, bradyarrhythmias predominate at 1232 to 1233 hours, followed by a final bradycardic arrest at 1308 hours. (Reproduced by permission of the authors and the *British Heart Journal* from Pool J, et al: Br Heart J *40*:627–629, 1978.)

group, 11 individuals (18%) had bradycardic arrests; four had complete heart block with slow fascicular or idioventricular escape rhythms and the other seven had abrupt asystole. In a more select group of hospitalized patients undergoing ambulatory ECG monitoring, Luu et al[5] reported sudden death in 21 individuals with severe congestive heart failure referred for cardiac transplantation. Surprisingly, primary ventricular tachyarrhythmias accounted for only 38% (8/21) of cardiac arrests in these patients, while bradycardia or electromechanical dissociation accounted for 62% (13/21). Fifty-four percent (7/13) of those patients with bradyarrhythmic deaths had no clear precipitating cause. Among the remainder, ischemia or electrolyte abnormalities were implicated.

In trying to arrive at an annual estimate of bradycardic death in the United States, the estimated 11% of all sudden deaths provided by Myerberg et al[1] seems to be the most reliable figure, as it includes only those cases in which the documented bradyarrhythmia at the time of out-of-hospital sudden death could reasonably be assumed to be causal. If we extrapolate this 11% to the estimated 300,000 sudden deaths per year in the United States, the overall incidence of "bradycardic sudden death syndrome" may be estimated to be approximately 33,000 per year. Furthermore, based on the report by Luu et al,[5] we can conclude that patients with very severe left ventricular dysfunction and congestive heart failure compose an important high-risk subgroup. In these latter patients, the proportion of bradycardic sudden deaths is much higher than 11% and may be greater than 50%.

MORTALITY ASSOCIATED WITH BRADYCARDIC CARDIAC ARREST

The mortality for patients with bradycardic cardiac arrest is generally reported to be higher than for those with tachycardia, whether the arrest occurred in the hospital or in the field.[4,6,7] For instance, among the 11 bradycardic arrests reported by Olshausen et al[4] the mortality was 100% vs. 74% among 50 patients with tachyarrhythmic cardiac arrest. It should be noted, however, that the patients with bradycardia tended to be older (71 vs. 64 years, $p < 0.01$), and of those whose medications were known, all (6/6) were taking drugs known to facilitate bradyarrhythmias (e.g., β-blockers, calcium channel blockers, or amiodarone). Six of the patients with bradycardic arrest died in their sleep or otherwise at rest. In the other five, circumstances at the time of death were unknown.

Kempf and Josephson[6] reviewed ambulatory ECG monitoring tapes on 27 outpatients with sudden death, of whom seven died from bradycardia. Although only two (10%) of 20 patients with ventricular tachycardia (VT) or ventricular fibrillation (VF) were resuscitated in this series, none of three patients with bradyarrhythmia were resuscitated. Of the bradycardic arrest patients, four had complete heart block with a slow fascicular rhythm or idioventricular rhythm and the other three had asystole. Bradyarrhythmia was similarly associated with a 100% mortality in the series reported by Panidis and Morganroth.[7] Of 14 inpatients and one outpatient monitored during a cardiac arrest episode, three had bradycardia (all had complete heart block), and all three died. By contrast, among patients with cardiac arrest of tachyarrhythmia origin, four (33%) of 12 survived hospitalization, although late mortality was high.

MECHANISMS OF BRADYCARDIC SUDDEN DEATH

Table 28-1 summarizes the conditions most often associated with bradycardic sudden death syndrome. In the last analysis, the mechanism of the asystolic or bradycardic event in most cases is failure of adequate automaticity of subsidiary cardiac pacemaker tissue in the absence of sinus node function. In the remaining instances, electromechanical dissociation is an important contributing factor. As described by Luu et al,[5] bradycardic/asystolic cardiac arrest is more prevalent in patients with very severely diseased hearts, and therefore may occur in the setting of a diffusely compromised His-Purkinje network. However, the impact of the multiple medications that these patients tend to be taking and the frequent presence of concomitant organ system disease are confounding factors. Thus, when drugs or metabolic derangements intervene to decrease the slope of phase 4 automaticity in pacemaker tissues (e.g., hyperkalemia), there is further compromise to the system.[8,9] Examples of such derangements include renal failure, acidosis, anoxia, potassium oversupplementation, trauma, and hypothermia. Hyperkalemic tissue is more susceptible to overdrive suppression, so that short runs of supraventricular tachycardia or VT in the presence of good ventriculoatrial conduction may provoke profound sinus arrest or more severe bradyarrhythmias. Such arrhythmias can be fatal directly; or the resultant tissue hypoxia and acidosis can lower fibrillation threshold sufficiently to provoke a catastrophic tachydysrhythmia.

Bradycardia After Electrical Cardioversion

Bradycardia or asystole following direct current cardioversion and defibrillation have been well described.[10,11] The presumed mechanism is overdrive suppression of the sinus node and subsidiary pacemakers or atrioventricular (AV) block. Waldecker et al[10] found the latter to be absent following cardioversion from atrial fibrillation, but present in 11 of 100 cases with VT or VF. In most cases, these bradydysrhythmias are transient phenomena and resolve without sequelae. For instance, in patients receiving shocks from an implantable cardioverter-defibrillator (ICD), prolonged heart block and prolonged asystole seem to be uncommon.[12] Niazi et al[12] reported a mean duration of asystole following defibrillation of less than 1.5 seconds, both clinically and in the operating room at the time of device implantation. There was no significant increase seen in those patients taking amiodarone. Concomitant coronary artery bypass grafting lengthened the duration minimally. Nonetheless, death due to asystole has been documented in one patient with an ICD following direct-current shock delivered appropriately by the device.[13] Newer ICDs have backup bradycardia pacing capabilities, which should obviate this problem. In our experience, postshock pacing is observed in the first one to four cycles in approximately 20% of patients undergo-

Table 28-1
Mechanisms of Bradycardic/Asystolic Sudden Death

Ischemic coronary syndromes
Abnormal neural control
  Hypotension/bradycardia syndrome (neurally mediated or cardioneurogenic syndromes)
    Fear-paralysis reflex
    Diving reflex
    Psychosocial stress (voodoo death)
  Aortic stenosis
  Sleep apnea syndrome
  Sudden infant death syndrome
  Athletic heart syndrome
Conduction system abnormalities
Artificial pacemaker failure
Electrolyte abnormalities

ing intraoperative device testing. Nonetheless, in the presence of severe left ventricular dysfunction, bradyarrhythmia with electromechanical dissociation may still be anticipated to occur in some patients.

Cardiac Autonomic Neural Control: Bradyarrhythmic Death Provoked by Fear or Anxiety

Any consideration of bradycardic sudden death not associated with acute coronary syndromes must include mechanisms of abnormal neural control. This term is a broad umbrella, covering a wide variety of syndromes and clinical situations ranging from aortic stenosis to voodoo death. Some of these are noteworthy for primary bradycardia/asystole, while in others the bradycardic/asystolic episode precipitates a fatal tachyarrhythmia.

Engel[14] reviewed circumstances associated with 170 sudden deaths occurring in individuals thought to be medically stable but under extremes of psychosocial stress. Reports of these deaths were derived either from the lay press or had been sent to him by interested colleagues. The attendant life situations were those of grief, fear, joy, and relief. Corroborating medical evidence was sparse, with only 16 reports being accompanied by additional information from credible sources. However, in those latter cases, many had no evidence for catastrophic anatomical pathology.

The mechanisms for death in such cases are only conjectural. In the laboratory, Miller and Caul[15] demonstrated that bradycardia, not tachycardia, was the response precipitated by feelings of helplessness in monkeys exposed to random positive or negative stimuli preceded by a warning signal. Corley et al[16] produced tachycardia giving way to bradycardia, and VF in monkeys exposed to helpless situations. The bradycardia was accompanied by QT-interval prolongation and T-wave inversion. Richter[17] reported bradycardic deaths in rats immersed in turbulent water with a prevalence of nearly 100% if the whiskers were shorn, suggesting helplessness through disorientation. These results were confirmed by several other groups.[18–20] In humans, Burrell[21] made detailed observations of Bantu tribespeople of South Africa during the 1950s, at a time before they had significant contact with white civilization and when they still clung rigidly to a centuries-old traditional life-style. Children were taught early to suppress displays of emotions. Stoicism was a societal more. For example, despite judicial flogging, Burrell[21] documented heart rates in flogging victims to be unaltered, suggesting remarkable autonomic control. Wishful death was part of this culture, especially in the aging male whose perceived usefulness to the family unit had waned. Burrell[21] reported patients with illnesses from which they were expected to recover who discharged themselves from the hospital, walked many miles back to their homes, then died suddenly shortly after arriving. In addition, sorcery and black magic were deep preoccupations. Several men were observed to die promptly after the prescription of the curse. The implication of all this was that these people had rather extraordinary vagal tone at baseline that could be augmented, willfully or by fear, to levels sufficient to cause death.

Kaada[22] writes extensively of what he terms the "fear paralysis reflex," whereby threat-induced fear elicits immediate motor and autonomic paralysis ("freezing"), accompanied by profound bradycardia that may itself result in death or may precipitate a fatal tachydysrhythmia. There is also apnea in expiration, a reduction in muscular tone, and no outcry. Helplessness and hopelessness are important features of the reflex induction and are incumbent to the situation wherein the victim views his plight as inescapable or insoluble and is unable to cope with it. Kaada[22] lists the stimuli that in animals may provoke this response: confrontation with a predator, restraint of movement (preventing flight), loss of support, unexpected and sudden noises, distress, and alarm calls. The response is markedly attenuated in the company of another of the same species, particularly if there has been bonding, as in parent–offspring bonding.

The fear paralysis reflex has been demonstrated in several animal species and has a peak incidence very early in life, antedating completion of neocortex development. In monkeys, it peaks at age 2–4 months, paralleling the peak incidence of sudden infant death syndrome in humans. Presumably, neocortical influences supervene over its induction later in life, but it could theoretically be released by various kinds of disinhibition in adulthood.

Although asystolic cardiac arrest of an autonomically mediated origin appears to be relatively rare in Western society, there is indirect evidence that such events do occur (Fig. 28–2). For instance, Milstein et al[23] reported observations in six survivors of a suspected asystolic sudden death event. All patients underwent detailed hemodynamic evaluation and conventional electrophysiological studies, all of which were nondiagnostic. Tilt-table testing was then undertaken, with findings in these six patients (group 1) compared to those from two control groups: six syncope patients with normal conventional electrophysiological evaluation but demonstrable neurally me-

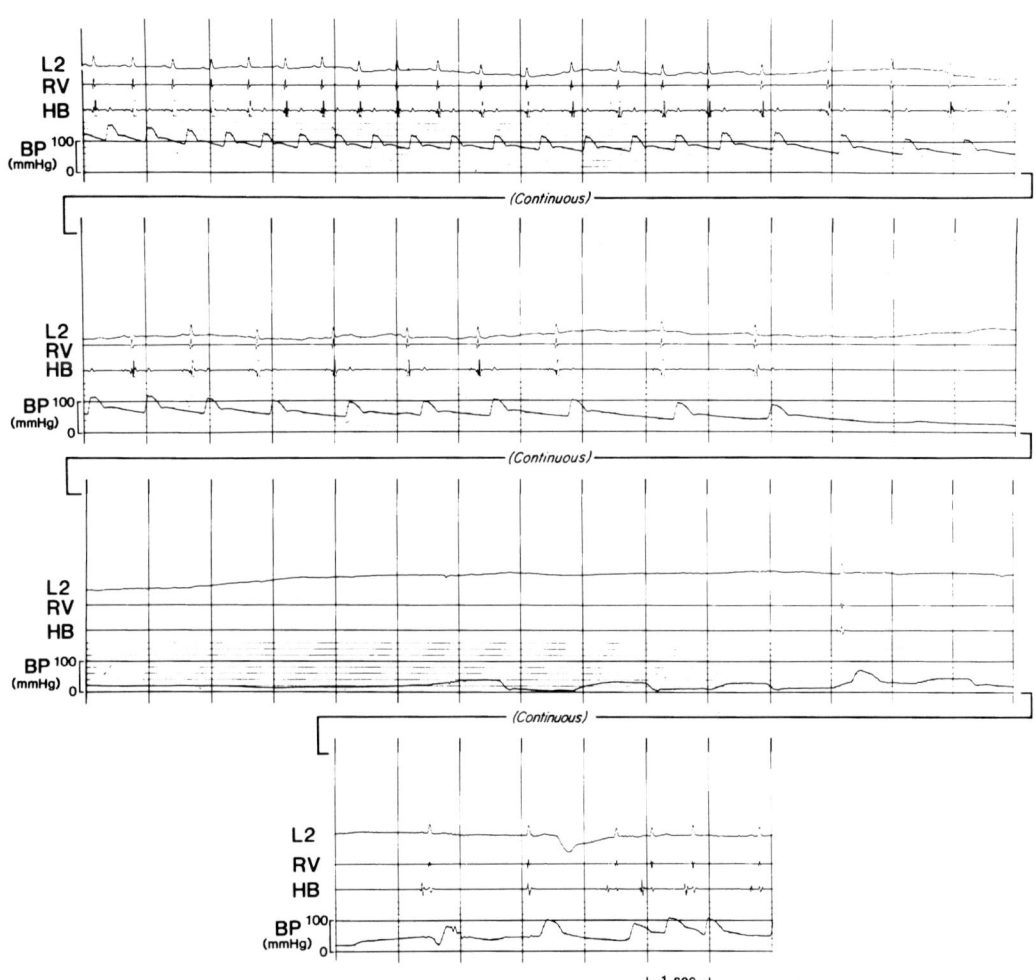

Fig. 28–2. Recording of a tilt-table induced asystolic event in an individual with a history of recurrent syncope, in whom one episode of severe cardiovascular collapse was documented electrocardiographically to be associated with a 22-second asystolic spell. All panels are continuous and depict a lead II electrocardiogram (L2), intracardiac electrograms from the right ventricular apex (RV) and His bundle region (HB), and an intra-arterial pressure recording. The tracing begins at 2 minutes into an 80-degree upright tilt test procedure. Gradual diminution of blood pressure is accompanied by a 16-second asystolic episode. The patient recovered spontaneously when returned to the supine position. (Reproduced by permission of the authors and the *Journal of the American College of Cardiology* from Milstein S, et al: J Am Coll Cardiol *14:*1626–1632, 1989.[26])

diated hypotension-bradycardia (group 2), and six patients with syncope in whom conventional electrophysiological evaluation provided a presumptive diagnosis (group 3).

During head-up tilt testing group 1 and 2 patients exhibited similar tilt-induced drops in mean arterial pressure and heart rate. By contrast, group 3 patients manifested only a moderate drop of arterial pressure and had an increase of heart rate. These findings support the notion that asystole and cardiovascular collapse on a neurally mediated basis may account for at least a small number of sudden death episodes each year. Furthermore, because management of a neurally mediated bradycardic event is dramatically different from that of tachyarrhythmia-related sudden death episodes, careful consideration should be given to neurally mediated bradycardic mechanisms when conventional electrophysiological studies fail to confirm susceptibility to VT or VF in sudden death survivors.

Aortic Stenosis

Sudden death associated with aortic stenosis is probably most often multifactoral, reflecting not only the impact of autonomic disturbances (discussed below) but also the severity of the valvular and myocardial disease, as well as any coexisting coronary artery lesions. Thus, ventricular tachyarrhythmias and conduction system disturbances are not unexpected and may result in sudden cardiovascular collapse. However, of particular interest in regard to bradyarrhythmic etiologies of sudden death is the potential for neurally mediated hypotension-bradycardia to be the cause of death in certain patients. Thus, in the setting of increased inotropic drive (e.g., exercise), peripheral vasodilation and bradycardia may be triggered by neural traffic from left ventricular mechanoreceptors as discussed earlier for other forms of neurally mediated syncope.[24-26] By way of example, in the report by Schwartz et al,[27] ECG findings in patients with prolonged syncopal episodes (>40 seconds) revealed ventricular asystole in some cases. In others, ventricular tachyarrhythmias were documented. Clearly, given the often severe degree of left ventricular hypertrophy and scarring, and possibly concomitant coronary artery disease as well in aortic stenosis patients, it would not be surprising for a sufficiently severe episode of hypotension-bradycardia to evolve into VF. The initial documented arrhythmia diagnosis may then be misleading in some of these cases.

Sudden Infant Death Syndrome

Sudden infant death syndrome (SIDS) annually affects 7000 U.S. infants 2–4 months of age.[28] The mechanism of death remains largely speculative, but it seems likely that there is a diverse spectrum of pathophysiology rather than one cause. Primary apnea, infant botulism, long QT syndrome with torsade de pointes leading to VF, sinus bradycardia, and the fear paralysis reflex have been variously implicated.

A report by Colan et al[29] noted bradycardia as the only significant cardiac arrhythmia in a survey of 1699 babies at high risk for SIDS (i.e., those with a history of near-SIDS, a sibling with previous SIDS, or who were premature). Sixty (4%) of the high-risk infants had heart rates less than 60 beats/min on at least one 12-hour ambulatory ECG. Only 12 of those infants were full term, making bradycardia the only cardiac rhythm abnormality for which prematurity was a risk factor. None of the babies had Wolff-Parkinson-White syndrome, long QT syndrome, or a widened QRS duration.

Valdes-Dapena[30] suggests that SIDS is a biphasic process, with intrauterine events influencing development in such a way as to confer a susceptibility for SIDS on affected infants when they are confronted with a challenge after birth (such as a respiratory infection). This is supported by data showing that in fact infants with SIDS are not the same developmentally as control subjects matched for gestational age, race, and socioeconomic status. This hypothesis is similar in nature to that of Kaada,[22] who links the end of the peak incidence of the fear paralysis reflex in animals to the development of the neocortex, as though something has retarded the maturation of inhibitory mechanisms until the latter stages of this process.

Apnea-Bradycardia and Sleep Apnea Syndromes

Apneic episodes in young infants are probably associated with immaturity of brain stem respiratory centers and may be closely related to SIDS. When apnea is prolonged (>10 seconds), severe bradycardia may also occur, probably mediated through chemoreflexes.[31] The frequency with which such a mechanism results in death is unknown.

In older patients, sleep is frequently associated with bradyarrhythmias.[32,33] As a rule these are believed to be benign. However, bradycardia is even more prevalent in association with the sleep apnea syndrome,[34,35] and consequently it is reasonable to assume that unexpected deaths in this setting may be suspected of being due to bradyarrhythmias in some instances. In others, bradycardia may facilitate development of ventricular tachyarrhythmias by a "pause-dependent" mechanism. Currently, attention has been focused primarily on ventricular ectopy and tachyarrhythmias as a complication of sleep apnea syndrome. However, little is known of the mechanisms of sudden death in this circumstance,[36] and consequently the possible contribution of bradyarrhythmias is at best speculative.

Bradyarrhythmic Death Associated with Acute Myocardial Infarction

Although second-degree or complete heart block is associated with increased mortality in patients with both inferior and anterior myocardial infarction (MI), the fatality is usually due to severe left ventricular involvement and a consequent tachyarrhythmia. Bradyarrhythmias are only rarely a direct cause of sudden death episodes in hospitalized patients with acute ischemic syndromes. Furthermore, these patients with evident conduction system disturbances tend to be managed quite effectively by temporary pacing, although the subsequent prognosis may nonetheless be poor owing to severe myocardial damage and susceptibility to ventricular tachyarrhythmias.[37-39] Electromechanical dissociation may also be associated with bradycardia. Perhaps of greatest concern, however, are the bradyarrhythmias associated with drug therapy (e.g., β-adrenergic blockers, lidocaine). For example, in the ISIS-1 trial,[40] bradycardia/asystole was associated with cause of death in ten atenolol-treated patients versus three placebo-treated patients. Although the ISIS-1 differences were not statistically significant, the trend is of concern. Thus β-adrenergic blockers may reduce the incidence of tachyarrhythmias, but bradycardia-related deaths may become a more serious problem.

SUMMARY

Bradyarrhythmias are a relatively infrequent cause of sudden death, accounting for an estimated 11% of all sudden deaths in the United States. However, several important settings (e.g., neurally mediated hypotension-bradycardia syndromes, apnea-bradycardia syndrome) may be associated with sudden death in the prime of life and therefore are particularly devastating. Additionally, bradyarrhythmic episodes are usually unexpected even in patients with known heart disease. Consequently, appropriate resuscitative measures (e.g., transthoracic pacing) often are not immediately applied or are not available. The result may contribute in part to an even higher mortality than is associated with tachyarrhythmia-related sudden cardiovascular collapse. Finally, the impact of bradyarrhythmias on sudden death is difficult to measure. In many cases an initial bradycardia may rapidly lead to inadequate coronary artery perfusion, myocardial ischemia, and VT or VF. As a result, the importance of a bradyarrhythmic origin of a sudden death episode may remain both underappreciated and inadequately protected against.

ACKNOWLEDGMENT

The authors thank Barry L. S. Detloff for technical assistance.

REFERENCES

1. Myerburg RJ, Conde CA, Sung RJ, et al: Clinical electrophysiologic and hemodynamic profile of patients resuscitated from prehospital cardiac arrest. Am J Med 68:568, 1980.
2. Iseri LT, Humphrey SB, Siner EJ: Prehospital brady-asystolic cardiac arrest. Ann Intern Med 88:741-745, 1978.

3. Bayés de Luna AB, Coumel P, Leclercq JF: Ambulatory sudden cardiac death: Mechanisms of production of fatal arrhythmia. Am Heart J *117:*151–159, 1989.
4. Olshausen KV, Witt T, Pop T, Treese N, Bethge K-P, Meyer J: Sudden cardiac death while wearing a Holter monitor. Am J Cardiol *57:*381–386, 1991.
5. Luu M, Stevenson MD, Stevenson LW, Baron K, Walden J: Diverse mechanisms of unexpected cardiac arrest in advanced heart failure. Circulation *80:*1675–1680, 1989.
6. Kempf FC, Josephson ME: Cardiac arrest recorded on ambulatory electrocardiograms. Am J Cardiol *53:*1577–1582, 1984.
7. Panidis IIP, Morganroth J: Sudden death in hospitalized patients: Cardiac rhythm disturbances detected by ambulatory electrocardiographic monitoring. J Am Col Cardiol *2:*798–805, 1983.
8. Vassalle M: Cardiac pacemaker potentials at different extra- and intracellular K^+ concentrations. Am J Physiol *208:*770, 1965.
9. Vassalle M: On the mechanism underlying cardiac standstill: Factors determining success or failure of escape pacemakers in the heart. J Am Coll Cardiol *5(suppl B):*35, 1985.
10. Waldecker B, Brugada P, Zehender M, Stevenson W, Wellens HJJ: Dysrhythmias after direct-current cardioversion. Am J Cardiol *57:*120, 1986.
11. Weaver WD, Cobb LA, Copass MK, Hallstrom AP: Ventricular defibrillation: A comparative trial using 175-J and 320-J shocks. N Engl J Med *307:*1101, 1982.
12. Niazi II, Kadri N, Mahmud R, et al: Absence of significant postdefibrillation bradyarrhythmias in patients with automatic implantable defibrillators. Am Heart J *115:*830, 1988.
13. Khastgir T, Aarons D, Veltri EP: Sudden bradyarrhythmic death in patients with the implantable cardioverter-defibrillator: Report of two cases. PACE *14:*395, 1991.
14. Engel GL: Psychologic stress, vasodepressor (vasovagal) syncope, and sudden death. Ann Intern Med *89:*403, 1978.
15. Miller RE, Caul WF: Influences of uncertainty on conditioned heart rates of monkeys. Physiol Behav *4:*975–980, 1969.
16. Corley CK, Greenhoot J, Mauk HP, et al: Abnormalities of cardiac rhythm associated with environmental stress. Fed Proc *29:*517, 1970.
17. Richter C: On the phenomenon of unexplained sudden death in animals and man. Psychosom Med *19:*191–198, 1957.
18. Binik YM, Theriault G, Shustack B: Sudden death in the laboratory rat: Cardiac function, sensory, and experimental factors in swimming deaths. Psychosom Med *39:*82, 1977.
19. Lynch JJ, Katcher AH: Human handling and sudden death in laboratory rats. J Nerv Ment Dis *159:*362–365, 1974.
20. Rosillini RA, Binik TM, Swligman MEP: Sudden death in the laboratory rat. Psychosom Med *38(1):*55–58, 1976.
21. Burrell RJW: The possible bearing of curse death and other factors in Bantu culture on the etiology of myocardial infarction. In James TN, Keyes JW (eds): The Etiology of Myocardial Infarction. Boston, Little, Brown, 1963.
22. Kaada B: Possible role of the fear paralysis reflex in sudden cardiac death. In Refsum H, Sulg IA, Rasmussen K (eds): Heart and Brain, Brain and Heart. Berlin, Springer-Verlag, 1989.
23. Milstein S, Beutikoffer J, Lesser J, et al: Cardiac asystole: A manifestation of neurally mediated hypotension-bradycardia. J Am Coll Cardiol *14(7):*1626, 1989.
24. Johnson AM: Aortic stenosis, sudden death, and left ventricular baroreceptors. Br Heart J *33:*1–5, 1971.
25. Mark AL, Kioschos JM, Abboud FM, Heistad DD, Schmid PG: Abnormal vascular responses to exercise in patients with aortic stenosis. J Clin Invest *63:*395–402, 1979.
26. Grech ED, Ramsdale DR: Exertional syncope in aortic stenosis: Evidence to support inappropriate left ventricular baroreceptor response. Am Heart J *121:*603–606, 1991.
27. Schwartz LS, Goldfischer J, Sprague GJ, Schwartz SP: Syncope and sudden death in aortic stenosis. Am J Cardiol *23:*647–658, 1969.
28. Valdes-Dapena MA: Sudden infant death syndrome: A review of the medical literature 1974–79. Pediatrics *93:*597–614, 1980.
29. Colan SD, Liberthson RR, Cahen L, Shannon DC, Kelly DH: Incidence and significance of primary abnormalities of cardiac rhythm in infants at high risk for sudden infant death syndrome. Pediatr Cardiol *5:*267, 1984.
30. Valdes-Dapena MA: Are some sudden crib deaths sudden cardiac deaths? J Am Coll Cardiol *5(suppl B):*113B, 1985.
31. Fenichel GM, Olson BJ, Fitzpatrick JE: Heart rate changes in convulsive and nonconvulsive neonatal apnea. Ann Neurol *7:*577–582, 1980.
32. Tilkian AG, Guilleminault C, Schroeder JS, et al: Sleep-induced apnea syndrome: Prevalence of cardiac arrhythmias and their reversal after tracheostomy. Am J Med *63:*348–358, 1977.
33. Brodsky M, Wu D, Denes P, Kanakis C, Rosen KM: Arrhythmias documented by 24 hour continuous electrocardiographic moni-

toring in 50 male medical students without apparent heart disease. Am J Cardiol 29: 390–395, 1977.
34. Guilleminault C, Connolly SJ, Winkle RA: Cardiac arrhythmia and conduction disturbances during sleep in 400 patients with sleep apnea syndrome. Am J Cardiol 52: 490–494, 1983.
35. Guilleminault C, Partinen M (eds): Obstructive Sleep Apnea Syndrome: Clinical Research and Treatment. New York, Raven, 1990.
36. Seppälä T, Partinen M, Pentillä A, Aspholm R, Tiainen E, Kaukianen A: Sudden death and sleeping history among Finnish men. J Int Med 229:23, 1990.
37. Hindman MC, Wagner GS, Jaro M, et al: The clinical significance of bundle branch block complicating acute myocardial infarction: 2. Indications for temporary and permanent pacemaker insertion. Circulation 58(4):689–699, 1978.
38. Hauler R, Liek I, Liem KL, Durrer D: Long term prognosis in patients with bundle branch block complicating acute anteroseptal infarction. Am J Cardiol 49:1581, 1982.
39. Barold SS, Ffalkoff MD, Onol S, Vaughan MJ, Heinle RA: Atrioventricular block in acute myocardial infarction: New developments. In Barold SS, Mugica J (eds): New Perspectives in Cardiac Pacing. Mt. Kisco, NY, Futura, 1991, pp. 3–21.
40. ISIS-1 Collaborative Group: Mechanisms for the early mortality reduction production reduced by beta-blockade started early in acute myocardial infarction, IFIF-1. Lancet i:921–923, 1988.

E
Out-of-Hospital Management Strategies

29

Results of Large-Scale Studies with β-Adrenergic-Blocking Drugs and Other Non-Antiarrhythmic Agents for the Prevention of Sudden Cardiac Death

JOSEF WIDERHORN
SHAHBUDIN H. RAHIMTOOLA

The one thing certain about life is death.
(An old Asian saying)

Sudden cardiac death (SCD) is said to be the major health problem in the United States, but is it that important a problem? Since death is inevitable, sudden death may not be an undesirable mode of exit. In general, about 50% of deaths in cardiovascular disorders are sudden, but only about 50% of sudden deaths are unexpected. Thus, the area of concern should be narrowed to *unexpected* sudden deaths. Furthermore, with the graying of America and the recognition that about 80% of all cardiovascular deaths occur in those aged 65 years or older, one needs to realize that if a 90-year-old person, even if apparently healthy, dies suddenly and unexpectedly, such a mode of death may not necessarily be undesirable. Therefore, the major issue with sudden death perhaps should be the problem of *premature unexpected sudden death*. Since most if not all studies of sudden death have so far not addressed this issue, our review will obviously not be able to address this important aspect of sudden death.

During the last four decades, major advances in identifying patients at risk have been made and various strategies to prevent and treat the high-risk population have been developed. In addition, even though many questions are still unanswered, our understanding of various pathophysiological mechanisms involved in SCD has increased considerably. A major step in the understanding of neurohumoral mechanisms involved in sudden death was made by Ahlquist in 1948 with the introduction of the concept of selective adrenergic stimulation and blockade through a series of specific receptors.[1] However, progress was slow until 1960, when the first competitive β-adrenergic-blocking drugs were developed, and Black et al[2,3] demonstrated that the effects of the sympathetic nervous system could be counteracted with an antagonist of β receptors. The therapeutic potential of the β-adrenergic-blocking compounds was immediately recognized and an extensive investigation led to the development of many new agents with different pharmacological properties and to their widespread use for various cardiovascular disorders, especially for the treatment of hypertension and ischemic heart disease. β-adrenergic-blocking drugs have been evaluated for the treatment of arrhythmias and for the prevention of SCD, particularly in post-myocardial infarction (MI) patients.

CLINICAL STUDIES WITH β-ADRENERGIC-BLOCKING DRUGS IN POST-MYOCARDIAL INFARCTION PATIENTS

Twenty-five years ago, propranolol was tested in several small studies with limited follow-up.[4–8] With the exception of the study by Snow and Manc,[7] these studies did not show a significant improvement in survival. However, the encouraging results reported by Snow and Manc,[7,8] even though their study was small and uncontrolled, drew attention to the potential of this new class of drugs. Since then, a large number of β-adrenergic-blocking agents have been synthesized and numerous studies have been performed during the early as well as the delayed post-MI period to assess their effects in this patient population.

Early Intervention Trials with Short- or Long-Term Follow-up

Limited Size Trials

In the acute phase trials, therapy with a β-blocker was started within 72 hours of the onset of symptoms of MI. These studies were mainly designed to assess the effects of a β-blocker on infarct size and immediate in-hospital mortality. Various β-adrenergic drugs (propranolol, tinolol, practolol, alprenol, oxprenol, metoprolol, atenolol, sotalol, acetabutol) were given orally or intravenously (IV) followed by short- or long-term oral therapy. These trials are summarized elsewhere.[9,10] With the exception of two major early intervention (<24 hours) studies[11,12] in which more than 1000 patients were enrolled, most of these studies were conducted on a small number of patients and did not show convincing evidence of a reduction in mortality. The inability to show a reduction in in-hospital mortality in the early intervention randomized trials with β-blockers is likely due to multiple factors, including flaws in study design, correct β-blocker dose, timing of intervention,[10] baseline heart rate and attainment of the target heart rate,[13] the subset of patients analyzed, and, most important, inadequate sample size. The mortality in the subset of population considered suitable for β-blocker therapy (patients without heart failure, cardiogenic shock, or bradyarrhythmias) post-MI is relatively low. Furthermore, a a reduction in infarct size and in the incidence of arrhythmias may not necessarily translate to an improved survival. Therefore, in order to show a reduction in mortality of 20–30%, more than 10,000 patients may need to be randomized. Because the smaller studies are less likely to have enough statistical power, further analysis will be restricted to large or megatrials (>1000 patients).

Large or Megatrials

The first among the large studies of early intervention following MI was reported by Hjalmarson et al[11] A total of 1395 patients were randomly assigned in double-blind fashion to IV metoprolol (given immediately after arrival in the hospital) followed by oral treatment, or to placebo. The mean interval between the onset of pain and the start of therapy was 11.3 hours. The reduction in total mortality was 36%, an actual reduction of 4%; the benefit was seen at 3 months but not at 1 week (Table 29-1). The beneficial effect on survival was maintained for up to 2 years but was not present at 5 years.[14,15] The episodes of ventricular tachycardia (VT) and ventricular fibrillation (VF) were also significantly reduced in the metoprolol treatment group. Subgroup analysis indicated that the survival benefit was present in metoprolol-treated patients with an initial heart rate above 70 beats/min.

The largest early intervention trial of β-blockade in acute MI was the First Intervention Study of Infarct Survival (ISIS-1).[12] In this study, 16,027 patients were randomly assigned to treatment with IV atenolol, 5–10 mg, followed by 100 mg/day orally for 7 days, or to placebo. Atenolol was administrated within 12 hours of onset of symptoms. The vascular mortality during the 7 days of the study was significantly lower ($p < 0.04$) in the treatment group, 3.9% (313/8037), than in the placebo group, 4.6% (365/7990). The 15% reduction in mortality had a wide 95% confidence interval and was mainly due to lower rates of cardiac rupture and electromechanical dissociation. The latter was presumably due to the lower rate of cardiac rupture in the atenolol treatment group. This difference in mortality was maintained for 1 year. A reduction of 15%

Table 29-1
Summary of the Randomized Placebo-Controlled Early Intervention Trials Post Myocardial Infarction with β-Adrenergic-Blocking Drugs with More Than 1,000 Patients

Trial	No. of Pts.	Entry Time, hr (mean)	β-Blocker	Dose	Follow-up	Total Mortality (1 wk) β-Blocker: No. of Deaths/No. of Pts. (%)	Total Mortality (1 wk) Placebo: No. of Deaths/No. of Pts. (%)	p Value	Total Mortality (3 mo) β-Blocker: No. of Deaths/No. of Pts. (%)	Total Mortality (3 mo) Placebo: No. of Deaths/No. of Pts. (%)	p Value	Total Mortality During Follow-Up β-Blocker: No. of Deaths/No. of Pts. (%)	Total Mortality During Follow-Up Placebo: No. of Deaths/No. of Pts. (%)	p Value	No. of Pts. Benefited/100 Treated Pts.
Göteborg[11]	1,395	<48 (11.3)	Metoprolol	15 mg IV + 200 mg/day	24 mo	18/698 (3.0)	23/697 (3.0)	NS	40/698 (5.7)	62/697 (8.9)	0.024	92/698 (13.2)	120/697 (17.2)	0.043	4.0
ISIS-1[12]	16,027	<12 (5.1)	Atenolol	5–10 mg IV + 100 mg/day	12 mo	317/8,037 (3.9)	365/7,990 (4.6)	0.04				691/8,037 (10.7)	703/7,990 (12)	0.01	1.3
MIAMI[15]	5,778	<24 (6.7)	Metoprolol	15 mg IV + 200 mg/day	15 days	74/2,877 (3.0)	87/2,901 (3.0)	NS				123/2,877 (4.3)	142/2,901 (4.9)	NS	—

NOTE: The mortality rates reported were at 24 months for the Göteborg study, 12 months for the ISIS-1 trial, and 15 days for the MIAMI trial.

in mortality is very small, even though it is statistically significant; the actual reduction in mortality was 0.7% (3.9% vs. 4.6%). In other words, it is necessary to treat approximately 150 patients in order to avoid one death during the first 7 days after an MI.

The beneficial effect on overall survival seen in the Göteborg and ISIS-1 trials could not be confirmed in another megatrial, the Metoprolol in Acute Myocardial Infarction (MIAMI) study.[16] In the MIAMI trial, 5778 patients were randomly assigned in double-blind fashion to receive metoprolol, 15 mg IV, followed by oral therapy, 200 mg/day, or placebo. After 15 days there were 123 deaths (4.3%) in the metoprolol-treated group versus 142 deaths (4.9%) in the placebo group; the 13% reduction in mortality was not statistically significant. However, a retrospective subgroup analysis showed that the treatment was beneficial in 2038 high-risk patients (30% of the study population), in whom mortality was reduced from 8.5% to 6% by metoprolol ($p = 0.03$).

Metoprolol has recently been tested again in the Thrombolysis in Myocardial Infarction (TIMI) Phase II trial[17] as an adjunct to thrombolytic therapy with tissue plasminogen activator (tPA) and prophylactic percutaneous transluminal coronary angioplasty (PTCA). The 3262 patients treated with tPA within the first 4 hours of the onset of pain were randomly assigned to an invasive strategy (PTCA) or to conservative management. A subgroup of 1390 patients was randomly assigned to early IV metoprolol (15 mg) followed by oral therapy with metoprolol, or to deferred therapy, with metoprolol to start on day 6 post MI. The end points of the β-blockade trial were resting and exercise radionuclide ejection fractions (EFs) both at discharge from the hospital and at 6 weeks, total mortality, reinfarction, and recurrent ischemic events. There were no between-group differences in mortality at both 6 and 42 days post MI. Similarly, early or deferred treatment with metoprolol had no effect on resting or exercise EF both prior to discharge and at 6 weeks. However, recurrent ischemia and nonfatal reinfarction rates were lower in the immediate treatment group ($p = 0.005$ and $p = 0.02$, respectively). Subgroup analysis revealed that patients treated within 2 hours of the onset of symptoms and patients in the low-risk group had a lower incidence of death or recurrent MI within 42 days than patients randomized to deferred therapy ($p = 0.01$ and $p = 0.007$, respectively).

Arrhythmias

Hjalmarson et al[11] reported a decrease in the frequency of ventricular fibrillation (VF) in the metoprolol group compared to the placebo group (0.9% vs. 2.4%, $p < 0.035$) (Table 29-2). A similar reduction has been observed for episodes of VT (2% vs. 3.7%, $p < 0.076$). Contrary to the results obtained in the Göteborg trial,[14] the incidence of VF was not reduced in the treatment group in the ISIS-1 and MIAMI trials (Table 29-2).[12,16] In ISIS-1, the incidence of VF was 2.4% in the atenolol treatment group and 2.5% in the placebo group; in the MIAMI trial, VF was seen in 1.7% of treated patients versus 1.8% of controls. Interestingly, in another smaller trial (735 patients)[18] that used the nonselective β-blocker propranolol, the frequency of VF was 0.8% (2/364) in the treated group versus 5.7% (14/371) in patients given placebo ($p = 0.006$). The discrepancy between this study's results and those of previous trials[16] may be explained by early entry into the study (2.5 hours, vs. 5.1 and 6.7 hours in ISIS-1[12] and MIAMI,[16] respectively) and by a possibly better efficacy of nonselective β-blockers in blunting the epinephrine-induced influx of potassium into cells and therefore in preventing the occurrence of

Table 29-2
Prevalence of Ventricular Fibrillation and Ventricular Tachycardia in the Major Early Intervention Trials

Trial	VT/VF		
	β-Blocker: No. of Pts. (%)	Placebo: No. of Pts. (%)	p Value
Göteborg[11]	VT 14 (2)	VT 26 (3.7)	0.076
	VF 6 (0.9)	VF 17 (2.4)	0.035
ISIS-1[12]	VF 189 (2.4)	198 (2.5)	NS
MIAMI[15]	VT 37 (1.3)	VT 40 (1.4)	NS
	VF 48 (1.7)	VF 52 (1.8)	

hypokalemia. In some animal models, propranolol had antifibrillatory properties that were not observed with atenolol.[19] However, in a comparative study of the antifibrillatory efficacy of five β-blockers, the antifibrillatory effects of propranolol were similar to those of metoprolol.[20]

In the Göteborg trial,[14] the incidence of supraventricular tachycardia (SVT) was lower in the treatment group ($p < 0.001$), while there was no difference between the subgroups for the occurrence of atrial fibrillation or flutter. However, in the MIAMI trial, SVT and atrial fibrillation/flutter occurred significantly less frequently in the treatment group ($p < 0.001$ and $p < 0.01$, respectively).

Delayed Intervention Trials With Long-Term Follow-Up

Since early 1970, a plethora of delayed entry, long-term trials have been performed; some have had small sample sizes and others were uncontrolled. A review of most of these trials, except the most recent ones, was published elsewhere.[10,21] Similar to the above analysis of early intervention trials we will restrict this review to trials with more than 1000 patients enrolled (Table 29–3).[22–24,27,30–34] The entry windows in these delayed entry studies ranged between 5 and 28 days.

Large and Megatrials

The first among the delayed entry megatrials was the Multicenter International Study,[22,23] which began in 1972 and was terminated prematurely because of the occurrence of serious oculocutaneous and peritoneal reactions to practolol. The 3038 patients were randomized within 7 to 28 days after MI to practolol, $β_1$-selective β-blockers with intrinsic sympathomimetic activity, or placebo. Patients were treated for a mean of 12 months and, in some centers, up to 3 years. Even though the confidence limits were very wide, there was a significant reduction in overall mortality (47 vs. 73 deaths, $p < 0.02$) and of deaths occurring within 2 hours (30 vs. 52, $p < 0.02$). Retrospective subgroup analysis showed a significant reduction in mortality in patients with anterior but not inferior infarction, in patients with diastolic blood pressure ≤ 78 mm Hg, and in patients with initial heart rates of more than 100 beats/min. However, this study had many problems related to design and statistical analysis. The analysis was not by "intention to treat"; when the excluded randomized patients were included in the analysis, the results were no longer significant.

The Norwegian Multicenter Study Group[24] enrolled 1884 patients in a randomized, placebo-controlled study with oral timolol given 7–28 days after MI. The follow-up was between 12 and 33 months, with a mean of 17 months. There was a reduction of total mortality (98 vs. 152 deaths, 10.6% vs. 17.5%, $p < 0.001$) and of sudden death mortality (deaths within 24 hours, 47 vs. 95, $p < 0.0001$) in the intervention group. The analysis was by "intention to treat," and the results had narrow confidence limits, making the results of this study very powerful. In distinction to the practolol study,[22,23] a beneficial result was noted in all infarcts (anterior and inferior) and all risk groups. In addition, the reinfarction rate was significantly reduced at 33 months of follow-up (14.4% vs. 20.1%, $p = 0.0006$). Analysis of the cohort of 732 patients aged 65–75 years[25] also revealed a significant reduction in overall mortality ($p < 0.05$), total cardiac death ($p < 0.01$), sudden death ($p < 0.05$), and reinfarction ($p < 0.01$) in the treated group. This suggests that older patients may also benefit from β-blocker treatment after MI.[25] More striking is that the beneficial results on mortality in the timolol treatment group persisted for up to 6 years after randomization; the cumulative mortality rates were 26.4% in the treated group versus 32.3% in the placebo group ($p = 0.0028$).[26] However, the final report[26] demonstrated that the beneficial effects of β-blockade were seen in men but not in women, in those aged 65 years or older but not in those less than 65 years, and in the high-risk group but not in the low-risk group. Furthermore, β-blockade no longer had a beneficial effect on reinfarction.

In 1977, the National Heart, Lung and Blood Institute (NHLBI) sponsored the Beta-Blocker Heart Attack Trial (BHAT).[27] During a 27-month interval, 2837 patients were randomly assigned to propranolol (1916 patients) or placebo (1921 patients) 5

Table 29-3
Summary of Randomized Placebo-Controlled Delayed Intervention Trials Post Myocardial Infarction with β-Adrenergic-Blocking Drugs with More Than 1,000 Patients

Trial	No. of Pts.	Entry Time	β-Blocker	Daily Dose	Average Follow-up	Total Mortality During Follow-up				Sudden Death*			
						β-Blocker: No. of Deaths/ No. of Pts. (%)	Placebo: No. of Deaths/ No. of Pts. (%)	p Value	No. of Pts. Benefited per 100 Treated Pts.	β-Blocker: No. of Deaths (%)	Placebo: No. of Deaths (%)	p Value	No. of Pts. Benefited per 100 Treated Pts.
Multicenter International Study[22,23]	3,038	7–28 d	Practolol	400 mg	14 mo	47/1,524 (3.1)	75/1,514 (4.8)	0.02	1.7	30 (2.0)	52 (3.4)	0.02	1.4
Norwegian International Study[24]	1,884	7–28 d	Timolol	20 mg	17 mo	98/945 (10.6)	152/939 (17.5)	0.0003	6.9	47 (7.7)	95 (13.9)	0.0001	6.2
BHAT[27]	3,837	5–21 d	Propranolol	180–240 mg	25 mo	138/1,916 (7.2)	188/1,921 (9.8)	0.005	2.6	64 (3.3)	89 (4.6)	0.05	1.3
Julian et al[32]	1,456	5–14 d	Sotalol	320 mg	12 mo	64/873 (7.3)	52/583 (8.9)	NS	—	25 (2.9)	14 (2.4)	NS	—
EIS[33,34]	1,741	14–31 d	Oxprenolol (slow release)	320 mg	12 mo	57/858 (6.6)	45/883 (5.1)	NS	—	25 (2.9)	24 (2.7)	NS	—
Taylor et al[35]	1,103	1–90 mo	Oxprenolol	40 mg	48 mo	60/632 (9.5)	48/471 (10.2)	NS	—	33 (5.3)	25 (5.2)	NS	—
LIT[36]	2,395	6–16 d	Lopressor	200 mg	12 mo	65/1,195 (5.4)	62/1,200 (5.2)	NS	—	14 (1.2)	20 (1.7)	NS	—

NOTE: Sudden death rates reported in the table are the deaths that occurred within 1 hour in references 27, 32, 33, and 36; within <2 hours for references 22 and 23; and within 24 hours in references 24 and 35.

to 21 days after MI. The average follow-up was 25 months. The total mortality was 7.2% in the treated group versus 9.8% in the placebo group ($p < 0.01$), i.e., a reduction in mortality of 26% and an actual reduction of 2.6% after a follow-up of 3 years. SCD (death within 1 month) paralleled the total mortality: 3.3% in the propranolol-treated group versus 4.6% in the placebo group ($p < 0.05$). Like timolol, propranolol, a nonselective β-blocker without intrinsic sympathomimetic activity, reduced total and sudden death mortality regardless of patient age or site of infarction. In fact, because of this beneficial drug effect and the previously published timolol study, the study was stopped 9 months ahead of schedule. The occurrence of nonfatal myocardial reinfarction was also reduced by 16% in the treatment group. An interesting finding in the BHAT study was that the difference in mortality between the treated group and the placebo group occurred during the sleeping hours (10 P.M. to 7 A.M., 21% vs. 34%, $p < 0.05$); the other circumstances surrounding death did not differ between groups.[28,29] However, the beneficial effect of propranolol was seen only in the high-risk group[30] and in smokers.[31]

Julian et al[32] studied the effect of sotalol, a β-blocker with Class III antiarrhythmic activity, in 1456 patients, 60% of whom were randomized to sotalol and 40% to placebo. The difference in total and sudden death mortality in the two groups was not significant, although a trend was noted in the sotalol group (18% reduction in mortality). However, there was a significant reduction of reinfarction, 27%.

Oxprenolol, a β-blocker with intrinsic sympathomimetic activity, has been tested in patients who have sustained an MI, with less encouraging results.[33–35] In the European Infarction Study (EIS),[33,34] 1741 patients were randomly assigned to slow-release oxprenolol, 320 mg/day (858 patients), or to placebo (883 patients). During 1 year of follow-up, there was a difference in cumulative mortality of 30.4% in favor of the placebo group ($p = $ NS). The difference in mortality clustered in the group of patients who were 65–69 years of age; in patients younger than 65 years, the mortality was no different. Another oxprenolol study[35] enrolled 1103 male patients who had sustained an MI 1–90 months previously. The patients were randomly assigned to 40 mg of oxprenolol (632 patients) or placebo (471 patients) and followed up for 6–84 months (mean, 48 months). There was no significant difference in total mortality between the two randomized groups. However, in the subgroup of 417 patients in whom therapy had been started within 4 months after infarction, oxprenolol increased the cumulative survival rate from 77% to 95% ($p < 0.001$). In the 274 patients in whom treatment was started between 5 and 12 months after infarction, the survival rate was similar, while in the 412 patients who were enrolled in the trial between 1 and 7½ years after infarction, oxprenolol significantly reduced the 6-year survival, from 92% to 79% ($p = 0.002$). The increased mortality in the latter group mainly occurred late after withdrawal from active treatment. In any case, this retrospective subgroup analysis should be interpreted cautiously.

In another study, the Lopressor Intervention Trial (LIT),[36] 2395 patients were randomized between 6 and 16 days post MI to metoprolol, 200 mg/day (1195 patients), or to placebo (1200 patients). The 12-month mortality was no different between the two randomized groups (5.4% vs. 5.2%, $p = $ NS, 95% confidence limits were -49% to $+25\%$). The sudden-death count was 14 in the metoprolol group and 20 in the placebo group. Owing to the low event rate in the placebo group (5.2%), the power of the study was too low to detect a reduction in mortality, and therefore the results were inconclusive.

Arrhythmias

The effect of β-blockade on arrhythmias in patients post-MI has been investigated in four of the seven above described studies.[32,37–39] In all of these studies, 24-hour ambulatory electrocardiographic (ECG) monitoring had been performed at the time of recruitment into the study and during follow-up in a subgroup of the study population. In the BHAT study,[38] 24-hour ECG monitoring was performed in 3279 of 3837 patients at baseline and after 6 weeks of therapy in a random sample of 27% of the study population. In the latter subset of 826 patients, an increase in prevalence of ventricular arrhythmias at 6 weeks was noted; this increase was blunted in the propranolol-treated group. At baseline, 8.1% of the patients receiving placebo and 7.2% of those taking propranolol had two or more PVCs/hr and at least one run of VT or couplets. After 6 weeks, ventricular arrhythmias were noted in 25.6% of patients in the placebo group versus 14.6% of patients in the propranolol group. Therefore, there was a 40% reduction in ventricular arrhythmias in the treated group, which was statistically significant (Z = 3.95). Ventricular ectopic activity was higher in patients with prior MI and congestive heart failure and was an independent predictor of mortality in both the treated and placebo groups.[40,41] Similar results were noted in the timolol[35] and sotalol[30] trials, but not in the oxprenolol[39] trial. In the EIS trial,[39] 736 patients underwent 24-hour ECG monitoring at baseline and after enrollment in the study at mean times of 10 days and 3, 6, and 12 months. During the 1-year follow-up period, the prevalence of ventricular arrhythmias did not change significantly in either treatment group. A decrease in the frequency of multiform ventricular extrasystoles was noted at 3 and 6 months but not at 1 year.

SUMMARY AND CLINICAL IMPLICATIONS

Even though the mortality benefit from early intervention trials with β-blockade issue is not completely resolved, at least two large trials[11,12] showed a decrease in total mortality. In addition, the early administration of β-adrenergic-blocking drugs may have had positive effects on infarct size,[11,16,42,43] chest pain,[11,16,42] arrhythmias,[11,16,42] recurrent ischemia,[17] and reinfarction rates.[11,17]

A favorable effect on survival was observed at least in two major delayed intervention, randomized, placebo-controlled studies.[24,27] These data are in agreement with the Beta-Blocker Pooling Project (BBPP) Research Group finding of a 24% reduction in overall mortality in patients treated with β-blockers[44] and with the findings of other reviews.[9,10,21]

Although the body of knowledge regarding the treatment of patients who have sustained an MI has increased rapidly, many questions remain unanswered. These questions include the following: (1) Is therapy with β-blockade beneficial to all postinfarction patients, and if not, in which subgroups of patients is it the most or the least beneficial? (2) Is the beneficial effect a class effect or an individual effect? (3) What is the ideal timing for intervention? (4) How long should the patient be treated? (5) Is the long-term treatment cost-effective?

Although in some studies[24,27] subgroup analysis indicated a beneficial effect for patients in all of the risk groups, the patients who would benefit most are those in the high-risk group, while the benefit in low-risk patients is, at best, marginal and highly controversial.[45–49] In fact, it appears that patients younger than age 50 who have a low mortality in control groups (3.5%) do not benefit from long-term β-blockade.[44] The maximum benefit was seen in the age group 50–59 years (37% reduction in mortality) and, in one study, in older patients (65–75 years old).[25] The benefit is also more evident in patients with previous infarcts, large infarcts, mild heart failure, and myocardial ischemia.[24,27] In the BHAT study,[50] propranolol decreased the incidence of sudden death by 47% in patients who had previous heart failure versus 13% in patients without it. A similar favorable action was noted in patients with cardiac enlargement in the Norwegian timolol study,[24,51] but not in the EIS trial.[33,34] These data were confirmed by the BBPP Research Groups meta-analysis.[44] It appears that patients at low risk (those less than 50–60 years old, women, those with a first infarction, those with good left ventricular function, those with no evidence of ischemia or arrhythmia, and nonsmokers) may not benefit from long-term β-blocker therapy.[45,46,48]

The beneficial effect on survival has been documented with various β_1-selective and nonselective β-blockers[11,12,24,27] but not with β-blockers that have intrinsic sympathomimetic activity.[33–35] Therefore, the beneficial effect on survival appears to be a class effect and is most probably related to β-blockade and not to other drug properties. The choice of β-blockers should be tailored to the individual patient and to the clinical situation. The pharmacokinetic properties and side effect profile are important considerations in the choice of β-blocker for clinical use. The dose of β-blockers should be adjusted to lower the resting heart rate and to blunt the response to exercise. Another issue is the timing of intervention. The TIMI Phase II trial revealed no difference in mortality between early or delayed intervention; this was true regardless of reperfusion data. Both early[11,12] and delayed[15,27] entry clinical trials revealed a reduction in mortality and additional beneficial effects on reinfarction rates, chest pain, infarct size, and arrhythmias. The doctrine, "time is muscle," applies to both thrombolytic and β-blocker therapy in order to have an effect on myocardial salvage.[11,16,42,43] If β-blockade cannot be given early for various reasons, delayed administration (5–21 days post infarction) and long-term therapy may favorably affect the survival and reinfarction rates.

The optimal duration of treatment with β-blocker therapy is not certain. A study[26] indicated that the benefit on survival present at 2 years[24] is maintained up to 6 years' follow-up in some subgroups of patients, even after the drug has been withdrawn. In another study, patients withdrawing from metoprolol treatment had an increase in mortality.[52] Furthermore, the mortality benefit seen at 2 years in the Göteborg trial[14] did not persist at 5 years.[15] Therefore, the therapy, if given, should be continued for at least 2 years. The cost-effectiveness of long-term β-blocker therapy compares favorably with that of coronary artery bypass surgery and the medical treatment of hypertension.[53,54] The adverse effects in most trials were mild and occurred in approximately 10–20% of patients. In the BHAT study[27] only bronchospasm, cold hands and feet, tiredness, and diarrhea occurred significantly more frequently in the propranolol group. The occurrence of new congestive heart failure was equal in either randomized group (6.7%). A relatively low prevalence of side effects was also seen in the Göteborg,[11] ISSI-1,[12] and Norwegian timolol[24] trials.

In conclusion, even though the value of β-blocker therapy in the thrombolytic era is unknown, we believe that routine β-blocker therapy is clinically indicated in high-risk patients after MI who are not successfully revascularized and in whom there is no contraindication to β-blocker therapy.

CLINICAL TRIALS WITH β-ADRENERGIC-BLOCKING DRUGS FOR THE TREATMENT OF HYPERTENSION

Even mild hypertension is associated with a significant increase in the incidence of stroke and coronary heart disease.[55,56] Since the risk for coronary heart disease and for cardiac death (sudden and nonsudden) are increased in the hypertensive population, it would be expected that aggressive treatment of hypertension would decrease this risk. However, several studies[57] failed to show clear protection against cardiac death. The reasons for lack of effect on coronary heart disease are not completely clear. It is possible that the side effects of diuretics, which were used in most trials (such as lowering potassium and magnesium levels, elevating lipid levels, and altering glucose tolerance), may have counteracted the beneficial effects derived from lowering the blood pressure. A logical approach would be to substitute β-blockers, which, in addition to their effects on blood pressure, also have anti-ischemic and anti-arrhythmic properties. Several trials[58–62] have explored this hypothesis; however, with the exception of one trial,[61,62] no benefits could be demonstrated.

In the Medical Research Council (MRC) trial,[58] 17,354 patients (men and women) were randomized to propranolol or bendrofluazide or placebo tablets. Even though the incidence of stroke was reduced in the treatment groups, the overall rate of coronary events was no different between the treated and placebo groups or between the propranolol and bendrofluazide groups. Retrospective subgroup analysis showed that nonsmoking men in the propranolol group had a lower incidence of coronary events.

The International Prospective Primary Prevention Study in Hypertension (IPPPSH) randomized 6357 men and women to treatment with oxprenolol or placebo.[59] However, supplementary drugs including other β-blockers were used in both groups as deemed necessary to lower the blood pressure. The incidence of sudden death, MI, and stroke was similar in both groups.

In contrast to the MRC[58] and IPPPSH[59]

trials, the Heart Attack Primary Prevention in Hypertension (HAPPHY) trial[60] enrolled only men with high diastolic blood pressure (100–130 mm Hg). Patients were randomized to treatment with β-blockers (atenolol or metoprolol, 3297 patients) or thiazide diuretics (bendrofluazide or hydrochlorothiazide, 3272 patients). Also in this study, the total mortality and coronary heart disease events (fatal and nonfatal) did not differ significantly. Because there was no randomization of the two β-blockers, no valid conclusion could be drawn regarding any differences between atenolol and metoprolol groups. The metoprolol arm of the HAPPHY study was continued until 1987 (the HAPPHY study was terminated on December 31, 1985) and the study was named MAPHY (Metoprolol Atherosclerosis Prevention in Hypertensives).[61-63] The MAPHY trial randomized 3234 hypertensive males (diastolic BP = 100–130 mm Hg) to metoprolol (1609 patients) or to thiazide diuretics (bendroflumethiazide or hydrochlorothiazide, 1609 patients). At a mean follow-up of 4.2 years, the total and cardiovascular mortality were significantly reduced in the metoprolol group ($p = 0.028$ and $p = 0.012$, respectively). The relative risk for coronary events was 0.58, with a 95% confidence interval of 0.41 to 0.80. The risk for nonfatal coronary events (MI) was also decreased significantly in the metoprolol group ($p = 0.0034$). The beneficial results were maintained until the end of the study at 10.8 years (relative risk = 0.76, 95% confidence interval = 0.58–0.98).[63] Of the cardiovascular deaths, 78% were classified as sudden (occurred within 24 hours after the onset of symptoms). Again, there were significantly fewer sudden deaths in the metoprolol group than in the diuretic group (32 vs. 45, $p = 0.47$). In addition, the total mortality was significantly lower in smokers randomized to metoprolol than in smokers randomized to diuretics ($p = 0.013$).

The results of the MAPHY trial[61-63] are strikingly different from the results obtained in previous trials.[58-60] In the MRC and IPPPSH trials, both men and women were enrolled, and subgroup analysis indicated that in men, the relative risk was lower in patients treated with β-blockers. In addition, 60% of the patients enrolled in the oxprenolol arm of the IPPPSH trial also received a diuretic, which may have altered the beneficial effect of the β-blocker. In the MAPHY study only men, who have a higher risk for coronary events than women, were enrolled. In addition, the diastolic blood pressure entry criterion was higher in the MAPHY trial (100–130 mm Hg, vs. 90–109 mm Hg in the MRC trial or 100–125 mm Hg in the IPPPSH trial). However, the MAPHY trial has drawn considerable criticism for not being a truly separate trial from the HAPPHY trial and for the methods used in statistical analysis, which may invalidate the results.[64-67] In addition, the results of the atenolol arm in the HAPPHY trial have not yet been published.

Even though there is controversy regarding the superiority of β-blockers over diuretics in the treatment of hypertension, the real unanswered issue is the effect of either therapy on coronary events in the population studied. In an overview of 14 randomized trials of antihypertensive drugs,[68] the proportional reduction in total coronary heart disease (14%, $p < 0.01$) was lower than that observed for stroke. In addition, the 11% reduction in fatal coronary heart disease was not significant. The results of the MRC trial, which compared treatment with β-blockers/diuretics with placebo, appear to confirm the above finding. Unfortunately, the lack of a placebo group in the HAPPHY and MAPHY trials left this issue unresolved.

Importantly, the current role of another major class of antihypertensive agents (Ca^{2+} channel entry blocking agents and angiotensin-converting enzyme inhibitors) needs to be kept in mind.

POTENTIAL MECHANISMS INVOLVED IN THE PREVENTION OF SUDDEN CARDIAC DEATH BY β-ADRENERGIC-BLOCKING DRUGS

The sympathetic nervous system and circulating catecholamine levels are major factors involved in the mechanism of SCD. Increased sympathetic stimulation and measured circulating levels of catecholamines may produce or exacerbate potentially lethal arrhythmias and have unfavorable consequences of myocardial ischemia.

Table 29-4
Megatrials with β-Blockers for the Treatment of Hypertension

Trial	No. of Pts.	Drug	Mean Follow-Up (yr)	Coronary Heart Disease Mortality, % Reduction in	No. of Pts. Benefited per 100 Treated Pts.
MRC[58]	17,354	Propranolol/diuretic vs. placebo	4.9	NR	—
IPPPSH[59]	6,357	Oxprenolol vs. placebo	4.1	NR	—
HAPPHY[60]	6,569	Atenolol/metoprolol vs. diuretics	3.8	NR	—
MAPHY[61–63]	3,234	Metoprolol vs. diuretics	4.2	15 ($p = 0.048$)	0.4

NOTE: The coronary heart disease mortality reported in the table included deaths due to myocardial infarction or coronary sudden death. The reduction in total mortality (cardiovascular and noncardiovascular) was 20% ($p = 0.028$) and the reduction in cardiovascular mortality (fatal coronary heart disease, sudden death, pulmonary embolism, fatal stroke, heart failure, and aortic aneurysm) was 26% ($p = 0.012$). NR = no reduction.

The potential beneficial effects of β-blockers on the incidence of sudden death are probably related to their antiarrhythmic and anti-ischemic effects. The antiarrhythmic properties of β-blockers are mainly related to their counteracting effects on the adrenergic system. Therefore, β-blockers may control arrhythmias produced by enhanced automaticity (arrhythmia in MI, digoxin toxicity, etc.) and also those due to re-entry. The second antiarrhythmic mechanism of certain β-blockers is the "quinidine-like" membrane-stabilizing effect. This second mechanism is mostly seen at higher serum concentrations of β-blockers and probably is not the responsible one in common clinical situations. In one study[69] in which propranolol effectively suppressed ventricular arrhythmias in up to 70% of patients, 40% of the patients required blood concentrations of 150–1000 mg/mL. These concentrations are in excess of those required for β-adrenoreceptor blockade (25–150 mg/mL). Therefore, even though the antiarrhythmic response to propranolol commonly occurs at β-blocker concentrations, other additional electrophysiological effects seen at higher concentrations may contribute to antiarrhythmic efficacy.[70,71] Furthermore, the electrophysiological effects of β-blockers, which confer their antiarrhythmic properties, are different when these agents are given IV in the acute situation and when they are given orally over the long term.[62,72] In fact, Edmonsson and Olsson[73] reported that whereas short-term administration of metoprolol did not produce repolarization changes, long-term treatment was associated with prolongation of monophasic action potential duration and refractoriness.

However, in the common clinical setting, the major antiarrhythmic mechanism is β-blockade.[74–77] This is substantiated by effective antiarrhythmic activity possessed by β-blockers such as atenolol, practolol, and timolol, which lack membrane-stabilizing properties. In addition, the d-isomer of propranolol, which has membrane-stabilizing properties but only minimal β-blockade effects, is ineffective in suppressing arrhythmias.[76] These antiarrhythmic effects mediated through β-blockade may occur locally, at the cardiac level, at the CNS/autonomic system level, or peripherally, such as the counteraction of catecholamine-induced intracellular transmembrane potassium influx[77,78] or the reduction of lipolysis and free fatty acid production.[79]

The beneficial effects on mortality observed in various trials of β-blockers post-MI[11,12,22,24,27] probably result from a combination of various mechanisms. There is evidence that β-blockers are effective in suppressing ventricular arrhythmias in patients with various underlying heart diseases.[75] In post-MI trials, the incidence of ventricular ectopy increased during the first 6 weeks post MI in both treated and placebo groups; however, in the treated group, these increases were blunted.[38] A similar effect was seen in the Norwegian timolol study[37]: the incidence of postinfarction ventricular ectopy increased significantly in the placebo group but not in the timolol group. However, as noted by the investigators in the timolol trial,[37] the modest reduction in ventricular arrhythmias could not explain the marked reduction in mortality. Furthermore, the beneficial effect was also noted in the treated group of patients who did not have ventricular arrhythmias.[24,37,38] Therefore, other mechanisms more powerful than suppression of ventricular ectopy must have been responsible in these trials. Among these mechanisms, the prevention of VF may have played an important role in increasing survival in the treated groups. This has been clearly shown in the Göteburg[11] and Norris[18] trials but not in the ISIS-1[12] and MIAMI[15] trials. β-blockers have been shown to increase the defibrillatory thresholds in both ischemic and nonischemic myocardium.[20] These antifibrillatory properties may not be entirely mediated through a β-blockade mechanism.[80] Interruption of stellate ganglionic impulses accounted for part of the augmentation in the threshold for VF.[20] Therefore, the effect on survival may have been due to an increased level of vagal inhibition which through various mechanisms (lower heart rates, increased defibrillation threshold, etc.) may prevent SCD.[81] In fact, in a recent analysis[13] the beneficial β-blocker effect noted in post-MI trials was related to a quantitative reduction in heart rate, which may be due to both sympathetic blockade and an increased vagal tone. The lower heart rate probably contributed to the antiischemic and antifibrillatory effects of β-blockers.

The anti-ischemic effects and prevention of reinfarction are other important mechanisms in the prevention of sudden death. In some trials, the reinfarction rates were lower in the β-blocker group.[11,17,25] In the ISIS-1 study, atenolol decreased the incidence of cardiac rupture and of electromechanical dissociation that presumably was the result of cardiac rupture.[12] Therefore, hemodynamic factors (lower wall stress, lower afterload) may have contributed to the protection conferred by β-blockers in the post-MI patients.

ROLE OF VASODILATOR THERAPY IN PREVENTING SUDDEN CARDIAC DEATH IN PATIENTS WITH CHRONIC CONGESTIVE HEART FAILURE

SCD is common in patients with chronic heart failure, accounting for approximately 50–70% of total cardiac mortality.[82] Sudden unexpected death has traditionally been attributed to lethal ventricular arrhythmias. However, even though this may be true for a large proportion of deaths, recent data show that at least some of these unexpected deaths are due to bradyarrhythmias or to electromechanical dissociation.[83]

Prevalence and Pathogenesis of Ventricular Arrhythmias

Patients with chronic congestive heart failure have a high prevalence of ventricular arrhythmias.[84–105] In various studies, the prevalence of complex ventricular ectopy ranged from 71% to 98% and the frequency of nonsustained VT ranged from 39% to 80%. The prevalence of arrhythmias increases with the severity of left ventricular dysfunction. The prevalence of nonsustained VT was less than 10% in patients who were in New York Heart Association (NYHA) functional Class I and was 70% in patients who were in NYHA Class IV.[86]

The pathogenesis of arrhythmias in patients with heart failure is multifactorial and has not been fully elucidated. Multiple factors may act concomitantly; however, in the individual patient one or more mechanisms appear to be predominant (Table 29-5). The arrhythmogenic substrate is very rich in patients with heart failure. Dilation, hypertrophy, aneurysms, scarring, and various abnormalities at the cellular level may easily sustain re-entry, increased automaticity, and triggered activity. Among the modulating factors, ischemia may play an important role because of the large numbers of patients with heart failure due to coronary artery disease. However, other factors must

Table 29–5
Factors Involved in the Pathogenesis of Arrhythmias in Heart Failure

Ischemia
Electrolyte imbalance
  Hypokalemia
  Hypomagnesemia
Neurohormonal imbalance
  Sympathetic tone
  Renin-angiotensin
  Circulating catecholamines
Structural abnormalities
  Hypertrophy
  Dilation
  Aneurysm
  Scars
Drugs
  Digoxin
  Diuretics
  Inotropes
  Vasodilators
  Antiarrhythmics

be of equal importance because the prevalence of arrhythmias is quite uniform among various groups of patients with heart failure of different etiologies. Neurohumoral abnormalities typically seen in the presence of heart failure are potent arrhythmogenic factors. High levels of sympathetic activation and of circulating catecholamines, alone or in combination with hemodynamic factors, electrolyte abnormalities, and pharmacological factors, may all be contributory in the genesis of lethal arrhythmias.

Prevalence of Sudden Cardiac Death

The prevalence of SCD is variable in various studies and may range anywhere from 22% to 86%.[87–90,94,97–99,102] Mortality was found to be higher in patients with underlying coronary artery disease in two studies.[87,106] However, it is not clear if this increase in total mortality was due to a higher incidence of sudden death. Furthermore, the increase in mortality in patients with underlying coronary heart disease could not be confirmed in other studies.[84,88] There is a dissociation between the prevalence of ventricular arrhythmias and the incidence of SCD among the various classes of heart failure.[86] The total mortality per year ranges from 12% to 15% for NYHA Class I and may reach 60% for Class IV. The sudden-death mortality accounts for 50–60% of total mortality in patients in NYHA Classes I and II but only 20–30% in patients in NYHA Class IV.[84]

Relationship Between Ventricular Arrhythmias and Sudden Cardiac Death

It appears that the incidence of ventricular arrhythmia rises in parallel with the worsening of left ventricular dysfunction, while the incidence of SCD does the opposite; the majority of patients with NYHA Class IV heart failure are dying because of progressive heart failure.[107] The relationship between the frequency of complex ventricular ectopy and mortality is unclear.[88–90,95,97,98,101–105] It appears that the frequency of ventricular ectopy is, at best, a weak predictor for SCD but a better predictor of total mortality. Therefore, the high incidence of nonsustained ventricular arrhythmia is probably a marker of the severity of left ventricular dysfunction.

Large Trials with Vasodilators in Patients with Congestive Heart Failure

A large number of studies using various vasodilators have been performed; however, these studies were of small size and short duration and had not enough statistical power to assess the effect of treatment on survival.[106] In 1980, a Veteran Administrative Cooperative Study (V-HeFT I) was initiated to determine the value of vasodilators in prolonging survival in patients with NYHA Class II and III heart failure (Table 29-6).[108,109] A total of 642 men with chronic heart failure treated with digoxin and diuretic were randomized to additional treatment with placebo, prazosin (20 mg/day), or the combination of hydralazine (300 mg/day) with isosorbide dinitrate (160 mg/day). The average follow-up was 2.3 years. Over the whole period of the study, the difference in mortality was *not* significant.[110] However, the cumulative mortality at 2-year follow-up was 25.6% in the hydralazine-isosorbide dinitrate (ISDN) and 34.3% in the placebo group, with a reduction in mortality of 25% ($p < 0.028$ on Cox regression analysis but $p = 0.053$ on the log-rank test). The incidence of sudden death was 44% of total mortality and was presumed to be due to

Table 29-6
Large Randomized Placebo-Controlled Trials with Vasodilators in Patients with Chronic Congestive Heart Failure

Study	No. of Pts.	NYHA Functional Class	Drug (No. of Pts.)	Follow-Up (mo)	Total Mortality Placebo (%)	Total Mortality Treatment (%)	p Value	No. of Pts. Benefited per 100 Treated Pts.	Sudden Cardiac Death Treatment (%)	Sudden Cardiac Death Placebo (%)	p Value
V-HeFT-I[108]	359	II, III	ISDN + HYD (106) vs. placebo (273)	24	25.6	34.3	0.028 (0.053)*	8.7	NA	NA	NA
CONSENSUS[107]	253	IV	Enalapril (127) vs. placebo (126)	36	36.2	46.9	NA	10.7			
				6	26.0	44.0	0.002	18.0			
				12	36.0	46.0	0.001	10.0	11	11	NS
SOLVD[113]	2,569	II, III	Enalapril (1,285) vs. placebo (1,284)	48	35.2	39.7	0.036	4.5	8.2	8.8	NS

Abbreviations: HYD, hydralazine; ISDN, isosorbide dinitrate; NA, not available; NS, not significant.
* Cox life-table regression model yielded $p < 0.028$; however, the log-rank statistic yielded $p = 0.053$.

arrhythmia.[111] The ISDN-hydralazine combination reduced the incidence of sudden death as compared to placebo.[111] The total mortality was higher in patients with underlying coronary heart disease with a history of antiarrhythmic therapy and with low EFs.[109] The high incidence of arrhythmia (VPCs, couplets = 81%; nonsustained VT = 28%) had no prognostic value.[84,109]

In the V-HeFT II study,[112] the combination of ISDN-hydralazine was compared with enalapril in 804 men who were already receiving digoxin and diuretic therapy. Most of those enrolled were in NYHA Class II or III (only 6% were in Class I). The mortality at 2 years was significantly lower in the enalapril group (18% vs. 25%, $p = 0.016$), with a reduction in mortality of 28%. The reduction of mortality in the enalapril group was due to a lower incidence of SCD when compared to that in the ISDN-hydralazine group (with no warning, 16% vs. 25%, $p = 0.015$; with warning, 7% vs. 12%, $p = 0.032$). The classification of sudden death was done by a single investigator and brings up the issue of potential bias. The 25% mortality in the ISDN-hydralazine group was similar to that seen in the V-HeFT I study (26%), and in the V-HeFT I study the benefit of ISDN-hydralazine was, at best, of borderline statistical significance. The authors speculated that the added benefit of enalapril as compared to the ISDN-hydralazine combination may be due to a nonvasodilator mechanism. However, it is possible that the lower efficacy of the ISDN-hydralazine combination may have been due to its untoward effects on neurohormonal factors and not only to an additional protective effect of enalapril. This hypothesis is supported by the data obtained by Daly et al.[113] This study compared the effects of hydralazine, nitrates, and captopril on circulatory norepinephrine and net myocardial release of norepinephrine in patients with heart failure. The arterial norepinephrine and net myocardial norepinephrine release after the administration of hydralazine and nitrates tended to increase, whereas a relatively lower arterial norepinephrine and myocardial epinephrine release occurred with captopril.

The reduction in SCD seen in the V-HeFT I and II studies was not seen in the other two trials,[107,114] despite a striking benefit on mortality in the latter two trials. In the Cooperative North Scandinavian Enalapril Survival Study (CONSENSUS) trial,[107] 253 patients in NYHA Class IV due to heart failure were randomized to enalapril or placebo. The mortality was reduced in the enalapril arm of the study by 40% at 6 months (26% vs. 44%, $p = 0.002$) and by 31% at 1 year (36% vs. 52%, $p = 0.001$). However, the number of SCDs was similar in both arms of the study.

Enalapril was again compared with placebo in patients in NYHA Classes II and III due to heart failure in a much larger study.[114] The Studies of Left Ventricular Dysfunction (SOLVD) investigators enrolled 2569 patients and followed them up for 48 months. The results of this study confirmed that enalapril reduced the mortality of patients in NYHA Classes II and III due to heart failure. The largest reduction in mortality occurred among deaths attributed to progressive congestive heart failure. The number of deaths due to arrhythmia was similar in the two arms of the study.

The mechanisms involved in the reduction of mortality in patients with heart failure treated with enalapril is not clear. Its superiority over the combination of ISDN-hydralazine[112] may suggest that mechanisms other than vasodilation could be operating in these patients. Some authors have suggested that enalapril may reduce ventricular arrhythmias in patients with heart failure.[115,116] However, these studies were small, and the findings could not be confirmed in larger studies.[86,117] A subset of patients in the CONSENSUS study[86] underwent 24-hour ECG monitoring at baseline and again after 6 weeks of treatment. There was no difference in the incidence of arrhythmia between the survivors and those who died. Furthermore, 70% of the patients had nonsustained VT at baseline; at 6 months, no correlation between mortality and nonsustained VT could be found. In another double-blind, parallel placebo-controlled trial[117] directed to assess the effect of enalapril on ventricular arrhythmias in 153 patients with heart failure, no difference was found between the two groups at 4 and 12 months' follow-up. Therefore, it appears that enalapril may be devoid of antiarrhythmic activity. The beneficial effect of enalapril may be due to its effects on neurohormonal imbalance. Higher serum and total body potassium levels and lower levels of plasma norepinephrine have been reported for both captopril and enalapril.[118,119]

In conclusion, vasodilator therapy is an effective form of treatment in patients with chronic heart failure; ACE inhibitors appear to be superior to other vasodilators. Despite the beneficial effect on total mortality, the effects of ACE inhibitors on SCD are still conflicting. Further investigation is necessary to elucidate the role of ACE inhibitor therapy in preventing or reducing SCD.

REFERENCES

1. Ahlquist RP: Study of adrenotropic receptors. Am J Physiol 153:586–598, 1948.
2. Black JW, Stephenson JS: Pharmacology of new adrenergic beta-receptor-blocking compound (netholide). Lancet ii:311–314, 1962.
3. Black JW, Crowther AF, Shanks RG, Smith LH, Dornhorst AC: New adrenergic beta receptor agonist. Lancet i:1080–1084, 1964.
4. Multicenter Trial of Propranolol in Acute Myocardial Infarction. Lancet ii:551–555, 1965.
5. Balcon R, Jewith DE, Daries JPH, Oram J: A controlled trial of propranolol in myocardial infarction. Lancet 2:917–920, 1966.
6. Norris RM, Coughey DE, Scott PJ: Trial of propranolol in acute myocardial infarction. Br Med J ii:398–400, 1968.
7. Snow PJD, Manc MD: Effect of propranolol on myocardial infarction. Lancet ii:551–555, 1965.
8. Snow PJD: Treatment of acute myocardial infarction with propranolol. Am J Cardiol 18:458–462, 1966.
9. May GS: A review of acute-phase beta blocker trials in patients with myocardial infarction. Circulation 67(suppl I):I-21–I-25, 1983.
10. Yusuf S, Peto R, Lewis J, Collins R, Sleight P: Beta blockade during and after myocardial infarction: An overview of randomized trials. Prog Cardiovasc Dis 5:335–371, 1985.
11. Hjalmarson A, Elmfeldt D, Herlitz J, et al: Effect on mortality of metoprolol in acute myocardial infarction: A double-blind randomized trial. Lancet ii:823–827, 1981.
12. ISIS-1 (First International Study of Infarct Survival) Collaborative Group: Randomized trial of intravenous atenolol among 16,027 cases of suspected acute myocardial infarction: ISIS-1. Lancet ii:57–66, 1986.
13. Kjekshus JK: Importance of heart rate in determining beta-blocker efficacy in acute and long-term acute myocardial infarction intervention trials. Am J Cardiol 57:43F–49F, 1986.
14. Herlitz J, Elmfeldt D, Holmberg S, et al: Göteborg Metoprolol Trial: Mortality and causes of death. Am J Cardiol 53:9D–14D, 1984.
15. Herlitz J, Hjalmarson A, Swedberg K, Ryden L, Waagstein F: Effects on mortality during five years after early intervention with metoprolol in suspected acute myocardial infarction. Acta Med Scand 223:227–231, 1988.
16. MIAMI Trial Research Group: Metoprolol in Acute Myocardial Infarction (MIAMI): A randomized, placebo controlled international trial. Eur Heart J 6:199–226, 1985.
17. TIMI Study Group: Comparison of invasive and conservative strategies after treatment with intravenous tissue plasminogen activator in acute myocardial infarction: Results of the Thrombolysis in Myocardial Infarction (TIMI) phase II trial. N Engl J Med 320:618–627, 1989.
18. Norris RM, Barnaby PF, Brown MA, et al: Prevention of ventricular fibrillation during acute myocardial infarction by intravenous propranolol. Lancet i:883–886, 1984.
19. Lube WF, Muller CA, Worthington M, McFadyen EL, Opie LH: Influence of propranolol isomers and atenolol on myocardial cyclic AMP, high energy phosphates and vulnerability to fibrillation after coronary artery ligation in the isolated rat heart. Cardiovasc Res 15:690–699, 1981.
20. Anderson JL, Rodier HE, Green LS: Comparative effects of beta-adrenergic blocking drugs on experimental ventricular fibrillation threshold. Am J Cardiol 51:1196–1202, 1983.
21. May GS: A review of long-term beta blocker trials in survivors of myocardial infarction. Circulation 67(suppl I):I-46–I-49, 1983.
22. Multicenter International Study: Improvement of prognosis of myocardial infarction by long-term beta-adrenoreceptor blockade using practolol. Br Med J 3:735–740, 1975.
23. Multicenter International Study: Reduction in mortality after myocardial infarction with long-term beta-adrenoreceptor blockade: Supplementary report. Br Med J 2:419–425, 1977.
24. Norwegian Multicenter Study Group: Timolol-induced reduction in mortality and reinfarction in patients surviving myocardial

infarction. N Engl J Med *304:*801–807, 1981.
25. Gundersen T, Abrahamsen AM, Kjekshus J, Ronmerik PK, for the Norwegian Multicenter Study Group: Timolol-related reduction in mortality and reinfarction in patients age 65–75 years surviving acute myocardial infarction. Circulation *66:*1179–1184, 1982.
26. Pedersen TR, for the Norwegian Multicenter Study Group: Six-year follow-up of the Norwegian multicenter study on timolol after acute myocardial infarction. N Engl J Med *313:*1055–1058, 1985.
27. Beta-Blocker Heart Attack Trial Research Group: A randomized trial of propranolol in patients with myocardial infarction: I. Mortality results. JAMA *247:*1707–1717, 1982.
28. Peters RW, Byington R, Arensberg D, et al: Mortality in the Beta Blocker Heart Attack Trial: Circumstances surrounding death. J Chronic Dis *40:*75–82, 1987.
29. Peters RW, Muller JE, Goldstein S, et al: Propanolol and the morning increase in frequency of sudden cardiac death (BHAT study). Am J Cardiol *63:*1518–1520, 1989.
30. Furberg CD, Hawkins CM, Lichstein E, for the Beta-Blocker Heart Attack Trial Study Group: Effect of propranolol in postinfarction patients with mechanical or electrical complications. Circulation *69:*761–765, 1984.
31. Jafri SM, Tilley BC, Peters R, Schultz LR, Goldstein S: Effects of cigarette smoking and propranolol in survivors of acute myocardial infarction. Am J Cardiol *65:* 271–276, 1990.
32. Julian DG, Prescott RJ, Jackson FS, Szekely P: A controlled trial of sotalol for one year after myocardial infarction. Lancet *i:* 1142, 1982.
33. European Infarction Study Group: European Infarction Study (EIS): A secondary prevention study with slow release oxprenolol after myocardial infarction. Eur Heart J *3:*583–586, 1982.
34. European Infarction Study Group: European Infarction Study (EIS): A secondary prevention study with slow release oxprenolol after myocardial infarction. Eur Heart J *5:*189–202, 1984.
35. Taylor SH, Silke B, Ebbutt A, Sutton GC, Pront BJ, Burley DM: A long-term prevention study with oxprenol in coronary heart disease. N Engl J Med *307:*1293–1301, 1982.
36. Lopressor Intervention Trial: Multicenter study of metoprolol in survivors of acute myocardial infarction. Eur Heart J *8:* 1056–1064, 1987.
37. Von der Lippe G, Lung-Johansen P, Kjekshus J: Effect of timolol on late ventricular arrhythmias after myocardial infarction. Acta Med Scand *651(suppl):*253–258, 1981.
38. Lichstein E, Morganroth J, Horrist R, Hubble E, for the BHAT Study Group: Effect of propranolol or ventricular arrhythmias: The beta-blocker heart attack trial experience. Circulation *65(suppl I):*I-5–I-10, 1983.
39. Bethge KP, Andersen D, Boissel JP, et al: Effect of oxprenol on ventricular arrhythmias: The European Infarction Study experience. J Am Coll Cardiol *6:*963–972, 1985.
40. Kotis BJ, Byington R, Friedman LM, et al, for the BHAT Study Group: Prognostic significance of ventricular ectopic activity in survivors of myocardial infarction. J Am Coll Cardiol *10:*231–242, 1987.
41. Kostis JD, Wilson AC, Sanders MR, Byington RP, for the BHAT Study Group: Prognostic significance of ventricular ectopic activity in survivors of acute myocardial infarction who receive propranolol. Am J Cardiol *61:*975–978, 1988.
42. Yusuf S, Sleight P, Rossi P, et al: Reduction of infarct size, arrhythmias and chest pain by early intravenous beta blockade in suspected acute myocardial infarction. Circulation *67(suppl):*I-32–I-41, 1983.
43. International Collaborative Study Group: Reduction of infarct size with early use of timolol during acute myocardial infarction. N Engl J Med *310:*9–15, 1984.
44. Beta-Blocker Pooling Project Research Group: The Beta-Blocker Pooling Project (BBPP): Subgroup findings from randomized trials in post infarction patients. Eur Heart J *9:*8–16, 1988.
45. Norris RM: β-adrenoreceptor blockers: An update on their role in myocardial infarction. Drugs *29:*97–104, 1985.
46. Griggs TR, Wagner GS, Beltes LS: Beta-adrenergic blocking agents after myocardial infarction: An undocumented need in patients at lowest risk. J Am Coll Cardiol *1:*1530–1533, 1983.
47. Chamberlain DA: Beta-adrenoreceptor antagonist after myocardial infarction: Where are we now? Br Heart J *49:*105–110, 1983.
48. Ahumada GG: Identification of patients who do not require beta antagonists after myocardial infarction. Am J Med *76:* 900–904, 1984.
49. Frishman WH, Furberg CD, Friedewald WT: Beta-adrenergic blockade for survivors of acute myocardial infarction. N Engl J Med *310:*830–836, 1984.
50. Chadda K, Goldstein S, Byington R, Curb JD: Effect of propranolol after acute myo-

cardial infarction in patients with congestive heart failure. Circulation 73:503–510, 1986.
51. Gundersen T: Secondary prevention after myocardial infarction: Subgroup analysis of patients at risk in the Norwegian timolol multicenter study. Clin Cardiol 8:253–265, 1985.
52. Olsson G, Olden A, Johansson R, Sjögren A, Rehnqvist N: Prognosis after withdrawal of chronic post infarction metoprolol treatment: A 27 year follow-up. Eur Heart J 9:365–372, 1988.
53. Goldman L, Sia B, Cook EF, Rutherford JD, Weinstein M: Cost and effectiveness of routine therapy with long-term beta-adrenergic antagonists after acute myocardial infarction. N Engl J Med 319:152–157, 1988.
54. Olsson G, Levin LA, Rehnqvist N: Economic consequences of post infarction prophylaxis with β blockers: Cost effectiveness of metoprolol. Br Med J 294:339–342, 1987.
55. MacMahon S, Peto R, Cutler J, et al: Blood pressure and coronary heart disease: Part I. Prolonged differences in blood pressure. Prospective observational studies corrected for the regressional dilution bias. Lancet 335:765–774, 1990.
56. Multiple Risk Factor Intervention Trial (MRFIT) Research Group: Baseline post electrocardiographic abnormalities, antihypertensive treatment and mortality in the Multiple Risk Factor Intervention Trial. Am J Cardiol 55:1–15, 1985.
57. Culter JA, MacMahon SW, Furberg CD: Controlled clinical trials of drug treatment for hypertension. Hypertension 13(suppl I):I-36–I-44, 1989.
58. Medical Research Council Working Party: MRC trial of treatment of mild hypertension: Principal results. Br Med J 291:91–104, 1985.
59. IPPPSH Collaborative Group: Cardiovascular risk and risk factors in a randomized trial of treatment based on the beta blocker oxprenolol: The International Perspective Primary Prevention Study in Hypertension (IPPPSH). J Hypertens 3:379–392, 1985.
60. Wilhemssen L, Berglund G, Elmfeldt D, et al, and the Heart Attack Primary Prevention in Hypertension Trial Research Group (HAPPHY): Beta-blockers versus diuretics in hypertensive men: Main results from HAPPHY trial. J Hypertension 5:561–572, 1987.
61. Wikstrand J, Warnold I, Olsson G, et al: Primary prevention with metoprolol in patients with hypertension: Mortality results from MAPHY study. JAMA 259:1976–1982, 1988.
62. Olsson G, Tuomilehto J, Berglund G, et al, for the MAPHY Study Group: Primary prevention of sudden cardiac death in hypertensive patients: Mortality results from MAPHY study. Am J Hypertens 4:151–158, 1991.
63. Wikstrand J, Warnold I, Tuomilehto J, et al: Metoprolol versus thiazide diuretics in hypertension: Morbidity results from MAPHY study. Hypertens 17:579–588, 1991.
64. Primary prevention with metoprolol in patients with hypertension [letter]. JAMA 260:1713–1716, 1988.
65. Moser M, Sheps S: Confusing messages from the newest of the β-blocker/diuretic hypertension trials: The Metoprolol Atherosclerosis Prevention in Hypertension trials. Arch Intern Med 149:2174–2175, 1989.
66. MAPHY, and the two arms of HAPPHY: Letters to the editor. JAMA 262:3272–3274, 1989.
67. Kaplan NM: Critical comments on recent literature: SCRAAPHY about MAPHY from HAPPHY. Am J Hypertens 1:428–430, 1988.
68. Collins R, Peto R, MacMahon S, Hebert P, et al: Blood pressure, stroke and coronary heart disease: Part 2. Short-term reduction in blood pressure. Overview of randomized drug trials in their epidemiologic context. Lancet 335:827–838, 1990.
69. Woosley R, Kornhauser D, Smith R, et al: Suppression of chronic ventricular arrhythmias with propranolol. Circulation 60:819–827, 1979.
70. Duff H, Mitchell B, Wyse G: Antiarrhythmic efficacy of propranolol: Comparison of low and high serum concentrations. J Am Coll Cardiol 8:959–965, 1986.
71. Raine AFG, Vaughan-Williams EM: Adaptation to prolonged β-blockade on rabbit atrial, Purkinje, and ventricular potentiates and papillary muscle contraction. Circ Res 48:804–812, 1981.
72. Venditti FJ, Garan H, Ruskin J: Electrophysiologic effects of beta blockers in ventricular arrhythmias. Am J Cardiol 60:3D–9D, 1987.
73. Edmonsson N, Olsson SD: Effects of acute and chronic beta receptor blockade on ventricular repolarization in man. Br Heart J 45:628–636, 1982.
74. Pratt C, Lichstein E: Ventricular antiarrhythmic effects of beta adrenergic blocking drugs: A review of mechanisms and clinical studies. J Clin Pharmacol 22:335–347, 1982.
75. Morganroth J: Antiarrhythmic effects of

beta-adrenergic blocking agents in benign or potentially lethal ventricular arrhythmias. Am J Cardiol 60:10D–14D, 1987.
76. Barrett AM, Cullum VA: The biological properties of the optical isomers of propranolol and their effect on cardiac arrhythmias. Br J Pharmacol 34:43–55, 1968.
77. Brown MJ, Brown DC, Murphy MB: Hypokalemia from beta$_2$ receptor stimulation by circulating epinephrine. N Engl J Med 39:1414–1419, 1983.
78. Nordehaug JE, Johannenssen KA, von der Lippe G, et al: Effect of timolol on changes in serum potassium concentration during acute myocardial infarction. Br Heart J 53:388–393, 1985.
79. Frishman WH: β-adrenergic blockade in the prevention of sudden cardiac death. In Kostis JB, Saunder M (eds): Wilex-Liss, 1990, pp 139–153.
80. Patterson E, Lucchesi BR: Antifibrillatory properties of beta-adrenergic receptor antagonists, nodolol, sotalol, atenolol and propranolol in the anesthetized dog. Pharmacology 28:121–129, 1984.
81. Eckberg DL: Beta blockade may prolong life in post-infarction patients in part by increasing vagal inhibition. Med Hypoth 15:421–432, 1984.
82. Oakley C: Genesis of arrhythmias in the failing heart and therapeutic implication. Am J Cardiol 67:26C–28C, 1991.
83. Luu M, Stevenson WG, Stevenson LW, Baron K, Wolden J: Diverse mechanisms of unexpected cardiac arrest in advanced heart failure. Circulation 80:1675–1680, 1959.
84. Francis G: Development of arrhythmias in the patients with congestive heart failure: Pathophysiology, procedure and prognosis. Am J Cardiol 57:3B–7B, 1986.
85. Massie BM, Conway M: Survival of patients with congestive heart failure: Post, present and future prospects. Circulation 75(suppl IV):IV-11–IV-19, 1987.
86. Kjekshus J: Arrhythmias in mortality in congestive heart failure. Am J Cardiol 65:42-I–48-I, 1990.
87. Franciosa JA, Wilen M, Ziesche S, Cohn JN: Survival in men with severe chronic left ventricular failure due to either coronary heart disease or idiopathic dilated cardiomyopathy. Am J Cardiol 51:832–836, 1983.
88. Wilson JR, Schwartz S, St. John Sutton M, et al: Prognosis in severe heart failure: Relation to hemodynamic measurements and ventricular ectopic activity. J Am Coll Cardiol 2:403–410, 1983.
89. Meinertz T, Hofmann T, Kasper W, et al: Significance of ventricular arrhythmias in idiopathic dilated cardiomyopathy. Am J Cardiol 53:902–907, 1984.
90. Chakko CS, Gheorghiade M: Ventricular arrhythmias in severe heart failure: Incidence, significance and effectiveness of antiarrhythmic therapy. Am Heart J 109:497–504, 1985.
91. Maskin CS, Siskind SJ, LeJemtel TH: High prevalence of nonsustained ventricular tachycardia in severe congestive heart failure. Am Heart J 107:896–901, 1984.
92. Cleland JGF, Dargie HJ, Ford I: Mortality in heart failure: Clinical variables of prognostic value. Br Heart J 58:572–582, 1987.
93. Nicolic G, Bishop RL, Singh JB: Sudden death recorded during Holter monitoring. Circulation 66:218–225, 1982.
94. Huang SK, Messer JV, Denes P: Significance of ventricular tachycardia in idiopathic dilated cardiomyopathy: Observations in 35 patients. Am J Cardiol 51:507:512, 1983.
95. Bigger JT: Why patients with congestive heart failure die: Arrhythmias and sudden cardiac death. Circulation 75:28–35, 1987.
96. Ikegawa T, Chino M, Hasegawa H, et al: Prognostic significance of 24 hour ambulatory electrocardiographic monitoring in patients with dilative cardiomyopathy: A prospective study. Clin Cardiol 10:78–82, 1987.
97. Von Olshausen K, Schafer A, Mehmel HC, Schwarz F, Senges J, Kubler W: Ventricular arrhythmias in idiopathic dilated cardiomyopathy. Br Heart J 51:195–201, 1984.
98. Holmes J, Kubo SH, Cody RJ, Kligfield P: Arrhythmias in ischemic and nonischemic dilated cardiomyopathy: Prediction of mortality by ambulatory electrocardiography. Am J Cardiol 55:146–151, 1985.
99. Sakurai T, Kawai C: Sudden death in idiopathic cardiomyopathy: Jpn Circ J 47:581–585, 1983.
100. Poll DS, Marchlinsky FE, Buxton AE, Doherty JU, Waxman HL, Josephson ME: Sustained ventricular tachycardia in patients with idiopathic dilated cardiomyopathy: Electrophysiologic testing and lack of response to antiarrhythmic drug therapy. Circulation 70:451–456, 1984.
101. Unverferth DV, Magorien RD, Moeschberger ML, Baker PB, Fetters JK, Leier CV: Factors influencing the one-year mortality of dilated cardiomyopathy. Am J Cardiol 54:147–152, 1984.
102. Gradman A, Deedwania P, Cody R, et al, for the Captopril-Digoxin Study Group: Predictors of total mortality and sudden death in mild to moderate heart failure. J Am Coll Cardiol 14:564–570, 1989.

103. Francis GS: Should asymptomatic ventricular arrhythmias in patients with congestive heart failure be treated with antiarrhythmic drugs? I. Introduction. J Am Coll Cardiol 12:274–276, 1988.
104. Chatterjee K: Should asymptomatic ventricular arrhythmias in patients with congestive heart failure be treated with antiarrhythmic drugs? II. Protagonist's viewpoint. J Am Coll Cardiol 12:276–278, 1988.
105. Prystowsky EN: Should asymptomatic ventricular arrhythmias in patients with congestive heart failure be treated with antiarrhythmic drugs? III. Antagonist's viewpoint. J Am Coll Cardiol 12:280–283, 1988.
106. Furberg CD, Yusuf S: Effect of drug therapy on survival inchronic congestive heart failure. Am J Cardiol 62:41A–45A, 1988.
107. CONSENSUS Trial Study Group: Effects of enalapril on mortality in severe congestive heart failure: results of the Cooperative North Scandinavian Enalapril Survival Study (CONSENSUS). N Engl J Med 316: 1429–1435, 1987.
108. Cohn JN, Archibald DG, Ziesche S, et al: Results of a Veterans Administration Cooperative Study: Effect of vasodilator therapy on mortality in chronic congestive heart failure. N Engl J Med 314:1547–1552, 1986.
109. Cohn JN, Archibald DG, Francis GS, et al: Veterans Administration Cooperative Study on Vasodilator Therapy of Heart Failure: Influence of prerandomization variables on the reduction of mortality by treatment with hydralazine and isosorbide dinitrate. Circulation 75(suppl IV):IV-49, 1987.
110. Rahimtoola SH: The pharmacologic treatment of chronic congestive heart failure. Circulation 80:693–699, 1989.
111. Cohn J: Mechanisms in heart failure and the role of angiotensin-converting enzyme inhibition. Am J Cardiol 66:2D–6D, 1990.
112. Cohn JN, Johnson G, Ziesche S, et al: A comparison of enalapril with hydralazine-isosorbide dinitrate in the treatment of chronic congestive heart failure. N Engl J Med 325:303–310, 1991.
113. Daly P, Roulean JL, Cousineu D, Burgess JH, Chatterjee K: Effects of captopril and hydralazine plus isosorbide dinitrate on myocardia sympathetic tone in patients with severe congestive heart failure. Br Heart J 56:12–18, 1986.
114. SOLVD Investigators: Effect of enalapril on survival in patients with reduced left ventricular ejection fractions and congestive heart failure. N Engl J Med 325: 293–302, 1991.
115. Webster MWI, Fitzpatrick A, Nicholls G, Ikram H, Wells E: Effects of enalapril on ventricular arrhythmias in congestive heart failure. Am J Cardiol 56:566–569, 1985.
116. Cleland JGF, Dargie HJ: Arrhythmias, catecholamines and electrolytes. Am J Cardiol 52:55A–59A, 1988.
117. Pratt C, Gardner M, Pepine C, et al, for the SOLVD Investigators: Lack of long-term ventricular arrhythmia reduction by enalapril in heart failure patients: A double blind, parallel placebo control trial [abstract]. Circulation 84(suppl II):II-348, 1991.
118. Cleland JGJ, Dargie HJ, Hodsmon GP, et al: Captopril in heart failure: A double blind controlled clinical trial. Br Heart J 52: 530–535, 1984.
119. Cleland JGF, Dargie HJ, Ball GS, et al: Effect of enalapril on heart failure: A double blind study of effects on exercise performance, renal function, hormones and metabolic state. Br Heart J 54:305–312, 1985.

30

Results of the Cardiac Arrhythmia Suppression Trial

RAYMOND L. WOOSLEY

CLINICAL AND SCIENTIFIC RATIONALE OF CAST

In the middle of the twentieth century, electrocardiographic (ECG) monitoring during acute myocardial infarction (MI) led to the concept of "warning arrhythmias" as harbingers of ventricular fibrillation (VF). Analyzing ECG data taped in the coronary care unit (CCU), Lown and Wolfe[1] predicted that there should be a relationship between the frequency and complexity of ventricular arrhythmias and the incidence of VF. The Lown grading system for ventricular arrhythmias became the basis for what has been termed the "PVC hypothesis." The hypothesis in its simplest form is that premature ventricular complexes (PVCs) are triggers for VF and that higher PVC frequency is associated with greater risk for sudden death. Simultaneously, ambulatory monitoring of cardiac rhythm was being developed by Holter.[2] As recorders became smaller, the technology rapidly improved and clinical studies began to examine the possible relationship between ambient ventricular arrhythmias and sudden cardiac death (SCD). Large clinical trials in patients with prior MI found that asymptomatic ventricular arrhythmias that were detected during ambulatory monitoring identified patients at an increased risk of sudden and, interestingly, nonsudden death.[3] There was a positive correlation between the risk of sudden death and the frequency and complexity of PVCs. A standard terminology based on the correlation between arrhythmias and sudden death in discrete populations was subsequently adopted by clinical researchers.[4] Asymptomatic ventricular arrhythmias in the absence of structural heart disease were termed "benign," whereas those same arrhythmias in a person with a history of ischemic heart disease were declared "potentially lethal" because they identified a patient at increased risk of sudden death. Arrhythmias such as recurrent ventricular tachycardia (VT) and/or VF were termed "malignant" because they are usually very symptomatic and often led to premature death.

Meanwhile, physicians in the 1960s observed that lidocaine was very effective at suppressing PVCs occurring in the CCU, and the pharmaceutical industry began research programs to develop orally effective agents that could be used for chronic oral therapy of arrhythmias. With the availability of ambulatory monitoring and newly developed computers able to rapidly quantify the frequency of PVCs, suppression of PVCs became a target of antiarrhythmic drug studies.[5] Because it could more easily be measured, the suppression of asymptomatic PVCs became a surrogate end point for clinical drug efficacy. The Lown group of investigators assessed PVC suppression during repeated periods of ambulatory monitoring and exercise testing and recommended this form of "acute drug testing" to guide therapy for patients with symptomatic ventricular arrhythmias.[6] Because the presence of PVCs was known to be a risk factor for sudden death, because PVCs could be readily quantified using ambulatory monitoring, and because orally active antiarrhythmic drugs were available, physicians concluded that it was necessary to reduce the risk of sudden death by suppressing PVCs. Extensive surveys of physician practice patterns documented the widespread practice of prescribing antiarrhythmic drugs to suppress PVCs in patients with ischemic heart disease.[7,8]

The usual practice of physicians was to obtain a 24-hour ambulatory ECG recording 7–14 days after an MI. If high-frequency PVCs (variously defined) or complex PVCs (couplets or runs of VT) were detected, antiarrhythmic therapy was considered essential for these "potentially lethal arrhythmias."[4] During drug therapy a second ambulatory ECG was recorded, and if the arrhythmia appeared to be suppressed, the patients were continued on this therapy indefinitely. Studies by Morganroth et al[9] gave guidelines for determining whether drug therapy had produced a statistically significant change in arrhythmia frequency. The issue of "clinically significant suppression" was rarely raised.

The practice of treating asymptomatic PVCs was supported by the uncontrolled reports of antiarrhythmic drugs being effective in preventing arrhythmia recurrence in patients with recurrent sustained VT induced by programmed ventricular stimulation.[10,11] These reports observed fewer symptomatic recurrences and fewer episodes of sudden death in the group of patients for whom a drug could be found that suppressed induction of VT. Because of the highly symptomatic nature of the arrhythmias in these populations, placebo-controlled studies were not feasible. However, the experience in this population was extrapolated to most other clinical settings, especially those involving patients with a history of ischemic heart disease. Vlay surveyed cardiologists in 65 academic centers and found that 50–90% prescribed antiarrhythmic drugs for patients with PVCs and any form of structural heart disease.[7] Ten percent of physicians felt that PVCs should be suppressed even in patients without structural heart disease. In the 1980s, the rationale of suppressing the risk factor, in this case PVCs, in the hope of reducing sudden death was indirectly given support by the finding of improved mortality through the treatment of other risk factors such as hypertension and hypercholesterolemia.

THE CARDIAC ARRHYTHMIA PILOT STUDY (CAPS)

Scientists at the National Institutes of Health (NIH) recognized the potential folly in the logic being used for antiarrhythmic drug therapy and called for an investigation of the value of antiarrhythmic therapy for asymptomatic arrhythmias. The problem was complicated by the fact that the clinical environment was changing rapidly. New technologies, such as signal-averaged ECGs and programmed ventricular stimulation, were being developed and applied broadly. Many new drugs were becoming available for clinical use, but basic information about these or even about the conventional antiarrhythmic drugs was often missing. Ultimately, the National Heart, Lung and Blood Institute (NHLBI) decided to conduct a pilot study to obtain some of the information that would be needed to design a much larger study evaluating the clinical merit of what had become common clinical practice, PVC suppression. Ten clinical centers and a coordinating center successfully competed for a participating role in the planning and execution of a pilot study. The pilot study, commonly referred to as CAPS, for Cardiac Arrhythmia Pilot Study, was begun in 1983. The objectives of CAPS were to obtain the information necessary for the possible future conduct of a trial to evaluate the ability of antiarrhythmic drugs to reduce SCD. However, at that time there was no single agent known that was uniformly effective at suppressing ventricular arrhythmias or that could be tolerated by a large fraction of patients for 1 or more years, the period considered to encompass the highest risk of sudden death. Therefore, CAPS sought to find a therapeutic strategy that would reduce arrhythmia frequency in asymptomatic patients with an acceptably low prevalence of adverse effects. The study was designed to find methods to evaluate drug efficacy and to determine the feasibility of recruiting and maintaining patients on drug therapy.

Eighteen drugs or drug combinations were considered as candidates for the trial. The investigators decided that it would be essential to have several drugs in the study since no single drug appeared to be uniformly effective in suppressing PVCs. There was also concern that none of the more effective or better tolerated drugs had been tested in patients with a prior MI, i.e., the likely target population. Neither overall response rate nor dose response had been established in this population.

The selection of a drug or drugs to be evaluated in CAPS was a difficult and controversial part of the protocol design. Many of the co-investigators designing the study desired that one of the established drugs such as quinidine, disopyramide, or procainamide be included. However, none of these drugs was included because of the prior published experience in which the rate of adverse effects caused excessive withdrawals that would threaten the power to detect a beneficial effect on mortality. The investigators chose encainide and flecainide as prototypic agents for the potent sodium channel blocking drugs. Each had proved capable of a high degree of arrhythmia suppression in patients with stable, high-frequency PVCs. They were selected over many other agents because it appeared that they would soon be marketed and, according to the limited comparative data available at that time, they appeared to be tolerated far better than conventional agents. In order to include drugs with a possibly different mechanism of action, moricizine and imipramine were chosen as the other two agents to be compared to placebo. Moricizine, a phenothiazine, had a very favorable side effect profile, and imipramine had a large clinical experience in the treatment of depression. There was appeal to the possibility that these drugs might be "CNS-acting" drugs.

It was decided that 500 patients with recent MI would be enrolled in a placebo-controlled evaluation of 1 year of therapy that suppressed PVCs. Entry criteria required that the patients had previously experienced a fully documented MI within 6–60 days. Also, the patients had to have frequent asymptomatic ventricular arrhythmias and reasonably good ventricular function. Patients with marked reduction in ventricular performance (ejection fraction < 0.20) were excluded because there was very little experience with these drugs in patients with reduced ventricular function and because of growing concern about the negative inotropic actions of related drugs such as disopyramide. Because neither the pharmacokinetics nor the safety of these drugs had been established in the elderly, patients 75 years of age or older were excluded.

There was a great deal of concern about the ability to measure an antiarrhythmic effect. In order to reduce the risk that random changes in arrhythmia frequency could mimic response to a drug, patients with high-frequency arrhythmia were selected. After PVCs were detected on a screening ambulatory 24-hour ECG a baseline 24-hour ambulatory ECG was performed, and only patients with ≥ 10 PVCs/hr or ≥ 5 episodes of unsustained VT (3–9 consecutive PVCs with a rate ≥ 100/min) qualified. Patients with ≥ 10 consecutive PVCs were excluded because there was concern that they should not be given placebo and that many physicians would want to treat them with antiarrhythmic drugs.

Patients who qualified were randomized to receive either placebo or one of the four drugs in double-blind fashion. Because it had become clinical practice to use ambulatory monitoring to evaluate the response to these and similar agents, the response of each patient was evaluated by repeated monitoring for 24 hours at steady state for each dosage of the drug. Patients randomized to receive placebo remained on placebo regardless of their monitoring results. The coordinating center for the study controlled dose titration and directed investigators to increase the dosage if necessary, even for patients receiving placebo. Up to three dose levels of the first drug were permitted to be given if necessary. Titration of response continued until efficacy (defined as $\geq 70\%$ reduction in PVC and $>90\%$ reduction in unsustained VT) was observed during analysis of repeat ambulatory ECG recordings. If suppression was not possible with the first drug or if the patients were intolerant or developed "proarrhythmia" (defined below), they could receive one of the two agents in the other general class. The coordinating center instructed the investigators to stop titration if suppression or proarrhythmia was observed and to have the subjects continue on their "effective" dose or placebo for 1 year of evaluation. Patients were seen every 3 months for repeat ambulatory ECG monitoring and evaluation of tolerance and compliance.

CAPS was one of the first clinical studies to employ a rigorous definition of proarrhythmia. It was based on the previously determined relationship between baseline arrhythmia frequency and arrhythmia variability observed in a similar clinical population. It required a three- to tenfold increase in PVC frequency and a return to baseline after discontinuation of drug therapy.

After successfully enrolling and following 500 patients for at least 1 year, the CAPS investigators reached the following conclusions[12]:

1. It was feasible to identify and enroll patients after MI with the frequency of asymptomatic ventricular arrhythmias that had been previously identified as a risk factor for a moderate increase in sudden death.
2. A statistically significant reduction in ventricular arrhythmia frequency could be accomplished with three of the four drugs.
3. Three of the four drugs were well tolerated, and patient compliance with therapy was at an acceptable level throughout the study.
4. The frequency of proarrhythmic events with each drug was low and could not be distinguished from that due to random increases in arrhythmia frequency in the placebo group.
5. Congestive heart failure occurred frequently and had to be considered in the design of future studies.
6. A full study to test the hypothesis that suppression of ventricular arrhythmias in patients with prior MI was feasible and should be initiated.

CARDIAC ARRHYTHMIA SUPPRESSION TRIAL (CAST)

After reviewing the results of CAPS, the NHLBI called for proposals to compete for participation in an international multicenter test of this hypothesis. Twenty-seven sites and a coordinating center were chosen to design the study, now known as the Cardiac Arrhythmia Suppression Trial (CAST). Patient enrollment began in June 1987. Because several hospitals and co-investigators participated at each site, the planning and protocol design was performed by a group of approximately 100 cardiologists, clinical pharmacologists, biostatisticians, and experts in clinical trial design. Several of the sites had participated in the Beta Blocker Heart Attack Trial (BHAT), CAPS, or other similar studies, and all were experienced clinical investigators. Numerous committees were formed to seek a consensus on the many difficult issues to be faced in designing and conducting the study. Limited funding and concerns for patient safety often dictated critical aspects of the protocol design.

Design of CAST

The investigators designed CAST in response to several primary considerations. Their first task (not a simple one) was to agree on the hypothesis to be tested. Many wanted to conduct a BHAT-like study and simply give drug or placebo in random order to patients with ventricular arrhythmias and compare mortality in the two groups. This would be a test of the hypothesis that antiarrhythmic drugs reduce mortality. However, the data from CAPS indicated that up to 30% of patients would not have a reduction in their arrhythmia and this could potentially obscure any improvement in mortality. Another consideration was that the study should mimic clinical practice so that the results would be directly applicable to patient care. Also, because the study designers wanted to be able to extrapolate the results of the study to any drug that was able to suppress ventricular ectopy in patients with a recent MI, the decision was made to test a suppression hypothesis, namely, that suppression of ventricular ectopy (by any one of several drugs) would reduce the incidence of sudden death. In fact, the study evaluated a strategy and not simply a drug.

The selection of drugs for CAST was a difficult and complex task that has been described in detail by Greene et al.[13] The Drug

Selection Committee in CAST reviewed conventional and investigational agents, employing a variety of scientific and practical considerations. It was their desire to evaluate several drugs that would possibly act by different mechanisms. They also wanted to evaluate drugs that were likely to be available for clinical use in the future. This meant that any investigational drug chosen had to be relatively far along in development. Many investigators wanted to include an established and familiar drug such as quinidine or procainamide. However, careful review of previous studies indicated that neither of these drugs had the requisite response rate (PVC suppression) or tolerability to enable randomization of the requisite number of patients (4400) in the time allotted for completion of enrollment (3 years). Therefore, other drugs and combinations were considered for inclusion. The following factors were considered: the total number of patients treated with the drug in the past, the duration of exposure (safety), the magnitude of the experience with the drug in patients like those to be enrolled in CAST (post-MI with reduced ejection fraction), expected withdrawal due to congestive heart failure, proarrhythmic potential, and confounding factors such as risk of organ toxicity or ancillary actions that would confound interpretation of the results (β-blocking activity). Many investigators felt that amiodarone should be included in the study. However, for many investigators its known toxicity made its use difficult to justify in a patient population in which it lacked any previously proven clinical benefit. Furthermore, the investigators recognized that its half-life varies from 13 to 103 days and that this would make titration very difficult if not impossible. Most patients would be out of the highest-risk period before the drug reached steady state. Its multiple actions such as β-blockade would confound interpretation of the suppression hypothesis and therefore prevent extrapolation to other drugs that might suppress ventricular arrhythmias.

Finally, the investigators chose the three drugs that appeared to have the greatest degree of efficacy in suppressing arrhythmias and the best tolerance in the CAPS study, the only controlled comparison available. These were encainide, flecainide, and moricizine. Although moricizine had slightly lower efficacy in CAPS, a low rate of side effects made it an attractive choice. Imipramine was not chosen because of its lower efficacy and the high incidence of intolerable side effects seen in CAPS. At that time, there was limited clinical experience with these drugs in patients with severe ventricular dysfunction. Likewise, at that time the proarrhythmic potential of all antiarrhythmic drugs was just becoming appreciated. However, in the only placebo-controlled experience available—i.e., CAPS—the proarrhythmic effects of encainide and flecainide could not be distinguished from placebo effects. Also, when the experience in CAPS patients with the lowest ejection fraction was examined, the incidence of worsening of congestive heart failure after administration of encainide and moricizine was no different from that seen with placebo. Yet for flecainide, there was a disturbing trend toward an increased incidence of worsening of congestive heart failure that was addressed in the design of CAST.

In CAPS the incidence of sudden death in the year following MI was lower than anticipated. There were only 50 deaths in the group of 500 patients in CAPS. In order to maintain power to detect an improvement in mortality due to an intervention, the enrollment criteria for CAST had to be narrowed to include a group with an increased risk for sudden death. In CAPS, there were no deaths in the group with normal ejection fraction (>0.55). Therefore, all patients in CAST were required to have an ejection fraction less than 0.55.

Patients 79 years of age or younger with a documented MI within the prior 6 days to 2 years were eligible for screening. Because of the lower frequency of deaths after the first 3 months following an MI, the ventricular ejection function criterion was reduced to ≤ 0.40 for those enrolled 90 days to 2 years after their infarctions. Those enrolled in the 6- to 89-day window had to have an ejection fraction of ≤ 0.55.

Because these criteria would likely restrict enrollment rates, the requirement for arrhythmia frequency was made lower than in CAPS and included any patient who had ≥ 6 PVCs/hr and could include any run of VT that was asymptomatic and ≤ 15 consecutive beats in length. Allowing a lower frequency of PVCs increased the risk that random variations in PVC frequency could mimic a drug-induced suppression. Therefore, an average frequency of ≥6 PVCs/hr was required on each of two 24-hour ambulatory ECG recordings for enrollment. Also, there was no lower limit on ejection fraction as long as the patients were not in congestive heart failure at the time of enrollment.

Because of the suppression hypothesis, the CAPS trial design was not appropriate for CAST. First, the placebo group in CAPS included some people who never responded, and deaths in that group would decrease the power to detect an improvement in mortality. Second, the treatment group would contain some nonresponders and would require their conversion to therapy with a second drug, as was done in CAPS.

Because the placebo-controlled experience in CAPS did not detect any harm from the drugs and it was cumbersome to maintain the blind, CAST began with an open-titration phase to identify responders whose PVCs were suppressed by ≥80% and had ≥90% suppression of VT episodes (slightly stricter criteria than in CAPS). Patients whose PVCs were suppressed were randomly assigned to remain on the effective drug identified during titration or switched to an identical placebo. Randomized patients were to be followed for 3–5 years, depending on when they were enrolled.

The primary end point for CAST was an arrhythmic death or resuscitated cardiac arrest. A secondary end point was total mortality or resuscitated cardiac arrest. Arrhythmic death was defined as instantaneous death in the absence of severe congestive heart failure or shock, unwitnessed death without a preceding change in symptoms for which no other cause could be ascribed, or documented cardiac arrest. The anticipated mortality due to sudden death in the CAST population was estimated to be approximately 11% in the 3 years of follow-up. This estimate was based on the clinical trial data that were available at the time CAST was being planned and included the experience in CAPS, BHAT, and the data from the Multicenter Post-infarction Group reported by Bigger et al.[14] These estimates were used to calculate a sample size for the study. In order to have a power projection of 0.85 with an alpha level of 0.025, a sample size of 4400 randomized patients was required to detect a 30% reduction in the 3-year estimate of sudden death. Because CAST was testing the hypothesis that suppression would either benefit or cause no change in mortality, a one-sided test for change was utilized. Although everyone in CAST recognized that the drugs could be harmful, that was not part of the primary hypothesis. Prospective statistical boundaries for benefit and harm were established prior to the beginning of CAST, and a Data and Safety Monitoring Committee (composed of non-CAST participants) was appointed to follow the progress of the study.

The high incidence of heart failure in patients receiving flecainide in CAPS was a concern because CAST would enroll patients with a much lower ejection fraction. Therefore it was decided that only those patients with an ejection fraction of ≥0.30 would receive flecainide. Patients in that category were randomized to receive either encainide or flecainide in open titration. However, those with an ejection fraction <0.30 were randomized to receive either encainide or moricizine during open titration. This allowed a direct comparison of two drugs, and the investigators anticipated dropping one of the drugs in either group if efficacy was unacceptably low or if adverse effects were excessive. Likewise, the investigators planned to add other drugs later in the study if new data made one or more drugs appear equivalent to or better than the drugs being tested.

The experience in CAPS indicated that therapy with these agents should be titrated beginning with a low and well-tolerated dose. To reach greater than a 50% response rate, one would have to be able to titrate the dosage higher in some patients. However, it was unlikely that many patients would respond to or tolerate titration to a higher third dosage. The experience in CAPS also indicated that some patients who failed to respond to one antiarrhythmic drug had an equal chance of responding to a second drug. For that reason, patients who failed to respond or were intolerant to the first drug could receive a second agent and be re-evaluated. Those with an ejection fraction of ≥0.30 were allowed to receive all three drugs if necessary. Based on the experience in CAPS, most patients should respond to the first or second dosage of the first drug, and titration should usually be completed in 10–20 days.

Enrollment in CAST began in June 1987 and the progress was closely followed by the Data and Safety Monitoring Committee. In April 1989 the Committee notified the NHLBI that two of the drugs should be removed from CAST because it was likely that they were causing harm and, in the time remaining in the study, it was unlikely that they would ever be able to demonstrate a beneficial effect on mortality.[15] The committee's recommendation was couched in such conservative terms because the study was designed to test for a reduction in mortality, not the harm that was observed. For this reason, the calculation of a p value for the magnitude of harm is, in the strictest sense, inappropriate. Figure 30-1 compares the actuarial probability of freedom from death or cardiac arrest in the 1498 patients receiving encainide or flecainide (lower line) or the corresponding placebo (upper line).[15] There was a 3.6-fold greater incidence of sudden death and/or cardiac arrest in the patients whose initial arrhythmias were suppressed by encainide or flecainide compared to the group randomized to placebo. Although only a small number of patients had been treated with moricizine, harm was not apparent in the group, and the Data and Safety Monitoring Committee recommended that the NHLBI continue the study with moricizine and perhaps other drugs that might have become available since CAST began.

Because of the alarming results of CAST, every effort was made to examine factors that might have predisposed to the toxicity. However, the harm was found in every subset examined: those with or without β-blocker therapy, with or without a calcium channel blocker, with or without digitalis, with ejection fractions above or below 0.3, or those enrolled less than or more than 90 days following their heat attack. There was also controversy over whether the harm was inherent to Class 1C drugs or could be expected from the other antiarrhythmic drugs. Shortly after CAST was reported, Hine et al published a meta-analysis of all available clinical trials with antiarrhythmic drugs and concluded that the harm was apparent with all classes of antiarrhythmic drugs that had been tested.[16] At that time there was only a limited experience with amiodarone, so no conclusion was reached,

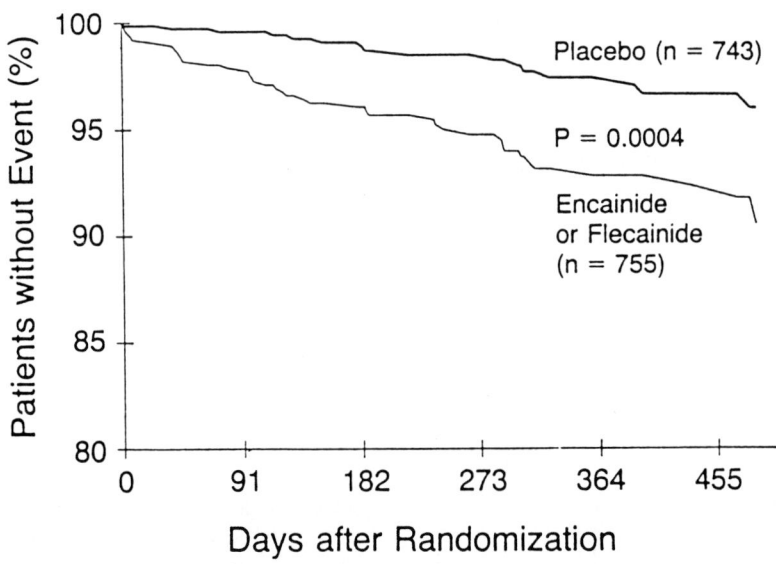

Fig. 30–1. Actuarial probabilities of freedom from death or cardiac arrest due to arrhythmias in 1498 patients receiving encainide or flecainide or corresponding placebo. (Reproduced by permission of the publisher from Echt DS, et al: N Engl J Med *324*:781–788, 1991.[18])

and ultimately several clinical trials with amiodarone have begun.

There has been a great deal of speculation about the mechanism of the increased mortality seen in CAST. The time course of the occurrence of deaths in CAST (shown in Fig. 30-1) is relatively constant and indicates that the harm is unlike the arrhythmia worsening that occurs early after initiating antiarrhythmic therapy. The time course has led several authors to hypothesize that the deaths may be due to an adverse interaction of the drugs with randomly occurring ischemic events.[17,18] This hypothesis is supported by several lines of indirect evidence. As shown in Table 30-1, there were fewer cases of nonfatal MI and new or worsened angina in the CAST treatment arm randomized to encainide or flecainide.[18] One possible interpretation is that the drugs converted nonfatal MI and anginal events to *fatal* events. In retrospect, the sodium channel blocking drugs have not been effective in arrhythmia models that involved myocardial ischemia. Nattel et al reported that pretreatment with aprindine caused an increased incidence of VT or VF in dogs during coronary occlusion.[19] Similar results were obtained with lidocaine in an ischemic pig model.[20] Dawson et al[21] found that the major active metabolite of encainide, O-demethyl encainide (ODE), reduced the threshold for electrical fibrillation in dogs with prior MI. Kou et al have found that flecainide was either ineffective or increased the rate of serious arrhythmias in their model of ischemia in the setting of prior infarction.[22] In sum, there seems to be a remarkable consistency of results when sodium channel blockers are evaluated in models that incorporate acute ischemia.

Many expressed concern about the low incidence of sudden death in CAST, and some unfamiliar with the protocol mistakenly concluded that CAST enrolled patients with a low risk of sudden death. In fact, when the mortality in the entire population enrolled in CAST is considered instead of just that in the randomized portion of the study, the incidence is very close to the anticipated rate for this population.[23] The data in the randomized follow-up portion of the study indicate that successful suppression of arrhythmias by an antiarrhythmic drug identifies a population of patients with a very good prognosis.

CAST-II

Following the directions of the Data and Safety Monitoring Committee, the investigators in CAST modified the design of CAST-II. After reviewing the available drugs, the investigators concluded that no new drugs should be added. However, in order to increase the response rate with moricizine, a third higher dosage was added. Since there were no cases of sudden arrhythmic death in the patients enrolled more than 90 days after infarction, CAST-II only enrolled patients in the period from 4 to 90 days after infarction. Likewise, entry criteria were changed so that only patients with a left ventricular ejection fraction of ≤0.40 could be enrolled in CAST-II. Because of a concern for the number of deaths in the open label phase of CAST,[23] a double-blind phase was added to the first 2 weeks of the initial titration phase in CAST-II.

Again, in July 1991, CAST-II was interrupted prematurely because of an increased incidence of deaths and cardiac arrests in the group receiving active drug therapy during the early phase of the trial.[24] In this case, the harm was detected in the initial titration phase, as shown in Figure 30-2. There were 17 deaths or cardiac arrests in 665 patients treated with moricizine, compared to only three in 660 patients in the placebo group. Furthermore, there was only an 8% chance that moricizine could ever be found to have a beneficial effect on mortality in the second phase of CAST-II. As shown in Figure

Table 30-1
Nonfatal infarction and New Angina in CAST

Outcome	Placebo	Active Drug
Death and cardiac arrest	26	63
Nonfatal infarction	33	19
New/increasing angina	88	65
Total	147	147

Source: Echt DS, et al: N Engl J Med *324*: 781–788, 1991.[18] Adapted by permission.

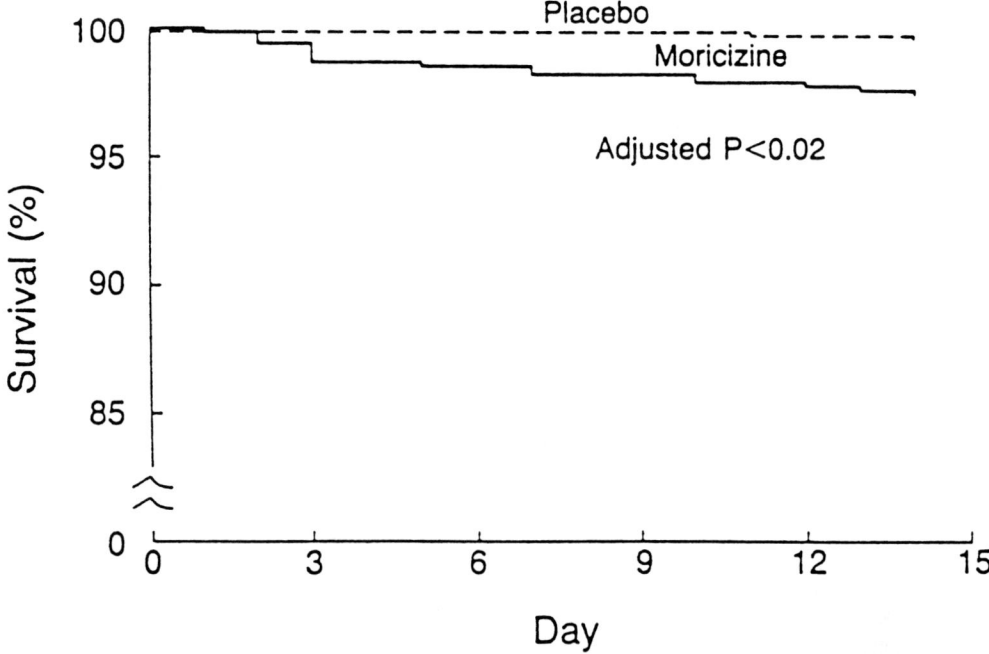

Fig. 30–2. Survival of patients during the first 14 days of treatment with moricizine or placebo. The end point was death or nonfatal cardiac arrest from any cause. The adjusted p value is based on the log-rank statistic and adjusted for sequential monitoring. (Reproduced by permission of the publisher from N Engl J Med 327:227–233, 1992.[24])

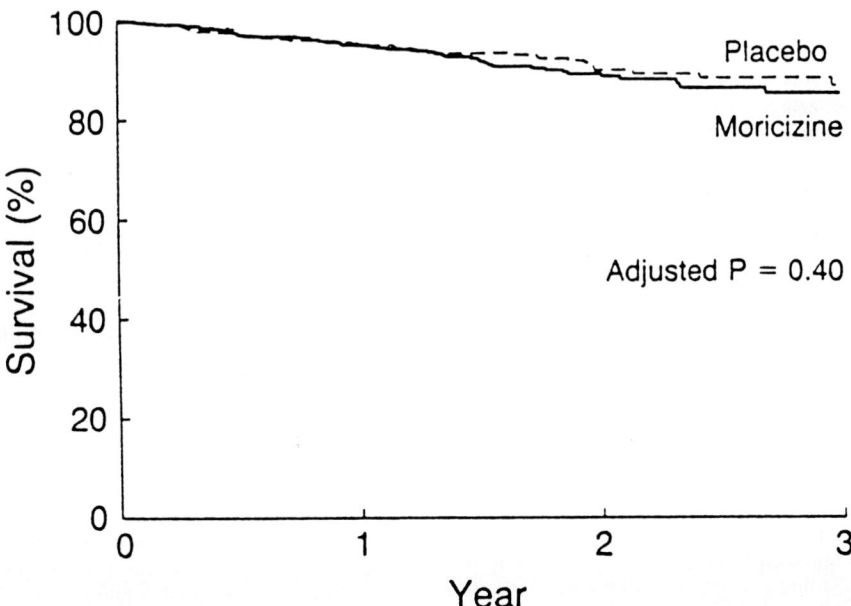

Fig. 30-3. Survival of patients in the long-term main study during treatment with moricizine or placebo after adequate suppression of PVCs with moricizine. The end point was death or nonfatal cardiac arrest due to arrhythmias. The adjusted p value is two-tailed. (Reproduced by permission of the publisher from N Engl J Med 327:227–233, 1992.[24])

30-3, there was a slowly developing trend for a greater number of deaths or cardiac arrests in the moricizine-treated group. Overall, the results of CAST-II were consistent with the results of CAST and the other studies of antiarrhythmic drugs.

SUMMARY

CAST and CAST-II epitomize the amazingly consistent experience with drugs that are antiarrhythmic by blocking sodium channels. The results of these trials have been either disappointing or alarming. With the failure of the PVC hypothesis, cardiologists now search for new, more reliable surrogates such as nonsustained VT, late potentials, heart rate variability, or inducible sustained VT using programmed stimulation. Hope continues that other classes of drugs may be able to reduce arrhythmic death. Several large clinical trials with amiodarone are under way in a variety of populations. Also, several pharmaceutical companies are developing drugs that block potassium channels in the hope that they will have only Class III activity and be devoid of the toxicity found with the drugs in CAST and CAST-II. However, because of the likelihood of only a small improvement in mortality and the known potential for harm with amiodarone and potassium channel blockers, large clinical trials will be essential to be sure that any benefit of therapy outweighs harm. However, it is unlikely that any major improvement in mortality will be found until we learn the mechanism of SCD and VF.

REFERENCES

1. Lown B, Wolf M: Approaches to sudden death from coronary heart disease. Circulation 44:130–142, 1971.
2. Holter NJ: New method for heart studies. Science 134:1214–1220, 1961.
3. Moss AJ, Davis HT, DeCamilla J, Bayer LW: Ventricular ectopic beats and their relation to sudden and nonsudden cardiac death after myocardial infarction. Circulation 60: 998–1003, 1979.
4. Morganroth J: Premature ventricular complexes. JAMA 252(5):673–676, 1984.
5. Higgins SB, Woosley RL, Herrin CB, Compton JL, Harris TR: A mini-computer-based system for quantification of ventricular arrhythmias. In: Computers in Cardiology, 5th Conference. Long Beach, CA, IEEE Computer Society, 1978, pp 355–358.
6. Hirsowitz G, Podrid PJ, Lampert S, Stein J, Lown B: The role of beta blocking agents as adjunct therapy to membrane stabilizing drugs in malignant ventricular arrhythmia. Am Heart J 111:852–860, 1986.
7. Vlay SC: How the university cardiologist treats ventricular premature beats: A nationwide survey of 65 university medical centers. Am Heart J 110:904–912, 1985.
8. Morganroth J, Bigger JT Jr, Anderson JL: Treatment of ventricular arrhythmias by United States cardiologists: A survey before the Cardiac Arrhythmia Suppression Trial results were available. Am J Cardiol 65: 40–48, 1990.
9. Morganroth J, Michelson EL, Horowitz LN, Josephson M, Pearlman AS, Dunkman WB: Limitations of routine long term ambulatory electrocardiographic monitoring to assess ventricular ectopic frequency. Circulation 58:408, 1978.
10. Ruskin JN, Dimarco JP, Garan H: Out of hospital cardiac arrest: Electrophysiologic observations and selection of long term antiarrhythmic therapy. N Engl J Med 303: 607–613, 1980.
11. Mason JW, Winkle RA: Electrode-catheter arrhythmia induction in the selection and assessment of antiarrhythmic drug therapy for recurrent ventricular tachycardia. Circulation 58:971–985, 1978.
12. CAPS Investigators: Effects of encainide, flecainide, imipramine and moricizine on ventricular arrhythmias during the year after myocardial infarction. Am J Cardiol 61: 501–509, 1988.
13. Greene HL, Roden D, Katz RJ, et al, and the Cast Investigators: The Cardiac Arrhythmia Suppression Trial: First CAST . . . then Cast-II. J Am Coll Cardiol 19:894–898, 1992.
14. Bigger JT Jr, Fleiss JL, Kleiger R, Miller JP, Rolnitzky LM, and the Multicenter Postinfarction Group: The relationship between ventricular arrhythmias, left ventricular dysfunction and mortality in the two years after myocardial infarction. Circulation 69: 250–258, 1984.
15. CAST Investigators: Preliminary report: Effect of encainide and flecainide on mortality in a randomized trial of arrhythmia suppression after myocardial infarction. N Engl J Med 321:406–412, 1989.
16. Hine LK, Laird NM, Hewitt P, Chalmers TC: Meta-analysis of empirical long-term antiarrhythmic therapy after myocardial infarction. JAMA 262(21):3037–3040, 1989.

17. Woosley RL. Antiarrhythmic drugs: Annu Rev Pharmacol Toxicol *31:*427–455, 1991.
18. Echt DS, Liebson PR, Mitchell LB, et al: Mortality and morbidity in patients receiving encainide, flecainide, or placebo: The Cardiac Arrhythmia Suppression Trial. N Engl J Med *324:*781–788, 1991.
19. Nattel S, Pedersen DH, Zipes DP: Alterations in regional myocardial distribution and arrhythmogenic effects of aprindine produced by coronary artery occlusion in the dog. Cardiovasc Res *15:*80–85, 1981.
20. Carson DL, Cardinal R, Savard P, et al: Relationship between an arrhythmogenic action of lidocaine and its effects on excitation patterns in acutely ischemic porcine myocardium. J Cardiovasc Pharmacol *8:*126–136, 1986.
21. Dawson AK, Roden DM, Duff HJ, Woosley RL, Smith RF: DIfferential effects of O-demethyl encainide on induced and spontaneous arrhythmias in the conscious dog. Am J Cardiol *54:*654–658, 1984.
22. Kou H, Nelson SD, Lynch JJ, Montgomery DG, DiCarlo L, Lucchesi BR: Effect of flecainide acetate on prevention of electrical induction of ventricular tachycardia and occurrence of ischemic ventricular fibrillation during the early postmyocardial infarction period: Evaluation in a conscious canine model of sudden death. J Am Coll Cardiol *9:*359–365, 1987.
23. Epstein AE, Bigger JT Jr, Wyse DG, et al. Events in the Cardiac Arrhythmia Suppression Trial (CAST): Mortality in the entire population enrolled. J Am Coll Cardiol *18(1):* 14–19, 1991.
24. CAST-II Investigators: Effect of the antiarrhythmic agent moricizine on survival after myocardial infarction. N Engl J Med *327:* 227–233, 1992.

31

Community Experience in Treating Out-of-Hospital Cardiac Arrest

JOSEPH P. ORNATO
ANIL OM

A major goal of all emergency medical services (EMS) systems is to return men and women who have been victims of out-of-hospital cardiac arrest or other life-threatening emergencies to taxpayer status in the community. Most initial episodes of sudden unexpected cardiac arrhythmia death in adults occur in the home or workplace.[1-3] Although only 2–4% of all runs in a typical EMS system are due to cardiac arrest,[4] such calls represent a large proportion of the incidents in which field intervention can make a life-or-death difference in outcome. Effective EMS systems are vital to dealing with the problem of sudden cardiac death (SCD) because they can provide (1) initial rescue and a source of referral for electrophysiological testing and therapeutic intervention in patients who experience their first episode of pulseless ventricular tachycardia (VT) or fibrillation (VF); and (2) salvage of patients who sustain rearrest despite treatment.

Over 80% of patients who develop out-of-hospital, primary cardiac arrest during ambulatory electrocardiographic (ECG) monitoring have a ventricular tachyarrhythmia (VT degenerating rapidly to VF in 62%, torsade de pointes in 13%, and VF in 8%) as the initiating event.[5] By the time rescue personnel arrive on the scene (typically 5–10 minutes after the onset of collapse), less than 70% of patients are found to have a ventricular tachyarrhythmias; 31% have bradycardia or asystole.[6]

The outcome of field resuscitation is strongly influenced by the initial rhythm. In 352 out-of-hospital cardiac arrest patients reported by Myerburg et al,[6] 67% patients with VT and 23% with VF survived hospitalization. None of the patients who presented initially with a bradyarrhythmia survived. Similar observations have been made by others.[7-9] Pulseless bradyarrhythmias present on arrival of paramedics may be a marker for a prolonged down time interval or a more severe underlying disease process.[10] Because ventricular tachyarrhythmias represent the most common, potentially treatable mechanism of sudden cardiac arrest in adults, the best prehospital emergency cardiac care programs have been designed to ensure that rapid defibrillation can be delivered when needed to as many patients as possible.

This chapter reviews the ways in which the EMS system design and function can maximize survival from out-of-hospital cardiac arrest.

THE "CHAIN OF SURVIVAL" CONCEPT

Survival from pulseless VT or VF is inversely related to the interval between onset and termination of the arrhythmia.[11] The best chances for survival occur when cardiopulmonary resuscitation (CPR) can be initiated within the first 4 minutes of arrest

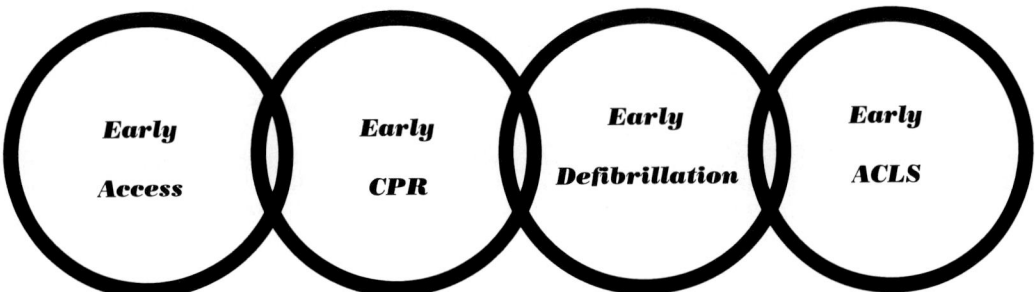

Fig. 31–1. Sequence of events in emergency cardiac care to optimize survival from out-of-hospital cardiac arrest.

and advanced cardiac life support (ACLS), including defibrillation, is delivered within the first 8 minutes.[12] The American Heart Association's Emergency Cardiac Care Committee and its Advanced Cardiac Life Support Subcommittee coined the phrase "chain of survival" in 1991 to describe a sequence of events that should occur in most out-of-hospital cardiac arrest cases to maximize the odds of successful resuscitation.[12] This ideal sequence includes early recognition of the problem and activation of the EMS system by a bystander, early CPR, rapid provision of defibrillation for patients who need it, and ACLS (e.g., intubation, administration of medications).[13] Schematically, this sequence can be depicted by a "chain of survival" (Fig. 31–1).

Early Access to the EMS System

Because most out-of-hospital cardiac arrests occur suddenly and without immediate premonitory symptoms, the victim rarely activates the EMS system prior to collapse. Bystanders can play a key role by alerting the community EMS system to the presence of a potential cardiac emergency. All too often, the untrained citizen only further delays treatment by attempting to inform relatives, call the neighbors, or contact the patient's personal physician instead of calling the local emergency telephone number.[14,15]

Before the EMS rescuers can aid the victim, the bystander must recognize that there is a problem, locate a telephone, make a correct call, and give accurate and precise information to the dispatcher. Once the alarm has been sounded, rescuers must travel to the scene, physically arrive at the patient's side, and perform an initial, cursory assessment. Public education can significantly improve the behavior of bystanders when a cardiac emergency occurs in the community. Citizens can be trained to quickly summon help and to initiate lifesaving CPR. For example, bystanders in Seattle initiated CPR in only 5% of cardiac arrests in 1970–71, but by 1976, 34% of cardiac arrest victims were receiving bystander CPR as a result of a widespread, pioneering, public education campaign.[16] Since then, the American Heart Association and the American Red Cross have trained millions of citizens to recognize cardiac emergencies, call for help, and perform CPR.[17,18]

Availability of a simple three-digit emergency number (911 in the United States) can avoid confusion and delay in activating the EMS system. This has been well documented in Minneapolis, where the percentage of emergency callers who could activate the EMS system in less than 1 minute rose from 63% before to 82% after institution of a 911 number.[19] Surprisingly, only two states currently have 911 available everywhere within their borders. One community in North Carolina lists 85 different emergency numbers in the local telephone book.[20,21] The American Heart Association has recommended that all communities implement an enhanced 911 system that displays the caller's location automatically on the dispatcher's terminal when the call is received.[13]

Early Cardiopulmonary Resuscitation

The next link in the chain is early initiation of CPR, preferably by bystanders. With rare exceptions (e.g., Milwaukee), EMS system response time characteristics are not good enough to provide CPR within the first few minutes of the patient's collapse.[22,23] One way to ensure initiation of early CPR is to educate and train a "critical mass" of the general population. The effectiveness of such training has varied widely. In Seattle, approximately 50% of the population has been trained to perform CPR,[24] while in Minneapolis only 23% of adults surveyed have received such training.[25] In smaller cities and in less affluent areas, the number of citizens trained is often much lower. What percentage of adults needs to be trained in CPR to provide reasonable protection in the community is difficult to determine with certainty. As a rule of thumb, the American Heart Association recommends that at least 20% of the adult population be trained in basic CPR to reduce mortality from out-of-hospital cardiac arrest.[26]

There are a number of problems with training the public to perform CPR. First, the wrong rescuers have been trained. The typical cardiac arrest victim is male, aged 60–65 years, and usually arrests at home, often in the presence of a spouse of similar age.[27] Most citizens who have taken CPR training are under age 30; typically, fewer than 10% live with family members known to have heart disease.[28] Most citizens who have received CPR training never actually witness or participate in managing a cardiac arrest; conversely, bystanders who witness a cardiac arrest usually do not know how to perform CPR.[25,29] For example, only 10% of CPR-trained citizens in Minneapolis have witnessed an arrest, while only 30% of citizens present at the site of a cardiac arrest were trained in CPR.[25] The majority of lay persons who attempt to perform CPR out-of-hospital are actually connected to the health professions by work or avocation.[30] The best solution to the problem may be to target CPR training to high-risk individuals, such as middle-aged persons, residents and staff of senior centers, and family members (particularly the spouse) of patients who are survivors of myocardial infarction or cardiac arrest or who have other risk factors for cardiac arrest.[28,31,32]

Skill retention is also a problem because CPR is a psychomotor technique that deteriorates rapidly over time unless practiced or used. In Belgium, 46% of bystanders who performed CPR forgot to perform mouth-to-mouth breathing; chest compressions were not done 17% of the time.[33] It is important for lay persons or health care professionals who perform CPR infrequently to receive at least annual reinforcement. However, only about 20% of trainees return for annual training in the United States.[25,29] Irrational fear of communicable disease, particularly infection with the human immunodeficiency virus (HIV), that is disproportionate to the known minimal risk of disease transmission is already beginning to influence the likelihood that trained rescuers will actually perform mouth-to-mouth ventilation on strangers.[34]

Is bystander CPR effective? Virtually all U.S. studies have shown that initiation of bystander CPR within 4 minutes of the patient's collapse results in up to a 12-fold improvement in the odds for survival (Fig. 31–2).[13] The mechanism by which early CPR improves outcome is unclear but may relate to CPR's ability to keep coarse VF from degenerating to asystole for a few extra minutes until rescuers arrive. In Seattle, when bystanders started CPR early, 80% of victims were in VF on arrival of the paramedic unit; without early CPR, only 68% of victims were in VF.[35] The presence of VF at the time of EMS arrival is a dependent variable in analyses of survival data[1,36] (i.e., the chance of restoring spontaneous circulation is higher when VF is present).[37] In Houston, 40% of pulseless VT or VF patients were discharged from the hospital when bystanders initiated CPR, as compared to only 19% when no bystander CPR was performed.[36]

EARLY DEFIBRILATION

The rationale for the use of early defibrillation stems from four observations: (1) ventricular tachyarrhythmias are the commonest cause of sudden, out-of-hospital cardiac arrest in adults, (2) defibrillation is the most effective treatment for pulseless ventricular tachyarrhythmias, (3) the effectiveness of defibrillation diminishes rapidly over time, and (4) unless treated promptly,

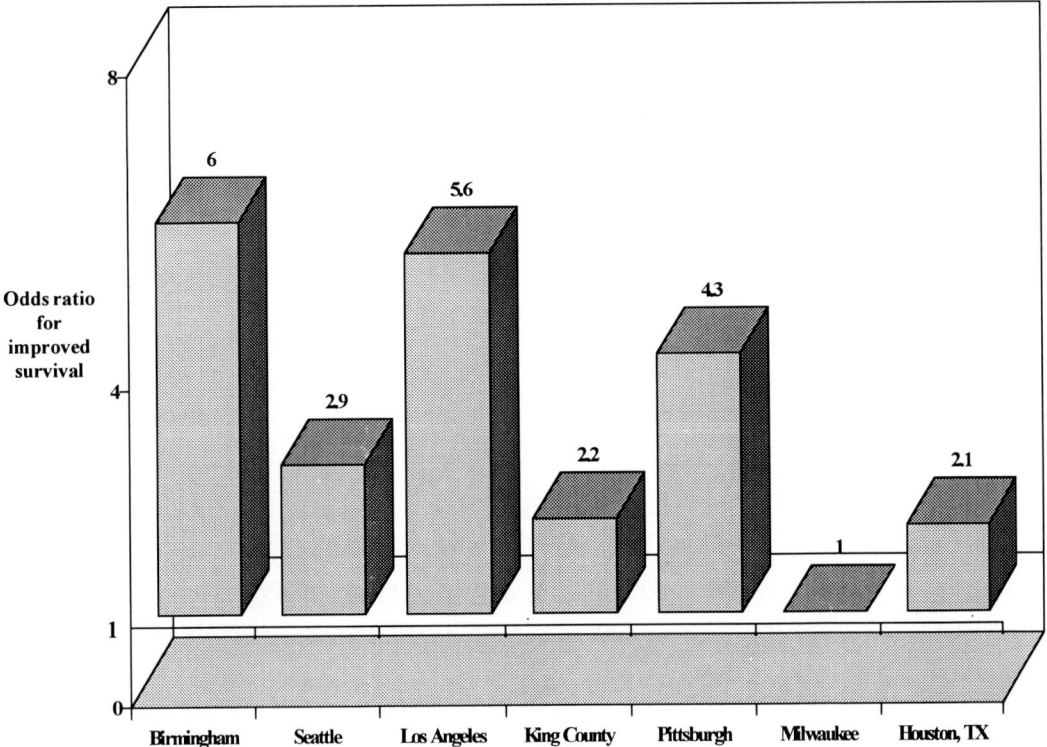

Fig. 31-2. Odds ratios favor better survival when bystanders perform CPR before arrival of the paramedic unit.[13]

VF becomes less coarse and eventually converts to fine VF or asystole.

The best outcomes from sudden arrhythmic cardiac arrest in adults have been reported from cardiac rehabilitation programs, where defibrillation can be performed within the first minute or two. Typically, 85–90% of patients are resuscitated and return to their prearrest neurological status.[38–40] Survival from out-of-hospital cardiac arrest treated by EMS personnel has been considerably lower, averaging 15–20% or less, with a maximum survival of 30%, depending on the EMS system configuration (Fig. 31-3).[41]

The best survival is attained in EMS systems that have first-responding firefighters or emergency medical technicians (EMTs) who are trained and equipped to defibrillate, along with fully trained paramedics. Rescue crews in the more numerous, first-responding tier who can provide first aid (including CPR) and defibrillate typically arrive on the scene within 2–4 minutes; paramedics, who can intubate and give medications, usually are on scene within 4–8 minutes of dispatch.

Unfortunately, not all communities have yet implemented such a comprehensive, tiered EMS system. Many systems, particularly in suburban or rural areas, have only EMTs who are neither trained nor equipped to defibrillate. For such areas, adding rapid defibrillation capability offers a cost-effective alternative that can significantly improve survival from out-of-hospital VF or pulseless VT.[42] In King County, Washington, the survival rate of patients in VF increased from 7% to 26% after an early defibrillation program was started.[43] Other areas have had similar results (Fig. 31-4).[13]

The American Heart Association has recently issued a position statement advocating the widespread implementation of rapid defibrillation programs throughout the nation. The American Heart Association endorses the position that:

All emergency personnel should be trained and permitted to operate an appropriately

VF Survival

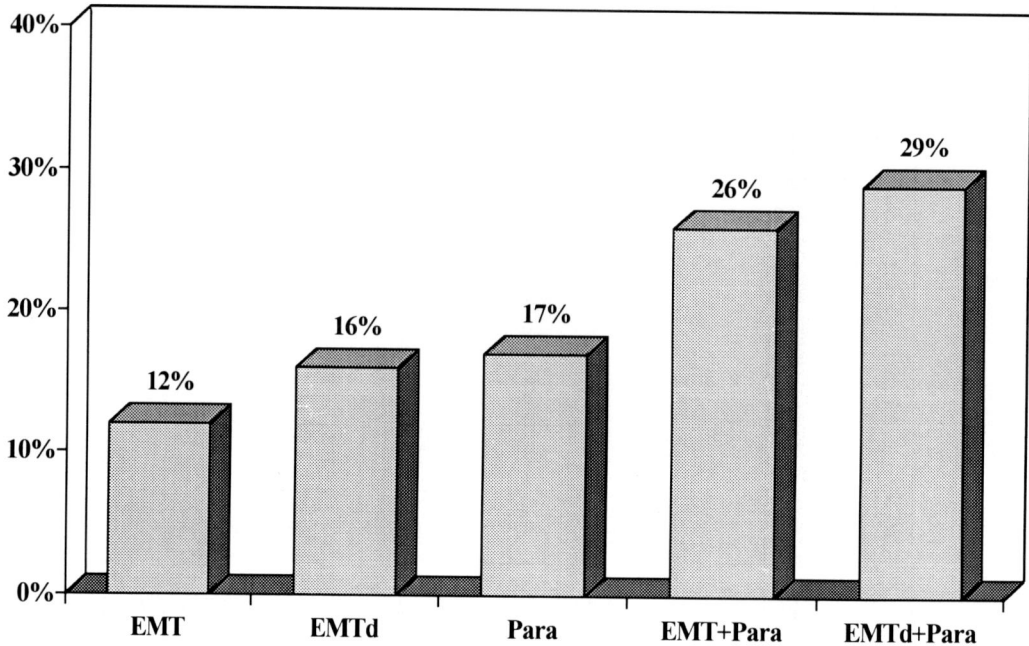

Fig. 31–3. Effect of EMS system design on survival from out-of-hospital VF. EMT, emergency medical technician; EMTd, authorized and equipped to defibrillate.[41]

maintained defibrillator if their professional activities require that they respond to persons experiencing cardiac arrest. This includes all first responding emergency personnel, both hospital and nonhospital (e.g., emergency medical technicians (EMTs), non-EMT first responders, fire fighters, volunteer emergency personnel, physicians, nurses, and paramedics).

To further facilitate early defibrillation, it is essential that a defibrillator be immediately available to emergency personnel responding to a cardiac arrest. Therefore, all emergency ambulances and other emergency vehicles that respond to or transport cardiac patients should be equipped with a defibrillator.[44]

More novel strategies have also been tried to increase the availability of rapid defibrillation in the community. For example, in England many patients call and receive a house call from their general practitioners when they develop symptoms such as chest pain. Approximately 5% of these patients develop cardiac arrest after the physician arrives.[45,46] The British Heart Foundation recently supplied 78 defibrillators to 25 general practices. Within the first year of the program, 9(68%) of 13 patients with cardiac arrest who went into VF immediately prior to or in the presence of the physicians were successfully resuscitated out-of-hospital, and 6 patients survived to hospital discharge.[47] Other approaches involving the training of family members of high-risk patients or community workers in the use of automated external defibrillators (AEDs) have met with variable success. Eisenberg et al trained family members of 59 patients who had survived out-of-hospital cardiac arrest in King County, Washington.[48] Only six of the ten cardiac arrests that occurred in these patients were defibrillated successfully, and only one patient survived for a few months and sustained new neurological impairment. In contrast, Swenson et al reported three successful resuscitations out of five cardiac arrests in 48 patients whose families had been trained to use an AED.[49]

Somewhat more encouraging results have been obtained when community first-responders have been trained to use AEDs. For example, 160 security officers were

VF Survival

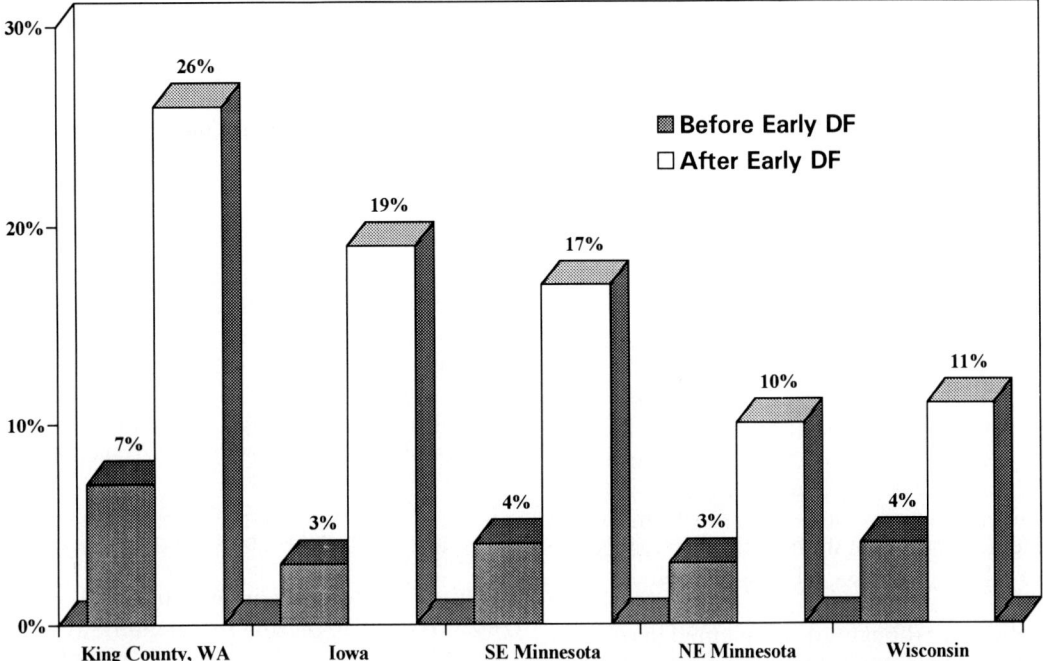

Fig. 31–4. Survival before (open boxes) and after (shaded boxes) implementation of EMT defibrillation programs.

trained to use these devices at Vancouver's World Expo 1986. Five cardiac arrests occurred among the 22.1 million visitors. The AED was correctly applied in all cases by security personnel. In two cases, the initial rhythm was VF and defibrillation was successful. Both patients had a pulse and were regaining consciousness by the time EMS personnel arrived on the scene.[50] Other experimental approaches to rapid defibrillation in the workplace include use on commercial aircraft, British rail stations, oil platforms in the North sea, electricity plants, passenger cruise ships, and merchant marine vessels.[51–53]

Early ACLS

Physicians provide prehospital ACLS by staffing specially equipped ambulances in many countries (e.g., western Europe, Scandinavia, Canada). In the United States, intermediate-level EMTs or full paramedics provide prehospital ACLS intervention (e.g., defibrillation or synchronized cardioversion, endotracheal intubation, intravenous (IV) fluid therapy, drug administration). Intermediate EMTs (often called cardiac technicians) typically receive several hundred hours of training; paramedics usually receive 1000 or more hours. Adding field ACLS capability appears to favorably affect survival from out-of-hospital cardiac arrest (see Fig. 31–3).

Some EMS systems have upgraded all ambulances to ACLS status to eliminate the possibility that dispatchers might send a basic life support unit on a call that needs a higher level of care. In Kansas City, Missouri, 11% of nonemergency calls that were thought to require only basic life support by the dispatcher actually needed ACLS intervention prior to hospital arrival.[54] An "all-ACLS" system eliminates the potential "failure point" in the 911 center because there is no triage of calls to an ACLS or basic cardiac life support (BCLS) response. Existing BCLS ambulances or first-responding vehicles can be upgraded to automated defibrillation capability with minimal expense. Automated defibrillators cost approximately $5000–8000 and require only 2–4 hours of additional training for first responders or EMTs. This is a nominal expense compared with the cost of a typical ambulance ($50,000–100,000) or fire truck ($250,000–500,000). In Richmond, Virginia, the upgrading from a half BCLS/half ACLS system to an all-ACLS system added less than 1% to the cost of ambulance service (only $2.88 per patient transported).[55]

DRUG THERAPY DURING RESUSCITATION

Beyond defibrillation, field endotracheal intubation and drug therapy improve oxygenation and coronary and cerebral perfusion pressure, and help to stabilize the cardiac rhythm. The most important medications used in the field for arrests due to VF or pulseless VT include epinephrine, lidocaine, and bretylium. Sodium bicarbonate, once thought to be essential in resuscitation, is no longer indicated for routine use early in resuscitation because it paradoxically lowers intramyocardial pH by shifting carbon dioxide intracellularly and does not appear to improve survival.[17,56]

Epinephrine

Intravenous epinephrine is the traditional vasopressor used during cardiac arrest, but recently the dosage has come into question. A dosage of 0.5–1.0 mg given as an IV bolus every 5 minutes has been standard in adults since the 1960s, but reported improvement in hemodynamics and increases in coronary and cerebral blood flow in animals with higher doses of epinephrine[57,58] have led many clinicians to use boluses higher than 1 mg (typically 0.2 mg/kg, which appears to be the optimal dose in animals) during CPR.

Gonzalez et al demonstrated a dose-dependent vasopressor response to 1-, 3-, and 5-mg bolus doses of epinephrine during controlled mechanical CPR in humans.[59] Paradis et al demonstrated that there is a significant increase in coronary perfusion pressure with high-dose epinephrine (0.2 mg/kg) as compared to standard-dose epinephrine during CPR in 32 patients.[60] All patients had initially received standard-dose epinephrine, and if there was no establishment of spontaneous rhythm, high-dose epinephrine was given. Despite the significant increase in coronary perfusion pressure, the outcome of patients who received high-dose epinephrine was still grim. Only four patients returned to spontaneous circulation; all remained comatose and died within 48 hours. However, patients in this study received only basic life support (CPR) in the field and were not given high-dose epinephrine until 25 ± 8 (mean ± SD) minutes after arrival at the emergency department. It is unclear whether results of this study can be generalized. In another study, reported by Callaham et al, 33 patients received high-dose epinephrine and 35 standard-dose epinephrine during CPR.[61] Although no adverse effects were noted with the use of high-dose epinephrine, there was no difference between groups in the hospital discharge rate or the patients' neurological status. However, conclusions must be drawn cautiously from this nonrandomized, retrospective study in which clinicians were allowed to choose the dose of epinephrine. Since patients who did not survive for at least 6 hours were excluded from analysis, lethal complications were not counted.[62]

Certain theoretical limitations of high-dose epinephrine are obvious. Some clinicians and scientists have expressed concern that high-dose epinephrine may be detrimental, especially during ischemia or VF. Since a fibrillating heart consumes oxygen at a rapid rate, high-dose epinephrine could theoretically increase oxygen demand more than it enhances oxygen delivery during CPR.[63–67] Such an adverse effect has already been noted in animal models, resulting in rapid depletion of myocardial adenosine triphosphate and impairment of left ventricular function following the return of spontaneous circulation.[68,69] Thus, until several large multicenter prospective trials now in progress are completed, the jury is still out on the optimal dose of epinephrine for use in clinical resuscitation.[62]

Lidocaine and Bretylium

Lidocaine and bretylium are widely used to treat VF or pulseless VT that is refractory to multiple defibrillation attempts, CPR, intubation, and epinephrine. There is still great uncertainty as to which should be given first, or whether either drug favorably affects the outcome of resuscitation in humans.[70] Lidocaine is generally recommended first because it, unlike bretylium, does not decrease systemic vascular resistance and therefore should not decrease coronary perfusion pressure.[17] Unlike bretylium, lidocaine increases the defibrillation energy requirement in dogs.[71]

Prehospital clinical trials have not demonstrated superiority of one drug over the other. Haynes et al randomized 146 victims of out-of-hospital cardiac arrest in VF to receive either lidocaine ($n = 72$) or bretylium ($n = 74$).[72] A spontaneous rhythm was obtained in 66/74 (89%) and 67/72 (93%) of patients receiving bretylium and lidocaine, respectively. However, the number of patients admitted to the hospital and discharged home was not significantly different between groups. Lack of superiority of one or the other drug was also noted by Olson et al.[73] Synergism between bretylium and lidocaine has been noted in canine models of VF, but no clinical trials have confirmed whether a similar effect occurs in humans.[74]

Amiodarone

Preliminary anecdotal case series reporting on the use of IV amiodarone in refractory VF or pulseless VT are encouraging, but no prospective controlled clinical trials have yet been conducted.[75-77] Chapman and Boyd reported on two patients with recurrent VF who were stabilized and survived following IV amiodarone after failing to respond to multiple other antiarrhythmic drugs.[75] Similar results were noted by Klein et al in 13 patients with VT which was refractory to at least three prior antiarrhythmic agents; 11 patients had also failed multiple DC countershocks.[76] But the most interesting series was reported by Williams et al, in which 11 of 14 patients initially survived prolonged resuscitation that lasted for at least 30 minutes (mean of 75 ± 9 minutes) before amiodarone was administered; 8 of the patients survived to hospital discharge and were maintained on oral amiodarone.[77] The potential value of IV amiodarone in out-of-hospital resuscitation remains to be determined.

BRADYASYSTOLIC CARDIAC ARREST

With the exception of patients who are bradyasystolic due to increased vagal tone (vasovagal syncope, respiratory arrest), survival is rare (1–3%) in patients whose initial rhythm is pulseless bradycardia or asystole since these rhythms tend to be a marker for a prolonged down time interval. Although widely recommended and used in an attempt to restore AV conduction and to stimulate intrinsic electrical activity, there is little objective evidence that 1-mg IV doses of atropine (up to a total vagolytic dose of 2 mg) are of benefit during bradycardiac or asystolic arrest (asystole or pulseless idioventricular rhythm).[78-81] Pacing externally in the field (or intravenously after arrival at the hospital) is also frequently tried but is rarely successful in altering long-term survival.[82-84]

ELECTROMECHANICAL DISSOCIATION

As with bradyasystole, patients who initially have organized electrical activity but no effective circulation (i.e., no pulse or blood pressure) have an extremely poor prognosis. There are many possible causes for electromechanical dissociation, but the final common physiological pathway may involve myocardial ischemia and dysfunction due to intramyocardial increases in carbon dioxide.[85,86] Field protocols generally direct paramedics to detect and empirically attempt to treat the few potentially correctable causes of electromechanical dissociation (e.g., hypovolemia, tension pneumothorax, pericardial tamponade, acidosis, and hypoxemia).

OUTCOME STUDIES IN OUT-OF-HOSPITAL CARDIAC ARREST

Survival results from out-of-hospital resuscitation of adults in cardiac arrest have varied widely. For example, Eisenberg et al reviewed published results of out-of-hospital resuscitation from 29 cities and found that the percentage of patients surviving to hospital discharge varied widely.[41] Repre-

Table 31-1
Representative Results from Published Studies of Cardiac Arrest Survival

Study	No.	% Witnessed	% Bystander	BLS Time (min)	ALS Time (min)	% in VF	% Surviving	% of VF Survivors
Iowa[87]	110	70	20	6	No ALS	58	11	19
Minnesota[88]	100	70	50	4	No ALS	51	6	12
Israel[89]	2995	82	8	Not reported	6	28	7	15
Los Angeles[90]	300	41	35	Not reported	5	45	10	14
Milwaukee[91]	1905	100	31	2	5	52	16	23
Seattle[92]	687	79	36	4	9	40	14	30
King County[93]	4068	55	54	4	10	52	18	29

sentative data from seven different EMS systems are presented in Table 31-1.[87-93]

The major problem in attempting to determine the relative importance of EMS system design, training, and medical protocols in affecting outcome from out-of-hospital cardiac arrest has been the lack of uniformity in record keeping and reporting methodology between EMS systems. In 1990, representative volunteers from the American Heart Association, the European Resuscitation Council, the Canadian Heart and Stroke Foundation, and the Australian Resuscitation Council met and developed an international consensus document that provides a template for reporting data on out-of-hospital cardiac arrest outcome research.[94]

SUMMARY

Survival from out-of-hospital cardiac arrest is possible if there is a well-organized, community approach to the problem. Although most cities have at least some form of advanced life support service available, very few cities have complete coverage within their borders.[55] Improving EMS services nationwide and fully implementing the "chain of survival" concept could save an additional 100,000-200,000 Americans each year.[13] Implementation of 911 service nationwide and upgrading every ambulance and first-responding vehicle to rapid defibrillation capability should be considered an urgent priority in all communities. Finally, the public must be trained to recognize the warning signs of a heart attack, to call for help immediately, and to initiate CPR when a cardiac arrest occurs.

REFERENCES

1. Bossaert L, Van Hoeyweghen R, Cerebral Resuscitation Study Group: Bystander cardiopulmonary resuscitation (CPR) in out-of-hospital cardiac arrest. Resuscitation 17(suppl):S55-S69, 1989.
2. Cobb LA, Hallstrom AP: Community-based cardiopulmonary resuscitation: What have we learned? Ann NY Acad Sci 382:330-342, 1982.
3. Litwin PE, Eisenberg MS, Hallstrom AP, Cummins RO: The location of collapse and its effect on survival from cardiac arrest. Ann Emerg Med 16:787-791, 1987.
4. Ornato JP, McNeill SE, Craren EJ, Nelson NM: Limitation on effectiveness of rapid defibrillation by emergency medical technicians in a rural setting. Ann Emerg Med 13:1096-1099, 1984.
5. Bayés de Luna A, Coumel P, Leclercq JF: Ambulatory sudden cardiac death: Mechanisms of production of fatal arrhythmia on the basis of data from 157 cases. Am Heart J 117:151-159, 1989.
6. Myerburg RJ, Conde CA, Sung RJ, et al: Clinical, electrophysiologic and hemody-

namic profile of patients resuscitated from prehospital cardiac arrest. Am J Med 68:568, 1980.
8. Hinkle LE, Argyros DC, Hayes JC, Robinson T, Alonso DR: Pathogenesis of an unexpected sudden death: Role of early cycle ventricular contractions. Am J Cardiol 39: 873, 1977.
9. Klein RC, Vera Z, Mason DT, DeMaria AN, Awan NA, Amsterdam EA: Ambulatory Holter monitor documentation of ventricular tachyarrhythmias as mechanisms of sudden death in patients with coronary artery disease [abstract]. Clin Res 27:7A, 1979.
10. Schaffer WA, Cobb LA: Recurrent ventricular fibrillation and modes of death in survivors of out-of-hospital ventricular fibrillation. N Engl J Med 293:260, 1975.
11. Weaver WD, Cobb LA, Hallstrom AP, Fahrenbruch C, Copass MK, Ray R: Factors influencing survival after out-of-hospital cardiac arrest. J Am Coll Cardiol 7:754, 1986.
12. Eisenberg MS, Bergner L, Hallstrom A: Cardiac resuscitation in the community: Importance of rapid provision and implications for program planning. JAMA 241: 1905–1907, 1979.
13. Cummins RO, Ornato JP, Thies WH, Pepe PE: Improving survival from sudden cardiac arrest: The "chain of survival" concept. Circulation 83:1832–1847, 1991.
14. Walters G, Gluckman F: Planning a pre-hospital cardiac resuscitation programme: An analysis of community and system factors in London. J R Coll Physicians Lond 23:107, 1989.
15. Stults KR: Phone first. J Emerg Med Serv 12:78, 1987.
16. Alvarez H, Cobb LA: Experience with CPR training of the general public. In: Proceedings of the National Conference on Standards for Cardiopulmonary Resuscitation and Emergency Cardiac Care. Dallas, American Heart Association, 1975, p 33.
17. American Heart Association: Standards and guidelines for cardiopulmonary resuscitation (CPR) and emergency cardiac care (ECC). JAMA 255:2905, 1986.
18. American Red Cross: Adult CPR. Boston, American National Red Cross, 1987.
19. Mayron R, Long RS, Ruiz E: The 911 emergency telephone number: Impact on emergency medical systems access in a metropolitan area. Am J Emerg Med 2:491–493, 1984.
20. Hunt RC, Allison EJ Jr, Yates JG III: The need for improved emergency medical services in Pitt county. NC Med J 47:39–42, 1986.
21. Hunt RC, McCabe JB, Hamilton GC, Krohmer JR: Influence of emergency medical services systems and prehospital defibrillation on survival of sudden cardiac death victims. Am J Emerg Med 7:68–82, 1989.
22. Thompson BM, Stueven HA, Mateer JR, Aprahamian CC, Tucker JF, Darin JC: Comparison of clinical CPR studies in Milwaukee and elsewhere in the United States. Ann Emerg Med 14:750–754, 1985.
23. Kowalski R, Thompson BM, Horwitz L, Stueven H, Aprahamian C, Darin JC: Bystander CPR in prehospital coarse ventricular fibrillation. Ann Emerg Med 13: 1016–1020, 1984.
24. Cobb LA, Werner JA, Trobaugh GB: Sudden cardiac death: 1. A decade's experience with out-of-hospital resuscitation. Mod Concepts Cardiovasc Dis 49:31, 1980.
25. Murphy RJ, Luepker RV, Jacobs DR Jr, Gillum RF, Folsom AR, Blackburn H: Citizen cardiopulmonary resuscitation training and use in a metropolitan area: The Minnesota Heart Survey. Am J Public Health 74: 513–515, 1985.
26. Selby ML, Kautz JA, Moore TJ, et al: Indicators of response to a mass media CPR recruitment campaign. Am J Public Health 72: 1039, 1982.
27. Litwin PE, Eisenberg MS, Hallstrom AP, Cummins RO: The location of collapse and its effect on survival from cardiac arrest. Ann Emerg Med 16:787–791, 1987.
28. Mandel LP, Cobb LA: CPR training in the community. Ann Emerg Med 14:669–671, 1985.
29. Gombeski WR Jr, Effron DM, Ramirez AG, Moore TJ: Impact on retention: Comparison of two CPR training programs. Am J Public Health 72:849–852, 1982.
30. Muelleman RL, Ornato JP: Factors affecting the likelihood that CPR will be used by trained rescuers. Neb Med J 70:172–177, 1985.
31. St. Louis P, Carter WB, Eisenberg MS: Prescribing CPR: A survey of physicians. Am J Public Health 72:1158–1160, 1982.
32. Goldberg RJ: Physicians and CPR training in high-risk family members. Am J Public Health 77:671–672, 1987.
33. Bossaert L, Van Hoeyweghen R, and the Cerebral Resuscitation Study Group: Evaluation of cardiopulmonary resuscitation (CPR) techniques. Resuscitation 17(suppl): S99, 1989.
34. Ornato JP, Hallagan LF, McMahon SB, Peeples EH, Rostafinski AG: Attitudes of BCLS instructors about mouth-to-mouth resuscitation during the AIDS epidemic. Ann Emerg Med 19:151–156, 1990.
35. Jakobsson J, Nyquist O, Rehnquist N: Cardiac arrest in Stockholm with special refer-

ence to the ambulance organization. Acta Med Scand 222:117, 1987.
36. Pepe P: Advanced cardiac life support: State of the art. In Vincent JL (ed): Emergency and Intensive Care. Berlin, Springer-Verlag, 1990, p 565.
37. Pepe P: Presumptive diagnosis of death versus whom to resuscitate. In Kuehl A (ed): EMS Medical Director's Handbook for the National Association of EMS Physicians. St. Louis, CV Mosby, 1989, p 275.
38. Van Camp SP, Peterson RA: Cardiovascular complications of outpatient cardiac rehabilitation programs. JAMA 256:1160, 1986.
39. Haskell WL: Cardiovascular complications during exercise training in cardiac patients. Circulation 57:920, 1978.
40. Hossack KF, Hartwig R: Cardiac arrest associated with supervised cardiac rehabilitation. J Cardiac Rehab 2:402, 1982.
41. Eisenberg MS, Horwood BT, Cummins RO, Reynolds-Haertie R, Hearne TR: Cardiac arrest and resuscitation: A tale of 29 cities. Ann Emerg Med 19:179–186, 1990.
42. Ornato JP, McNeill SE, Craren EJ, Nelson NM: Limitations on effectiveness of rapid defibrillation by emergency medical technicians in a rural setting. Ann Emerg Med 13:1096–1099, 1984.
43. Eisenberg MS, Copass MK, Hallstrom AP, et al: Treatment of out-of-hospital cardiac arrest with rapid defibrillation by emergency medical technicians. N Engl J Med 302:1379–1383, 1980.
44. Kerber RE: Statement on early defibrillation from the Emergency Cardiac Care Committee, American Heart Association. Circulation 83:2233, 1991.
45. Rawlins DC: Study of the management of suspected cardiac infarction by British immediate care doctors. Br Med J 294:352–354, 1981.
46. Pai GR, Haites NE, Rawles JM: One thousand heart attacks in Grampian: The place of cardiopulmonary resuscitation in general practice. Br Med J 294:352–354, 1987.
47. Colquhoun MC: Use of defibrillators by general practitioners. Br Med J 297:336–337, 1988.
48. Eisenberg MS, Moore J, Cummins RO, et al: Use of the automatic external defibrillator in home of survivors of out-of-hospital ventricular fibrillation. Am J Cardiol 63:443–446, 1989.
49. Swenson RD, Hill DL, Martin JS, Wirkus M, Weaver WD: Automatic external defibrillators used by family members to treat cardiac arrest [abstract]. Circulation 76(suppl IV):IV-463, 1987.
50. Weaver WD, Sutherland K, Wirkus MJ, Bachman R: Emergency medical care requirements for large public assemblies and a new strategy for managing cardiac arrest in this setting. Ann Emerg Med 18:155–160, 1989.
52. Cummins RO: From concept to standard-of-care? Review of the clinical experience with automated external defibrillators. Ann Emerg Med 18:1269–1275, 1989.
53. Chadda KD, Kammerer RJ, Kuphal J, Miller K: Successful defibrillation in the industrial, recreational, and corporate settings by laypersons [abstract]. Circulation 76(suppl IV):IV-12, 1987.
54. Wilson BD, Graton MC, Overton J, Watson W: Unexpected ALS procedures on non-emergency ambulance calls: The value of a single tier system. Prehosp Disaster Med 6:382, 1991.
55. Ornato JP, Racht EM, Fitch JJ, Berry JF: The need for ALS in urban and suburban EMS systems. Ann Emerg Med 19:151–152, 1990.
56. Ornato JP, Gonzalez ER, Jaffe AS: Cardiovascular drug use in cardiopulmonary resuscitation. In Messerli FH (ed): Cardiovascular Drug Therapy. Philadelphia, WB Saunders, 1990, pp 121–138.
57. Brown CG, Werman HA, Davis EA, Hamlin R, Hobson J, Ashton JA: Comparative effect of graded doses of epinephrine on regional brain blood flow during CPR in a swine model. Ann Emerg Med 15:1138–1144, 1986.
58. Brown CG, Werman HA, Davis EA, Hobson J, Hamlin RL: The effect of graded doses of epinephrine during cardiopulmonary resuscitation on regional myocardial blood flow in a swine model. Circulation 75:491–497, 1987.
59. Gonzalez ER, Ornato JP, Garnett AR, Levine R, Young DS, Racht EM: Dose-dependent vasopressor response to epinephrine during CPR in humans. Ann Emerg Med 18:920–926, 1989.
60. Paradis NA, Martin GB, Rosenberg J, et al: The effect of stand- and high-dose epinephrine on coronary perfusion pressure during prolonged cardiopulmonary resuscitation. JAMA 265:1139–1144, 1991.
61. Callaham M, Barton CW, Kayser S: Potential complications of high-dose epinephrine therapy in patients resuscitated from cardiac arrest. JAMA 265:1117–1122, 1991.
62. Ornato JP: High-dose epinephrine during resuscitation: A word of caution [editorial]. JAMA 265:1160–1161, 1991.
63. McKeever WP, Gregg DE, Canney PC: Oxygen uptake of the nonworking left ventricle. Cir Res 6:612–623, 1958.
64. Monroe RG, French G: Ventricular pres-

sure-volume relationships and oxygen consumption in fibrillation and arrest. Circ Res 8:260–266, 1960.
65. Kohn RM: Myocardial oxygen uptake during ventricular fibrillation and electromechanical dissociation. Am J Cardiol 11:483–486, 1963.
66. Brown CG, Taylor RB, Werman HA, Luu T, Spittler G, Hamlin RL: Effect of standard doses of epinephrine on myocardial oxygen delivery and utilization during cardiopulmonary resuscitation. Crit Care Med 16:536–539, 1988.
67. Brown CG, Werman HA: Adrenergic agonists during cardiopulmonary resuscitation. Resuscitation 19:1–16, 1990.
68. Ditchey RV, Lindenfeld J: Failure of epinephrine to improve the balance between myocardial oxygen supply and demand during closed-chest resuscitation in dogs. Circulation 78:382–389, 1988.
69. Midei MG, Sugiura S, Maughan WI, Sagawa K, Weisfeldt ML, Guerci AD: Preservation of ventricular function by treatment of ventricular fibrillation with phenylephrine. J Am Coll Cardiol 16:489–494, 1990.
70. Weaver WD, Fahrenbruch CE, Johnson DD, Hallstrom AP, Cobb LA, Copass MK: Effect of epinephrine and lidocaine therapy on outcome after cardiac arrest due to ventricular fibrillation. Circulation 82:2027–2034, 1990.
71. Chow MSS, Kluger J, Lawrence R, Fieldman A: The effects of lidocaine and bretylium on the defibrillation threshold during cardiac arrest and cardiopulmonary resuscitation. Proc Soc Exp Biol Med 182:63, 1986.
72. Haynes RE, Chinn TL, Copass MK, Cobb LA: Comparison of bretylium tosylate and lidocaine in the management of out-of-hospital ventricular fibrillation: A randomized clinical trial. Am J Cardiol 48:353, 1981.
73. Olson DW, Thompson BM, Darin JC, Milbrath MH: A randomized comparison of bretylium tosylate and lidocaine in resuscitation of patients from out-of-hospital ventricular fibrillation in a paramedic system. Ann Emerg Med 13:807, 1984.
74. Hanyok JJ, Chow MSS, Kluger J, Fieldman A: Antifibrillatory effects of high dose bretylium and a lidocaine-bretylium combination during cardiopulmonary resuscitation. Crit Care Med 16:691, 1988.
75. Chapman JR, Boyd MJ: Intravenous amiodarone in ventricular fibrillation. Br Med J 282:951–952, 1981.
76. Klein RC, Machell C, Rushforth N, Standefur J. Efficacy of intravenous amiodarone as short-term treatment for refractory ventricular tachycardia. Amer Heart J 115:96–101, 1988.
77. Williams ML, Woelfel A, Cascio WE, Simpson RJ, Gettes LS, Foster FR: Intravenous amiodarone during prolonged resuscitation from cardiac arrest. Ann Intern Med 110:839–842, 1989.
78. Myerburg RJ, Estes D, Zaman L, et al: Outcome of resuscitation from bradyarrhythmia or asystolic prehospital cardiac arrest. J Am Coll Cardiol 4:1118, 1984.
79. Stueven HA, Tonsfeldt DJ, Thompson BM, et al: Atropine in asystole: Human studies. Ann Emerg Med 13:815, 1984.
80. Coon GA, Colinton JE, Ruiz E: Use of atropine for bradysystolic prehospital cardiac arrest. Ann Emeg Med 10:462–467, 1981.
81. Iseri LT, Humphrey SB, Siner EJ: Pre-hospital bradyasystolic cardiac arrest. Ann Intern Med 88:741–745, 1978.
82. Ornato JP, Carveth WL, Windle JR: Pacemaker insertion for prehospital bradyasystolic cardiac arrest. Ann Emerg Med 13:101, 1984.
83. Zoll PM, Zoll RH, Falk RH, et al: External noninvasive temporary cardiac pacing: Clinical trials. Circulation 71:937, 1984.
84. Falk RH, Jacobs L, Sinclair A, et al: External noninvasive cardiac pacing in out-of-hospital cardiac arrest. Crit Care Med 11:779, 1983.
85. Weisfeldt ML, Bishop RL, Greene HL: Effects of pH and pCO_2 on performance of ischemic myocardium. In Roy P, Rona G (eds): International Study Group for Research in Cardiac Metabolism: The Metabolism of Contraction. Recent Advances in Studies on Cardiac Structure and Metabolism, vol X. Baltimore, University of Maryland Press, 1975, p 355.
86. Ewy GA: Defining electromechanical dissociation. Ann Emerg Med 13:830, 1984.
87. Stults KR, Brown DD, Schug VL, et al: Prehospital defibrillation performed by emergency medical technicians in rural communities. N Engl J Med 301:219–223, 1984.
88. Vukov LF, White RD, Bachman JW, et al: New perspectives on rural EMT defibrillation. Ann Emerg Med 17:318–321, 1988.
89. Eisenberg MS, Hadas E, Nuri I, et al: Sudden cardiac arrest in Israel: Factors associated with successful resuscitation. Am J Emerg Med 6:319–323, 1988.
90. Guzy PM, Pearce LM, Greenfield S: The survival benefit of bystander cardiopulmonary resuscitation in a paramedic served metropolitan area. Am J Public Health 73:766–769, 1983.
91. Stueven H, Troiano P, Thompson B, et al: Bystander/first responder CPR: Ten years

experience in a paramedic system. Ann Emerg Med 15:707–710, 1986.
92. Weaver WD, Cobb LA, Fahrenbruch CE, et al: Use of the automatic external defibrillator in the management of out-of-hospital cardiac arrest. N Engl J Med 319:661–666, 1988.
93. Eisenberg MS, Hallstrom AP, Copass MK, et al: Treatment of ventricular fibrillation with emergency medical technician defibrillation and paramedic services. JAMA 251:1723–1726, 1984.
94. Cummins RO, Chamberlain DA, Abramson NS, et al: Recommended guidelines for uniform reporting of data from out-of-hospital cardiac arrest: The Utstein style. Ann Emerg Med 20:861–874, 1991.

F
Work-up and Assessment of Risk for Sudden Cardiac Death

32

Patients with Cardiac Arrest and Documented Ventricular Fibrillation

STEFAN OSSWALD
THOMAS G. TROUTON
SEAN O'NUNAIN
JEREMY N. RUSKIN

The incidence of sudden cardiac death (SCD) in the United States is estimated to range from 300,000 to 400,000 per year,[1-3] and SCD accounts for approximately 50% of all cardiovascular deaths. Most of these unexpected deaths are the first manifestation of cardiac disease.[4] Based on whole-population figures they result in an incidence of 1–2/1000 population per year (0.1–0.2%). With the widespread use of cardiopulmonary resuscitation and advanced cardiac life support, including out-of-hospital defibrillation by emergency personnel, up to 30% of victims survive an out-of-hospital cardiac arrest.[5,6] The percentage of survivors varies from 2% to 44%, depending on the reporting center, the primary documented arrhythmia, and differences in the definition of SCD.[7,8] In early series, long-term survival following resuscitation from SCD was characterized by high recurrence rates (30% at 1 year and 45% at 2 years),[9-11] but this has improved significantly over the past decade,[12] mainly because of accurate risk assessment for recurrence of SCD, the more aggressive treatment of ischemia, and the introduction of the cardioverter-defibrillator.[13,14]

Despite a long-term reduction in sudden death rates with the implantable cardioverter-defibrillator (ICD), the high costs of this treatment modality make a careful risk-benefit assessment mandatory. With the widespread use of device therapy and the broadening of clinical indications, the estimated costs per life-year saved may be rising despite increasing device longevity and shorter hospital stays (resulting from the increased use of nonthoracotomy lead systems).[15] Therefore, the primary goal of risk stratification is to select appropriate high-risk patients for ICD implantation; a related goal is to define subgroups in whom an ICD is not needed. Ultimately, risk stratification may become the tool with which to select patients who would benefit most from this therapy in terms of life-years saved, if escalating costs demand more restrictive indications.[15]

PATHOPHYSIOLOGY OF FATAL ARRHYTHMIAS IN CARDIAC ARREST SURVIVORS

SCD is usually defined as an unexpected death that occurs within 1 hour after onset of cardiac symptoms and includes arrhythmic as well as nonarrhythmic causes (e.g., electromechanical dissociation, acute infarction with cardiogenic shock, pulmonary embolism, aortic dissection, and the like). Clinically it is helpful to divide arrhythmic SCD into three categories: (1) primary ventricular tachyarrhythmias, (2) secondary ventricular tachyarrhythmias (due to supraventricular tachyarrhythmias with fast atrioventricular [AV] conduction or accessory pathway conduction), and (3) bradyarrhythmias and asystole. Regardless of the underlying heart disease, ventricular fibrillation (VF) is associated with the best short-term survival to hospital admission[7,16] and accounts for the greatest proportion of survivors of out-of-hospital cardiac arrest. VF is the first documented rhythm in 60–85% of patients resuscitated from SCD[17,18] and is found even more frequently if the underlying heart disease is coronary artery disease (CAD).[12] Data from Holter monitoring have shown that rapid ventricular tachycardia (VT) is most commonly the initial arrhythmia, followed by degeneration to polymorphic VT and VF.[18,19] Secondary VF arrests, in the presence of ventricular pre-excitation and a rapidly conducting accessory pathway with antegrade refractory periods shorter than 260 msec, are found in younger patients and are usually exercise related[20]; however, it is estimated that the absolute incidence of SCD due to Wolff-Parkinson-White syndrome is extremely low and affects probably only 1/1000 patients with this syndrome. Patients with SCD due to complete heart block and asystole have a very poor short-term prognosis and usually die before hospital admission.[16] The underlying pathology is usually severe conduction system disease, which may be exaggerated by overdrive suppression after cessation of intermittent supraventricular arrhythmias.[21,22] Fatal asystole is often associated with the use of negative dromotropic drugs that potentiate pre-existing conduction abnormalities and/or suppress lifesaving escape rhythms. Conversely, asystole has also been reported to be the initial arrhythmia responsible for spontaneous VF in some patients.[23–25] Bradyarrhythmias, asystole, and electromechanical dissociation are more frequently found as causes of SCD in patients with severe congestive heart failure.[26]

STRUCTURAL CARDIAC ABNORMALITIES FOUND IN CARDIAC ARREST SURVIVORS

The first step in the clinical evaluation of cardiac arrest survivors is assessment of the underlying structural heart disease, which is highly age dependent. The most commonly encountered structural cardiac abnormality in cardiac arrest survivors older than 40 years is CAD, which is present in 65–80% of this group.[12,14,16,25,27–39] The prevalence of CAD in autopsy series is even higher.[40] Dilated cardiomyopathy is found in approximately 10–15% of patients over 40 years of age and includes various forms of idiopathic dilated cardiomyopathy, inflammatory myocarditis (e.g., viral myocarditis and postinflammatory myocardial fibrosis, sarcoid, Chagas's disease) and infiltrative cardiomyopathies (amyloidosis, hemochromatosis). Hypertrophic cardiomyopathy, either primary or secondary, is frequently found in combination with CAD and is an independent predictor of risk for SCD.[41,42] At autopsy, patients with CAD and SCD had a higher incidence of ventricular hypertrophy than patients with CAD alone, who died from other causes.[43] Patients with valvular heart disease usually comprise those with calcific aortic stenosis and left ventricular (LV) hypertrophy and are typically elderly patients (>70 years), whereas mitral valve prolapse syndrome is more frequently found in younger women. Malignant ventricular tachyarrhythmias and SCD associated with mitral valve prolapse, however, are thought to develop when hemodynamically significant mitral regurgitation and LV dilation are present and, therefore, tend to occur during the later course of this disease.[44,45]

In younger patients (<40 years), who frequently suffer cardiac arrest in the setting of physical exertion, hypertrophic cardiomyopathy with or without outflow tract obstruction is frequently encountered. Regardless of the underlying etiology, hypertrophic cardiomyopathy often affects children and young adults aged 10–35 years.[46–48] Congenital abnormalities, such as the Wolff-Parkinson-White syndrome with rapid antegrade conduction over the accessory pathway during atrial fibrillation,[20] anomalies of coronary arteries,[49] right ventricular dysplasia, congenital heart disease (e.g., repaired tetralogy of Fallot or transposition of the great arteries), the long QT interval syndromes, and mitral valve prolapse, are less common causes of SCD in this patient group. Rheumatic heart disease, which still has a high prevalence in nonindustrialized countries, and other forms of infiltrative myocarditis have the potential for malignant ventricular arrhythmias; however, they are more frequently associated with conduction system disease and heart block than with primary ventricular arrhythmias.

In a minority of cardiac arrest survivors (5–10%) no structural heart disease can be identified and other triggers such as coronary vasospasm, severe electrolyte abnormalities (e.g., hypokalemia, hypomagnesemia, hyperkalemia), proarrhythmic drug effects (e.g., antiarrhythmics, antidepressants, antihistaminics), or substance abuse (e.g., cocaine, amphetamines) must be considered.[50,51] Finally, there is a small number of cardiac arrest survivors in whom neither structural heart disease nor other triggers can be identified, suggesting that primary VF may occur in the normal heart.[52]

GENERAL CLINICAL EVALUATION OF CARDIAC ARREST SURVIVORS

The initial management of cardiac arrest survivors is usually characterized by a variable stabilization period in an intensive care unit with continuous rhythm monitoring. A considerable number of patients remain unstable, accounting for the high early in-hospital mortality of up to 50–60%.[16] One third of these patients die from cardiogenic shock or congestive heart failure, whereas recurrent cardiac arrhythmias account for only 5–10% of early deaths. Other reasons for early mortality are respiratory complications, sepsis, and hypoxic brain damage without recovery. In some of these unstable patients aggressive interventions such as intra-aortic balloon pumping, acute angioplasty, or coronary bypass surgery may be necessary. Neurological recovery from hypoxic encephalopathy is usually fairly rapid when full recovery is achieved. In a study of 457 cardiac arrest survivors, 39% remained comatose within 4 days of admission and accounted for 80% of all deaths.[53] Of those patients who subsequently recovered from coma, 25% were conscious on admission to the hospital and 92% were conscious by the third day. Two thirds of all survivors recovered without neurological deficit, whereas in another third mild deficits persisted. Early recovery of consciousness and blood glucose levels below 300 mg/dl on admission were predictive of a favorable outcome, while coma persisting 3 days after admission was associated with a poor prognosis.[54]

Once patients have survived this critical period, all those without significant remaining neurological impairment should undergo full cardiac evaluation unless there are other contraindications (e.g., terminal illness). There is no age limitation, since elderly patients in particular may have correctable cardiac disorders such as aortic stenosis or complete heart block. With a careful cardiovascular examination that includes chest x-ray and serial electrocardiographic (ECG) and CPK/CK-MB analysis, acute or chronic CAD, congestive heart failure, hypertrophic cardiomyopathy, and other conditions such as Wolff-Parkinson-White syndrome or the long QT syndrome can be identified. The clinical examination should focus on the extent of generalized atherosclerosis, in particular on cerebrovascular atherosclerosis, which together with heart rate and pump function is an important determinant of the hemodynamic consequences of tachyarrhythmias. A thorough history from the patient and witnesses can often identify possible triggering mechanisms, which may give hints to the pathophysiological mechanisms of arrhythmogenesis and underlying heart disease (e.g., preceding angina pectoris, SCD in the setting of physical exertion, etc.). sometimes the family history is suggestive of genetically determined disorders manifesting as SCD such as the long QT syndrome,[55] hypertrophic cardiomyopathy,[56] the familial form of dilated cardiomyopathy, arrhythmogenic right ventricular dysplasia,[57] and familial SCD without cardiomyopathy.[58,59]

Electrolyte abnormalities (hypokalemia or hypomagnesemia) are quite commonly found in cardiac arrest survivors and may play a triggering role in arrhythmogenesis. However, hypokalemia after resuscitation may represent a secondary phenomenon related to a catecholamine-induced potassium shift into skeletal muscles, sometimes exaggerated by respiratory alkalosis due to mechanical hyperventilation during CPR.[60] Conversely, severe hyperkalemia, which may occur in the setting of pre-existing renal failure and/or therapy with angiotensin-converting enzyme drugs in combination with potassium-sparing diuretics or prostaglandin inhibitors, is a well-established cause of lethal conduction abnormalities and also VT.[61,62] Metabolic acidosis, severe muscle injury (crush syndrome), and shock may contribute to an increased extracellular potassium concentration via cell membrane leakage. This potassium shift lowers the negative transmembrane resting potential and spontaneous phase 4 depolarization, resulting in conduction block and suppression of automaticity.[63] Furthermore, a proarrhythmic effect of certain drugs (e.g., digoxin, antiarrhythmics, antihistamines)[64,65] and intoxication with psychotropic drugs (tricyclic antidepressants, amphetamines, and recreational substance abuse [e.g., cocaine]) should always be considered[50,51] and the appropriate plasma level measurements and toxicology screening tests performed.[64]

Based on this clinical approach, the age-dependent prevalence of underlying heart disease, and the first documented rhythm, the etiology of SCD can usually be assigned to one of the following categories: (1) ischemic heart disease, (2) nonischemic heart disease, or (3) no overt heart disease. These categories are helpful for decision-making and the choice of further noninvasive and invasive investigations.

NONINVASIVE LABORATORY EVALUATIONS

Assessment of Left Ventricular Function

LV function is the strongest independent predictor for recurrence and long-term survival after out-of-hospital cardiac arrest[29,66,67] and is also predictive of successful suppression of inducible ventricular arrhythmias during serial drug testing.[29,38,68] For noninvasive assessment of LV ejection fraction (LVEF), echocardiography and radionuclide ventriculography are commonly employed. Newer techniques such as magnetic resonance imaging[69] or positron emission tomography are currently being evaluated for this purpose. In a study of 154 SCD survivors, LVEF at rest, assessed by exercise radionuclide ventriculography, was the only independent predictor of long-term outcome[70]: the 5-year mortality in the subgroup of 45 patients with normal LVEF (> 0.50) was only 4%, compared to almost 70% for the group with an LVEF < 0.35. Moderately impaired LV function (LVEF of 0.35–0.50) was associated with a 5-year mortality of 48%.[70] Wall motion abnormalities at rest or during exercise as well as a further decrease in the ejection fraction during exercise were not independent predictors of survival in this study.[70]

Ambulatory Holter Monitoring

Holter monitoring is commonly used for noninvasive evaluation of cardiac arrest survivors and reveals ventricular premature beats or nonsustained VT in up to 50–70%.[12,71] The incidence of sustained VT and VF recorded by ambulatory monitoring is extremely low, reflected in a less than 10% in-hospital recurrence rate of SCD.[16] However, Holter data from documented SCD episodes have generated important insights into the modes of arrhythmia initiation in victims of SCD, demonstrating that VF is frequently triggered by VT and is rarely the primary arrhythmia.[72–74] Although ischemic ST changes immediately before the fatal event have been postulated by some,[75] Holter data from other studies do not support this hypothesis.[73]

The role of complex ventricular ectopy as a direct trigger for subsequent SCD remains unclear. Complex ventricular ectopy and nonsustained VT after cardiac arrest and after myocardial infarction (MI) have been shown to be associated with a higher incidence of SCD.[12,71,76,77] More recent studies addressing the issue of LV dysfunction have shown that ventricular ectopy after MI is predictive of SCD only in patients with impaired LV function.[67,78] Early studies with empirical antiarrhythmic treatment of ventricular ectopy showed no difference in the rate of recurrent cardiac arrest.[9,11] In a later study documenting successful suppression of ventricular ectopy in 52% of patients, the recurrence rate of SCD was 5% after 1 year and 29% after 5 years, as compared to 19% and 48% in patients with nonsuppressed ventricular ectopic activity.[30] However, after correcting for LV function, the presence of ventricular ectopy and the effect of drug suppression were no longer predictive. These data suggest that Holter-documented complex ventricular ectopy and its suppressibility by antiarrhythmic treatment are a marker of LV dysfunction but have no direct impact on the recurrence of SCD. Recent observations from the Cardiac Arrhythmia Suppression Trial (CAST) where a population at low risk for SCD has been investigated showed that effective arrhythmia suppression with encainide or flecainide was associated with a threefold excess mortality.[79] Treatment with moricizine resulted in an increase in early fatal proarrhythmia and no benefit over placebo in long-term survival. Thus, the current view of ventricular ectopy and nonsustained VT in patients resuscitated from SCD is still controversial; these arrhythmias may be a marker of underlying cardiac disease rather than the cause of increased mortality.

Signal-Averaged Electrocardiogram

Late potentials recorded in the terminal phase of the filtered QRS complex by the signal-averaged ECG, thought to represent an arrhythmogenic anatomical substrate, have also been reported to be predictive of spontaneous arrhythmic events. Most evidence for the prognostic value of late potentials has been derived from large prospective screening studies after MI. The incidence of abnormal signal-averaged ECG findings or late potentials 1 month after acute MI is 24–44%[80–83] and is associated with a 16.7–28.9% incidence of subsequent arrhythmic events (SCD, VF, or VF) during a mean follow-up of 7.5–14 months, compared to only 0.8–3.5% among patients with normal signal-averaged ECG findings. The combination of LV dysfunction as assessed by radionuclide ventriculography and the signal-averaged ECG provides a sensitive tool for detecting high-risk patients after MI. In two prospective studies, patients with an LVEF <0.40 and abnormal findings on signal-averaged ECG experienced a 34–36% arrhythmic event rate (SCD, VF, or VT) within the first year following MI, whereas none of the patients with a normal EF and a normal signal-average ECG suffered arrhythmic events (negative predictive accuracy = 100%).[81,82] The prognostic value of the signal-averaged ECG is less well defined in patients with nonischemic heart disease. However, it seems that a filtered QRS width > 120 msec and late potentials (amplitude < 40 μV, duration > 38 msec) might also be predictive of a negative outcome in patients with dilated cardiomyopathy,[84,85] but with a lower specificity and sensitivity than in patients with ischemic heart disease. In patients with hypertrophic cardiomyopathy the signal-averaged ECG is abnormal in 15–20%. The predictive value for SCD, however, is not proven in this condition.[86] The prognostic value of the signal-averaged ECG in the heterogeneous group of cardiac arrest survivors is not yet established, but it seems to be less frequently positive when the documented arrhythmia is VF as compared to sustained VT.[87,88]

Exercise Stress Testing

Exercise testing with scintigraphy has been used to assess overt or silent ischemia. Both exercise thallium stress testing and exercise radionuclide ventriculography have a sensitivity and specificity in the range of 80–95% for the detection of ischemia, depending on the extent of CAD. Thallium scintigraphy has the limitation that diffuse three-vessel disease with symmetrically diminished uptake may be missed. With exercise radionuclide ventriculography, significant three-vessel disease usually manifests as a decrease in LVEF during exercise of more than 0.05. The latter method has the additional advantage that an accurate assessment of LV function is obtained at the same time. Exercise testing itself rarely provokes arrhythmias in this patient population and is not useful for guidance of antiarrhythmic therapy.

Assessment of Autonomic Nervous Influence on the Cardiovascular System

Other more investigational methods for noninvasive risk stratification in cardiac arrest survivors include heart rate variability (HRV) and determination of baroreceptor reflex sensitivity, which both reflect the influence of autonomic tone on the cardiovascular system. HRV has been shown to correlate inversely with long-term outcome after MI. In a study of 808 survivors of acute MI, mortality was 34% during a mean follow-up period of 31 months if HRV was less than 50 msec, compared to 12% in patients with HRV of more than 100 msec.[89] Other data suggest that HRV is also decreased in patients with overt congestive heart failure, impaired LV function, and increasing age. Baroreceptor reflex sensitivity as a measure of autonomic tone has proven to be a powerful predictor of ischemia-induced VF after healed experimental MI.[90] Direct comparison of these techniques has shown that each measures different aspects of parasympathetic innervation and that the information gained from the two studies is complementary.[91]

The value of different combinations of noninvasive methods for risk stratification after MI, such as signal-averaged ECG, HRV, and Holter monitoring[92] or HRV and baroreceptor reflex sensitivity[93] for the prediction of SCD, has been prospectively assessed, but the current role of such strategies in the evaluation of cardiac arrest survivors remains to be determined.

INVASIVE LABORATORY EVALUATIONS

Cardiac Catheterization and Coronary Angiography

Cardiac catheterization (coronary angiography with left and right heart hemodynamics and left ventriculography) is usually the first and most efficient invasive test for assessment of heart disease in patients who have sustained cardiac arrest.[94] Younger patients with no obvious structural heart disease should not be exempted, for coronary angiography may detect rare entities such as aberrant origins of coronary arteries and other vascular anomalies.[49] In cases of dilated cardiomyopathy, right ventricular endomyocardial biopsy may provide further information but usually shows only nonspecific intersitial infiltrates and fibrosis. Acute myocarditis with muscle cell necrosis is rarely seen. The most powerful predictor of recurrent cardiac arrest and nonsudden cardiac death is the LVEF.[29,66,67] In a study of 166 cardiac arrest survivors, an LVEF < 0.30 was associated with a 2.6-fold increased risk of recurrent cardiac arrest and a 4.3-fold increased risk of cardiac death.[29]

The prevalence of CAD in this series was 74% (three-vessel CAD: 61%, two-vessel CAD: 20%, one-vessel CAD: 18%) and an LV aneurysm was present in 28%. Neither coronary anatomy nor the presence of an LV aneurysm was predictive of recurrent cardiac arrest. These findings were confirmed by the Coronary Artery Surgery Study (CASS), which included 19,946 patients with CAD who were randomly assigned to either surgical or medical treatment. Over a mean follow-up of 5 years, 2,445 patients died (12.2%), and 761 of them died suddenly (3.8%). The overall incidence of SCD was lower in the surgically treated group (2.5% vs. 4.7%) despite similar coronary anatomy and LV function in the surgically and medically treated groups, suggesting a favorable impact of surgical revascularization on the long-term incidence of SCD.[95] For both treatment groups, hemodynamic and angiographic findings at baseline showed no differences between patients who died suddenly and those who died of other causes. In the medically treated group, univariate comparison of clinical parameters revealed that SCD was more frequently associated with male sex, digitalis therapy, and the absence of unstable angina. In the surgically treated group, SCD was associated with male sex and less frequent use of antianginal medication (β-adrenoceptor blockers or nitrate treatment). In conclusion, this large prospective trial of patients at low risk of SCD could not define hemodynamic or angiographic parameters that were predictive of the mode of death and that prospectively identified patients at high risk for SCD.[95,96]

PROGRAMMED ELECTRICAL STIMULATION

Prognostic Impact of Inducible Ventricular Arrhythmias in Cardiac Arrest Survivors

After definition of the underlying heart disease and treatment of possibly reversible factors such as ischemia, electrolyte imbalance, congestive heart failure, and discontinuation of possibly proarrhythmic drugs, electrophysiological evaluation has become the most important tool for risk stratification and selection of therapy in cardiac arrest survivors.[14,29,94,97] The incidence of CAD in large series of cardiac arrest survivors ranges from 60% to 75%, and sustained ventricular arrhythmias are inducible in 50–70% using programmed electrical stimulation (PES) in the baseline, drug-free state.[25,29,31,33,34,36-39] Sustained monomorphic VT is induced at PES in approximately 40–50% of patients and tends to be more frequently induced in patients with prior MI or depressed LV function,[34,98] whereas polymorphic VT and VF are found in 10–20%. However, in 30–50% only nonsustained VT or no arrhythmia is inducible (Table 32-1).

The incidence of induced sustained arrhythmias at baseline PES depends on the underlying heart disease, the degree of LV dysfunction, the presenting arrhythmia, and the aggressiveness of the programmed stimulation protocol used. Several studies have addressed this issue, both in patients presenting with VT and in those presenting with VF. In patients presenting with VT, most studies have found a high sensitivity and reproducibility (approximately 90%) in the induction of ventricular arrhythmias using PES, irrespective of the protocol used.[36,99-101] Prior MI and prior clinical VT predict the induction of VT at PES (VT inducible in 91% if both are present, vs. 13% if both are absent) but are not predictive for the induction of VF.[99]

In cardiac arrest survivors, however, the incidence and specificity of arrhythmia induction are lower than in patients presenting with VT. A comparative study of two different PES protocols using double and triple extrastimuli techniques in 196 cardiac arrest survivors and 46 control patients yielded a twofold increase in the induction of monomorphic VT (21% vs. 40%, $p < 0.001$) and VF (8% vs. 19%, $p < 0.004$) if triple extrastimuli were used instead of double extrastimuli,[37] a finding similar to that found in patients presenting with VT.[102] In contrast to patients presenting with VT, in whom a significant correlation between the induction of nonspecific VF and short coupling intervals has been found,[103] this study did not find such a relationship in cardiac arrest survivors.[37] When triple extrastimuli were applied at the shortest possible coupling interval, VF was never induced in con-

Table 32–1.
Incidence of Inducible Ventricular Arrhythmias at Baseline Electrophysiological Study in Survivors of Cardiac Arrest

Study	n	CAD (%)	Protocol (No. of Extrastimuli)	MVT (%)	VF/PVT (%)	NSVT (%)	None (%)
Roy et al, 1983[34]	119	71	2–3	38	23	9	30
Swerdlow et al, 1987[37]	196	69	3	40	19	11	30
Eldar et al, 1987[31]	108	61	3	38	10	21	31
Wilber et al, 1988[29]	166	75	2–3	37	15	27	21
Freedman et al, 1988[36]	150	67	3	55	15	5	25
Hays et al, 1989[25]	100	64	3	40	29	—	31
Furukawa et al, 1989[39]	101	(100*)	4	45	14	17	25
Poole et al, 1990[38]	241	69	3	27	16	14	43
Powell et al, 1993[14]	331	72	3	38	15	16	31
		61–75%		27–55%	10–29%	5–27%	21–43%

Abbreviations: CAD, prevalence of coronary artery disease in the patient population; MVT, sustained monomorphic ventricular tachycardia (VT); VF, ventricular fibrillation; PVT, sustained polymorphic VT; NSVT, nonsustained VT; None, no inducible ventricular arrhythmia.
* Study analyzed electrophysiological findings in 101 patients with CAD out of 142 cardiac arrest survivors (71% prevalence of CAD).

trol patients (0% vs. 19%) despite the use of shorter coupling intervals than those necessary for VF induction in cardiac arrest survivors.[37] In fact, there was a significant correlation between the induction of VF and the incidence of VF as the presenting arrhythmia. Using a similar stimulation protocol, it has been reported in another study that VF was inducible in up to 25% of cardiac arrest survivors as compared to only 3% in patients presenting with monomorphic VT.[104] These data suggest that VF induction in patients whose presenting arrhythmia is VF may be a specific result, in contrast to VF induction in patients presenting with recurrent VT, which is considered to be a nonspecific finding and a function of the aggressiveness of the protocol use.[103,105,106] In the evaluation of cardiac arrest survivors, stimulation protocols employing up to triple extrastimuli at two drive cycle lengths and two different right ventricular sites have become standard for most laboratories.[107]

Apart from the stimulation protocol used, the prognostic value of PES depends largely on the nature and extent of underlying structural heart disease, and its role is best established in patients with CAD whose presenting arrhythmia is monomorphic VT.[99,100,106,108,109] The role of PES is less well established in patients with sustained ventricular arrhythmias and dilated cardiomyopathy[110,111] or hypertrophic cardiomyopathy.[112-114] The role of PES for risk stratification and therapy guidance in survivors of out-of-hospital cardiac arrest has been extensively studied. However, owing to the heterogeneity of underlying heart disease in this population, different definitions of inducibility and noninducibility and differences in the therapeutic management (e.g., incidence of implanted ICDs), the predictive accuracy of PES in this setting is difficult to assess and to compare between studies. In order to obtain comparable data in future trials, guidelines for uniform reporting of data in survivors of out-of-hospital cardiac arrest have recently been proposed by the Utstein conference.[115] Currently published data still lack this uniformity and are further complicated by the fact that most studies of cardiac arrest survivors do not report separate results for ischemic and nonischemic heart disease. CAD usually accounts for the majority of patients (60–75%) in published studies.

In this heterogeneous population of cardiac arrest survivors, it has been shown that induction of arrhythmias at baseline PES is predictive of total cardiac mortality but does not predict recurrent cardiac arrest.[29,38] Persistent inducibility of VT or VF on antiarrhythmic drugs, however, is strongly predictive of both total cardiac mortality and recurrent cardiac arrest.[29,39] In the study of Wilber et al.,[29] the rate of recurrent cardiac arrest in patients with inducible VT or VF that was suppressed by drugs during serial electrophysiological testing was 6% after 1 year and 15% after 3 years of follow-up, as compared to 33% and 50%, respectively, in patients whose arrhythmias were not suppressed by drugs. Both persistently inducible arrhythmias and reduced LVEF were independent predictors of a poor outcome (Fig. 32-1). The relative risk for recurrent cardiac arrest was increased fourfold when ventricular arrhythmias were persistently inducible at PES, 2.6-fold when severe LV dysfunction (EF $\leq$ 0.30) was present, and 4.2-fold in the absence of surgical revascularization. Persistent inducibility of ventricular arrhythmias and severe LV dysfunction were found to interact in a multiplicative way, resulting in a 10-fold increased risk for recurrent cardiac arrest if both risk factors were present. A more recent study, which assessed long-term outcome in 217 survivors of out-of-hospital cardiac arrest in relation to their antiarrhythmic regimen, showed comparable results.[116] In this study, patients were classified either as having no inducible arrhythmias at baseline PES (37%), as drug responders with inducible but drug-suppressed arrhythmias (24%), or as nonresponders with persistently inducible arrhythmias (39%). Most patients in the last group received an ICD (53%) or were given amiodarone (42%). Twenty-three (28%) of 81 patients without inducible arrhythmias at baseline received an ICD, whereas none of the drug responders did initially. Overall survival and SCD-free survival for either group was not different at 2 years and 5 years, respectively, despite an almost twofold increase in the incidence of arrhythmic events in nonresponders as compared to drug responders and noninducible patients,

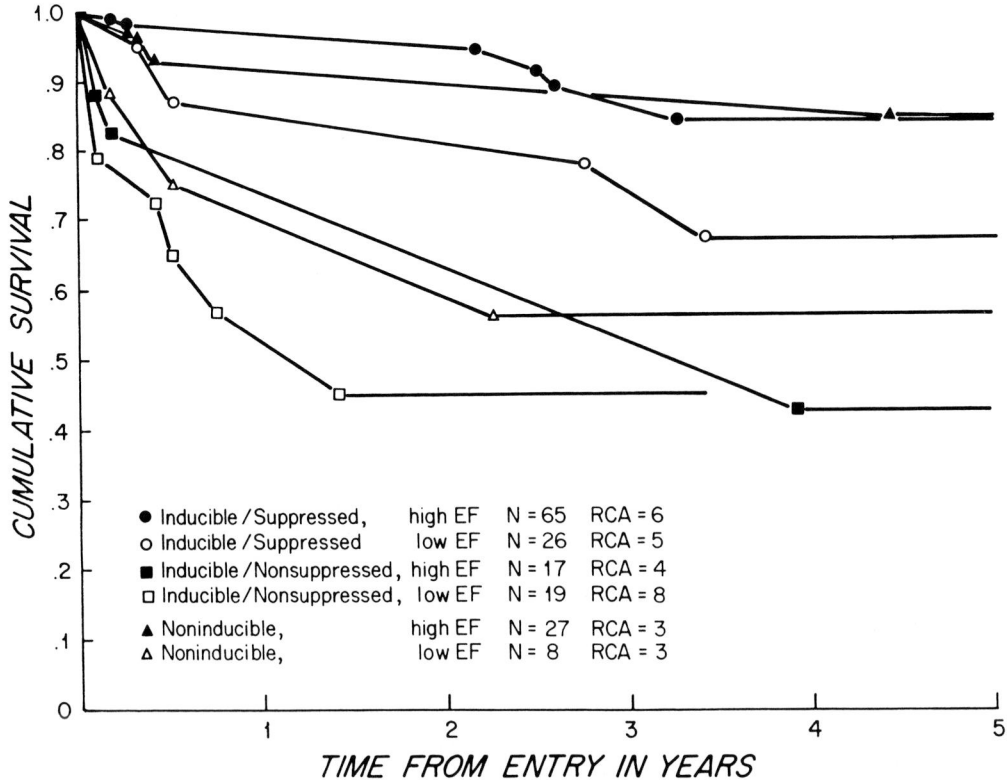

Fig. 32–1. Cumulative survival without recurrent cardiac arrest is shown in relation to electrophysiological study results and left ventricular ejection fraction (EF). High = EF > 30%. Low = EF ≤ 30%. Inducible/suppressed, patients with inducible drug-suppressed ventricular arrhythmias; N, number of patients; RCA, number of recurrent cardiac arrests. (Reproduced by permission of the *New England Journal of Medicine* from Wilber DJ, et al: N Engl J Med *318*:19–24, 1988.[29])

respectively. Comparison of clinical baseline characteristics revealed a higher incidence of nonischemic heart disease and a significantly higher LVEF in patients without inducible arrhythmias (LVEF 0.41 ± 0.15 in patients without inducible arrhythmias, vs. 0.36 ± 0.11 in drug responders and 0.32 + 0.13 in nonresponders). However, the overall mortality in patients with no inducible arrhythmias was not better than that of drug responders or nonresponders and approached 35% at 5 years. The relatively favorable outcome of nonresponders may be partially explained by the more frequent use of ICD and amiodarone therapy in this group as compared to drug responders and patients with no inducible arrhythmias at baseline PES.[116]

Several studies examined the predictive value of PES in survivors of out-of-hospital cardiac arrest with CAD as the underlying anatomical substrate.[39,117] Furukawa and coworkers reported a study of 101 patients with chronic CAD (71%) out of a population of 142 survivors of out-of-hospital cardiac arrest. In this study, ventricular arrhythmias (VT, VF, and nonsustained VT) were inducible in 76 (75%) of 101 patients at baseline PES and were successfully suppressed by antiarrhythmic drug therapy in 32 (42%) of 76 patients. In patients with induced arrhythmias that were not suppressed by drugs the rate of recurrent cardiac arrest was approximately 35% at 2 years, which was significantly higher than in patients without inducible arrhythmias at baseline PES (9% at 2 years) or with inducible arrhythmias that were suppressed by drugs (10% at 2 years). LV dysfunction, defined as LVEF < 0.35, was the strongest independent predictor of recurrent cardiac arrest within the first 6 months (11.2%), whereas the presence of persistently inducible arrhythmias was highly predictive of recurrent cardiac arrest after the first 6 months of follow-up.[39] These findings confirm the earlier findings of Wilber et al[29] and underscore the time dependence of risk factors and predictors of SCD. In a smaller study of 56 patients with chronic CAD and out-of-hospital cardiac arrest,[117] monomorphic VT was inducible in 22 (39%) and was suppressed by PES-guided drug therapy in 11 (50%) of the 22. The actuarial recurrence rate of SCD at 2 years was 31% in patients with suppressed arrhythmias and was similar to that of empirically treated patients without inducible monomorphic VT (26%). Patients without inducible sustained monomorphic VT and corrected precipitants of out-of-hospital cardiac arrest (ischemia, $n = 7/9$ and proarrhythmia, $n = 2/9$) had no recurrence of SCD at 2 years. In the 11 patients with monomorphic VT that was not suppressed by PES-guided drug therapy (nonresponders) and who were treated with ICD implantation (10 patients) or endocardial resection (one patient) the SCD recurrence rate at 2 years was 11%, comparable to that of patients without inducible monomorphic VT who were treated with ICDs (7% recurrence of SCD at 2 years). Although the size of this study is too small to estimate the predictive accuracy of electrophysiological testing, it underscores the importance of treating reversible precipitants, particularly ischemia, in this high-risk patient population.[117]

The predictive value of PES in cardiac arrest survivors with nonischemic heart disease remains controversial. A prospective study of patients with dilated cardiomyopathy and congestive heart failure showed only a 20% sensitivity of PES for prediction of SCD.[118] In another study of 47 patients with dilated cardiomyopathy and a mean LVEV 0.28 ± 0.09, monomorphic VT was reliably inducible in patients who presented clinically with this arrhythmia (13/13 patients) and its suppression by PES-guided drug therapy was associated with a good long-term prognosis. However, in patients who presented with VF or nonsustained VT, neither induction of VT nor of VF was predictive of long-term outcome or recurrent SCD.[111] Correspondingly, the absence of inducible arrhythmias was not associated with a favorable outcome, and it was concluded that the risk of SCD could not be predicted by PES in patients with dilated cardiomyopathy if the clinical and induced arrhythmias were not VT.[111]

In general it appears that patients with inducible arrhythmias at baseline PES usually have worse LV function than those without inducible arrhythmias. Inducible arrhythmias in patients with severely impaired LV function are less likely to be suppressed by antiarrhythmic drugs. In most studies, the incidence of implanted ICDs is highest in the subgroup of patients who present with inducible arrhythmias that are not suppressed by PES-guided drug therapy. Irrespective of underlying disease and state of arrhythmia inducibility, patients with impaired LV function remain at high risk for SCD. Patients with preserved LV function and CAD have a good prognosis if a triggering factor such as ischemia can be corrected and the inducible arrhythmia is not monomorphic VT. Patients with preserved LV function and inducible arrhythmias that are suppressed by drugs also have a good prognosis if the underlying heart disease is CAD, but their outcome remains uncertain if the underlying disease is not CAD.

Prognostic Impact of Noninducibility at Baseline PES

Most studies define noninducibility as six or fewer ventricular beats during PES. Conversely, the definition of nonsustained VT is variable, and in some studies the definitions of nonsustained VT and absence of inducible arrhythmias overlap, thus complicating interpretation.

In the study of Wilber et al, patients with no inducible arrhythmias at baseline PES (<5 beats) had a recurrence rate of cardiac arrest of 13% at 1 year, 15% at 2 years, and 16% at 3 years of follow-up.[29] The recurrence rate of SCD was lower if LV function was preserved (LVEF ≥ 0.30; recurrent cardiac arrest 8% at 1 years and 13% at 3 years), but was very high if the LVEF was poor (LVEF < 0.30: recurrent cardiac arrest 25% at 1 year and 44% at 3 years).[29] In the study of Fogoros et al,[116] patients without inducible arrhythmias at baseline PES

(<10 beats) had a comparable risk of recurrent cardiac arrest of 4% at 1 year, 8% at 2 years, and 11% at 3 years.[116] In contrast to these studies, recent data from our own laboratory comparing the long-term survival of 228 survivors of out-of-hospital cardiac arrest with inducible arrhythmias with survival in 103 survivors without inducible arrhythmias at baseline PES revealed a cardiac mortality of 4.8% at 1 year and 6.8% at 3 years for patients without inducible arrhythmias as compared to 7.9% at 1 year and 15.8% at 3 years in patients with inducible arrhythmias at baseline PES.[119] The seemingly better results of this study in comparison to those reported by Fogoros et al may be explained by a higher incidence of implanted ICDs in patients without inducible arrhythmias (50% vs. 11%) and a mildly better LVEF (0.47 ± 2 vs. 0.41 ± 0.15). However, the beneficial effect of implanting ICDs in survivors of out-of-hospital cardiac arrest with no inducible arrhythmias at baseline PES has been questioned in a recent study that compared 99 patients with an ICD to 95 patients without an ICD.[120] Long-term overall survival was equal for both groups (90% at 2 years) despite a significant reduction in SCD in the ICD group (2% vs. 9% at 2 years, $p = 0.04$). These findings raise the possibility that the benefit of reducing SCD with ICD therapy may be offset by an operative mortality of 3% and associated long-term morbidity of this therapy when applied to a low-risk group.

The inability to induce any ventricular arrhythmia at baseline PES is generally associated with better LV function, a lower incidence of CAD, and a better long-term outcome. The extent of LV impairment in patients without inducible arrhythmias is the strongest determinant of recurrent cardiac arrest and total mortality. Patients with no inducible arrhythmias and advanced CAD with preserved LV function who undergo revascularization have an excellent prognosis. Patients with significantly impaired LV function irrespective of the underlying disease remain at high risk for SCD and are, based on currently available data, best managed with ICD therapy. The outcome in patients with preserved function and nonischemic heart disease or CAD without correctable factors (ischemia, proarrhythmia) is still uncertain. The results of prospective trials are awaited.

CARDIAC ARREST SURVIVORS WITH SPECIFIC CONDITIONS

In the era of the ICD, the question of whether all cardiac arrest survivors with documented VF should undergo ICD implantation or whether there is still an indication for electrophysiological evaluation has become a challenging topic. Our current approach to this question depends mainly on the underlying heart disease, LV function, and the presence of correctable precipitants of cardiac arrest such as ischemia, but our approach may change in the future as the results of ongoing prospective trials of ICD therapy in different subgroups of patients provide new insights into the risk-cost-benefit ratio of this therapy.

Ischemic Heart Disease

Apart from CAD, which accounts for 70–80% of cardiac arrests, ischemic heart disease also includes syndromes of relative myocardial ischemia such as coronary artery spasm and small-vessel disease (syndrome X) and, to some extent, aspects of hypertrophic cardiomyopathy. All these syndromes share (1) the potential for relative ischemia, and (2) an anatomical substrate in the form of different degrees of scarring or interstitial fibrosis, both of which are responsible for abnormal cellular electrophysiological properties and electrical heterogeneity of the myocardium as a whole.

Role of Myocardial Infarction

A new Q-wave MI serving as the trigger for VF is found in 15–20% of all cardiac arrest survivors.[10,121] The occurrence of VF within the first 24–48 hours after the onset of a new Q-wave infarct is not associated with a worse outcome, and the long-term incidence of SCD is not increased compared to uncomplicated infarcts.[122-124] Correspondingly, evaluation of this patient group should not differ from routine assessment after MI.[125] More difficult to define is the prognostic impact of non-Q-wave infarction and elevated cardiac enzyme levels after resuscitation. As differentiation between a primary ischemic event and secondary resuscitation-related myocardial necrosis can be extremely difficult, this heterogeneous group is usually evaluated in the same way as cardiac arrest survivors without evidence of myocardial necrosis.[121,125]

The effect of prior MI as the potential for arrhythmogenesis is best reflected in the extent of impairment of LV function, as discussed earlier.[27,29,126] Patients with prior MI have a higher incidence of inducible VT than other arrhythmias,[99,116] which supports the concept that VT is more likely to occur in patients with severely impaired LV function, whereas patients presenting with VF frequently have a less abnormal ventricular substrate.[121] This concept is based on the observations that patients presenting with VT usually have a lower LVEF[121] and a higher percentage of late and fractionated signals during endocardial mapping than patients presenting with primary VF.[127,128] Furthermore, if sustained ventricular arrhythmias are induced by comparable modes of initiation at PES, mean tachycardia cycle length tends to be shorter in patients presenting with SCD than in those with hemodynamically tolerated VT.[100] Indirect evidence for this concept is provided by the observation that the signal-averaged ECG more frequently shows late potentials in patients with hemodynamically tolerated VT (85%) than in patients with aborted SCD (55%).[86,121] These observations favor the hypothesis that VT and VF share a qualitatively similar substrate, but that this substrate is quantitatively less represented in patients with primary VF.[121,129]

Role of Reversible Ischemia

From autopsy studies of patients with fatal MI, Schuster and Bulkley identified a high-risk subgroup of patients with a high mortality who had severe CAD and symptoms of angina and ECG changes suggesting ongoing ischemia.[130] In a subsequent prospective clinical study of 70 such high-risk patients, 40 patients died within 6 months of recurrent infarction and 47% of these deaths were sudden.[131] These authors hypothesized that postinfarction angina identified a high-risk population who could benefit from surgical intervention.[131] It has now been shown that the risk of recurrent cardiac arrest is reduced in cardiac arrest survivors subsequently treated by coronary artery bypass grafting.[126,132] Kelly et al have used PES to examine the effect of CABG surgery on inducible ventricular arrhythmias in patients with life-threatening ventricular arrhythmias and in cardiac arrest survivors.[133] In this study, coronary revascularization abolished inducible ventricular arrhythmias in a substantial proportion, predominantly when the induced arrhythmia was VF. Inducible monomorphic VT was only rarely abolished.[133]

Role of Epidemiological and Environmental Factors

Large prospective population studies reveal that risk factors such as smoking, systolic blood pressure, serum cholesterol, weight, vital capacity, heart rate, and ECG abnormalities are predictive of an increased risk of SCD in subjects free of overt CAD, but that in the presence of CAD they no longer predict the risk for sudden death.[41,42] Male sex seems to be an independent but less powerful risk factor.[134]

Epidemiological data have also shown a circadian variability in acute coronary events, including MI and SCD, with the highest incidence in the early morning hours and the lowest incidence during the night.[135,136] The circadian distribution of SCD suggests an important role of the autonomic nervous system, which is dominated by sympathetic activity in the early morning hours after awakening.[137] The heightened sympathetic activity is associated with increased plasma catecholamines, an increase in heart rate and blood pressure, and an increase in platelet aggregability but diminished fibrinolytic activity.[138] In patients receiving β-adrenoceptor-blocking agents after MI this early morning peak of SCD is suppressed.[139] Whether sympathetic stimulation acts via ischemia or as an independent factor remains unclear. Although no circadian variability of arrhythmias induced by PES could be proven,[140] experimental data have shown that ventricular arrhythmias in a canine model of acute superimposed on chronic myocardial ischemia are significantly reduced by left stellectomy, suggesting an independent arrhythmogenic effect of sympathetic stimulation.[141] Other models of sympathetic stimulation by environmental stress factors have shown a significantly decreased vulnerability to ventricular arrhythmias after stress adaptation, which is reflected biochemically as a decrease in phosphorylase activity.[142,143] In conclusion, sympathetic stimulation in the setting of stable CAD seems to act as a potent trigger of SCD, either with or without ischemia, whereas pharmacological and surgical sympathetic denervation has a protective effect. Ischemia itself, as a trigger or as a result of ventricular arrhythmia, has a propensity to cause deterioration in well-organized VT to disorganized VF.[144]

The concept of arrhythmogenesis proposed by Myerburg et al[145,146] incorporates all these factors in a single model in which ventricular arrhythmias result from the interaction of structural abnormalities and functional factors, which operate as triggers. The occurrence of ventricular arrhythmias in this model depends on the extent of pre-existing structural abnormalities as well as the severity of the triggering factors. An important feature of this model is the time dependence of the interaction of the structural and functional factors, implying that risk stratification and treatment require regular reassessment.

Nonischemic Heart Disease

This group of conditions is very heterogeneous but consists mainly of idiopathic dilated cardiomyopathy, hypertrophic cardiomyopathy, the long QT interval syndromes (LQTS), and other congenital anomalies. Common features in this population are younger age, better LV function, and an equal sex distribution. More important, when currently applied techniques for risk stratification are used in this patient population, they prove to be less sensitive and less specific than in patients with ischemic heart disease.

Idiopathic Dilated Cardiomyopathy

Patients with idiopathic dilated cardiomyopathy have a high incidence of SCD and commonly exhibit nonsustained VT (20–60%) on Holter monitoring.[147,148] The role of signal-averaged ECG in stratifying patients at risk for SCD is not determined.

There is some evidence that the presence of late potentials on the signal-averaged ECG and a filtered QRS with > 120 msec are predictive of arrhythmic events.[84,85] Earlier studies, however, found that signal-averaged ECG was not useful in discriminating patients with idiopathic dilated cardiomyopathy who presented with ventricular arrhythmias from those who did not,[149] or in predicting subsequent SCD.[150] The results of PES in patients with idiopathic dilated cardiomyopathy are also very variable, and sustained monomorphic VT is inducible in only a minority of patients, usually those who present clinically with this arrhythmia.[111,149] Suppression of monomorphic VT with antiarrhythmic drugs seems to be associated with a favorable outcome. However, in patients presenting with idiopathic dilated cardiomyopathy with inducible arrhythmias other than VT, programmed stimulation may not be appropriate to guide antiarrhythmic drug therapy.[111] Two trials of ICD therapy in patients with idiopathic dilated cardiomyopathy, the European Dilated Cardiomyopathy Study and the Defibrillator Implantation as Bridge to Later Transplant (DEFIBRILAT) trial, are currently under way and will help to define nonpharmacological treatment strategies in this population in the future.

Hypertrophic Cardiomyopathy

SCD in patients with hypertrophic cardiomyopathy is usually found in younger age groups, with a high incidence in young adults aged 10–35 years[46–48] and with familial clustering.[151] Although a relationship between wall thickness and subsequent SCD has been described,[151] the prognostic value of echocardiography for risk prediction is low. Hemodynamic parameters seem not to correlate with the potential for fatal arrhythmias and are not useful for risk stratification for arrhythmic events.[152–154] Nonsustained VT on Holter monitoring was found to be associated with a subsequent sudden death rate of up to 8% per year in two earlier studies.[153,155] In a more recent study of patients with hypertrophic cardiomyopathy, nonsustained VT in the absence of hemodynamic symptoms (syncope) and inducible arrhythmias at PES was not associated with an adverse short-term prognosis.[156] However, if patients with hypertrophic cardiomyopathy have experienced an episode of out-of-hospital cardiac arrest or syncope of uncertain origin, a high incidence of inducible arrhythmias and conduction system abnormalities is usually found at PES.[113,114,156,157] In a study of 230 patients with hypertrophic cardiomyopathy, sustained ventricular arrhythmias, predominantly polymorphic VT, were induced by PES in 36%, whereas supraventricular arrhythmias were found in 14% and conduction system abnormalities in 43% of patients.[156] Multivariate analysis of clinical, hemodynamic, and electrophysiological parameters revealed that sustained ventricular arrhythmias induced by PES and a history of aborted SCD were independent predictors of recurrent cardiac arrest. At the moment it is not known whether pharmacological or surgical interventions or ICD implantation can reduce the risk for SCD in hypertrophic cardiomyopathy. A recent study of 30 cardiac arrest survivors with hypertrophic cardiomyopathy, in two thirds of whom sustained ventricular arrhythmias were inducible by PES, suggests that ICD implantation may be beneficial.[158]

Idiopathic Long QT Interval Syndrome

Survivors of out-of-hospital cardiac arrest with idiopathic LQTS are at a high risk of recurrent SCD, which is estimated to approach 1% per year.[159] In patients with this syndrome without a history of cardiac arrest, the prediction of risk for SCD is difficult, although a history of SCD in a first-degree relative,[159] T-wave alternans, extreme QT prolongation (>540 msec) or AV block in the neonatal period are predictive for SCD in some studies.[159–161] The signal-averaged ECG is not useful in this population since late potentials are not characteristic of LQTS. Electrophysiological evaluation also is not helpful, because induction of ventricular arrhythmias is rare and has no prognostic value. Lack of shortening of the QT interval in response to catecholamine infusion during atrial pacing may be helpful in some cases when the diagnosis is uncertain but has no utility in evaluating the risk for recurrent cardiac arrest.

CARDIAC ARREST SURVIVORS WITH NO OVERT STRUCTURAL HEART DISEASE

In a study of 43 patients out of 1195 cardiac arrest survivors, who had an EF >0.50 and no significant CAD, 16% suffered recurrent cardiac arrest during a mean follow-up period of 8 years.[162] Localized wall motion abnormalities detected on echocardiography and abnormalities of the 12-lead ECG were associated with a significant increase in long-term mortality, resulting in a 5-year mortality of 30% if the ECG was abnormal compared to only 3% if the ECG showed no significant abnormality. A recent review of the world literature reported a total 54 survivors of out-of-hospital cardiac arrest with "normal" hearts,[163] and it was concluded that the prognostic value of PES in these patients is not established. However, it seems that VF is inducible in a high proportion of these patients and may represent a specific end point.[52,163]

SUMMARY

Patients who present with out-of-hospital cardiac arrest are generally at high risk for recurrent cardiac arrest (10–50% at 2 years). The goals of risk assessment are to identify patients with correctable factors that will improve outcome if adequately treated (e.g., coronary bypass surgery after ischemia-related cardiac arrest) and to quantify the risk for recurrence of SCD for subsets of patients based on the type and severity of underlying heart disease and, in particular, the degree of LV dysfunction. For patients at highest risk of recurrence, ICD therapy is usually recommended. However, with current methods of risk stratification, a substantial proportion of survivors of out-of-hospital cardiac arrest are identified as having an intermediate or even indeterminate risk. Although ICD therapy is offered to many of these patients at present, the choice of the most appropriate therapy in the future awaits further refinement of risk stratification and the results of ongoing prospective trials on the role of the ICD and antiarrhythmic drugs such as amiodarone in specific patient subsets.

REFERENCES

1. Myerburg RJ, Castellanos A: Cardiac arrest and sudden cardiac death. In Braunwald E (ed): Heart Disease, 4th ed. 1992, pp. 756–789.
2. Myerburg RJ: Sudden cardiac death: Epidemiology, causes, and mechanisms. Cardiology 2:2–9, 1987.
3. Gillum RF: Sudden coronary death in the United States. Circulation 79:756–765, 1989.
4. Epstein SE, Quyymi AA, Bonow RO: Sudden cardiac death without warning: Possible mechanisms and implications for screening asymptomatic populations [see comments]. N Engl J Med 321:320–324, 1989.
5. Eisenberg MS, Copass MK, Hallstrom AP, et al: Treatment of out-of-hospital cardiac arrest with rapid defibrillation by emergency medical technicians. N Engl J Med 302:1379–1383, 1980.
6. Thompson RG, Hallstom AP, Cobb LA, et al: Bystander-initiated cardiopulmonary resuscitation in the management of ventricular fibrillation. Ann Intern Med 90:737–741, 1979.
7. Eisenberg MS, Cummins RO, Damon S, et al: Survival rates from out-of-hospital cardiac arrest: Recommendations for uniform definitions and data to report. Ann Emerg Med 19:1249–1259, 1990.
8. Eisenberg MS, Cummins RO, Larsen MP: Numerators, denominators, and survival rates: Reporting survival from out-of-hospital cardiac arrest. Am J Emerg Med 9:544–546, 1991.
9. Liberthson RR, Nagel EL, Hirschmann JC, et al: Prehospital ventricular fibrillation: Prognosis and follow-up course. N Engl J Med 291:317–321, 1974.
10. Cobb LA, Baum RS, Alvarez IH, et al: Survival after resuscitation from out-of-hospital ventricular fibrillation: 4 years follow up. Circulation 51, 52(suppl III):III-223–III-228, 1975.
11. Baum RS, Alvarez IH, Cobb LA, et al: Survival after resuscitation from out-of-hospital ventricular fibrillation. Circulation 50:1231–1235, 1974.
12. Myerburg RJ, Kessler KM, Estes D, et al: Long-term survival after prehospital cardiac arrest: Analysis of outcome during an 8 year study. Circulation 70:538–546, 1984.
13. Hargrove WC, Josephson ME, Marchlinski FE, et al: Surgical decisions in the management of sudden cardiac death and malignant ventricular arrhythmias: Subendocardial resection, the automatic internal defibrillator, or both. J Thorac Cardiovasc Surg 97:923–928, 1989.
14. Powell AC, Fuchs T, Finkelstein DM, et al: Influence of the automatic implantable cardioverter-defibrillator on the long-term prognosis of survivors of out-of-hospital cardiac arrest. Circulation 88:1083–1092, 1993.
15. Anderson MH, Camm AJ: Implications for present and future applications of the implantable cardioverter-defibrillator resulting from the use of a simple model of cost efficacy. Br Heart J 69:83–92, 1993.
16. Myerburg RJ, Conde CA, Sung RJ, et al: Clinical, electrophysiologic and hemodynamic profile of patients resuscitated from prehospital cardiac arrest. Am J Med 68:568–576, 1980.
17. Liberthson RR, Nagel EL, Hirschman JC, et al: Pathophysiologic observations in prehospital ventricular fibrillation and sudden cardiac death. Circulation 49:790–798, 1974.
18. Bayés de Luna A, Coumel P, Leclercq JF: Ambulatory sudden cardiac death: Mechanisms of production of fatal arrhythmia on the basis of data from 157 cases. Am Heart J 117:151–159, 1989.
19. Paridis IP, Morganroth J: Sudden death in hospitalized patients: Cardiac rhythm disturbances detected by ambulatory electrocardiographic monitoring. J Am Coll Cardiol 2:798–805, 1983.
20. Klein GJ, Bashore TM, Sellers TD, et al: Ventricular fibrillation in the Wolff-Parkinson-White syndrome. N Engl J Med 301:1080–1085, 1979.
21. Greenberg HM: Bradycardia at onset of sudden death: Potential mechanisms. Ann NY Acad Sci 427:241–252, 1984.
22. Bardy GH, Packer DL, German LD, et al: Utility of electrophysiologic studies in the management of tachycardia, sudden death, and syncope. Ann NY Acad Sci 427:16–38, 1984.
23. Surawicz B, Reddy CP: Tachy-bradycardia syndrome. In Surawicz B, Reddy CP, Prystowski EN (eds): Boston, Martinus Nijhoff, 1984, pp 199–211.
24. Savage HR, Kissane JQ, Becher EL, et al: Analysis of ambulatory electrocardiograms in 14 patients who experienced sudden cardiac death during monitoring. Clin Cardiol 10:621–632, 1987.
25. Hays LJ, Lerman BB, DiMarco JP: Nonventricular arrhythmias as precursors of ventricular fibrillation in patients with out-of-hospital cardiac arrest. Am Heart J 118:53–57, 1989.
26. Luu M, Stevenson WG, Stevenson LW, et

al: Diverse mechanisms of unexpected cardiac arrest in advanced heart failure. Circulation 80:1675–1680, 1989.
27. Wilber DJ, Garan H, Ruskin JN: Electrophysiologic testing in survivors of cardiac arrest. Circulation 75(suppl III):III-146–III-150, 1987.
28. Ruskin JN: Role of invasive electrophysiological testing in the evaluation and treatment of patients at high risk for sudden cardiac death. Circulation 85(suppl I):I-152–I-159, 1992.
29. Wilber DJ, Garan H, Finkelstein D, et al: Out-of-hospital cardiac arrest: Use of electrophysiological testing in the prediction of long-term outcome. N Engl J Med 318:19–24, 1988.
30. Lampert S, Lown B, Graboys TB, et al: Determinants of survival in patients with malignant ventricular arrhythmia associated with coronary artery disease. Am J Cardiol 61:791–797, 1988.
31. Eldar M, Sauve MJ, Scheinman MM: Electrophysiologic testing and follow-up of patients with aborted sudden death. J Am Coll Cardiol 10:291–298, 1987.
32. Morady F, DiCarlo L, Winston S, et al: Clinical features and prognosis of patients with out of hospital cardiac arrest and a normal electrophysiologic study. J Am Coll Cardiol 4:39–44, 1984.
33. Skale BT, Miles WM, Heger JJ, et al: Survivors of cardiac arrest: Prevention of recurrence by drug therapy as predicted by electrophysiologic testing or electrocardiographic monitoring. Am J Cardiol 57:113–119, 1986.
34. Roy D, Waxman HL, Kienzle MG, et al: Clinical characteristics and long-term follow-up in 119 survivors of cardiac arrest: Relation to inducibility at electrophysiologic testing. Am J Cardiol 52:969–974, 1983.
35. Benditt DG, Benson DWJ, Klein GJ, et al: Prevention of recurrent sudden cardiac arrest: Role of provocative electropharmacologic testing. J Am Coll Cardiol 2:418–425, 1983.
36. Freedman RA, Swerdlow CD, Soderholm DV, et al: Prognostic significance of arrhythmia inducibility or noninducibility at initial electrophysiologic study in survivors of cardiac arrest. Am J Cardiol 61:578–582, 1988.
37. Swerdlow CD, Bardy GH, McAnulty J, et al: Determinants of induced ventricular arrhythmias in survivor of out-of-hospital ventricular fibrillation. Circulation 76:1053–1060, 1987.
38. Poole JE, Mathisen TL, Kudenchuck PJ, et al: Long-term outcome in patients who survived out-of-hospital ventricular fibrillation and who undergo electrophysiologic studies: Evaluation by electrophysiologic subgroups. J Am Coll Cardiol 16:657–665, 1990.
39. Furukawa T, Rozanski J, Nogami A, et al: Time-dependent risk of and predictors for cardiac arrest recurrent in survivors of out-of-hospital cardiac arrest with chronic coronary artery disease. Circulation 80:599–608, 1989.
40. Reichenbach DD, Moss NS, Meyer E: Pathology of the heart in sudden cardiac death. Am J Cardiol 39:865–872, 1977.
41. Kannel WB, Thomas HEJ: Sudden coronary death: The Framingham study. Ann NY Acad Sci 382:3–21, 1982.
42. Kannel WB, Schatzkin A: Sudden death: Lessons from subsets in population studies. J Am Coll Cardiol 5:141B–149B, 1985.
43. Perper JA, Kuller LH, Copper M, et al: Arteriosclerosis of coronary arteries in sudden unexpected deaths. Circulation 52(suppl 3):27–33, 1975.
44. Pocock WA, Bosman CK, Chesler E, et al: Sudden death in primary mitral valve prolapse. Am Heart J 107:378–382, 1984.
45. Barlow JB, Pocock WA, Marcus R, et al: Risk groups among patients with mitral-valve prolapse syndrome. N Engl J Med 321:1051–1052, 1989.
46. Maron BJ, Henry WL, Clark CL, et al: Asymmetric septal hypertrophy in childhood. Circulation 53:9–19, 1976.
47. Maron BJ, Roberts WC, Epstein SE, et al: Sudden death in hypertrophic cardiomyopathy: A profile of 78 patients. Circulation 65:1388–1394, 1982.
48. Maron BJ, Bonow RO, Cannon IRO, et al: Hypertrophic cardiomyopathy: Interrelations of clinical manifestations, pathophysiology, and therapy. N Engl J Med 316:780–789, 1987.
49. Liberthson RR, Dinsmore RE, Fallon JT, et al: Aberrant coronary artery origin from the aorta: Report of 18 patients, review of the literature, and delineation of natural history and management. Circulation 59:748–754, 1979.
50. Sherief HT, Carpentier RG: Electrophysiological mechanisms of cocaine-induced cardiac arrest: A possible cause of sudden cardiac death. J Electrocardiol 24:247–255, 1991.
51. Pallasch TJ, McCarthy FM, Jastak JT: Cocaine and sudden cardiac death. J Oral Maxillofac Surg 47:1188–1191, 1989.
52. Wellens HJ, Lemery R, Smeets JL, et al: Sudden arrhythmic death without overt

heart disease. Circulation 85(suppl 1):I-92-I-97, 1992.
53. Longstreth WTJ, Diehr P, Inui TS: Prediction of awakening after out-of-hospital cardiac arrest. N Engl J Med 308:1378–1382, 1983.
54. Longstreth WTJ: Prognostic significance of neurologic examination and glycemia after cardiac arrest. Resuscitation 17(suppl): S175–S179, 1989.
55. Garza LA, Vick RL, Nora JJ, et al: Heritable QT-prolongation without deafness. Circulation 41:39–48, 1970.
56. Clark CL, Henry WL, Epstein SE, et al: Familial prevalence and transmission of idiopathic hypertrophic subaortic stenosis. N Engl J Med 289:709, 1973.
57. Smeeton WM, Smith WM: Sudden death due to a cardiomyopathy predominantly affecting the right ventricle—right ventricular dysplasia. Med Sci Law 27:207–212, 1987.
58. Green JR, Korovetz MJ, Shanklin DR, et al: Sudden unexpected death in three generations. Arch Intern Med 124:359–363, 1969.
59. Brookfield L, Bharati S, Denes P, et al: Familial sudden death: Report of a case and review of the literature. Chest 94:989–993, 1988.
60. Salerno DM, Asinger RW, Elsperger J, et al: Frequency of hypokalemia after successfully resuscitated out-of-hospital cardiac arrest compared with that in acute myocardial infarction. Am J Cardiol 59: 84–88, 1987.
61. McIvor ME, Cummings CE, Mower MM, et al: Sudden cardiac death from acute fluoride intoxication: The role of potassium. Ann Emerg Med 16:777–781, 1987.
62. Hultgren HN, Swenson R, Wettach G: Cardiac arrest due to oral potassium administration. Am J Med 58:139–142, 1975.
63. Vassalle M: On the mechanisms underlying cardiac standstill: Factors determining success or failure of escape pacemakers in the heart. J Am Coll Cardiol 5(suppl B): B35–B42, 1985.
64. Olson DS, Stueven HA, Teresi JL, et al: Digoxin levels in prehospital sudden-death syndrome. J Clin Pharmacol 27:184–186, 1987.
65. Ruskin JN, McGovern B, Garan H, et al: Antiarrhythmic drugs: A possible cause of out-of-hospital cardiac arrest. N Engl J Med 309:1302–1306, 1983.
66. Swerdlow CD, Winkle RA, Mason JW, et al: Determinants of survival in patients with ventricular arrhythmias. N Engl J Med 308: 1436–1442, 1983.
67. Bigger JT, Fleiss JL, Kleiger R, et al: The relationships among ventricular arrhythmias, left ventricular dysfunction, and mortality in the 2 years after myocardial infarction. Circulation 69:250–258, 1984.
68. Kuchar DL, Rottman J, Berger E, et al: Prediction of successful suppression of sustained ventricular tachyarrhythmias by serial drug testing from data derived at the initial electrophysiologic study. J Am Coll Cardiol 12:982–988, 1989.
69. Wagner S, Buser P, Auffermann W, et al: Cine magnetic resonance imaging: Tomographic analysis of left ventricular function. Cardiol Clin 7:651–659, 1989.
70. Ritchie JL, Hallstrom AP, Troubaugh JC, et al: Out-of-hospital sudden coronary death: Rest and exercise radionuclide left ventricular function in survivors. Am J Cardiol 55:645–651, 1985.
71. Weaver WD, Cobb LA, Hallstrom AP: Ambulatory arrhythmias in resuscitated victims of cardiac arrest. Circulation 66: 212–218, 1982.
72. Bayés de Luna A, Coumel P, Leclercq JF: Ambulatory sudden cardiac death: Mechanisms of production of fatal arrhythmia on the basis of data from 157 cases. Am Heart J 117:151–159, 1989.
73. Kempf FCJ, Josephson ME: Cardiac arrest recorded on ambulatory electrocardiograms. Am J Cardiol 53:1577–1582, 1984.
74. Pratt CM, Francis MJ, Luck GC, et al: Analysis of ambulatory electrocardiograms in 15 patients during spontaneous ventricular fibrillation with special reference to preceding arrhythmic events. J Am Coll Cardiol 2:789–797, 1983.
75. Meissner MD, Morganroth J: Silent myocardial ischemia as a mechanism of sudden cardiac death. Cardiol Clin 4:593–605, 1986.
76. Rapaport E: Sudden cardiac death. Am J Cardiol 62:31–61, 1988.
77. Rapaport E, Remedios P: The high risk patient after recovery from myocardial infarction. J Am Coll Cardiol 1:391–400, 1983.
78. Mukharji J, Rude RE, Poole WK, et al: The MILLIS study group: Risk factors for sudden death after acute myocardial infarction. Two year follow-up. Am J Cardiol 54: 31–36, 1984.
79. CAST Investigators: Preliminary report: Effect of encainide and flecainide on mortality in a randomized trial of arrhythmia suppression after myocardial infarction. N Engl J Med 321:406–412, 1989.
80. Breithardt G, Schwarzmaier M, Borgreffe M, et al: Prognostic significance of late ventricular potentials after acute myocardial infarction. Eur Heart J 4:487–495, 1987.

81. Gomes JA, Winters SL, Stewart D, et al: A new noninvasive index to predict sustained ventricular tachycardia and sudden death in the first year after myocardial infarction: Based on signal-averaged electrocardiogram, radionuclide ejection fraction and Holter monitoring. J Am Coll Cardiol 10:349–357, 1987.
82. Kuchar DL, Thorburn CW, Sammel NL: Prediction of serious arrhythmic events after myocardial infarction: Signal-averaged electrocardiogram, Holter monitoring and radionuclide ventriculography. J Am Coll Cardiol 9:531–538, 1987.
83. Deniss AR, Richard DA, Cody DV, et al: Prognostic significance of ventricular tachycardia and fibrillation induced at programmed stimulation and delayed potentials on the signal-averaged electrocardiograms of survivors of acute myocardial infarction. Circulation 74:731–745, 1986.
84. Ohnishi Y, Inoue T, Fukuzaki H: Value of the signal-averaged electrocardiogram as a predictor of sudden death in myocardial infarction and dilated cardiomyopathy. Jpn Circ J 54:127–136, 1990.
85. Mancini DM, Wong KL, Simson MB, et al: Prognostic value of abnormal signal-averaged electrocardiogram in patients with nonischemic congestive cardiomyopathy. Circulation 87:1083–1092, 1993.
86. Simson MB: Noninvasive identification of patients at high risk for sudden cardiac death: Signal-averaged electrocardiography. Circulation 51(suppl I):I-145–I-151, 1992.
87. Freedman RA, Gillis AM, Keren A, et al: Signal-averaged electrocardiographic late potentials in patients with ventricular fibrillation or ventricular tachycardia: Correlation with clinical arrhythmia and electrophysiological study. Am J Cardiol 55:1350–1353, 1985.
88. Dolack LG, Callahan DB, Bardy GH, et al: Signal averaged electrocardiographic late potentials in resuscitated survivors of out-of-hospital ventricular fibrillation. Am J Cardiol 65:1102–1104, 1990.
89. Kleiger RE, Miller P, Bigger JT, et al: Decreased heart rate variability and its association with increased mortality after acute myocardial infarction. Am J Cardiol 59:256–262, 1987.
90. Schwartz PJ, Vanoli E, Stramba BM, et al: Autonomic mechanisms and sudden death: New insights from analysis of baroreceptor reflexes in conscious dogs with and without a myocardial infarction. Circulation 78:969–979, 1988.
91. Bigger TJ, LaRovere MT, Steinmann RC, et al: Comparison of baroreflex sensitivity and heart period variability in patients after acute myocardial infarction. J Am Coll Cardiol 14:1511–1518, 1989.
92. Farell TG, Bashir Y, Cripps T, et al: Risk stratification for arrhythmic events in postinfarction patients based on heart rate variability, ambulatory electrocardiographic variables and signal averaged electrocardiogram. J Am Coll Cardiol 18:687–697, 1991.
93. Schwartz PJ, La Rovere MT, Vanoli E: Autonomic nervous system and sudden cardiac death: Experimental basis and clinical observations for post-myocardial infarction risk stratification. Circulation 85(suppl I):I-77–I-91, 1992.
94. Akhtar M, Garan H, Lehmann MH, et al: Sudden cardiac death: Management of high-risk patients. Ann Intern Med 114:499–512, 1991.
95. Holmes DRJ, Davis K, Gersh BJ, et al: Risk factor profiles of patients with sudden cardiac death and death from other cardiac causes: A report from the Coronary Artery Surgery Study (CASS). J Am Coll Cardiol 13:524–530, 1989.
96. Holmes DRJ, Davis KB, Mock MB, et al: The effect of medical and surgical treatment on subsequent sudden cardiac death in patients with coronary artery disease: A report from the Coronary Artery Surgery Study. Circulation 73:1254–1263, 1986.
97. Ruskin JN, DiMarco JP, Garan H: Out-of-hospital cardiac arrest: Electrophysiologic observations and selection of long-term antiarrhythmic therapy. N Engl J Med 303:607–613, 1980.
98. Wilber DJ, Kelly E, Garan H, et al: Determinants of inducible ventricular arrhythmias in survivors of out-of-hospital cardiac arrest [abstract]. Circulation 74(suppl II):II-482, 1986.
99. Schoenfeld MH, McGovern BA, Garan H, et al: Determinants of the outcome of electrophysiologic study in patients with ventricular arrhythmias. J Am Coll Cardiol 6:298–306, 1985.
100. Buxton AE, Waxman HL, Marchlinski FE, et al: Role of triple extrastimuli during electrophysiologic study of patients with documented sustained ventricular tachyarrhythmias. Circulation 69:532–540, 1984.
101. Mann E, Luck JC, Griffin JC, et al: Induction of clinical ventricular tachycardia using programmed stimulation: Value of third and fourth extrastimuli. Am J Cardiol 52:501–506, 1983.
102. Rosenbaum MS, Wilber DJ, Finkelstein D, et al: Immediate reproducibility of electri-

cally induced sustained monomorphic ventricular tachycardia before and during antiarrhythmic therapy. J Am Coll Cardiol 17: 133–138, 1991.
103. Morady F, DiCarlo L, Baerman JM, et al: Comparison of coupling intervals that induce clinical and non-clinical forms of ventricular tachycardia during programmed stimulation. Am J Cardiol 57:1269–1273, 1986.
104. Adhar GC, Larson LW, Bardy GH, et al: Sustained ventricular arrhythmias: Differences between survivors of cardiac arrest and patients with recurrent sustained ventricular tachycardia. J Am Coll Cardiol 12: 159–165, 1988.
105. DiCarlo LAJ, Morady F, Schwartz AB, et al: Clinical significance of ventricular fibrillation-flutter induced by ventricular programmed stimulation. Am Heart J 5: 959–963, 1985.
106. Brugada P, Green M, Abdollah H, et al: Significance of ventricular arrhythmias initiated by programmed ventricular stimulation: The importance of the type of ventricular arrhythmia induced and the number of premature stimuli required. Circulation 69: 87–92, 1984.
107. Fisher JD, Kim SG, Ferrick KJ, et al: Programmed electrical stimulation of the ventricle: An efficient, sensitive and specific protocol. PACE 15:435–450, 1992.
108. Mason JW, Winkle RA: Electrode-catheter arrhythmia induction in the selection and assessment of antiarrhythmic drug therapy for recurrent ventricular tachycardia. Circulation 58:986–997, 1978.
109. Morady F, DiCarlo L, Winston S, et al: A prospective comparison of triple extrastimuli and left ventricular stimulation in studies of ventricular tachycardia induction. Circulation 70:52–57, 1984.
110. Poll DS, Marchlinski FE, Buxton AE, et al: Sustained ventricular tachycardia in patients with iodiopathic dilated cardiomyopathy: Electrophysiologic testing and lack of response in antiarrhythmic drug therapy. Circulation 70:451–456, 1984.
111. Poll DS, Marchlinski FE, Buxton AE, et al: Usefulness of programmed stimulation in idiopathic dilated cardiomyopathy. Am J Cardiol 58:992–997, 1986.
112. Fananapazir L, Tracy CM, Leon MB: Electrophysiologic abnormalities in patients with hypertrophic cardiomyopathy: A consecutive analysis of 155 patients. Circulation 80:1259–1268, 1989.
113. Fananapazir L, Epstein SE: Hemodynamic and electrophysiologic evaluation of patients with hypertrophic cardiomyopathy surviving cardiac arrest. Am J Cardiol 67: 280–287, 1991.
114. Kuck KH, Kunze KP, Schluter M, et al: Programmed electrical stimulation in hypertrophic cardiomyopathy: Results in patients with and without cardiac arrest or syncope. Eur Heart J 9:177–185, 1988.
115. Cummins RO, Chamberlain DA, Abramson NS, et al: AHA Medical/Scientific Statement: Special Report: Recommended Guidelines for Uniform Reporting of Data From Out-of-Hospital Cardiac Arrest. The Utstein Style: A Statement for Health Professionals From a Task Force of the American Heart Association, the European Resuscitation Council, the Heart and Stroke Foundation of Canada, and the Australian Resuscitation Council. Circulation 84:960–975, 1991.
116. Fogoros RN, Elson JJ, Bonnet CA, et al: Long-term outcome of survivors of cardiac arrest whose therapy is guided by electrophysiologic testing. J Am Coll Cardiol 19: 780–788, 1991.
117. Sousa J, Rosenheck S, Calkins H, et al: Results of electrophysiologic testing and long-term prognosis in patients with coronary artery disease and aborted sudden death. Am Heart J 122:1001–1006, 1991.
118. Kron J, Hart M, Schual BS, et al: Idiopathic dilated cardiomyopathy: Role of programmed electrical stimulation and Holter monitoring in predicting those at risk of sudden death. Chest 93:85–90, 1988.
119. Trouton TG, Powell AC, Krishnan S, et al: Inducibility of ventricular arrhythmias at baseline electrophysiologic study in cardiac arrest survivors [abstract]. J Am Coll Cardiol 21:327A, 1993.
120. Crandall BG, Morris CD, Cutler JE, et al: Implantable cardiover-defibrillator therapy in survivors of out-of-hospital cardiac arrest without inducible arrhythmias. J Am Coll Cardiol 21:1186–1192, 1993.
121. Hurwitz JL, Josephson ME: Sudden cardiac death in patients with chronic coronary heart disease. Circulation 85(suppl I): I-43–I-49, 1992.
122. Volpi A, Cavalli A, Franzosi MG, et al: One-year prognosis of primary ventricular fibrillation complicated myocardial infarction. Am J Cardiol 63:1174–1178, 1989.
123. Goldberg R, Szklo M, Tonascia JA, et al: Acute myocardial infarction: Prognosis complicated by ventricular fibrillation or cardiac arrest. JAMA 241:2024–2027, 1979.
124. Weaver WD, Cobb LA, Hallstrom AP: Characteristics of survivors of exertion- and nonexertion-related cardiac arrest: Value of subsequent exercise testing. Am J Cardiol 50:671–676, 1982.

125. Brooks R, McGovern BA, Garan H, et al: Current treatment of patients surviving out-of-hospital cardiac arrest. JAMA 265:762–768, 1991.
126. Tresch DD, Wetherbee JN, Siegel R, et al: Long-term follow-up of survivors of prehospital sudden cardiac death treated with coronary bypass surgery. Am Heart J 110:1139–1145, 1985.
127. Cassidy DM, Vassallo JA, Buxton AE, et al: the value of catheter mapping during sinus rhythm to localize site of origin of ventricular tachycardia. Circulation 69:1103–1110, 1984.
128. Kadish AH, Rosenthal ME, Vassallo JA, et al: Sinus mapping in patients with cardiac arrest and coronary disease-results and correlation with outcome. PACE 12:301–310, 1989.
129. Cassidy DM, Vassallo JA, Miller JM, et al: Endocardial catheter mapping in patients in sinus rhythm: Relation to underlying heart disease and ventricular arrhythmias. Circulation 73:645–652, 1986.
130. Schuster EH, Bulkley BH: Ischemia at a distance after acute myocardial infarction: A cause of early postinfarction angina. Circulation 62:509–515, 1980.
131. Schuster EH, Bulkley BH: Early post-infarction angina: ischemia at a distance and ischemia in the infarct zone. N Engl J Med 305:1101–1105, 1981.
132. Every NR, Fahrenbruch CE, Hallstrom AP, et al: Influence of coronary bypass surgery on subsequent outcome of patients resuscitated from out-of-hospital cardiac arrest. J Am Coll Cardiol 19:1435–1439, 1992.
133. Kelly P, Ruskin JN, Vlahakes GJ, et al: Surgical coronary revascularization in survivors of prehospital cardiac arrest: Its effect on inducible ventricular arrhythmias and long-term survival. J Am Coll Cardiol 15:267–273, 1990.
134. Vaitkus PT, Kindwall KE, Miller JM, et al: Influence of gender on inducibility of ventricular arrhythmias in survivors of cardiac arrest with coronary artery disease. Am J Cardiol 67:537–539, 1991.
135. Muller JE, Ludmer PL, Willich SN, et al: Circadian variation in the frequency of sudden cardiac death. Circulation 75:131–138, 1987.
136. Willich SN, Levy D, Rocco MB, et al: Circadian variation in the incidence of sudden cardiac death in the Framingham Heart Study population. Am J Cardiol 60:801–806, 1987.
137. Willich SN, Goldberg RJ, Maclure M, et al: Increased onset of sudden cardiac death in the first three hours after awakening. Am J Cardiol 70:65–68, 1992.
138. Muller JE, Tofler GH, Stone PH: Circadian variation and trigger of onset of acute cardiovascular disease. Circulation 79:733–743, 1989.
139. Peters RW, Muller JE, Goldstein S, et al: Propranolol and the morning increase in the frequency of sudden cardiac death (BHAT Study). Am J Cardiol 63:1518–1520, 1989.
140. McClelland J, Halperin B, Kudenchuk P, et al: Circadian variation in ventricular electrical instability associated with coronary artery disease. Am J Cardiol 65:250–258, 1990.
141. Schwartz PJ, Billman GE, Stone HL: Autonomic mechanisms in ventricular fibrillation induced by myocardial ischemia during exercise in dogs with healed myocardial infarction: An experimental preparation for sudden cardiac death. Circulation 69:790–800, 1984.
142. Parker GW, Michael LH, Entman ML: An animal model to examine the response to environmental stress as a factor in sudden cardiac death. Am J Cardiol 60:18, 1987.
143. Skinner JE, Beder SC, Entman ML: Psychological stress activates phophorylase in the heart of the conscious pig without increasing heart rate and blood pressure. Proc Natl Acad Sci USA 80:4513–4517, 1983.
144. Morady F, DiCarlo LAJ, Krol RB, et al: Role of myocardial ischemia during programmed stimulation in survivors of cardiac arrest with coronary artery disease. J Am Coll Cardiol 9:1004–1012, 1987.
145. Myerburg RJ, Kessler KM, Bassett AL, et al: A biological approach to sudden cardiac death: Structure, function and cause. Am J Cardiol 63:1512–1516, 1989.
146. Myerburg RJ, Kessler KM, Castellanos A: Sudden cardiac death: Structure, function, and time-dependence of risk. Circulation 85(suppl I):I-2–I-10, 1992.
147. Meinertz T, Hofmann T, Kaspar W, et al: Significance of arrhythmias in idiopathic dilated cardiomyopathy. Am J Cardiol 53:902–907, 1984.
148. Unverferth DV, Magorien RD, Moeschberger ML: Factors influencing the one-year mortality of dilated cardiomyopathy. Am J Cardiol 51:507–512, 1984.
149. Breithardt G, Borgreffe M, Karbenn U, et al: Prevalence of late potentials in patients with and without ventricular tachycardia: Correlation with angiographic findings. Am J Cardiol 49:1932–1939, 1982.
150. Meinertz T, Treese N, Kaspar W, et al: Determinants of prognosis in idiopathic dilated cardiomyopathy as determined by programmed electrical stimulation. Am J Cardiol 56:337–341, 1985.

151. Spirito P, Maron BJ: Relation between extent of left ventricular hypertrophy and occurrence of sudden cardiac death in hypertrophic cardiomyopathy. J Am Coll Cardiol 15:1521–1526, 1990.
152. McKenna WJ, Deanfield J, Faruqui A, et al: Prognosis in hypertrophic cardiomyopathy: Role of age and clinical, electrocardiographic and hemodynamic parameters. Am J Cardiol 47:532–538, 1981.
153. McKenna WJ, Camm AJ: Sudden death in hypertrophic cardiomyopathy: Assessment of patients at risk. Circulation 80:1489–1492, 1989.
154. Maron BJ, Roberts WC, Edwards JE: Sudden death in patients with hypertrophic cardiomyopathy: Characterization of 26 patients without functional limitation. Am J Cardiol 41:803–810, 1978.
155. Maron BJ, Savage DA, Wolfson JK, et al: Prognostic significance of 24 hour ambulatory electrocardiographic monitoring in patients with hypertrophic cardiomyopathy: A prospective study. Am J Cardiol 48:252–257, 1981.
156. Fananapazir L, Chang AC, Epstein SE, et al: Prognostic determinants in hypertrophic cardiomyopathy. Circulation 86:730–740, 1992.
157. Watson RM, Schwartz JL, Maron BJ, et al: Inducible polymorphic ventricular tachycardia and ventricular fibrillation in a subgroup of patients with hypertrophic cardiomyopathy at high risk for sudden death. J Am Coll Cardiol 10:761–774, 1987.
158. Fananapazir L, Leon MB, Bonow RO, et al: Sudden death during empiric amiodarone therapy in symptomatic hypertrophic cardiomyopathy. Am J Cardiol 67:169–174, 1991.
159. Moss AJ, Schwartz PJ, Crampton RS, et al: The long QT syndrome: Prospective longitudinal study of 328 families. Circulation 84:1136–1144, 1991.
160. Weintraub RG, Gow RM, Wilkinson JM: The congenital long QT syndromes in childhood. J Am Coll Cardiol 16:674–680, 1990.
161. Schwartz PJ, Locati E, Priori J, et al: The long QT syndrome. In Zipes DP, Jallife P (eds): Cardiac Electrophysiology. Philadelphia, WB Saunders, 1990, pp 589–605.
162. Kudenchuck PJ, Cobb LA. Greene HL, et al: Late outcome of survivors of out-of-hospital cardiac arrest with left ventricular ejection fractions greater than 50% and without significant coronary artery disease. Am J Cardiol 67:704–708, 1991.
163. Viskin S, Belhassen B: Idiopathic ventricular fibrillation. Am Heart J 120:661–671, 1990.

33

Patients with Nonsustained Ventricular Tachycardia

ALFRED E. BUXTON

The presence of nonsustained ventricular tachycardia (VT) (runs of three or more consecutive premature ventricular complexes at rates above 100 beats/min, terminating spontaneously within 30 seconds) has been recognized as a marker of increased risk for sudden death in patients with recent myocardial infarction (MI) for two decades. Interest in this arrhythmia initially arose when it was noted frequently in the minutes immediately preceding episodes of primary ventricular fibrillation (VF) in patients with acute MI.[1,2] Subsequently a number of studies documented an association between nonsustained VT occurring in the late hospital phase of infarction and sudden death after hospital discharge.[3-10] Other studies then examined the relation between this arrhythmia and sudden death in patients without coronary artery disease. It has become increasingly clear that the prognostic significance of nonsustained VT depends on the clinical setting in which it occurs. This chapter reviews the relation between nonsustained VT and sudden death in the setting of various types of cardiac disease. We will examine various techniques that have been used to quantify the risk for sudden death in each case.

QUANTITATIVE RISK OF SUDDEN DEATH FOR PATIENTS WITH NONSUSTAINED VENTRICULAR TACHYCARDIA

Asymptomatic patients in whom nonsustained VT is discovered fortuitously without evidence of structural heart disease or a family history of sudden death (e.g., in association with one of the long QT syndromes) are at very low risk for sudden death and do not require further investigation.[11] In contrast, in almost every group of patients studied who have evidence of structural heart disease, nonsustained VT identifies a subgroup at increased risk for sudden death. However, in most disease states examined, the presence of nonsustained VT is a marker for patients at equally increased risk for nonsudden cardiac death. Thus, the specificity of nonsustained VT as a predictor for *sudden* cardiac death (SCD) is questionable. We will concentrate on three types of heart disease that have been studied extensively: hypertrophic cardiomyopathy, idiopathic dilated cardiomyopathy, and coronary artery disease.

Hypertrophic Cardiomyopathy

Nonsustained VT is found in approximately 20% of patients with hypertrophic cardiomyopathy.[12-16] Two studies have examined the relation between nonsustained VT and sudden death in patients with hypertrophic cardiomyopathy.[17,18] Each study included only patients without symptoms of arrhythmias. Together, a total of 185 patients were studied, with a mean follow-up of 30–36 months. A total of 14 cardiac deaths occurred, all but one of which were classified as sudden. The risk of sudden death was 7- to 12-fold higher in the patients with nonsustained VT on Holter monitoring than in those without the arrhythmia. However, since all but one of the deaths were sudden in the patients with and without nonsustained VT, the specificity of this arrhythmia as a predictor of sudden death in this population is uncertain. Although the negative predictive value of the Holter results (i.e., the likelihood of sudden death in patients without nonsustained VT) was 97–98%, the positive predictive value (i.e, the likelihood of sudden death in patients with nonsustained VT) was modest, at 21–24%. We can conclude, then, that nonsustained VT is a relatively sensitive predictor of the risk of SCD in patients with hypertrophic cardiomyopathy, but its accuracy as a clinical predictor is unclear at this time.

Idiopathic Dilated Cardiomyopathy

Nonsustained VT also occurs frequently in patients with idiopathic dilated cardiomyopathy. In this context it has been documented in approximately 50% of patients by means of 24-hour ambulatory monitoring.[19–24] In this disease the relationship between asymptomatic arrhythmias found on electrocardiographic (ECG) monitoring and sudden death is less clear than in the case of hypertrophic cardiomyopathy. Three studies involving a total of 173 patients have prospectively evaluated this relationship, with a mean follow-up of 30–36 months.[20,23,24] A total of 49 cardiac deaths occurred, of which 20 (41%) were classified as sudden. In contrast to the situation seen with hypertrophic cardiomyopathy, the risk of sudden death in patients with nonsustained VT (10%) did not exceed that in patients without nonsustained VT (13%). Only 26% of the cardiac deaths were sudden in the patients with nonsustained VT, compared to 63% in patients without VT. Furthermore, the sensitivity of nonsustained VT as a predictor of sudden death was only 40% (8 of 20 deaths). Thus, in patients with idiopathic dilated cardiomyopathy, nonsustained VT is both insensitive and nonspecific as a predictor of SCD.

Coronary Artery Disease

The prevalence and prognostic significance of nonsustained VT in patients with coronary artery disease depend on the time that monitoring is performed relative to the acute MI. Although the highest prevalence is found in patients during the acute phase of infarction (almost 50%),[5,25] nonsustained VT occurring at this time does not carry long-term prognostic significance.[5] In contrast, nonsustained VT can be documented in 10–20% of patients 2–4 weeks after the onset of infarction.[3–10] When it is discovered at this time there is a clear association with risk for late sudden death. Four studies have specifically examined this relationship in a total of 1736 patients monitored for 6–24 hours and followed up for 12–48 months.[6,8–10] A total of 200 cardiac deaths occurred, of which 126 (63%) were sudden. The risk of sudden death in the patients with nonsustained VT (14%) was approximately twice that of the patients without VT (6%). The sensitivity of nonsustained VT as marker for sudden death was 31% (39 of 126 deaths). Sudden death accounted for 60% of the cardiac deaths in the patients with nonsustained VT and for 64% of the cardiac deaths in patients without nonsustained VT. Thus, the documentation of nonsustained VT in patients with recent infarction identifies a population at relatively high risk of sudden death. However, the Holter finding itself is not specifically predictive of SCD, and is only moderately sensitive.

In summary, the discovery of nonsustained VT in patients with hypertrophic cardiomyopathy, or in patients with coronary artery disease and recent MI, identifies populations at significantly increased risk of sudden death. Although this finding is useful for targeting populations for study, it lacks sufficient precision to allow the practitioner to make therapeutic decisions when dealing with individual patients. For patients with idiopathic dilated cardiomyopathy, nonsustained VT does not carry any useful prognostic information beyond indicating a population of patients more likely to die (either suddenly or nonsuddenly).

SPECIALIZED TESTING TO IDENTIFY RISK IN INDIVIDUAL PATIENTS

These limitations of long-term ECG monitoring have led investigators to examine other techniques capable of providing information that carries greater clinical utility. The three that have received the most attention are exercise testing, programmed stimulation, and signal averaging of the surface ECG.

Exercise Testing

Exercise testing has been examined in patients with hypertrophic cardiomyopathy and in patients with coronary artery disease. In both cases it lacks sensitivity, inducing ventricular tachyarrhythmias in a minority of patients.[12,26,27] Although exercise testing has proved useful in the evaluation of the postinfarction patients for the prediction of those liable to develop recurrent ischemic events after infarction, it does not identify patients specifically at risk for (arrhythmia-mediated) SCD.[28] We are not aware of any studies specifically studying the provocation of arrhythmias by exercise in patients with idiopathic dilated cardiomyopathy.

Electrophysiological Testing

Since Wellens demonstrated two decades ago that programmed electrical stimulation could reproduce monomorphic sustained VT in patients with previously documented episodes, use of this modality has rapidly proliferated.[29] Although the technique was initially used to study the mechanisms causing sustained VT, it was subsequently found useful to guide both pharmacological and surgical therapy. Later studies demonstrated that in many patients resuscitated from out-of-hospital cardiac arrest, especially those with coronary artery disease and prior MI, monomorphic sustained VT could be induced. Uncontrolled studies suggested that therapy aimed at suppressing these inducible arrhythmias was effective in preventing recurrent cardiac arrest. These observations, and the discovery from fortuitous ECG recordings obtained at the onset of spontaneous cardiac arrests that such events were most often initiated by VT (even if VF later ensued), suggested that programmed stimulation might be applied prospectively to populations known to be at high risk for sudden death. Several studies (with conflicting results) examined the ability of programmed stimulation to identify patients with recent MI at risk of late SCD. At the same time, a number of studies have applied programmed stimulation to a wide variety of patients with spontaneous episodes of nonsustained VT. Initially, we studied such patients in a manner similar to the initial studies of patients with spontaneous sustained VT, in an attempt to define arrhythmia mechanisms.[30,31] We and others then prospectively evaluated the ability of the results of programmed stimulation to provide prognostically useful information.[32,41] The rationale behind such studies is as follows: (1) The potential outcomes of programmed stimulation include no inducible arrhythmia, inducible nonsustained VT, and inducible sustained VT. (2) The patients with no inducible arrhythmia and those with only nonsustained inducible VT should be at relatively low risk for arrhythmically mediated sudden death (one would not expect programmed stimulation to predict patients at risk of sudden death precipitated by acute ischemia). (3) Patients with sustained induced VT should be the group at highest risk for sudden death. (4) Only patients with sustained induced tachycardias would be candidates for antiarrhythmic therapy. (5) Antiarrhythmic therapy that prevented the inducible sustained tachycardias should markedly reduce the risk of sudden death in these patients.

Our initial studies of programmed stimulation in patients with nonsustained VT revealed that the results of programmed stimulation were directly related to the presence and type of anatomical heart disease.[30] Sustained monomorphic VT was rarely induced in patients with structurally normal hearts or in patients with noncoronary heart disease. Subsequent studies have revealed inducible monomorphic sustained VT in 0–10% of patients with idiopathic dilated cardiomyopathy.[42–45] Inducible tachycardia has not been related to a history of syncope in such patients.[42–45] We did not find any relation between a history of syncope and inducible VT in patients with coronary artery disease,[30] although another group found a negative relationship between the two factors.[38] In asymptomatic patients with hypertrophic cardiomyopathy and nonsustained VT, inducible VT (polymorphic in most cases) has been reported in 21–56%.[46,47] Of note, a history of syncope in patients with hypertrophic cardiomyopathy appears to significantly increase the chance of inducing VT.[46,47] These observations stand in marked contrast to the results obtained when programmed stimulation is applied to patients with nonsustained VT and coronary artery disease. In this population, monomorphic sustained VT has been induced in 30–50%.[30,33–40] Series that included patients with syncope did not differ significantly in the rate of inducible VT from those excluding patients with a history of syncope.

The likelihood of inducing VT in patients with coronary artery disease is clearly related to the stimulation protocol used and to the extent of left ventricular (LV) dysfunction. Stimulation protocols limited to a maximum of two ventricular extrastimuli have yielded induction rates of 20–30%.[33,38,41] With protocols utilizing three extrastimuli, up to 55% of patients will have inducible monomorphic sustained VT.[33–37,39,40,48] Induction rates rise with increasing degrees of LV dysfunction.[48] In 107 consecutive patients with coronary artery disease and spontaneous nonsustained VT, we have found inducible monomorphic sustained VT in 37% of patients with an LV ejection fraction ≤ 0.40 versus 19% of patients with ejection fraction > 0.40 (unpublished data). Others have induced sustained VT in as many as 50% of patients with ejection fractions ≤ 0.40.[48] We have also noted a significantly greater chance of inducing sustained VT in patients with LV aneurysms.[30]

In view of the differences in prognostic significance of nonsustained VT, and the results of programmed stimulation in relation to underlying heart disease, it should be clear that any investigation of the prognostic utility of such a technique either must be limited to a homogeneous group of patients or must be designed to allow statistically appropriate analysis of subgroups of patients based on the type of heart disease. Unfortunately, many authors have reported outcome results based on heterogeneous patient groups, which makes logical analysis difficult. In addition, because of assumptions about the significance of the results of programmed stimulation (noted earlier), there are as yet no published controlled studies of this technique in any patient population. That is, the majority of reported patients who have had sustained (and in some cases, even nonsustained) VT induced have been given antiarrhythmic therapy. Nonetheless, a large body of observational data now exists that permits some conclusions to be drawn.

No prospective analyses of the prognostic significance of programmed stimulation in patients with hypertrophic cardiomyopathy have been reported. Two retrospective analyses from the same laboratory suggest a greater chance of inducing sustained VTs (both uniform and polymorphic) in patients evaluated after cardiac arrest than in patients studied because of syncope, presyncope, asymptomatic nonsustained VT, or a family history of sudden death.[46,47] The majority of induced tachycardias were polymorphic, the specificity of which is uncertain. Inducible ventricular tachyarrhythmias were more often found in patients with a history of cardiac arrest or syncope who had nonsustained VT on 24–48 hours of Holter monitoring. This correlation was not observed in patients evaluated for the other indications noted above. Thus, the prognostic utility of electrophysiological studies in asymptomatic patients with nonsustained VT and hypertrophic cardiomyopathy is not known at this time.

Five studies reported to date have evaluated the utility of programmed stimulation to predict sudden death in patients with idiopathic dilated cardiomyopathy without prior symptomatic ventricular tachyarrhythmias.[42–45,48] Unfortunately, two of the studies used stimulation protocols employing a maximum of two ventricular extrastimuli, a technique that appears to markedly decrease the yield of inducible arrhythmias.[42–45] Additionally, only two of the reports permit analysis of outcome in relation to the presence of spontaneous nonsustained VT and inducible VT.[44,48] However, as noted previously, inducible sustained VT is both uncommon in this population and not clearly related to the presence of spontaneous nonsustained VT. Overall, the relation of sudden death during follow-up (12–19 months) to inducible ventricular tachyarrhythmias can be evaluated in 97 patients. Uniform sustained VT was induced in 4 patients, of whom 1 died suddenly. Polymorphic sustained VT was induced in 8 patients, of whom 2 died suddenly. No sustained tachycardia was induced in 85 patients, of whom 16 died suddenly. Thus, 25% of patients with inducible sustained tachyarrhythmias died suddenly, versus 18% of patients without inducible tachycardia, and the majority of sudden deaths occurred in patients without inducible tachycardias. We would conclude that programmed stimulation lacks adequate sensitivity and specificity to be clinically useful as a predictive test in patients with idiopathic dilated cardiomyopathy.

Twelve published studies that we are aware of have examined the relationship between arrhythmias induced by programmed stimulation, antiarrhythmic therapy, and SCD in patients with spontaneous nonsustained VT and coronary artery disease.[33–41,48–50] The results of most are difficult to interpret because of a number of factors: inclusion of patients with multiple types of heart disease with failure to stratify the results by heart disease,[33,40] use of stimulation protocols employing only two ventricular extrastimuli, which, as noted above, severely compromises the sensitivity of the study in this patient population,[33,38,41] retrospective analysis,[37] failure to state criteria for treatment,[49,50] failure to state whether induced VT was uniform or polymorphic,[49,50] inclusion of patients with complex forms of ventricular ectopy other than nonsustained VT (couplets, multiform premature complexes),[33,37,41] and atypical definitions of sustained VT.[50] When studies with the above limitations are eliminated, four studies involving a total of 230 patients remain for analysis.[34,36,39,48] All used similar stimulation protocols involving three ventricular extrastimuli, all intended to judge antiarrhythmic efficacy by programmed stimulation, and each report permits analysis of outcome in relation to the presence or absence of inducible VT at the time of hospital discharge. Two of the reports included patients without regard for LV function,[34,36] a third included only patients with an ejection fraction < 0.40,[39] while for the fourth, we include only patients with an ejection fraction < 0.40 in this analysis, because patients with an ejection fraction ≥ 0.40 were grouped with noncoronary patients, preventing analysis of the coronary patients.[48] Of note, these studies antedated the use of implantable cardioverter-defibrillators in this patient population.

Sustained monomorphic VT was induced in 43–50% of patients in these reports, and 43–75% responded to drug therapy, as judged from programmed stimulation. After mean follow-up times ranging from 14 to 28 months, arrhythmic events (almost all being sudden death or cardiac arrest rather than sustained VT) occurred in 10–23% of patients. The mean negative predictive value (the percent of patients free of events who had no sustained tachycardia induced at the baseline study and who were discharged without antiarrhythmic therapy) was 91% (range, 79–96%). As noted previously, the true positive predictive value of inducible VT (the chance of an arrhythmic event developing in patients with inducible tachycardia) cannot be determined, as almost every patient with inducible sustained tachycardia received antiarrhythmic drugs. However, some idea of the risk of sudden death and of the effect of antiarrhythmic therapy guided by programmed stimulation can be obtained by examining the outcome in patients discharged without inducible VT versus those discharged with persistently inducible tachycardia on empirical therapy. The arrhythmic event rates in patients discharged without inducible tachycardia ranged from 0 to 11% (mean, 7%). In contrast, the arrhythmic event rates in patients discharged on empirical therapy ranged from 7% to 88% (mean, 45%). The major limitations to interpreting these data are obviously: (1) Some of the arrhythmic events in the treated patients undoubtedly resulted from "proarrhythmic" episodes. (2) Therefore, we cannot be certain of the real risk to the patients with inducible tachycardia had they been left untreated. Nonetheless, we can reasonably conclude from these studies that programmed stimulation is capable of identifying a relatively low-risk population that is unlikely to benefit from antiarrhythmic therapy—those patients without inducible sustained monomorphic VT on the baseline electrophysiological study (in the absence of antiarrhythmic drugs). In addition, it seems likely that those patients with inducible sustained VT are at significantly higher risk of sudden death. Several multicenter trials now in progress are attempting to define the risk of sudden death in patients with inducible tachycardia, and to quantify the benefits of antiarrhythmic therapy guided by programmed stimulation.

Signal-Averaged Electrocardiography

The recognition that VT initiated many if not most out-of-hospital cardiac arrests, and the demonstration that re-entry within the myocardium was the mechanism underlying most clinical sustained VTs, led to the development of techniques capable of detecting evidence of the physiological requisites for re-entry in patients. One such requirement, slow conduction of electrical impulses, has been studied extensively. Evidence of slow conduction and delayed activation in localized areas of myocardial tissue can be seen during activation mapping, both during sinus rhythm and during VT in patients with VT.[51-53] Signal averaging of the surface ECG is a technique that can detect abnormally slowed conduction and delayed myocardial activation noninvasively.

Signal averaging permits high-level amplification of very low-level signals (such as those resulting from areas of slowed conduction) while at the same time avoiding amplification of noise. It is performed during sinus rhythm using a variety of methods. The technique that has been applied most often in patients with nonsustained VT is called ensemble or time domain analysis. Usually 150–200 sinus complexes are recorded from orthogonal (x, y, z) leads. The signals from each lead are averaged, then high-pass filtered (in order to eliminate low-frequency signals caused by the repolarization phase of the action potential), and then combined into a vector magnitude, or "filtered QRS complex."[54] The parameters measured from the filtered QRS complex are its duration (determined automatically by computer algorithm), the amplitude of the terminal 40 msec of the filtered QRS complex, and the duration of the low-level signals (<40 μV) in the terminal portion of the filtered QRS complex.

A number of studies have now examined the relationship of signal-averaged ECG abnormalities to spontaneous (asymptomatic) ventricular arrhythmias. The studies may be divided into two types: studies correlating the signal-averaged ECG with ventricular arrhythmias induced by programmed stimulation,[55-59] and those examining the prognostic significance of signal-averaged ECG abnormalities.[57,60] We first reported findings of the signal-averaged ECG in a heterogeneous group of patients with nonsustained VT.[61] This study demonstrated a good correlation of ECG abnormalities with inducible VT. However, because sustained monomorphic VT was induced almost exclusively in patients with coronary artery disease and prior MI, it became obvious that in order to determine the true value of the signal-averaging technique, we would have to restrict the analysis to a homogeneous group of patients with coronary artery disease.

We then performed analyses of signal-averaged ECGs only in patients who had coronary heart disease and spontaneous nonsustained VT.[56,58] The larger study examined 50 patients, 19 of whom had a prior anterior and 31 a prior inferior infarction.[58] Twenty-four of the patients had sustained monomorphic VT inducible by programmed stimulation in the absence of antiarrhythmic agents. Although the filtered QRS duration was significantly longer in the patients with inducible tachycardia, the amplitude of the last 40 msec of the QRS complex did not correlate with inducibility of tachycardia. In addition, we found a significant influence of infarction site on the results of the signal-averaged ECG: patients with inferior infarctions had significantly longer filtered QRS durations and a lower amplitude of the terminal portion of the QRS complex than patients with anterior infarctions. Furthermore, while the filtered QRS duration was significantly longer in patients with than in those without inducible tachycardia after inferior infarction, this parameter did not distinguish those with inducible tachycardia after anterior infarction. The amplitude of the terminal portion of the filtered QRS complex did not distinguish patients with inducible tachycardia from those without it after infarction at either location.

Our group also examined the signal-averaged ECG in 16 patients without a history of sustained VT or fibrillation and nonischemic dilated cardiomyopathy.[55] Eleven of these 16 patients had documented nonsustained VT. Five of the 11 patients with nonsustained VT had one or more abnormal parameters on the signal-averaged ECG, and two of these patients had inducible sustained VT.[62]

Two other groups have correlated the signal-averaged ECG with inducibility of VT in heterogeneous populations of patients with nonsustained VT.[57,59] Both groups found the signal-averaged ECG to be abnormal significantly more often in patients with inducible monomorphic VT than in those without inducible tachycardia. These studies did not find any correlation between the signal-averaged ECG results and infarct site.

Overall, these studies suggest a high degree of sensitivity but only moderate specificity of an abnormal signal-averaged ECG for identifying patients with inducible VT. At this time, the most useful aspect of the test appears to be its high negative predictive value: patients with normal results have a low probability of having inducible sustained monomorphic VT.

The prognostic significance of signal-averaged ECG abnormalities has also been examined in two uncontrolled prospective studies involving patients with both cardiomyopathies and coronary artery disease.[57,60] The prevalence of signal-averaged abnormalities ranged from 26–42%. After average follow-ups of 17–30 months, two and six patients, respectively, experienced sudden death. Abnormalities of the signal-averaged ECG were present in 50 and 100% of the patients dying suddenly. The positive predictive accuracy of an abnormal signal-averaged ECG ranged from 9 to 13%, but the significance of these figures is unclear because all patients in these studies underwent electrophysiological testing, and patients with inducible VT received therapy guided by serial drug testing. Thus, the prognostic significance of the signal-average ECG cannot be evaluated independently of inducible VT on the basis of published information. Presumably, the treatments given to patients prevented some sudden deaths that would have occurred in patients with abnormal signal-averaged ECGs. If these populations had remained untreated, the positive predictive accuracy likely would have been higher. The prognostic significance of a normal signal-averaged ECG in this population seems clearer. The majority of these ECGs occurred in patients without inducible tachyarrhythmias, and these patients did not receive antiarrhythmic therapy. The negative predictive value of the signal-averaged ECG in the two studies was 96–100%.

SUMMARY

Nonsustained VT is one marker of the risk for sudden death in patients with structural heart disease. The risk of sudden death in patients with this arrhythmia depends on the type and severity of the underlying heart disease. The discovery of this arrhythmia in patients with coronary artery disease identifies a population of patients at high risk, but it does not carry a high enough predictive accuracy to define individual patients likely to benefit from antiarrhythmic therapy. In other words, an association exists between spontaneous nonsustained VT and SCD, but causality has not been demonstrated. The signal-averaged ECG and invasive electrophysiological tests appear to be capable of identifying with much higher degrees of accuracy the risk for sudden death in patients with coronary artery disease and will likely play complementary roles in patient care. However, prospective, controlled trials are needed to determine whether the information provided by these technologies, when combined with available antiarrhythmic therapies, will result in a decrease in the incidence of sudden death.

REFERENCES

1. El-Sherif N, Myerburg RJ, Scherlag BJ, et al: Electrocardiographic antecedents of primary ventricular fibrillation: Value of the R-on-T phenomenon in myocardial infarction. Br Heart J 38:415, 1976.
2. Lie KI, Wellens HJJ, Downar E, Durrer D: Observations on patients with primary ventricular fibrillation complicating acute myocardial infarction. Circulation. 52:755, 1975.
3. Vismara LA, Amsterdam EA, Mason DT: Relation of ventricular arrhythmias in the late hospital phase of acute myocardial infarction to sudden death after hospital discharge. Am J Med 59:6, 1975.
4. Schulze RA, Rouleau J, Rigo P, Bowers S, Strauss HW, Pitt B: Ventricular arrhythmias in the late hospital phase of acute myocardial infarction: Relation to left ventricular func-

tion detected by gated cardiac blood pool scanning. Circulation 52:1006, 1975.
5. de Soyza N, Bennett FA, Murphy ML, Bissett JK, Kane JJ: The relationship of paroxysmal ventricular tachycardia complicating the acute phase and ventricular arrhythmia during the late hospital phase of myocardial infarction to long-term survival. Am J Med 64:377, 1978.
6. Anderson KP, DeCamilla J, Moss AJ: Clinical significance of ventricular tachycardia (3 beats or longer) detected during ambulatory monitoring after myocardial infarction. Circulation 57:890, 1978.
7. Cats VM, Lie KI, Van Capelle FJ, Durrer D: Limitations of 24-hour ambulatory electrocardiographic recording in predicting coronary events after acute myocardial infarction. Am J Cardiol 44:1257, 1979.
8. Kleiger RE, Miller JP, Thanavaro S, Province MA, Martin TF, Oliver GC: Relationship between clinical features of acute myocardial infarction and ventricular runs 2 weeks to 1 year after infarction. Circulation 63:64, 1981.
9. Bigger JT, Weld FM, Rolnitzky LM: Prevalence, characteristics and significance of ventricular tachycardia (three or more complexes) detected with ambulatory electrocardiographic recording in the late hospital phase of acute myocardial infarction. Am J Cardiol 48:815, 1981.
10. Bigger JT, Fleiss JL, Kleiger R, Miller JP, Rolnitzky LM, the Multicenter Post-Infarction Research Group: The relationships among ventricular arrhythmias, left ventricular dysfunction, and mortality in the 2 years after myocardial infarction. Circulation 69:250, 1984.
11. Kennedy HL, Whitlock JA, Sprague MK, Kennedy LJ, Buckingham TA, Goldbert RJ: Long-term follow-up of asymptomatic healthy subjects with frequent and complex ventricular ectopy. N Engl J Med 312:193, 1985.
12. Savage DD, Seides SF, Maron BJ, Myers DJ, Epstein SE: Prevalence of arrhythmias during 24-hour electrocardiographic monitoring and exercise testing in patients with obstructive and nonobstructive hypertrophic cardiomyopathy. Circulation 59:866, 1979.
13. Mulrow JP, Healy MJ, McKenna WJ, Krikler S: Variability of ventricular arrhythmias in hypertrophic cardiomyopathy and implications for treatment. Am J Cardiol 58:615, 1986.
14. Frank MJ, Watkins LO, Prisant LM, Stefadouros MA, Abdulla AM: Potentially lethal arrhythmias and their management in hypertrophic cardiomyopathy. Am J Cardiol 53:1608, 1984.
15. Newman H, Sugrue D, Oakley CM, Goodwin JF, McKenna WJ: Relation of left ventricular function and prognosis in hypertrophic cardiomyopathy: An angiographic study. J Am Coll Cardiol 5:1064, 1985.
16. Spirito P, Watson RM, Maron BJ: Relation between extent of left ventricular hypertrophy and occurrence of ventricular tachycardia in hypertrophic cardiomyopathy. Am J Cardiol 60:1137, 1987.
17. Maron BJ, Savage DD, Wolfson JK, Epstein SE: Prognostic significance of 24 hour ambulatory electrocardiographic monitoring in patients with hypertrophic cardiomyopathy: A prospective study. Am J Cardiol 48:252, 1981.
18. McKenna WJ, England D, Doi YL, Deanfield JE, Oakley C, Goodwin JF: Arrhythmia in hypertrophic cardiomyopathy: I. Influence on prognosis. Br Heart J 46:168, 1981.
19. Suyama A, Anan T, Araki H, Takeshita A, Nakamura M: Prevalence of ventricular tachycardia in patients with different underlying heart disease: A study by Holter ECG monitoring. Am Heart J 112:44, 1986.
20. Huang SK, Messer JV, Denes P: Significance of ventricular tachycardia in idiopathic dilated cardiomyopathy: Observation in 35 patients. Am J Cardiol 51:507, 1983.
21. Unverferth DV, Magorien RD, Moeschberger ML, Baker PB, Fetters JK, Leier CV: Factors influencing the one-year mortality of dilated cardiomyopathy. Am J Cardiol 54:147, 1984.
22. Holmes J, Kubo SH, Cody RJ, Kligfield P: Arrhythmias in ischemic and nonischemic dilated cardiomyopathy: Prediction of mortality by ambulatory electrocardiography. Am J Cardiol 55:146, 1985.
23. Neri R, Mestroni L, Salvi A, Camerini F: Arrhythmias in dilated cardiomyopathy. Postgrad Med J 62:593, 1986.
24. Olshausen KV, Stienen U, Math D, Schwarz F, Kubler W, Meyer J: Long-term prognostic significance of ventricular arrhythmias in idiopathic dilated cardiomyopathy. Am J Cardiol 61:146, 1988.
25. Campbell RW, Murray A, Julian DG: Ventricular arrhythmias in first 12 hours of acute myocardial infarction: Natural history study. Br Heart J 46:351, 1981.
26. McKenna WJ, Chetty S, Oakley CM, Goodwin JF: Arrhythmia in hypertrophic cardiomyopathy: Exercise and 48 hour ambulatory electrocardiographic assessment with and without beta adrenergic blocking therapy. Am J Cardiol 45:10, 1980.
27. Califf RM, McKinnis RA, McNeer JF, et al:

Prognostic value of ventricular arrhythmias associated with treadmill exercise testing in patients studied with cardiac catheterization for suspected ischemic heart disease. Am Coll Cardiol 6:1060, 1983.
28. Théroux P, Waters DD, Halphen C, Debaisieux JC, Mizgala HF: Prognostic value of exercise testing soon after myocardial infarction. N Engl J Med 301:341, 1979.
29. Wellens HJ, Schuilenburg RM, Durrer D: Electrical stimulation of the heart in patients with ventricular tachycardia. Circulation 46:216, 1972.
30. Buxton AE, Waxman HL, Marchlinski FE, Josephson ME: Electrophysiologic studies in nonsustained ventricular tachycardia: Relation to underlying heart disease. Am J Cardiol 53:985, 1983.
31. Buxton AE, Waxman HL, Marchlinski FE, Josephson ME: Electropharmacology of nonsustained ventricular tachycardia: Effects of class I antiarrhythmic agents, verapamil and propranolol. Am J Cardiol 53:738, 1984.
32. Buxton AE, Marchlinski FE, Waxman HL, Flores BT, Cassidy DM, Josephson ME: Prognostic factors in nonsustained ventricular tachycardia. Am J Cardiol 53:1275, 1984.
33. Gomes JA, Hariman RI, Kang PS, El-Sherif N, Chowdhry I, Lyons J: Programmed electrical stimulation in patients with high-grade ventricular ectopy: Electrophysiologic findings and prognosis for survival. Circulation 70:43, 1984.
34. Buxton AE, Marchlinski FE, Flores BT, Miller JM, Doherty JU, Josephson ME: Nonsustained ventricular tachycardia in patients with coronary artery disease: Role of electrophysiologic study. Circulation 75:1178, 1987.
35. Kharsa MH, Gold RL, Moore H, Yazaki Yoshizumi, Haffajee CI, Alpert JS: Long-term outcome following programmed electrical stimulation in patients with high-grade ventricular ectopy. PACE 11:603, 1988.
36. Klein RC, Machell C: Use of electrophysiologic testing in patients with nonsustained ventricular tachycardia: Prognostic and therapeutic implications. J Am Coll Cardiol 14:155, 1989.
37. Kowey PR, Waxman HL, Greenspon A, et al, and the Philadelphia Arrhythmia Group: Value of electrophysiologic testing in patients with previous myocardial infarction and nonsustained ventricular tachycardia. Am J Cardiol 65:594, 1990.
38. Manolis AS, Estes NAM: Value of programmed ventricular stimulation in the evaluation and management of patients with nonsustained ventricular tachycardia associated with coronary artery disease. Am J Cardiol 65:201, 1990.
39. Wilber DJ, Olshansky B, Moran JF, Scanlon PJ: Electrophysiological testing and nonsustained ventricular tachycardia: Use and limitations in patients with coronary artery disease and impaired ventricular function. Circulation 82:350, 1990.
40. Turitto G, Fontaine JM, Ursell S, Caref EB, Bekheit S, El-Sherif N: Risk stratification and management of patients with organic heart disease and nonsustained ventricular tachycardia: Role of programmed stimulation, left ventricular ejection fraction, and the signal-averaged electrocardiogram. Am J Med 88:35, 1990.
41. Zheutlin TA, Roth H, Chua W, et al: Programmed electrical stimulation to determine the need for antiarrhythmic therapy in patients with complex ventricular ectopic activity. Am Heart J 111:860, 1986.
42. Meinertz T, Treese N, Kasper W, et al: Determinants of prognosis in idiopathic dilated cardiomyopathy as determined by programmed electrical stimulation. Am J Cardiol 56:337, 1985.
43. Das SK, Morady F, Di Carlo L, et al: Prognostic usefulness of programmed ventricular stimulation in idiopathic dilated cardiomyopathy without symptomatic ventricular arrhythmias. Am J Cardiol 58:998, 1986.
44. Poll DS, Marchlinski FE, Buxton AE, Josephson ME: Usefulness of programmed stimulation in idiopathic dilated cardiomyopathy. Am J Cardiol 58:992, 1986.
45. Stamato NJ, O'Connell JB, Murdock DK, et al: The response of patients with complex ventricular arrhythmias secondary to dilated cardiomyopathy to programmed electrical stimulation. Am Heart J 112:505, 1986.
46. Watson RM, Schwartz JL, Maron BJ, Tucker E, Rosing DR, Josephson ME: Inducible polymorphic ventricular tachycardia and ventricular fibrillation in a subgroup of patients with hypertrophic cardiomyopathy at high risk for sudden death. J Am Coll Cardiol 10:761, 1987.
47. Fananapazir L, Tracy CM, Leon MB, et al: Electrophysiologic abnormalities in patients with hypertrophic cardiomyopathy: A consecutive analysis in 155 patients. Circulation 80:1259, 1989.
48. Hammill SC, Trusty JM, Wood DL, et al: Influence of ventricular function and presence or absence of coronary artery disease on results of electrophysiologic testing for asymptomatic nonsustained ventricular tachycardia. Am J Cardiol 65:722, 1990.
49. Veltri EP, Platia EV, Griffith LSC, Reid PR: Programmed electrical stimulation and long-

term follow-up in asymptomatic, nonsustained ventricular tachycardia. Am J Cardiol 56:309, 1985.
50. Sulpizi AM, Friehling TD, Kowey PR: Value of electrophysiologic testing in patients with nonsustained ventricular tachycardia. Am J Cardiol 59:841, 1987.
51. Cassidy DM, Vassallo JA, Miller JM, et al: Endocardial catheter mapping in patients in sinus rhythm: Relationship to underlying heart disease and ventricular arrhythmias. Circulation 73:645, 1986.
52. Vassallo JA, Cassidy DM, Marchlinski FE, Miller JM, Buxton AE, Josephson ME: Abnormalities of endocardial activation pattern in patients with previous healed myocardial infarction and ventricular tachycardia. Am J Cardiol 58:479, 1986.
53. Josephson ME, Horowitz LN, Farshidi A: Continuous local electrical activity. Circulation 57:659, 1978.
54. Simson MB: Identification of patients with ventricular tachycardia after myocardial infarction from signals in the terminal QRS complex. Circulation 64:235, 1981.
55. Poll DS, Marchlinski FE, Falcone RA, Josephson ME, Simson MB: Abnormal signal-averaged electrocardiograms in patients with nonischemic congestive cardiomyopathy: Relationship to sustained ventricular tachyarrhythmias. Circulation 72:1308, 1985.
56. Buxton AE, Simson MB, Falcone RA, Marchlinski FE, Doherty JU, Josephson ME: Results of signal-averaged electrocardiography and electrophysiologic study in patients with nonsustained ventricular tachycardia after healing of acute myocardial infarction. Am J Cardiol 60:80, 1987.
57. Winters SL, Stewart D, Targonski A, Gomes AJ: Role of signal averaging of surface QRS complex in selecting patients with nonsustained ventricular tachycardia and high grade ventricular arrhythmias for programmed ventricular stimulation. J Am Coll Cardiol 12:148, 1988.
58. Buxton AE, Britton N, Simson MB: Application of the signal-averaged electrocardiogram in patients with nonsustained ventricular tachycardia after myocardial infarction: Implications for prediction of sudden cardiac death risk. J Electrocardiol S40, 1988.
59. Turitto G, Fontaine JM, Ursell SN, Caref EB, Henkin R, El-Sherif N: Value of the signal-averaged electrocardiogram as a predictor of the results of programmed stimulation in nonsustained ventricular tachycardia. Am J Cardiol 61:1272, 1988.
60. Turitto G, Fontaine JM, Ursell S, Caref EB, Bekheit S, El-Sherif N: Risk stratification and management of patients with organic heart disease and nonsustained ventricular tachycardia: Role of programmed stimulation, left ventricular ejection fraction, and the signal-average electrocardiogram. Am J Med 88:1–35N, 1990.
61. Buxton AE, Simson MB, et al: Signal averaged ECG in patients with nonsustained ventricular arrhythmias [abstract]. J Am Coll Cardiol 3:495, 1984.
62. Marchlinski FE: Personal communication. July, 1992.

34

Hemodynamically Tolerated Sustained Ventricular Tachycardia: Clinical Features and Risk of Sudden Death During Follow-up

MARC D. MEISSNER
TIMOTHY J. LESSMEIER
RUSSELL T. STEINMAN
MICHAEL H. LEHMANN

Sustained ventricular tachycardia (VT), even when associated with relatively mild symptoms, is commonly considered to be an ominous arrhythmia. Holter recordings have certainly demonstrated that sustained VT often serves as a precursor to ventricular fibrillation (VF) and sudden death.[1-6] Data from a number of studies,[7-13] however, suggest that patients who develop sustained VT not associated with syncope or cardiac arrest are less likely to suffer a lethal arrhythmia recurrence than are those patients with poorly tolerated sustained VT or VF. These and other observations suggested to us the need for a standardized approach to grading symptoms associated with ventricular tachyarrhythmias (Table 34–1).[14]

Unfortunately, there is no uniform definition in the literature for the term "hemodynamically tolerated." Although some investigators have included a criterion of supine mean arterial pressure greater than 65 mm Hg,[15,16] we will use the term "hemodynamically tolerated" simply to refer to sustained VT (lasting ≥30 sec) with symptoms limited to Classes I and II (Table 34–1). We recognize that the latter symptoms may be associated with relative hypotension. The sustained VTs under discussion are known or assumed to be predominantly monomorphic in appearance.

The fact that hemodynamically tolerated sustained VT may have distinct immediate and long-term clinical implications argues for the importance of considering this tachyarrhythmia as a separate entity. In this chapter, we will discuss hemodynamically tolerated sustained VT as it relates to sudden cardiac death (SCD) in patients both with and without coronary artery disease (CAD). The current management implications of hemodynamically tolerated sustained VT are discussed in Chapter 42.

MAGNITUDE OF THE PROBLEM

The prevalence of hemodynamically tolerated sustained VT in the general population is unknown; even an accurate estimate of the size of this subset among patients with sustained VT is not readily available. Several factors may account for the difficulty in obtaining such an estimate from the literature: (1) the lack of a standardized approach to grading arrhythmia-related symptoms, (2) frequent nonreporting of symptoms or hemodynamic status during VT, and (3) a probable selection bias toward un-

Table 34–1
Proposed Four-Tier System for Grading the Severity of Symptoms Caused by Ventricular Tachyarrhythmias*

Class I	Asymptomatic or symptoms limited to palpitations or fluttering
Class II	Lightheadedness, dizziness, chest pain, or dyspnea
Class III	Syncope or altered mental status or other evidence of significant secondary end-organ dysfunction (including pulmonary edema, acute myocardial infarction, low-output state, or stroke)
Class IV	Cardiac arrest (absent pulse and respiration)

SOURCE: Lehmann MH, et al: Am J Cardiol 67: 1421–1423, 1991.[14] Reproduced by permission.
* It is assumed that the tachyarrhythmias are documented, ideally by electrocardiographic recordings, or at least attested to by medical or paraprofessional personnel.

derrepresentation, reflecting a lesser likelihood of referral to investigative centers because of either the milder nature of symptoms or misdiagnosis of the arrhythmia.[17–24] Despite these limitations, pooled data from the electrophysiological literature indicate that roughly half of the cases of sustained VT referred for treatment are hemodynamically tolerated.[7–9,12,13,16,19,21,25–31] This figure, however, is not readily extrapolated to the general population of patients with sustained VT since those with very rapid, poorly tolerated VTs might experience cardiac arrest before they can be evaluated.

Determinants of Hemodynamic Status During Sustained VT

Among the multiple factors that contribute to the ultimate hemodynamic expression of sustained VT,[12,32–36] rate is certainly an important one. Although as a general rule slower VT rates are better tolerated than faster ones,[19,33,34] a considerable overlap can exist between well and poorly tolerated rates, not only among different patients but even in the same individual (with multiple sustained VT morphologies).[27,33,37] The contribution of VT rate to symptom status receives some indirect support from the demonstration of improved patient tolerance of a given VT after the rate has been significantly slowed by antiarrhythmic agents such as amiodarone.[16,27,28,33] Nonetheless, worsening of symptoms despite a slower tachycardia has also been described.[38]

A host of hemodynamic factors may alter the rate threshold at which VT becomes poorly tolerated. Impairment in both systolic and diastolic left ventricular (LV) function may occur acutely at the onset of sustained VT and worsen during the arrhythmia.[34] Reduced LV systolic pressure in VT has been shown to correlate with faster VT rates,[34] which tend to limit diastolic filling.[32] Moreover, abnormalities in myocardial contractility during sustained VT may occur secondary to changes in heart rate per se.[39,40]

Mechanisms of hemodynamic compromise may vary according to underlying LV function. Lima et al.[32] observed that patients with an LV ejection fraction (EF) $\leq$ 0.40 developed severe incoordination of ventricular contraction and relaxation during sustained VT as a result of an abnormal electrical activation sequence, a concept supported by other studies[36]; however, patients with normal or near-normal ventricular function (EF $\geq$ 0.50) developed incomplete relaxation or interruption of diastolic filling during sustained VT.[32]

The role of underlying LV function as a determinant of symptom production during sustained VT is still not well defined, with some studies documenting more severe symptoms in patients with reduced LVEF or pre-existing congestive heart failure history[12] but others failing to confirm these associations.[19,33] Additional factors that may be relevant to symptom status during VT include secondary myocardial ischemia (with attendant contractile dysfunction[41–43] and possibly mitral regurgitation[44]), nonphysiological atrioventricular sequence,[35] and maladaptive blood pressure responses following VT onset.[33]

Given the multiplicity of factors involved, only comprehensive studies with large numbers of patients and multivariate analyses are likely to identify the independent determinants of hemodynamic response to sustained VT.

Electrocardiographic Recognition of Sustained VT

The fact that patients presenting with sustained VT need not be hemodynamically compromised has contributed to misdiagnosis and mistreatment of patients presenting with well-tolerated wide QRS tachycardia.[7-13] Hence, we have listed in Table 34-2 a number of electrocardiographic (ECG) criteria[23,45,46] that favor the diagnosis of VT in the setting of wide QRS tachycardia.

It cannot be overemphasized, however, that regardless of specific ECG features, VT should be considered the most likely diagnosis in an adult patient presenting with hemodynamically tolerated regular wide QRS tachycardia, especially in the setting of prior myocardial infarction (MI)[22] or other structural heart disease.[22-24]

Table 34-2
Electrocardiographic Criteria Suggestive of VT as the Basis for Wide-QRS-Complex Tachycardia*

1. Atrioventricular dissociation
2. Second-degree ventriculoatrial block
3. QRS duration >0.14 sec with a right bundle-branch block pattern†
4. QRS duration >0.16 sec with a left bundle-branch block pattern‡
5. Positive QRS concordance in the precordial leads
6. Extreme left axis deviation (between -90 degrees and ± 180 degrees)
7. Combination of left bundle-branch block pattern and right axis deviation
8. In patients with pre-existing bundle-branch block, a different QRS pattern compared to baseline ECG
9. Absence of an RS complex in all precordial leads
10. RS interval (onset of R wave to deepest part of S wave) > 100 msec when RS complex is present in one or more precordial leads

* See references 23, 45, and 46. It should be noted that QRS duration during VT is typically ≥0.12 sec but may be as short as 0.09 sec.[47]
† Predominantly positive QRS complex in V_1.
‡ Predominantly negative QRS complex in V_1.

HEMODYNAMICALLY TOLERATED SUSTAINED VT IN PATIENTS WITH CAD

Few data are available regarding clinical characteristics and outcomes specifically in patients with hemodynamically tolerated sustained VT and CAD. This is probably due to several factors, including (1) the rarity of studies prospectively designed to address this group of patients, (2) the heterogeneous causes of cardiac disease in published series, (3) the lack of precise identification of each patient with reference to hemodynamic status during VT, (4) with rare exception,[13] lack of follow-up and actuarial data to define outcomes in these patients, and (5) lack of systematic comparisons to an otherwise similar cohort of patients with poorly tolerated VT. Even with these methodological problems, however, it is possible to formulate a reasonable clinical and prognostic characterization of patients with CAD and hemodynamically tolerated VT.

Clinical Presentation and Electrophysiological Findings in Patients with CAD

A middle-aged man with a prior MI is the typical clinical profile of a CAD patient who presents with hemodynamically tolerated sustained VT. Indeed, some 85% of the patients are men[23,24] with a mean age in the early 60s[13,21,23,24] and a history of previous infarction in at least 70–85% of cases.[21,23,24] Mean LVEF is typically about 0.34.[13,21,24] One half to three fourths of the patients are taking oral antiarrhythmic medication at presentation.[13,21] VT often begins while the patient is at rest[24] and lasts for a mean of 6.4 hours (range, ½ to 24 hours) prior to medical evaluation.[24] In various studies the mean VT rate ranges from 170 to 192 beats/min, with maximal rates as high as 240–270 beats/min.[20,21,23,24] Mean systolic blood pressure during VT is usually above 100 mm Hg.[21,24]

In patients with CAD who present with hemodynamically tolerated sustained VT, electrophysiological testing reveals inducible sustained VT in a mean of 97% (range, 88–100%) of patients,[7,9,12,13,24,30] very similar to the inducibility rate observed in patients presenting with poorly tolerated sustained VT.[48] Whereas sustained VT is the most commonly induced arrhythmia, "nonclinical" uniform VT morphologies may be induced in up to 53% of cases.[24,29] The fact that these latter sustained VTs may be faster (and potentially less well tolerated) than the presenting arrhythmia[24] highlights the importance of electrophysiological testing as part of the baseline evaluation in patients with hemodynamically tolerated sustained VT.

Outcome in Patients with CAD

Most recent studies (all retrospective) suggest that patients with a history of cardiac arrest related to sustained ventricular tachyarrhythmia are more prone to sudden death than patients with a history of relatively well-tolerated (i.e., symptom class I or II [Table 34–1]) sustained VT.[7–13] However, several problems with the literature make it difficult to neatly analyze and summarize outcomes in patients with hemodynamically tolerated sustained VT, especially the nonuniformity in reporting of patient characteristics and outcome events and the inconsistent use of actuarial analysis. Within these limitations, we will review outcomes for two different but analogous patient groups: those presenting with spontaneous hemodynamically tolerated sustained VT, and those presenting with various sustained ventricular tachyarrhythmias for which electrophysiologically guided antiarrhythmic therapy was instituted that resulted in inducible hemodynamically sustained VT at discharge.

CAD Patients Presenting with Spontaneous Hemodynamically Tolerated Sustained VT

One study has systematically analyzed outcome (with actuarial analysis) specifically in patients with CAD who presented with hemodynamically tolerated sustained monomorphic VT (Table 34–3).[13] The population in that study consisted of 75 such patients whose mean age was 63 years (range, 39–84 years) with a mean LVEF of 0.34 (range, 0.11–0.60). Eighty-eight percent of these patients who underwent baseline electrophysiological studies had inducible sustained ventricular tachyarrhythmias.

Suppression by antiarrhythmic agents or VT surgery was achieved in 15% and 13% of the patients, respectively. Patients in whom suppression was not achieved received amiodarone (56%), conventional agents (21%), or sotalol (12%), or underwent arrhythmia surgery (2%) or implantable cardioverter-defibrillator (ICD) implantation (9%). During a mean follow-up of 34 ± 26 months, there were no sudden deaths (or appropriate ICD discharges) in the suppressed group, as compared to cumulative 1- and 4-year sudden death rates of 7% and 13%, respectively, in the group in which tachyarrhythmias were not suppressed. These outcomes are significantly better than those that have been reported for cardiac arrest survivors treated by electrophysiologically guided therapy (cumulative 4-year sudden death rate of approximately 10% for suppressed vs. 43% for nonsuppressed patients).[50]

In a report of outcomes for 200 post-MI patients who experienced VT or VF, Brugada et al observed that "Patients with a single myocardial infarction, NYHA Class I or II, and *well-tolerated VT* greater than two months after myocardial infarction, had an excellent prognosis. . . . Only one of 55 patients (2%) died of nonsudden cardiac death. No patients died suddenly."[11] However, outcomes in this VT group were not specifically compared to those of otherwise similar patients with poorly tolerated VT, thus limiting the usefulness of the prognostic information in this study.

It is difficult to derive precise information about patients with CAD and hemodynamically tolerated sustained VT from studies that include patients with cardiac diagnoses other than CAD. However, since patients with CAD compose the great majority of these study populations,[7–9,12,15,16,28,51] it is not unreasonable to assume that many of the observations in the studies reviewed below are relevant to patients with CAD.

In a nonrandomized retrospective study, Leclercq et al investigated life expectancy in 295 patients followed up for more than 5 years after a first episode of sustained monomorphic VT (treated primarily with medication).[26] Patients with ischemic and nonischemic (e.g., dilated) cardiomyopathies and LVEF > 0.30 had a significantly higher cumulative cardiac mortality rate at 10 years when the initial VT presentation was with

Table 34-3
Summary of Outcomes in Patients Presenting with Spontaneous Hemodynamically Tolerated Sustained Ventricular Tachycardia in the Setting of Coronary Artery Disease*

Study	No. of Pts.	Pts. with CAD No. (%)	Pts. with HT-Sust. VT No. (%)	Antiarrhythmic Treatment	Mean LVEF† (%)	Actuarial Analysis Provided for Pts. with HT-Sust. VT	Mean F/U (mo)†	Outcome in Pts. with HT-Sust. VT
Steinman et al,[13]	75	75 (100)	75 (100)	Yes	34	Yes	34 ± 26	SD mortality (arrhythmia suppressed): 0% over F/U period SD mortality (arrhythmia nonsuppressed): 7% at 1 yr; 13% at 4 yr
Leclercq et al[26]	295	156 (53)	79‡	Yes	NA	Yes	61 ± 40	SD mortality (estimated)§ LVEF > 30%: 1% at 1 yr; 5% at 2 yr; 8% at 4 yr LVEF ≤ 30%: 10% at 1 yr; 13% at 2 yr; 17% at 4 yr
Gottlieb et al[9]	158	130 (82)	62 (39)	Yes	35	No	22	SD mortality (tolerated VT both spont. and on amiodarone): 2% SD mortality (tolerated VT spont. only): 10% SD mortality (tolerated VT only on amiodarone): 17%
Saxon et al[12]	121	91 (75)	48 (40)	Yes	39 ± 15 (H)	Yes	32 ± 26 (H)	SD mortality: 2 ± 2% at 1 yr; 9 ± 5% at 2 yr; 13 ± 6% at both 3 and 4 yr Total mortality: 33 ± 8% overall death rate at 4 yr
Fogoros et al[7]	78	63 (81)	28 (36)	Yes	32 ± 12 (H)	Yes	19 ± 13 (H)	SD mortality: 0% at 6 mo; 5% (0–15)¶ at 1 yr; 5% (0–15)¶ at 2 yr VT recurrence: 34% (16–52)¶ at 6 mo; 39% (19–54)¶ at 1 yr; 53% (31–75)¶ at 2 yr
Wilensky et al[25]	97	NA	49 (51)	Yes‖	NA	No	17 ± 12	SD in 7/16 VT pts. SD or recurrent VT in 16/42 VT pts.

Abbreviations: CA, cardiac arrest; CAD, coronary artery disease; F/U, follow-up; H, hemodynamically stable patients only; HT-Sust. VT, hemodynamically tolerated sustained VT; LVEF, left ventricular ejection fraction; NA, data not available; Pts, Patients; SD, sudden death; Spont, spontaneously; VT, ventricular tachycardia; yr, year(s)

* Predominantly, but not exclusively, patients with CAD (see text for discussion). The proportion of patients presenting with spontaneous hemodynamically tolerated sustained VT varies among the series.
† For all patients, unless otherwise specified by "(H)".
‡ Includes only those patients among group I (n = 156) and II (n = 55) combined, i.e., ischemic and nonischemic LV cardiomyopathies, respectively.
§ Based on authors' comments that approximately 60% of actuarial cardiac mortality was due to SCD. Numbers rounded to nearest whole.
‖ Except two patients.
¶ 95% confidence intervals.

rather than without syncope (61% vs. 29%, respectively; $p < 0.001$). The findings were similar though less pronounced in patients whose LVEF was ≤ 0.30: a 5-year cardiac mortality of 67% for the syncope groups versus a 39% mortality for the nonsyncope groups ($p < 0.05$). Based on the authors' statement that approximately 60% of cardiac mortality was due to SCD, actuarial sudden death rates for the patients with nonsyncopal sustained VT may be estimated at 14% and 17% at 5 and 10 years, respectively, for patients with LVEF > 0.30, and 23% and 36% at 5 and 10 years, respectively, for patients with LVEF ≤ 0.30.[26] However, the strength of these data is limited by at least two observations: (1) In patients whose LVEF was > 0.30, 5–7 year survival free of cardiac death was virtually identical in patients presenting with and without syncope. (2) The number of patients available for follow-up beyond 5 years was small in the group that showed marked survival differences at 10 years.[26]

One preliminary report compared the clinical outcomes of 62 patients presenting with hemodynamically tolerated sustained VT with outcomes in 96 patients presenting with VF or "nontolerated" VT treated with amiodarone.[9] CAD (remote MI) was present in 82% of patients. Mean age for the entire population was 60 ± 11 years and mean LVEF was 0.30 ± 0.16. The mean LVEF and the proportion of patients with CAD were similar in both groups (i.e., tolerated and nontolerated arrhythmia) (C. Gottlieb, pers. comm.). During a 22-month follow-up period, cardiac arrest occurred more frequently in patients presenting with a nontolerated rather than tolerated arrhythmia (34% vs. 10%, respectively, if the arrhythmia remained inducible and nontolerated on amiodarone, compared to 17% vs. 2%, respectively, if the arrhythmia was either noninducible or inducible but tolerated on amiodarone).[9]

Saxon et al retrospectively analyzed clinical characteristics and outcomes according to presenting symptoms in three subgroups of 121 patients with documented spontaneous or induced sustained VT or VF.[12] Antiarrhythmic medications (no details provided) were discontinued for ≥ 48 hours prior to electrophysiological study. Forty-eight (40%) patients, 75% of whom had CAD, presented with palpitations only. Their mean induced VT rate was significantly slower (188 beats/min [range, 145–267]) than that of patients presenting with syncope or cardiac arrest (204 beats/min [range, 166–264] and 251 beats/min [range, 198–343], respectively). Sustained polymorphic VT was induced significantly more frequently in patients with cardiac arrest than in those with palpitations (28% vs. 12.5%, respectively), although there was no significant difference in arrhythmia inducibility between the palpitation and syncope groups. LVEF was significantly lower in patients presenting with cardiac arrest or syncope than in those with palpitations (0.31 ± 0.14 and 0.30 ± 0.11 vs. 0.39 ± 0.15, respectively). Treatment, which varied both within and among subgroups, consisted of antiarrhythmic medication, antitachycardia surgery, or ICD. A significantly better sudden death-free survival rate was observed in the palpitation group: $91 \pm 5\%$ and $87 \pm 6\%$ at 2 and 4 years, respectively, vs. $72 \pm 8\%$ and $59 \pm 11\%$ in the cardiac arrest group.[12] However, since a multivariate analysis was not performed, it cannot be determined whether these differences in survival were independent of the significant differences in LVEF and in treatment among these groups.

In another study, Fogoros et al analyzed arrhythmia outcomes in an amiodarone-treated group of 28 patients (with CAD in 82%) who presented with only lightheadedness or dizziness during sustained monomorphic VT.[7] Following treatment, their actuarial sudden death risk was significantly lower than that of a similar cohort of patients who differed only in that their VT presentation was with syncope. Moreover, there was only one sudden death among the 13 first recurrences, compared to seven of nine fatal initial recurrences in the syncope group, despite a similar actuarial risk for recurrent ventricular tachyarrhythmias for up to 24 months of follow-up. Sudden death mortality was 5% at 2 years for patients presenting with well-tolerated VT.[7]

In contrast to these studies, Wilensky et al reported in preliminary form that mode of presentation (i.e., syncope, VT, or sudden death) in patients with inducible sustained monomorphic VT did not predict the likelihood of lethal or nonlethal recurrences in

80 of 97 such patients for whom follow-up data were available.[25] Interpretation of these data is limited, however, as the authors did not state whether multivariate analysis was performed.

In summary, actuarial data from most studies suggest that among patients with CAD who present with spontaneous hemodynamically tolerated sustained VT and who are treated primarily medically, the following ranges (upper limits) for sudden death mortality are observed: 0–10% at 1 year and 8–18% at 4 years, with the highest mortality rates largely confined to patients with nonsuppressed arrhythmia and/or poor LV function.[7,13,26] These figures contrast with average recurrent cardiac arrest rates of 13% and 25% at 1 and 4 years, respectively, in CAD patients receiving electrophysiologically guided therapy following an episode of aborted sudden death. The recurrence rates are even higher for such patients in the setting of LVEF < 0.30 or nonsuppression of inducible VT.[50]

CAD Patients with Inducible Sustained VT Rendered Hemodynamically Tolerated by Antiarrhythmic Therapy

In contrast to the foregoing studies, others have examined outcomes in relation to symptom status during induced sustained VT following electrophysiologically guided antiarrhythmic treatment in patients who presented with a variety of sustained ventricular tachyarrhythmias (Table 34-4). Although results of such studies cannot be directly extrapolated to spontaneous sustained VT, they are relevant to the notion that hemodynamic stabilization (by pharmacological means) of an inducible sustained VT may help to protect the patient from sudden death by rendering recurrences well tolerated. Indeed, the great majority of such patients survive their recurrences.[8,27–29]

Horowitz et al performed electrophysiological studies on 100 patients who had symptomatic sustained ventricular tachyarrhythmias complicating CAD.[27] Among the 80 patients in whom VT was inducible after amiodarone loading, cardiovascular collapse occurred in 30%, and half of these patients subsequently died suddenly. In stark contrast, there were no sudden deaths among 56 patients in whom slower induced VT did not produce severe symptoms. Others have also observed relatively low sudden death rates among patients with drug-slowed, tolerated VT.[8,29]

However, the beneficial result of hemodynamic tolerance of inducible sustained VT following antiarrhythmic therapy is not always correlated with drug-induced slowing of VT. Thus, Waller et al[28] observed that patients who were only mildly symptomatic during VT had a significantly lower nonactuarial sudden death mortality (25% over the follow-up period) than those who experienced severe symptoms despite greater VT slowing (39%).[28] Another study by the same group reported a discordance in some patients between symptom severity and the rate of induced VT following drug therapy.[38]

Thus, patients with inducible sustained VT rendered hemodynamically tolerated by antiarrhythmic drugs are at low to moderate risk for SCD. Slower VT rates following drug therapy are generally but not invariably associated with better outcomes.

Pathophysiological Differences Between Patients with CAD Presenting with Hemodynamically Tolerated Sustained VT and Those Presenting with Cardiac Arrest

There appears to be a pathophysiological basis for suggesting that hemodynamically well-tolerated VT may have a less ominous prognosis than non-infarction-related cardiac arrest, which commonly results from rapid—ostensibly poorly tolerated—sustained monomorphic VT that culminates in VF.[52] Extent of coronary arterial stenoses was found to be similar in most[51,53–55] but not all[56] studies of patients with sustained VT compared to those with cardiac arrest, although the former patients had experienced a prior MI more often,[51,53] generally with more extensive scarring.[56] The extent of electrophysiological abnormalities in patients with tolerated sustained monomorphic VT are more severe than in cardiac arrest survivors, as assessed by endocardial catheter mapping,[53,57] intraoperative epicardial mapping,[54] electrophysiological studies,[51,56,58] and signal-averaged ECG.[54,56,59] Sustained monomorphic VT is

Table 34-4
Summary of Outcomes in Patients with Inducible Hemodynamically Tolerated Sustained VT as a Result of Electrophysiologically Guided Antiarrhythmic Therapy for Sustained VT or VF in the setting of Coronary Artery Disease*

Study	No. of Pts.	Pts. with CAD No.	Pts. with CAD (%)	Pts. with HT-Sust. VT No.	Pts. with HT-Sust. VT (%)	Antiarrhythmic Treatment	Mean LVEF† (%)	Actuarial Analysis Provided for Pts. with HT-Sust. VT	Mean F/U (mo)†	Outcome in Pts. with HT-Sust. VT
Horowitz et al[27]	100	100	(100)	56	(56)	Yes	25	No	12‡	HT-Sust. VT recurrence: 26/56 pts. (46%) over F/U period Total mortality: 0% over F/U period
Kadish et al[8]	121	102	(84)	57	(47)	Yes	35 ± 17	Yes	27	SD mortality: 5% at 1 yr
Waller et al[28]	258	210	(81)	143§	(55)	Yes	29	No	24	SD mortality: 36/143 pts. (25%) over F/U period VT or VF recurrence: 70/143 pts. (50%) over F/U period Total mortality: 44/143 (31%) over F/U period
				51∥ ("stable" subset)				Yes	~20	SD mortality: 4% at both 1 and 2 yr VT recurrence: 32% at 1 yr 39% at 2 yr Total mortality: 6% at 1 yr 18% at 2 yr
Krafchek et al[29]	45	45	(100)	12	(27)	Yes	25 ± 11	No	17 ± 13	SD mortality: 0% over F/U period HT-Sust. VT recurrences: 10/12 pts. (83%) over F/U period

Abbreviations as in Table 34-3.
* Predominantly, but not exclusively, patients with CAD (see text for discussion). The proportion of patients presenting with spontaneous hemodynamically tolerated sustained VT varies among series.
† For all patients.
‡ For their group 2 patients (i.e., VT still inducible on amiodarone).
§ Combination of VT patients with mild symptoms ($n = 97$) and those with VT cycle length increase < 100 msec and mild symptoms ($n = 46$).
∥ Their group 2 patients only (i.e., ≥100 msec antiarrhythmic drug-induced increase in sustained VT cycle length, and absence of severe symptoms).

induced more frequently (94%) in patients who present with that arrhythmia[48,53] than in cardiac arrest survivors (only 73%),[53,60] in whom polymorphic VT is more commonly induced.[53,55,56,58,59] Moreover, when sustained VT is induced, the rate tends to be slower in those presenting with sustained VT than in those who have had a cardiac arrest.[51,53,56]

Thus, CAD patients with sustained VT tend to have more extensive scarring with larger anatomical/functional obstacles that are more likely to support stable re-entrant circuits (with better tolerated VT) than patients who have survived a cardiac arrest.

HEMODYNAMICALLY TOLERATED SUSTAINED VT IN PATIENTS WITHOUT CAD

There are few accurate data regarding hemodynamically tolerated sustained VT in the absence of CAD, probably in part because of the methodological problems discussed earlier. In addition, knowledge from the literature regarding SCD in such patients is significantly limited by any or all of the following factors: (1) imprecise or poor characterization of VT—for example, use of the modified Lown classification,[61] which does not distinguish between sustained and nonsustained forms; (2) "lumping" of diverse types of ventricular tachyarrhythmia; and (3) imprecision in relating sudden death outcome data to patients with specific arrhythmias, e.g., sustained VT. In spite of these limitations, it can be roughly estimated that hemodynamically tolerated sustained VT may occur in approximately 25% (range, 13–40%) of all non-CAD patients presenting with sustained VT.[12,62]

Sustained monomorphic VT unassociated with CAD may be observed in two main contexts: (1) underlying cardiac disease presumed to be etiologic for VT (e.g., dilated cardiomyopathy, right ventricular dysplasia, hypertrophic cardiomyopathy, and postoperative congenital heart disease), found in about 70% (range, 26–82%) of non-CAD patients with sustained VT,[26,62–65] and (2) no overt structural cardiac abnormality, in which setting VT is termed "idiopathic" or "primary," although attempts have been made to identify subtypes (e.g., catecholamine-sensitive VT).

Hemodynamically Tolerated Sustained VT in the Setting of Overt Cardiomyopathy

Idiopathic Dilated Cardiomyopathy

Sudden death is a significant clinical problem in patients with idiopathic dilated cardiomyopathy.[65–76] A very crude sudden death rate of 16% was observed during follow-up periods of 2 months to 10 years among a total of 278 patients, a variable proportion of whom had spontaneous VT, frequently nonsustained.[63,65–70,72,75]

Idiopathic dilated cardiomyopathy is the underlying cardiac abnormality in 3–15% (mean, 9%) of all patients presenting with sustained VT.[63,65,67] Whereas nonsustained VT has been detected in 42–60% (mean, 49%) of patients with idiopathic dilated cardiomyopathy undergoing routine 24-hour ambulatory ECG,[66,68,69] sustained VT was noted in 6% of such patients in one study.[77] Unfortunately, the above-mentioned methodological limitations in the literature do not allow a meaningful estimate of SCD rates in patients with idiopathic dilated cardiomyopathy and spontaneous hemodynamically tolerated sustained VT. Suppression of inducible sustained VT by electrophysiologically guided drug therapy may be protective[73] but does not necessarily prevent sudden death.[67]

Hypertrophic Cardiomyopathy

SCD is a known complication of hypertrophic cardiomyopathy.[78] In pooled data from several studies, roughly 7% of 322 affected individuals (many treated surgically or medically) died suddenly during a 1-week to 7-year follow-up period.[79–83] Although children and young adults ages 10–35 years are the most common victims of SCD,[78,79,84–89] older patients are not entirely spared.[89]

VT, predominantly nonsustained or noncharacterized, has been observed in 5–57% (mean, 28%) of patients with hypertrophic cardiomyopathy who have undergone ambulatory ECG (Holter) monitoring.[79–83,90–96] Earlier studies suggested that demonstration of (primarily nonsustained) VT on prolonged Holter monitoring predicted a significantly higher 3-year sudden death mortality than that in patients without VT (25% vs. 5%, respectively).[79,80] However, there is still no well-established causal relation between VT and sudden death in patients with hypertrophic cardiomyopathy, as attested to by the weak relation between nonsustained VT and sudden death in young patients, who should be at greater risk.[82] Regrettably, there are also no systematic data regarding hemodynamically sustained monomorphic VT in patients with hypertrophic cardiomyopathy.

Arrhythmogenic Right Ventricular Dysplasia

Arrhythmogenic right ventricular dysplasia is the term used to describe a rare form of predominantly right ventricular cardiomyopathy of unknown etiology whose principal manifestation is VT, usually exhibiting left-bundle-branch block morphology.[97-99] The typical patient is a young or middle-aged man[97] whose symptoms during VT typically range from palpitations to syncope, but may include cardiac arrest.[97-99]

A crude SCD rate of 2% was observed during a 1- to 28-year follow-up period among a total of 164 patients with arrhythmogenic right ventricular dysplasia, a variable proportion of whom had sustained and/or nonsustained VT, many of them treated, as reported in eight studies.[63-65,98,99-102] Data for patients presenting specifically with hemodynamically tolerated sustained VT are very limited; there were no SCDs during a 2.5—22-year follow-up period among a total of only nine such reported patients, aged 1–67 years, whose VT rates ranged from 120 to 260 beats/min.[98,99,101]

Postoperative Congenital Heart Disease

Little specific information is available from the literature regarding hemodynamically tolerated sustained VT following surgical treatment of congenital heart disease. Sudden cardiac death is a well-known late complication in patients following repair of tetralogy of Fallot.[103-108] Although sustained VT has also been described as a sequel to this surgery,[109-111] neither the prevalence of hemodynamically tolerated sustained VT nor its possible relation to sudden death (if any) is well defined.[107]

Hemodynamically Tolerated Sustained VT in the Absence of Overt Heart Disease

Gross evidence of structural heart disease is lacking in about 12% (range, 6–24%) of all patients—and in 25% (range, 14–74%) of non-CAD patients—presenting with sustained VT.[62-65] The VT in this setting, therefore, has been termed "idiopathic." However, occult pathological and/or hemodynamic abnormalities have frequently been detected in such patients,[112,113] thus raising doubts about the legitimacy of the designation "idiopathic" in many instances.

There were no SCDs among a total of 129 mostly medically treated patients with idiopathic VT (rates of 130–260 beats/min) during follow-up periods ranging from 2 months to 5 years as reported in seven different studies.[63-65,114-117] These reports included 18 patients with known hemodynamically tolerated sustained VT. Most patients were young and the VT resolved spontaneously in a few. However, the prognosis may be less favorable in some cases.[118] The lack of symptom description during VT and the presenting occult cardiac abnormalities in some patients are limitations in some of these reports.

Although no uniform subcategorization of patients with idiopathic VT has emerged, VT morphology, site of VT origin, catecholamine sensitivity, and response to pharmacological agents have been used to categorize these patients.

Repetitive monomorphic VT characteristically exhibits a left bundle-branch block and inferior axis morphology. Endocardial mapping typically has shown the earliest ventricular activation during tachycardia to occur at the right ventricular outflow tract on the interventricular septum.[119,120] This arrhythmia occurs predominantly in younger patients free of obvious structural heart disease, and may be provoked by exercise or catecholamines. No SCDs occurred among 70 patients with repetitive monomorphic VT during a follow-up period of 3–90 months in three studies.[119-121] The VT was known to be hemodynamically tolerated in eight of 78 patients reported in three studies.[119,121,122] No sudden deaths occurred during a 3–72-month follow-up period in five of these patients for whom data were provided.[119,121]

Right bundle-branch block morphology with left axis deviation characterizes another morphologically distinct type of idiopathic sustained VT that characteristically maps to the left ventricle and is generally responsive to verapamil.[123–127] This VT was known to be hemodynamically tolerated in a total of 24 of 33 patients in five reports,[123–127] with no SCDs occurring in eight patients for whom short- and longer-term data were provided.[123,124]

Catecholamine-sensitive VT, which may be due to cAMP-mediated triggered activity,[128] has been observed in subjects both with and without apparent heart disease.[129–131] Among a total of 37 patients with catecholamine-sensitive VT (30% with no structural heart disease), 25 (68%) were sustained.[128–131] During a 15-month follow-up period, there were no SCDs among eight patients with sustained VT that was definitely (four patients)[129–131] or probably (four patients)[128] hemodynamically tolerated.

SUMMARY

Clinical manifestations of sustained VT can range from absence of symptoms to cardiac arrest. Hemodynamically tolerated sustained VT accounts for approximately 50% of cases of sustained VT referred for electrophysiological evaluation. Although slower VTs tend to be better tolerated, rate is but one of many determinants of the hemodynamic expression of sustained VT. Independent of suggestive ECG features (see Table 34–2), sustained VT should be considered the most likely diagnosis in an adult patient presenting with hemodynamically tolerated regular wide QRS tachycardia, especially in the setting of prior infarction or other structural heart disease.

Among patients with CAD, hemodynamically tolerated sustained monomorphic VT is typically seen in middle-aged men with prior MI, frequently in the setting of chronic antiarrhythmic drug administration. Outcome data specifically pertaining to patients with hemodynamically tolerated sustained VT in CAD are limited. Nevertheless, most available information supports the notion that CAD patients with spontaneous hemodynamically tolerated sustained VT face a relatively lower short- and long-term sudden death mortality (Table 24–3) than patients presenting with cardiac arrest. When sustained monomorphic VT is not associated with cardiac arrest, it remains to be seen whether lesser grades of symptom severity (e.g., Classes I–III in Table 34–1) correlate with prognosis.[132]

Sustained monomorphic VT unassociated with CAD may occur in the context of other underlying cardiac diseases (e.g., cardiomyopathy arrhythmogenic right ventricular dysplasia, postoperative congenital heart disease, etc.) or in the absence of overt structural heart disease (i.e., "idiopathic" variety). The latter has also been categorized on the basis of morphology, site of origin, and response to catecholamines and/or pharmacological agents. Despite a known incidence of sudden death in most cardiomyopathies (idiopathic dilated and hypertrophic) and following surgical repair of tetralogy of Fallot, information regarding outcomes of patients with hemodynamically tolerated sustained VT in the setting of these conditions is extremely limited. Hemodynamically tolerated sustained VT appears to carry a good prognosis in patients with arrhythmogenic right ventricular dysplasia. The incidence of sudden death is generally extremely low in patients with hemodynamically tolerated sustained VT in the absence of structural heart disease.

Our understanding of the topic reviewed in this chapter is currently limited by widespread inconsistencies in data reporting and analysis. Prospective studies using precise and standardized nomenclature to characterize arrhythmias and symptoms are needed to better define clinical and electrophysiological characteristics and actuarial outcomes in CAD and non-CAD patients with hemodynamically tolerated sustained VT.

REFERENCES

1. Nikolic G, Bishop RL, Singh JB: Sudden death recorded during Holter monitoring. Circulation 66:218–225, 1982.
2. Pratt CM, Francis MJ, Luck JC, Wyndham

CR, Miller RR, Quinones MA: Analysis of ambulatory electrocardiograms in 15 patients during spontaneous ventricular fibrillation with special reference to preceding arrhythmic events. J Am Coll Cardiol 2: 789–797, 1983.
3. Panidis IP, Morganroth J: Sudden death in hospitalized patients: Cardiac rhythm disturbances detected by ambulatory electrocardiographic monitoring. J Am Coll Cardiol 2:798–805, 1983.
4. Kempf FC, Josephson ME: Cardiac arrest recorded on ambulatory electrocardiograms. Am J Cardiol 53:1577–1582, 1984.
5. Milner PG, Platia EV, Reid PR, Griffith LS: Ambulatory electrocardiographic recordings at the time of fatal cardiac arrest. Am J Cardiol 56:588–592, 1985.
6. Olshausen KV, Witt T, Pop T, Treese N, Bethge KP, Meyer J: Sudden cardiac death while wearing a Holter monitor. Am J Cardiol 67:381–386, 1991.
7. Fogoros RN, Fiedler SB, Elson JJ: The automatic implantable cardioverter-defibrillator in drug-refractory ventricular tachyarrhythmias. Ann Intern Med 107:635–641, 1987.
8. Kadish AH, Buxton AE, Waxman HL, Flores B, Josephson ME, Marchlinski FE: Usefulness of electrophysiologic study to determine the clinical tolerance of arrhythmia recurrences during amiodarone therapy. J Am Coll Cardiol 10:90–96, 1987.
9. Gottlieb CD, Berger MD, Miller JM, et al: What is an acceptable risk for cardiac arrest patients treated with amiodarone? [abstract]. Circulation 78:II-500, 1988.
10. Herre JM, Sauve MJ, Malone P, et al: Long term results of amiodarone therapy in patients with recurrent sustained ventricular tachycardia or ventricular fibrillation. J Am Coll Cardiol 13:442–449, 1989.
11. Brugada P, Talajic M, Smeets J, Mulleneers R, Wellens HJJ: The value of the clinical history to assess prognosis of patients with ventricular tachycardia or ventricular fibrillation after myocardial infarction. Eur Heart J 10:747–752, 1989.
12. Saxon LA, Uretz EF, Denes P: Significance of the clinical presentation in ventricular tachycardia/fibrillation. Am Heart J 118:695–701, 1989.
13. Steinman RT, Lehmann MH, Zheutlin T, et al: Long-term outcome of electrophysiologically-guided therapy for hemodynamically-tolerated sustained ventricular tachycardia in coronary artery disease [abstract]. J Am Coll Cardiol 15:123A, 1990.
14. Lehmann MH, Steinman RT, Meissner MD, Schuger CD, Mosteller RD, Nabih MA: Need for a standardized approach to grading symptoms associated with ventricular tachyarrhythmias. Am J Cardiol 67: 1421–1423, 1991.
15. Rosenheck S, Sousa J, Calkins H, et al: Comparison of the results of electrophysiologic testing after short-term and long-term treatment with amiodarone in patients with ventricular tachycardia. Am Heart J 121: 1693–1698, 1991.
16. Marchlinski FE, Buxton AE, Miller MJ, Vassallo JA, Flores BT, Josephson ME: Amiodarone versus amiodarone and a type IA agent for treatment of patients with rapid ventricular tachycardia. Circulation 74:1037–1043, 1986.
17. Morady F, Baerman JM, DiCarlo LA Jr, DeBuitleir M, Krol RB, Wahr DW: A prevalent misconception regarding wide-complex tachycardias. JAMA 254:2790–2792, 1985.
18. Dancy M, Camm AJ, Ward D: Misdiagnosis of chronic recurrent ventricular tachycardia. Lancet ii:320–323, 1985.
19. Morady F, Shen EN, Bhandari A, Schwartz AB, Scheinman MM: Clinical symptoms in patients with sustained ventricular tachycardia. West J Med 142: 341–344, 1985.
20. Stewart RB, Bardy GH, Greene HL: Wide complex tachycardia: Misdiagnosis and outcome after emergent therapy. Ann Intern Med 104:766–771, 1986.
21. Buxton AE, Marchlinski FE, Doherty JU, Flores B, Josephson ME: Hazards of intravenous verapamil for sustained ventricular tachycardia. Am J Cardiol 59:1107–1110, 1987.
22. Tchou P, Young P, Mahmud R, Denker S, Jazayeri M, Akhtar M: Useful clinical criteria for the diagnosis of ventricular tachycardia. Am J Med 84:53–56, 1988.
23. Akhtar M, Shenasa M, Jazayeri M, Caceres J, Tchou PJ: Wide QRS complex tachycardia: Reappraisal of a common clinical problem. Ann Intern Med 109:905–912, 1988.
24. Steinman RT, Herrera C, Schuger CD, Lehmann MH: Wide QRS tachycardia in the conscious adult. JAMA 261: 1013–1016, 1989.
25. Wilensky RL, Klein LS, Miles WM, Fineberg N, Zipes DP: Presenting symptoms do not predict long-term outcome in patients with sustained ventricular tachycardia [abstract]. PACE 13:562, 1990.
26. Leclercq JF, Leenhardt A, Ruta I, et al: Esperance de vie apres une premiere crise de tachycardie ventriculaire monomorphe soutenue. Arch Mal Coeur 84:1789–1796, 1991.

27. Horowitz LN, Greenspan AM, Spielman SR, et al: Usefulness of electrophysiologic testing in evaluation of amiodarone therapy for sustained ventricular tachyarrhythmias associated with coronary heart disease. Am J Cardiol 55:367–371, 1985.
28. Waller TJ, Kay HR, Spielman SR, Kutalek SP, Greenspan AM, Horowitz LN: Reduction in sudden death and total mortality by antiarrhythmic therapy evaluated by electrophysiologic drug testing: Criteria of efficacy in patients with sustained ventricular tachyarrhythmia. J Am Coll Cardiol 10:83–89, 1987.
29. Krafchek J, Lin HT, Beckman KJ, et al: Cumulative effects of amiodarone on inducibility of ventricular tachycardia: Implications for electrophysiological testing. PACE 11:434–444, 1988.
30. Buxton AE, Waxman HL, Marchlinski FE, Untereker WJ, Waspe LE, Josephson ME: Role of triple extrastimuli during electrophysiologic study of patients with documented sustained ventricular tachyarrhythmias. Circulation 69:532–540, 1984.
31. Miller JM, Marchlinski FE, Buxton AE, Josephson ME: Relationship between the 12-lead electrocardiogram during ventricular tachycardia and endocardial site of origin in patients with coronary artery disease. Circulation 77:759–766, 1988.
32. Lima JAC, Weiss JL, Guzman PA, Weisfeldt ML, Reid PR, Traill TA: Incomplete filling and incoordinate contraction as mechanisms of hypotension during ventricular tachycardia in man. Circulation 68:928–938, 1983.
33. Hamer AWF, Rubin SA, Peter T, Mandel WJ: Factors that predict syncope during ventricular tachycardia in patients. Am Heart J 107:997–1005, 1984.
34. Saksena S, Ciccone JM, Craelius W, Pantopoulos D, Rothbart ST, Werres R: Studies on left ventricular function during sustained ventricular tachycardia. J Am Coll Cardiol 4:501–508, 1984.
35. Hamer AW, Zaher CA, Rubin SA, Peter T, Mandel WJ: Hemodynamic benefits of synchronized 1:1 atrial pacing during sustained ventricular tachycardia with severely depressed ventricular function in coronary heart disease. Am J Cardiol 55:990–994, 1985.
36. Raichlen JS, Links JM, Reid PR: Effect of electrical activation site on left ventricular performance in ventricular tachycardia patients with coronary heart disease. Am J Cardiol 55:84–88, 1985.
37. Callans DJ, Marchlinski FE, Josephson ME: Heart rate criteria alone may fail to distinguish well and poorly tolerated ventricular tachycardia [abstract]. PACE 14:(Pt II):709, 1991.
38. Rae AP, Kay HR, Horowitz LN, Spielman SR, Greenspan AM: Proarrhythmic effects of antiarrhythmic drugs in patients with malignant ventricular arrhythmias evaluated by electrophysiologic testing. J Am Coll Cardiol 12:131–139, 1988.
39. Koch-Weser J, Blinks JR: The influence of the interval between beats on myocardial contractility. Pharmacol Rev 15:601, 1963.
40. Pidgeon J, Lab M, Seed A, Elzinga G, Papadoyannis D, Noble MIM: The contractile state of cat and dog heart in relation to the interval between beats. Circ Res 47:559, 1980.
41. Gibson DG, Prewitt TA, Brown DJ: Analysis of left ventricular wall movement during isovolumic relaxation and its relation to coronary artery disease. Br Heart J 38:1010, 1976.
42. Gibson DG, Traill TA, Brown DJ: Changes in left ventricular free wall thickness in patients with ischemic heart disease. Br Heart J 39:1312, 1977.
43. Traill TA, Gibson DG: Left ventricular relaxation and filling: Study by echocardiography. Prog Cardiol 8:39, 1979.
44. Hunt D, Burdeslaw JA, Baxley WA: Left ventricular volumes during ventricular tachycardia, first post-tachycardia beat, and subsequent beats in normal rhythm. Br Heart J 36:148, 1974.
45. Dongas J, Lehmann MH, Mahmud R, Denker S, Soni J, Akhtar M: Value of preexisting bundle branch block in the electrocardiographic differentiation of supraventricular from ventricular origin of wide QRS tachycardia. Am J Cardiol 55:717–721, 1985.
46. Brugada P, Brugada J, Mont L, Smeets J, Andries EW: A new approach to the differential diagnosis of a regular tachycardia with a wide QRS complex. Circulation 83:1649–1659, 1991.
47. Hayes JJ, Stewart RB, Greene HL, Bardy GH: Narrow QRS ventricular tachycardia. Ann Intern Med 114:460–463, 1991.
48. Berger MD, Waxman HL, Buxton AE, Marchlinski FE, Josephson ME: Spontaneous compared with induced onset of sustained ventricular tachycardia. Circulation 78:885–892, 1988.
49. Rosenbaum MS, Wilber DJ, Finkelstein D, Ruskin JN, Garan H: Immediate reproducibility of electrically induced sustained monomorphic ventricular tachycardia before and during antiarrhythmic therapy. J Am Coll Cardiol 17:133–138, 1991.

50. Furukawa T, Rozauski JJ, Nogami A, Moroe K, Gosselin AJ, Lister JW: Time dependent risk of and predictors for cardiac arrest recurrence in survivors of out-of-hospital cardiac arrest with chronic coronary artery disease. Circulation 80: 599–608, 1989.
51. Adhar GC, Larson LW, Bardy GH, Greene HL: Sustained ventricular arrhythmias: Differences between survivors of cardiac arrest and patients with recurrent sustained ventricular tachycardia. J Am Coll Cardiol 12:159–165, 1988.
52. Meissner MD, Akhtar M, Lehmann MH: Nonischemic sudden tachyarrhythmic death in atherosclerotic heart disease. Circulation 84:905–912, 1991.
53. Vaitkus PT, Kindwall E, Marchlinski FE, Miller JM, Buxton AE, Josephson ME: Differences in electrophysiological substrate in patients with coronary artery disease and cardiac arrest or ventricular tachycardia: Insights from endocardial mapping and signal-averaged electrocardiography. Circulation 84:672–678, 1991.
54. Denniss AR, Ross DL, Richards DA, et al: Difference between patients with ventricular tachycardia and ventricular fibrillation as assessed by signal-averaged electrocardiogram, radionuclide ventriculography and cardiac mapping. J Am Coll Cardiol 11:276–283, 1988.
55. Dolack GL, Callahan DB, Bardy GH, Greene HL: Signal-averaged electrocardiographic late potentials in resuscitated survivors of out-of-hospital ventricular fibrillation. Am J Cardiol 65:1102–1104, 1990.
56. Stevenson WG, Brugada P, Waldecker B, Zehender M, Wellens HJJ: Clinical, angiographic, and electrophysiologic findings in patients with aborted sudden death as compared with patients with sustained ventricular tachycardia after myocardial infarction. Circulation 71:1146–1152, 1985.
57. Cassidy DM, Vassallo JM, Miller JM, et al: Endocardial catheter mapping in patients in sinus rhythm: Relationship to underlying heart disease and ventricular arrhythmias. Circulation 73:645–652, 1986.
58. Schoenfeld MH, McGovern B, Garan H, Kelly E, Grant G, Ruskin JN: Determinants of the outcome of electrophysiologic study in patients with ventricular tachyarrhythmias. J Am Coll Cardiol 6:298–306, 1985.
59. Freedman RA, Gillis AM, Keren A, Soderholm-Difatte V, Mason JW: Signal-averaged electrocardiographic late potentials in patients with ventricular fibrillation or ventricular tachycardia: Correlation with clinical arrhythmia and electrophysiologic study. Am J Cardiol 55:1350–1353, 1985.
60. Akhtar M, Garan H, Lehmann MH, Troup PJ: Sudden cardiac death: Management of high-risk patients. Ann Intern Med 114:499–512, 1991.
61. Ryan M, Lown B, Horn H: Comparison of ventricular ectopic activity during 24-hour monitoring and exercise testing in patients with coronary heart disease. N Engl J Med 292:224–229, 1975.
62. Naccarelli GV, Prystowsky EN, Jackman WM, Heger JJ, Rahilly GT, Zipes DP: Role of electrophysiologic testing in managing patients who have ventricular tachycardia unrelated to coronary artery disease. Am J Cardiol 50:165–171, 1982.
63. Reiter MJ, Smith WM, Gallagher JJ: Clinical spectrum of ventricular tachycardia with left bundle branch morphology. Am J Cardiol 51:113–121, 1983.
64. Trappe HJ, Brugada P, Talajic M, et al: Prognosis of patients with ventricular tachycardia and ventricular fibrillation: Role of the underlying etiology. J Am Coll Cardiol 12:166–174, 1988.
65. Leclercq JF, Coumel P, Denjoy I, et al: Long-term follow-up after sustained monomorphic ventricular tachycardia: Causes, pump failure, and empiric antiarrhythmic therapy that modify survival. Am Heart J 121:1685–1692, 1991.
66. Huang SK, Messer JV, Denes P: Significance of ventricular tachycardia in idiopathic dilated cardiomyopathy: Observations in 35 patients. Am J Cardiol 51:507–512, 1983.
67. Poll DS, Marchlinski FE, Buxton AE, Doherty JU, Waxman HL, Josephson ME: Sustained ventricular tachycardia in patients with idiopathic dilated cardiomyopathy: Electrophysiologic testing and lack of response to antiarrhythmic drug therapy. Circulation 70:451–456, 1984.
68. Meinertz T, Hofmann T, Kasper Q, et al: Significance of ventricular arrhythmias in idiopathic dilated cardiomyopathy. Am J Cardiol 53:902–907, 1984.
69. von Olshausen K, Schafer A, Mehmel HC, Schwarz F, Senges J, Kubler W: Ventricular arrhythmias in idiopathic dilated cardiomyopathy. Br Heart J 51:195–201, 1984.
70. Das SK, Morady F, DiCarlo L Jr, et al: Prognostic usefulness of programmed ventricular stimulation in idiopathic dilated cardiomyopathy without symptomatic ventricular arrhythmias. Am J Cardiol 58:998–1000, 1986.
71. Nikutta P, Daniel W, Bossaller C, Hausmann D: Sudden and non-sudden death in

dilated cardiomyopathy: Are there differences in left ventricular function impairment? [abstract]. Circulation 74(suppl II): 203A, 1986.
72. Stevenson LW, Fowler MB, Schroeder JS, Stevenson WG, Dracup KA, Fond V: Poor survival of patients with idiopathic cardiomyopathy considered too well for transplantation. Am J Med 83:871–876, 1987.
73. Liem LB, Swerdlow CD: Value of electropharmacologic testing in idiopathic dilated cardiomyopathy and sustained ventricular tachyarrhythmias. Am J Cardiol 62: 611–616, 1988.
74. Kron J, Hart M, Schual-Berke S, Niles NR, Hosenpud JD, McAnulty JH: Idiopathic dilated cardiomyopathy: Role of programmed electrical stimulation and holter monitoring in predicting those at risk of sudden death. Chest 93:85–90, 1988.
75. Milner PG, DiMarco JP, Lerman BB: Electrophysiological evaluation of sustained ventricular tachyarrhythmias in idiopathic dilated cardiomyopathy. PACE 11: 562–568, 1988.
76. Middlekauff HR, Stevenson WG, Woo MA, Moser DK, Stevenson LW: Comparison of frequency of late potentials in idiopathic dilated cardiomyopathy and ischemic cardiomyopathy with advanced congestive heart failure and their usefulness in predicting sudden death. Am J Cardiol 66:1113–1117, 1990.
77. Unverferth DV, Magorien RD, Moeschberger ML, Baker PB, Fetters JK, Leier CV: Factors influencing the one-year mortality of dilated cardiomyopathy. Am J Cardiol 54:147–152, 1984.
78. Maron BJ, Roberts WC, Epstein SE: Sudden death in hypertrophic cardiomyopathy: A profile of 78 patients. Circulation 65: 1388–1394, 1982.
79. McKenna WJ, England D, Doi YL, Deanfield JE, Oakley C, Goodwin JF: Arrhythmia in hypertrophic cardiomyopathy: I. Influence on prognosis. Br Heart J 46: 168–172, 1981.
80. Maron BJ, Savage DD, Wolfson JK, Epstein SE: Prognostic significance of 24 hour ambulatory electrocardiographic monitoring in patients with hypertrophic cardiomyopathy: A prospective study. Am J Cardiol 48:252–257, 1981.
81. Kowey PR, Eisenberg R, Engel TR: Sustained arrhythmias in hypertrophic obstructive cardiomyopathy. N Engl J Med 310:1566–1569, 1984.
82. McKenna WJ, Franklin RCG, Nihoyannopoulos P, et al: Arrhythmia and prognosis in infants, children and adolescents with hypertrophic cardiomyopathy. J Am Coll Cardiol 11:147–153, 1988.
83. Lazzeroni E, Domenicucci S, Finardi A, et al: Severity of arrhythmias and extent of hypertrophy in hypertrophic cardiomyopathy. Am Heart J 118;734–738, 1989.
84. Swan DA, Bell B, Oakley CM, Goodwin JF: Analysis of symptomatic course and prognosis and treatment of hypertrophic obstructive cardiomyopathy. Br Heart J 33: 671–685, 1971.
85. Adelman AG, Wigle ED, Ranganathan N, et al: The clinical course in muscular subaortic stenosis: A retrospective and prospective study of 60 hemodynamically proved cases. Ann Intern Med 77:515–525, 1972.
86. Shah PM, Adelman AG, Wigler ED, et al: The natural (and unnatural) history of hypertrophic cardiomyopathy. Circ Res 34/ 35(suppl II):II-179–II-195, 1973.
87. Maron BJ, Henry WL, Clark CE, Redwood DR, Roberts WC, Epstein SE: Asymmetric septal hypertrophy in childhood. Circulation 53:9–19, 1976.
88. Maron BJ, Bonow RO, Cannon RO III, Leon MB, Epstein SE: Hypertrophic cardiomyopathy: Interrelations of clinical manifestations, pathophysiology, and therapy. N Engl J Med 316:780–852, 1987.
89. Spirito P, Chiarella F, Carratino L, Zoni-Berisso M, Bellotti P, Vecchio C: Clinical course and prognosis of hypertrophic cardiomyopathy in an outpatient population. N Engl J Med 320:749–755, 1989.
90. Savage DD, Seides SF, Maron BJ, Meyers DJ, Epstein SE: Prevalence of arrhythmias during 24-hour electrocardiographic monitoring and exercise testing in patients with obstructive and nonobstructive hypertrophic cardiomyopathy. Circulation 59:866, 1979.
91. Canedo MI, Frank MJ, Abdulla AM: Rhythm disturbances in hypertrophic cardiomyopathy: Prevalence, relation to symptoms and management. Am J Cardiol 45:848, 1980.
92. Bjarnoson I, Herdarsen T, Jonsson S: Cardiac arrhythmias in hypertrophic cardiomyopathy. Br Heart J 48:198, 1982.
93. Shapiro LM, Zezvlka A: Hypertrophic cardiomyopathy: A common disease with a good prognosis. Br Heart J 50:530, 1983.
94. Frank MJ, Watkins LO, Prisant ML, Stefadourous MA, Abdulla AM: Potentially lethal arrhythmias and their management in hypertrophic cardiomyopathy. Am J Cardiol 53:1608, 1984.
95. Schiavone WA, Maloney JD, Lever HM, Castle LW, Sterba R, Morant V: Electro-

physiologic studies of patients with hypertrophic cardiomyopathy presenting with syncope of undetermined etiology. PACE 9:476–481, 1986.
96. Fananapazir L, Tracy CM, Leon MB, et al: Electrophysiologic abnormalities in patients with hypertrophic cardiomyopathy: A consecutive analysis in 55 patients. Circulation 80:1259–1268, 1989.
97. Marcus FI, Fontaine GH, Guiraudon G, et al: Right ventricular dysplasia: A report of 24 adult cases. Circulation 65:384–398, 1982.
98. Marcus FI, Fontaine GH, Frank R, Gallagher JJ, Reiter MJ: Long-term follow-up in patients with arrhythmogenic right ventricular disease. Eur Heart J 10:68–73, 1989.
99. Dungan WT, Garson A Jr, Gillette PC: Arrhythmogenic right ventricular dysplasia: A cause of ventricular tachycardia in children with apparently normal hearts. Am Heart J 102:745–750, 1981.
100. Rossi P, Massumi A, Gillette P, Hall RJ: Arrhythmogenic right ventricular dysplasia: Clinical features, diagnostic techniques, and current management. Am Heart J 103:415–420, 1982.
101. Blomstrom-Lundqvist C, Sabel KG, Olsson SB: A long term follow up of 15 patients with arrhythmogenic right ventricular dysplasia. Br Heart J 58:477–488, 1987.
102. Furlanello F, Bettini R, Bertoldi A, et al: Arrhythmia patterns in athletes with arrhythmogenic right ventricular dysplasia. Eur Heart J 10:16–19, 1989.
103. Quattlebaum TG, Varghese J, Neill CA, Donahoo JS: Sudden death among postoperative patients with tetralogy of Fallot: A follow-up study of 243 patients for an average of twelve years. Circulation 54: 289–291, 1976.
104. Gillette PC, Yeoman MA, Mullins CE, McNamara DG: Sudden death after repair of tetralogy of Fallot: Electrocardiographic and electrophysiologic abnormalities. Circulation 56:566–570, 1977.
105. Garson A Jr, Nihill MR, McNamara DG, Cooley DA: Status of the adult and adolescent after repair of tetralogy of Fallot. Circulation 59:1232–1240, 1979.
106. Kavey REW, Blackman MS, Sondheimer HM: Incidence and severity of chronic ventricular dysrhythmias after repair of tetralogy of Fallot. Am Heart J 103:342–350, 1982.
107. Garson A Jr, Randall DC, Gillette PC, et al: Prevention of sudden death after repair of tetralogy of Fallot: Treatment of ventricular arrhythmias. J Am Coll Cardiol 6: 221–227, 1985.
108. Chandar JS, Wolff GS, Garson A Jr, et al: Ventricular arrhythmias in postoperative tetralogy of Fallot. Am J Cardiol 65: 655–661, 1990.
109. Horowitz LN, Vetter VL, Harken AH, Josephson ME: Electrophysiologic characteristics of sustained ventricular tachycardia occurring after repair of tetralogy of Fallot. Am J Cardiol 46:446–452, 1980.
110. Kugler JD, Pinsky WW, Cheatham JP, Hofschire PJ, Mooring PK, Fleming WH: Sustained ventricular tachycardia after repair of tetralogy of Fallot: New electrophysiologic findings. Am J Cardiol 51: 1137–1143, 1983.
111. Deal BJ, Scagliotti D, Miller SM, Gallastegui JL, Hariman RJ, Levitsky S: Electrophysiologic drug testing in symptomatic ventricular arrhythmias after repair of tetralogy of Fallot. Am J Cardiol 59: 1380–1385, 1987.
112. Strain JE, Grose RM, Factor SM, Fisher JD: Results of endomyocardial biopsy in patients with spontaneous ventricular tachycardia but without apparent structural heart disease. Circulation 68:1171–1181, 1983.
113. Vignola PA, Aonuma K, Swaye PS, et al: Lymphocytic myocarditis presenting as unexplained ventricular arrhythmias: Diagnosis with endomyocardial biopsy and response to immunosuppression. J Am Coll Cardiol 4:812–819, 1984.
114. Hernandez A, Strauss A, Kleiger RE, Goldring D: Idiopathic paroxysmal ventricular tachycardia in infants and children. J Pediatr 86:182–188, 1975.
115. Bergdahl DM, Stevenson JG, Kawabori I, Guntheroth WG: Prognosis in primary ventricular tachycardia in the pediatric patient. Circulation 62:897–901, 1980.
116. Garson A, Gillette PC, Porter CJ, McNamara DG: Ventricular tachycardia in children with a normal heart [abstract]. Circulation 66:II-170, 1982.
117. Lemery R, Brugada P, Della Bella P, Dugernier T, van den Dool A, Wellens HJJ: Nonischemic ventricular tachycardia: Clinical course and long-term follow-up in patients without clinically overt heart disease. Circulation 79:990–999, 1989.
118. Deal BJ, Miller SM, Scagliotti D, Prechel D, Gallastegui JL, Hariman RJ: Ventricular tachycardia in a young population without overt heart disease. Circulation 73: 1111–1118, 1986.
119. Buxton AE, Waxman HL, Marchlinski FE, Simson MB, Cassidy D, Josephson ME: Right ventricular tachycardia: Clinical and electrophysiologic characteristics. Circulation 68:917–927, 1983.

120. Buxton AE, Marchlinski FE, Doherty JU, et al: Repetitive, monomorphic ventricular tachycardia: Clinical and electrophysiologic characteristics in patients with and patients without organic heart disease. Am J Cardiol 54:997–1002, 1984.
121. Rahilly GT, Prystowsky EN, Zipes DP, Naccarelli GV, Jackman WM, Heger JJ: Clinical and electrophysiologic findings in patients with repetitive monomorphic ventricular tachycardia and otherwise normal electrocardiogram. Am J Cardiol 50: 459–468, 1982.
122. Zimmermann M, Maisonblanche P, Cauchemez B, Leclercq JF, Coumel P: Determinants of the spontaneous ectopic activity in repetitive monomorphic idiopathic ventricular tachycardia. J Am Coll Cardiol 7:1219–1227, 1986.
123. Lin FC, Finley CD, Rahimtoola SH, Wu D: Idiopathic paroxysmal ventricular tachycardia with a QRS pattern of right bundle branch block and left axis deviation: A unique clinical entity with specific properties. Am J Cardiol 52:95–100, 1983.
124. German LD, Packer DL, Bardy GH, Gallagher JJ: Ventricular tachycardia induced by atrial stimulation in patients without symptomatic cardiac disease. Am J Cardiol 52:1202–1207, 1983.
125. Belhassen B, Shapira I, Pelleg A, Copperman I, Kauli N, Laniado S: Idiopathic recurrent sustained ventricular tachycardia responsive to verapamil: An ECG-electrophysiologic entity. Am Heart J 108: 1034–1037, 1984.
126. Strasberg B, Kusniec J, Lewin RF, Sclarovsky S, Arditti A, Agmon J: An unusual ventricular tachycardia responsive to verapamil. Am Heart J 111:190–192, 1986.
127. Ohe T, Shimomura K, Aihara N, et al: Idiopathic sustained left ventricular tachycardia: Clinical and electrophysiologic characteristics. Circulation 77:560–568, 1988.
128. Lerman BB, Belardinelli L, West A, Berne RM, DiMarco JP: Adenosine-sensitive ventricular tachycardia: Evidence suggesting cyclic AMP-medicated triggered activity. Circulation 74:270–280, 1986.
129. Sung RJ, Shen EN, Morady F, Scheinman MM, Hess D, Botvinick EH: Electrophysiologic mechanism of exercise-induced sustained ventricular tachycardia. Am J Cardiol 51:525–530, 1983.
130. Woelfel A, Foster JR, McAllister RG Jr, Simpson RJ Jr, Gettes LS: Efficacy of verapamil in exercise-induced ventricular tachycardia. Am J Cardiol 56:292–297, 1985.
131. Vlay SC: Catecholamine-sensitive ventricular tachycardia. Am Heart J 114:455–461, 1987.
132. Larsen G, Walance C, Griffith K, Kron J, Cutler J, McAnulty J: Is sustained ventricular tachycardia without hemodynamic impairment a less dangerous form of ventricular tachycardia? J Am Coll Cardiol 19: 282A, 1992.

35

Post Infarction High Risk of Sudden Death

J. ANTHONY GOMES
STEPHEN L. WINTERS
JOHN IP

The cause of death in patients who survive an acute myocardial infarction (MI) is likely due to a variety of factors, including reinfarction resulting in heart failure and/or a fatal ventricular tachyarrhythmia or bradyarrhythmia; cardiac rupture; and a primary ventricular tachyarrhythmia. Several out-of-hospital resuscitation studies[1-11] have demonstrated that the majority of patients who succumb to sudden cardiac death (SCD) have a rapid, sustained ventricular tachycardia (VT) that degenerates into ventricular fibrillation (VF). Often the VT that degenerates into VF is rapid with rates above 200 beats/min or of the torsade de pointes type, initiated by ventricular premature depolarizations (VPDs) that produce a short–long cycle sequence.[10,11] On the other hand, bradyarrhythmia as a cause of sudden death is seen in a minority of patients, accounting for 5–10%. The propensity for induction of sustained ventricular tachyarrhythmias in the laboratory in the majority of patients with coronary artery disease who survive an episode of out-of-hospital cardiac arrest lends further credence to the opening statement.[12] Factors that produce the ultimate fatal event remain incompletely understood but likely include the presence of a substrate characterized by slow and inhomogeneous propagation of conduction, ischemia, drugs, VPD, autonomic factors, and as yet unknown local factors.[10,11]

The institution of coronary care units, the use of intravenous and oral β-adrenergic blocking agents, and the more recent use of thrombolytic agents have resulted in a significant decline in post-MI mortality.[13-24] Whereas in 1966, the 1-year mortality of patients surviving an acute MI was 14%, today, in the era of thrombolytic therapy, the mortality is in the range of 3–5%, or a 64% reduction in mortality.[13] More than 50% of the patients, however, will die suddenly.

It is likely that mortality will continue to be high in subsets of patients who are older, have multiple infarctions, have significant left ventricular (LV) dysfunction, and have ventricular arrhythmias, as well as in those who do not undergo thrombolysis. Thus it is of clinical relevance to risk stratify patients so that preventive and therapeutic strategies can be applied to high-risk patients who sustain an acute MI. This chapter reviews the selection of and therapeutic approach to high-risk patients who have sustained an acute MI.

PATIENTS AT HIGH RISK AFTER MYOCARDIAL INFARCTION

Patients at high risk following an MI can be categorized into three groups: (1) those who develop sustained VT or VF within 48 hours post infarction, (2) those who develop sustained VT or VF more than 48 hours post infarction, and (3) those who have significant LV dysfunction, late potentials, abnormal heart rate variability, and high grades of ventricular ectopy.

Sustained VT/VF Within 48 Hours Post MI

The mortality of patients who develop sustained VT/VF within 48 hours of acute MI depends on the presence or absence of heart failure, even in the setting of anterior wall MI. In the absence of significant LV failure the 1-year mortality is low in patients with early VF. In-hospital mortality is high among patients with significant heart failure.[25] Aggressive therapy of heart failure, revascularization, and cardiac transplantation are the only possible therapeutic approaches that have the potential of altering survival in such patients.

Sustained VT/VF More Than 48 Hours Post-MI

The majority of these patients have hemodynamically significant ventricular tachyarrhythmia occurring 8 to 60 days post MI (mean, 13 ± 9 days). In a study[26] of 108 patients, of whom 32 (group I) had a sustained ventricular tachyarrhythmia 8–60 days post MI and 76 (group II) did not have an arrhythmia and served as the control group, the predictors of sustained ventricular arrhythmias were assessed utilizing univariate and multivariate analysis. The most significant variables that separated group I patients from group II in the univariate analysis (Table 35–1) included sex; a late potential-I on the signal-averaged electrocardiogram (ECG), defined as an abnormal signal-averaged QRS complex and/or an abnormal duration of low-amplitude signals of <40 μV and/or an abnormal root mean square voltage (RMS-40) in the terminal QRS complex; late potential-II, defined as an abnormal signal-averaged QRS complex and an abnormal RMS-40; ejection fraction; frequency and characteristics of VPDs; the presence of bundle-branch block; and the presence of dyskinesis. No significant between-group differences were found for age, site of MI, and the presence or absence of an aneurysm, although a higher proportion of patient (31%) had an LV aneurysm on radionuclide angiography in group I than in group II (18%). Stepwise logistic regression analysis of variables found significant in the univariate analysis revealed that late potentials-II χ^2 = 16.07, p = 0.001) and ejection fraction (χ^2 = 10.09, p = 0.001) were most significantly related to the occurrence of malignant ventricular tachyarrhythmias late after MI. The observation made in this study suggest that sustained malignant ventricular arrhythmias late post MI are the result of the formation of a substrate, likely owing to histological changes in either zones of infarction or the periinfarct area, as noted by the presence of late potentials in these patients, rather than the occurrence of acute myocardial ischemia. Furthermore, this study suggests that two noninvasive tests, the signal-averaged ECG and assessment of LV function, are very useful in selecting a high-risk subset of patients at risk for late malignant ventricular arrhythmias.

Table 35–1
Variables of Significance in the Univariate Model

Variable	χ^2	p Value
Sex	10.302	<0.001
Late potential-I	10.756	<0.005
Late potential-II	22.63	<0.0001
Ejection fraction	14.93	<0.001
VPDs < 10/hr	6.7	<0.03
VPDs > 10/hr	5.9	<0.05
Couplets	7.79	<0.02
Nonsustained VT	7.73	<0.02
Bundle-branch block	5.83	<0.01
Dyskinesis	5.92	<0.05

SOURCE: Gomes JA, et al: J Am Coll Cardiol 17: 320, 1991. Reproduced by permission.

MANAGEMENT AND SURVIVAL OF PATIENTS WITH MALIGNANT VENTRICULAR ARRHYTHMIAS LATE POST MYOCARDIAL INFARCTION

Mortality is high in patients with malignant ventricular tachyarrhythmias late post MI. The long-term survivals in these patients reported in ten different studies since the 1970s to 1990 are listed in Table 35–2. Whereas in the 1970s and 1980s the long-term survival was dismal (17–67%), there was a remarkable improvement in the late 1980s. This improvement in survival was related to an improvement in therapy.

Table 35-2
Survival of Patients With Malignant VT Late Post-MI

Study	Year	No. of Pts.	Long-Term Survival	Follow-up
Wilson and Adgey[27]*	1974	105	53%	36
Wellens et al[28]*	1982	30	17%	4
Marchlinski et al[29]†	1983	12	67%	12
Garan et al[33]‡	1984	10	70%	21
DiMarco et al[34]*	1985	24	87%	15
DiMarco et al[34]‡	1985	21	90%	18
Kleiman et al[35]†	1988	87	59%	26
Landymore et al[36]‡	1990	26	85%	43
Bourke et al[37]‡	1990	27	70%	32
Willems et al[38]*	1990	390	66%	21
Gomes et al[26]†	1990	32	91%	20

* Medical therapy.
† Medical and surgical therapy.
‡ Surgical therapy.

Patients who sustain malignant ventricular arrhythmias late after an MI should be treated aggressively with electrophysiologically guided therapy, including of antiarrhythmic drug therapy, surgery consisting of endocardial resection and coronary revascularization, and implantation of a cardioverter-defibrillator.

A poor survival was noted in the past with the use of empirical antiarrhythmic drug therapy; additionally, the surgical mortality was high in such patients. In 1974, Wilson and Adgey[27] reported a 57% rate of survival to hospital discharge and a 57% survival rate of hospital survivors for 36 months in 105 patients. In 1982, Wellens and coworkers[28] reported a dismal 17% survival over 4 months in 30 patients. Marchlinski et al[29] reported a 67% survival over 12 months, an improvement over the previous two studies, utilizing both medical therapy and surgery. However, the surgical mortality remained high. Thus Marchlinski reported a 41% operative mortality in 12 patients, Lie et al[30] reported a 50% operative mortality for aneurysmectomy or infarctectomy or both, Wald et al[31] reported a mortality of 37% in 16 patients, and Buda et al[32] reported an operative mortality of 60% in the perioperative period in patients whose MI occurred less than 6 weeks before surgery, implying that early surgery was associated with a high surgical risk. Subsequently a better survival was noted for surgery in these patients. In 1984 Garan et al[33] reported a 70% survival in ten patients followed for 21 months for surgical therapy. These patients had failed antiarrhythmic drug therapy. DiMarco et al[34] in 1985 reported an 87% survival in 26 patients who were treated with medical therapy and followed up for 15 months and a 90% survival in 21 patients treated surgically at an 18 month follow-up. They reported a 16% surgical mortality, a substantial decline from that seen in earlier studies. Kleiman and coworkers[35] reported their results in 87 patients who had sustained ventricular tachyarrhythmia occurring 3 days to 90 days post MI. The long-term survival was 59% at 26 months. In their study there was no significant difference in survival between medically treated patients (49%) and surgically treated patients (61%). A marked improvement in early postoperative survival was noted in patients treated after 1981, in comparison with those treated before 1981 (96% vs. 31%). The better surgical survival in the second half of the study was attributed to improvement in surgical techniques. Landymore et al[36] in 1990 reported results in 26 patients with drug-resistant VT who underwent endocardial resection. An 80% survival rate was noted in 32 patients. However, there was a 12% 30-day mortality and a 19% late mortality. Their study suggested that although endocardial resection is effective in preventing drug-resistant malignant sustained VT following acute MI, it is associated with a rather high perioperative mortality in patients without a well-demonstrated aneurysm and a severely depressed ejection fraction. Bourke et al[37] reported surgical results in 27 patients with drug-refractory VT occurring within 60 days after MI. They reported a 70% survival over 21 months. Additionally, they reported a 29.6% mortality within 30 days of map-guided endocardial resection. Of interest, emergency surgery was associated with a higher early mortality of 43%, in contrast to planned surgery (15%).

Willems et al[38] in 1990 reported the results of a large multicenter prospective study in 390 patients with late post-MI sustained symptomatic VT/VF. A 66% survival was noted for a 21-month follow-up period. Five variables were determined as independent prognostic factors in those patients whose VT/VF occurred less than 6 weeks after MI. These variables included age less than 70 years, Killip Class III or IV in the subacute phase of infarction, cardiac arrest during the arrhythmias, anterior MI, and multiple infarctions. They also noted that mortality varied according to risk category. Risk was determined on the basis of multivariate analysis. This analysis identified the following variables as predictors of total mortality: Q-wave infarction, cardiac arrest during the index arrhythmia, Killip Class III or IV in the subacute phase of infarction, and multiple infarctions. The observed mortality was 12% for 243 patients in the lowest risk group, 28% for 92 patients in the intermediate risk group, and 55% in 55 patients in the highest risk group. The poor long-term survival noted in this multicenter study was likely related to the following: (1) non-electrophysiologically guided therapy at most centers; (2) parallel drug testing in some centers; (3) an empirical approach to antiarrhythmic therapy in some centers; (4) surgical therapy and devices such as the implantable defibrillator were used late in the course of therapy in patients who were refractory to antiarrhythmic drug therapy; and (5) the approach to therapy was not standardized among collaborating centers.

Gomes et al[26] recently reported their observations on treatment and survival in a total of 32 patients with episodes of sustained VT/VF 8–60 days post MI. An additional 76 patients without sustained ventricular arrhythmias served as controls. Of the 32 patients, 28 had one to four episodes of VT, one patient had more than 10 episodes, two patients had more than 30 episodes, and one had incessant VT. Seven (22%) of 32 patients had an unstable course with frequent hemodynamically compromising VT recalcitrant to drug therapy and requiring repeated cardioversion. Antiarrhythmic therapy guided by invasive testing was the main modality of therapy in 14 (44%) of the 32 patients; 14 (44%) underwent surgery consisting of endocardial resection with or without focal cryoablation in 12 patients and revascularization surgery in two patients without intraoperative or perioperative mortality. Revascularization surgery was performed additionally in 10 of 12 patients who had endocardial resection. The automatic implantable cardioverter-defibrillator (AICD) was used in four patients, one of whom continued to have inducible VT postoperatively. Patients who underwent map-guided surgery and implantation of an AICD had failed a mean of three drug trials.

In 41% of patients the arrhythmias were rendered noninducible. The drugs used in these patients include a Class 1A/1B drug in five patients and a Class III agent, amiodarone or sotalol, in ten patients. Six patients (19%) were placed on β-blockers, including sotalol, which has β-blocker properties). Of 12 patients who underwent endocardial resection, the arrhythmia was noninducible postoperatively in ten (83%). Of the seven unstable patients, four underwent surgery, and all four survived. Of the remaining three patients who were treated with drugs, two died while in the hospital. Of the four patients who had an AICD implanted, three were discharged on antiarrhythmic therapy and two of the four patients have had appropriate shocks. However, the role of the AICD is difficult to determine from this study since only four patients had an AICD implanted.

During a follow-up period of 20 ± 14 months, five (15.6%) patients with sustained VT/VF had an arrhythmic event and four (9.3%) died a cardiac-related death. All of the five patients who had an arrhythmic event were on drug therapy. None of the patients who had undergone surgery had an arrhythmic event. Six of the 76 patients without late sustained VT (i.e., the control group) died. The long-term actuarial arrhythmia-free survival and total survival were not significantly different between patients with late VT versus the control group.

Our study noted a good long-term survival in patients with sustained malignant ventricular tachyarrhythmias late post MI; surprisingly, survival was not different from survival in a control group of patients with significantly better LV function. These observations on survival suggest that current aggressive management, including surgery directed at the arrhythmic substrate, revascularization surgery, and the use of Class III antiarrhythmic agents such as amiodarone and sotalol, can appreciably alter the long-term survival of these very high-risk patients, which in the past was dismal. The results of our study also indicate that the majority of these patients will not respond to antiarrhythmic drug therapy as the sole modality of therapy. Thus, when a patient presents with a sustained malignant ventricular tachyarrhythmia late post infarction, coronary angiography should be promptly performed should surgery be necessary. In some of these patients, VT is recurrent and recalcitrant to IV and oral drugs, including IV amiodarone, and the only lifesaving treatment is surgical resection of the substrate. Thus, we recommend that patients who have had more than two episodes of spontaneous sustained VT/VF on drug therapy and those who have failed three or more drug trials on the basis of inducibility should be considered for early surgery. The decision for surgery should also be based on coronary anatomy and LV geometry and function. On the other hand, the absence of a well-demarcated aneurysm or severe LV dysfunction (LVEF < 0.30) is not a contraindication to surgery at our institution. The role of the AICD in this patient population remains poorly defined. At our institution, AICDs are considered for the following patients: (1) patients who are poor candidates for surgery and who remain inducible on antiarrhythmic drug therapy; (2) patients with single-vessel coronary artery disease (i.e., the infarct artery) without an aneurysm and who remain inducible; and (3) patients who undergo blind (i.e., non-map-guided) surgery and who have posterior inferior scars. The latter two factors are predictors of surgical failure.

ASYMPTOMATIC HIGH-RISK PATIENTS

A variety of noninvasive and invasive tests have been used to risk stratify asymptomatic patients following an MI. The role of 24-hour Holter monitoring, LV dysfunction, signal-averaged ECG, heart rate variability, combined noninvasive algorithms, and programmed electrical stimulation and treatment strategies will be reviewed.

Prognostic Significance of Asymptomatic Ventricular Arrhythmias and LV Function

Over the last two decades, 24-hour Holter monitoring has been used to assess the frequency and characteristics of VPDs as well as their prognostic significance. Table 35–3 summarizes the observations of five large studies[39–43] totaling 5671 patients who were followed up for an average of 29 months. In these studies ventricular arrhythmias were categorized according to their frequency and characteristics. For the purpose of this discussion, a positive Holter recording will be defined as the presence of frequent VPDs (>10/hr), couplets, or runs of nonsustained VT, and a negative Holter recording will be defined as the absence of VPDs (or <10 VPDs/hr). The incidence of sudden cardiac death ranged from 8% to 15% (mean, 11%) in patients with a positive Holter recording, whereas it was 3–6% (mean, 4%) in patients with a negative Holter recording. It is noteworthy that total cardiac death was also twice as high in patients with ventricular arrhythmias as in those without. Despite these important observations, the use of asymptomatic VPDs on a 24-hour Holter was important inherent limitations. These include: (1) A low sensitivity and specificity (Table 35–4). (2) The ideal time for performing a 24-Holter is controversial. The frequency of VPDs peaks 6–8 weeks post-infarction;

Table 35–3
Relationship Between Ventricular Arrhythmias Recorded on a 24-Hour Holter and Sudden Cardiac Death in Survivors of Acute Myocardial Infarction

Study	No. of Pts.	Follow-up (mos)	Positive Holter Recording		Negative Holter Recording	
			No. of Pts.	SCD No. (%)	No. of Pts.	SCD No. (%)
Ruberman et al[39]	1739	42	462	68 (15)	1277	71 (6)
Moss et al[40]	940	36	216	23 (11)	724	32 (4)
Mukharji et al[41]	533	18	78	10 (13)	455	19 (4)
Bigger et al[42]	819	24	245	30 (12)	574	24 (4)
Kostis et al[43]	1640	25	665	51 (8)	975	25 (3)
Total	5671	29	1666	182 (11)	4005	171 (4)

however, most Holter studies were performed 10–21 days post infarction. Additionally, obtaining a 24-hour Holter 8 weeks post-infarction may indeed be too late since a majority of arrhythmic events occur in the first 3 months post-infarction. (3) Prognosis may be different in patients with Q-wave versus non-Q-wave infarction. (4) The relationship between ventricular arrhythmias and LV dysfunction. Although it seems now clear that the presence of asymptomatic ventricular arrhythmias is associated with an independent risk for SCD, the presence of ventricular arrhythmias is association with LV dysfunction carries the highest risk (Table 35–5). Thus, it is justifiable to risk stratification utilizing both tests, rather than one test alone.

Prognostic Significance of the Signal-Averaged ECG

In the last decade several prospective studies have assessed the prognostic significance of the signal-averaged ECG following MI. Table 35–6 summarizes the results of six large prospective studies[44] comprising a total of 1068 patients who had signal-averaged ECGs recorded from 6 days to as long as 6 weeks post MI, for a mean follow-up period of approximately 11 months. The method of defining late potentials as well as the recording techniques in these studies deferred substantially. Nonetheless, all studies showed that patients who had late potentials post-MI had a significantly higher arrhythmic event rate than patients without-

Table 35–4
Sensitivity and Specificity of the Frequency and Characteristics of VPDs for Predicting Sudden Cardiac Death

Definition	Prevalence (%)	Sudden Cardiac Death	
		Sensitivity (%)	Specificity (%)
Any VPD	84	92	16
>10 VPD/hr	13	95	88
Repetitive VPD	20	34	81
>10/hr or repetitive	26	43	75
Multiform	33	62	69
>10/hr, pairs, and multiform	7	16	93
>10/hr, pairs, or multiform	41	67	60

Source: Data from Kostis et al.[43]

Table 35-5
Sudden Cardiac Death in Relation to Left Ventricular Function
and Ventricular Arrhythmias

	Schulze et al[44]		Mukharji et al[41]	
Category	No. (%) of Pts.	SCD (%)	No. (%) of Pts.	SCD (%)
Low or no VA + normal EF	33 (41)	0	314 (59)	2
Low or no VA + abnormal EF	19 (23)	0	141 (26)	10
VA + normal EF	3 (4)	0	38 (7)	8
VA + abnormal EF	26 (32)	31	40 (8)	18

Abbreviations: VA, ventricular arrhythmia; EF, ejection fraction.

late potentials. Arrhythmic events were defined as the occurrence of sustained VT or SCD. Thus, during a mean follow-up period of 11 months, 20% of patients with late potentials had an arrhythmic event, whereas only 3% of patients without late potentials had events.

Breithardt et al[45] studied a total of 132 patients up to 6 weeks following MI. Their study was qualitative in terms of defining the occurrence of late potentials. Forty-five percent of patients had late potentials and 55% did not. Patients with late potentials had a 12% arrhythmic event rate, whereas only 3% without late potentials had arrhythmic events. This difference was significant at $p < 0.05$. Of interest, the incidence of sustained ventricular arrhythmias was 5% in patients with late potentials of <40 msec whereas it was 25% in patients with late potentials of ≥40 msec.

Denniss and coworkers[46] studied a total of 306 patients. They defined the presence of late potentials as an abnormal QRS duration of >120 msec. They noted late potentials in 26% of patients. During a follow-up period of 12 months, 19% of patients with late potentials had an arrhythmic event, in contrast to 4% without late potentials. This difference was highly significant at $p < 0.001$. The presence of late potentials was strongly associated with inducibility of VT in the electrophysiology laboratory.

Kuchar and coworkers[47] studied a total of 200 patients post-MI. According to their definition the presence of a filtered QRS duration > 120 msec or an RMS-40 of <20 μV defined the presence of an abnormal signal-averaged ECG or the presence of late potentials. In their study, 39% of patients had late potentials and 61% did not. During a follow-up period of 14 months, 17% of patients with late potentials had an arrhythmic event, in contrast to 1% of patients without late po-

Table 35-6
Prospective Studies of the Significance of Late Potentials (LP)
Post Myocardial Infarction

Study	No. of Pts.	LP +	LP −	Follow-up (mo)	Event Rate (%) LP +	Event Rate (%) LP −	p Value
Breidthardt et al[45]	132	45%	55%	15 ± 10	12	3	<0.05
Denniss et al[46]	306	26%	74%	12	19	4	<0.001
Kuchar et al[47]	200	39%	61%	14	17	1	<0.001
Gomes et al[48]	115	42%	58%	14 ± 8	27	4	<0.001
Cripps et al[49]	159	24%	76%	12 ± 6	26	1	<0.001
El-Sherif et al[50]	156	25%	75%	12	23	3	<0.001
Total	1068	32%	68%	11	20	3	—

tentials. This difference was highly significant at $p < 0.001$.

Gomes and coworkers[48] studied 115 patients post-MI. Late potentials were defined as the presence of either an abnormal signal-averaged QRS complex of >114 msec and/or an abnormal RMS-40 of <20 µV and/or an abnormal duration of low-amplitude signals of >38 msec. They recorded late potentials in 42% of patients. They noted an arrhythmic event rate of 27% in patients with late potentials and 4% in patients without late potentials. This difference was highly significant at $p < 0.001$.

Cripps and coworkers[49] studied a total of 139 patients, again utilizing a quantitative approach. They noted late potentials in 24% of patients. The arrhythmic event rate was 26% in patients with late potentials and 1% in patients without late potentials.

El-Sherif and co-workers[50] studied a total of 156 patients post-MI, utilizing a quantitative definition for late potentials. They noted late potentials in 25% of patients. During a follow-up period of 12 months they noted a 23% arrhythmic event rate in patients with late potentials, whereas those without had a 3% arrhythmic event rate. This difference was highly significant at $p < 0.001$. They also observed that the highest correlation between late potentials and arrhythmic event was seen when the signal-averaged ECG was obtained 6–30 days following the MI. They reported that the signal-averaged ECGs recorded before 5 days and after 1 month did not correlate with the occurrence of an arrhythmic event.

Clearly, the sensitivity and specificity of the signal-averaged ECG in predicting arrhythmic events depend on the definition of what constitutes late potentials. When an abnormal signal-averaged ECG was defined as any one abnormal quantitative variable, the sensitivity for an arrhythmic event was 81% and specificity was 65%, utilizing a 40-Hz high-pass filter. When it was defined as two or more variables, sensitivity was 69% and the specificity was 80%. When late potentials were defined as the occurrence of prolonged QRS complex of >114 msec as well as an abnormal voltage in the terminal 40 msec, then the specificity increased to 95% and the sensitivity dropped to 56%. However, this combination provided the highest positive predictive value, 58%.

Independent prognostic value of late potentials after MI has been reported in several studies. Kuchar and coworkers[51] noted that a signal-averaged ECG defined as an abnormal RMS-40 of <20 mV or a filtered QRS complex of >120 msec at 40-Hz high-pass filtering and the ejection fraction were independently related to the occurrence of an arrhythmic event by using multivariable regression analysis. In their study the frequency and characteristics of VPDs on 24-hour Holter monitoring were not independently related to an event.

Gomes et al[52] studied 102 patients post-MI by utilizing the Cox regression analysis. They noted that ejection fraction and the presence of late potentials, defined as one or more abnormal quantitative variables, and the occurrence of nonsustained VT, defined as more than or equal to three VPDs in a sequence on 24-hour Holter monitoring, were independently related to an arrhythmic event. They also studied the prognostic value of 27 clinical and noninvasive variables that included three quantitative variables: the duration of the signal-averaged QRS complex, the duration of low-amplitude signals, and the voltage in the terminal 40 msec of the QRS complex at 25 Hz, as well as 40-Hz high-pass filtering; the results of 24-hour Holter monitor dichotomized at >10 VPDs/hr, <10 VPDs/hr couplets, runs of nonsustained VT as well as ejection fraction dichotomized as >40% or ≤40%, site of MI as well as the size of MI determined from CP values was used in the Cox model. The study showed that the signal-averaged QRS complex was the most important independent variable predictive of an arrhythmic event post-MI. This study pointed out that the signal-averaged QRS complex is an important variable and should be used in the definition of late potentials post MI. However, the signal-averaged ECG used alone for risk stratification has important limitations. These include the following.

1. The positive predictive value is low, ranging from 12% to 27%, although the negative predictive value is very high, 96–99%.

2. Time-dependent changes on the signal-averaged ECG[51] have been noted. Approximately 16% of abnormal recordings become normal at 6 weeks and 30% at 1 year when compared with recordings obtained before discharge from the hospital. Thus, it

seems that a recording taken prior to discharge may have utility in risk stratification for a 1-year period but may not have much utility subsequently. It is important to note likewise that an abnormal signal-averaged ECG in the setting of sustained VT following an MI does not normalize unless specific surgery to remove the arrhythmic substrate is performed.

3. The prognostic significance of the signal-averaged ECG may not be identical in patients with inferior and anterior MIs. In a study[52] of 99 patients, of whom 50 had an anterior wall MI and 49 had an inferior MI this question was assessed. Of the 99 patients, 35 had an arrhythmic event 8 days to 24 months after MI, whereas the remaining 64 patients had no arrhythmic events up to 24 months after the MI. These latter patients were used as controls. In this study the presence of late potentials was classified as late potential-I if any one abnormal signal-averaged parameter was present and late potential-II if an abnormal signal-averaged QRS duration was present in combination with an abnormal RMS-40.

The study showed that the sensitivity for predicting arrhythmic events for late potentials-I was only 56% and the specificity was 84% in patient with anterior wall MI. In contrast, in inferior wall MI, the sensitivity of late potential-I was 94% while the specificity was only 57%. When late potentials-II were assessed, at predicting an arrhythmic event, in patients with anterior wall MI the sensitivity dropped further to 39% but the specificity increased to 94%, whereas in inferior wall MI the sensitivity dropped slightly to 82% but the specificity improved markedly to 84%. Thus it seems clear that late potentials have a high predictive value in predicting arrhythmic events in patients who have sustained an inferior wall MI but not in patients with anterior wall MI.

In this regard the ejection fraction is superior in predicting arrhythmic events in patients with anterior MI. Thus, the ejection fraction is of greater clinical relevance than the absence of late potentials in anterior wall MI.

4. Relationship between late potentials and patency of the infarct related coronary artery. Recent studies[53-56] have demonstrated that reperfusion occurring spontaneously or following thrombolysis results in modulation of late potentials. The observations reported in four studies are summarized in Table 35–7. Gang and coworkers[53] originally assessed the presence of late potentials in patients undergoing successful or unsuccessful reperfusion after thrombolytic therapy with the use of recombinant tissue plasminogen activator (tPA). The signal-averaged ECG was obtained within 48 hours of the index infarction and the presence of late potentials was defined if all three parameters were normal.

Table 35–7
Relationship Between Late Potential and the Status of the Infarct-Related Coronary Artery

Treatment Group	Artery Patent (%)	Artery Closed (%)	p Value
Gang et al (tPA)[53]	0	33	0.02
Turitto et al (urokinase)[54]	7	15	NS
Vatterot et al (tPA)[55]	24	83	<0.04
Zimmerman et al (tPA)[56]	13	26	<0.05

No late potentials were noted in 38 patients who were given tPA in whom the infarct artery was patent, whereas the incidence of late potentials was 33% in those patients in whom the artery was closed. This difference was significant at $p < 0.02$. Gang et al also noted that in patients who did not receive tPA but in whom a patent coronary artery was demonstrated, the incidence of late potentials was only 14%, whereas it was 32% in those patients in whom the artery was closed.

Turito and coworkers[54] subsequently used urokinase to make the same observation. However, in their study the presence of late potentials was assessed 13 ± 2 days following the index infarction. They found no significant differences in patients with a patent coronary artery and those without a patent coronary artery. However, a higher percentage of patients with patent coronary arteries had no late potentials, in comparison with patients with a closed coronary artery.

Vatterot and coworkers[55] reported their findings in a total of 124 consecutive patients with acute MI receiving thrombolytic agents or percutaneous transluminal coronary angioplasty. These authors made some very important observations. They again found a significantly lower incidence of late potentials in patients with a patent coronary artery (20%) than in patients with a closed coronary artery (71%). Of 48 patients who received thrombolytic agents 4 hours after the onset of symptoms, 24% of patients with an open coronary artery had late potentials, whereas 83% of patients with a closed coronary artery had late potentials. This difference was significant at $p < 0.04$.

Utilizing multivariable analysis, these investigators noted that the most powerful predictor of late potentials was a closed infarct related artery followed by MI and age of the patient. Of considerable importance was the observation that the ejection fraction was not significantly different and was not an independent predictor of late potentials in patients receiving thrombolysis. Their study also noted that the QRS duration at 40-Hz high-pass filtering was the most powerful independent predictor of vascular patency. This observation concurred with previous observations that the QRS duration at 40 Hz is the best predictor of an arrhythmic event following MI relative to other clinical and noninvasive variables.

Prognostic Significance of Heart Rate Variability

Recently, heart rate variability has been used as a noninvasive index of autonomic balance in man. That heart rate variability is decreased in patients with MI was first suggested by Schneider and Costiloe.[57] Subsequently, several investigators[58-60] have reported a poor survival in patients with decreased heart rate variability post-MI.

The value of heart rate variability, 24-hour Holter monitoring, and the signal-averaged ECG was assessed in predicting arrhythmic events in 416 patients surviving an MI by Farrell, et al.[60] Impaired heart rate variability, defined as <20 msec, late potentials, ventricular ectopic activity, repetitive forms, ejection fraction, and Killip classification were significant independent predictors of an arrhythmic event in the univariate model. When these univariate predictors were assessed in the Cox regression model, only heart rate variability followed by the presence of late potentials and repetitive forms remained as independent predictors for an arrhythmic event. The other variables and ejection fraction did not add significantly to the model. What is surprising is the observation that the use of thrombolytic therapy did not affect heart rate variability, ejection fraction, the incidence of late potentials, and Holter monitoring results, yet the incidence of death was lower in patients receiving thrombolytic therapy.

These investigators noted that, using heart rate variability and late potential combination, they obtained a sensitivity of 58%, a positive rate of accuracy of 33%, and a relative risk of 18.5%. The combination of heart rate variability, late potentials, and repetitive forms had an even higher predictive accuracy of 58% and a relative risk of 23.5% but a sensitivity of only 29% (Table 35–8).

Utilizing the Kaplan–Meyer survivorship analysis they noted that patients with an abnormal heart rate variability of less than 20 msec and late potentials, the arrhythmia-free survival was about 62% for a 2-year period, whereas it was approximately 98% for the same period in patients with normal heart rate variability and no late potentials. This difference in survival was highly significant at $p = 0.0001$. Needless to say, these interesting observations need confirmation. Nonetheless, the observations in this study suggest that future strategies should use at least the combination of heart rate variability and late potentials and possibly ejection fraction and Holter monitoring to risk categorize the patients into the highest risk category. High-risk patients, who account for about 10% of the post-MI population, should be targeted for interventional therapy. In contrast, in patients in whom heart rate variability is normal and there are no late potentials and no significant LV dysfunction, the arrhythmic event rate is extremely low and no further intervention should be required. It is important to keep in mind, however, that a substantial proportion of events post-MI may be related to reinfarction or ischemia. The occurrence of ischemia cannot be assessed by any of these noninvasive tests. Therefore, exercise testing for the detection of significant ischemia

Table 35-8
Combination of Noninvasive Variables for Prediction of Arrhythmic Events

	Relative Risk (95% CI)	Positive Predictive Accuracy (%)	Negative Predictive Accuracy (%)
HRV < 20 msec + LP	18.5	33	93
HRV < 20 msec + VE10	12.6	34	96
HRV < 20 msec + REP	15.0	43	77
HRV < 20 msec + EF < 0.40	6.3	22	91
EF < 0.40 + LP	4.7	19	94
EF < 0.40 + VE10	5.9	19	94
EF < 0.40 + REP	5.2	15	95
EF < 0.40 + LP + VE10	6.9	28	97
HRV < 20 msec + LP + VE10	13.9	43	96
HRV < 20 msec + LP + REP	23.5	58	95

Source: Farrell TG, et al: J Am Coll Cardiol 18:687–697, 1991. Modified by permission.
Abbreviations: HRV, heart rate variability; EF, ejection fraction; LP, late potential; VE10, > or = 10 VPDs/hr; REP, repetitive pattern.

will require therapeutic interventions such as anti-ischemia therapy with drugs or revascularization inclusive of angioplasty and coronary artery bypass surgery.

ROLE OF INVASIVE ELECTROPHYSIOLOGICAL STUDY FOR RISK STRATIFICATION

The role of an invasive electrophysiological study for risk stratification in asymptomatic people post MI remains highly controversial. Some studies show that it has prognostic value, while others show that its role in prognostication is minimal. A variety of reasons could account for these diverse observations.

1. All studies have used a small cohort of patients.
2. A large number of studies have used a very low-risk population.
3. The follow-up has not been long enough and the stimulation protocol utilized has varied between studies.
4. The incidence of inducibility has varied from one study to the next.
5. The prognostic significance of inducibility of sustained monomorphic VTs versus the induction of VF seems to be quite different.

Table 35-9
Prognostic Significance of Inducible Sustained VT Versus Inducible VF

Study	Induced Response		Arrhythmic Events		
	Sust. VT (%)	VF (%)	Sust. VT (%)	VF (%)	Noninducible (%)
Denniss et al[61]	80 (20)	56 (14)	6 (7.5)*	2 (3.4)*	4 (1.5)*
Bhandari et al[62]	19 (25)	14 (19)	4 (21)	1 (7)	2 (4.6)
Cripps et al[63]	8 (11)	14 (19)	6 (75)	0 (0)	0 (0)
Bhandari et al[64]	10 (19)	6 (14)	5 (50)	1 (16)	1 (2.8)

Abbreviations: Sust., sustained; VT, ventricular tachycardia; VF, ventricular fibrillation.
* Frequency of sudden cardiac death only.

Table 35–9 summarizes the results of four studies[61–64] which assessed the induced response in relation to an arrhythmic event. As seen from these studies, the induction of sustained monomorphic VT seems to be more specific for an arrhythmic event than induction of VF. Nonetheless, the positive predictive value of electrophysiological testing is likely not appreciably higher than that of other noninvasive tests described above. Furthermore, electrophysiological testing is an invasive and relatively expensive test. Additionally, no studies have demonstrated that treatment with antiarrhythmic drugs with EP guidance in the asymptomatic population is associated with a better survival. Thus, routine electrophysiological testing for risk stratification post-MI in asymptomatic patients is not recommended at this time.

LONG-TERM ANTIARRHYTHMIC DRUG TRIALS IN SURVIVORS OF ACUTE MYOCARDIAL INFARCTION

The occurrence of asymptomatic ventricular arrhythmias post MI is associated with an independent risk of SCD. However, whether treatment of ventricular arrhythmias with antiarrhythmic drugs prevents the occurrence of SCD remains an unanswered question. In the meanwhile, studies using β-antiadrenergic blockers established that the treatment of patients post MI with β-blockers decreased the incidence of SCD significantly. Approximately ten large studies[65–74] have assessed survival of patients on long-term antiarrhythmic drug trials with the use of such drugs as procainamide, tocainide, phenytoin, aprindine, and mexiletine. More recently the Cardiac Arrhythmias Suppression Trial (CAST) study used encainide, flecainide, and moricizine in a placebo-controlled trial. The latter study was designed to establish whether suppression of the arrhythmia assessed on Holter monitoring would prevent SCD.

All previous studies before the CAST study showed no difference in survival between patients placed on drugs and those not treated with antiarrhythmic drugs. In fact, in all of those studies the mortality tended to be higher in the drug treatment group than in the no-drug-therapy group.

Of the 2309 patients initially enrolled in the CAST study, the arrhythmia was suppressed in 1727 patients by one of the three drugs. These patients were subsequently randomly assigned to receive one of the antiarrhythmic medications to suppress the arrhythmia or were placed on placebo. Of considerable interest was the observation that patients on antiarrhythmic drugs had a significantly higher event rate for SCD as well as total cardiac mortality than those who received placebo. The incidence of deaths from cardiac arrhythmias was 4.5% in the encainide and flecainide arm but only 1.2% in the placebo group. The overall cardiac mortality was 7.7% in the encainide and flecainide groups, compared with 3% in the placebo group. Because of these observations the encainide and flecainide arms of the study were discontinued; however, the moricizine arm was continued. More recently the moricizine arm was discontinued because patients in the moricizine group showed a higher mortality than the control group.

The results of the CAST study raised several important issues both for the academician and for the practitioner. The use of encainide, flecainide, and moricizine in suppressing VPDs as a therapeutic end point has been placed in question, although other antiarrhythmic agents, such as amiodarone, may be more effective in this regard. It also became clear that suppression of VPDs by antiarrhythmic drugs alone does not necessarily prevent the occurrence of SCD, as happened in the CAST study. Although this conclusion is valid, it may not be so for other drugs such as amiodarone or sotalol. The study focused greater awareness in the medical community regarding the use of antiarrhythmic agents. Finally, the observations in the CAST study emphasize the importance of risk stratification for the selection of the highest risk category of patients to undergo interventional therapy.

FUTURE DIRECTIONS

Studies need to be designed in high-risk patients to assess the role of electrophysiologically guided antiarrhythmic therapy, the role of drugs such as amiodarone and sotalol, and the role of AICDs. It is possible that in these high-risk patients, prophylactic antiarrhythmic therapy may not be the wisest choice for preventing SCD. In this regard, a search for anti-SCD drugs may be preferable over one for antiarrhythmic drugs. Antiarrhythmic drug therapy has a high proarrhythmic rate in high-risk patients with severe LV dysfunction. This may negate any beneficial effects of antiarrhythmic drug therapy. The latter reasoning, however, seems not necessarily to be the case in patients who have symptomatic sustained VT in the setting of coronary artery disease who are treated with EP guided therapy. Nonetheless, recent studies have pointed out that even in this patient population, the best survival free of arrhythmic death is obtained with the use of implanted defibrillators and surgery directed at the substrate as well as revascularization rather than the use of antiarrhythmic drug therapy alone.

REFERENCES

1. Lieberthson RR, Nagel EL, Hirschman JC, Nussenfeld SR: Prehospital ventricular defibrillation: Prognosis and follow-up course. N Engl J Med 291:317–321, 1974.
2. Baum RS, Alvarez A III, Cobb LA: Survival after resuscitation from out-of-hospital ventricular fibrillation. Circulation 50:1231–1235, 1974.
3. Goldstein S, Landis JR, Leighton R, et al: Characteristics of the resuscitated out-of-hospital cardiac arrest victim with coronary artery disease. Circulation 64:977–984, 1981.
4. Myerberg RJ, Kessler KM, Estes D, et al: Long-term survival after prehospital cardiac arrest: Analysis of outcome during an 8-year study. Circulation 70:538–546, 1984.
5. Nikolic G, Bishop RL, Singh J: Sudden death recorded during Holter monitoring. Circulation 66:218–225, 1982.
6. Panidis IP, Morganroth J: Sudden death in hospitalized patients: Cardiac rhythm disturbances detected by ambulatory electrocardiographic monitoring. J Am Coll Cardiol 2:798–805, 1983.
7. Pratt CM, Francis MJ, Luck JC, Wyndham CR, Miller RR, Quinones MA: Analysis of ambulatory electrocardiograms in 15 patients during spontaneous ventricular fibrillation with special reference to preceding arrhythmic events. J Am Coll Cardiol 2:789–797, 1983.
8. Kempf FC, Josephson ME: Cardiac arrest recorded on ambulatory electrocardiograms. Am J Cardiol 53:1577–1582, 1984.
9. Roelandt J, Klootwijk P, Lubsen J, Janse MJ: Sudden death during long-term ambulatory monitoring. Eur Heart J 5:7–20, 1984.
10. Leclercq JF, Maisonblanche P, Cauchemez B, Coumel P: Respective role of sympathetic tone and of cardiac pauses in the genesis of 62 cases of ventricular fibrillation recorded during Holter monitoring. Eur Heart J 9:1276–1283, 1988.
11. Gomes JA, Alexopoulos D, Winters SL, Deshmukh P, Fuster V, Suh K: The role of silent ischemia, the arrhythmic substrate and the short-long sequence in the genesis of sudden cardiac death. J Am Coll Cardiol 14:1618, 1989.
12. Ruskin JN, DiMasco JP, Garan H: Out-of-hospital cardiac arrest: Electrophysiologic observation and selection of long term antiarrhythmic therapy. N Engl J Med 303:607, 1980.
13. Norris RM: The changing natural history and Prognosis of Acute myocardial infarction. In Gersh BJ, Rahimtoola SH (eds): Acute Myocardial Infarction. New York, Elsevier, 1991, pp 87–97.
14. Norwegian Multicenter Study Group: Timolol-induced reduction in mortality and reinfarction in patients surviving acute myocardial infarction. N Engl J Med 304:801–807, 1981.
15. Beta-Blocker Heart Attack Research Group: A randomized trial of propranolol in patients with acute myocardial infarction. JAMA 247:1717–1724, 1982.
16. Beta-Blocker Pooling Project Research Group: Subgroup findings from randomized trials in post infarction patients. Eur Heart J 9:8–16, 1988.
17. ISIS-2 (Second International Study of Infarct Survival) Collaborative Group: Randomized trial of intravenous streptokinase, oral aspirin, both, or neither among 17,187 cases of suspected acute myocardial infarction: ISIS 2. Lancet ii:349–359, 1988.
18. Muller DW, Topol EJ, George BS, et al: Long-term follow-up in the Thrombolysis and Angioplasty in Acute Myocardial Infarction (TAMI) trials: Comparison of trials with thrombolysis alone. Circulation 80(suppl II):II-520, 1989.
19. GISSI Trial Group: Long-term effects of intravenous thrombolysis in acute myocardial infarction: Final report of the GISSI study. Lancet ii:871–874, 1987.
20. Williams DO, Braunwald E, Knatterud G, et al: The Thrombolysis in Myocardial Infarction (TIMI) trial: Outcome at one year

of patients randomized to either invasive or conservative management. Circulation 80(suppl II):II–519, 1989.
21. Schroder R, Neuhaus KL, Leizorovicz A, et al: A prospective placebo-controlled double-blind multicenter trial of streptokinase in acute myocardial infarction (ISAM): Long-term mortality and morbidity. J Am Coll Cardiol 9:197–203, 1987.
22. Simoons ML, Arnold A: One year follow-up of rt-PA without and with immediate PTCA. Circulation 80(suppl II):II–520, 1980.
23. Van de Werf F, Arnold AE: The European Co-operative rt-PA vs Placebo trial: 1 year follow-up. Circulation 80(suppl II):II–520, 1989.
24. Dalen JE, Gore GM, Braunwald F, et al: Six and twelve month follow-up of the phase I Thrombolysis in Myocardial Infarction (TIMI) trial. Am J Cardiol 62:179–185, 1988.
25. Tofler GH, Stone PH, Muller JE, and the MILIS Study Group: Prognosis after cardiac arrest due to ventricular tachycardia or ventricular fibrillation associated with acute myocardial infarction (MILIS study) Am J Cardiol 60:755–761, 1987.
26. Gomes JA, Winters SL, Ergin A, et al: The clinical and electrophysiologic determinants, treatment and survival of patients with sustained malignant ventricular tachyarrhythmias late post-myocardial infarction. J Am Coll Cardiol 17:320, 1990.
27. Wilson C, Adgey AAJ: Survival of patients with late ventricular fibrillation after acute myocardial infarction. Lancet ii:124, 1974.
28. Wellens HJJ, Bar FWH, Vanagt EJDM, Brugada P: Medical treatment of ventricular tachycardia: Consideration in the selection of patients for surgical therapy. Am J Cardiol 49:186–193, 1982.
29. Marchlinski FE, Waxman HL, Buxton AE, Josephson ME: Sustained ventricular tachycardia during the early post-infarction period: Electrophysiologic findings and prognosis for survival. J Am Coll Cardiol 2:40–50, 1983.
30. Lie KI, Liem KL, Schuilenberg RM, David GK, Durrer D: Early identification of patients developing late in-hospital ventricular fibrillation after discharge from the coronary care unit. Am J Cardiol 41:974, 1978.
31. Wald RW, Waxman MB, Carey PN, Gunstenson J, Goldman BS: Management of intractable ventricular tachyarrhythmias after myocardial infarction. Am J Cardiol 44:329, 1979.
32. Buda AJ, Stinson EB, Harrison DC: Surgery for life-threatening ventricular tachyarrhythmias. Am J Cardiol 44:329–338, 1979.
33. Garan H, Ruskin JN, DiMarco JP, McGovern B, Levine H, Buckler MJ: Refractory ventricular tachycardia complicating recovery from acute myocardial infarction: Treatment with map-guided infarctectomy. Am J J 107:571, 1984.
34. DiMarco JP, Lerman BB, Kron IL, Sellers TD: Sustained ventricular tachyarrhythmias within 2 months of acute myocardial infarction: Results of medical and surgical therapy in patients resuscitated from the initial episode. J Am Coll Cardiol 6:759–768, 1985.
35. Kleiman RB, Miller JM, Buxton AE, Josephson ME, Marchlinski FE: Prognosis following sustained ventricular tachycardia occurring early after myocardial infarction. Am J Cardiol 62:528–533, 1988.
36. Landymore RW, Gardner MA, McIntyre AJ, Barker RA: Surgical intervention for drug-resistant ventricular tachycardia. J Am Coll Cardiol 16:37–41, 1990.
37. Bourke JP, Hilton CJ, McComb JM, et al: Surgery for control of recurrent life-threatening ventricular tachyarrhythmias within 2 months of myocardial infarction. J Am Coll Cardiol 16:42–48, 1990.
38. Willems AR, Tijssen JGP, Van Capelle FJL, et al: Determinants of prognosis in symptomatic ventricular tachycardia or ventricular fibrillation late after myocardial infarction. J Am Coll Cardiol 16:521–530, 1990.
39. Ruberman W, Weinblatt E, Goldberg JD, et al: Ventricular premature beats and mortality after acute myocardial infarction. N Engl J Med 297:750–757, 1977.
40. Moss AJ, Davis HT, DeCamilla J, Bayer LW: Ventricular ectopic beats and their relation to sudden and nonsudden cardiac death after myocardial infarction. Circulation 60:998–1003, 1979.
41. Mukharji J, Rude RE, Poole WK, et al, and the MILIS Study Group: Risk factors for sudden death after acute myocardial infarction: Two-year follow-up. Am J Cardiol 54:31–36, 1984.
42. Bigger J, Fleiss JL, Kleiger K, et al, and the Multicenter Post-infarction Research Group: The relationship between ventricular arrhythmias, left ventricular dysfunction and mortality in the two years after dysfunction and mortality in the two years after myocardial infarction. Circulation 69:250–258, 1984.
43. Kostis JB, Byington R, Friedman LM, et al: Prognostic significance of ventricular ectopic activity in survivors of acute myocardial infarction. J Am Coll Cardiol 10:231–242, 1987.
44. Schulze RA Jr, Strauss HW, Pitt B: Sudden death in the year following myocardial infarction: Relation to ventricular premature

contractions in the late hospital phase and left ventricular ejection fraction. Am J Med 62:192–195, 1977.
45. Breithardt G, Borggrefe M, Haarten K: Role of programmed ventricular stimulation and non-invasive recording of ventricular late potentials for the identification of patients at risk of ventricular arrhythmias after acute myocardial infarction. In Zipes DP, Jalife J (eds): Cardiac Electrophysiology and Arrhythmias. Orlando, FL, Grune & Stratton, 1984, pp 553–561.
46. Denniss AR, Richards DA, Cody DV, et al: Prognostic significance of ventricular tachycardia and fibrillation induced at programmed stimulation and delayed potentials detected on the signal-averaged electrocardiograms of survivors of acute myocardial infarction. Circulation 74:731–745, 1986.
47. Kuchar DL, Thorburn CW, Samuel NL: Late potentials detected after myocardial infarction: Natural history and prognostic significance. Circulation 74:1280–1289, 1986.
48. Gomes JA, Winters SL, Martinson M, et al: The prognostic significance of quantitative signal-averaged variables relative to clinical variables, site of myocardial infarction, ejection reaction and ventricular premature beats: A prospective study. J Am Coll Cardiol 1:377–384, 1988.
49. Cripps T, Bennett ED, Camm AJ, Ward DE: High-gain signal-averaged electrocardiogram combined with 24-hours monitoring in patients early after myocardial infarction for bedside prediction of arrhythmic events. Br Heart J 60:181, 1989.
50. El-Sherif N, Ursell SN, Bekheit S, et al: Prognostic significance of the signal averaged electrocardiogram depends on the time of recording in the post-infarction period. Am Heart J 118:256–264, 1989.
51. Kuchar DL, Samuel L, Thorburn C: Natural history and prognostic significance of late potentials up to 5 years after myocardial infarction. J Am Coll Cardiol 15:724, 1990.
52. Gomes JA, Winters L: The prognostic significance of the signal-averaged electrocardiogram in the infarct survivor. In Gersh BJ, Rahimtoola SA (eds): Acute Myocardial Infarction. New York, Elsevier, 1991.
53. Gang E, Lew AS, Hong M, et al: Decreased incidence of late potentials after successful thrombolytic therapy of myocardial infarction. N Engl J Med 321:712–716, 1989.
54. Turitto G, Risa AL, Zanchi E, Prate L: The signal-average electrocardiogram and ventricular arrhythmias after thrombolysis for acute myocardial infarction. J Am Coll Cardiol 15:1270–1276, 1990.
55. Vatterot PJ, Hammill SC, Bailey WR, Wiltgen CM, Gersh BJ: Late potentials on signal-averaged electrocardiograms and patency of the infarct-related artery in survivors of acute myocardial infarction. J Am Coll Cardiol 17:330, 1991.
56. Zimmerman M, Adamec R, Ciaroni S, Malbois F, Tieche R: Reduction in the frequency of ventricular late potentials after acute myocardial infarction by early thrombolytic therapy. Am J Cardiol 67:697–703, 1991.
57. Schneider RA, Costiloe JP: Relationship of sinus arrhythmic to age and its prognostic significance in ischemia heart disease. Clin Res 13:219, 1965.
58. Wolf MM, Varigos GA, Hunt D, Sloman G: Sinus arrhythmia in acute myocardial infarction. Med J Aust 2:52–55, 1978.
59. Kleiger RE, Miller JP, Brigs JT Jr, Moss AJ, and the Multicenter Post-Infarction Research Group: Decreased heart rate variability and its association with increased mortality after myocardial infarction. Am J Cardiol 60:86–89, 1987.
60. Farrell TG, Bashier Y, Cripps T, et al: Risk stratification for arrhythmic events in post infarction patients based on heart rate variability, ambulatory electrocardiographic variables and the signal averaged electrocardiogram. J Am Coll Cardiol 18:687–697, 1991.
61. Denniss AR, Richards DA, Cody DV, et al: Prognostic significance of ventricular tachycardia and fibrillation induced at programmed stimulation and delayed potentials detected on the signal-averaged electrocardiograms of survivors of acute myocardial infarction. Circulation 74:731–745, 1986.
62. Bhandari AK, Hong R, Kotlewski A, et al: Prognostic significance of programmed ventricular stimulation in survivors of acute myocardial infarction. Br Heart J 61:410–416, 1989.
63. Cripps T, Bennett ED, Camm AJ, Ward DE: Inducibility of sustained monomorphic ventricular tachycardia as a prognostic indicator in survivors of recent myocardial infarction: A prospective evaluation in relation to other prognostic variables. J Am Coll Cardiol 14:289–296, 1989.
64. Bhandari A, Hong R, Kotlewski A, et al: Prognostic significance of programmed stimulation in high risk patients surviving acute myocardial infarction [abstract]. J Am Coll Cardiol 11:6A, 1988.
65. Kosowsky BD, Taylor J, Lown B, et al: Long-term use of procainamide following acute myocardial infarction. Circulation 47:1204–1210, 1973.
66. Collaborative Group: Phenytoin after recovery from myocardial infarction: Controlled

trial in 568 patient. Lancet *ii:*1055–1057, 1971.
67. Peter T, Ross D, Duffield A, et al: Effect on survival after myocardial infarction of long-term treatment with phenytoin. Br Heart J *40:*1356–1360, 178.
68. Bastian BC, Macfarlane PW, McLauchlan JH, et al: A prospective randomized trial of tocainide in patients following myocardial infarction. Am Heart J *100:*1017–1022, 1980.
69. Ryden L, Arnman K, Conradson TB, et al: Prophylaxis of ventricular tachyarrhythmias with intravenous and oral tocainide in patient with and recovering from acute myocardial infarction. Am Heart J *100:*1006–1012, 1980.
70. Chamberlain DA, Jewitt DE, Julian DG, et al: Oral mexiletine in high-risk patients after myocardial infarction. Lancet *ii:*1234–1327, 1980.
71. IMPACT Research Group: International Mexiletine and Placebo Antiarrhythmic Coronary Trial: Report on arrhythmia and other findings. J Am Coll Cardiol *6:*1148–1163, 1984.
72. Gottlieb SM, Achuff SC, Mellits ED, et al: Prophylactic antiarrhythmic therapy of high risk survivors of myocardial infarction: Lower mortality at 1 month but not a 1 year. Circulation *75:*L792–799, 1987.
73. Cardiac Arrhythmia Pilot Study (CAPS) Investigators: Effect of encainide, flecainide, imipramine and moricizine on ventricular arrhythmias during the year after acute myocardial infarction: The CAPS. Am J Cardiol *61:*501–509, 1988.
74. Cardiac Arrhythmia Suppression Trial (CAST) Investigators: Preliminary report: Effect of encainide and flecainide on mortality in a randomized trail of arrhythmia suppression after myocardial infarction. N Engl J Med *321:*406–412, 1989.

G
Therapeutic Options and Assessment of Efficacy

36

Coronary Artery Surgery for the Prevention and Treatment of Sudden Cardiac Death

ROBERT A. O'ROURKE

The role of coronary artery bypass graft (CABG) surgery in the prevention of sudden cardiac death (SCD) and the management of survivors has not been well defined.[1] Considering the frequency of subsequent restenosis following initially successful coronary angioplasty, the usefulness of this method of myocardial revascularization in patients who present with SCD is even more problematic.[1] This chapter discusses the incidence of coronary artery disease in deaths due to cardiac arrhythmias, the common occurrence of myocardial ischemia as an inciting factor, the reduced prevalence of sudden death in coronary artery disease patients after myocardial revascularization, and the role of CABG surgery in preventing *recurrent* sudden death.

CARDIAC PATHOLOGY IN SUDDEN CARDIAC DEATH

Clinical evidence of cardiac disease is present in 90% of patients with death due to arrhythmias.[2] The commonest pathological finding in patients with SCD is severe atherosclerosis of several coronary arteries.[3] In postmortem studies, associated ventricular damage from previous myocardial infarction (MI) is a frequent finding in victims of SCD. Most nonsurvivors of sudden death have multivessel coronary artery disease, with about 50% also having evidence of one or more prior *healed* MIs.[4] Acute coronary artery thrombosis with *recent acute* MI is observed in fewer than 30% of patients with SCD.[5] However, pathological examination of the coronary arteries frequently shows complicated atherosclerotic lesions with intraluminal thrombi and/or plaque fissuring, usually at the site of a pre-existing area of fixed stenosis. In an autopsy study of 220 patients with SCD, Lieberthson and associates[6] reported a >75% coronary artery stenosis in 94% of victims, a 60% prevalence of three-vessel coronary artery disease, and a 44% prevalence of old MI. Fifty-eight percent had acute coronary artery occlusion, 32% of whom had coronary artery thrombosis and 56% a ruptured plaque. An acute MI was present in 27%. More recently, Davis and Thomas[7] reported "major thrombi" in 44 of 100 consecutive autopsies performed in patients with ischemic heart disease and sudden death. Arteriographic studies of cardiac arrest survivors also report a high prevalence of long, diffusely irregular coronary artery segments that may provide the substrate for coronary thrombosis as the triggering event for arrhythmia.[8]

In a study by Wilber et al,[9] 125 (75%) of 166 survivors of out-of-hospital cardiac arrests had coronary artery disease unassociated with acute MI. Arteriography showed three-vessel coronary artery stenosis in 60%, two-vessel disease in 20%, and single-vessel disease in 20% of patients. The

---

An earlier version of this chapter appeared as an overview in a supplement to *Circulation* 85:I2–I10, 1992.

mean left ventricular ejection fraction averaged 0.41. Thus, the typical pathological substrate for SCD is severe epicardial coronary artery disease with or without old MI. Moreover, in the Coronary Artery Surgical Study (CASS) registry,[10] there was no difference in clinicopathological characteristics between patients who had a sudden versus a nonsudden cardiac death.

MYOCARDIAL ISCHEMIA AS A PRECIPITATING FACTOR

Several clinical observations support a role for acute myocardial ischemia at least as a contributing factor to SCD.[11] The Framingham study results indicate a circadian variation in the incidence of SCD that is consistent with the morning increase in catecholamines, platelet aggregability, and the incidence of unstable angina and nonfatal MI.[12] Also, symptoms or signs suggesting myocardial ischemia, angina pectoris, or a documented MI precede 30–50% of cardiac arrests in patients with coronary artery disease.[13]

In an important dog study of acute ischemia superimposed on recent MI, Garan et al[14] showed that *spontaneous* ventricular arrhythmias in postinfarction dogs were the result of ischemia, whereas total infarct size correlated with electrically induced but not with spontaneously occurring arrhythmias.

With the high incidence of severe coronary artery stenoses in survivors and nonsurvivors of SCD, it is not surprising that a precise definition of the role of acute myocardial ischemia in episodes of cardiac arrest is often impossible. In patients with ischemic heart disease the extent and severity of coronary atherosclerosis and the probability of recurrent myocardial ischemia are important determinants of the risk for sudden death. Most studies indicate that the extent of impaired left ventricular systolic function, as assessed by the ejection fraction, is the most powerful independent determinant of risk for subsequent sudden death in patients with coronary artery disease.[11,15] Frequent and repetitive ventricular arrhythmias, particularly nonsustained ventricular tachycardia (VT), are also associated with an increased risk for SCD.[16] Unfortunately, a fatal ventricular arrhythmia may be the first symptomatic manifestation of coronary artery disease in approximately 50% of patients who experience SCD.[3]

Other diseases of the coronary arteries may also cause SCD. An anomalous origin of a coronary artery, particularly if the artery courses between the pulmonary artery and aorta, may result in acute myocardial ischemia and fatal arrhythmia.[1] Spasm with or without fixed coronary artery stenosis may also produce acute, sometimes fatal, myocardial ischemia. Less common disorders of the coronary arteries that can cause sudden death include dissection, trauma, embolism, and arteritis.[17]

Although many potential mechanisms may be responsible for cardiac arrest and sudden death, there is likely a complex interaction between triggering events such as worsened ischemia, hypoxia, acidosis, electrolyte imbalance, stimulation of the sympathetic nervous system, and cardiac and noncardiac drugs and chronic susceptibility to arrhythmias due to prior ventricular scarring.[11] Several possible contributing factors should be considered when planning future preventive treatment for specific survivors of SCD.

It is likely that the prevention or reduction of myocardial ischemia would decrease the incidence of sudden death in patients with coronary artery disease who have either symptomatic or silent myocardial ischemia. This postulate is supported by the decreased incidence of sudden death in patients with documented myocardial ischemia who undergo CABG surgery.

PRIMARY AND SECONDARY PREVENTION OF SUDDEN CARDIAC DEATH

The assessment and management of patients at greater risk for sudden death may be separated into two major categories: the primary prevention of SCD in patients with heart disease who are at high risk, and the secondary prevention of recurrent cardiac arrest and sudden death in patients who have been successfully resuscitated from an episode of cardiac arrest.[1] Few data are available on the primary prevention of SCD in patients with structural heart disease, including the high percentage of such patients with coronary artery disease. However, clinical trials using β-blocking drugs in patients after MI, and CABG in patients with stable coronary artery disease, have shown a reduced incidence in both sudden and total cardiac mortality after intervention.[18-21] Although the exact mechanisms by which these therapies decrease sudden death are poorly documented, the prevention of recurrent episodes of acute myocardial ischemia is a likely factor.[1]

As mentioned previously, it is often useful to consider acute precipitating events such as ischemia and/or thrombosis in terms of treating transient phenomena as well as a fixed anatomical substrate (e.g., healed MI, severe coronary artery stenosis) that makes the patient chronically subject to arrhythmias.[1] The relative importance of acute factors versus the role of a fixed anatomical predisposition to arrhythmias is often difficult to determine.[11] In general, the best approach to management employs both efforts to correct transient initiating factors, whenever possible, and also to modify the fixed cardiac substrate upon which these triggers act.[1]

DIAGNOSTIC ASSESSMENT

The cardiac evaluation for survivors of SCD usually includes a noninvasive (radionuclide ventriculography or two-dimensional echocardiography) or invasive assessment of left ventricular function prior to or at the time of coronary arteriography. In general, all survivors of an out-of-hospital cardiac arrest unassociated with a new MI should undergo a detailed anatomical and functional cardiac evaluation.[1] With rare exceptions, diagnostic cardiac catheterization with coronary arteriography, left ventricular cineangiography, and hemodynamic assessment is indicated.[11] In patients with coronary artery disease, assessment for inducible myocardial ischemia such as with ECG–exercise testing or with exercise or dipyridamole-thallium myocardial perfusion imaging or two-dimensional echocardiographic assessment of wall motion and function adds useful information concerning the physiological importance of coronary artery stenoses as a cause of myocardial ischemia.[3] Any decision regarding the optimal course of treatment will be greatly influenced by the coronary and ventricular angiographic findings. After obtaining information concerning the presence and extent of coronary artery stenosis, global and regional ventricular function, and the presence or absence of ventricular aneurysms, the physician can consider therapeutic options in a logical manner.[11] The demonstration of severe coronary artery disease, especially left main or advanced multivessel disease, generally warrants surgical revascularization, which is often effective when used alone in survivors without inducible VT. Less severe coronary artery disease often is managed with aggressive anti-ischemic medical therapy or percutaneous transluminal coronary angioplasty (PTCA).[1]

REDUCED PREVALENCE OF SUDDEN DEATH AFTER CORONARY ARTERY BYPASS GRAFT SURGERY

There is certainly a place for surgical myocardial revascularization in the prevention of sudden death. Four hundred fifty-two (26%) of the 1725 deaths were sudden among the 13,476 patients in the Coronary Artery Surgical Study (CASS) registry, all of whom had significant coronary artery disease, operable vessels, and no significant valvular disease[14]; the mean follow-up averaged 4.6 years. The incidence of sudden death during follow-up was 5.2% in patients assigned to medical therapy as compared to 1.8% in those assigned to surgical therapy (Fig. 36–1). When a history of congestive heart failure was present, the prevalence of SCD was statistically less with surgical treatment in patients with two- or three-vessel coronary artery stenoses (Fig. 36–2).[19] In patients with a history of congestive heart failure, the difference in favor of surgical therapy was even greater (Fig. 36–3).[19]

In another CASS report,[20] the SCD rate in 160 patients with a left ventricular ejection fraction of 0.35 to 0.45 was three times higher in patients randomized to medial therapy than in patients treated with CABG surgery; the duration of follow-up averaged 7 years.

In the prospective randomized European Coronary Surgery Study, there was a signif-

534   Sudden Cardiac Death

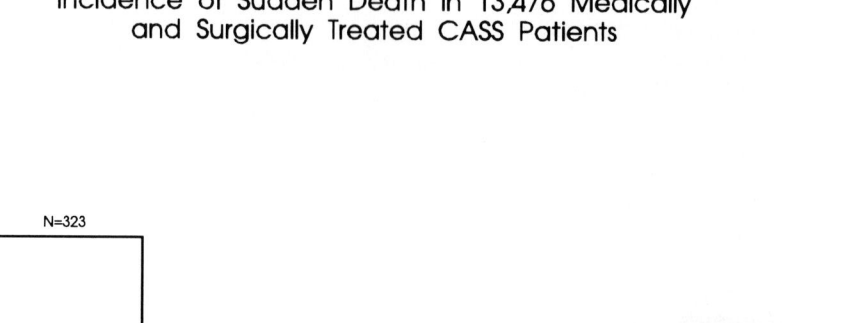

Fig. 36–1. Incidence of sudden death in patients assigned to medical therapy (5.2%), surgical therapy (1.8%), or both (3.4%) in CASS (Coronary Artery Surgical Study). (Plotted from data in Holmes DR, et al: Circulation 73:1254–1263, 1986.[19])

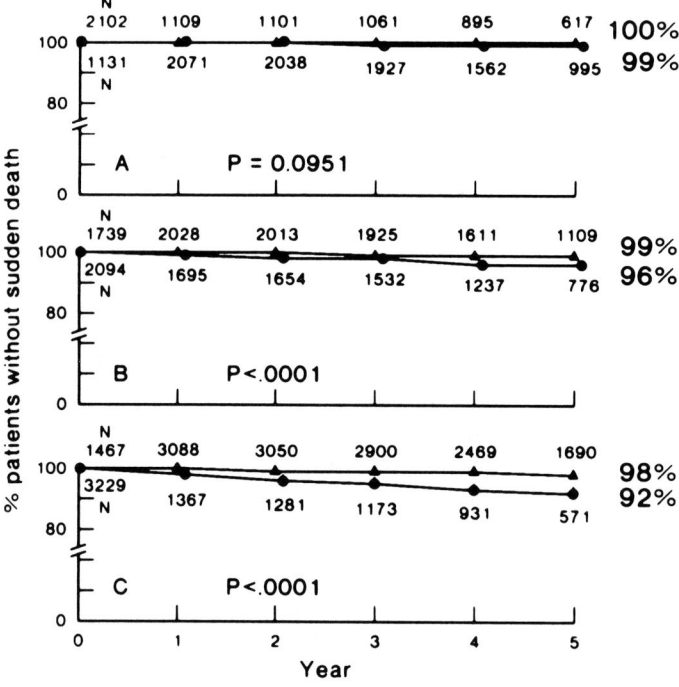

Fig. 36–2. Percentage of patients without sudden death in surgically treated group (▲) compared with that in medically treated group (●). *None* had a history of congestive failure. *A*, patients with one-vessel disease; *B*, patients with two-vessel disease; *C*, patients with three-vessel disease; and N, number of patients. (Reproduced with permission from Holmes DR, et al: Circulation 73:1254–1263, 1986.[19])

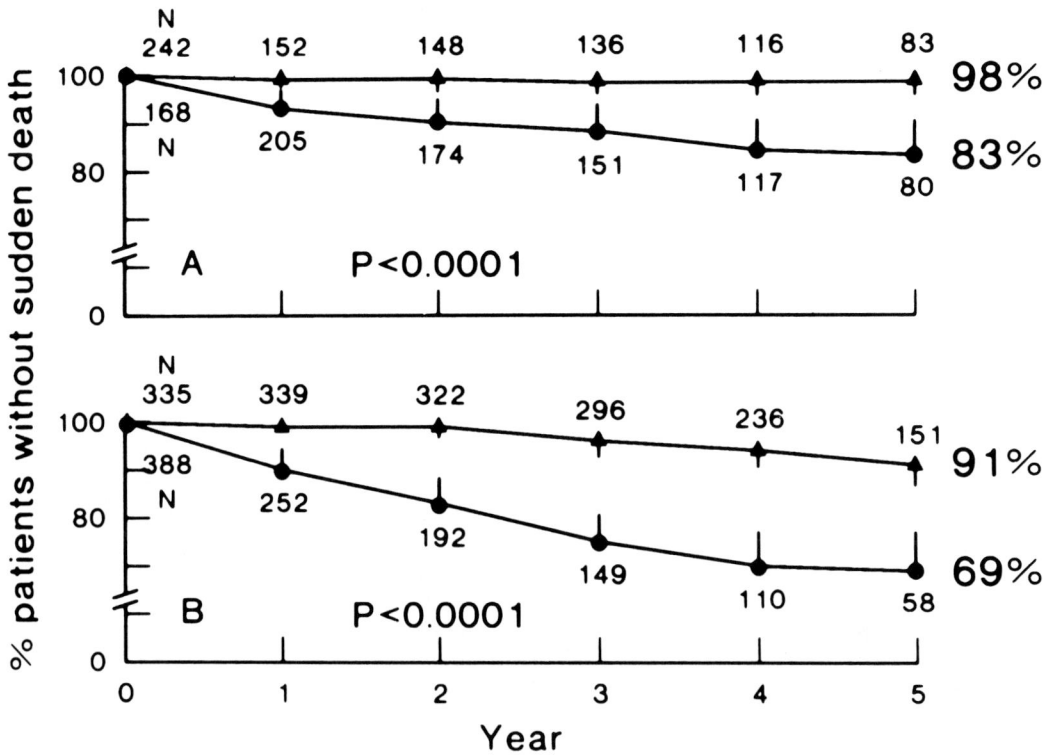

Fig. 36–3. Percentage of patients without sudden death in surgically treated group (▲) compared with that in medically treated group (●). *All* had a history of heart failure. *A*, patients with two-vessel disease; *B*, patients with three-vessel disease; N, number of patients. (Reproduced with permission from Holmes DR, et al: Circulation *73:*1254–1263, 1986.[19])

icant decrease in the cumulative risk of sudden death at 8 years of follow-up in patients assigned to surgical therapy (3%) as compared to those assigned to medical treatment (9%) (Fig. 36–4).[21]

The report of Weiner and associates from the CASS registry,[22] further indicates that most groups of patients with ischemia during exercise testing have the same likelihood of developing an acute MI or sudden death whether the exercise-induced ischemia was silent or symptomatic. An important exception were patients in the three-vessel coronary artery disease subgroup where the risk appeared higher for those with *silent* ischemia during exercise (Figs. 36–5 and 36–6).[22] Myocardial revascularization also is likely to decrease the occurrence of SCD in patients with exercise-induced silent but definite myocardial ischemia.

ROLE OF MYOCARDIAL REVASCULARIZATION IN PREVENTING RECURRENT SUDDEN DEATH

Despite the lack of available control data, CABG also seems to be beneficial in patients with prior episodes of cardiac arrest, with coronary artery surgery alone being most effective in patients without preoperative inducible VT during electrophysiological testing. Tresch et al[23] reported favorable outcomes in most of 49 survivors of prehospital cardiac arrest patients who were treated with CABG surgery; the 5-year survival rate was 72%. In a recent report from the University of Washington[23a] concerning 265 patients who were followed for up to 18 years after resuscitation from out-of-hospital cardiac arrest, CABG surgery significantly reduced the incidence of subsequent cardiac arrests during follow-up. Swerdlow

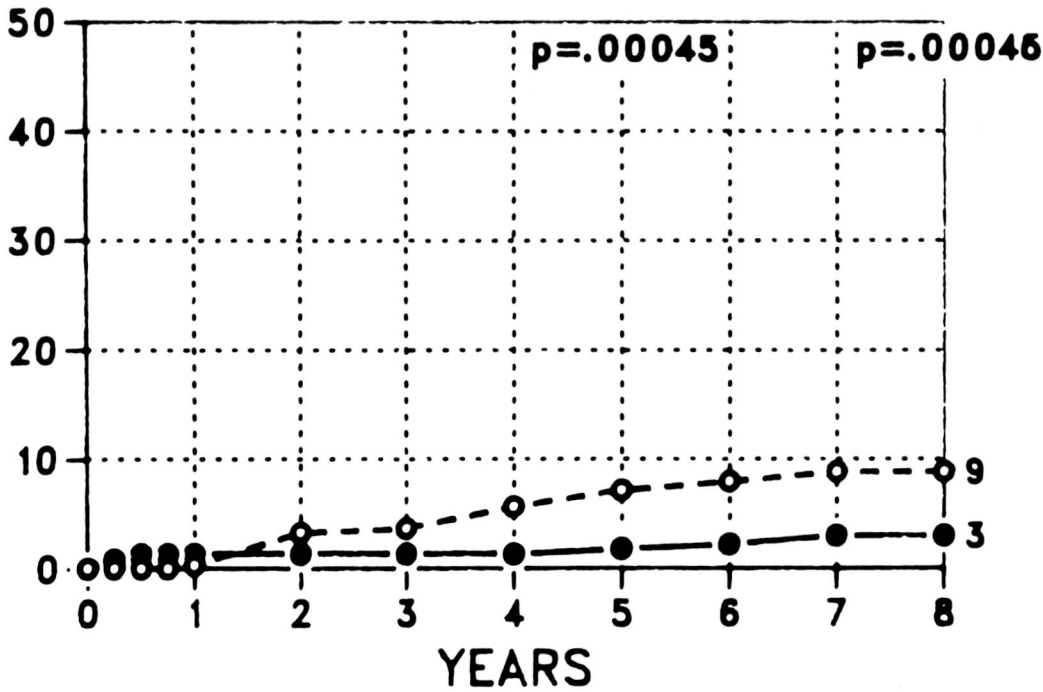

Fig. 36–4. Cumulative risk of sudden cardiac death in patients assigned to medical (○) vs. surgical therapy (●). (Reproduced with permission from Varnauskas E, and the European Surgical Study Group: Circulation 72(suppl V):V90–V101, 1985.[21]).

et al,[24] Morady et al,[25] and Kehoe et al[26] reported a low postoperative mortality rate in a combined total of 28 cardiac arrest survivors *without inducible arrhythmias* who underwent surgical myocardial revascularization. However, the results with anti-ischemic drug therapy in similar patients were also good. In the previously mentioned report by Wilber et al[9] of the long-term follow-up of 166 survivors of SCD without an acute MI, cardiac surgery was an independent predictor of a favorable outcome. Of note, 27 of the 34 surgically treated patients in that series underwent myocardial revascularization only.

Less information is available specifically concerning the effects of revascularization in patients *with inducible ventricular arrhythmias*. Kelly and associates[27] reported the suppression of inducible ventricular tachyarrhythmias after CABG surgery in 14 of 31 patients. On multivariant analysis, the induction of ventricular fibrillation (VF) at the preoperative electrophysiological study was the only significant predictor of the suppression of inducible ventricular arrhythmias by coronary surgery. By contrast, inducible VT persisted in 80% of patients in whom preoperative electrophysiological testing induced this arrhythmia. Kron et al[28] reported that revascularization alone was effective in five of eight cardiac arrest survivors who had either polymorphic VT or VF (but *not* sustained monomorphic VT) inducible at a preoperative electrophysiological study.

Importantly, recurrent monomorphic VT usually is not controlled by myocardial revascularization alone, and direct excision or ablation of the tissue responsible for the tachycardia usually is required when a surgical approach is chosen.[29,30] Alternatively, an implantable defibrillator may be the therapy selected (discussed in other chapters in greater detail).

Considering all the information currently

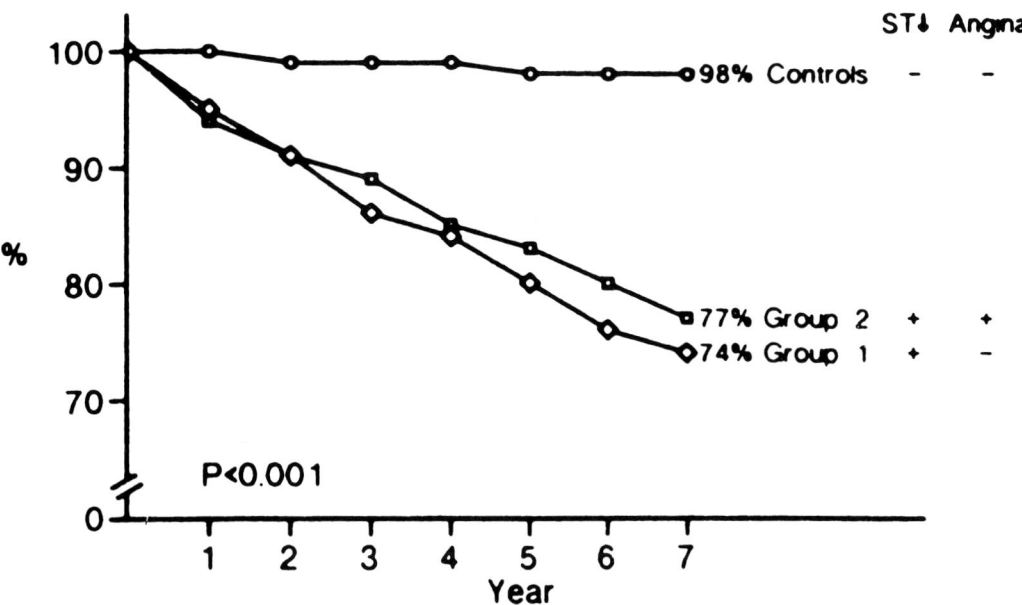

Fig. 36–5. Cumulative 7-year probability of remaining free of myocardial infarction and sudden death among group 1 (silent ST ↓ with exercise) and group 2 (pain + ST ↓ with exercise) and among 1019 patients without coronary artery disease or a positive exercise test. The control patients had substantially fewer events. (Reproduced with permission from Weiner DA, et al: Am J Cardiol 62: 1155–1158, 1988.[22]).

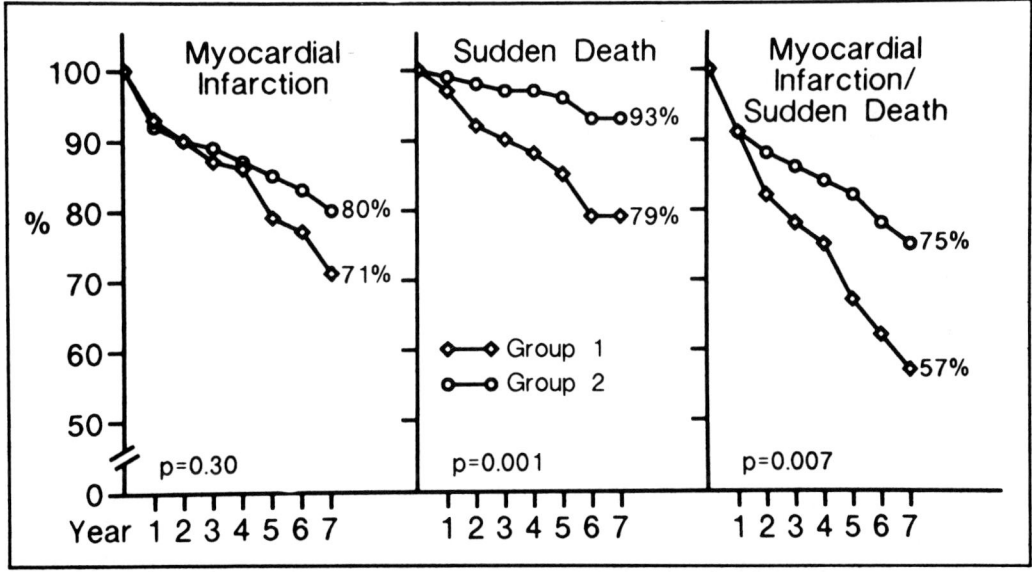

Fig. 36–6. Cumulative 7-year probability of remaining free of infarction, sudden death, and the combined end points among patients without (group 1) or with (group 2) angina during exercise-induced ST-segment depression. All had three-vessel disease. Sudden death and combined end points were more frequent among group 1 patients. (Reproduced with permission from Weiner DA, et al: Am J Cardiol 62:1155–1158, 1988.[22])

available, surgical myocardial revascularization should be considered as part of the therapeutic approach to most patients resuscitated from cardiac arrest, especially those with suspected or definite episodes of acute myocardial ischemia. Pre- and postoperative electrophysiological testing is usually indicated.[3]

Coronary artery surgery should be considered as primary therapy for survivors of sudden death with critical coronary artery stenosis, significant regions of myocardium at risk, and no inducible ventricular arrhythmias at electrophysiological study.[9] In patients with inducible polymorphic VT or VF, postoperative testing is essential since fewer than half of these patients will have their arrhythmias suppressed by myocardial revascularization alone.[1,3]

It should be emphasized that patients with sustained monomorphic VT at electrophysiological study and scars due to prior MI will usually *not* be treated successfully with coronary artery surgery alone; a direct surgical approach, defibrillator implantation, and/or postoperative antiarrhythmic therapy usually will be necessary.

These conclusions concerning the role of revascularization apply only when CABG surgery is the method employed. Similar data concerning revascularization using either angioplasty or when thrombolysis reopens an infarct vessel are not available. However, Stack et al[31] reported a low rate of SCD after early intravenous thrombolytic therapy followed by emergency coronary angioplasty. In that study, 94% of 342 patients underwent successful reperfusion. There were only eight cardiac deaths after discharge, for a 1-year survival rate of 98% among the 304 patients who survived to hospital discharge.

In the 1988 ACC/AHA guidelines for PTCA, there was general agreement that coronary angioplasty is justified (Class I indication) for patients with appropriate single-vessel or multivessel coronary artery disease who "have been resuscitated from cardiac arrest or from sustained ventricular tachycardia in the absence of acute myocardial infarction."[32] However, since there is an average restenosis rate of 30% during the first 6 months after PTCA and since the restenosis may or may not be associated with chest pain, the risk of recurrent SCD likely will be greater in such patients treated with PTCA than in similar patients who have undergone CABG surgery. Thus, if a patient's initial manifestation of myocardial ischemia is VF, a general recommendation for PTCA as the appropriate sole therapy for this patient cannot be justified at this time.[1]

SUMMARY

The usually pathological finding in SCD is extensive atherosclerotic coronary artery disease. Clinical observations indicate that acute myocardial ischemia is often a contributing factor.

Clinical trials using β-blockers in postinfarction patients and surgical myocardial revascularization in patients with chronic ischemic heart disease have demonstrated a reduction in both sudden and total cardiac deaths after intervention.

Knowledge of the presence and extent of coronary artery disease, the severity of regional and global left ventricular dysfunction, the formation of ventricular aneurysms, and the presence or absence of spontaneous or inducible ischemia has great implications for effective therapeutic management.

Coronary artery surgery should be considered as primary therapy in patients with critical coronary artery stenosis, significant regions of myocardium at risk, and no inducible ventricular arrhythmias at electrophysiological testing. In survivors of sudden death with preoperative inducible polymorphic VT or VF, repeat electrophysiological testing after surgery is essential since only 50% will be suppressed by revascularization surgery alone. In patients with sustained monomorphic VT on electrophysiological testing and scars due to prior MI, CABG surgery alone will usually not be successful in preventing postoperative induction of the same arrhythmia.

Currently, there are no data to support PTCA as the *sole* therapy for post-SCD patients who have inducible VT or VF on electrophysiological testing.

REFERENCES

1. O'Rourke RA: Role of myocardial revascularization in sudden cardiac death. Circulation 85(suppl I):I-2–I-10, 1992.

2. Hinkle LE, Thaler HT: Clinical classification of cardiac deaths. Circulation 65: 457–464, 1982.
3. Ruskin JN, McGovern B, Garan H: Sudden death. In Stein JH (ed): Internal Medicine, 3rd ed. Boston, Little, Brown, 1990, pp 108–112.
4. Barbour DJ, Warnes CA, Roberts WC: Cardiac findings associated with sudden death secondary to atherosclerotic coronary artery disease: Comparison of patients with and those without previous angina pectoris and/or healed myocardial infarction. Circulation 75(suppl 2):9–11, 1987.
5. Baum RS, Alvarez H III, Cobb LA: Survival after resuscitation from out-of-hospital ventricular fibrillation. Circulation 50: 1231–1235, 1974.
6. Lieberthson RR, Nagel EL, Hirschman JC, Nussenfield SR, Blackbourne BD, Davis JH: Pathophysiologic observations in prehospital ventricular fibrillation and sudden cardiac death. Circulation 499:790–798, 1974.
7. Davis MJ, Thomas A: Thrombosis and acute coronary artery lesions in sudden cardiac ischemic death. N Engl J Med 310:1137–1140, 1984.
8. Stevenson WG, Wiener I, Yeatman L, Wohlgelernter D, Weiss JN: Complicated atherosclerotic lesions: A potential cause of ischemic ventricular arrhythmias in cardiac arrest survivors who do not have inducible ventricular tachycardia? Am Heart J 116: 1–6, 1988.
9. Wilber DJ, Garan H, Finkelstein D, et al: Out-of-hospital cardiac arrest: Use of electrophysiologic testing in the prediction of long-term outcome. N Engl J Med 318: 19–24, 1988.
10. Holmes DR, Davis K, Gersh BJ, Mock MB, Pettinger MB, Coronary Artery Surgery Study (CASS): Risk factor profiles of patients with sudden cardiac death and death from other cardiac causes. A report from the Coronary Artery Surgery Study (CASS). J Am Coll Cardiol 13:524–531, 1989.
11. DiMarco JP, Haines DE: Sudden cardiac death. Curr Probl Cardiol 15:185–232, 1990.
12. Willich SN, Levy D, Roco MB, Tofler GH, Stone PH, Muller JE: Circadian variation in the incidence of sudden cardiac death in the Framingham Heart Study population. Am J Cardiol 60:801–806, 1987.
13. Marcus FI, Cobb LA, Edwards JE, et al: Mechanism of death and prevalence of myocardial ischemic symptoms in the terminal event after acute myocardial infarction. Am J Cardiol 61:8–15, 1988.
14. Garan H, McComb JM, Ruskin JN: Spontaneous and electrically induced ventricular arrhythmias during acute ischemia superimposed on 2 week old canine myocardial infarction. J Am Coll Cardiol 11:603–611, 1988.
15. Ritchie JL, Hallstrom AP, Trobaugh GB, et al: Out of hospital sudden coronary artery death: Rest and exercise radionuclide left ventricular function in survivors. Am J Cardiol 55:645–651, 1985.
16. Bigger JT, Fleiss JL, Kleiger R, Miller JP, Rolnitzky LM: The relationships among ventricular arrhythmias, left ventricular dysfunction and mortality in the 2 years after myocardial infarction. Circulation 69: 250–258, 1984.
17. Crawford MH, O'Rourke RA: The role of cardiac catheterization in patients after myocardial infarction. Cardiol Clin 2:105–111, 1984.
18. Beta Blocker Heart Attack Trial Research Group: A randomized trial of propranolol in patients with acute myocardial infarction: I. Mortality results. JAMA 247:1707–1714, 1982.
19. Holmes DR, Davis KB, Mock MB, et al: The effect of medical and surgical treatment on subsequent sudden cardiac death in patients with coronary artery disease: A report from the Coronary Artery Surgery Study. Circulation 73:1254–1263, 1986.
20. Passamani E, Davis KB, Gillespie MJ, Killip T: A randomized trial of coronary artery bypass surgery: Survival of patients with a low ejection fraction. N Engl J Med 312: 1665–1671, 1985.
21. Varnauskas E, and the European Coronary Surgery Study Group: Survival, myocardial infarction and employment status in a prospective randomized study of coronary bypass surgery. Circulation 72(suppl V): V90–V101, 1985.
22. Weiner DA, Ryan TS, McCabe CH, et al: Risk of developing an acute myocardial infarction or sudden death in patients with exercise-induced silent myocardial ischemia: A report from the Coronary Artery Surgery Study (CASS) registry. Am J Cardiol 62: 1155–1158, 1988.
23. Tresch DD, Wetherbee JN, Siegel R, Troup PJ, Keelan MH Jr, Orlinger GN: Long-term follow-up of survivors of prehospital sudden cardiac death treated with coronary bypass surgery. Am Heart J 110:1139–1145, 1985.
23a. Every NR, Fahrenbrach CE, Hallstrom AP, Weaver WD, Cobb LA: Influence of coronary bypass surgery on subsequent outcome of patients resuscitated from out of hospital cardiac arrest. J Am Coll Cardiol 19: 1435–1438, 1992.

24. Swerdlow CD, Freedman RA, Peterson J, Clay D: Determinants of prognosis in ventricular tachyarrhythmia patients without induced sustained arrhythmias. Am Heart J 111:433–438, 1986.
25. Morady F, DiCarlo L, Winston S, Davis JC, Scheinman MN: Clinical features and prognosis of patients with out of hospital cardiac arrest and a normal electrophysiologic study. J Am Coll Cardiol 4:39–44, 1984.
26. Kehoe R, Tommaso C, Zheutlin T, et al: Factors determining programmed stimulation responses and long-term arrhythmic outcome in survivors of ventricular fibrillation with ischemic heart disease. Am Heart J 116:355–363, 1988.
27. Kelly P, Ruskin JN, Vlahakes GJ, Buckley MJ Jr, Freeman CS, Garan H: Surgical coronary revascularization in survivors of prehospital cardiac arrest: Its effects on ventricular arrhythmias and long-term survival. J Am Coll Cardiol 15:267–273, 1990.
28. Kron IL, Lerman BB, Haines DE, Flanagan TL, DiMarco JP: Coronary bypass grafting in patients with ventricular fibrillation. Ann Thorac Surg 48:85–89, 1989.
29. Ricks WB, Winkle RA, Shumway NE, Harrison DC: Surgical management of life-threatening ventricular arrhythmias in patients with coronary artery disease. Circulation 56:38–42, 1977.
30. Buda AJ, Stinson EB, Harrison DC: Surgery for life-threatening ventricular tachyarrhythmias. Am J Cardiol 44:1171–1177, 1979.
31. Stack RS, Califf RM, Hinohara T, et al: Survival and cardiac event rates in the first year after emergency coronary angioplasty for acute myocardial infarction. J Am Coll Cardiol 11:1141–1149, 1988.
32. Ryan TJ, Faxon DP, Gunnar RM, et al: Guidelines for percutaneous transluminal coronary angioplasty: A report of the American College of Cardiology/American Heart Association Task Force on Assessment of Diagnostic and Therapeutic Cardiovascular Procedures. Circulation 78:486–502, 1988.

37
Role of Noninvasive Techniques to Guide Drug Therapy in High-Risk Cases

SUSAN O'DONOGHUE
EDWARD PLATIA

The prevention of sudden death in patients who have survived cardiac arrest or who are believed to be at high risk remains one of the major challenges facing cardiologists. Twenty years ago the tools available for identifying high-risk patients and evaluating response to therapy were fairly limited. The technological triumphs of the past two decades might have been expected to put this elusive goal within our grasp. Notably, the introduction of ambulatory monitoring techniques by Holter in 1961 provided a practical means of evaluating the heart rhythm in a qualitative and quantitative fashion. Since most sudden deaths are due to ventricular tachycardia (VT) and fibrillation (VF), it made intuitive sense to focus on ambient ventricular arrhythmias and their response to interventions in an attempt to reduce the incidence of sudden death. This rationale led to the widespread use of what has come to be known as the noninvasive approach to managing ventricular arrhythmias. This approach includes long-term ambulatory electrocardiographic (ECG) monitoring and exercise testing to help determine risk and to guide therapy. There are two major assumptions inherent in the noninvasive approach: (1) that ventricular ectopic activity is a trigger for, or at least a marker of, sustained ventricular arrhythmias, and thus identifies the patient at risk, and (2) that suppression of ventricular ectopic activity as ascertained by noninvasive techniques will prevent the occurrence or recurrence of lethal events.

This chapter examines the data relevant to these two assumptions and the current verdict regarding the use of noninvasive techniques to guide drug therapy.

AMBULATORY ELECTROCARDIOGRAPHIC MONITORING

The use of ambulatory monitoring for the evaluation and treatment of patients with ventricular arrhythmias has several attractive features. It is widely available and relatively inexpensive, and the data are relatively easy to interpret. It yields quantitative and qualitative information regarding the heart rhythm and can be performed while the patient carries out his usual daily activities. Repeat studies during long-term follow-up provide information on the progression or stability of any detected arrhythmia. Symptoms that the patient experiences during the period of recording can be correlated with the simultaneous heart rhythm recording.

It is a matter of pure chance, and therefore relatively unusual, for an episode of sustained VT or VF to be recorded during ambulatory monitoring. Therefore, it is primarily premature ventricular complexes (PVCs) and nonsustained VT that are quantitated and used to evaluate drug therapy. It becomes crucial, then, to have a working classification of arrhythmias which bears prognostic significance, to understand the natural variability of ventricular ectopy as measured by ambulatory monitoring, and to devise a definition of suppression and proarrhythmia in response to drug therapy.

CLASSIFICATION OF VENTRICULAR ARRHYTHMIAS

In 1971 Lown and Wolf presented a grading system for PVCs based on frequency and the presence of "complex" forms—multiform PVCs, couplets, salvos, and R-on-T complexes.[1] The rationale for the classification was based on observations made in the coronary care unit with patients hospitalized for acute myocardial infarction (MI). The cause of sudden death in this setting was usually VF, and such patients often experienced certain PVC forms, thus characterized as high grade, prior to developing VF. A modified version of the Lown classification became widely adopted and was employed in innumerable studies of chronic ischemic heart disease and other patient populations (Table 37–1). The shortcomings of the Lown classification were acknowledged by Lown at the time of its introduction, and further limitations to its practical application were later described.[2] Multiform complexes and R-on-T phenomena were found to have no independent prognostic significance, and more recent large studies have focused on the quantitative assessment of PVCs and the presence or absence of nonsustained VT.

The absence of established norms or a standard classification for ventricular arrhythmias contributes to, and is a reflection of, the difficulty of assessing their prognostic significance. It is reasonably well established that complex ventricular arrhythmias can occur in apparently normal hearts and have little or no prognostic significance. In the setting of heart disease, particularly coronary disease, the presence of frequent PVCs or nonsustained VT is associated with an increased mortality.[3-12] However, many of the studies that demonstrated this association could not clearly separate the influence of ventricular arrhythmias from that of reduced ejection fraction. Two large multicenter trials have concluded that ventricular arrhythmias are an independent predictor of mortality. The Multicenter Investigation of the Limitation of Infarct Size (MILIS) followed 532 patients for up to 24 months following infarction. Twenty-four-hour monitoring was performed on day 10 post infarction.[13] Multivariate analysis demonstrated that the presence of PVCs of ≥10/hr was the strongest single predictor of sudden death independent of left ventricular (LV) function, which was the second most predictive variable. Importantly, among 280 survivors reclassified 6 months post infarction, neither frequent PVCs nor LV dysfunction predicted sudden death over the subsequent 18 months. The Multicenter Post-Infarction Research Group (MPIP) examined the relationships among ventricular arrhythmias, LV dysfunction, and mortality in 766 patients, again utilizing predischarge 24-hour ambulatory monitoring.[14] LV dysfunction, nonsustained VT, and PVCs of ≥3/hr were found to have independent prognostic significance. LV dysfunction was a better predictor of mortality in the first 6 months post infarction, whereas the presence of ventricular arrhythmias was a better predictor of late mortality (Table 37–2).

Some controversy remains regarding interpretation of the data from MILIS and MPIP.[15] The relationship between ventricular arrhythmias and LV function in chronic coronary disease was examined by Califf et al.[16] Three hundred ninety-five patients referred for cardiac catheterization were evaluated with 24-hour ambulatory ECG. Ventricular arrhythmias, as classified by the modified Lown grading system, did not con-

Table 37–1
Lown Classification of Ventricular Arrhythmia

Lown Grade	Definition
0	No ventricular premature depolarizations (VPDs)
1	<30 VPDs/hr
2	≥30 VPDs/hr
3	Multiform VPDs
4A	Paired VPDs
4B	≥3 consecutive VPDs
5	R-on-T VPDsn(R-V/QT < 1.0)

Table 37-2
Independent Contribution of Left Ventricular Dysfunction and Ventricular Arrhythmias to Death Early (<6 mo) and Late After Myocardial Infarction

Factor	Hazard Ratio* 0–6 mo	>6 mo	Z Ratio†	p value
LVEF <0.30	5.4	1.9	2.8	<0.01
1–3 VPDs/hr	0.8	2.0	1.2	NS
≥3 VPDs/hr	1.2	3.7	2.2	<0.05
Paired VPDs	1.1	3.8	1.8	<0.10
VPD runs	1.8	2.0	0.3	NS

* Ratio of the instantanous probability of dying per unit time for patients with the factor to that for patients without the factor.
† Critical ratio comparing two hazard ratios.

tribute independent prognostic information. Ejection fraction was more useful in identifying patients at high risk of sudden death.

It is clear that many factors contribute to the risk of sudden death, and therefore it should not be surprising that simply categorizing ventricular arrhythmias by ambulatory monitoring is of limited value. Bigger suggested classifying ventricular arrhythmias as malignant, potentially malignant, or benign.[17] This type of classification acknowledges the importance of both substrate and trigger in the genesis of lethal arrhythmias.

VARIABILITY OF VENTRICULAR ARRHYTHMIAS

Many investigators have examined the temporal variability of ventricular arrhythmias and the resulting influence on both risk stratification and the evaluation of drug therapy. Morganroth et al found that in 15 stable patients with various cardiac disorders, the spontaneous variation in PVC frequency was 48% from hour to hour, 23% from day to day, and 37% between repeated 3-day monitoring periods.[18] It was suggested that when a 24-hour monitoring period was used, an 83% reduction in PVC frequency was required to distinguish a true therapeutic effect from spontaneous or biological variability. In a similar analysis, Michelson and Morganroth reported that a 65% decrease in mean hourly frequency of VT was needed to demonstrate therapeutic effect.[19] Pratt et al examined spontaneous variability during 4 consecutive days of recording.[20] In addition to confirming the presence of significant day-to-day variability, the study found that patients with coronary artery disease have significantly greater variability in PVC frequency than patients without coronary disease. Furthermore, patients with ten or more runs of VT had significant hourly variability, and therefore an 85% reduction in VT was required to distinguish drug effect from spontaneous variability. In the presence of five or fewer VT runs, even 100% suppression may be the result of variability alone. Many other investigators have employed efficacy criteria based on similar analyses.[21–24] The suppression criteria adopted by the Cardiac Arrhythmia Suppression Trial (CAST) were an 80% reduction in PVCs and a 90% reduction in ventricular runs.

In addition to hourly and daily variability, ventricular arrhythmias exhibit long-term biological variability. This is particularly pertinent in the postinfarction setting. Several studies have chronicled the natural history of ventricular arrhythmias following MI.[25,26] Klieger et al provided Holter data from 289 survivors of infarction at 2 weeks, at monthly intervals of 6 months, and then at 9 and 12 months.[27] Nonsustained VT was least prevalent at 2 weeks post infarction, most prevalent at 1 month, and leveled off after 3 months (Fig. 37–1). Thus, the early postinfarction period may be particularly treacherous from the standpoint of meaningful interpretation of Holter data. Even patients with chronic "stable" ventricular ectopy can exhibit significant long-term variability. Pratt et al reported on 26 patients with symptomatic, complex "non-life-threatening" ventricular arrhythmias.[28] Compared to the initial ambulatory ECG recording, a second recording made a mean of 17 months later showed 50% reduction in PVCs and an 83% reduction in VT. Over one third of patients appeared to have therapeutic efficacy during this second placebo period.

Short- and long-term variability in the fre-

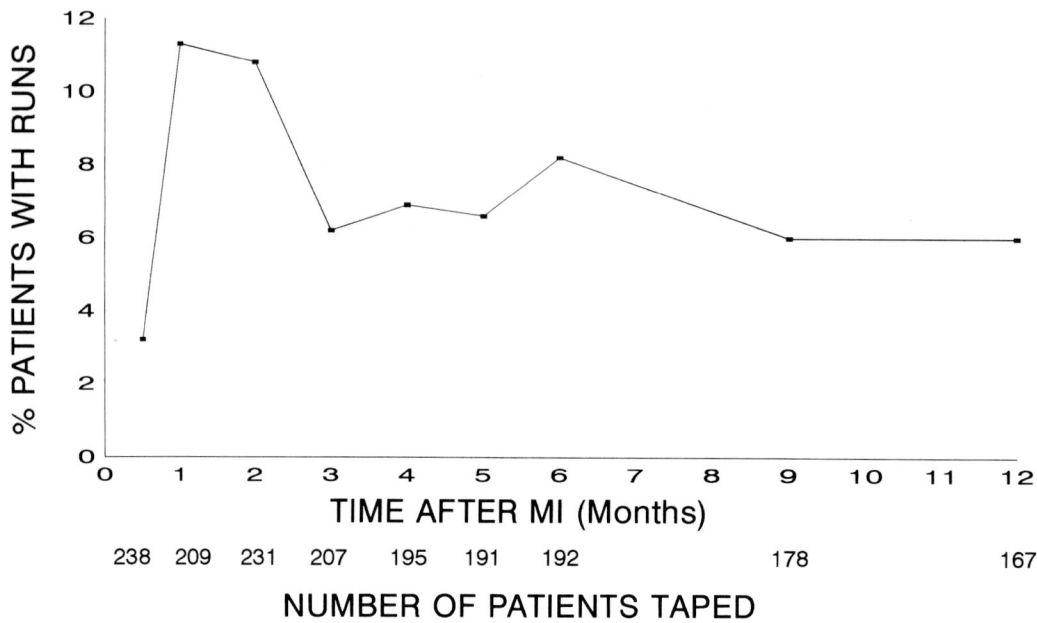

Fig. 37–1. Percentage of patients with ventricular runs and time after myocardial infarction (MI). The frequency of ventricular runs is lowest at 2 weeks, becomes highest at 1 month, decreases, and then levels off 2–12 months after MI.

quency of ventricular arrhythmias must be taken into account when managing individual patients as well as in the design of clinical trials.

DEFINITION OF PROARRHYTHMIA

It is well known that antiarrhythmic agents can result in the appearance of new arrhythmias or aggravate pre-existing ones. Virtually any form of bradyarrhythmia or tachyarrhythmia may be caused by an "antiarrhythmic" agent. Criteria proposed for the definition of ventricular proarrhythmia are shown in Table 37–3.[29] The distinction between proarrhythmia and lack of drug efficacy can be exceedingly difficult when a patient exhibits increased frequency of PVCs or VT during drug therapy. Ironically, those patients at highest risk for spontaneous sustained ventricular arrhythmias are the most likely to have a proarrhythmic response, and also the most likely to demonstrate drug inefficacy.[30–32] Velebit et al reported on 155 patients who underwent 48 hours of baseline ambulatory ECG monitoring followed by serial drug testing.[33] In this group, which had a high density of ventricular arrhythmias and relatively little hourly variability, proarrhythmia could be defined as a fourfold increase in PVC frequency or a tenfold increase in repetitive forms. The extrapolation of this definition of proarrhythmia to patients whose baseline variability has not been established or who have a lower frequency of arrhythmia is tenuous

Table 37–3
Criteria for Ventricular Proarrhythmia

Torsades de pointes with QT prolongation

New onset of sustained, uniform ventricular tachycardia (conversion of nonsustained ventricular tachycardia to sustained ventricular tachycardia)

New, multiform, sustained ventricular premature complexes or repetitive forms

Responses to programmed electrical stimulation:
    Conversion of nonsustained to sustained ventricular tachycardia
    Increased rate of ventricular tachycardia
    Initiation of ventricular tachycardia with fewer premature stimuli

Table 37-4
Definitions of Proarrhythmic Effects in the Cardiac Arrhythmia Suppression Trial

A. Increase in Ventricular Premature Complex (VPC) Frequency

Baseline Frequency (Average VPCs/hr)	Increase Required to Declare Proarrhythmia* (Average VPCs/hr)
10	10×
30	7×
100	4×
300	3×
1000	2×

B. Increase in Unsustained Ventricular Tachycardia (VT)

Baseline Frequency (Episodes of VT/Day)	Frequency Required to Declare Proarrhythmia
<5	>50 episodes/day
≥5	>10× increase

C. New sustained VT
D. New torsades de pointes VT

*Multipliers obtained from the empirical formula: $y = \exp[3.118 + 0.646 (\ln[x])]$, where x = baseline VPCs/hr.

at best. The criteria for definition of ventricular proarrhythmia adopted by the CAST investigators are shown in Table 37–4.

EXERCISE TESTING

Exercise testing has long been used as an adjunct to ambulatory monitoring in the evaluation and treatment of ventricular arrhythmias. There is a sound physiological basis for the belief that exercise testing can provide additional useful clinical information. Exercise is accompanied by autonomic, electrophysiological, hemodynamic, and metabolic alterations that can directly or indirectly provoke arrhythmias (Fig. 37–2).[34]

There are two ways in which exercise testing can be used to evaluate the response of ventricular arrhythmias to drug therapy. The first involves defining effective therapy by demonstrating suppression of ventricular arrhythmias during exercise testing. Lown,

Graboys and colleagues found that in their experience, 10–15% of patients with a history of sustained ventricular tachyarrhythmia had spontaneous arrhythmia during exercise testing but not during ambulatory ECG recordings.[35,36] They also reported that 15% of patients whose arrhythmia appeared to be controlled on ambulatory monitoring still had repetitive ventricular arrhythmias induced by exercise. This would support the usefulness of exercise testing in evaluating drug efficacy. However, there are data showing significant variability in exercise-induced ventricular arrhythmias.[37,38] Even patients with prior sustained ventricular arrhythmias may not exhibit complex ventricular ectopy during exercise testing. Therefore, the presence and reproducibility of exercise-related arrhythmias should be established before exercise testing is considered as a therapeutic end point.

The second reason to perform exercise testing in assessing antiarrhythmic drug therapy is to look for evidence of proarrhythmia or adverse hemodynamic drug effects. Exercise-provoked proarrhythmia may be secondary to ischemia, which can alter conduction velocity and promote reentrant VT. Alternatively, the arrhythmia aggravation may relate to the primary autonomic and concomitant electrophysiological changes that accompany exercise. Slater and colleagues reported a group of patients in whom exercise testing yielded evidence of proarrhythmia despite apparent suppression of ectopy on ambulatory monitoring.[32]

Although exercise testing has been recommended as part of arrhythmia management for all patients, its exact role remains to be defined, particularly when used in conjunction with electrophysiological testing.

CLINICAL EXPERIENCE WITH THE NONINVASIVE APPROACH

The most compelling data regarding therapy of sustained ventricular tachyarrhythmias utilizing the noninvasive approach are that of Graboys et al, reported in 1982.[23] Their methods and results will be recounted in some detail, because this publication laid the groundwork for much of clinical practice in recent years. Their study included

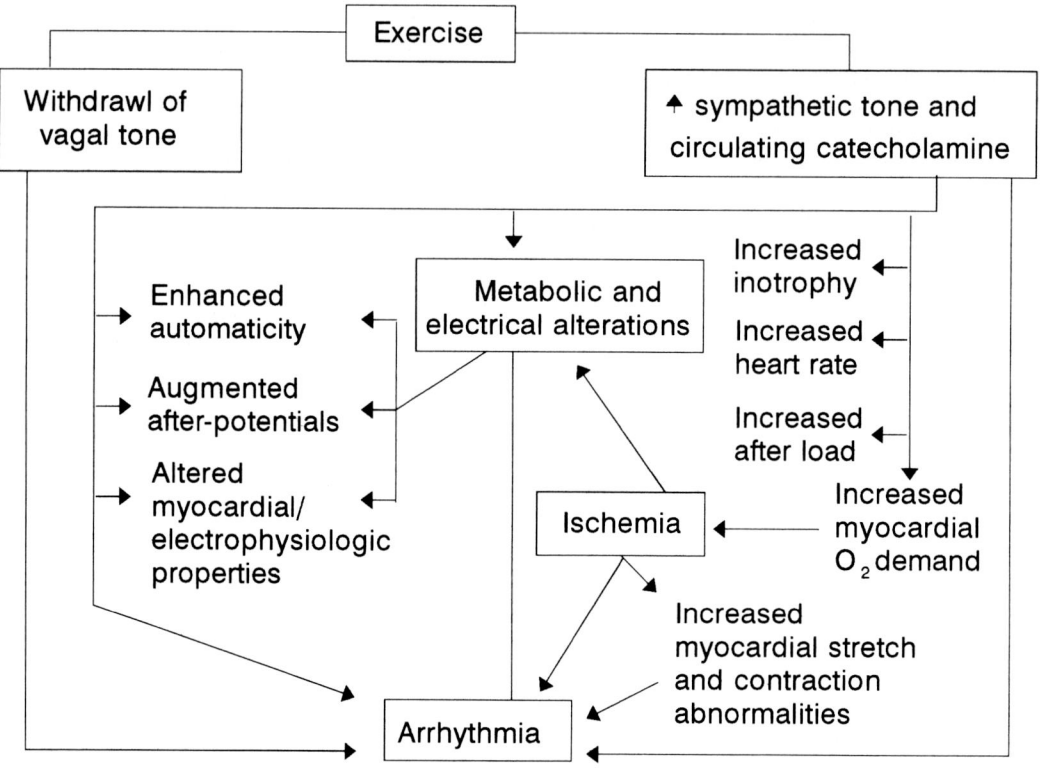

Fig. 37–2. Role of exercise testing to induce arrhythmia. With exercise there are changes in autonomic tone, especially an increase in sympathetic neural inputs to the heart and circulating catecholamines. These changes cause important direct and indirect effects that can induce arrhythmia.

123 patients with one or more episodes of sustained, hemodynamically compromising VT or VF. Initial evaluation included 48 hours of continuous ECG monitoring in the drug-free state, as well as a baseline exercise treadmill test (performed in 60 patients). This was followed by acute drug testing, which consisted of a control period utilizing monitoring and bicycle ergometry and subsequent administration of single large oral doses of antiarrhythmic agents, with bicycle ergometry and monitoring then repeated. Blood sampling for drug concentration was carried out at frequent intervals. Each patient underwent an acute drug test every 24 hours, for an average of six drug tests. The second phase of drug testing employed maintenance oral doses for 48–96 hours, accompanied by 24-hour monitoring and exercise testing. Drugs that had appeared effective during acute testing as well as drugs that could not be tested in a single large dose were used in this second phase.

Successful therapy was defined as abolition of grades 4B and 5 ectopy, 90% reduction in grade 4A, and >50% reduction in total PVCs by both ambulatory monitoring and exercise testing. Once an effective response was demonstrated, two of the drugs tested were generally selected for maintenance therapy. The average hospital stay to define effective therapy was 17 days. With this protocol, effective therapy was identified in 79.7% of patients. During a follow-up of 29 months, the annual sudden death rate was 2.3% in patients in whom therapy was deemed effective and 43% in patients in whom successful therapy was not identified.

Several important issues must be addressed regarding these data. First, the extremely low mortality observed in the group with effective drug therapy has not been successfully reproduced, possibly because other investigators have used less rigorous noninvasive testing.[39,40] The patient population in the Graboys study may have been biased toward those with a high density of ambient arrhythmias, in whom a noninvasive end point might be most reliable. The study also included a fairly large proportion of patients (44%) with normal LV function. It must also be noted that the study design did not allow the investigators to determine whether (1) the drug therapy that suppressed ventricular ectopy resulted in a reduction in sudden death, or (2) the ability to suppress ventricular ectopy identified patients who have a low risk of recurrent events. The fact that many of the patients had already had recurrent events supports the former interpretation. However, this interpretative limitation applies to all nonrandomized trials.

Innumerable studies have demonstrated the ability of Class I antiarrhythmic agents to suppress ventricular arrhythmias. The relative efficacy of the various agents was reviewed in a recent meta-analysis.[41] The evidence that drugs could suppress ventricular arrhythmias, along with the persuasive logic of the "PVC hypothesis," led to widespread use of Class I agents guided by noninvasive end points. It is important to recognize that the common clinical practice of placing a patient on one antiarrhythmic drug and performing 24-hour ambulatory ECG monitoring to demonstrate suppression is not the equivalent of the noninvasive approach as reported by Graboys et al. Furthermore, randomized trials have been unable to demonstrate a beneficial effect on mortality from use of Class I antiarrhythmic agents. Furberg[42] reviewed the six largest randomized trials reported before March 1983 (Table 37–5), and Yusuf and Teo have provided a more recent review of the available large randomized trials.[43] There are many limitations of the various study designs that may have contributed to the lack of demonstrable benefit. Many trials did not use presence of ventricular arrhythmias as an entry criterion, did not titrate drug therapy, or did not demonstrate suppression. Most utilized a single antiarrhythmic agent rather than carrying out serial testing, and sudden death mortality was not separated from total mortality. Most clinical trials have included predominantly patients who are not in the highest-risk subgroups, and thus a true beneficial effect for some of the patients might be masked by lack of benefit or harm to enrolled low-risk patients. The results of CAST, which tested the PVC hypothesis in a large trial without these design flaws, are discussed elsewhere in this volume.

Demonstrating benefit in the highest-risk subgroups in a randomized trial will be difficult because of ethical constraints regarding a "no-treatment" arm in cardiac arrest survivors. The introduction of drug testing using electrophysiological studies effectively shifted emphasis away from the noninvasive approach for the highest-risk patients. Because electrophysiological testing errs on the side of overpredicting drug failure, whereas ambulatory monitoring overpredicts drug success, the invasive approach has been considered more prudent.[39,40,44] The availability and success of implantable cardioverter-defibrillators have further undermined the role of, and evaluation by, the noninvasive approach.

There are recent and ongoing randomized

Table 37–5
Long-Term Trial of Antiarrhythmics: Mortality Results

	No. Randomized		No. of Deaths		% Mortality		
Trial	Control	Intervention	Control	Intervention	Control	Intervention	p Value*
Collaborative group	285	283	26	23	9.1	8.1	0.75
Peter et al	76	74	14	18	18.4	24.3	0.49
Ryden et al	56	56	5	5	8.9	8.9	1.0
Bastian et al	74	72	3	4	4.1	5.6	0.97
Chamberlain et al	163	181	19	24	11.7	13.3	0.78
Hagemeijer et al	149	151	18	11	12.1	7.3	0.25

* p values computed for χ^2 test comparing the proportion of deaths in each group.

trials that should provide some information regarding the comparative efficacy of the various treatment approaches. The Electrophysiological Study versus Electrocardiographic Monitoring (ESVEM) trial compared the predictive accuracy of the noninvasive approach and electrophysiological testing for prevention of recurrent ventricular tachyarrhythmias by antiarrhythmic drugs.[45,46] Qualifying entry criteria included a clinical history of at least 15 seconds of documented ventricular tachycardia or fibrillation, or unmonitored syncope. Patients were eligible for enrollment if they averaged at least 10 PVCs per hour by 48-hour Holter monitoring and had inducible ventricular tachycardia by electrophysiological study. Patients were then randomly assigned to undergo serial testing of up to six antiarrhythmic drugs by either the noninvasive approach (Holter monitoring plus exercise testing), or electrophysiological study.

Of 2103 patients enrolled in the study, 486 were randomized, and 296 ultimately received a drug predicted to be effective. Seventy-seven percent of the Holter monitoring group received a prediction of efficacy, versus 45% of the electrophysiologic study group. After 1 year, there were fewer arrhythmia recurrences in the electrophysiological study group. However, over a 6-year follow-up period there were 150 arrhythmia recurrences and 34 arrhythmic deaths among the 296 patients, with no difference in actuarial probabilities of events in the two study groups.

These high event rates suggest that neither approach by itself has an acceptable predictive accuracy for high-risk patients, especially in the era of implantable defibrillators. The ESVEM patient population had a high density of ambient ventricular arrhythmia (average 330 PVCs/hr; 85% with nonsustained VT by Holter monitoring), while only 21% of patients initially presented with cardiac arrest. These clinical characteristics may be the result of selection bias, and must be considered before extrapolating ESVEM results to other types of patients. Whether ESVEM is an indictment of serial drug testing by electrophysiologic testing is unclear. In reality, the complementary data provided by telemetry monitoring and electrophysiologic testing are used to guide patient therapy. Electrophysiologic testing is undertaken only if a particular antiarrhythmic drug appears to suppress ambient VT, which was not the case in ESVEM. Finally, the generally accepted protocol for electrophysiologic testing is significantly more rigorous than that employed in ESVEM. This may account in part for the relatively high percent prediction of efficacy and recurrence rate seen in the EPS limb of ESVEM. Brugada's "parallel study," although not a randomized trial, may also provide insights into the prognostic significance of both invasive and noninvasive techniques.[47]

AMBULATORY MONITORING AND AMIODARONE THERAPY

The unique pharmacodynamics of amiodarone make its efficacy more difficult to evaluate using electrophysiological testing than that of other antiarrhythmic agents. Therefore particular attention has been given to the role of ambulatory monitoring in patients treated with amiodarone. Several investigators have determined that both the positive and negative predictive values of ambulatory monitoring are reasonably good (Table 37–6).[48] Of particular importance, the likelihood that suppression of complex ventricular arrhythmia by ambulatory monitoring portends a good clinical outcome is greater for amiodarone than for Class I antiarrhythmic drugs. Thus ambulatory monitoring may have a special role in guiding therapy with amiodarone. However, it must be cautioned that for patients without sufficient complex ventricular arrhythmias during baseline monitoring, the prognostic value of ambulatory monitoring during amiodarone treatment is uncertain, since "suppression" cannot be demonstrated.

AMBULATORY MONITORING IN IDIOPATHIC DILATED CARDIOMYOPATHY

Idiopathic dilated cardiomyopathy is the third most common cause of congestive heart failure in the United States. The prognosis is related to the degree of ventricular

Table 37-6
Amiodarone Therapy Guided by Holter Monitoring

	No. of Pts. Evaluated	Mean Follow-up (mo)	Rec. and/or SCD Not Predicted by Holter	Rec. and/or SCD Predicted by Holter	Sensitivity (%)	Specificity (%)	Positive Predictive Value (%)	Negative Predictive Value (%)
Veltri (1986)	52	11	3/34	12/18	80	84	67	91
Marchlinski (1985)	74	11	6/34	11/21	65	74	52	82
Nademanee (1982)	13	12	0/13	—	—	—	—	—
Sokoloff (1986)	107	14	16/53	9/27	36	67	33	70
Kim (1987)	80	19	—	—	47	75	39	80
					31	94	71	75
					44	88	54	82
					42	93	67	82

Abbreviations: Rec., recurrence; SCD, sudden cardiac death.

dysfunction, the presence of symptoms, and the presence of complex ventricular ectopy. Many of the studies reporting on clinical outcome in congestive heart failure include patients with coronary disease as well as nonischemic cardiomyopathies. There are, however, a number of studies confined to patients with idiopathic dilated cardiomyopathy that have examined the relationship between ventricular arrhythmias and survival. Huang and associates followed up 35 patients for between 4 and 74 months, and compared patients with and without nonsustained VT at baseline.[49] No association was demonstrated between ventricular arrhythmias and survival; however, there were only two sudden deaths during follow-up, the patient group without VT had poorer functional status, and no multivariate analysis was performed. In a group of 69 patients, Unverforth and colleagues reported a 35% mortality at 1 year, with most deaths considered sudden.[50] Ventricular arrhythmias were an independent prognostic factor. In contrast, Von Olshausen and associates found no correlation between ventricular arrhythmias on ambulatory monitoring and survival in 60 patients. However, only three sudden deaths occurred in this study, which included many patients with an ejection fraction between 0.40 and 0.55.[51] Meinertz and coworkers reported an association between frequent nonsustained VT and sudden death in seventy-four patients,[52] and Romeo and colleagues found complex ventricular arrhythmias to be the only independent predictor of sudden death in 104 patients.

Despite the reasonably well-established relationship between ventricular arrhythmias and sudden death in patients with idiopathic dilated cardiomyopathy, there is as yet no evidence that antiarrhythmic drug therapy guided by the noninvasive approach can reduce the risk of sudden death. No study has been carried out comparing antiarrhythmic therapy to no therapy using suppression of ventricular arrhythmia as an end point. A small comparative study that did not evaluate suppression found no benefit to the use of antiarrhythmic drug therapy.[53] There are ongoing trials evaluating the efficacy of amiodarone in idiopathic dilated cardiomyopathy.

THE NONINVASIVE APPROACH IN HYPERTROPHIC CARDIOMYOPATHY

The majority of deaths due to hypertrophic cardiomyopathy are sudden and likely due to tachyarrhythmias. Several studies have identified nonsustained VT as one of the risk factors for sudden death in this population.[54-56] Medical therapy has included β-blockade, calcium channel blockade, disopyramide, and amiodarone. These agents have been used for their hemodynamic effects as well as for antiarrhythmic properties. Although there is good evidence for symptomatic and hemodynamic benefit, no randomized trials are available comparing drug therapy to placebo with regard to survival. A small controlled study demonstrated suppression of nonsustained VT by disopyramide, and ongoing trials should determine its effect on survival.[57] McKenna and colleagues have demonstrated suppression of ventricular ectopy by amiodarone, and in uncontrolled studies have suggested improved survival on amiodarone.[58-60] These findings are in contrast to these of Leon and coworkers, who found an increased incidence of sudden death with amiodarone therapy.[61] A randomized trial seems warranted in light of the potential toxicity of amiodarone and the young age of many patients with hypertrophic cardiomyopathy.

SUMMARY

In the past two decades, knowledge regarding the mechanisms involved in sudden death and the risk factors for various patient populations has expanded considerably. The development of ambulatory ECG monitoring techniques provided a tool that has become widely used in an attempt to identify patients at risk and to guide antiarrhythmic drug therapy. Yet there is no evidence that this strategy has resulted in lower patient mortality. In fact, data from the CAST study, as well as that inferred from the large number of smaller uncontrolled studies, suggest that the risk to patients may outweigh the benefit. Why? Perhaps the high-risk patient must be more selectively defined, so that adverse effects in patients who do not need treatment do not obscure the favorable response in patients who should be treated. Perhaps Class I antiarrhythmic drugs have too many unfavorable or unpredictable effects to be truly valuable in preventing sudden death. Almost certainly, widespread de facto acceptance of the "PVC hypothesis," with its compelling logic and simplicity, has fostered continued use of antiarrhythmic drugs because they suppress PVCs.

The genesis of lethal ventricular arrhythmias is a complex, multifactorial process. In the presence of a suitable substrate, usually in the form of damaged myocardium, triggering arrhythmias, autonomic influences, ischemia, electrolyte abnormalities, and a myriad of other subtle influences may conspire to initiate the fatal arrhythmia. It is therefore not surprising that identifying effective drug therapy is difficult, and why therapy that appears effective should prove ineffective. Yet the clinician still must determine whether and how to treat individual patients. Table 37-7 outlines potential roles of noninvasive testing for which there are some supportive data. Within the realm of identification of high-risk patients, noninvasive testing is useful in the setting of coronary disease, idiopathic dilated cardiomyopathy, and hypertrophic cardiomyopathy. There are insufficient data regarding prognostic value in other entities, such as restrictive cardiomyopathy, mitral valve prolapse, and heart failure due to valvular heart disease. For patients with coronary disease,

Table 37-7
Role of Noninvasive Techniques in the Management of Ventricular Arrhythmias

	Ambulatory Electrocardiographic Monitoring	Exercise Testing
Identification of high-risk pt.		
Coronary artery disease	+	+
Idiopathic dilated cardiomyopathy	+	?
Hypertrophic cardiomyopathy	+	+
Evaluation of drug therapy		
Class 1 agents		
Detection of proarrhythmia	+	+
Efficacy (prevention of sudden death)	?	?
Suppression of exercise-mediated VT	?	+
Amiodarone		
Efficacy (prevention of sudden death)	+	?

noninvasive indices, which include ejection fraction and signal-averaged ECGs, can clearly select a subgroup at very high risk for sudden death.[62,63] However, risk stratification benefits patients only if it results in therapy that can reduce that risk. The only drug therapy known to reduce the risk of sudden death in coronary disease is β-blockade, and its effect is not directly dependent on the presence or suppression of PVCs. Therefore, the true value of noninvasive testing for risk stratification is dependent on the development of additional treatment strategies of proven efficacy. Since Class I antiarrhythmic drug therapy guided by noninvasive techniques has not proved to reduce the incidence of sudden death and has potential adverse effects, it cannot be recommended.

For patients who have already survived an episode of sustained ventricular tachyarrhythmia in the absence of reversible cause, risk stratification is no longer the issue. It seems prudent to guide the treatment of such patients with the most rigorous of assessments. Since invasive-guided therapy has a higher negative predictive value than noninvasive techniques, this approach has become widely recommended. Ongoing trials will compare the effectiveness of various treatment strategies. The precise role of noninvasive techniques as an adjunct to the invasive approach is not yet well defined. It is reasonable to believe that the two approaches will provide additive information. Certainly ambulatory monitoring and exercise testing are useful in detecting ischemia-related proarrhythmia or late proarrhythmia.

REFERENCES

1. Lown B, Wolf M: Approaches to sudden death from coronary heart disease. Circulation 43:130–142, 1971.
2. Bigger JT Jr, Weld FM: Analysis of prognostic significance of ventricular arrhythmias after myocardial infarction: Shortcomings of Lown grading system. Br Heart J 45:717–724, 1981.
3. Kennedy HL, Pescarmona JE, Bouch RJ, Goldberg RJ: Coronary artery status of apparently healthy subjects with frequent and complex ventricular ectopy. Ann Intern Med 92:179–185, 1980.
4. Brodsky M, Wu D, Denes P, Kanakis C, Rosen KM: Arrhythmias documented by 24 hour continuous electrocardiographic monitoring in 50 male medical students without apparent heart disease. Am J Cardiol 39:390–395, 1977.
5. Hinkle LE, Carver ST, Argyros DC: The prognostic significance of ventricular premature contractions in healthy people and in people with coronary heart disease. Acta Cardiol 43:5–32, 1974.
6. Kostis JB, McCrone K, Moreya AE, et al: Premature ventricular complexes in the absence of identifiable heart disease. Circulation 63:1351–1356, 1981.
7. Kotler MN, Tabatznik B, Mower MM, Tominaga S: Prognostic significance of ventricular ectopic beats with respect to sudden death in the late postinfarction period. Circulation 47:959–966, 1973.
8. Ruberman W, Weinblatt E, Goldberg JD, Frank CW, Shapiro S: Ventricular premature beats and mortality after myocardial infarction. N Engl J Med 297:750–757, 1977.
9. Bigger JT, Weld FM: Analysis of prognostic significance of ventricular arrhythmias after myocardial infarction. Br Heart J 45:717–724, 1981.
10. Moss AJ, Davis HT, DeCamilla J, Bayer LW: Ventricular ectopic beats and their relation to sudden and nonsudden cardiac death after myocardial infarction. Circulation 60:998–1003, 1978.
11. Anderson KP, DeCamilla J, Moss AJ: Clinical significance of ventricular tachycardia (3 beats or longer) detected during ambulatory monitoring after myocardial infarction. Circulation 57:890–897, 1978.
12. Bigger JT Jr, Weld FM, Rolnitzky LM: Prevalence, characteristics, and significance of ventricular tachycardia (three or more complexes) detected with ambulatory electrocardiographic recording in the late hospital phase of acute myocardial infarction. Am J Cardiol 48:815–823, 1981.
13. Mukharji J, Rude RE, Poole K, et al: Risk factors for sudden death after acute myocardial infarction: Two-year follow-up. Am J Cardiol 54:31–36, 1984.
14. Bigger JT, Fleiss JL, Klieger R, et al: The relationships among ventricular arrhythmias, left ventricular dysfunction, and mortality in the 2 years after myocardial infarction. Circulation 69:250–258, 1984.
15. Surawicz B: Prognosis of ventricular arrhythmias in relation to sudden cardiac death: Therapeutic implications. J Am Coll Cardiol 10:435–437, 1987.
16. Califf RM, McKinnis RA, Burks J, et al: Prognostic implications of ventricular ar-

rhythmias during 24 hour ambulatory monitoring in patients undergoing cardiac catheterization for coronary artery disease. Am J Cardiol 50:23–31, 1982.
17. Bigger JT: Definition of benign versus malignant ventricular arrhythmias: Targets for treatment. Am J Cardiol 52:47C–54C, 1983.
18. Morganroth J, Michelson EL, Horowitz LN: Limitations of routine long-term electrocardiographic monitoring to assess ventricular ectopy. Circulation 58:408–414, 1978.
19. Michelson EL, Morganroth J: Spontaneous variability of complex ventricular arrhythmias detected by long-term electrocardiographic recording. Circulation 61:690–695, 1980.
20. Pratt CM, Slymen DJ, Wierman AM, et al: Analysis of the spontaneous variability of ventricular arrhythmias: Consecutive ambulatory electrocardiographic recordings of ventricular tachycardia. Am J Cardiol 56:67–72, 1985.
21. Sami M, Kraemer H, Harrison DC, et al: A new method for evaluating antiarrhythmic drug efficacy. Circulation 62:1172–1179, 1980.
22. Mitchell LB, Duff HJ, Maryari DE, Wyse DG: A randomized clinical trial of noninvasive and invasive approaches to drug therapy of ventricular tachycardia. N Engl J Med 317:1682–1687, 1987.
23. Graboys TB, Lown B, Podrid PJ, DeSilva R: Long-term survival of patients with malignant ventricular arrhythmias treated with antiarrhythmic drugs. Am J Cardiol 50:437–443, 1982.
24. Kim SG, Seiden SW, Matos JA, Waspe JE, Fisher JD: Discordance between ambulatory monitoring and programmed stimulation in assessing efficacy of Class IA antiarrhythmic agents in patients with ventricular tachycardia. J Am Coll Cardiol 6:539–544, 1985.
25. Bigger JT Jr, Weld FM, Coromilas J, Rolnitzky LM, DeTurk WE: Prevalence and significance of arrhythmias in 24-hour ECG recordings made within one month of acute myocardial infarction. In Kulbertus HE, Wellens HJJ (eds): The first year after a myocardial infarction. Mt. Kisko, NY, Futura, 1983; pp 161–175.
26. Lichstein E, Morganroth J, Harrist R, for the BHA Study Group: Effect of propranolol on ventricular arrhythmia: The Beta-Blocker Heart Attack Trial experience. Circulation 67(suppl I):I-5–I-10, 1983.
27. Klieger RE, Miller JP, Thanavaro S, et al: Relationship between clinical features of acute myocardial infarction and ventricular runs two weeks to one year following infarction. Circulation 63:64–70, 1981.
28. Pratt CM, Delclos G, Wierman AM, et al: The changing baseline of complex ventricular arrhythmias. N Engl J Med 313:1444–1449, 1985.
29. Horowitz LN, Zipes DP, Bigger T Jr, et al: Proarrhythmia, arrhythmogenesis or aggravation of arrhythmia: A status report 1987. Am J Cardiol 59:54E–56E, 1987.
30. Ruskin JN, McGoven B, Garan H, DiMarco JP, Kelly E: Antiarrhythmic drugs: A possible cause of out-of-hospital cardiac arrest. N Engl J Med 6:424–428, 1983.
31. Rae AP, Jay HR, Horowitz LN, Spielman SR, Greenspon AM: Proarrhythmic effects of antiarrhythmic drugs in patients with malignant ventricular arrhythmias evaluated by electrophysiologic testing. J Am Coll Cardiol 12:131–139, 1988.
32. Slater W, Lampert S, Podrid PJ, Lown B: Clinical predictors of arrhythmia worsening by antiarrhythmic drugs. Am J Cardiol 61:349–353, 1988.
33. Velebit V, Podrid P, Lown B, Cohen BH, Graboys TB: Aggravation and provocation of ventricular arrhythmias by antiarrhythmic drugs. Circulation 65:886–894, 1982.
34. Podrid PJ, Venditti FJ, Levine PA, Klein MD: The role of exercise testing in evaluation of arrhythmias. Am J Cardiol 62:24H–33H, 1988.
35. Lown B, Podrid PJ, DeSilva RA, Graboys TB: Sudden cardiac death: Management of the patient at risk. Curr Probl Cardiol 4:1–62, 1980.
36. Graboys TB: Limitations of ambulatory ECG recording to assess therapy in the individual patient. In Wenger NK, Mock MB, Ringvist I (eds): Ambulatory Electrocardiographic Recording. Chicago, Year Book Medical, 1981; pp 367–377.
37. Faris JV, McHenry PC, Jordan JW, Morris SN: Prevalence and reproducibility of exercise-induced ventricular arrhythmias during maximal exercise testing in normal men. Am J Cardiol 37:617–622, 1976.
38. Sheps DS, Ernst JC, Briese FR, et al: Decreased frequency of exercise-induced ventricular ectopic activity in the second of two consecutive treadmill tests. Circulation 55:892–895, 1977.
39. Platia EV, Reid PR: Comparison of programmed electrical stimulation and ambulatory electrocardiographic (Holter) monitoring in the management of ventricular tachycardia and ventricular fibrillation. J Am Coll Cardiol 4:493–500, 1984.
40. Mitchell LB, Duff HJ, Maryari DE, Wyse DG: A randomized clinical trial of noninvasive and invasive approaches to drug therapy of ventricular tachycardia. N Engl J Med 317:1682–1687, 1987.

41. Salerno D, Gillingham KJ, Berry DA, Hodges M: A comparison of antiarrhythmic drugs for the suppression of ventricular ectopic depolarizations: A meta-analysis. Am Heart J 120:340-353, 1990.
42. Furberg CD: Effect of antiarrhythmic drugs on mortality after myocardial infarction. Am J Cardiol 52:32C-36C, 1983.
43. Yusuf S, Teo KK: Approaches to prevention of sudden death: Need for fundamental reevaluation. J Cardiovasc Electrophysiol 2: S233-S239, 1991.
44. Kim SG: Values and limitations of programmed stimulation and ambulatory monitoring in the management of ventricular tachycardia. Am J Cardiol 62:7I-12I, 1988.
45. Mason JW, ESVEM Investigators: A comparison of electrophysiologic testing with Holter monitoring to predict antiarrhythmic drug efficacy for ventricular tachyarrhythmias. N Engl J Med 329:445-451, 1993.
46. Ward DE, Camm AJ: Dangerous ventricular arrhythmias—can we predict drug efficacy? (editorial). N Engl J Med 329:498-499, 1993.
47. Brugada P, Lemery R, Talajic M, Bella PD, Wellens HJJ: Treatment of patients with ventricular tachycardia or ventricular fibrillation: First lessons from the "parallel study." In Brugada P, Wellens HJJ (eds): Cardiac Arrhythmias: Where to Go From Here? Mount Kisco, NY, Futura, 1987; pp 457-470.
48. Gottlieb C, Josephson ME: The preference of programmed stimulation-guided therapy for sustained ventricular arrhythmia. In Brugada P, Wellens HJJ (eds): Cardiac Arrhythmias: Where to Go From Here? Mount Kisco, NY, Futura, 1987; pp 421-434.
49. Huang SK, Messer JV, Denes P: Significance of ventricular tachycardia in idiopathic dilated cardiomyopathy: Observations in 35 patients. Am J Cardiol 51: 507-512, 1983.
50. Unverforth DV, Magorien RD, Moeschbarger ML, et al: Factors influencing the one-year mortality of dilated cardiomyopathy. Am J Cardiol 54:147-152, 1984.
51. Von Olshausen K, Schafer A, Mehmal HC, et al: Ventricular arrhythmias in idiopathic dilated cardiomyopathy. Br Heart J 51: 195-201, 1984.
52. Meinertz T, Hofmann T, Kasper W, et al: Significance of ventricular arrhythmias in idiopathic dilated cardiomyopathy. Am J Cardiol 53:902-907, 1984.
53. Chakko S, Gheorghiade M: Ventricular arrhythmias in severe heart failure: Incidence, significance, and effectiveness of antiarrhythmic therapy. Am Heart J 109:497-504, 1985.
54. Savage D, Seides S, Maron B, Myers D, Epstein S: Prevalence of arrhythmias during 24 hour electrocardiographic monitoring and exercise testing in patients with obstructive and nonobstructive hypertrophic cardiomyopathy. Circulation 59:866-875, 1979.
55. Maron B, Savage D, Wolfson J, Epstein S: Prognostic significance of 24 hour ambulatory electrocardiographic monitoring in patients with hypertrophic cardiomyopathy: A prospective study. Am J Cardiol 48:252-257, 1981.
56. McKenna W, England D, Doi Y, et al: Arrhythmia in hypertrophic cardiomyopathy: I. Influence on prognosis. Br Heart J 46: 168-172, 1981.
57. Pollick C: Disopyramide in hypertrophic cardiomyopathy: II. Noninvasive assessment after oral administration. Am J Cardiol 62:1252-1255, 1988.
58. McKenna W, Harris L, Perez G, et al: Arrhythmias in hypertrophic cardiomyopathy: II. Comparison of amiodarone and verapamil in treatment. Br Heart J 46:173-178, 1981.
59. McKenna W, Oakley C, Krikler D, Goodwin J: Improved survival with amiodarone in patients with hypertrophic cardiomyopathy and ventricular tachycardia. Br Heart J 53: 412-416, 1985.
60. McKenna W, Adams K, Polonieki J, et al: Long-term survival with amiodarone in patients with hypertrophic cardiomyopathy and ventricular tachycardia. Circulation 80(suppl II):II-7, 1989.
61. Leon M, Tracy C, Winkler J, Berganio C, Bonow R, Epstein S: Amiodarone does not prevent, and may increase, sudden death in patients with hypertrophic cardiomyopathy. Circulation 76(suppl IV):IV-248, 1987.
62. Gomes JA, Winters SL, Martinson M, et al: The prognostic significance of quantitative signal-averaged variables relative to clinical variables, site of myocardial infarction, ejection fraction, and ventricular premature beats: A prospective study. J Am Coll Cardiol 13:377-384, 1989.
63. Breithardt G, Martinez-Rubio A, Borggrefe M: Correlation between programmed ventricular stimulation and signal-averaged electrocardiograms in the identification of patients at high risk for serious ventricular arrhythmias. PACE 13:685-691, 1990.

38

Serial Electrophysiological-Electropharmacological Testing in Survivors of Cardiac Arrest

ERIC N. PRYSTOWSKY
TIMOTHY K. KNILANS

For many years antiarrhythmic drugs have been the primary therapy administered to cardiac arrest survivors to prevent recurrence of sustained ventricular tachyarrhythmia. Progressive advances in technology of the implantable cardioverter-defibrillator coupled with many scientific publications demonstrating its effectiveness in preventing sudden death in patients previously resuscitated from an episode of cardiac arrest have elevated the implantable cardioverter-defibrillator to first-line treatment in many instances. Thus, it is important to review the role of antiarrhythmic drug therapy for cardiac arrest survivors, including primary therapy to prevent recurrences of sustained ventricular tachycardia (VT) or fibrillation (VF) as well as secondary treatment in patients with an implantable cardioverter-defibrillator. Many published studies report on patients with sustained monomorphic VT as well as cardiac arrest survivors, but for the purpose of this chapter, only data from studies dealing solely with cardiac arrest victims are reviewed.

CANDIDATES FOR SERIAL ELECTROPHYSIOLOGICAL-ELECTROPHARMACOLOGICAL TESTING

Patients eligible for serial electrophysiological-electropharmacological testing must have a ventricular tachyarrhythmia induced at control study to guide drug efficacy.[1] In our opinion, only sustained ventricular tachyarrhythmias should be used to guide serial drug testing. It has been known for many years that induction of sustained VT or VF depends not only on the type of heart disease the patient has but also on the presenting clinical arrhythmia.[2,3] In general, patients who have coronary artery disease are more likely to have an arrhythmia induced than those with no heart disease or cardiomyopathy, and induction rates are higher with sustained monomorphic VT than in patients who have been resuscitated from cardiac arrest.[2,3]

The results of electrophysiological testing in 1473 survivors of cardiac arrest are summarized in Table 38–1.[4-16] None of these patients had a cardiac arrest associated with an acute myocardial infarction (MI). Seventy-one percent of patients had coronary artery disease, and the programmed electrical stimulation protocols used varied somewhat among the investigators. In most cases three ventricular extrastimuli were used and more than one ventricular site was chosen for testing. Undoubtedly differences in protocol design account for some of the variations in arrhythmias initiated and the total percentage of patients who had an inducible arrhythmia. Regardless, sustained ventricular tachyarrhythmias were induced in 719

Table 38–1
Inducibility of Ventricular Tachyarrhythmias in Survivors of Cardiac Arrest

Study	PES Protocol (No. of VES)	No. of Pts.	CAD (%)	No. of MVT-S	No. of PVT/VF	No. of VT-NS	No. of Non-inducible	Non-inducible and VT-NS (%)
Roy et al[4]	2 or 3	119	71	45	27	11	36	40
Benditt et al[5]	4	31	65	25†	—	2	4	19
Raviele et al[6]	2	10	91	8	1	1	0	10
Stevenson et al[7]	3	15	100	7	4	—	4‡	27
Skale et al[8]	2 or 3	58	55	41§	2	—	15	—
Swerdlow et al[9]	3	140	69	56	27	16	41	41
Eldar et al[10]	3	108	61	41	11	23	33	52
Wilber et al[11]	2 or 3	166	75	61	25	45	35	48
Freedman et al[12]	3	150	67	82	23	8	37	30
Kehoe et al[13]	2	38	100	17	4	1	16	45
Hays et al[14]	3	100	64	40	29	0	31	31
Poole et al[15]	2 to 4	241	69	66	39	34	102	56
Fogoros et al[16]	3	217	70	—‖	—	—	81	37
Prystowsky*	3	80	87	26	12	—	42‡	53
Total	—	1473	71%	515 (41%)	204 (16%)	141 (11%)	477 (32%)	10–56%

Abbreviations: PES, programmed electrical stimulation; CAD, coronary artery disease; MVT-S, monomorphic sustained ventricular tachycardia; PVT, polymorphic sustained ventricular tachycardia; VF, ventricular fibrillation; VT-NS, nonsustained ventricular tachycardia; VES, ventricular extrastimuli.
* Consecutive series of patients, 1988–91.
† MVT-S vs. PVT not specified.
‡ Includes VT-NS.
§ MVT-S vs. VT-NS not specified.
‖ Inducibility not differentiated between MVT-S, PVT/VF, and VT-NS.

patients, and 41% had sustained monomorphic VT and 16% had VF or sustained polymorphic VT initiated. Nonsustained VT was initiated in some patients, but we would not recommend that this arrhythmia be used to guide serial drug testing.

An ongoing controversy has been whether to accept initiation of VF at control electrophysiological study as an arrhythmia against which to judge drug efficacy.[16] This is especially true if VF is initiated using triple ventricular extrastimuli, which has a decreased specificity.[1] Those who argue in favor of using induction of VF at baseline study to judge drug efficacy give as evidence that VF is often the clinical arrhythmia identified at resuscitation of cardiac arrest victims. The opposing argument accepts VF as a clinical arrhythmia but recognizes that initiation of VF can be a nonspecific finding. This issue still remains unsettled, but we currently allow the use of induced VF during control study as an index arrhythmia to guide drug testing. Of note, Buxton and colleagues[17] have suggested that if inducible VF at control study converts to sustained monomorphic VT initiated in the cause of antiarrhythmic drug treatment, the VF most likely represents a true positive result. These data are intriguing but require further investigation.

Serial electrophysiological-electropharmacological testing has been evaluated in several studies of cardiac arrest survivors.[4–6,8,10–13,15] Because differences in pacing protocols, definitions of suppressibility, and use of amiodarone in patients who have not responded to other drug trials are present in the studies, exact comparisons among the trials are difficult to perform. The use of amiodarone in many patients and the fact that inducible sustained ventricular arrhythmia during amiodarone therapy does not necessarily augur a poor prognosis[18] make it particularly difficult to evaluate results from many of these investigations. Regardless, the majority of data demonstrate that during drug treatment noninducibility of ventricular tachyarrhythmias compared with continued inducibility confers a better prognosis regarding freedom from recurrent cardiac arrest in this patient group.[4,5,8,10-13]

Differences of opinion regarding the usefulness of serial electrophysiological drug testing in survivors of cardiac arrest are highlighted in two large series of patients with divergent results.[11,15] Wilber et al[11] evaluated results in 166 cardiac arrest survivors. They reported recurrent cardiac arrest in 11 (12%) of 91 patients in whom inducible VF or VT was suppressed by treatment (83 patients received drugs), in 12 (33%) of 36 patients who had continued initiation of VT, and in 6 (17%) of 35 patients who had no inducible VF or VT at initial control electrophysiological study. Univariate analysis showed persistence of inducible VT during treatment, a left ventricular ejection fraction (LVEF) of ≤0.30, and absence of coronary artery revascularization or endocardial resection as significant variables related to recurrent cardiac arrest. In particular, continued inducibility of VT independent of LVEF or cardiac surgery was associated with approximately a fourfold increase in recurrent cardiac arrest. Further evaluation demonstrated that LVEF as a covariable was important in patients who had no inducible arrhythmia during therapy. The 1-year incidence of cardiac arrest was 14% for patients with an LVEF of ≤0.30, and approximately 1–2% for those with an LVEF of >0.30. These latter data are of particular importance and demonstrate that factors other than inducibility should be taken into account during serial electrophysiological-pharmacological testing.

Contrary data were published by Poole and colleagues.[15] During serial electrophysiological drug testing in 92 patients who had documented VF at the time of cardiac arrest, successful suppression of tachyarrhythmias was noted in 19 (36%) of 56 patients with VT and 25 (69%) of 36 patients with VF initiated at control study. Follow-up data revealed that the arrhythmia-free survival did not differ between patients in whom the arrhythmia was suppressed and those in whom it was still induced. Of note, 71% of patients who still had inducible ventricular tachyarrhythmias during treatment with a Class I antiarrhythmic drug were discharged receiving amiodarone without a repeat electrophysiological test. In addition, the authors[15] define successful suppression of inducible arrhythmias during drug testing as the inability to initiate a sustained ventricular tachyarrhythmia. Using this definition, initiation of long runs consisting of many seconds of nonsustained VT could be considered a success, which would be defined as a failure by many other investigators.

In summary, although differences are apparent between investigators regarding the role of serial electrophysiological-electropharmacological testing in survivors of cardiac arrest, the majority of data do support the use of this methodology.

ALTERNATIVE METHODS TO JUDGE DRUG EFFICACY

Empirical Approach

We discourage the use of empirical drug selection to treat cardiac arrest survivors, for this method has resulted in a relatively high rate of cardiac arrest recurrence.[19-22] Liberthson et al[19] noted that 10 of 29 cardiac arrest survivors treated empirically died suddenly during follow-up. Myerburg et al[21] demonstrated a 10% rate of recurrent cardiac arrest in the first year and a 5% recurrence rate in the second, third, and fourth years of follow-up during chronic antiarrhythmic drug therapy in patients with cardiac arrest. These authors did not use specific invasive or noninvasive antiarrhythmic suppression criteria, but did use plasma drug levels as a "therapeutic" guide.

Noninvasive Testing

Lown and Graboys[23] have advocated the use of serial Holter monitoring and exercise testing to guide efficacy of antiarrhythmic drug treatment. Their approach is rigorous and consists of testing during a loading and maintenance phase of drug treatment using specific criteria for reduction in ventricular arrhythmia. Using this approach they reported the annual incidence of sudden death during follow-up in patients with effective compared with ineffective therapy to be 2.3% and 43.6%, respectively.[23] They often used two antiarrhythmic drugs in their study to provide a so-called fail-safe program of drug protection, and details regarding the various drug combinations employed are not clearly delineated in their report.

A comparison of noninvasive and invasive methods to guide drug therapy was performed by Mitchell et al,[24] who noted that invasive testing predicted drug efficacy better than the use of noninvasive methods. However, recently reported results from the Electrophysiologic Study Versus Electrocardiographic Monitoring (ESVEM) trial demonstrated no significant difference in recurrence of arrhythmias between therapy guided by invasive and noninvasive methods.[25] Importantly, patients were entered into the ESVEM trial only if they had both sufficient spontaneous ventricular arrhythmia to guide drug therapy as well as inducible sustained ventricular tachyarrhythmias at control testing.[25] In this regard, it is relatively common for cardiac arrest survivors to have insufficient spontaneous ventricular arrhythmias to guide drug treatment.[8,24,25] Further, neither the study by Mitchell et al[24] nor ESVEM[25] contained a sufficient number of survivors of cardiac arrest to form a definitive opinion. We still prefer the use of electrophysiologically guided treatment in patients in whom antiarrhythmic drugs are given as primary therapy.

Amiodarone Therapy

The results of amiodarone therapy are a conundrum remaining to be elucidated. It has been known for many years that initiation of VT during amiodarone therapy does not preclude a favorable clinical response.[18,26-31] We think that results of electrophysiological testing with amiodarone are useful to define high-risk candidates for recurrent ventricular tachyarrhythmias, although this is somewhat controversial. In patients who are rendered noninducible, the prognosis is much better than in those in whom tachycardia can still be initiated during amiodarone treatment.[26,28-31] Further, an easier mode of tachycardia initiation during drug treatment compared with control electrophysiological study predicts arrhythmia recurrence.[27] Finally, cardiac arrest recurrences are noted in those individuals in whom the induced arrhythmia is hemodynamically unstable, whereas nonfatal recurrences usually occur in patients in whom the induced sustained tachycardia is stable at electrophysiological testing.[28]

We discourage the use of empirical amiodarone treatment in an era in which implantable cardioverter-defibrillators appear to offer a far better prognosis. Fogoros et al[32] employed empirical treatment with amiodarone in 29 patients with a history of hemodynamically unstable sustained VT or cardiac arrest, and they noted that the actuarial risk for sudden cardiac death (SCD) was 31% at 1-year follow-up. Herre et al[33] treated 427 patients with empirical amiodarone, with follow-up of ≤98 months. Patients who entered the study had either cardiac arrest or sustained VT prior to drug treatment. At 1 year the SCD rate was 9% and the incidence of SCD was significantly higher in those patients who had an LVEF of <0.40. Particularly important was the fact that the patients who presented with cardiac arrest were 3.14 times as likely to have SCD during follow-up compared with patients who had sustained VT as their initial arrhythmia. Thus, these and other data show that empirical amiodarone treatment does not confer as good a long-term prognosis in cardiac arrest victims as does an implanted cardioverter-defibrillator, in which 1-year SCD rates usually are less than 3%.

ANTIARRHYTHMIC DRUG CANDIDATES

Antiarrhythmic drugs may be given as primary therapy to prevent recurrences of VT or VF in cardiac arrest survivors, or as secondary treatment to prevent arrhythmias, for example, nonsustained VT or atrial fibrillation, that occur in patients in whom a cardioverter-defibrillator has been implanted. Drugs may also be given to patients with an implantable cardioverter-defibrillator to slow the VT rate so that antitachycardia pacing techniques may be applied, to decrease the episodes of recurrent sustained ventricular tachyarrhythmias, or to slow the rate of VT enough to allow consciousness to be maintained prior to delivery of a shock to restore sinus rhythm.

Figure 38–1 demonstrates our current approach to cardiac arrest survivors regarding use of antiarrhythmic drugs as primary therapy.[16] Since we utilize electrophysiological testing to guide drug therapy, patients will be offered antiarrhythmic drug treatment only if sustained VT or VF is initiated at control study. Recent data suggest a relatively high recurrence rate in patients who have suppressible VT or VF during drug treatment but in whom an LVEF of <0.30 is present,[11] and we no longer recommend serial testing in these individuals (Fig. 38–1). Thus, primary antiarrhythmic drug treatment is offered to patients with inducible sustained VT or VF who have an LVEF ≥0.30. As with all algorithms, exceptions occur.

The scheme presented in Figure 38–1 applies to patients who have coronary artery disease. More data are known for this group of patients, and it is less clear whether patients with cardiomyopathy or other forms of heart disease are appropriate candidates for serial electrophysiological-pharmacological testing. Our present bias is to avoid drugs as first-line treatment in these patients, and we use implantable cardioverter-defibrillators as primary treatment as a general rule. In patients who have coronary artery disease, revascularization should be performed when necessary, even in patients considered for drug treatment. Recent studies suggest that coronary artery revascularization may prevent initiation of VF after surgery that was inducible prior to surgery, but initiation of sustained monomorphic VT is uncommonly altered with revascularization.[34,35]

In patients in whom serial electrophysiological-electropharmacological testing is utilized, one must decide when to discontinue drug trials if success has not been achieved. We[16] reviewed the results from serial drug testing in 74 survivors of cardiac

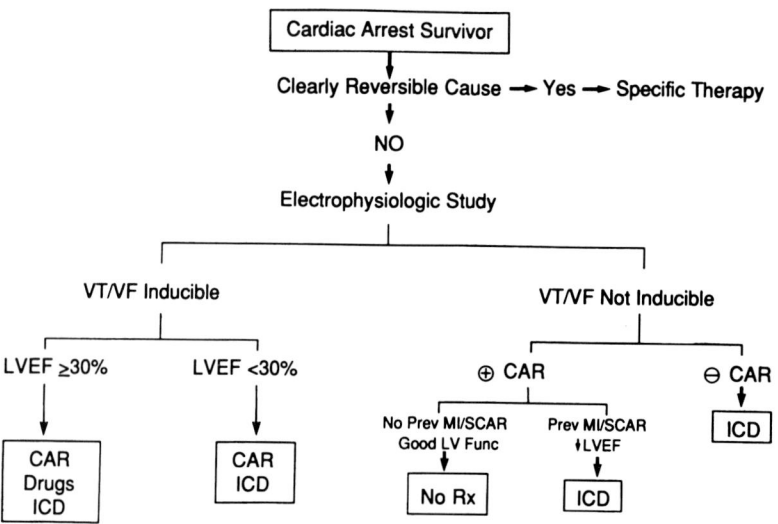

Fig. 38–1. Treatment strategy for survivors of cardiac arrest. Specific therapy should be given to patients with clearly reversible causes of cardiac arrest, for example, acute myocardial infarction. Electrophysiological study results then subdivide patients into two treatment group approaches. VT, ventricular tachycardia; VF, ventricular fibrillation; LVEF, left ventricular ejection fraction; CAR, coronary artery revascularization (+, yes; −, no); ICD, implantable cardioverter-defibrillator; Prev, previous; MI, myocardial infarction; LV Func, left ventricular function; Rx, treatment. See text for details. (Reproduced by permission of the American Heart Association from Knilans TK, and Prystowsky, EN: Circulation 85(suppl I):I-118–I-124, 1992.[16])

arrest, 51 of whom had coronary artery disease, at a time when implantable cardioverter-defibrillators were not readily available for general use. In 24 (32%) of 74 patients noninducibility occurred, and in the majority of patients a maximal beneficial effect was noted within two drug trials; it was very uncommon to identify a drug or drug combination thereafter that produced a desirable end point. Thus, our current approach for most patients is to attempt up to two drug trials and thereafter consider the patient for alternative nonpharmacological treatment.

ANTIARRHYTHMIC DRUG–IMPLANTABLE CARDIOVERTER-DEFIBRILLATOR INTERACTION

It is not uncommon for patients with an implantable cardioverter-defibrillator to receive antiarrhythmic drugs as secondary treatment. Animal data show that many of these agents can have an adverse effect to cause an increase in the defibrillation threshold. These effects often depend on the type of drug used. Encainide, flecainide, and propafenone tend to increase the defibrillation threshold, whereas fewer effects are noted with quinidine and procainamide.[36-40] Whereas Sotalol has been shown to decrease defibrillation threshold,[41] the results from amiodarone have been variable.[42-47]

A recent study of Jung et al[48] evaluated the long-term effects of antiarrhythmic drug therapy on internal defibrillation energy requirements. At a mean follow-up period of 24 ± 6 months the defibrillation threshold for all patients increased significantly ($p < 0.05$), from 14.2 ± 3.7 J at initial implantation to 18.3 ± 5.4 J at the time of device replacement. Eleven patients received chronic amiodarone treatment, and defibrillation thresholds increased in eight patients. Further, the defibrillation threshold was higher in patients who received amiodarone (21 ± 5 J) than in patients who received a Class I agent (14 ± 3 J) ($p < 0.05$). These preliminary results suggest that particular caution is necessary when amiodarone is administered to patients with an implantable cardioverter-defibrillator, especially in those patients in whom the defibrillation threshold safety margin was rather narrow at initial implantation. Re-evaluation of defibrillation thresholds is probably warranted in such circumstances.

REFERENCES

1. Prystowsky EN: Electrophysiologic-electropharmacologic testing in patients with ventricular arrhythmias. PACE *11*:225–251, 1988.
2. Naccarelli GV, Prystowsky EN, Jackman WM, Heger JJ, Rahilly GT, Zipes DP: Role of electrophysiologic testing in managing patients who have ventricular tachycardia unrelated to coronary artery disease. Am J Cardiol *50*:165–171, 1982.
3. Prystowsky EN, Miles WM, Evans JJ, et al: Induction of ventricular tachycardia during programmed electrical stimulation: Analysis of pacing methods. Circulation *73*:II-32–38, 1986.
4. Roy D, Waxman HL, Kienzle MG, Buxton AE, Marchlinski FE, Josephson ME: Clinical characteristics and long-term follow-up in 119 survivors of cardiac arrest: Relation to inducibility at electrophysiologic testing. Am J Cardiol *52*:969–974, 1983.
5. Benditt DG, Benson DW, Klein GJ, Pritzker MR, Kriett JM, Anderson RW: Prevention of recurrent sudden cardiac arrest: Role of provocative electropharmacologic testing. J Am Coll Cardiol *2*:418–425, 1983.
6. Raviele A, DiPede F, Delise P, Piccolo E: Value of serial electropharmacological testing in managing patients resuscitated from cardiac arrest. PACE *7*:850–860, 1984.
7. Stevenson WG, Brugada P, Waldecker B, Zehender M, Wellens HJJ: Clinical, angiographic, and electrophysiologic findings in patients with aborted sudden death as compared with patients with sustained ventricular tachycardia after myocardial infarction. Circulation *71*:1146–1152, 1985.
8. Skale BT, Miles WM, Heger JJ, Zipes DP, Prystowsky EN: Survivors of cardiac arrest: Prevention of recurrence by drug therapy as predicted by electrophysiologic testing or electrocardiographic monitoring. Am J Cardiol *57*:113–119, 1986.
9. Swerdlow CD, Bardy GH, McAnulty J, et al: Determinants of induced sustained arrhythmias in survivors of out-of-hospital ventricular fibrillation. Circulation *76*:1053–1060, 1987.
10. Eldar M, Sauve MJ, Scheinman MM: Electrophysiologic testing and follow-up of patients with aborted sudden death. J Am Coll Cardiol *10*:291–298, 1987.

11. Wilber DJ, Garan H, Finkelstein D, et al: Out-of-hospital cardiac arrest: Use of electrophysiologic testing in the prediction of long-term outcome. N Engl J Med *318:* 19–24, 1988.
12. Freedman RA, Swerdlow CD, Soderholm-Difatte V, Mason JW: Prognostic significance of arrhythmia inducibility or noninducibility at initial electrophysiologic study in survivors of cardiac arrest. Am J Cardiol *61:*578–582, 1988.
13. Kehoe R, Tommaso C, Zheutlin T, et al: Factors determining programmed stimulation responses and long-term arrhythmic outcome in survivors of ventricular fibrillation with ischemic heart disease. Am Heart J *116:*355–363, 1988.
14. Hays LJ, Lerman BB, DiMarco JP: Nonventricular arrhythmias as precursors of ventricular fibrillation in patients with out-of-hospital cardiac arrest. Am Heart J *118:*53–57, 1989.
15. Poole JE, Mathisen TL, Kudenchuk PJ, et al: Long-term outcome in patients who survive out of hospital ventricular fibrillation and undergo electrophysiologic studies: Evaluation by electrophysiologic subgroups. J Am Coll Cardiol *16:*657–665, 1990.
16. Knilans TK, Prystowsky EN: Antiarrhythmic drug therapy in the management of cardiac arrest survivors. Circulation *85:*I-118–I-124, 1992.
17. Buxton AE, Marchlinski FE, Miller JM, Rosenthal ME, Josephson ME: Role of procainamide in identifying clinically relevant polymorphic tachycardias. Circulation *78:* II-71(A), 1988.
18. Heger JJ, Prystowsky EN, Jackman WM, et al: Amiodarone: Clinical efficacy and electrophysiology during long-term therapy for recurrent ventricular tachycardia or ventricular fibrillation. N Engl J Med *305:*539–545, 1981.
19. Liberthson RR, Nagel EL, Hirschman JC, Nussenfeld SR: Prehospital ventricular defibrillation: Prognosis and follow-up course. N Engl J Med *291:*317–321, 1974.
20. Myerburg RJ, Conde C, Sheps DS, et al: Antiarrhythmic drug therapy in survivors of prehospital cardiac arrest: Comparison of effects on chronic ventricular arrhythmias and recurrent cardiac arrest. Circulation *59:* 855–863, 1979.
21. Myerburg RJ, Kessler KM, Estes D, et al: Long-term survival after prehospital cardiac arrest: Analysis of outcome during an 8 year study. Circulation *70:*538–546, 1984.
22. Moosvi AR, Goldstein S, Medendorp SV, et al: Effect of empiric antiarrhythmic therapy in resuscitated out-of-hospital cardiac arrest victims with coronary artery disease. Am J Cardiol *65:*1192–1197, 1990.
23. Lown B, Graboys TB: Management of patients with malignant ventricular arrhythmias. Am J Cardiol *39:*910–918, 1977.
24. Mitchell LB, Duff HJ, Manyari DE, Wyse DG: A randomized clinical trial of the noninvasive and invasive approaches to drug therapy of ventricular tachycardia. N Engl J Med *317:*1681–1687, 1987.
25. Mason JW, for the Electrophysiologic Study versus Electrocardiographic Monitoring (ESVEM) Investigators: A comparison of electrophysiologic testing with Holter monitoring to predict antiarrhythmic-drug efficacy for ventricular tachyarrhythmias. N Engl J Med *329:*445–451, 1993.
26. Heger JJ, Prystowsky EN, Miles WM, Zipes DP: Clinical experience with amiodarone for treatment of recurrent ventricular tachycardia and ventricular fibrillation. Br J Clin Pract *40:*4, No. 44, 1986.
27. Klein LW, Fineberg N, Heger JJ, et al: Prospective evaluation of a discriminant function for prediction of recurrent symptomatic ventricular tachycardia or ventricular fibrillation in coronary artery disease patients receiving amiodarone and having inducible ventricular tachycardia at electrophysiologic study. Am J Cardiol *61:*1024–1030, 1988.
28. Horowitz LN, Greenspan AM, Spielman SR, et al: Usefulness of electrophysiologic testing in evaluation of amiodarone therapy for sustained ventricular tachyarrhythmias associated with coronary heart disease. Am J Cardiol *55:*367–371, 1985.
29. Greene HL: The efficacy of amiodarone in the treatment of ventricular tachycardia or ventricular fibrillation. Prog Cardiovasc Dis *31:*319–354, 1989.
30. Fisher JD, Kim SG, Waspe LE, Johnston DR: Amiodarone: Value of programmed electrical stimulation and Holter monitoring. PACE *9:*422–435, 1986.
31. Borggrefe M, Breithardt G: Predictive value of electrophysiologic testing in the treatment of drug-refractory ventricular arrhythmias with amiodarone. Eur Heart J *7:*735–742, 1986.
32. Fogoros RN, Fiedler SB, Elson JJ: The automatic implantable cardioverter-defibrillator in drug-refractory ventricular tachyarrhythmias. Ann Intern Med *107:*635–641, 1987.
33. Herre JM, Sauve MJ, Malone P, et al: Long-term results of amiodarone therapy in patients with recurrent sustained ventricular tachycardia or ventricular fibrillation. J Am Coll Cardiol *13:*442–449, 1989.

34. Kelly P, Ruskin JN, Vlahakes GJ, Buckley MJ, Freeman CS, Garan H: Surgical coronary revascularization in survivors of prehospital cardiac arrest: Its effect on inducible ventricular arrhythmias and long-term survival. J Am Coll Cardiol 15:267–273, 1990.
35. Kron IL, Lerman BB, Haines DE, Flanagan TL, DiMarco JP: Coronary artery bypass grafting in patients with ventricular fibrillation. Ann Thorac Surg 48:85–89, 1989.
36. Fain ES, Dorian P, Davy JM, et al: Effects of encainide and its metabolites on energy requirements for defibrillation. Circulation 73:1334–1341, 1986.
37. Reiffel JA, Coromilas JM, Zimmerman JM, et al: Drug device interactions: Clinical considerations. PACE 8:369–373, 1985.
38. Peters W, Gang ES, Solingen S, et al: Acute effects of intravenous propafenone on the internal ventricular defibrillation energy requirements in the anesthetized dog [abstract]. J Am Coll Cardiol 17:129A, 1991.
39. Dawson AK, Steinberg MI, Shapland JE, et al: Effect of class I and class II drugs on current and energy required for internal defibrillation [abstract]. Circulation 72:III-383, 1985.
40. Marchlinski FE, Flores B: Effect of procainamide on the defibrillation threshold in man [abstract]. Circulation 78:II-154, 1988.
41. Wang M, Dorian P: DL and D sotalol decrease defibrillation energy requirements. PACE 12:1522–1529, 1989.
42. Fain ES, Lee JT, Winkle RA: Effects of acute intravenous and chronic oral amiodarone on defibrillation energy requirements. Am Heart J 114:8–17, 1987.
43. Williams ML, Woelfel A, Cascio WE, et al: Intravenous amiodarone during prolonged resuscitation from cardiac arrest. Ann Intern Med 110:839–842, 1989.
44. Fogoros RN: Amiodarone-induced refractoriness to cardioversion. Ann Intern Med 100:699–700, 1984.
45. Guarnieri T, Levine JH, Veltri EP, et al: Success of chronic defibrillation and the role of antiarrhythmic drugs with the automatic implantable cardioverter/defibrillator. Am J Cardiol 60:1061–1064, 1987.
46. Huang SKS, Tan de Guzman WL, Chenarides JG, et al: Effects of long-term amiodarone therapy on the defibrillation threshold and the rate of shocks of the implantable cardioverter-defibrillator. Am Heart J 122:720–727, 1991.
47. Frame LH: The effect of chronic oral and acute intravenous amiodarone administration on ventricular defibrillation threshold using implanted electrodes in dogs. PACE 12:339–346, 1989.
48. Jung W, Manz M, Luderitz B: Effects of antiarrhythmic drugs on defibrillation threshold in patients with the implantable cardioverter defibrillator. PACE 15:645–648, 1992.

39

Results of Surgery for Ventricular Tachycardia

RAMAN L. MITRA
PETRA VAN POL
JOHN M. MILLER
W. CLARK HARGROVE
MARK E. JOSEPHSON

Recurrent sustained ventricular tachycardia (VT) that is refractory to programmed stimulation-guided antiarrhythmic therapy accounts for up to 60% of patients with postinfarction VT.[1] Alternative therapeutic options that are currently available to prevent or treat potentially lethal arrhythmias in this group include:

1. Implantable cardioverter-defibrillators (ICDs) with or without antitachycardia pacing (ATP) (the ATP devices are investigational at the time of this writing)
2. Percutaneous catheter ablation of arrhythmogenic areas
3. Surgical ablation of arrhythmogenic areas
4. Amiodarone
5. Some combination of the above

While amiodarone is an effective antiarrhythmic agent, serious side effects (including potentially lethal pulmonary interstitial fibrosis) limit its use as a first-line agent, particularly in younger patients. Improved detection algorithms and expanded ATP programming of fourth-generation ICDs have increased their usefulness in the treatment of drug-refractory VT; however, these devices are still investigational and not generally available.

Furthermore, those patients who experience frequent episodes of VT despite maximal antiarrhythmic therapy are not ideal candidates for ICD implantation because of unacceptably frequent device discharges, which can lead to severe emotional and physical hardship for the patient and greatly reduce the battery life of the device. Only ablative therapy, whether surgical or by percutaneous catheter techniques, is potentially curative.

The last two decades have seen significant technical advances in surgical and catheter ablation of VT because of (1) a better understanding of the re-entrant mechanisms underlying postinfarction VT and the importance of identifying the site of origin of VT,[2-6] (2) improved pre- and intraoperative endocardial mapping techniques to guide surgery or catheter ablation,[7-12] and (3) use of primary or adjunctive cryotherapy or laser ablation.[13-16] This chapter summarizes the results of surgical treatment of VT resulting from coronary artery disease (CAD) at the Hospital of the University of Pennsylvania and examines the preoperative and operative variables affecting the success of the procedure. A comparison of our results with those from other institutions will be presented, and variables that may contribute to differences in the reported success rate of surgical ablation among multiple institutions will be discussed.

DEFINITIONS

Definitions used in this chapter include the following:

Sustained ventricular tachycardia: A uniform-morphology VT lasting more than 30 seconds or requiring earlier cardioversion because of hemodynamic compromise.

Primary surgical success: The absence of spontaneous or inducible VT or sudden death on long-term follow-up, without adjunctive antiarrhythmic drugs, after ablative surgical procedures.

Clinical success: The absence of spontaneous VT or sudden death after hospital discharge with or without adjunctive antiarrhythmic drugs, following ablative surgical procedures.

Operative death: Death occurring from any cause within 30 days of operation.

Site of origin of VT: Endocardial (rarely epicardial) site exhibiting earliest electrical activity during VT occurring more than 40 msec before the QRS and closest to mid-diastole and having a 1:1 association with each cycle of VT. The electrogram from this site should be demonstrated to be presystolic, i.e., maintaining a fixed relationship to the onset of the subsequent QRS complex, rather than a late "dead end" pathway. Diastolic bridging (electrical activity spanning throughout electrical diastole) and/or continuous activity at this site which is required for maintenance of VT are considered optimal.

Distinct VT morphologies: Comparison of VT-1 and VT-2 revealing either contralateral bundle-branch block morphology or more than 90 degrees of divergence of the frontal plane QRS axes.

Disparate sites of origin of VT: A distance of 5 cm or more between sites of origin of two distinct VTs.

Clinical VT: VT that has been documented to occur spontaneously.

PREOPERATIVE EVALUATION

VT may be deemed refractory to antiarrhythmic therapy because of either (1) ineffectiveness of drugs to suppress spontaneous episodes or render the arrhythmia noninducible or (2) intolerable side effects of an otherwise effective drug. A patient with such a VT should be considered for subendocardial resection (SER), implantation of an ICD, or both forms of therapy. The most important factor in determining whether such a patient is an appropriate candidate for surgical ablation is a well-defined pathophysiological substrate for VT, that is, scarring with or without an aneurysm.

All such patients should undergo preoperative angiographic/hemodynamic catheterization, including contrast ventriculography (preferably biplane) and electrophysiological studies for VT initiation, electropharmacological testing, and endocardial catheter mapping when feasible. Preoperative stimulation and endocardial mapping are important because up to 50% of clinical VTs may be noninducible or inadequately mapped intraoperatively.[17-21] Preoperative information regarding the sites of origin of VTs can reduce intraoperative mapping time and direct the surgeon to those areas that require ablation, particularly when disparate sites of origin are present.[17,22] Further, we and others have observed that up to 20% of VTs originate from endocardial regions that macroscopically appear normal and are more than 1–2 cm in distance from scar or aneurysmal tissue.[23] These areas would escape detection during a purely visually guided surgical procedure and therefore would increase the rate of surgical failure.

Our preoperative endocardial mapping scheme divides the endocardium into 12 zones (Fig. 39–1). Some 15 to 20 sites are usually mapped during VT, including those between numbered sites on the map (e.g., site 2-3 is a site between the apical and middle portion of the ventricular septum). We use filtered (50- to 400-Hz) bipolar signals (1-cm interelectrode distance) at variable gain. The onset of high-frequency activity is taken as the earliest component. Resetting and entrainment are used to distinguish early from late or "dead-end" paths.[24] Additional techniques used include pacing at the site of origin and determining if the return cycle following termination of pacing equals the VT cycle length.

In 5% of patients with CAD, programmed stimulation fails to induce clinical VT,[25] and in other cases hemodynamic instability during a readily inducible VT precludes extensive activation mapping. For these situa-

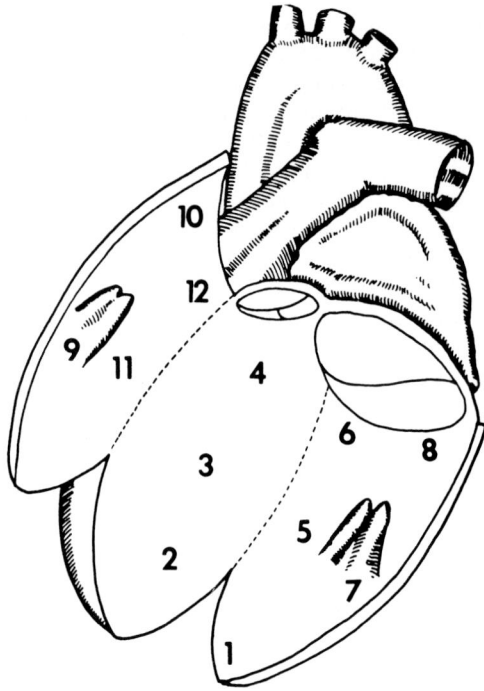

Fig. 39–1. Endocardial mapping scheme for the left ventricle.

tions, two indirect mapping techniques are possible: sinus mapping[26] and pace mapping.[27] A sinus map is obtained by recording endocardial electrograms from various sites during sinus rhythm. Abnormal areas are defined as electrograms having two of the following three characteristics: low amplitude (<3 mV), prolonged duration (>70 msec), or an amplitude/duration ratio of <0.45. By definition, fractionated electrograms have amplitudes <0.5 mV and durations >133 msec. Although sensitive for sites of origin of VT (86%), sinus mapping is not specific (46%), and thus these criteria for abnormal and fractionated sites have a low positive predictive accuracy for the site of origin.[28,29]

A pace map is obtained by identifying an endocardial site at which pacing during sinus rhythm (2× diastolic threshold and at or near the cycle length of the clinical or induced VT) produces a 12-lead electrocardiogram (ECG) morphology closely matching the 12-lead ECG of the clinical/induced VT. Such a match suggests that the pacing site is at or near the site of VT origin. Limitations of pace mapping include (1) the need for a 12-lead ECG of the spontaneous VT, which may not be available if the clinical VT is noninducible, and (2) the occurrence of a close pace-map match when pacing at a site near but not actually at the site of origin. The usefulness and limitations of the procedure have been previously described in detail.[30]

Other factors precluding catheter mapping include the presence of left ventricular (LV) thrombus, aortic stenosis, congestive heart failure during VT, a tortuous aorta, and an abdominal aortic aneurysm.

SURGICAL ABLATION VERSUS ICD IMPLANTATION

The status of LV function and clinical New York Heart Association (NYHA) class are the most important determinants in selecting surgery or an ICD. The experience at several institutions has shown that operative mortality is high in patients with poor preoperative LV function and approaches 30% or more in patients in NYHA Class III of IV or with an LVEF ≤ 0.20.[11,16–19,21–23,31–33] The leading cause of operative and long-term mortality in patients who have undergone surgery for VT is intractable heart failure rather than an arrhythmia. These patients would thus seem better served with ICD implantation, for which operative mortality is between 1% and 3%.[34,35] The use of nonthoracotomy lead system devices may further reduce the operative mortality of ICD implantation in these high-risk patients by obviating the need for a thoracotomy.

It should be mentioned that ventriculographic calculation of EF is not likely to be accurate in the presence of an aneurysm since the assumptions of ellipsoid ventricular geometry are not valid. Garan et al[21] examined the functional status of the nonaneurysmal ventricular segments and determined that poor systolic function in these areas was the only independent predictor of operative mortality. In our experience, however, we could not predict the operative outcome of patients with apical aneurysms who had a mean EF of 0.35 in the nonaneurysmal portions.[36]

OPERATIVE PROCEDURES

The operative procedure uses a median sternotomy approach followed by cannulation of the right atrium and ascending aorta and institution of normothermic (38° C) cardiopulmonary bypass. The LV is vented through the right superior pulmonary vein and access to the LV endocardium is obtained via an incision through the aneurysm or infarct/scar. Induction of sustained VT is then attempted via programmed stimuli delivered through fine stainless steel plunge electrodes in each ventricle. In the event of induction of only polymorphic VT, 500 mg of procainamide hydrochloride is administered IV as a bolus into the heart–lung machine in an attempt to "organize" ventricular activity. Endocardial mapping using a roving bi- or quadripolar electrode probe to sequentially map single individual sites is then performed during all morphologically distinct VTs. An attempt is made to initiate and map as many of the patient's VT morphologies as is possible. In approximately 90% of patients at least one morphology of VT can be mapped in this manner. The combination of preoperative catheter and intraoperative mapping has yielded a mean of two VTs per patient mapped (range, 1–11). After completion of mapping studies, SER, consisting of a 1–3-mm-thick resection of the site of origin with lateral margins of 1–1.5 cm on all sides, is performed at 37° C with the heart beating in patients with anterior wall aneurysms and under cold cardioplegia in patients with inferior infarctions. Confirmation of effective resection/ablation is performed by restimulation immediately after resection. Most of the endocardial scar is resected; however, the papillary muscles are generally spared unless directly implicated as arrhythmogenic areas by mapping studies. If uniform VT can still be initiated (15%), further cycles of mapping, resection/freezing, and restimulation are undertaken. Adjunctive cryoablation ($-70°$ C for 3 minutes with a 1.5-cm flat-head cryoprobe [Frigitronics Inc., Shelton, CT]) is used when disparate sites of origin are present or when sites of origin involve the papillary muscles.

Endocardial exposure is more difficult for VTs originating from the inferior and posterior segments of the LV; therefore, following endocardial mapping, the aorta is generally cross-clamped and cardioplegia generally is initiated prior to SER. Because some VTs appear to inscribe a macrore-entrant wave front around the perimeter of the infarct zone, extensive cryoablation is applied to the isthmus of myocardium between the basal edge of the incision and the mitral valve apparatus to optimize successful ablation of these VTs.[37]

In those patients in whom no mapping data are available (i.e., preoperative mapping was not performed and VT is not inducible intraoperatively), resection is based on visual demarcation of scar or indirect techniques like sinus mapping.

Additional procedures such as coronary artery bypass grafting, aneurysmectomy, and valve replacement are subsequently performed as indicated in specific cases. Currently patients undergo repeat programmed stimulation approximately 7–10 days postoperatively with stimulation from at least two right ventricular sites with triple ventricular extrastimuli. If more aggressive stimulation is required preoperatively for VT initiation, these methods are also employed at the postoperative electrophysiological study.

RESULTS

The patient profile of 343 consecutive patients who underwent SER at the Hospital of the University of Pennsylvania from October 1977 to June 1991 is shown in Table 39–1. The operative (30-day) mortality was 15% (52/343). The single most common cause of operative mortality was congestive heart failure (67%); of note, no deaths were attributed to a ventricular arrhythmia.

A number of categorical variables were analyzed to determine possible association with operative mortality (Table 39–2). Preoperative NYHA Class III or IV was the single most important factor in determining operative mortality. This was closely associated with an LVEF < 0.20. Emergency surgery, prior heart surgery, and multisite infarction were each associated with a significantly higher operative mortality if present as a preoperative characteristic. Prior use of amiodarone was not associated with a higher operative mortality in our series.

Table 39-1
Demographic Data on 343 Patients Undergoing Subendocardial Resection at the Hospital of the University of Pennsylvania Between October 1977 and June 1991

Characteristic	Value
Age (yr)	60 ± 9 (range, 37–81)
Sex	
Male	298 (83%)
Female	45 (17%)
Ejection fraction	0.28 ± 0.10
Number of diseased coronary arteries	2.1 ± 0.9
Infarction	
Anterior	222 (64%)
Inferior	85 (26%)
Ant. + inf.	30 (8%)
Lateral	6 (2%)
Number of VT morphologies	2.5 ± 1.5
Presence of LV aneurysm	75%

Of those patients surviving, 68% were cured by surgery alone, i.e., VTs were noninducible at postoperative electrophysiological study and did not recur spontaneously. An additional 22% were rendered noninducible following addition of antiarrhythmic therapy. Among survivors, the actuarial freedom from sudden death is 98% at 1 year, 97% at 2 years, and 96% at 5 years.

Among patients whose VT was not inducible postoperatively, late VT occurred in 6 patients (2%) and sudden death in 11 (3%). The importance of mapping on surgical outcome is shown in Figure 39-2. The surgical success rate is markedly enhanced, as a larger percentage of VTs are mapped, and the surgical success rate approaches 90% when 100% of VTs are mapped.

The improvement in outcome over time is due in part to improvements in mapping and surgical techniques, but may also be due to identification of patients who are better candidates for SER. The number of patients who have undergone SER at our institution now stands at 343. If this population is divided into sequential centiles, the primary success rate of operative survivors has increased from 64% to 81% from the first centile to the fourth. The clinical success rate has increased from 82% to 100%. It should be noted that the follow-up time in the fourth centile is the shortest (6 months to 2 years) and therefore may not reflect the long-term success rate.

DISCUSSION

Comparison of Surgical Ablative Procedures

Since Couch first reported LV aneurysmectomy as a technique for treating ventricular tachycardia,[38] the ability of ablative

Table 39-2
Preoperative Characteristics Affecting Mortality of Subendocardial Resection

Characteristic	Operative Mortality if Characteristic:		p Value
	Present	Absent	
Male sex	34/241 (14%)	9/41 (22%)	0.197
Age ≥ 60 yr	24/150 (16%)	15/124 (12%)	0.268
Emergency surgery	9/25 (36%)	33/257 (13%)	0.027*
Prior heart surgery	6/19 (32%)	37/263 (14%)	0.040*
Prior amiodarone use	8/87 (9%)	35/195 (18%)	0.144
NYHA Class III or IV	24/90 (27%)	19/192 (10%)	0.001*
EF ≤ 0.20	20/72 (28%)	22/184 (12%)	0.002*
Bypass grafts ≥ 3	13/57 (23%)	14/138 (10%)	0.020*
Cryoablation used	28/148 (19%)	15/134 (11%)	0.072
Multisite infarction (anterior + inferior)	9/23 (39%)	34/259 (13%)	0.019*

* Statistically significant at $p < 0.05$ level.

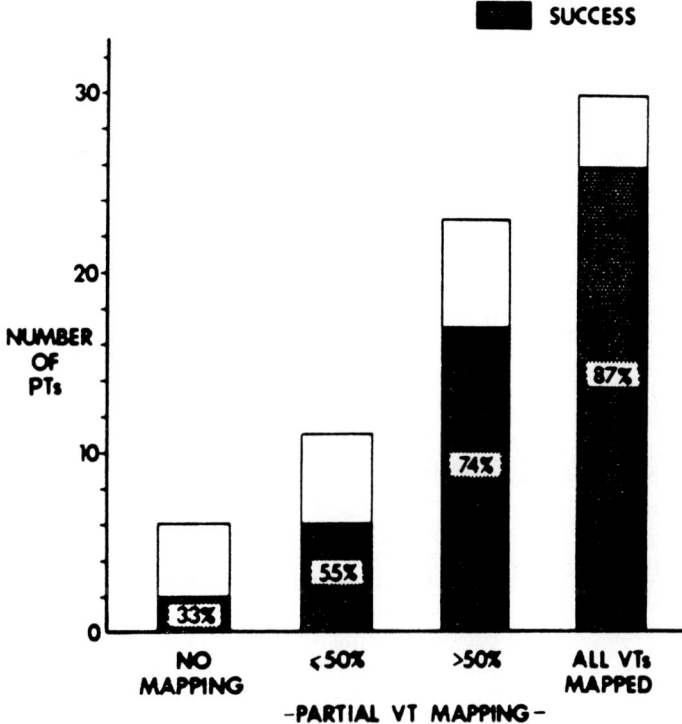

Fig. 39–2. Influence of endocardial mapping on the success of surgery for ventricular tachycardia.

surgery to cure VT has been recognized. Unfortunately, aneurysmectomy alone has not proved to be an effective technique for eliminating VT[39] and has been associated with a high operative mortality (>30%). A significant advance in VT surgery occurred in 1978 when Guiraudon et al[9] introduced the encircling endocardial ventriculotomy (EEV), while Josephson et al[8] described the technique of subendocardial resection in 1979. EEV as first described, however, was associated with a high postoperative incidence of LV dysfunction[31,32] and, as originally described, is rarely used in the United States. A modified or partial EEV, however, based on detailed intraoperative mapping to localize the origin of VT and thereby limit the extent of EEV, is still performed in Europe with operative mortality and success rates comparable to those of SER performed in the United States.[32] Use of cryotherapy alone or adjunctively with SER[13,14,40,41] as well as endo- and epicardial laser ablation[15,16,42] has been shown to be an effective means of improving surgical success in selected cases.

A comparison of results of surgery performed for VT at various institutions, however, is fraught with difficulties, for multiple reasons:

1. A lack of standard definitions and criteria to assess outcome. Although some investigators have considered the elimination of clinical VT to be a primary surgical success,[43] we consider the recurrence of any VT, whether spontaneous or induced postoperatively, to be a surgical failure. We also consider any death during follow-up that is not clearly attributable to a nonarrhythmic cause to be a clinical failure.

2. Differences in patient selection and profile can significantly affect the results of surgery. Most centers performing surgery for VT report the mean EF of patients undergoing the procedure to be about 0.30. In our cohort, the mean EF was 0.28 ±

0.10, with half of the patients having an EF < 0.25. The lowest operative mortality reported for SER currently stands at 6%[18]; the mean EF in this cohort was 0.34 ± 0.12. Although this figure is higher than our series, it is difficult to determine whether this difference is significant. Of note, 50% of our patients were referred from hospitals with cardiac surgical programs because of their high surgical risk.

In our experience, patients undergoing elective SER fare better than those undergoing emergency SER (operative mortality of 13% and 36%, respectively). Swerdlow et al[44] and Haines et al[18] also report a much higher operative mortality among patients taken to the operating room emergently.

3. The significance of success and failure rates must also account for the total number of patients in any given series. As of our last publication, 269 patients had undergone SER at the Hospital of the University of Pennsylvania, which represents the single largest series reported. This compares to 123 patients reported from Alabama,[31] 105 patients from Stanford,[44] 93 patients from Dusseldorf,[32] 80 patients from Baylor,[17] 65 from Duke-Barnes,[43] and 45 patients from Virginia.[18]

4. The aggressiveness of preoperative and intraoperative mapping is not the same at all institutions, although a number of investigators concur with our findings regarding the importance of preoperative mapping for a successful outcome.[17,18,23,31,32,43]

5. The lack of a standardized postoperative electrophysiological protocol, i.e., epicardial versus endocardial stimulation and number of extrastimuli, may also lead to differences in reported postoperative inducibility rates.

Although these differences make a comparative analysis difficult, most investigators currently agree that the following interventions greatly lessen the postoperative inducibility rates and increase the long-term surgical and clinical success:

1. Extensive preoperative mapping.
2. Sequential intraoperative mapping and resection of all inducible clinical VTs during normothermic cardiopulmonary bypass.
3. Application of cryoablation or laser ablation to VTs originating from the inferior wall, thereby obviating the need for mitral valve replacement unless hemodynamically indicated.

Map-Guided versus Visually Guided Resection

There have been no prospective studies comparing map-guided and visually guided SER at the same institution. Our experience has been a far greater success rate (88%) when all VTs are mapped than when none are mapped (56%). Swerdlow et al[44] reported a 25% postoperative inducibility rate in map-guided SER versus 64% in visually guided SER patients ($p < 0.001$). Similar observations have been reported by several other groups.[17,18,20,43] Recently, Landymore et al[45] reported a series of 26 patients who underwent extended SER with a 12% operative mortality and a 100% surgical cure rate (follow-up of 6–92 months; mean, 43). The late mortality was 19%. These authors felt, however, that an increased risk of postoperative ventricular septal defect was present owing to the extensive resection; therefore, they used a prophylactic Gore-Tex septal patch. No episodes of systemic thromboembolism were reported in their study. Nevertheless, this underscores the potential disadvantages of a more generalized procedure that results in greater structural alteration of the LV. Most series still favor map-guided resection. The mapping techniques also vary among institutions and may also account for reported differences in the efficacy of map-guided procedures.[43]

As mentioned previously, about 10–20% of VTs originate from normal-appearing endocardial tissue.[22,23] These areas would be missed during a visually guided resection, resulting in a lower success rate. Moreover, with VT early post MI, there is no visible scar to guide surgery.

Single Point Mapping versus Multiple Site Mapping

Our results thus far are generally based on single point (occasionally a 4-cm^2 plaque with 20 bipoles) mapping in the operating room. The mapping time was not significantly different in survivors versus nonsurvivors (45 ± 13 vs. 42 ± 12 minutes). Multisite computer-based mapping systems have a theoretical advantage by allowing rapid acquisition of data during VT; therefore, fewer cycles of VT would be required to determine the site of origin.[17,22,43,46] Branyas et al[46] demonstrated that single-beat analysis yielded a uniform, reproducible activation pattern when six consecutive beats of sustained monomorphic VT were recorded using a multipoint computer mapping system. Whether such a system would be useful if only nonsustained VT is inducible is yet to be demonstrated, since basing surgical resection on analysis of the activation pattern of nonsustained VT assumes that the activation sequence is the same as during sustained VT. The problem with nonsustained VT (even if the morphology is similar to a clinical or induced sustained VT) is that the activation pattern can change over a few beats until it "settles into" the activation pattern of sustained VT. This may not be observed if the nonsustained VT is too short in duration. Future studies will have to address this issue.

Other phenomena such as early presystolic sites with exit block and late dead-end potentials may be confused with the site of origin,[47] particularly if analysis is based on a few beats; therefore, the need for physician interaction to confirm the site of origin by an electrophysiologist is not obviated by these techniques. It appears that the primary impediment to mapping is not single versus multisite techniques as much as the inability to induce all relevant VTs.

Because the mortality rates of single site map-guided resection and visually guided resection are not significantly different (11.6% vs. 11.4%), it appears that the additional time of mapping does not meaningfully augment the operative mortality.[43]

As further developments continue with multisite computer-based mapping techniques, we will be able to determine the degree to which they improve surgical outcome.

Endocardial versus Epicardial Mapping

About 90% of VTs in man have been shown to have an earliest activation at an endocardial site, with centrifugal spread of electrical activity to the remainder of the heart.[48,49] The remaining 10% have either circular or continuous-loop patterns of activation or may originate from subepicardial sites. A subepicardial origin of VT has the distinct advantage of being amenable to ablative laser therapy or cryotherapy and obviates the need for ventriculotomy and cardiopulmonary bypass. This would be expected to lower surgical mortality. Recent reports on the use of neodymium:YAG laser epicardial photocoagulation have demonstrated promising efficacy of this technique.[42]

Role of Mitral Valve Modification or Replacement

The re-entrant circuits involving the inferior wall often involve the papillary muscle, which has led some groups to advocate excision of the papillary muscles and mitral valve replacement.[50,51] We have never observed the papillary muscle to be the site of origin of VT, although the subjacent free wall myocardium has been implicated. Hargrove et al,[37] using intraoperative mapping, have subsequently demonstrated the importance of the anular isthmus (ventricular muscle between the basal end of the ventriculotomy and the mitral valve anulus) as part of a macrore-entry circuit in VTs originating from the inferior wall. SER plus focal endocardial cryoablation of the anular isthmus resulted in a 93% surgical cure (operative mortality of 7% [1/15] and 13 of 14 noninducible). No patient required mitral valve replacement as a result of the surgical procedure.

Effect of Amiodarone Pretreatment on Surgical Outcome

The use of amiodarone prior to SER is still controversial. Both Cox[43] and Lawrie et al[17] reported a higher operative mortality in patients with a history of amiodarone use who had undergone SER. The findings of Hargrove and Miller (who also stratified for duration of amiodarone use) do not support this.[34] The reason for this discrepancy is not clear.

Surgical Ablation in the Era of the ICD

The availability of the ICD to treat ventricular tachyarrhythmias with an operative mortality of 1–3% raises the question of whether surgical ablation for VT (operative mortality of 15%) is still warranted. Several issues are pertinent to determining the answer to this question and include the following:

1. Operative mortality of SER greatly varies, depending on the preoperative status of the patient, and is significantly higher (approximately 30%) in patients in NYHA Class III or IV, in those requiring emergency surgery, and in those with an LVEF < 0.20. Until the recent availability of the ICD, surgical ablation was the only option to treat such patients, and therefore the operative mortality in part reflects the poor preoperative status of such patients rather than the actual mortality of an optimal cohort of carefully selected patients. There has also been a learning curve over the past 15 years at even the most experienced institutions with respect to both patient selection and operative technique. In more recent series and in our own experience with the last 100 patients, the operative mortality in properly selected patients is as low as 5–7%, with 90–100% clinical success.[18,34]

2. The incidence of sudden death is not significantly different between patients who have received an ICD and those who have undergone endocardial resection, and is approximately 5% at 5 years.[34]

3. The leading cause of immediate and long-term death in patients who have undergone SER is heart failure, reflecting the underlying cardiac disease.[17,22,43] This would not be affected by ICD therapy, as is evidenced by a 5-year survival rate of 60–70%[52,53] in patients with an LVEF < 0.40 compared to 60–70% for SER.[34,43] Of note is the contribution of a 15–20% operative mortality to the total mortality in the SER group, which may be lowered to 5% with proper patient selection.

4. Whereas SER provides a 90% or greater long-term freedom from arrhythmic events,[34,43] ICD patients must often continue on antiarrhythmic medications to decrease the number of episodes of VT or slow the rate sufficiently in order to minimize the frequency of device discharges or permit the possibility of ATP termination. Adverse psychological aspects experienced from device discharges are familiar to those caring for such patients. Problems with inappropriate discharges, lead fractures, and device infection requiring explanation have also been reported.[52–55]

There is no doubt that the ICD has offered a therapeutic option for patients who do not wish to undergo SER as well as for those who would be expected to have high operative mortality. The use of nonthoracotomy lead system devices may further reduce the operative mortality of ICD implantation in these high-risk patients by obviating the need for a thoracotomy. As pointed out by others,[35,43] the ICD may in fact lower the operative mortality of SER because those patients who have a high preoperative mortality risk can now be offered alternative treatment.

Defining the Ideal Candidate for Surgical Ablation

Based on the current literature, the ideal patient for SER is one who has suffered an anterior MI with formation of a discrete aneurysm; has one (mappable) and the same morphology of spontaneous and electrophysiologically induced VT; has normal to augmented contractile function in the non-aneurysmal segments of the LV; is in NYHA Class II or lower; and has no significant CAD aside from the infarct-related vessel. SER alone would have a high probability (90–100%) of curing this patient, with an operative mortality of less than 10% and perhaps as low as 5%. A prospective study examining the morbidity and mortality of surgical ablation versus ICD implantation in this patient population would appear warranted.

REFERENCES

1. Rae AP, Greenspan AM, Spielman SR, et al: Antiarrhythmic drug efficacy for ventricular tachyarrhythmias associated with coronary artery disease as assessed by electrophysiologic studies. Am J Cardiol 55:1494, 1985.
2. Wellens HJJ, Duren DR, Lie KI: Observation on mechanism of ventricular tachycardia in man. Circulation 54:237, 1975.
3. Akhtar M, Damato AN, Batsford WP, Ruskin JN, Ogunkelu JB, Vargas G: Demonstration of reentry within the His-Purkinje system in man. Circulation 50:1150, 1974.
4. Josephson ME, Horowitz LN, Farshidi A, Kastor JA: Recurrent sustained ventricular

tachycardia: I. Mechanisms. Circulation 57: 431, 1978.
5. Wit AL, Allessie MA, Bonke FIM, Lammers W, Smeets J, Fenoglio JJ: Electrophysiologic mapping to determine the mechanism of experimental ventricular tachycardia initiated by premature impulse: Experimental approach and initial results demonstrating reentrant excitation. Am J Cardiol 49:166, 1982.
6. de Bakker JMT, van Capelle FJL, Janse MJ, et al: Reentry as a cause of ventricular tachycardia in patients with chronic ischemic heart disease: Electrophysiologic and anatomic correlation. Circulation 77:589, 1988.
7. Wittig JH, Boineau JP: Surgical treatment of ventricular arrhythmias using epicardial, transmural, and endocardial mapping. Ann Thorac Surg 20:117, 1975.
8. Josephson ME, Horowitz LN, Farshidi A, Spear JF, Kastor JA, Moore EN: Recurrent sustained ventricular tachycardia: 2. Endocardial mapping. Circulation 57:440, 1978.
9. Guiraudon G, Fontaine G, Frank R, Escande G, Etievent P, Cabrol C: Encircling endocardial ventricuolotomy: A new surgical treatment for life-threatening ventricular tachycardias resistant to medical treatment following myocardial infarction. Ann Thorac Surg 26:438, 1978.
10. Josephson ME, Harken AH, Horowitz LN: Endocardial excision: A new surgical technique for the treatment of life-threatening ventricular tachycardias resistant to medical treatment following myocardial infarction. Circulation 60:1430, 1979.
11. Moran JM, Kehoe RF, Loeb JM, Lichtenthal PR, Sanders JH Jr, Michaelis LL: Extended endocardial resection for the treatment of ventricular tachycardia and ventricular fibrillation. Ann Thorac Surg 34:538, 1982.
12. Morady F, Frank R, Kou WH, et al: Identification and catheter ablation of the zone of slow conduction during ventricular tachycardia in humans. J Am Coll Cardiol 11:775, 1988.
13. Gallagher JJ, Anderson RW, Kasell J, et al: Cryoablation of drug-resistant ventricular tachycardia in a patient with a variant of scleroderma. Circulation 57:190, 1978.
14. Camm J, Ward DE, Cory-Pearce R, Rees GM, Spurrell RAJ: The successful cryosurgical treatment of paroxysmal ventricular tachycardia. Chest 75:612, 1979.
15. Selle JG, Svenson RH, Sealy WC, et al: Successful clinical laser ablation of ventricular tachycardia: A promising new therapeutic method. Ann Thorac Surg 42:380, 1986.
16. Svenson RH, Gallagher JJ, Selle JG, Zimmern SH, Fedor JM, Robicsek F: Successful intraoperative neodymium:YAG laser photocoagulation: A successful new map-guided technique for the intraoperative ablation of ventricular tachycardia. Circulation 76:1319, 1987.
17. Lawrie GM, Pacifico A, Kaushik R, Nahas C, Earle N: Factors predictive of results of direct ablative operations for drug-refractory ventricular tachycardia. J Thorac Cardiovasc Surg 101:44, 1991.
18. Haines DE, Lerman BB, Kron IL, DiMarco JP: Surgical ablation of ventricular tachycardia with sequential map-guided sebendocardial resection: Electrophysiologic assessment and long-term follow-up. Circulation 77:131, 1988.
19. Hunt GB, Ross DL: Comparison of effects of three anesthetic agents on induction of ventricular tachycardia in a canine model of myocardial infarction. Circulation 78:221, 1986.
20. Manolis AS, Rastegar H, Payne D, Cleveland R, Estes AM: Surgical therapy for drug-refractory ventricular tachycardia: Results with mapping-guided subendocardial resection. J Am Coll Cardiol 14:199, 1989.
21. Garan H, Nguyen K, McGovern B, Buckley M, Ruskin JN: Perioperative and long-term results after electrophysiologically directed ventricular surgery for recurrent ventricular tachycardia. J Am Coll Cardiol 8:201, 1986.
22. Miller JM, Kienzle MG, Harken AH, Josephson ME: Subendocardial resection for ventricular tachycardia: Predictors of surgical success. Circulation 70:624, 1984.
23. Krafchek J, Lawrie GM, Roberts R, Magro SA, Wyndham CRC: Surgical ablation of ventricular tachycardia: Improved results with a map-directed regional approach. Circulation 73:1239, 1986.
24. Almendral JM, Gottlieb CD, Rosenthal ME, et al: Entrainment of ventricular tachycardia: Explanation for the surface electrocardiogram phenomena by analysis of electrograms recorded within the tachycardia circuit. Circulation 77:569, 1988.
25. Gottlieb C, Josephson ME: The preference of programmed stimulation guided therapy for sustained VT. In Brugada P, Wellens HJJ (eds): Cardiac Arrhythmias: Where Do We Go From Here? Mt. Kisco, NY, Futura, 1987, p 721.
26. Waldo AL, Arciniegas JG, Klein H: Surgical treatment of life threatening ventricular arrhythmias: The role of intraoperative mapping and consideration of the presently avail-

able surgical techniques. Prog Cardiovasc Dis 23:247, 1981.
27. O'Keefe DB, Curry PVL, Prior AL, Yates AK, Deverall PB, Sowton E: Surgery for ventricular tachycardia using operative pace mapping. Br Heart J 43:116, 1980.
28. Kienzle MG, Miller JM, Falcone RA, Harken A, Josephson ME: Intraoperative endocardial mapping during sinus rhythm: Relationship to site of origin of ventricular tachycardia. Circulation 70:957, 1984.
29. Vassallo JA, Cassidy D, Simson MB, Buxton AE, Marchlinski FE, Josephson ME: Relation of late potentials to site of origin of ventricular tachycardia associated with coronary artery disease. Am J Cardiol 55:985, 1985.
30. Josephson ME, Waxman HL, Cain ME, Gardner MJ, Buxton AE: Ventricular activation during ventricular endocardial pacing: II. Role of pace-mapping to localize origin of ventricular tachycardia. Am J Cardiol 50:11, 1982.
31. McGiffin DC, Kirklin JK, Plumb VJ, et al: Relief of life threatening ventricular tachycardia after direct operations. Circulation 76(suppl V):V-93, 1987.
32. Ostermeyer J, Borggrefe M, Breithardt G, et al: Direct operations for the management of life-threatening ventricular tachycardia. J Thorac Cardiovasc Surg 94:848, 1987.
33. Yee ES, Scheinman MM, Griffin JC, Ebert PA: Surgical options for treating ventricular tachyarrhythmia and sudden death. J Thorac Cardiovasc Surg 94:866, 1987.
34. Hargrove WC, Miller JM: Risk stratification and management of patients with recurrent ventricular tachycardia and other malignant ventricular arrhythmias. Circulation 79(suppl I):I-178, 1989.
35. Kron IL, Haines DE, Tribble CG, et al: Operative risks of the implantable defibrillator versus endocardial resection. Ann Surg 211:600, 1990.
36. Martin JL, Untereker WJ, Harken AH, Horowitz LN, Josephson ME: Aneurysmectomy and endocardial resection for VT: Favorable hemodynamic and antiarrhythmic results in patients with global LV dysfunction. Am Heart J 103:960, 1982.
37. Hargrove WC, Miller JM, Vassallo JA, Josephson ME: Improved results in the operative management of ventricular tachycardia related to inferior wall infarction: Importance of the annular isthmus. J Thorac Cardiovasc Surg 92:726, 1986.
38. Couch OA Jr: Cardiac aneurysm with ventricular tachycardia and subsequent excision of aneurysm. Circulation 20:251, 1959.
39. Boineau JP, Cox JL: Rationale for a direct surgical approach to control ventricular arrhythmias. Am J Cardiol 49:381, 1982.
40. Klein GJ, Harrison L, Ideker RF, et al: Reaction of the myocardium to cryosurgery: Electrophysiology and arrhythmogenic potential. Circulation 59:364, 1979.
41. Page PL, Cardinal R, Senasa M, Kaltenbrunner W, Cossetts R, Nadeau R: Surgical treatment of ventricular tachycardia: Regional cryoablation guided by computerized epicardial and endocardial mapping. Circulation 80(suppl I):I-124, 1989.
42. Littmann L, Svenson RH, Gallagher JJ, et al: Functional role of the epicardium in postinfarction ventricular tachycardia. Circulation 83:1577, 1991.
43. Cox JL: Patient selection criteria and results of surgery for refractory ischemic ventricular tachycardia. Circulation 79(suppl I):I-163, 1989.
44. Swerdlow CD, Mason JW, Stinson EB, Oyer PE, Winkle RA, Derby GC: Results of operations for ventricular tachycardia in 105 patients. J Thorac Cardiovasc Surg 92:105, 1986.
45. Landymore RW, Gardner MA, McIntyre AJ, Barker RA: Surgical intervention for drug-resistant ventricular tachycardia. J Am Coll Cardiol 16:37, 1990.
46. Branyas NA, Cain ME, Cox JL, Cassidy DM: Transmural ventricular activation during consecutive cycles of sustained VT associated with coronary artery disease. Am J Cardiol 65:861, 1990.
47. Miller JM, Vassallo JA, Hargrove WC, Josephson ME: Intermittent failure of local conduction during ventricular tachycardia. Circulation 72:1286, 1985.
48. Horowitz LN, Josephson ME, Harken AH: Epicardial and endocardial activation during sustained ventricular tachycardia in man. Circulation 61:1227, 1980.
49. Miller JM, Harken AH, Hargrove WC, Josephson ME: Pattern of endocardial activation during sustained ventricular tachycardia. J Am Coll Cardiol 6:1280, 1985.
50. Moran JM, Kehoe RF, Loeb JM, et al: The role of papillary muscle resection and mitral valve replacement in the control of refractory ventricular arrhythmia. Circulation 68(suppl II):II-154, 1983.
51. Kron IL, DiMarco JP, Lerman BB, Nolan SP: Resection of scarred papillary muscles improves outcome after surgery for ventricular tachycardia. Ann Surg 203:658, 1986.
52. Akhtar M, Avitall B, Jazayeri M, et al: Role of implantable cardioverter defibrillator

therapy in the management of high-risk patients. Circulation *85(suppl I)*:I-131, 1992.
53. Marchlinski FE, Buxton AE, Flores BF: The automatic implantable cardioverter-defibrillator: Follow-up and complications. In El-Sherif N, et al (eds): Cardiac Pacing and Electrophysiology. New York, Grune & Stratton, 1990, p 743.
54. Echt DS, Armstrong K, Schmidt P: Clinical experience, complications and survival in 70 patients with the AICD. Circulation *71*:289, 1985.
55. Callans DJ, Hook BG, Kleiman RB, Marchlinski FE: Oversensing and undersensing errors in fourth generation implantable cardioverter-defibrillators. Circulation *84(suppl II)*:II-428, 1991.

40

Role of Catheter Ablation

MELVIN M. SCHEINMAN

Over the past decade, clinicians have made wider use of ablative procedures for the treatment of patients with cardiac arrhythmias. These techniques have proved to be especially important in the management of patients with supraventricular tachycardia (SVT) and are currently being applied to subsets of patients with ventricular tachycardia (VT). This chapter reviews the application of catheter ablative therapy in the treatment of patients with life-threatening cardiac arrhythmias.

The relationship of ventricular arrhythmias to sudden cardiac death (SCD) has been well established by prior epidemiological studies[1,2] and by ambulatory electrocardiographic (ECG) recordings of patients who have sustained SCD.[3,4] Less well appreciated is the relationship of SVT as a cause of SCD. Dr. Yin Shi Wang from our laboratory recently reviewed our experience with 290 consecutive patients with aborted sudden death referred to our medical center over a period of 11 years.[5] We found that 13 patients had documented or strong presumptive evidence of SVT as the cause of cardiac collapse. In that study, all patients had at least one episode of documented cardiac arrest due to ventricular fibrillation (VF). An effort was made to obtain all ECGs made prior to the cardiac arrest.

All 296 patients underwent electrophysiological studies to exclude an arrhythmic cause for the cardiac arrest. A sustained SVT was inducible in 40 patients. In 27 of the 40, a concurrent ventricular arrhythmia was also inducible. Because the supraventricular arrhythmia was not and the ventricular arrhythmia was associated with hemodynamic collapse, these 27 patients were excluded for analysis. Of the remaining 13 patients, 7 patients had a documented spontaneous SVT that deteriorated into VT and 10 of 13 had a hemodynamically unstable SVT inducible in the catheter laboratory.

SUPRAVENTRICULAR TACHYCARDIA AS A CAUSE OF SUDDEN DEATH IN PATIENTS WITHOUT EXTRANODAL BYPASS TRACTS

A total of 4 (30.8%) of 13 of our patients had atrial fibrillation or flutter associated with rapid ventricular response which preceded VF. All of these patients had structural heart disease, including hypertensive and/or coronary heart disease and severe obstructive pulmonary disease in one. For these patients, the mean shortest R-R interval during spontaneous atrial fibrillation has 223 ± 25 msec. During electrophysiological study all 4 had evidence of enhanced atrioventricular (AV) nodal conduction. One patient had evidence of an atrio-Hisian[6] and another of an atriofascicular bypass tract.[7] These patients had no evidence of an extranodal bypass tract and were treated with catheter ablation of the AV junction.

TECHNIQUE FOR CATHETER ABLATION OF THE ATRIOVENTRICULAR JUNCTION

The original technique described for catheter ablation of the AV junction involved application of high-energy direct-current shocks.[8] A multipolar electrode catheter is inserted across the tricuspid valve for recording the largest unipolar His bundle potential. In addition, an electrode catheter is inserted against the apex of the right ventricle to allow for temporary right ventricular pacing (Fig. 40–1). One or more shocks of 200–300 J are applied from the electrode catheter to an indifferent patch placed over the left scapula. After complete AV block is achieved, a permanent cardiac pacemaker is inserted. This technique has been modified so that radio-frequency energy is applied in preference to high-energy direct-current discharges.[9,10] The reason why radio-frequency energy has replaced direct-current shocks is because of less barotrauma, more homogeneous lesions, and obviation of the need of a general anesthetic agent.

The use of radio-frequency energy for catheter ablation of the AV junction has recently been summarized in a five-center study.[11] The results of this study are tabulated in Tables 40–1 through 40–3. Five of the most active centers performing catheter ablative procedures pooled their data. A total of 260 patients underwent attempted ablation of the AV junction with the use of radio-frequency energy. Complete AV block was achieved in 86–99%. Complications included two possibly procedure-related deaths and one postprocedure myocardial infarction (MI) (Table 40–1).

Evans et al[12] reported the results of direct-current ablation in 136 consecutive patients with drug-refractory supraventricular arrhythmia. Complete AV block was achieved in 82% of patients. In contrast to the results achieved with radio-frequency applications, they concluded that direct-current ablation carries a significant risk of death and was implicated as the cause of

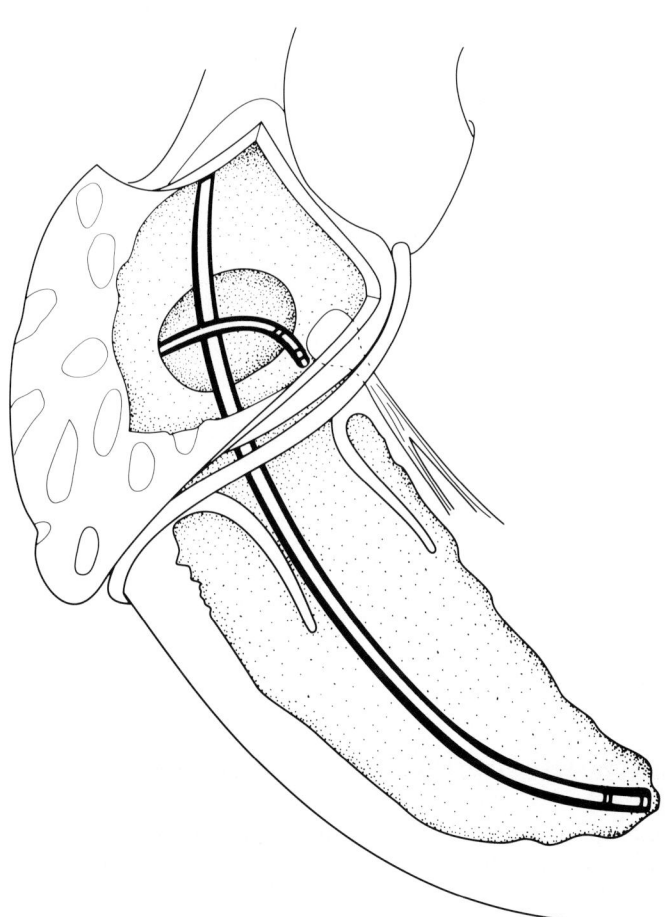

Fig. 40–1. Catheter positions for ablation of the atrioventricular junction. A standard electrode catheter is inserted into the apex of the right ventricle. A second catheter is positioned to record the largest His bundle potential associated with the largest atrial potential.

Table 40–1
Atrioventricular Junction Ablation

Center	No. of Pts.	Success Rate (%)	Complications (n)
A	30	99	EMD and death in patients with severe myocardial disease (1)
B	95	99	None
C	14	86	Myocardial infarction (1); sudden death (1)
D	66	98	Tamponade (1); groin hematoma (1); pericarditis (1)
E	55	95	Mild chest pain (4)

Table 40–2
Accessory Pathway Ablation

Center	No. of Pts.	Success Rate (%)	Complications (n)
A	247	99	Complete AV block (1); tamponade (1); pericarditis (1); groin hematoma (1); femoral artery pseudoaneurysm (1); right atrial clot (2); left atrial hematoma (1)
B	260	95	Left circumflex occlusion (1); left coronary artery spasm (1); TIA 1 wk post ablation (1); large pelvic hematoma (1); femoral artery pseudoaneurysm (1); aortic valve perforation, mild AI (1); complete AV block, permanent pacemaker (1)
C	98	88	Damage to congenitally fenestrated aortic valve (1); pulmonary embolus (1); AV block (1); pneumothorax (1); groin hematoma (1)
D	126	88	Tamponade (2); microembolus to foot (1); coronary artery spasm (1)
E	56	95	Mild to moderate chest pain (6)

Table 40–3
Atrioventricular Modification for Atrioventricular Node Re-entry Tachycardia

Center	No. of Pts.	Success Rate (%)	Complications (n)
A	57	99	AV block (1); pulmonary embolus (1)
B	130	85	Complete AV block (7)
C	41	85	AV block (4)
D	50	85	Complete AV block (6); leg deep vein thrombosis (1); pericardial effusion (asymptomatic) (1)
E	37	97	None

lethal arrhythmias in 5.1% of treated patients. It should be emphasized that these deaths occurred in patients with severely impaired ventricular function. It is not known whether the five-center study alluded to above had comparably ill patients. In any event, at this time it appears prudent to use radio-frequency rather than direct-current ablative therapy. The two energy forms appear to be equally effective, but radio-frequency energy appears to be associated with fewer side effects and obviates need for general anesthesia.

RATIONALE FOR USE OF CATHETER ABLATION OF THE ATRIOVENTRICULAR JUNCTION FOR PATIENTS WITH SUDDEN DEATH DUE TO SUPRAVENTRICULAR TACHYCARDIA

A review of our data base[5] showed that four patients resuscitated from aborted sudden death had atrial fibrillation (three patients) or atrial flutter (one patient) as the proximate arrhythmia prior to VF. These patients were also found to have enhanced AV conduction, with two patients showing evidence of atrio-Hisian or atriofascicular bypass tracts. Such patients may be entirely without symptoms until they develop atrial fibrillation or flutter, usually from concurrent unrelated cardiac disease. This arrhythmia, which is usually benign, may prove lethal in these patients because the normal AV nodal "filter" is short-circuited.[13,14] The same may explain the inefficacy of "AV nodal" blocking drugs such as digoxin, β-blockers, or calcium channel blockers. For patients with life-threatening arrhythmias resulting from atrial fibrillation, use of catheter ablative techniques appears to be the treatment of choice, for drug therapy may be of uncertain benefit in these patients. The chief drawback to applying AV junctional ablation is the need for lifelong pacing in these patients.

SUDDEN CARDIAC DEATH IN PATIENTS WITH THE WOLFF-PARKINSON-WHITE SYNDROME

In our experience, six (46%) of the 13 patients with cardiac arrest due to SVT had an accessory bypass tract.[5] In one patient with hypertrophic cardiomyopathy, VF followed an episode of orthodromic reciprocating tachycardia associated with a rapid ventricular response. The remaining five patients had VF after a documented episode of atrial fibrillation associated with a rapid ventricular rate. Only one of these patients presented with SCD as the initial manifestation of the Wolff-Parkinson-White syndrome.

Our observations confirm other prior reports of SCD in patients with the Wolff-Parkinson-White syndrome.[15] These patients characteristically have accessory pathways with short refractory periods (<270 msec) and, more important, with preexcited R-R intervals during atrial fibrillation of <250 msec. As reported earlier, sudden death is unusual as the presenting symptom in patients with the Wolff-Parkinson-White syndrome.[16] Most often, such patients have repeated episodes of tachycardia prior to the cardiac arrest. In addition, older patients must be carefully evaluated to exclude other possible causes, particularly coexisting VT in patients with coronary artery disease.[17]

The available data suggest that asymptomatic individuals with ventricular pre-excitation are at very low risk for sudden death. Noninvasive evaluation results suggesting the presence of pathways with poor antegrade function include the occurrence of spontaneous Mobitz type II AV block, loss of pre-excitation at a low heart rate (<120 beats/min) during exercise stress testing, and loss of ventricular pre-excitation with infusion of procainamide.[18,19] The use of non-invasive testing to assess for accessory pathway refractoriness has been challenged.[18] We believe that the risk for sudden death in asymptomatic individuals with pre-excitation is so low that invasive studies are not warranted except in very special circumstances (i.e., airline pilots, athletes, etc.).

RADIO-FREQUENCY ABLATION OF ACCESSORY PATHWAYS

Jackman et al[20] pioneered the use of radio-frequency techniques for ablation of accessory pathways in all locations. Approximately two thirds of accessory pathways

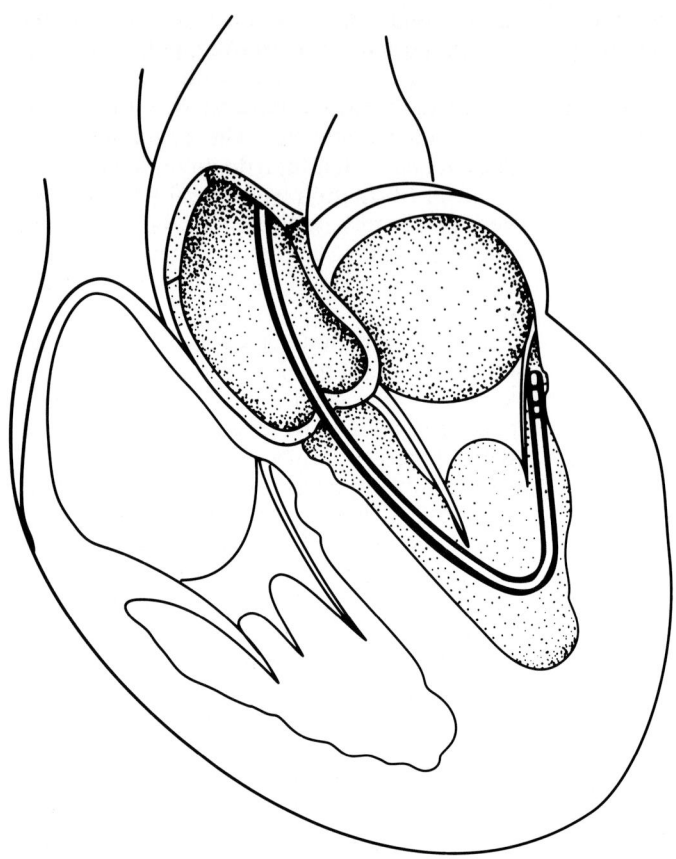

Fig. 40–2. Catheter position used for attempted ablation of left free wall accessory pathways. The catheter is wedged against the anulus over the site of earliest ventricular preexcitation.

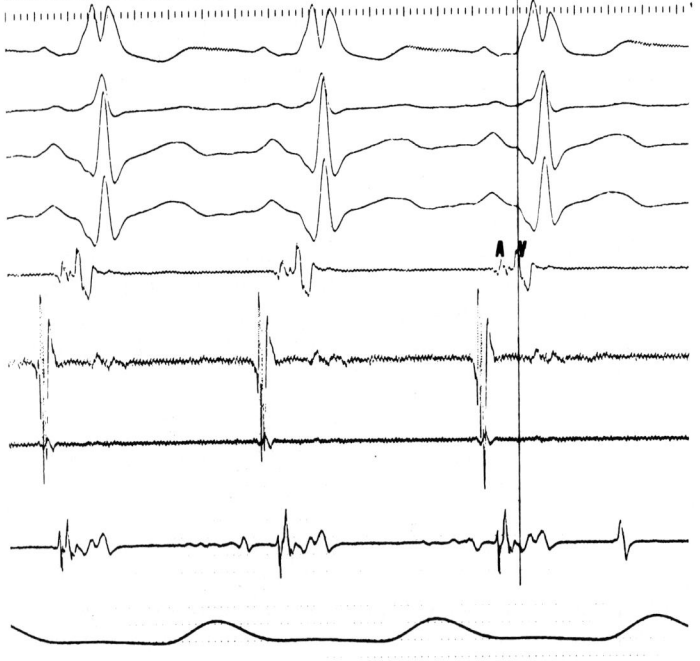

Fig. 40–3. Simultaneous V_1, I, II, and F surface recordings together with intracardiac recordings near the mitral anulus. The rove catheter (top intracardiac tracing) shows merging of the atrial (A) and ventricular (V) electrograms.

are found over the left free wall. Two techniques are currently used for ablation of these pathways. A retrograde aortic technique involves placement of the ablation catheter in close proximity to the mitral anulus in the putative location of the accessory pathway (Fig. 40–2). Application of radio-frequency energy (25–40 watts) is used to destroy the pathway. Prompt loss of pathway conduction (i.e., <10 complexes after initiation of radio-frequency current) is an excellent sign of long-term successful ablation. An alternative technique described by Swartz et al involves transseptal left atrial catheterization and ablation of the accessory pathway over the atrial aspect of the mitral anulus.[21] Either technique is associated with excellent efficacy and a low incidence of adverse effects. The catheter is positioned so that the atrial and ventricular electrograms are closely coupled (Fig. 40–3). Application of radio-frequency energy should result in prompt loss of pre-excitation (Fig. 40–4).

Approximately 25% of accessory pathways are located in the atrial septum. For purposes of catheter ablative therapy, these pathways are divided into anteroseptal (superior to the His bundle), midseptal (between the os of the coronary sinus and the His bundle), and posteroseptal (apical or just to the right or left of the coronary sinus os). The majority of septal accessory pathways may be ablated from a right heart approach. On occasion, a left heart approach is required for left posterior paraseptal pathways, and on rare occasions for left midseptal pathways.

Approximately 10% of accessory pathways are found on the right free wall. These pathways may be approached from either a femoral or subclavian vein approach. In some centers, an electrode catheter is inserted into the right coronary artery for more rapid identification of right free wall accessory pathways.[22]

The results and adverse effects of radio-frequency catheter ablative techniques have been recently summarized. Five of the largest centers in the United States have compiled their data, which are summarized in Table 40–2.

SUDDEN DEATH IN PATIENTS WITH ATRIOVENTRICULAR NODAL RE-ENTRY

In our series, we identified three patients with SCD due to AV nodal re-entry. One of these patients had a 50% right coronary lesion and a history of recurrent palpitations and chest pain. Ergonovine administration produced spasm in the right coronary artery and replicated her pain. The induced typical AV nodal re-entrant tachycardia replicated her pain pattern and was associated with marked ST-segment depression. All of these patients had typical AV nodal re-entry associated with a mean cycle length of 293.3 ± 20 msec. The induced tachycardia produced severe hypotension and required prompt termination by cardiac pacing.

SCD due to AV nodal re-entry appears to be quite rare. We could find only two prior reports of this association in the literature. Hays et al[23] found one instance (of 100 consecutive patients) of AV node re-entry as a cause of sudden death. An additional case was described by Benditt et al.[24]

RADIO-FREQUENCY ABLATION IN PATIENTS WITH ATRIOVENTRICULAR NODAL RE-ENTRY TACHYCARDIA

A number of groups have reported successful modification of the AV node, result-

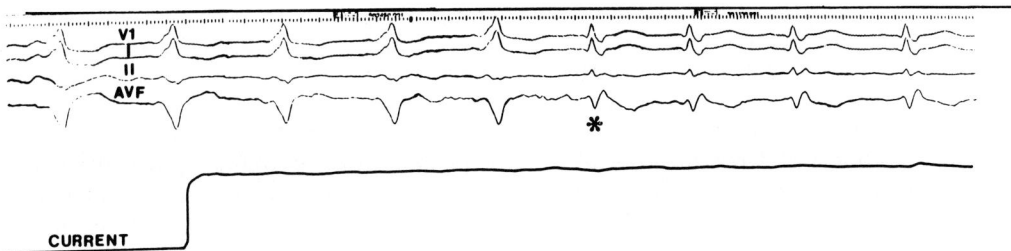

Fig. 40–4. Application of radiofrequency energy for patients shown in Figure 40–3. The surface tracings show disappearance of the delta wave soon after initiation of the radiofrequency current.

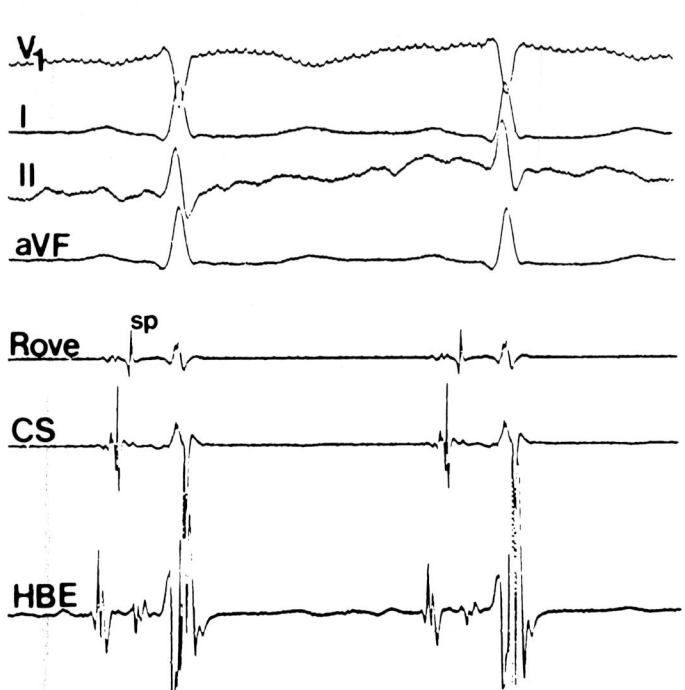

Fig. 40–5. Simultaneous surface and intracardiac recordings in a patient with atrioventricular nodal re-entrant tachycardia showing discrete slow pathway (SP) potential. Ablation in this region resulted in sole fast pathway conduction.

ing in tachycardia cure, but with preservation of normal AV nodal conduction. Initial reports described a technique using radiofrequency energy for ablation of the fast pathway. This technique was associated with a relatively high (8%) incidence of inadvertent complete AV block.[25] Others have reported use of a technique for slow pathway ablation that is not associated with inadvertent AV block. Slow pathway ablation involves placement of the ablation catheter between the os of the coronary sinus and the septal leaflet of the tricuspid valve. Roman et al have described inscription of a slow pathway potential in this region and use of this potential to target slow pathway ablation (Fig. 40–5).[26] As opposed to the fast pathway, which is reliably located just proximal to the His bundle, the slow pathway location appears to be more variable, with successful ablation occurring near the coronary sinus os, apical to the os, or in a midseptal location.[27,28] Current efforts are directed initially at slow pathway ablation because of excellent efficacy (>90%) and the very low risk of complete AV block. In selected very symptomatic individuals in whom slow pathway ablation fails, attempts at fast pathway ablation with its attendant risks may be warranted. The widest reported experience using radio-frequency ablation is detailed in Table 40–3.

VENTRICULAR TACHYCARDIA AND SUDDEN CARDIAC DEATH

The relationship between VT and SCD has been well established by prior epidemiological studies and documented by 24-hour Holter studies.[1–4] The risk of SCD in patients with nonsustained VT is discussed elsewhere in this text. There are no data on the natural history of sustained VT (i.e., tachycardia persisting for over 30 seconds) since this is recognized as a potentially malignant problem requiring active intervention. Attempted drug therapy of VT has been associated with a high incidence of SCD. Use of amiodarone (the most effective available antiarrhythmic agent), for example, is associated with a 9% incidence of sudden death in the first year and a roughly 3% annual incidence thereafter.[29] This has led to the increased use of device therapy for these patients.[30] Other nonpharmacological techniques involve use of cardiac electrosurgery[31] or catheter ablation.

TECHNIQUE OF CATHETER ABLATION FOR PATIENTS WITH VENTRICULAR TACHYCARDIA

Catheter ablation of VT foci remains the most demanding of catheter ablative procedures. The technique involves insertion of electrode catheters into both the right and left ventricles. Standard pacing techniques are used to initiate the tachycardia. The ablating catheter is moved to as many endocardial sites as possible during induced VT in order to define the earliest endocardial electrogram relative to surface ECG recordings (Fig. 40–6 and 40–7).[32] The latter defines the exit point of the VT focus. More recently, pacing techniques have been used to locate the critical slow zone necessary for initiation and maintenance of the tachycardia. Pacing from the putative VT site that results in a long delay between pacemaker spike and ventricular activation, together with a pace-mapped 12-lead ECG identical to the spontaneous VT, is strong evidence that pacing is initiated just proximal to or within the critical slow zone for maintenance of the tachycardia.[33] Once this zone is identified, then either high-energy direct-current shocks or radio-frequency energy is applied from the catheter to an indifferent chest patch. An alternative approach has been described for patients with VT localized to the ventricular septum. This approach involves insertion of catheters to the earliest endocardial breakthrough sites localized to the right and left sides of the septum. Energy is directed from the electrode catheter on one side of the septum to the other catheter in order to destroy the septal focus.[34] The pacing induction protocol is re-

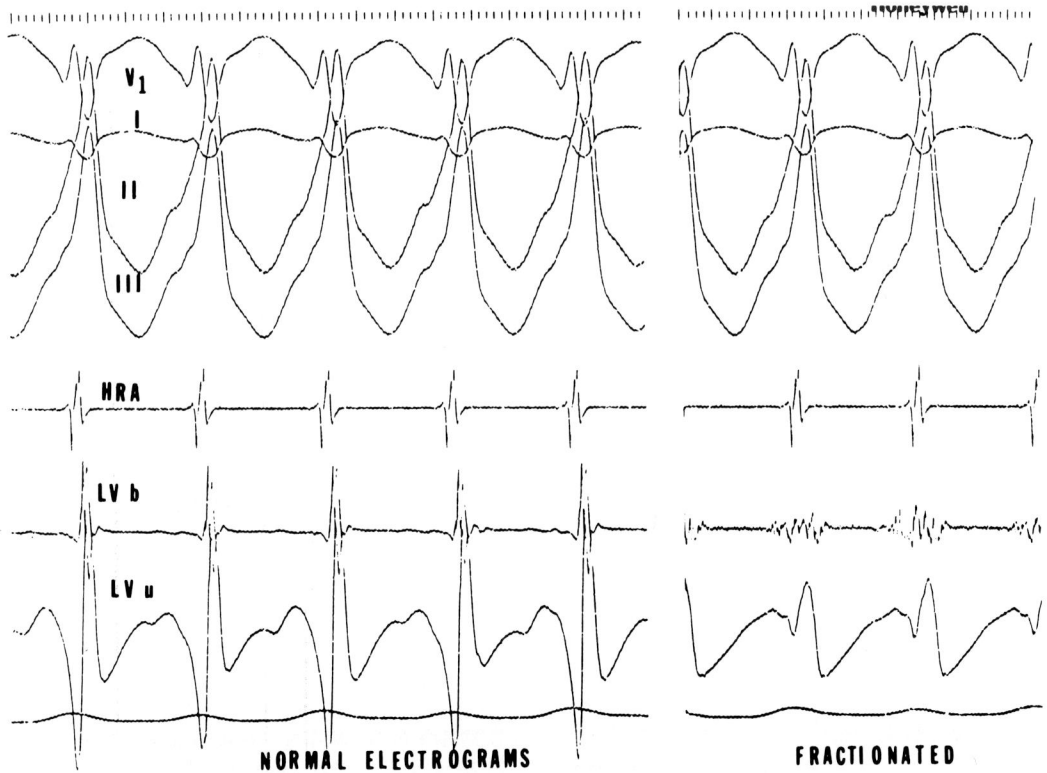

Fig. 40–6. *Right panel:* Examples of electrograms recorded from areas of normal ventricle during ventricular tachycardia in a patient with coronary artery disease. *Left panel:* Examples of fractionated electrograms recorded just prior to onset of surface ECG recording.

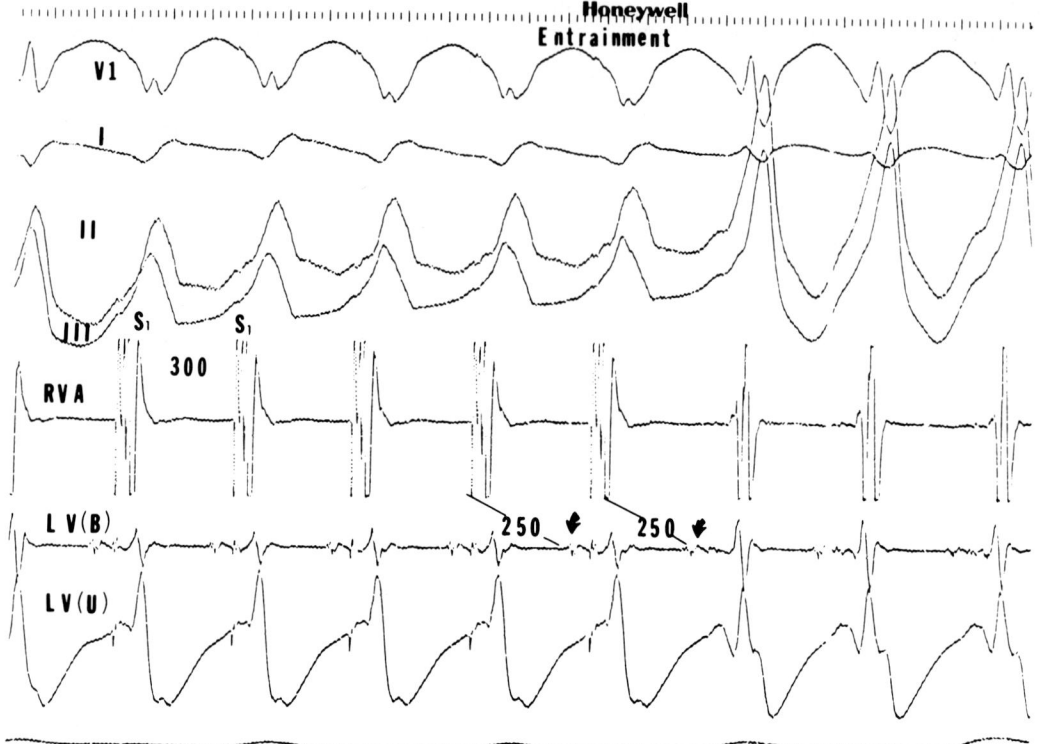

Fig. 40–7. Overdrive pacing showing entrainmment of tachycardia and mid-diastolic potential to the paced rate and emergence of mid-diastolic potential preceding the surface QRS after termination of pacing.

peated to determine whether the tachycardia is still inducible. If the tachycardia is not inducible, the procedure is terminated and the patient is observed for at least 24 hours in an intensive care setting.

RESULTS OF DIRECT-CURRENT CATHETER ABLATION FOR VENTRICULAR TACHYCARDIA

Use of direct-current shocks for ablation of VT foci was first introduced in man by Hartzler and Giorgi.[35] Since then a number of groups have described experience with this technique.[36–39] The largest experience to date was reported from a voluntary worldwide registry set up to monitor the efficacy and safety of ablative procedures.[40] In the final report of this registry, 164 patients underwent attempted catheter ablation using high-energy direct-current shock. Total efficacy, defined as tachycardia control without need for antiarrhythmic agents, was achieved in 18% of patients. Partial efficacy, defined as tachycardia control but requiring adjunctive drug therapy, was achieved in 41%. Serious adverse effects were common and included procedure-related deaths in 11 patients. These deaths were due to post-shock intractable ventricular arrhythmias, electromechanical dissociation, acute cardiac tamponade, or pump failure. Other serious nonfatal complications included cerebrovascular accidents, cardiac tamponade, and ventricular arrhythmia (Table 40–4). Late deaths occurred in 40 (24%); 16 patients died suddenly.

RADIO-FREQUENCY ABLATION FOR PATIENTS WITH VENTRICULAR TACHYCARDIA

There is limited experience with the use of radio-frequency energy for patients with

Table 40–4
Results of Attempted Ventricular Tachycardia Focus Ablation in 164 Patients
(Follow-up Interval = 12 ± 11 mo)

Clinical Response	No. (%) of Pts.
Group 1 No recurrent VT; taking no antiarrhythmic drugs	30 (18)
Group 2 No recurrent VT; antiarrhythmic drug therapy required	67 (41)
Group 3 Recurrent VT or unsuccessful (includes all patients with sudden death and procedure-related death)	67 (41)
Early Complications:	
Procedure-related death	1
Hypotension	10
Acute pulmonary edema	3
CVA or TIA	3
Pulmonary embolus	1
Cardiac tamponade	2
Pericarditis	4
Possible MI	1
Syncope	1
LV thrombus	1
Sepsis	2
Chest pain	2
New arrhythmias:	
Sustained, new morphology VT	2
Polymorphous VT/VF	1
Second-degree AV block (transient)	1
Third-degree AV block	3
New SVT	
VF 1 hr post ablation	
Mortality Statistics	
Total deaths	40 (24)
Procedure-related deaths	11
Death due to cardiogenic shock, possibly procedure related	1
SCD	16
Acute MI with shock at 2 wk	1
Death from CHF	6
Noncardiac deaths:	
GI bleed	1
CVA, possibly embolic	1
Suicide	1
Sepsis	1
Cancer	1

Abbreviations: VT, ventricular tachycardia, CVA, cerebrovascular aneurysm; TIA, transient ischemic attack; MI, myocardial infarction; LV, left ventricle; VF, ventricular fibrillation; SVT, supraventricular tachycardia; SCD, sudden cardiac death; CHF, congestive heart failure.

VT due to coronary artery disease or idiopathic cardiomyopathy. Radio-frequency ablation has been used in patients with right ventricular outflow tract tachycardia as well as for patients with bundle-branch re-entrant tachycardia. Patients with right ventricular outflow tract tachycardia present with VT of left bundle-branch block and inferior axis morphology.[41] These patients often have a history of exercise-induced tachycardia without evidence of associated cardiac disease. Tachycardia can often be initiated only after infusion of isoproterenol, with or without programmed stimulation. The outflow tract is carefully mapped in order to define the earliest endocardial breakthrough. In addition, pace mapping producing a QRS morphology identical to the spontaneous tachycardia is very helpful in locating the tachycardia site. Radio-frequency energy is applied to the putative site in an effort to ablate the VT focus. Very encouraging results have been reported by Klein, Miles et al.[42]

Bundle-branch re-entry is another tachycardia that has proved eminently amenable to radio-frequency ablation. This tachycardia characteristically occurs in patients with dilated cardiomyopathy associated with left intraventricular conduction delay.[43] The tachycardia is usually very rapid and is almost always associated with a history of syncope or aborted SCD. These patients usually have an intraventricular conduction delay with a prolonged HV interval (Fig. 40–8). This tachycardia is usually readily inducible by programmed stimulation, although in some patients VT initiation may be facilitated by programming a pause in the induction protocol.[44] The tachycardia mechanism usually involves antegrade conduction over the right bundle branch and retrograde conduction over the left bundle branch. A His deflection is recorded prior to the surface ECG recording with HV $\geq$ the spontaneously conducted complexes (Fig. 40–9). Bundle-branch re-entry must therefore be differentiated both from SVT and from myocardial VT with retrograde conduction to the His bundle. Since the right bundle branch is a critical component of the tachycardia circuit, catheter ablation of this structure has resulted in tachycardia cure.[45] The ablation catheter is positioned against the right ventricular summit in order to record the largest right bundle-branch potential. Radio-frequency energy is applied to this region for selective ablation of the right bundle branch.[44] To date, we have performed this procedure in 10 patients using radio-frequency energy without complications, nor have we found it necessary to provide chronic pacing for these patients. In our experience, 30% of patients will have coexisting inducible myocardial VT tachy-

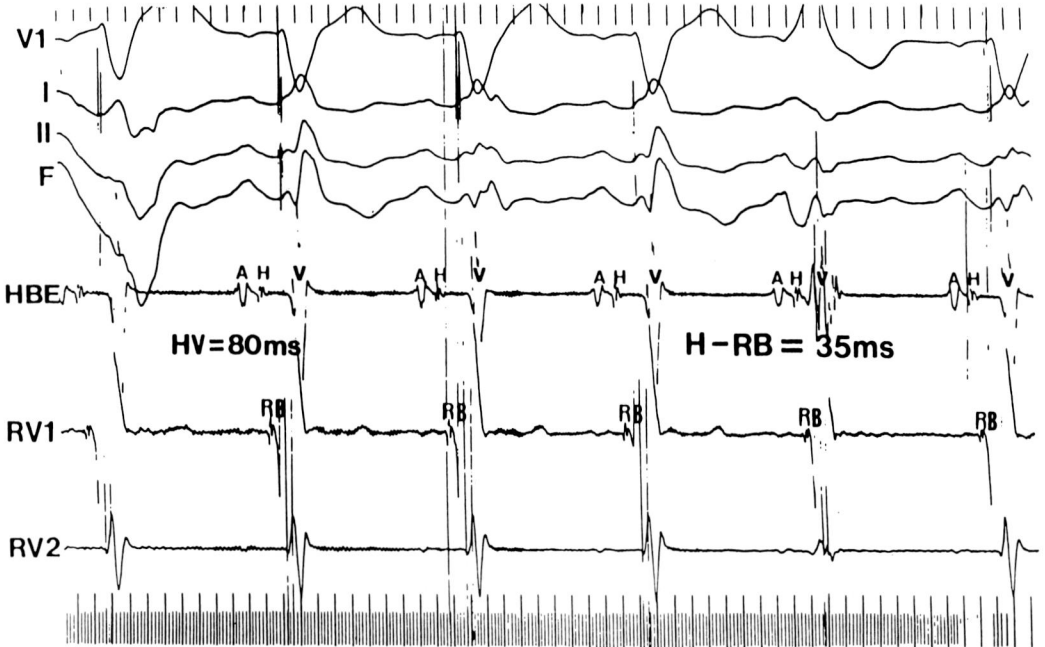

Fig. 40–8. Simultaneous surface and intracardiac recordings from the His bundle (HBE) and proximal right bundle (RV_1 and RV_2) during sinus rhythm in a patient with bundle-branch re-entrant tachycardia. The interval from the His bundle to the right bundle (H-RB) is 35 msec.

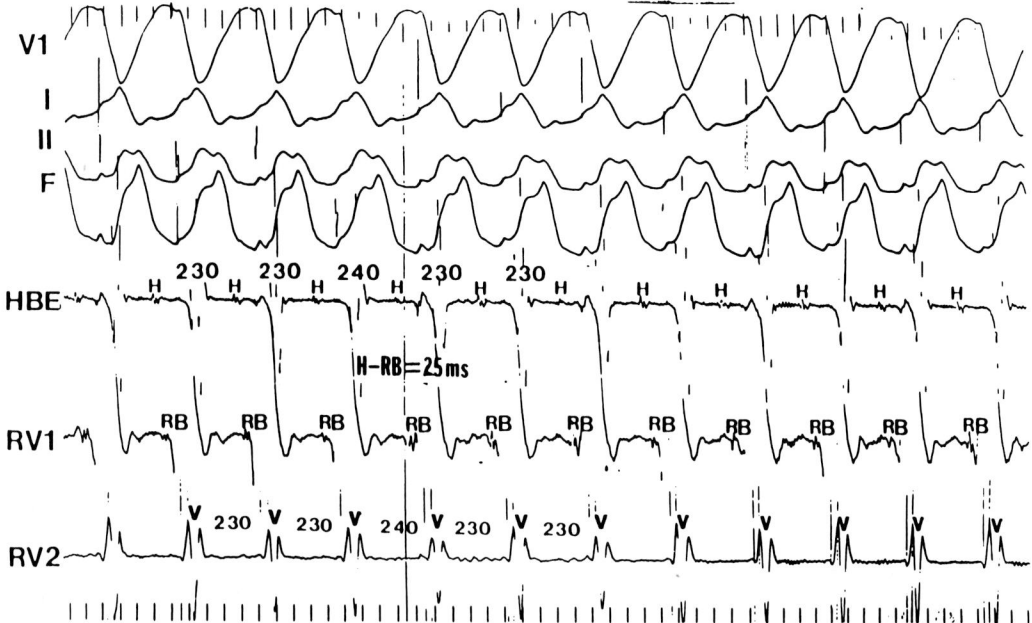

Fig. 40–9. Recordings during induced bundle-branch re-entrant tachycardia with His bundle preceding QRS complexes, together with shortening of the H-RB interval. The tachycardia was no longer inducible after ablation of the right bundle branch. Abbreviations are in Figure 40–8.

cardia and some of these patients may require concomitant drug therapy.[46]

SUMMARY

We have tried to integrate the role of catheter ablative procedures in the treatment of patients with cardiac arrest. We have found SVT to be the cause of SCD in approximately 5% of patients with SCD referred for cardiac electrophysiological studies. This is a minimum figure for SVT as a cause of SCD since those who are not resuscitated or those not referred for evaluation were omitted. Our experience highlights the importance of performing detailed electrophysiological studies for patients with SCD in order to properly diagnose the substrate for SVT. We have found that appropriate treatment of the tachycardia obviates the need for an automatic defibrillator. Moreover, in questionable cases where internal defibrillator therapy is thought to be required, control of the SVT is mandatory in order to avoid unnecessary discharges. Catheter ablative procedures are the treatment modalities of choice since they provide absolute control or cure of the arrhythmia. For patients with arrhythmias arising from atrial tissue (i.e., atrial fibrillation/flutter or atrial tachycardia), complete tachycardia control may be achieved by ablation of the AV junction. In contrast, tachycardia cure without the need for pacing is currently readily achievable by radio-frequency ablation of accessory pathways or with AV nodal modification procedures.

Catheter ablative procedures currently have a more limited role in patients with VT. This is particularly true for patients with VT due to myocardial disease, since the efficacy is relatively low and the potential for adverse effects (especially with the use of radio-frequency ablation) comparatively high. Catheter ablative techniques have been applied successfully in subsets of patients with VT. For example, they have become the therapy of choice for patients with bundle-branch re-entry and are being applied more widely in patients with right ventricular outflow tract tachycardia. Better mapping techniques, improved catheter design, and perhaps alternative energy sources will allow wider applications of ablative procedures for patients with VT.

REFERENCES

1. Eisenberg MS: The problem of sudden cardiac death. In Eisenberg MS, et al (eds): Sudden Cardiac Death in the Community. New York, Praeger, 1984.
2. Cobb LA, Werner JA, Trobengh GB: Sudden cardiac death: A decade's experience with out-of-hospital resuscitation. Mod Concepts Cardiovasc Dis 49:31, 1980.
3. Kramars MS, Black WH, Wells PJ: Sudden cardiac death: Etiologies, pathogenesis, and management. Disease-A-Month 36:381, 1989.
4. Bayés de Luna A, Coumel P, Leclercq J: Ambulatory sudden cardiac death: Mechanisms of production of fatal arrhythmia on the basis of data from 167 cases. Am Heart J 117:151, 1988.
5. Wang YS, Scheinman MM, Chien WW, Cohen TJ, Lesh MD, Griffin JC: Patients with supraventricular tachycardia presenting with aborted sudden death: Incidence, mechanism and long-term follow-up. J Am Coll Cardiol 18:1711, 1991.
6. Brechenmacher C, Courtadon M, Jorrde M, Yermia JC, Cheynel J, Voegtlin R: Syndrome de Wolff-Parkinson-White par association de fibres atrio-hissiennes et de fibres de mahaim: Confrontation entre l'electorphysiologie et l'histologie. Arch Mal Coeur 69:1275, 1976.
7. Kou WH, Morady F, deBuitleir MD, Nelson SD: Electrophysiologic demonstration of an atrio-fascicular accessory pathway. PACE 11:166, 1988.
8. Scheinman MM, Morady F, Hess DS, Gonzalez R: Catheter-induced ablation of the atrioventricular junction to control refractory supraventricular arrhythmias. JAMA 248:851, 1982.
9. Huang SK, Bharati S, Lev M, Marcus FI: Pathological and electrophysiological observations of chronic atrioventricular block induced by closed-chest catheter ablation with radiofrequency energy. J Am Coll Cardiol 7:131A, 1986.
10. Yeung-Lai-Wai JA, Alison JF, Lonergan L, Mohama R, Leather R, Kerr CR: High success rate of atrioventricular node ablation with radiofrequency energy. J Am Coll Cardiol 18:1753, 1991.
11. Scheinman MM, Akhtar M, Dreifus L, et al: North American Society of Pacing and Electrophysiology statement for catheter ablation for cardiac arrhythmias, personnel and facilities. PACE 15:715–721, 1992.
12. Evans GT Jr, Scheinman MM, Bardy G, et al: Predictors of in-hospital mortality after DC catheter ablation of atrioventricular junction: Results of a prospective, international, multicenter study. Circulation 84:1924, 1991.
13. Lown B, Ganong WF, Levine SA: The syndrome of short P-R interval, normal QRS complex and paroxysmal rapid heart action. Circulation 5:693, 1952.
14. Myerburg RJ, Sung RJ, Castellanos A: Ventricular tachycardia and ventricular fibrillation in patients with short P-R intervals and narrow QRS complexes. PACE 2:568, 1979.
15. Klein GJ, Bashore TM, Sellers TD, Pritchett EL, Smith WM, Gallagher JJ: Ventricular fibrillation in the Wolff-Parkinson-White syndrome. N Engl J Med 301:1080, 1979.
16. Gallagher JJ, Pritchett ELC, Sealy WC, et al: The preexcitation syndromes. Prog Cardiovasc Dis 2:285, 1978.
17. Lloyd EA, Hanes RN, Zipes DS, Heger JJ, Prystowsky EN: Syncope and ventricular tachycardia in patients with ventricular preexcitation. Am J Cardiol 52:79, 1983.
18. Sharma AD, Yee R, Guiraudon G, Klein GJ: Sensitivity and specificity of invasive and noninvasive testing for risk of sudden death in Wolff-Parkinson-White syndrome. J Am Coll Cardiol 10:373, 1987.
19. Gaita F, Giustetto C, Riccardi R, Mangiardi L, Brusca A: Stress and pharmacologic tests as methods to identify patients with Wolff-Parkinson-White syndrome at risk of sudden death. Am J Cardiol 64:487, 1989.
20. Jackman WM, Wang X, Friday KJ, et al: Catheter ablation of accessory atrioventricular pathways (Wolff-Parkinson-White syndrome) by radiofrequency current. N Engl J Med 324:1605, 1991.
21. Swartz J, Fletcher R, Cohen A, Weston L, Wish M, Jones J: Endocardial atrial catheter ablation of accessory pathways after intravascular localization [abstract]. PACE 13:527, 1990.
22. Lesh MD, Van Hare GF, Schamp DJ, et al: Curative radiofrequency catheter ablation for accessory pathways in all locations [abstract]. PACE 14:670, 1991.
23. Hays LJ, Lerman BB, DiMarco JP: Nonventricular arrhythmias as precursors of ventricular fibrillation in patients with out-of-hospital cardiac arrest. Am Heart J 118:53, 1989.
24. Benditt DG, Pritchett ELC, Smith WM, Wallace AG, Gallagher JJ: Characteristics of atrioventricular conduction and the spectrum of arrhythmias in Lown-Ganong-Levine syndrome. Circulation 57:454, 1978.

25. Lee MA, Morady F, Kadish A, et al: Catheter modification of the atrioventricular junction with radiofrequency energy for control of atrioventricular nodal reentry tachycardia. Circulation 83:827, 1991.
26. Roman CA, Wang X, Friday KJ, et al: Catheter technique for selective ablation of slow pathway in AV nodal reentrant tachycardia [abstract]. PACE 13:498, 1990.
27. Jazayeri MR, Hempe SL, Sra JS, et al: Selective transcatheter ablation of the fast and slow pathways using radiofrequency energy in patients with atrioventricular nodal reentrant tachycardia. Circulation 85:1318–1328, 1992.
28. Kay GN, Epstein AE, Dailey SM, Plumb VJ: Selective radiofrequency ablation of the slow pathway for the treatment of atrioventricular nodal reentrant tachycardia: Evidence of involvement of perinodal myocardium within the reentrant circuit. Circulation 85:1675–1688, 1992.
29. Herre JM, Sauve MJ, Malone P, et al: Long-term results of amiodarone therapy in patients with recurrent sustained ventricular tachycardia or ventricular fibrillation. J Am Coll Cardiol 13:442, 1989.
30. Mirowski M, et al: The automatic implantable defibrillator: New modality for treatment of life-threatening ventricular arrhythmias. PACE 5:384, 1982.
31. Miller JM, et al: Subendocardial resection for ventricular tachycardia: Predictors of surgical success. Circulation 70:624, 1984.
32. Marchlinski FE, et al: Localization of endocardial site for catheter ablation of ventricular tachycardia. In Fontaine G, Scheinman MM (eds): Ablation in Cardiac Arrhythmias. Mt. Kisco, NY, Futura, 1987.
33. Morady F, Frank R, Kou WH, et al: Identification and catheter ablation of a zone of slow conduction in the reentrant circuit of ventricular tachycardia in humans. J Am Coll Cardiol 11:775, 1988.
34. Winston SA, Davis JC, Morady F, et al: A new approach to electrode catheter ablation for ventricular tachycardia arising from the septum. Circulation 70:11, 1984.
35. Hartzler GO, Giorgi LV: Electrode catheter ablation of refractory focal ventricular tachycardia. J Am Coll Cardiol 2:1107, 1983.
36. Morady F, Scheinman MM, DiCarlo LA Jr, et al: Catheter ablation of ventricular tachycardia with intracardiac shocks: results in 39 patients. Circulation 75:1037, 1987.
37. Frank R, Fontaine G, Tonet JL, Grosgogeat Y: Long-term experience of fulguration for the treatment of ventricular tachycardia [abstract]. PACE 11:912, 1988.
38. Haissaguerre M, Warin JF, Lematayer P, Guillem JP, Blanchot P: Catheter ablation of ventricular tachycardia using high cumulative energy: Results in 28 patients with a mean follow-up of 27 months [abstract]. PACE 11:913, 1988.
39. Sellers TD, Dilorenzo D, Primerano P, et al: Catheter ablation of resistant ventricular tachycardia: Immediate results and long-term follow-up [abstract]. PACE 11:920, 1988.
40. Evans GT, Scheinman MM: The Percutaneous Cardiac Mapping and Ablation Registry: Final summary and results. PACE 11:1621–1626, 1988.
41. Lerman BB: Ventricular tachycardia unassociated with coronary artery disease. In Zipes DP, Rowlands DJ (eds): Progress in Cardiology. Philadelphia, Lea & Febiger, 1988.
42. Klein LS, Miles MW, Gering LE, Shih HT, Zipes DP: Radiofrequency catheter ablation of ventricular tachycardia in patients without structural heart disease [abstract]. J Am Coll Cardiol 17:91A, 1991.
43. Caceres J, Jazayeri M, McKinnie J, et al: Sustained bundle branch reentry as a mechanism of clinical tachycardia. Circulation 79:256–270, 1989.
44. Denker S, Lehmann M, Mahmud R, Gilberg C, Akhtar M: Facilitation of ventricular tachycardia induction with abrupt changes in ventricular cycle length. Am J Cardiol 53:508–515, 1984.
45. Langberg JJ, Desai J, Dullet N, Scheinman MM: Treatment of macroreentrant ventricular tachycardia with radiofrequency ablation of the right bundle branch. Am J Cardiol 63:1010–1013, 1989.
46. Cohen TJ, Chien WW, Lurie KG, et al: Radiofrequency catheter ablation for treatment of bundle branch reentrant ventricular tachycardia: results and long-term follow-up. J Am Coll Cardiol 18:1767–1773, 1991.

41

Role of Implantable Cardioverter-Defibrillators in the Management of Patients with Ventricular Tachycardia and Ventricular Fibrillation

MASOOD AKHTAR
MOHAMMAD JAZAYERI
JASBIR SRA
ANWER DHALA
SANJAY DESHPANDE
ZALMEN BLANCK
KATHI AXTELL

Ventricular tachycardia (VT) and ventricular fibrillation (VF) are the major precipitants of sudden cardiac death (SCD). Among the various therapeutic options available for prevention of VT/VF-related SCD, the implantable cardioverter-defibrillator (ICD) has emerged as the most effective.[1-13] The salient aspects of this technological advance, the appropriate patient population, and future directions in ICD therapy are reviewed here.

BACKGROUND

The ICD is the brainchild of Dr. Michael Mirowski, who conceived the idea and worked with Dr. Morton Mower to develop a functioning unit.[1] After extensive testing in animals, the first implantation of an ICD in a human took place in 1980. Food and Drug Administration (FDA) approval came in 1985, and since that time, the growth of ICD therapy has been phenomenal. In 1993, more than 15,000 unit implants are expected worldwide. The medical and economic impacts of this technology are obvious.

CURRENT STATUS AND TECHNOLOGY

At present, three manufacturers offer FDA-approved devices. These are the CPI Ventak (models 1550, 1555, 1600), the Medtronic pacemaker cardioverter-defibrillator PCD (model 7217B), and the Ventritex Cadence (model V-100). All of these systems employ implantation of epicardial patches (Fig. 41–1). Two patches are used in conjunction with the CPI and Ventritex devices, while up to three patches can be used for the Medtronic system. These patches are placed either intrapericardially or outside the pericardium in such a manner that when high-voltage current travels between the patches, the maximum amount of ventricular myocardium is within the electrical field. In addition to these high-voltage patch leads, separate bipolar sensing leads are used for detection of VT and VF. Two epicardial screw-in leads (Fig. 41–1) or a bipolar endocardial lead can be used for this purpose.

For patients not needing thoracotomy, the ICD can be employed in conjunction with nonthoracotomy leads (Fig. 41–2). We

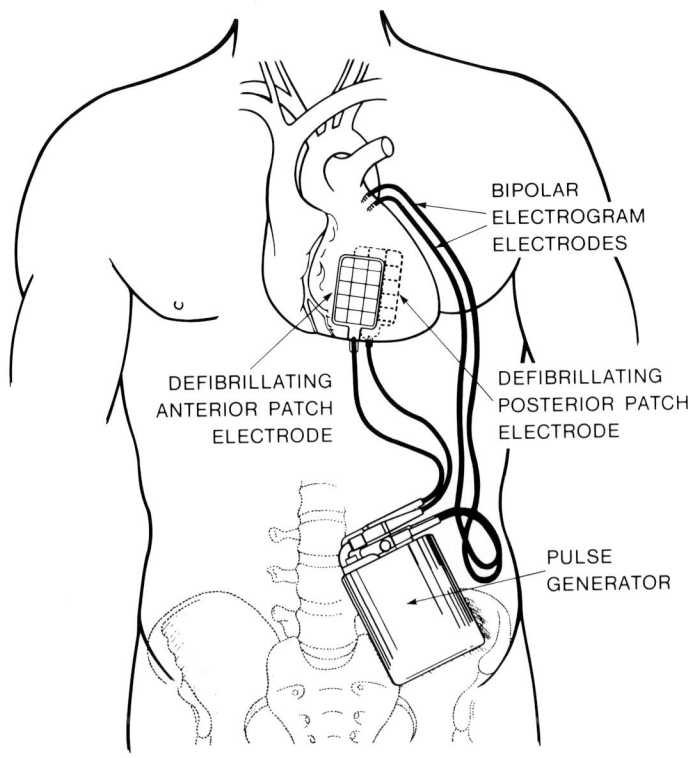

EPICARDIAL LEAD SYSTEM

Fig. 41–1. Epicardial placement of ICD system. The figure shows two epicardial patches and two screw-in epicardial leads for rate sensing. A bipolar endocardial lead can also be used for rate sensing. All four leads are tunneled and connected to the ICD generator placed in the abdominal pocket.

have used the CPI Endotak nonthoracotomy leads and the Medtronic PCD nonthoracotomy leads. The Endotak nonthoracotomy lead consists of an Endotak-C lead alone or as part of an endocardial and subcutaneous patch combination. The Endotak-C lead is placed in the right ventricle (RV) and performs bipolar rate sensing and cardioversion-defibrillation within the same lead. The porous tip is the rate-sensing cathode, while the RV spring electrode is the rate-sensing anode and shocking cathode. The superior vena cava (SVC) spring electrode on that same lead functions as the cardioversion-defibrillation anode. To ensure appropriate placement of these electrodes for various sized hearts, three Endotak-C lead lengths, 10, 13, or 16 cm distance between the distal and the SVC electrode and tip of the catheter, are available. When the subcutaneous patch is used in combination with the Endotak C, an AICD-Y connector is used for three-site defibrillation.

The PCD nonthoracotomy lead system consists of two or three leads. One lead is placed in the RV and has bipolar sensing, pacing, and cardioversion-defibrillation capabilities. The tip electrode is screw-in and can be used as a cathode for bipolar pacing. Proximal to this is the anodal ring electrode for bipolar sensing, and more proximally is a 5-cm-long coil used for cardioversion-defibrillation. Another lead with a 5-cm coil can be placed either in the coronary sinus or SVC, or both. For alternative lead configuration a subcutaneous patch can also be employed.

All three devices detect VT and VF by rate criteria, although a distinction from sinus tachycardia and atrial fibrillation can be made with programming of abrupt onset and rate stability to distinguish these forms of SVT from VT in the PCD model.

Once the detection criteria for VT/VF are met, the therapy choices are somewhat different. In the Ventak models there is no antitachycardia pacing (ATP) option, but the low-energy first shock strength can be programmed to be as low as 0.1 J in the Ventak 1600 model. For the 1550 model, the first

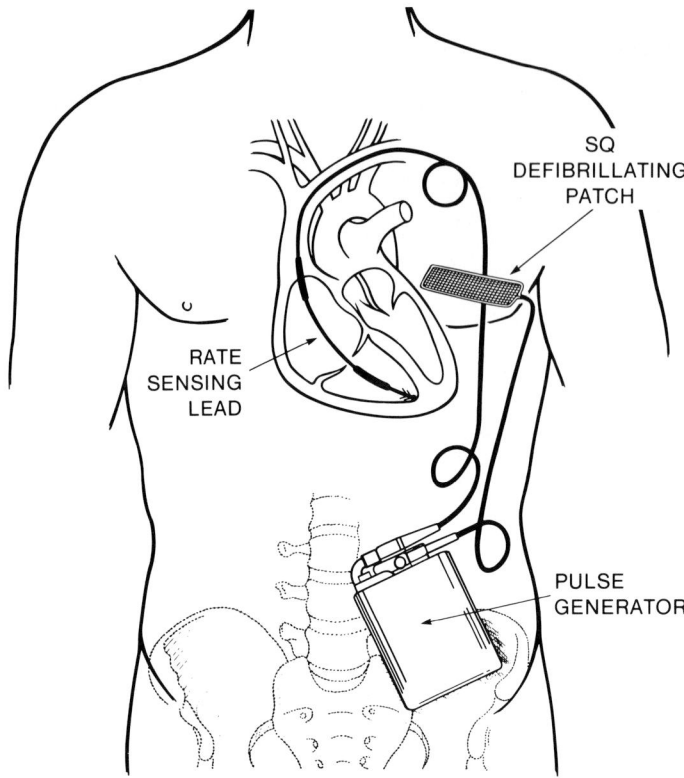

Fig. 41–2. Nonthoracotomy lead placement. The endocardial lead is placed in the right ventricular apex. Defibrillation is accomplished between one of the spring electrodes and the subcutaneous patch. Rate sensing occurs via a bipolar mechanism involving a tip electrode and spring combination. A variety of other lead and patch combinations can be used. See text for details.

shock can be 26 J. The maximum energy in all Ventak models is 30 J except for the 1555 model, where it can be 35 J and is nonprogrammable for all shocks. In the 1550 and 1600 models the second through fifth shocks are fixed at 30 J and are nonprogrammable.

The Medtronic PCD is a multiprogrammable device that delivers antitachycardia pacing (ATP), cardioversion, and defibrillation. Depending on the nature of the ventricular arrhythmia, the PCD can be programmed to deliver therapy in two different zones. For tachycardia detection the device can be programmed at cycle lengths ranging from 600 to 280 msec tachycardia detection interval. The number of intervals for detection can range from 4 to 52, as long as all beats have cycle lengths ≤ the tachycardia detection interval. The fibrillation detection interval range is 400–240 msec, and the number of intervals for detection can be 6–30 for this purpose; only 75% of the intervals need to meet the rate cut-off criteria. For distinction from SVT such as atrial fibrillation and sinus tachycardia stability (variation of 30–130 msec), an abrupt onset can be programmed. When activated, the stability criterion analyzes only those values of cycle lengths that fulfill the interval criterion. The device is deemed unstable when the difference between the current measured cycle length is at or above the programmable stability value. The sudden-onset criterion is met when the current interval falls below the programmed percentage of the average of the prior four beats.

Therapy with the PCD model can start with ATP either as a burst or autodecremental ramp pacing. For most, up to 15 sequences with up to 15 pulses in each sequence can be programmed. The initial sequence is a programmed percentage of the tachycardia cycle length and the first beat of the burst is calculated as a percentage of the tachycardia cycle length, and all intervals of a burst sequence are identical. Similarly, ramp pacing can be programmed up to 15 beats and 5 sequences. There is a programmable interval at the onset of ramp pacing between the tachycardia cycle length and ramp pacing, and there is an automatic programmable decrement with each successive cycle in the ramp. There are also automatic increases in the number of cycles after each unsuccessful sequence. Cardioversion energy can be programmed from 0.2 to 34 J, and defibrillation energy can be programmed up to a maximum energy output of 34 J.

Cardioversion and defibrillation pulses can be programmed as single, simultaneous, and sequentially timed pulses. The stored energy and width of the pulse can also be programmed. For cardioversion, the current pathway can be programmed for each therapy, but for all VF therapies the current pathway must remain the same. Bradycardia pacing in a VVI mode with rates between 30–90/min is also available for the PCD. Additionally, the PCD model can be used for noninvasive programmed electrical stimulation via the model 9710 programmer and can give data over time. The device retains 20 intervals just prior to the last detected VT or VF and 10 intervals following the last VT or VF therapy.

The Ventritex Cadence model V-100 has many of the same characteristics as the PCD but has some additional features, such as (1) a higher maximum shock strength of 40 J, (2) stored and retrievable electrograms, and (3) biphasic shock for cardioversion and defibrillation.

Once the leads and patches are placed, the pacing threshold and R-wave signals are evaluated from the rate-sensing leads. The defibrillation thresholds are then tested by induction of VF with alternating currents. A defibrillation threshold of less than 50% of the maximum voltage output capacity is considered adequate, although achievement of a defibrillation threshold of less than 5 J with epicardial patches is not uncommon in our experience. For a nonthoracotomy lead system defibrillation, a threshold of < 20 J is acceptable. Biphasic shock decreases the energy requirement for defibrillation and is quite useful in patients with high defibrillation thresholds, as is the availability of high-energy devices such as the Ventak 1555. All of the leads are then tunneled to the abdominal pocket and the functioning of the entire system (Fig. 41–1) is verified by induction of VF. Detection of VF by an ICD is followed by charging of the capacitor and then device discharge. A conversion to sinus or other supraventricular rhythms is the rule. However, a brief period of accelerated ventricular rhythm may be observed before the sinus rhythm is restored.

PREDISCHARGE TESTING AND PROGRAMMING

Patients with VF and a low defibrillation threshold during intraoperative testing with epicardial patches are not always tested prior to hospital discharge. However, all patients who receive nonthoracotomy lead systems and those with tiered therapy devices for VT should undergo predischarge testing under anesthesia. This permits reexamination of the defibrillation threshold, selection of ATP, and low-energy cardioversion option therapy. Most patients are discharged on no antiarrhythmic medication.

FOLLOW-UP

Patients are followed up in routine clinic visits at periodic intervals. In patients with nonthoracotomy lead systems, repeat testing at 4–8 weeks is important and those with high VF threshold (i.e., ≥20 J) are retested at 6 months. In patients who receive repeated shocks or in whom a change in arrhythmia status is noted, readmission and testing of the device is desirable. Antiarrhythmic medications are added to control SVT and frequent episodes of VT in some patients.

EFFECTIVENESS OF ICD IN PATIENTS WITH VT OR VF

There is little argument regarding the effectiveness of ICD in terminating VT or VF.[2–4,14–16] This has been proved repeatedly in the operating room at the time of initial implantation, on postoperative testing in the electrophysiology laboratory prior to discharge or follow-up analysis, and by electrocardiographic documentation during spontaneous VT/VF (Fig. 41–3) in ICD re-

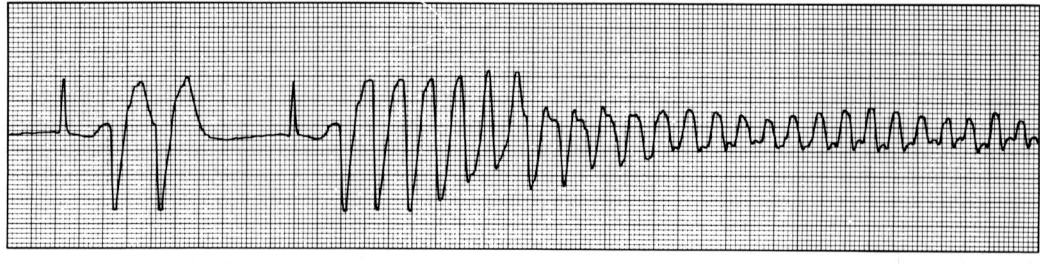
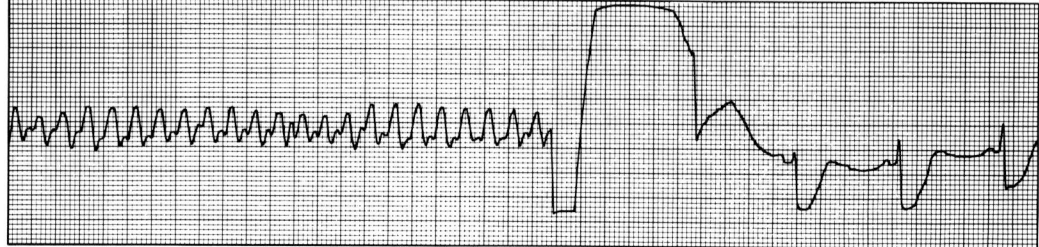

Fig. 41–3. Termination of ventricular tachycardia (VT) with ICD. Following onset of a rapid VT, the arrhythmia is promptly detected and an ICD shock is delivered, with resumption of sinus rhythm. Interestingly, the patient had no symptoms prior to the ICD shock. (Reproduced with permission from Tchou PJ, et al: Ann Intern Med 109:529, 1988.[14])

cipients. Furthermore, the benefits of ICD therapy in the prevention of SCD from VT/VF is also difficult to challenge at this time. The evidence includes (1) immediate amelioration of symptoms—syncope and near syncope—in the ICD population immediately following the shock, (2) a reduction in the incidence of SCD to less than 2% annually in most series of patients with an ICD, and (3) a statistically significant difference between actual and projected survival based on the assumption that the first ICD

Table 41–1
Clinical Experience with the Implantable Cardioverter-Defibrillator in 500 Patients

	LVEF < 0.30	0.30 ≤ LVEF ≤ 0.40	LVEF > 0.40
Patients (n)	206	162	132
Age (yr; mean ± SD)	62.9 ± 10.0	63.4 ± 10.0	60.3 ± 12.1
Sex (M/f)	167/39	128/34	102/29
LVEF (mean ± SD)	20.6 ± 4.7	34.5 ± 3.8	51.7 ± 7.5
Cardiovascular disease			
CAD	163	52	94
Myopathy	38	107	34
Other	5	3	4
NYHA class (n)			
I	20	52	94
II	154	107	34
III	32	3	4
Cause of death			
SCD	10 (4.9%)	6 (3.7%)	2 (1.5%)
Non-SCD	28 (13.6%)	12 (7.4%)	9 (6.8%)
Other	12 (5.8%)	14 (8.6%)	9 (6.8%)
Total	50	32	20

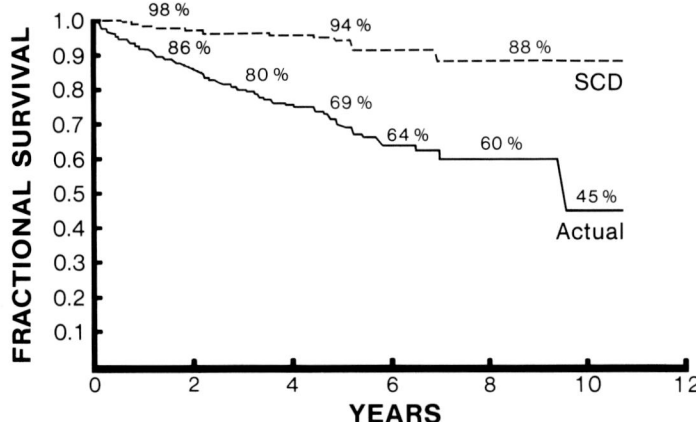

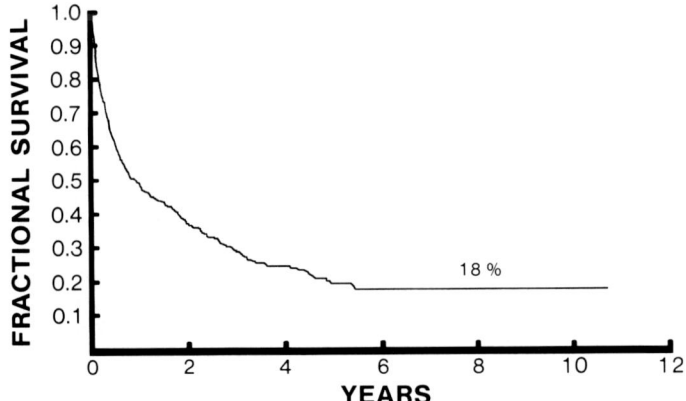

Fig. 41–4. Actual (top panel) and projected (bottom panel) survival curves are depicted. Note marked improvement in actual vs. projected survival. The differences between the two curves represent first ICD intervention in each patient and suggest that it was lifesaving.

shock is lifesaving. This benefit is statistically significant even if only 15% of the appropriate ICD shocks are lifesaving.[17] Figure 41–4 shows survival data in our initial 500 implantees, and Figure 41–5 depicts the same type of information in the subgroup of patients with left ventricular ejection fraction (LVEF) ≤0.30. Table 41–1 lists clinical characteristics of the same 500 patients.

SELECTION OF PATIENTS FOR ICD THERAPY

Since a variety of therapy options now exist for patients with VT/VF, one needs to define the role of such therapies in individual patients.[18] Other options include antiarrhythmic drugs, VT surgery, and catheter ablative techniques. Several issues must be addressed before making decisions regarding therapy selections.

Clinical Presentation

The prognosis regarding the recurrence of life-threatening arrhythmias is worse in patients who present with cardiac arrest than in those with hemodynamically stable VT. For cardiac arrest survivors (and to some

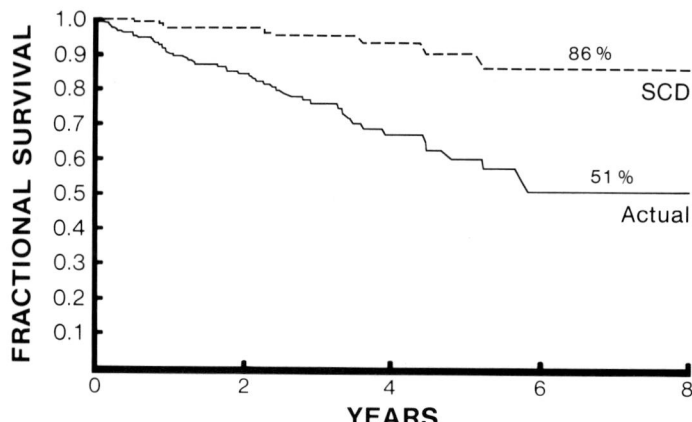

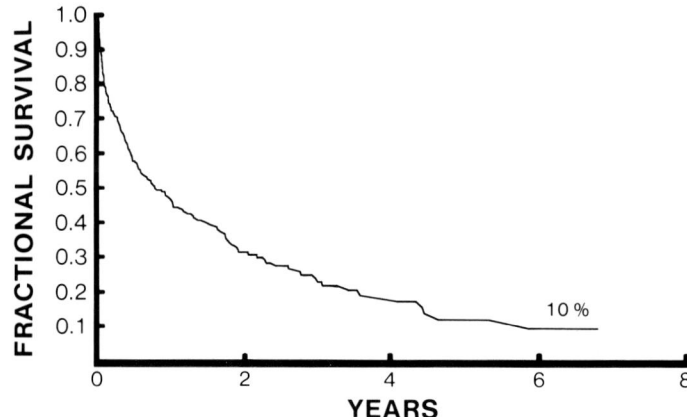

Fig. 41–5. (top panel) Actual survival of ICD patients with LVEF ≤ 30%. A significant improvement in survival, comparable to the projected survival (bottom panel), suggests that in this population, the main cause of death is arrhythmia against which the ICD provides protection.

extent, for patients with VT-related syncope), selection of an effective, definitive form of therapy is more crucial. Among the antiarrhythmic drugs, amiodarone and sotalol are the most effective agents at the present time. However, when amiodarone is compared to ICD, a better outcome is observed with ICD than with amiodarone during the first 3 years of follow-up.[19] In the experience of the same group, patients presenting with cardiac arrest had more than three times the recurrent cardiac arrest rate than those with less severe manifestations.[6] In general, patients presenting with hemodynamically stable VT can be safely treated with drugs, since the SCD rate in this population is substantially lower, even if the VT is not controlled.

Nature of the Underlying Substrate

The value of VT surgery and serial drug testing has primarily been examined in patients with chronic coronary artery disease, particularly in the setting of an old myocardial infarction (MI).[8–12,20–22] The reliability of drug testing in patients with hypertrophic or idiopathic dilated cardiomyopathy has not been convincingly demonstrated. Similarly, VT surgery is seldom offered to patients with noninfarction myocardial substrates. With the exception of monomorphic VT due to bundle-branch re-entry, where ablation of the right bundle or left bundle is curative, ICD therapy may be the only reliable treatment in patients with VT/VF who have dilated and hypertrophic forms of cardiomyopathy.[3]

Induced Arrhythmias

The reliability of drug testing is primarily of value in patients with inducible monomorphic VT.[21] When polymorphic VTs or VFs are initiated, their suppression may not accurately predict pharmacological control. Polymorphic VTs/VFs also do not provide reliable guidance toward ablation of focal pathology for the control of VT.

Left Ventricular Ejection Fraction

The value of this parameter powerfully influences the outcome in patients with VT-VF. There is an inverse relationship between the LVEF and both SCD and non-SCD. This kind of analysis is particularly important for therapy selection. For example, survivors of cardiac arrest with inducible VT suppressed on antiarrhythmic drugs have a 14% incidence of SCD at 1 year.[7] On the other hand, patients with well-preserved LV function have an acceptable outcome on antiarrhythmic drug therapy and are also better candidates for VT surgery. The risk of VT surgery is high when the LVEF drops below 0.20. In patients with poor LV function, therefore, neither drug therapy nor VT surgery seems desirable, and ICD therapy appears to be an appropriate alternative.

New York Heart Association Functional Class

The New York Heart Association functional class can not only significantly influence the overall cardiovascular survival, but may also impact the mode of death. Patients may be naturally preselected for pump failure–related death if they survive to functional class III or IV.[22] In these patients, VT surgery is too risky and ICD therapy may not prolong life and should be prescribed only if these patients are candidates for heart transplantation.[23] On the other hand, in individuals with an LVEF ≤ 0.30 but in NYHA Class I or II, the mechanism of cardiovascular death may be arrhythmic. These patients are likely to benefit from ICD therapy.[2,3]

It should be clear from the above that (1) ICD therapy is the most effective form of treatment for termination of VT/VF; (2) there is a larger pool of patients who can benefit from ICD relative to VT surgery; and (3) compared to antiarrhythmia drugs, ICD provides better and more reliable protection against arrhythmic SCD in patients with an LVEF ≤ 0.30 (the impact on SCD reduction by ICD in this population is exemplified by comparison to the results of the ESVEM trial, where a 10% rate of SCD was noted at 1 year in essentially a VT population[6]), in patients with a non-coronary artery substrate, in patients with inducible polymorphic VT or VF, and in patients without inducible VT/VF. A further advantage of ICD therapy becomes obvious if one examines the natural history of patients with SCD. The latter is of multifactorial origin where a variety of triggers, mostly acute, interact with chronic substrates to precipitate SCD. ICD therapy is the only form of broad-spectrum treatment that can terminate VT/VF regardless of these underlying mechanisms, substrates, or triggers. At present, no pharmacological antiarrhythmic agent can achieve this highly desirable goal.

PROBLEMS WITH ICD THERAPY

The common problems encountered in the ICD population are listed in Table 41–2. In our series, no intra- or perioperative deaths occurred in patients who received an ICD alone, and such mortality was less than 1% when concomitant open heart surgery was performed. Infection of the ICD system continues to remain a significant concern and often requires explantation. With nonthoracotomy lead systems, infections can be usually controlled without explantation of the system. If this observation pans out it will represent a major benefit of nonthoracotomy lead systems. Other problems are relatively uncommon and generally easy to manage.

Table 41-2
Complications in 500 Patients Receiving ICD Therapy

Complication	Patients No. (%)
Perioperative death	4 (0.8)
Pulmonary embolism	2 (0.4)
Perioperative MI	3 (0.6)
ARDS	4 (0.8)
Infections	8 (0.2)
Generator malfunction	20 (4.0)
Inappropriate sensing	30 (6.0)

Abbreviations: ICD, implantable cardioverter-defibrillator; MI, myocardial infarction; ARDS, adult respiratory distress syndrome.

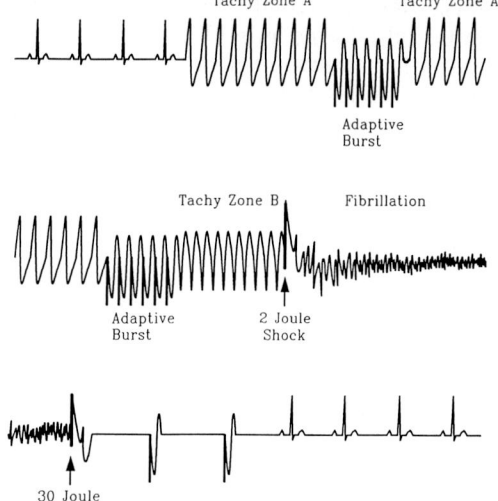

Fig. 41-6. Tiered therapy for ventricular tachyarrhythmia. *Top,* an episode of ventricular tachycardia develops and falls into zone A. The initial programmed therapy is an autodecremental adaptive burst. The initial pacing attempt fails to terminate ventricular tachycardia. *Middle,* after tachycardia redetection, a second, slightly faster burst is delivered that accelerates the tachycardia into zone B, for which the programmed therapy has a higher rate limit than in zone A. With the 2-J shock programmed for initial therapy in zone B, ventricular tachycardia degenerates to ventricular fibrillation. *Bottom,* fibrillation falls into an even faster zone called "fibrillation," for which a 30-J shock is programmed. The shock terminates the fibrillation, and sinus bradycardia follows. Demand bradycardia pacing ensues until sinus rhythm spontaneously recurs. (Reproduced with permission from Akhtar M, et al: Ann Intern Med *114*:449, 1991.[4])

FUTURE TRENDS IN ICD THERAPY

At present, all of the FDA-approved devices require a thoracotomy for the placement of epicardial patches. All of the existing devices provide excellent protection against SCD and have a superb track record for detecting and terminating VT/VF.

Although the ICD has effectively accomplished the basic task for which it was developed, the detection and termination of VT/VF, many additional features remain desirable. Clinical needs have shaped the newer developments in ICD therapy. Many of these newer and highly desirable features have already been incorporated into the current generation of approved and investigational models. These aspects of ICD therapy are elaborated below.

Tiered Therapy (Fig. 41-6)

These so-called antitachycardia devices provide a selection of several methods for termination of VT. When VT can be terminated with overdrive stimulation, antitachycardia pacing is selected as the initial therapy option (Fig. 41-7). The cycle length of pacing, duration, and so forth can be programmed and tested to confirm its efficacy. The selection of the pacing mode and the exact program varies among the different manufacturers, but from the available menus, VT termination can be accomplished regularly. In general, the pace-terminable VT is monomorphic, hemodynamically tolerable, with cycle lengths exceeding 250 msec. Overdrive termination can be applied frequently since it is seldom perceptible to the patient and there is minimal drain on the battery reserve. When ATP is ineffective or leads to rate acceleration, cardioversion and defibrillation shocks can be promptly delivered (Fig. 41-6).

With fast and hemodynamically unstable VT, low-energy cardioversion can be selected as the initial ICD intervention. Rapid polymorphic VT and VF are best managed by high-energy shock. The initial programmed energy setting depends on the defibrillation threshold tested at the time of implantation. The initial VT therapy and the final VF therapy settings are programmed prior to discharge and periodically tested for reliable long-term efficacy. It is anticipated that over time, the initial settings may require reprogramming because of changes in the substrate, rate of VT, pharmacological intervention, and so forth. Even the nature of VT could drastically change and require major alterations for effective termination. This is clearly one of the major advantages of programmable antitachycardia devices, allowing flexibility and tailoring of therapy to individual patient needs.

Storage of Data

The FDA-approved devices store information regarding one or more of the following: the number of ICD discharges delivered, status of the battery, programmed parameters, event recall, and intracardiac electrograms. The availability of intracardiac electrograms and the device responses in the form of marker channel displays are of great help. Individualized therapy will be difficult to deliver in the absence of reliable information regarding a patient's clinical VT/VF in the ambulatory environment. Nonetheless, these features do add a great deal of complexity to achieve the best possible results in ICD recipients.

Discrimination Between Supraventricular Tachycardia and Ventricular Tachycardia

For the most part, rate cutoff has been utilized to distinguish SVT from VT. In the

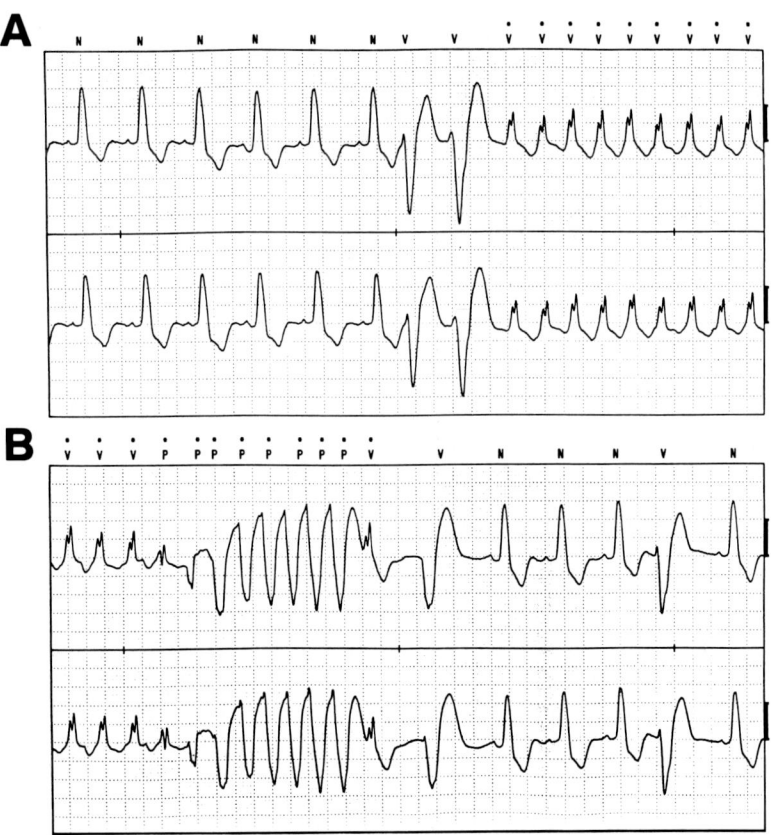

Fig. 41-7. Antitachycardia pacing. The response of new devices to ventricular tachycardia is noted. The tachycardia is sensed (**A**) and overdrive pacing therapy is delivered (**B**) with successful conversion to sinus rhythm. This form of therapy is usually imperceptible to the patient, particularly when the entire duration of event (i.e., the initial tachycardia and consequent antitachycardia pacing) is brief. (Reproduced with permission from Akhtar M, et al: Implantable cardioverter defibrillator therapy for prevention of sudden cardiac death. In Crawford MH (ed): Cardiac Arrhythmia and Related Syndromes. Cardiol Clin *11(1)*:97, 1993.)

event the SVT rates exceed the programmed value, antiarrhythmic drugs such a digitalis, β-blockers, or calcium channel blockers can be utilized to slow the SVT rate to below the rate cutoff. This would generally suffice. However, other features can now be programmed to facilitate separation between SVT and VT. These include sudden onset and rate stability. Sudden onset is designed to distinguish sinus tachycardia from VT. Because the sinus acceleration is gradual in most situations, an abrupt shortening of the R-R interval below a preset percentage compared to the underlying sinus cycle length is helpful in making the correct interpretation of the arrhythmia problem. The rate (R-R) stability criterion is for distinction between VT and atrial fibrillation. A percentage of R-R variations between consecutive cycles can be programmed and should help to avoid delivery of undesirable ICD shocks in the event of atrial fibrillation. The inappropriate shock delivery for SVT continues to be a problem in ICD recipients in approximately 10% of the cases when the rate criterion alone is utilized (table 41–2). Incorporation of sudden onset and rate stability has improved the precision of SVT versus VT detection to some extent. Ultimately, dual chamber sensing should streamline this separation further and ICD shocks will seldom be delivered for non-VT/VF rhythms.

Size of Generator

The currently approved and investigational devices still weigh more than 200 g and are therefore placed in abdominal pockets. The bulk of the generator size is to accommodate the capacitors and batteries, and a significant reduction in volume will require consideration of this aspect. Nonetheless, reduction of size is likely in the future and a generator weighing less than 150 g could be implanted in the pectoral region. This will be possible in the near future. However, the need for prolonged life, storage requirements, and possibly dual chamber sensing and pacing may hinder attempts at further miniaturization. It is also conceivable that several series of ICD generators may be developed. Some may be small, designed for limited shocks of high energy for termination of VF only, perhaps used as prophylactic devices. This type of device will be used for initial rescue in high-risk patients. Subsequently a more sophisticated system can be implanted, even using the pre-existing leads once the need for long-term ICD therapy is established.

Nonthoracotomy Implants

From the very beginning it was realized that cardiac defibrillation can be accomplished from an endocardial lead system implanted percutaneously. The development of the lead system to reliably accomplish this, however, has taken a significant amount of investigational work. Nonetheless, the nonthoracotomy lead systems currently under clinical investigation seem effective in more than 80% of cases, providing adequate defibrillation. With some exploration, one can find a satisfactory location for these leads, and it seems likely that nonthoracotomy defibrillation will become the standard technique in the years to come. At our institution, only the nonthoracotomy leads are used unless they are not available or the patient is undergoing concomitant open heart surgery. More than 100 nonthoracotomy lead systems have been attempted, with a success rate in excess of 80%. Acceptable defibrillation thresholds were found in more than 90% during the last 30 implants, suggesting an element of experience.

Cost Considerations

This is a rather important issue for all forms of high technology medical devices because of their expensive nature. There is little argument regarding the efficacy of ICD in terminating VT/VF, but it must be delivered in a cost-effective manner. In a relative sense, when compared with other medical interventions, the ICD therapy compares favorably.[24] The initial cost per life saved per year analysis was done at a time when the longevity of the generator was limited to less than 2 years. Since then, the anticipated life expectancy of an ICD system has doubled, effectively reducing the cost further. One of the main factors adding to ICD therapy cost is prior non-ICD interventions. Many of these patients undergo prolonged hospitalization with multiple drug testing and/or VT surgery before an ICD is prescribed. Early implantation is likely to reduce this cost, and this should be taken into consideration, particularly when non-ICD therapy is likely to fail. Competition among the various vendors may create competitive pricing and, hopefully, reduce the cost further.

REFERENCES

1. Mirowski M, et al: Standby automatic defibrillator: An approach to prevention of sudden coronary death. Arch Intern Med 126:158, 1970.
2. Lehmann MH, et al: The automatic implantable cardioverter defibrillator as antiarrhythmic treatment modality of choice for survivors of cardiac arrest unrelated to acute myocardial infarction. Am J Cardiol 62:803, 1988.
3. Akhtar M, et al: Role of implantable cardioverter defibrillator therapy in the management of high-risk patients. Circulation 85(I):I-131, 1992.
4. Akhtar M, et al: Sudden cardiac death: Management of high risk patients. Ann Intern Med 114:499, 1991.
5. Herre JM, et al: Long-term results of amiodarone therapy in patients with recurrent sustained ventricular tachycardia or ventricular fibrillation. J Am Coll Cardiol 13:442, 1989.
6. ESVEM Investigators. Incidence of drug efficacy predictions in the Electrophysiologic Study Versus Electrocardiographic Monitoring trial (ESVEM) [abstract]. J Am Coll Cardiol 19(3):387A, 1992.
7. Wilber DJ, et al: Out-of-hospital cardiac arrest: Use of electrophysiologic testing in the prediction of long-term outcome. N Engl J Med 318:19, 1988.
8. Hargrove WC, Miller JM: Risk stratification and management of patients with recurrent ventricular arrhythmias. Circulation 79(suppl I):I-178, 1989.
9. Caceres J, et al: Cryoablation of refractory sustained ventricular tachycardia due to coronary artery disease. Am J Cardiol 63:296, 1989.
10. Caceres J, et al: Efficacy of cryosurgery alone for refractory monomorphic sustained ventricular tachycardia due to inferior wall infarct. J Am Coll Cardiol 11:1254, 1988.
11. deBakker JMT, Janse MJ, Van Capelle FJL, Durrer D: Endocardial mapping by simultaneous recording of endocardial electrograms during cardiac surgery for ventricular aneurysm. J Am Coll Cardiol 2:947, 1983.
12. Miller JM, Kienzle MG, Harken AH, Josephson ME: Morphologically distinct sustained ventricular tachycardias in coronary artery disease: Significance and surgical results. J Am Coll Cardiol 4:1973, 1984.
13. Caceres J, et al: Sustained bundle branch reentry as a mechanism of clinical tachycardia. Circulation 79:256, 1989.
14. Tchou PJ, et al: Automatic implantable cardioverter defibrillators and survival of patients with left ventricular dysfunction and malignant ventricular arrhythmias. Ann Intern Med 109:529, 1988.
15. Winkle RA, et al: Long-term outcome with the automatic implantable cardioverter-defibrillator. J Am Coll Cardiol 13:1353, 1989.
16. Kelly PA, et al: The automatic implantable cardioverter defibrillator: Efficacy, complications and survival in patients with malignant ventricular arrhythmias. J Am Coll Cardiol 11:1278, 1988.
17. Deshpande S, et al: Is implantable cardioverter defibrillator intervention truly lifesaving in patients receiving such therapy? [abstract] J Am Coll Cardiol 19(3):208A, 1992.
18. Akhtar M, et al: Implantable cardioverter defibrillator therapy for prevention of sudden cardiac death in patients with ventricular tachycardia and ventricular fibrillation: ICD therapy in sudden cardiac death. PACE 16(II):511, 1993.
19. Newman D, et al: Survival after implantation of the cardioverter defibrillator. Am J Cardiol 69:899, 1992.
20. Miller JM, et al: Subendocardial resection for ventricular tachycardia: Predictors of surgical success. Circulation 70:624, 1984.
21. Horowitz LN, et al: Recurrent sustained ventricular tachycardia: 3. Role of the electrophysiologic study in selection of antiarrhythmic regimens. Circulation 58:986, 1978.
22. Packer M: Lack of relation between ventricular arrhythmias and sudden death in patients with chronic heart failure. Circulation 85(suppl I):I-50, 1992.
23. Jeevanandam V, et al: The implantable defibrillator: An electronic bridge to cardiac transplantation. Circulation 86(suppl II):II-276, 1992.
24. Kupperman M, et al: An analysis of the cost effectiveness of the implantable defibrillator. Circulation 81:91, 1990.

42

Comparison of Therapeutic Modalities for Preventing Sudden Cardiac Death in Patients with Sustained Ventricular Tachyarrhythmias

MICHAEL H. LEHMANN
RUSSELL T. STEINMAN
MARC D. MEISSNER

Patients who have survived known or suspected episodes of sustained ventricular tachyarrhythmias generally are at greater risk of sudden cardiac death (SCD) than is the general population. A whole host of therapies, both pharmacological and non-pharmacological, that have the potential to reduce mortality from tachyarrhythmic arrest are now available for such patients. Choosing among these various treatment modalities is sometimes a daunting task. Unfortunately, no randomized clinical trial results are available for comparing the effectiveness of one therapy over another. Until such data are forthcoming, the clinician caring for patients with sustained ventricular tachyarrhythmias can rely only on observational (mainly retrospective) studies. This chapter brings together information from these studies with the goal of developing a practical approach to selecting therapy.

Patients with sustained ventricular tachyarrhythmias constitute a heterogeneous group with differing underlying cardiac disease and a broad spectrum of clinical presentations, varying from palpitations at one end to cardiac arrest at the other.[1] We will first discuss the various therapies available for these patients and then focus on approaches to specific arrhythmia presentations, with special attention on potential modulating clinical factors.

OVERVIEW OF AVAILABLE THERAPIES

The major therapeutic options available for treating patients with sustained ventricular tachyarrhythmias are summarized in Table 42–1. It should be noted that although *suppressive* or *empirical antiarrhythmic therapy* will be mentioned in the discussion below, these therapeutic options were deliberately omitted from Table 42–1 because of potential major limitations in their application to patients with life-threatening sustained ventricular tachyarrhythmias. Such limitations include inadequate frequency or complexity of premature ventricular beats to provide a therapeutic end point in about 30% of cases[2,3] and common inability (without the use of electrophysiological testing) to detect unsuspected proarrhythmia, such as potential conversion of nonsustained to sustained monomorphic ventricular tachycardia (VT).[4] Consequently, most electrophysiologists do not consider suppressive or empirical antiarrhythmic therapy to be major therapeutic options in patients with sustained ventricular tachyarrhythmias, unless there are significant contraindications

Table 42–1
Therapies for Preventing Sudden Cardiac Death in Patients with Prior Sustained VT or VF

Therapy	Prerequisites	Advantages	Disadvantages
EP-guided drug therapy	Inducible sustained monomorphic VT	Simplicity of oral drug therapy	Need to consistently maintain adequate blood levels requires high patient compliance Side effects, possibly lethal (especially proarrhythmia)
VT surgery	Inducible sustained monomorphic VT	Possibility of "cure"	Risk of perioperative death (particularly in patients with poor LV function) greatly limits the number of appropriate candidates
Implantable cardioverter-defibrillator (ICD)	NYHA Class I/III	Excellent protection from sudden tachyarrhythmic death	Risk, albeit low, of perioperative death (increased in patients with LVEF < 0.30) Hardware-related complications (e.g., infection, lead fracture) "Inappropriate" shocks (i.e., triggered by sinus tachycardia or various atrial tachyarrhythmias)
Transcatheter ablation	Inducible monomorphic VT that is mappable	Possibility of "cure" (especially in bundle-branch re-entry[16])	Procedure-related morbidity/mortality Inadequate as sole therapy if there is coexistent nonmappable sustained VT, or multiple VT morphologies
Myocardial revascularization (surgery or PTCA)	To be considered *primary* therapy, the following triad must be present: 1) *No* inducible sustained monomorphic VT 2) Well-preserved LV function, ideally *without* prior scarring 3) Significant proximal CAD	Excellent protection from sudden tachyarrhythmic death if *all* prerequisites are met	Risk, albeit low, of perioperative death Inadequate as primary therapy if any prerequisite is not met
Cardiac transplantation	Criteria for placement on transplant waiting list	Cure	Possibility of sudden death while waiting for new heart Transplant-related mortality Possibility of organ rejection

Abbreviations: EP, electrophysiology; CAD, coronary artery disease; LV, left ventricular; LVEF, left ventricular ejection fraction; PTCA, percutaneous transluminal coronary angioplasty; VF, ventricular fibrillation; VT, ventricular tachycardia.

to the treatment modalities listed in Table 42–1. Results of the recently completed ESVEM (Electrophysiologic Study versus Electrocardiographic Monitoring) trial suggest that there may be a select subset of tachyarrhythmia patients (largely limited to those with sustained VT and frequent spontaneous premature ventricular complexes) whose survival is similar with either Holter- or electrophysiologically-guided drug selection, although actuarial incidence of arrhythmic events (which include resuscitated cardiac arrest) is substantial with either approach.[5]

Among available therapies, only *cardiac transplantation* is capable of providing an absolute cure, in that the arrhythmia-prone heart is replaced by one that is essentially normal. Such an ultimate type of treatment, however, is clearly reserved for patients with very advanced heart failure who meet transplant criteria. Relative cure may be achieved through *electrophysiologically guided VT surgery, transcatheter ablation,* and, under certain limited conditions, *myocardial revascularization (or PTCA).* These therapies either disrupt the re-entrant VT circuit (surgery or catheter ablation) or eliminate the basis for recurrent ischemia-mediated ventricular fibrillation (VF; revascularization/PTCA). None of these treatment modalities, however, halts progression of the underlying coronary or myocardial disease, which may give rise to a new arrhythmogenic substrate at some future time. Surgical ablation of VT using mechanical dissection,[6] local tissue freezing,[8,9] or laser-induced tissue vaporization[10] usually requires that the inducible monomorphic VT be sustained in order to precisely map the site of origin; otherwise, on-line computerized multipoint recording systems are required to construct the activation sequence from a limited number of beats.[11,12] The potentially high perioperative mortality associated with VT surgery[13-15] mandates very careful patient selection, greatly limiting the number of appropriate candidates to those individuals with well-preserved left ventricular function and mappable, well-localized VT foci.[13-15]

Transcatheter ablation of VT is probably most successful in the select subset of patients with sustained bundle-branch re-entrant VT, in whom interruption of this tachycardia circuit can be readily achieved by ablation of the right bundle.[16] The success rate of ablation is high and the complication rate lower for this type of sustained VT than for sustained VT originating in the myocardium.[17] However, because sustained bundle-branch re-entrant VT typically occurs in patients with extensive myocardial scarring and depressed left ventricular function,[18] it is likely that sustained VTs arising from diseased myocardium—and requiring additional therapies—may coexist with bundle-branch re-entry.[19]

In patients who have survived cardiac arrest unrelated to acute myocardial infarction (MI), *myocardial revascularization (surgery or PTCA)* may favorably affect prognosis[20] but can be considered potentially curative only if there is minimal or no myocardial scarring.[21,22] Revascularization has no *primary* role in the treatment of spontaneous or inducible sustained monomorphic VT (see below).[23,24]

For most high-risk patients with a history of sustained VT or VF, the therapeutic options are primarily reduced to a choice between *electrophysiologically guided drug therapy* or the *implantable cardioverter-defibrillator (ICD).* Although oral antiarrhythmic drug therapy has the advantage of ease of administration, suppression of inducible sustained VT with conventional agents is usually achieved in no more than about a third of patients.[25-28] Moreover, even when an effective regimen is found, lapses in patient compliance or intolerable side effects may result in subtherapeutic serum drug levels, an unacceptable situation in patients prone to cardiac arrest from sustained ventricular tachyarrhythmias. In these very high-risk patients, therefore, only agents with a long half-life, such as amiodarone, can provide the most consistent cardiac tissue concentrations over time. Unfortunately, the numerous, sometimes life-threatening side effects of this medication[29-31] limit the ability of many patients to continue on amiodarone in the dosage range (400 mg/day) usually required for adequate protection against recurrent life-threatening sustained ventricular tachyarrhythmias.

In contrast, while not preventing arrhythmia initiation, ICD therapy[32,33] can provide continuous protection against sudden death by effecting prompt electrical defibrillation or cardioversion as needed. It is thus no surprise that ICD therapy has emerged as perhaps the most significant recent advance in the treatment of patients known to be at significant risk of SCD.[34,35] The complexity and expense of this therapy, however, mandate that its utilization be carefully defined in relation to other treatment modalities.

PROTECTION FROM SUDDEN CARDIAC DEATH WITH ICD THERAPY VERSUS OTHER TREATMENT MODALITIES

The ability of the ICD to protect patients with sustained ventricular tachyarrhythmias from fatal recurrences is well documented in the literature. Indeed, data re-

Table 42-2
Two-Year Cumulative Actuarial Incidence (Determined by Meta-analysis) of Sudden Death and Total Mortality in Recipients of Automatic Cardioverter-Defibrillator Implants Requiring Thoracotomy

Study	Clinical Profile					Implantees (n)	Actual Deaths Over 2 Years*		2-Year Cumulative Actuarial Rates	
	Mean Age (yr)	Men (%)	ASHD (%)	Cardiac Arrest on Presentation† (%)	Mean LVEF (%)		Sudden (n)	Total (n)	Sudden Death (%)	Total Mortality (%)
Tchou et al[36]	60	73	76	≥77	37	70	1	5	2	7
Myerburg et al[37]	64	82	85	75	33	60	4	9	9	17
Winkle et al[38]	58	80	78	80	34	270	5	31	3	16
Manolis et al[39]	60	87	78	≥64	35	77	0	3	0	5
Kelly et al[40]	59	77	65	54	33	94	1	3	1	6
Troup et al[41]‡	60	86	75	≥66	33	165	8	22	7	16
Total						736	19	73		
Estimated summary statistics, mean									3.5	13.6
95% CI§									1.9 to 5.1	10.7 to 16.5

SOURCE: Lehmann MH: Ann Intern Med 114:499–512, 1991.[35] Reproduced by permission.
* Some published data were supplemented by personal communications with authors.
† The proportion of patients presenting with ventricular fibrillation was taken as a minimum value for the prevalence of cardiac arrest on presentation when cardiac arrest was not specified.
‡ Updated information was obtained (Troup PJ, pers. comm.)
§ The percentages are based on actuarial estimates of the number of patients at risk during the first and second years of follow-up;[42] 427 patients were "statistically withdrawn" over the 2-year period because of shorter follow-up or device explantation.

cently pooled from several studies[36-41] involving a total of 736 patients, most of whom were cardiac arrest survivors, have yielded a cumulative 2-year sudden death rate of only 3.5% (Table 42-2).[35] In a multicenter study of 876 ICD implantees, the cumulative 2-year sudden death rate was 6.6% (unpublished observations from ref. 43). Both these figures are considerably lower than the previously reported cumulative 2-year sudden death rates of 15–40% in cardiac arrest survivors.[44,45]

We[35] recently compared actuarial data in patients with sustained ventricular tachyarrhythmias (mostly cardiac arrest survivors) treated with ICD therapy and those undergoing alternative treatments.[2,13,31,46] The results of that comparison are given in Table 42-3, which shows a lower cumulative 2-year sudden death rate in ICD implantees versus that observed with all other treatment modalities except for VT surgery; however, the significantly greater operative risk associated with surgery for VT yields a significantly higher cumulative 2-year total mortality than that seen with ICD therapy. Although these data suggest a greater protective effect against sudden death afforded by ICD therapy, such a comparison must be interpreted very cautiously because of the retrospective nature of the data collection, selection bias, and likely heterogeneities in patient characteristics (although mean left ventricular ejection fractions [LVEFs] were comparable in the various series).

While most workers in the field acknowledge that ICD therapy has effectively set a new standard for protection against SCD, some investigators have recently questioned the validity of concluding that ICD therapy truly confers overall survival benefit.[47-49] These challengers argue that sudden death rates represent only one aspect of the assessment of ICD effectiveness; overall survival benefit with devices may be less impressive when the following factors are taken into account; (1) A perioperative (30-day) mortality for thoracotomy-requiring implants, in a broad spectrum of patients,

Table 42-3
Two-Year Cumulative Event Rates in Patients Receiving Various Antiarrhythmic Therapies for Sustained VT or VF

Study	Therapies	Patients (n)	Sudden Death (%)	Total Mortality
Tchou et al,[36] Myerburg et al,[37] Winkle et al,[38] Manolis et al,[39] Kelly et al,[40] Troup et al[41]	ICD (requiring thoracotomy)	736	3.5*	13.6*ǁ
Lampert et al[2]	PVC-directed therapy	161†	17	≥25
Herre et al[31]	Empirical amiodarone	427	12	34
Wilber et al[46]	EP-directed therapy	166‡	14	≥24
Hargrove and Miller[13]	Arrhythmia surgery	269	3.7§	37§ǁ

SOURCE: Lehman MH: Ann Intern Med *114:*499–512, 1991.[35] Reproduced by permission.
* Based on estimated summary cumulative event rates from Table 42-2.
† Includes patients with (52%) and without (48%) suppression of high-grade premature ventricular complexes (present in 73% of the study population).
‡ Includes patients with (79%) and without (21%) inducible ventricular tachycardia. In 28% of patients with the latter finding, the arrhythmia was not suppressed by surgery (done in 5% of all patients) or drugs.
§ Miller J., pers. comm.
ǁ Includes perioperative mortality.

which ranges from 0.7% to 5.5%,[37–40,50–56] averaging 3.1%,[52] and which appears to be considerably higher in the setting of poor left ventricular function (LVEF < 0.30, NYHA functional Classes III and IV).[52,53,57,58] (2) The occurrence of nonsudden tachyarrhythmic death.[59] (3) The significant total cardiac mortality rates that can be observed among ICD implantees.[53] (4) The possibility that nonshocked implantees may have intrinsically better outcomes than their counterparts who receive device discharges, thereby artificially buoying overall survival among ICD recipients.[47]

Although perioperative mortality is indeed an important issue, the risk of implant-related death is very low (approximately 1%) in patients with an LVEF >0.30.[53,58,60] Moreover, perioperative mortality associated with ICD implantation is likely to decline as nonthoracotomy-requiring devices become more available[61] and as postoperative management practices evolve; an example is the recent trend toward immediate device activation post implantation to avoid potentially lethal delays in resuscitation from perioperative cardiac arrest.[52] Tachyarrhythmic nonsudden death certainly occurs during long-term follow-up of ICD recipients; however, the actuarial incidence is quite low (cumulative rate of 1.4% at 5 years) (unpublished observations from ref. 43). While it is true that total cardiac mortality is significant among ICD recipients (24–30% cumulative incidence at 5 years),[38,43,50,54] the fact that the majority of implantees have received appropriate shocks months to years before succumbing to nonarrhythmic cardiac death strongly suggests that the lives of these individuals have been extended.[37,57,62] Such a beneficial effect of ICD therapy even appears to extend to patients with markedly reduced LVEF.[36,56,63] In addition, the contention that nonshocked patients may represent a lower-risk subset that dilutes the mortality data has not been substantiated in studies of large numbers of ICD recipients.[60,64]

The most serious criticism raised concerning ICD therapy is that despite protection from SCD, long-term actuarial survival, ranging from 26% to 40% at 5 years in several large series,[38,43,50,54,65] may be no better than that seen with drug or other therapies.[48] The unfortunate lack of prospective randomized controlled trials has left this controversy unresolved.

One indirect line of evidence for survival benefit with ICD therapy comes from the multicenter study of Epstein and coworkers[66] showing that among patients with high defibrillation thresholds, the survival rate was markedly higher in those individuals who nonetheless went on to generator implantation. However, the most direct evidence to date has been provided by the retrospective case-control study of Newman et al.[67] In that study, actuarial survival in 60 patients receiving ICD therapy for sustained ventricular tachyarrhythmias (59% associated with cardiac arrest) was compared with that of 120 non-device-treated controls matched for age, underlying heart disease, LVEF, presenting arrhythmia, and amiodarone therapy status. Mean LVEF in both groups was about 0.35 and follow-up was largely concurrent. At 3 years, the cumulative sudden death mortality was 15% in the ICD treatment group versus 37% in controls,[67] compatible with the superior protective effect of ICD therapy that was suggested previously by our review of the literature (see Table 42–3).[35] More important, Newman et al[67] observed that survival among ICD implantees was significantly better than among controls over a 5-year follow-up period (Cox proportional hazards model; $p < 0.05$). Figure 42–1, from that report, shows that there was clearly a sustained benefit in survival for at least 3 years among ICD-treated patients; the convergence in survival curves at 4 to 5 years is difficult to interpret, owing to the small numbers of patients followed out to that point in time. It is hoped that more definitive results will emerge from prospective randomized clinical trials, some of which are already ongoing in Canada and Europe.[68,69]

OUTCOME WITH ICD THERAPY AS A GOLD STANDARD FOR DEFINING THERAPEUTIC STRATEGIES TO PREVENT SUDDEN CARDIAC DEATH IN PATIENTS WITH SUSTAINED VENTRICULAR TACHYARRHYTHMIAS

Until more definitive data become available from prospective clinical trials, we

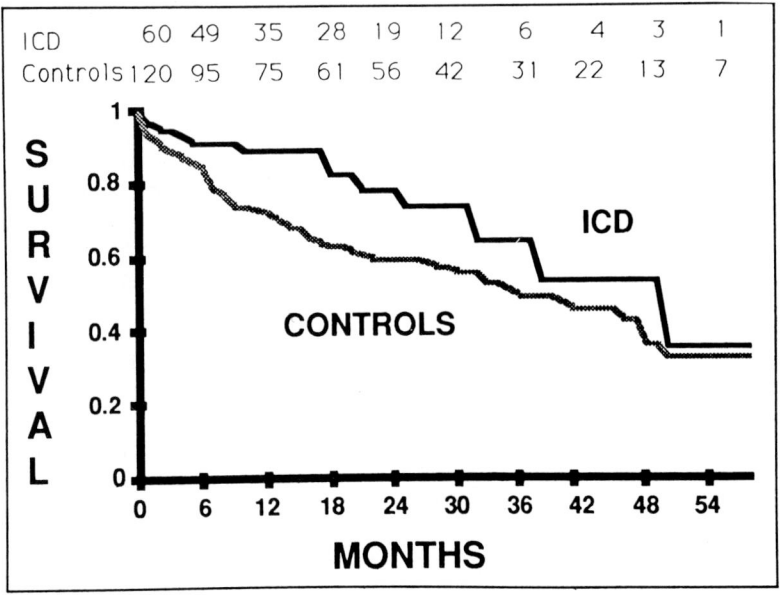

Fig. 42–1. Actuarial survival with ICD therapy vs. medical therapy in patients with sustained VT or VF. Upper solid curve describes the probability of survival in 60 patients treated with an implantable cardioverter-defibrillator (ICD). Lower shaded curve describes the probability of survival among the 120 medically treated matched controls. The numbers at the top of the graph refer to the number of patients available for follow-up in the ICD group (top row) and in the control group (bottom row) at 6-month intervals. By the Cox proportional hazards model there was a significant difference between the two survivorships when patients were followed to 60 months (one-sided test, $Z = -1.87$, $p < 0.05$). CONTROLS = controls matched to ICD cases. (Reproduced by permission of the *American Journal of Cardiology* from Newman D, et al: Am J Cardiol 69:899, 1992.[67])

Table 42–4
Suggested Actuarial-Based Approach for Determining the Role of ICD Therapy in Survivors of Sustained VT or VF*

Patient Group	Estimated 4-yr Cumulative Incidence of Sudden Death Without ICD Therapy	Relative Protection from Sudden Death with ICD vs. Other Therapies
Very high risk	≥20%	ICD definitely superior
Moderately high risk	10–20%	ICD generally superior, but patient subsets most likely to benefit need to be better defined
Low risk	≤10%	ICD comparable to other therapies

* Assumes that patients are in NYHA functional Class I–III and have sufficient compliance to permit adequate ICD follow-up.

must make optimal use of the knowledge that has already accumulated regarding the role of ICD versus other therapies in patients who have manifested sustained ventricular tachyarrhythmias. At least from the standpoint of preventing sudden death, the excellent results achieved with ICD therapy permit us to use these results as a gold standard to aid in stratifying therapies for patients at risk.

Table 42–5
Clinical Scenarios in Which ICD is the Primary Therapeutic Option

Patient Group	Comments
Very high risk of sudden death*	
• Resuscitated from cardiac arrest (VF or sustained VT) *or* syncope secondary to sustained monomorphic VT, with LVEF ≤ 0.30, *regardless* of VT inducibility or drug response	Assumes bundle-branch re-entry has been excluded as the sole cause of sustained monomorphic VT
• Resuscitated from cardiac arrest (VF or sustained VT) *or* syncope secondary to sustained monomorphic VT, with LVEF > 0.30 *and* drug-refractory inducible sustained monomorphic VT or VF	Assumes bundle-branch re-entry has been excluded as the sole cause of sustained monomorphic VT; also assumes long QT syndrome is not the cause of VT/VF
No established, reliable therapeutic alternative	
• Resuscitated from cardiac arrest (VF or sustained VT) *or* syncope secondary to sustained monomorphic VT, in the *absence* of inducible sustained monomorphic VT or VF	Assumes clinical conditions *other than* long QT syndrome (e.g., coronary artery disease or nonischemic [idiopathic dilated or hypertrophic obstructive] cardiomyopathy)

Source: Akhtar M, et al: Circulation 85(suppl I):I-131, 1992.[56] Modified by permission of the American Heart Association.
Note: In all of the above scenarios and in subsequent tables, if severe congestive heart failure is present, cardiac transplantation should be considered as an alternate option. It is also assumed in this and in subsequent tables that reversible causes, such as acute ischemia, electrolyte imbalance, and drug effects, are excluded and that a full pacing protocol is used before and after drug therapy. It is further assumed that sustained monomorphic VT provides a more reliable target for serial drug testing and VT ablation, and is usually amenable to overdrive termination.
* As actuarially defined in Table 42–4.

One possible scheme reflecting this approach is provided in Table 42–4, which focuses on actuarial sudden death mortality data at 4 years to help define the level of sudden death risk and the need for ICD therapy. It must be emphasized that the actuarial guidelines provided in Table 42–4 can only be considered approximations at the present time. Moreover, total cardiac and overall mortality considerations must also be taken into account; therefore, patients with a relatively short life expectancy (e.g., those with NYHA Class IV congestive heart failure) should *not* be evaluated according to these guidelines.

In order to be able fully to implement the therapy stratification proposed in Table 42–4, actuarial data are required for various patient populations, presenting arrhythmias, underlying ventricular function, and so on. Unfortunately, such information has not been systematically collected and analyzed. Consequently, we must make some clinically reasonable guesses regarding risk group assessment for particular patient subsets.

Table 42–6
Clinical Scenarios in Which ICD is a Major Therapeutic Option

Patient Group	Therapeutic Alternatives (Not Necessarily with Comparable Results)
Moderate risk for sudden death*	
• Inducible hypotensive sustained monomorphic VT in following settings:	Effective drug therapy or VT (or RB†) ablation
• CAD or IDCM, LVEF > 0.30, and history of VF or hypotensive sustained monomorphic VT	
• CAD or IDCM, and history of syncope	Effective drug therapy or VT (or RB†) ablation
• Inducible hemodynamically stable sustained monomorphic VT in patients with CAD or IDCM, tolerated spontaneous sustained monomorphic VT, and LVEF ≤ 0.30	Effective drug therapy or VT (or RB†) ablation
• Inducible hypotensive sustained monomorphic VT in patients with CAD and spontaneous nonsustained monomorphic VT associated with presyncope or syncope	Effective drug therapy or VT (or RB†) ablation
• Hypotensive recurrent polymorphic nonsustained VT *not* associated with prolonged QT or reversible causes (such as ischemia)	Effective drug therapy
• Resuscitated from cardiac arrest (VT/VF) or syncope, in long QT syndrome	β-blocker, pacemaker, or left stellate sympathectomy
Low risk for sudden death*	
• Inducible hemodynamically stable Sust. MVT in patients with CAD, LVEF > 0.30, and spontaneous, hemodynamically tolerated sustained monomorphic VT	Effective drug therapy or VT ablation

Source: Akhtar M, et al: Circulation 85(suppl I):I-131, 1992.[56] Modified and reproduced by permission of the American Heart Association.
Abbreviations: CAD, coronary artery disease; IDCM, idiopathic dilated cardiomyopathy; RB, right bundle; LVEF, left ventricular ejection fraction; VT, ventricular tachycardia; VF, ventricular fibrillation.
* As actuarially defined in Table 42–4.
† In setting of inducible sustained bundle-branch re-entry.

Table 42-7
Clinical Scenarios in Which ICD Therapy Is Not Indicated

Clinical Presentation	Therapeutic Alternative
Acute ischemia-mediated VT/VF, normal LV function, no inducible sustained monomorphic VT	Anti-ischemic therapy
Resuscitated from cardiac arrest with unequivocal toxic/metabolic etiology and no inducible sustained monomorphic VT	Eliminate precipitating factors
Incessant VT/VF unrelated to antiarrhythmic drugs	Effective drug therapy or VT ablation
VF secondary to AF in Wolff-Parkinson-White syndrome	Ablation of accessory pathway
Surgical/medical/psychiatric contraindications	Effective drug therapy or VT ablation

Source: Akhtar M, et al: Circulation *85(suppl I)*:I-131, 1992.[56] Modified and reproduced by permission of the American Heart Association.

Tables 42-5 and 42-6 offer a scheme for risk group assignment that is basically compatible with the treatment stratification concept we have outlined above. Table 42-5 includes clinical scenarios that generally correspond to the "very high risk" group of Table 42-4, for which ICD therapy represents an appropriate first-line treatment modality. Table 42-5 includes clinical scenarios corresponding to a mixture of the "moderately high risk" and "low risk" groups of Table 42-4, for which ICD therapy is certainly appropriate but not necessarily a superior treatment choice. For completeness, Table 42-7 is provided to indicate clinical settings in which ICD therapy is clearly *not* indicated. Within the context of these general guidelines, we will now discuss the role of ICD and other therapies in the management of patients with specific tachyarrhythmia presentations.

TACHYARRHYTHMIC CARDIAC ARREST WITHOUT ACUTE MYOCARDIAL INFARCTION IN THE SETTING OF CORONARY ARTERY DISEASE

Patients with coronary artery disease constitute the largest group of survivors of cardiac arrest in the absence of acute infarction.[46] Before discussing the roles of various treatment modalities, we will briefly mention pathophysiological considerations that provide the conceptual framework for therapy selection in these patients.

Whereas VF remains the major final common pathway to tachyarrhythmic cardiac arrest in patients with coronary artery disease, such a potentially lethal outcome can result from two major mechanistic pathways:[70] (1) *the ischemic route,* which precipitates VF either directly or indirectly (almost always via polymorphic VT); and (2) *the scar-related route,* which gives rise mainly to sustained monomorphic VT that, if rapid and poorly tolerated, degenerates to VF. Considerable experimental and clinical evidences support the concept that the scar-related route gives rise to sustained monomorphic VT by a variety of processes independent of acute ischemia.[70] Indeed, therapeutic interventions of an anti-ischemic nature have a very low likelihood of suppressing inducible sustained monomorphic VT related to prior myocardial scarring.[23,24] Following tachyarrhythmic cardiac arrest in the latter setting, therefore, anti-ischemic therapy must be viewed as largely adjunctive, with the important purpose of limiting or preventing future ischemic episodes that might precipitate sudden tachyarrhythmic death, either independently of, or synergistically with, the scar-related substrate.[20,71]

The importance of inducibility of sustained monomorphic VT and the extent of myocardial scarring (as reflected by the LVEF in predicting recurrent cardiac arrest) is documented in two large series.[46,72] The study of Furukawa et al[72] provides the

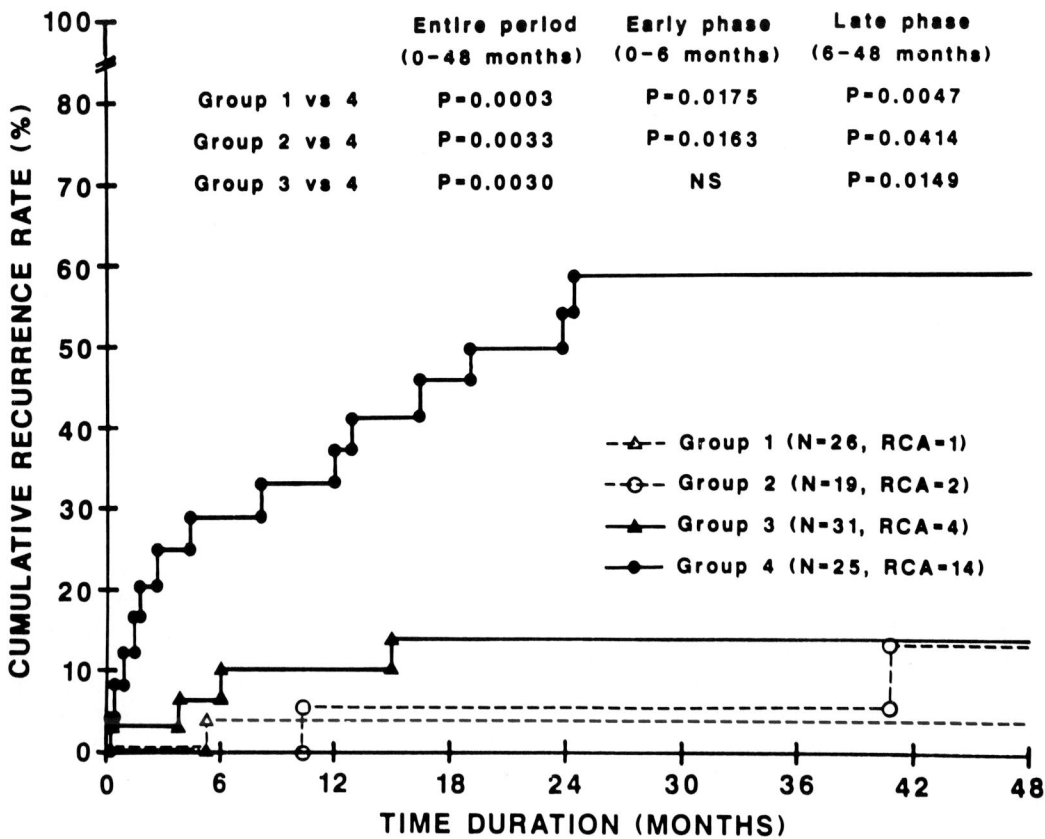

Fig. 42–2. Cumulative actuarial curve of cardiac arrest recurrence for each of four groups of coronary artery disease patients with a history of aborted sudden death. The curves were based on two multivariate predictors—an ejection fraction (LVEF) < 0.35 and persistent inducibility of ventricular tachyarrhythmias. Group 1, LVEF ≥ 0.35 and no persistent inducibility; group 2, LVEF ≥ 0.35 and persistent inducibility; group 3, LVEF < 0.35 and no persistent inducibility; group 4, LVEF < 0.35 and persistent inducibility. At the top of the panel, the cumulative recurrence rates during the entire period, the early phase, and the late phase of follow-up are compared. RCA, recurrence of cardiac arrest. (Reproduced by permission of the American Heart Association from Furukawa T, et al: Circulation 80:599, 1989.[72])

most precise information on this relationship in patients with tachyarrhythmic cardiac arrest in the setting of coronary artery disease. Actuarial data from that study (Fig. 42–2) indicate that, following antiarrhythmic medications, patients with an LVEF < 35 and persistently inducible sustained VT have a 50% chance of recurrent arrest within 2 years.[72] Hence, ICD implantation is strongly advised in these cases. Even when inducible sustained VT is suppressed, patients with an LVEF < 0.35 still face a moderately high risk of sudden death that would justify ICD therapy. For patients with an LVEF ≥ 0.35, studies with a large number of cases and long-term follow-up are needed to determine how outcome following suppression of inducible sustained VT by drugs compares with results of ICD therapy.

Anti-ischemic therapy alone is likely to benefit only a minority, some 10–15%, of coronary artery disease patients who survive tachyarrhythmic cardiac arrest unrelated to acute infarction.[21,22,46,72] Such patients are individuals with minimal or no myocardial scarring and no inducible sustained monomorphic VT, but with angiographic or scintigraphic studies supporting the likely presence of significant ischemically jeopardized myocardium, especially in tandem with a history of chest pain just prior to collapse.

TACHYARRHYTHMIC ARREST IN THE ABSENCE OF CORONARY ARTERY DISEASE

Detailed actuarial data regarding cumulative incidence of sudden death, analogous to that of Figure 42–2, are not readily available in patients without coronary artery disease who survive a tachyarrhythmic cardiac arrest. It is known, however, that patients with either idiopathic dilated cardiomyopathy[73,74] or hypertrophic cardiomyopathy[75] face a significant risk of subsequent sudden death following an aborted tachyarrhythmic cardiac arrest. The low rate of inducibility of sustained monomorphic VT in these patients[3] deprives the physician of a suitable therapeutic end point for use of antiarrhythmic medication, even if one were to assume that such therapy would be truly protective against recurrent cardiac arrest. In the absence of inducible sustained VT, ICD therapy represents the most reasonable choice in these patients.[76] Regardless of the presence or absence of inducible sustained VT, VF survivors with idiopathic dilated cardiomyopathy have a low sudden death rate with ICD therapy.[76a] Cardiac transplantation can provide a more long-term solution to the arrhythmic and hemodynamic problems in appropriate candidates with idiopathic dilated cardiomyopathy, but the risk of recurrent cardiac arrest while patients await a new heart may still require ICD implantation as a "bridge to transplant."[77,78]

Individuals with "primary electrical disease," who develop VF in the absence of gross structural cardiac abnormalities, likely harbor some type of arrhythmic substrate (presumably microscopic) that puts them at risk for recurrent cardiac arrest.[79–82] The fact that such individuals often lack inducible sustained monomorphic VT limits the ability of programmed ventricular stimulation to provide an end-point for drug therapy. ICD implantation in these patients is therefore justifiable; indeed, appropriate device discharges have been documented during long-term follow-up of implantees with primary electrical disease.[82] Favorable results have also been reported with the use of quinidine in patients who have inducible polymorphic VT or VF,[83] but worldwide experience with this approach is limited and longer-term follow-up in these relatively young individuals is needed in order to better define the treatment modalities most likely to prevent sudden death.

In patients who have survived an episode of VF on the basis of congenital long-QT syndrome, ICD therapy has occasionally been employed to provide protection against fatal recurrences,[84] although the success of β-blocker therapy,[85] sometimes in conjunction with permanent pacemaker implantation,[86,87] and left stellate sympathectomy[88] have constituted the conventional therapeutic approaches for this condition. It is unclear, however, whether ICD therapy should be relegated to the status of treatment-of-last-resort or, instead, merits more aggressive utilization in these relatively young, high risk individuals, who may not be as fortunate to survive another cardiac arrest.

SUSTAINED MONOMORPHIC VT ASSOCIATED WITH SYNCOPE

In the presence of organic heart disease it is probably prudent to view the occurrence of syncope during sustained monomorphic VT as a "self-aborted" cardiac arrest. At the very least, recurrence of such a symptomatic tachyarrhythmia could result in serious injury or even death on a secondary basis. The extent to which the conceptual analogy between syncope and aborted cardiac arrest can be extended to prognosis, however, is not clear. Perhaps the most relevant data available to date are those of Leclercq et al,[89] who reported actuarial survival in a retrospective series of (mainly medically treated) patients with either coronary artery disease or nonischemic dilated cardiomyopathy who presented with sustained monomorphic VT. For patients with an LVEF ≤ 0.30, cumulative cardiac mortality at 5 years was 67% in the 35 individuals manifesting syncope, versus 37% in those 58 without significant hemodynamic compromise during VT ($p < 0.05$).[89] Because approximately 60% of cardiac deaths in that study were sudden,[90] it can be estimated that the cumulative actuarial incidence of sudden death in patients with an LVEF ≤ 0.30 was about 32% at 4 years after an episode of sustained VT with syncope. When the same statistical reasoning is applied to those patients from Leclercq's series with an identical arrhythmic presentation but an LVEF > 0.30, the 4-year cumulative sudden death incidence was only about 11%. From the perspective of Table 42–4, such calculations suggest that patients presenting with sustained monomorphic VT associated with syncope in the setting of organic heart disease and significantly reduced LVEF (≤ 0.30) warrant strong consideration for ICD therapy; when the LVEF is >0.30 alternative therapies may provide protection from sudden death comparable to that of an ICD.

Leclercq et al[90] have also reported that patients with organic heart disease and sustained VT, including those with syncope, may benefit from the addition of β-blocker therapy. The basis for such benefit (protection from ischemia, attenuation of sympathetic stimulation or amelioration of congestive heart failure in some cases, etc.) remains unclear and deserves further investigation.

Special mention should be made of bundle-branch re-entry, which must always be considered a potential mechanism for rapid sustained monomorphic VT associated with syncope in a patient with poor left ventricular function, particularly when an intraventricular conduction abnormality is present with a prolonged His-to-ventricle (HV) interval.[16,18,19] Careful electrophysiological analysis of the induced VT is critical to the diagnosis.[16,18] Tachycardia cure by transcatheter ablation of the right bundle[16] is generally felt to be the treatment of choice, but additional therapies, including ICD implantation, may be required if there are coexistent inducible poorly tolerated sustained VTs.[19]

In the absence of organic heart disease, sustained VT is very uncommon, and, when it occurs, is typically hemodynamically well tolerated. Thus, little information is available for making therapeutic recommendations in patients without overt organic heart disease who develop sustained VT associated with syncope. Transcatheter radiofrequency ablation merits serious consideration if such VTs are inducible and have a readily identifiable site of origin, especially when localized to the right ventricular outflow tract.[91] In patients for whom such therapy is not practical or feasible, electrophysiologically guided selection of antiarrhythmic medication (which might include calcium channel blockers or a β-blocker, in cases of exercise-induced VT) is a valid alternative in compliant patients. ICD therapy should probably be reserved for patients not responsive to or intolerant of other therapies, or those individuals whose type of employment is such that symptomatic VT recurrences also could jeopardize the lives of others.

HEMODYNAMICALLY TOLERATED SUSTAINED MONOMORPHIC VT

A review of the available literature concerning this entity has already been presented. At the present time, it appears that in patients who present with this arrhythmia in the setting of coronary artery disease, treatment with antiarrhythmic drug therapy results in a sudden death rate lower than that reported in similarly treated cardiac arrest survivors, but roughly comparable to that associated with ICD therapy. Thus, in patients with coronary artery disease and hemodynamically tolerated sustained monomorphic VT, a variety of therapies other than antitachycardia pacing or very low-energy cardioversion (ICD therapy) may be considered, including electrophysiologically guided drug therapy, VT ablative surgery in low-operative-risk cases, and transcatheter radiofrequency ablation in selected patients with readily mappable VTs.

In patients with hemodynamically tolerated sustained monomorphic VT associated with idiopathic dilated cardiomyopathy, a similar broad range of therapeutic options may be considered when sustained VT can be replicated by programmed ventricular stimulation. In the absence of such VT inducibility, ICD therapy or empirical treatment with amiodarone may have to be considered on an individualized basis.

Sudden death is a rare outcome in patients without organic heart disease (or even those with right ventricular dysplasia) who present with hemodynamically tolerated sustained monomorphic VT. Hence, a wide range of antiarrhythmic treatment modalities may be considered, with drugs or transcatheter radiofrequency ablation (when feasible) generally being preferred, and antitachycardia pacing (ICD therapy) reserved for refractory cases.

POLYMORPHIC VT IN THE ABSENCE OF QT PROLONGATION

There are no reports describing a large clinical experience with this entity. In patients with coronary artery disease, this tachyarrhythmia should be considered possible evidence of recurrent myocardial ischemia and treated as such.[92-94] In the absence of coronary artery disease, polymorphic VT (sustained or nonsustained) without QT prolongation, when associated with dizziness or syncope, should probably be viewed as a prefibrillatory arrhythmia that could precipitate cardiac arrest.[95,96] Hence, in the absence of treatable causes, and until a benefit from antiarrhythmic drug therapy can be demonstrated, ICD implantation merits strong consideration as a therapeutic option.

SYNCOPE OF UNKNOWN ORIGIN

As difficult as it is to obtain definitive information regarding preferred therapeutic management in patients with a history of sustained ventricular tachyarrhythmias, the data are even more murky with regard to patients who are suspected of having such arrhythmias as the basis for syncope of unknown origin. Since electrocardiographic (ECG) recordings during the syncopal spell are lacking, it is never even certain whether one is dealing with an arrhythmia in the first place, let alone a tachyarrhythmia or bradyarrhythmia. Accordingly, before embarking on an antiarrhythmic program in such patients, it is crucial to assess the risk for development of sustained ventricular tachyarrhythmias by integrating clinical data with the results of diagnostic studies.

In the absence of organic heart disease there is a low likelihood of sudden death during follow-up,[97,98] and treatment directed at sustained ventricular tachyarrhythmias is rarely required. Tilt-table testing is likely to be of greatest benefit in these cases because of the ability of this procedure to unmask neurocardiac syncope, which is amenable to medical therapy.[99-101]

On the other hand, syncope in the setting of organic heart disease can be a harbinger of cardiac arrest.[97,102] In a study of patients with an LVEF $<$ 0.30 and syncope, the cumulative incidence of SCD was about 30% at 1 year.[102] The proportion of these deaths due to sustained ventricular tachyarrhythmias is not well defined but is probably at least in the neighborhood of 40%.[103] Although sustained monomorphic VT is inducible in some 56% of patients with organic heart disease and syncope,[101] there are no definitive studies that prove that suppression of such inducible sustained VT prolongs life. Until such studies are performed, it is probably most prudent to approach inducible sustained monomorphic VT in the setting of organic heart disease and syncope of unknown origin *as if* it were the causative arrhythmia. ICD therapy can certainly be justified in such a setting (especially when LVEF is $\leq$0.30),[101] although there is as yet no consensus on this point[34]; thus, a variety of pharmacological and nonpharmacological treatment modalities (described earlier) aimed at eradicating putative spontaneous episodes of sustained VT may be considered.

FUTURE DIRECTIONS

In patients with known or suspected sustained ventricular tachyarrhythmias, the most pressing need is the design and execution of studies—ideally, randomized clinical trials—which will provide detailed outcome information on the results of different therapeutic interventions.[68] Also remaining to be defined is the extent to which outcome varies as a function of different clinical parameters, including presenting arrhythmia, type of organic heart disease, left ventricular function, and so forth.

Besides the need to further clarify the role of ICD therapy in patients with known or suspected sustained ventricular tachyarrhythmias, attention must be turned to the larger group of high-risk cardiac patients who have not yet had an arrhythmic event but who may possibly benefit from prophylactic ICD implantation. These patients include those with coronary artery disease and a low LVEF, either soon after MI[104,105] or on a more chronic basis.[106,107] Prospective ICD trials in such patients are already under way[108] or in the process of being designed.[109]

REFERENCES

1. Lehmann MH, Steinman RT, Meissner MD, Schuger CD, Mosteller RD, Nabih MA: Need for a standardized approach to grading symptoms associated with ventricular tachyarrhythmias [editorial]. Am J Cardiol 67:1421, 1991.
2. Lampert S, Lown B, Graboys TB, Podrid PJ, Blatt C: Determinants of survival in patients with malignant ventricular arrhythmia associated with coronary artery disease. Am J Cardiol 61:791, 1988.
3. Skale BT, Miles WM, Heger JJ, Zipes DP, Prystowsky EN: Survivors of cardiac arrest: Prevention of recurrence by drug therapy as predicted by electrophysiologic testing or electrocardiographic monitoring. Am J Cardiol 57:113, 1986.
4. Buxton AE, Josephson ME: Role of electrophysiologic studies in identifying arrhythmogenic properties of antiarrhythmic drugs. Circulation 73(suppl II):II-67, 1986.
5. Mason JW: A comparison of electrophysiologic testing with holter monitoring to predict antiarrhythmic-drug efficacy for ventricular tachyarrhythmias. N Engl J Med 329:445, 1993.
6. Guiraudon G, Fontaine G, Frank R, Escande G, Etievent P, Cabrol C: Encircling endocardial ventriculotomy: A new surgical treatment for life-threatening ventricular tachycardias resistant to medical treatment following myocardial infarction. Ann Thorac Surg 26:438, 1978.
7. Josephson ME, Harken AH, Horowitz LN: Endocardial excision: A new surgical technique for the treatment of recurrent ventricular tachycardia. Circulation 60:1430, 1979.
8. Guiraudon GM, Klein GJ, Vermeulen FE, Yee R, Van Hemel NM: Encircling endocardial cryoablation: A technique for surgical treatment of ventricular tachycardia after myocardial infarction [abstract]. Circulation 68(suppl III):III-176, 1983.
9. Caceres J, Akhtar M, Werner P, et al: Cryoablation of refractory sustained ventricular tachycardia due to coronary artery disease. Am J Cardiol 63:296, 1989.
10. Svenson RH, Littman L, Gallagher JJ, et al: Termination of ventricular tachycardia with epicardial laser photocoagulation: A clinical comparison with patients undergoing successful endocardial photocoagulation alone. J Am Coll Cardiol 15:63, 1990.
11. Downar E, Harris L, Mickelborough LL, Shaikh N, Parson ID: Endocardial mapping of ventricular tachycardia in the intact human ventricle: Evidence for a reentrant mechanism. J Am Coll Cardiol 11:783, 1988.
12. Lawrie GM, Pacifico A, Kaushik R, Nahas C, Earle N: Factors predictive of results of direct ablative operations for drug-refractory ventricular tachycardia: Analysis of 80 patients. J Thorac Cardiovasc Surg 101:44, 1991.
13. Hargrove WC, Miller JM: Risk stratification and management of patients with recurrent ventricular tachycardia and other malignant ventricular arrhythmias. Circulation 79(suppl I):178, 1989.
14. Cox JL: Patient selection criteria and results of surgery for refractory ischemic ventricular tachycardia. Circulation 79(suppl I):163, 1989.
15. DiMarco JP: Management of sudden cardiac death survivors. Circulation 85(suppl I):I-125, 1992.
16. Tchou P, Jazayeri M, Denker S, Dongas J, Caceres J, Akhtar M: Transcatheter electrical ablation of right bundle branch: A method of treating macroreentrant ventricular tachycardia attributed to bundle branch reentry. Circulation 78:246, 1988.
17. Morady, Scheinman MM, DiCarlo LA Jr, et al: Catheter ablation of ventricular tachycardia with intracardiac shocks: Results in 33 patients. Circulation 75:1037, 1987.
18. Caceres J, Jazayeri M, McKinnie J, et al: Sustained bundle branch reentry as a mechanism of clinical tachycardia. Circulation 79:256, 1989.
19. Van Wyhe GG, Bailin SJ, Wickemeyer WJ, Rough RR, McGaughey MD, Johnson WB: Prospective search for bundle branch reentrant ventricular tachycardia; High incidence (22%) and frequent association with non bundle branch reentrant ventricular tachycardia [abstract]. Circulation 84(suppl II):II-318, 1991.
20. O'Rourke RA: Role of myocardial revascularization in sudden cardiac death. Circulation 85(suppl I):I-112, 1992.
21. Morady F, DiCarlo L, Winston S, Davis JC, Scheinman MM: Clinical features and prognosis of patients with out of hospital

cardiac arrest and a normal electrophysiologic study. J Am Coll Cardiol 4:39, 1984.
22. Kehoe RF, Tommaso C, Zheutlin TA, et al: Factors determining programmed stimulation responses and long-term arrhythmic outcome in survivors of ventricular fibrillation with ischemic heart disease. Am Heart J 116:355, 1988.
23. Kelly P, Ruskin J, Vlahakes G, Buckley MJ, Freeman CS, Garan H: Surgical coronary revascularization in survivors of prehospital cardiac arrest: Its effect on ventricular arrhythmia inducibility and long term survival. J Am Coll Cardiol 15:267, 1990.
24. Costeas XF, Hill PE, DiMarco JP, Schoenfeld MH: Surgical revascularization and the management of life-threatening ventricular tachyarrhythmias: Lack of efficacy in inducible sustained monomorphic ventricular tachycardia [abstract]. PACE 15:595, 1992.
25. Spielman SR, Schwartz JS, McCarthy DM, et al: Predictors of the success or failure of medical therapy in patients with chronic recurrent sustained ventricular tachycardia: A discriminant analysis. J Am Coll Cardiol 1:401, 1983.
26. Swerdlow CD, Gong G, Echt DS, et al: Clinical factors predicting successful electrophysiologic-pharmacologic study in patients with ventricular tachycardia. J Am Coll Cardiol 1:409, 1983.
27. Rae AP, Greenspan AM, Spielman SR, et al: Antiarrhythmic drug efficacy for ventricular tachyarrhythmias associated with coronary artery disease as assessed by electrophysiologic studies. Am J Cardiol 55:1494, 1985.
28. Knilans TK, Prystowsky EN: Antiarrhythmic drug therapy in the management of cardiac arrest survivors. Circulation 85(suppl I):I-118, 1992.
29. Fogoros RN, Anderson KP, Winkle RA, Swerdlow CD, Mason JW: Amiodarone: Clinical efficacy and toxicity in 96 patients with recurrent, drug-refractory arrhythmias. Circulation 68:88, 1983.
30. Raeder EA, Podrid PJ, Lown B: Side effects and complications of amiodarone therapy. Am Heart J 109:975, 1985.
31. Herre JM, Sauve MJ, Malone P, et al: Long-term results of amiodarone therapy in patients with recurrent sustained ventricular tachycardia or ventricular fibrillation. J Am Coll Cardiol 13:442, 1989.
32. Mirowski M, Mower MM, Staewen WS, et al: Standby automatic defibrillator: An approach to prevention of sudden coronary death. Arch Intern Med 126:158, 1970.
33. Mirowski M, Reid PR, Mower MM, et al: Termination of malignant ventricular arrhythmias with an implanted automatic defibrillator in human beings. N Engl J Med 303:322, 1980.
34. Lehmann MH, Saksena S: NASPE policy statement: Implantable cardioverter defibrillators in cardiovascular practice. Report of the Policy Conference of the North American Society of Pacing and Electrophysiology. PACE 14:969, 1991.
35. Lehmann MH: The results of device therapy in high risk patients. In Akhtar M, Garan H, Lehmann MH, Troup PJ (eds): Sudden Cardiac Death: Management of High-Risk Patients. Ann Intern Med 114:499–512, 1991.
36. Tchou PJ, Kadri N, Anderson J, Caceres JA, Jazayeri M, Akhtar M: Automatic implantable cardioverter defibrillators and survival of patients with left ventricular dysfunction and malignant ventricular arrhythmias. Ann Intern Med 109:529, 1988.
37. Myerburg RJ, Luceri RM, Thurer R, et al: Time to first shock and clinical outcome in patients receiving an automatic implantable cardioverter-defibrillator. J Am Coll Cardiol 14:508, 1989.
38. Winkle RA, Mead RH, Ruder MA, et al: Long-term outcome with the automatic implantable cardioverter-defibrillator. J Am Coll Cardiol 13:1353, 1989.
39. Manolis AS, Tan-DeGuzman W, Lee MA, et al: Clinical experience in seventy-seven patients with the automatic implantable cardioverter defibrillator. Am Heart J 118:445, 1989.
40. Kelly PA, Cannom DS, Garan H, et al: The automatic implantable cardioverter-defibrillator: Efficacy, complications and survival in patients with malignant ventricular arrhythmias. J Am Coll Cardiol 11:1278, 1988.
41. Troup P, Chapman P, Wetherbee MD, et al: Mortality Associated with the AICD [abstract]. PACE 12:688, 1989. (Updated and additional relevant material provided by P. Troup, pers. comm.)
42. Kleinbaum DG, Kupper LL, Morgenstern H: Epidemiologic Research: Principles and Quantitative Methods. New York, Van Nostrand Reinhold, 1982, p 96.
43. Lehman MH, Thomas A, Jackson K, et al: Long-term outcome with implantable cardioverter defibrillator therapy in a multicenter investigator-edited database [abstract]. Circulation 82:III-166, 1990.
44. Myerburg RJ, Kessler KM, Estes D, et al: Long-term survival after prehospital cardiac arrest: Analysis of outcome during an 8 year study. Circulation 70:538, 1984.
45. Bau RS, Alvarez H III, Cobb LA: Survival

after resuscitation from out-of-hospital ventricular fibrillation. Circulation 50:1231, 1974.
46. Wilber DJ, Garan H, Finkelstein D, et al: Out-of-hospital cardiac arrest: Use of electrophysiologic testing in the prediction of long-term outcome. N Engl J Med 318:19, 1988.
47. Furman S: AICD benefit [editorial]. PACE 12:399, 1989.
48. Fisher JD, Brodman R, Kim SG, Ferrick KJ, Roth JA: VT/VF: 60/60 protection. PACE 13:218, 1990.
49. Kim SG, Fisher JD, Furman S, et al: Benefits of implantable defibrillators are overestimated by sudden death rates and better represented by the total arrhythmic death rate. J Am Coll Cardiol 17:1587, 1991.
50. Edel TB, Maloney JD, Moore S, et al: Six-year clinical experience with the automatic implantable cardioverter defibrillator. PACE 14:1850, 1991.
51. Gartman DM, Bardy GH, Allen M, Misbach GA, Ivey TD: Short-term morbidity and mortality of implantation of automatic implantable cardioverter-defibrillator. J Thorac Cardiovasc Surg 100:353, 1990.
52. Mosteller RD, Lehmann MH, Thomas AC, Jackson K, and Participating Investigators: Operative mortality with implantation of the automatic cardioverter-defibrillator. Am J Cardiol 68:1340, 1991.
53. Kim SG, Fisher JD, Choue CW, et al: Influence of left ventricular function on outcome of patients treated with implantable defibrillators. Circulation 85:1304, 1992.
54. Cohen TJ, Reid PR, Mower MM, et al: The automatic implantable cardioverter-defibrillator: Long-term clinical experience and outcome at a hospital without an open-heart surgery program. Arch Intern Med 152:65, 1992.
55. Saksena S, Stout R, Poliseno M, Krol RB, Mehta D, Worldwide Guardian 4210 Phase I Investigators: Tachycardia detection and treatment with a third-generation implantable cardioverter-defibrillator: An international experience. J Am Coll Cardiol [in press].
56. Akhtar M, Avitall B, Jazayeri M, et al: Role of implantable cardioverter defibrillator therapy in the management of high-risk patients. Circulation 85(suppl I):I-131, 1992.
57. Levine JH, Mellits ED, Baumgardner RA, et al: Predictors of first discharge and subsequent survival in patients with automatic implantable cardioverter-defibrillators. Circulation 84:558, 1991.
58. Gohn D, Edel T, Pollard C, Firstenberg M, et al: Determinants of operative mortality in implantable cardioverter defibrillators [abstract]. J Am Coll Cardiol 17(suppl A): 86A, 1991.
59. Guarnieri T, Levine JH, Griffith LSC, Veltri EP: When "sudden cardiac death" is not so sudden: Lessons learned from the automatic implantable defibrillator. Am Heart J 115:205, 1988.
60. Lessmeier T, Lehmann MH, Fromm B, et al: What results can be expected from implantable cardioverter-defibrillator therapy in coronary artery disease patients presenting exclusively with ventricular fibrillation? [abstract]. J Am Coll Cardiol 19:208A, 1992.
61. Lehmann MH, Mitchell LB, Saksena S, Sakun V, Worldwide PCD Investigators: Operative (30-day) mortality with transvenous vs. epicardial ICD implantation: An intention-to-treat analysis [abstract]. Circulation [in press].
62. Fogoros RN, Elson JJ, Bonnet CA: Survival of patients who have received appropriate shocks from their implantable defibrillators. PACE 14:1842, 1991.
63. Fogoros RN, Elson JJ, Bonnet CA, Fiedler SB, Burkholder JA: Efficacy of the automatic implantable cardioverter-defibrillator in prolonging survival in patients with severe underlying cardiac disease. J Am Coll Cardiol 16:381, 1990.
64. Gross JN, Song SL, Buckingham T, Furman S, the Bilitch Registry Group: Influence of clinical characteristics and shock occurrence on ICD patient outcome: A multicenter report. PACE 14:1881, 1991.
65. Song SL: The Bilitch Report: Performance of implantable cardiac rhythm management devices. PACE 15(pt 1):475, 1992.
66. Epstein AE, Ellenbogen KA, Kirk KA, Kay GN, Dailey SM, Plumb VJ, and the High Defibrillation Threshold Investigators: Clinical characteristics and outcome of patients with high defibrillation thresholds: A multicenter study. Circulation 86: 1206, 1992.
67. Newman D, Sauve MJ, Herre J, et al: Survival after implantation of the cardioverter defibrillator. Am J Cardiol 69:899, 1992.
68. Connolly SJ, Yusuf S: Evaluation of the implantable cardioverter defibrillator in survivors of cardiac arrest: The need for randomized trials [editorial]. Am J Cardiol 69: 959, 1992.
69. Kuck KH, Siebels J, Schneider M, et al: Preliminary results of a randomized trial, AICD vs. drugs [abstract]. Rev Eur Tech Biomed 12:110, 1990.
70. Meissner MD, Akhtar M, Lehmann MH: Nonischemic sudden tachyarrhythmic

death in atherosclerotic heart disease: Pathophysiologic and clinical correlates. Circulation 84:905, 1991.
71. Cobb LA, Hallstrom AP, Weaver WD, Trobaugh GB, Greene HL: Considerations in the long-term management of survivors of cardiac arrest. Ann NY Acad Sci 432: 247, 1984.
72. Furukawa T, Rozanski JJ, Nogami A, Moroe K, Gosselin AJ, Lister JW: Time-dependent risk of and predictors for cardiac arrest recurrence in survivors of out-of-hospital cardiac arrest with chronic coronary artery disease. Circulation 80:599, 1989.
73. Stevenson WG, Middlekauff HR, Stevenson LW, Saxon LA, Woo MA, Moser D: Significance of aborted cardiac arrest and sustained ventricular tachycardia in patients referred for treatment therapy of advanced heart failure. Am Heart J 124:123, 1992.
74. Fazio G, Veltri EP, Tomaselli G, Lewis R, Griffith LSC, Guarnieri T: Long-term follow-up of patients with nonischemic dilated cardiomyopathy and ventricular tachyarrhythmias treated with implantable cardioverter defibrillators. PACE 14:1905, 1991.
75. Cecchi F, Maron BJ, Epstein SE: Long-term outcome of patients with hypertrophic cardiomyopathy successfully resuscitated after cardiac arrest. J Am Coll Cardiol 13: 1283, 1989.
76. Fogoros RN, Elson JJ, Bonnet CA, Fiedler SB, Chenarides JG: Long-term outcome of survivors of cardiac arrest whose therapy is guided by electrophysiologic testing. J Am Coll Cardiol 19:780, 1992.
76a. Lessmeier T, Lehmann MH, Steinman RT, et al: Outcome with implantable cardioverter defibrillator therapy for survivors of ventricular fibrillation secondary to idiopathic dilated cardiomyopathy or coronary artery disease without myocardial infarction. Am J Cardiol 73:911, 1993.
77. Bolling SF, Deeb GM, Morady F, et al: Automatic internal cardioverter defibrillator: A bridge to heart transplantation. J Heart Lung Transplant 10:562, 1991.
78. Haverich A, Troster J, Wahlers T, Fieguth HG, Klein H: The automatic implantable cardioverter defibrillator (AICD) as a bridge to heart transplantation. PACE 15(pt III):701, 1992.
79. Lemery R, Brugada P, Bella PD, Dugernier T, Wellens HJJ: Ventricular fibrillation in six adults without overt heart disease. J Am Coll Cardiol 13:911, 1989.
80. Wever EF, Hauer RN, Oomen A, Bakker PF, Robles de Medina EO: Unfavorable outcome in patients with primary electrical disease who survived cardiac arrest [abstract]. Circulation 84:II-20, 1991.
81. Roelke M, Powell AC, Liberthson RR, et al: Electrophysiologic observations and long-term follow-up in eleven patients with idiopathic ventricular fibrillation [abstract]. J Am Coll Cardiol 19:283A, 1992.
82. Meissner MD, Lehmann MH, Steinman RT, et al: Ventricular fibrillation in patients without significant structural heart disease: A multicenter experience with implantable cardioverter-defibrillator therapy. J Am Coll Cardiol 21:1406, 1993.
83. Belhassen B, Shapira I, Shoshani D, Paredes A, Miller H, Laniado S: Idiopathic ventricular fibrillation: Inducibility and beneficial effects of class I antiarrhythmic agents. Circulation 75:809, 1987.
84. Kron J, Oliver RP, Norsted S, Silka MJ: The automatic implantable cardioverter-defibrillator in young patients. J Am Coll Cardiol 16:896, 1990.
85. Schwartz PJ, Locati E: The idiopathic long QT syndrome: Pathogenetic mechanisms and therapy. Eur Heart J 6:103D, 1985.
86. Eldar M, Griffin JC, Abbott JA, et al: Permanent cardiac pacing in patients with the long QT syndrome. J Am Coll Cardiol 10: 600, 1987.
87. Moss AJ, et al: Efficacy of permanent pacing in the management of high-risk patients with long QT syndrome. Circulation 84: 1524, 1991.
88. Schwartz, et al: Left cardiac sympathetic denervation in the therapy of congenital long QT syndrome. Circulation 84:503, 1991.
89. Leclercq JF, Leenhardt A, Ruta I, et al: Espérance de vie après une premiere crise de tachycardie ventriculaire monomorphe soutenue. Arch Mal Coeur 84:1789, 1991.
90. Leclercq JF, Coumel P, Denjoy I, et al: Long-term follow-up after sustained monomorphic ventricular tachycardia: Causes, pump failure, and empiric antiarrhythmic therapy that modify survival. Am Heart J 121:1685, 1991.
91. Klein LS, Shih HT, Hackett FK, Zipes DP, Miles WM: Radiofrequency catheter ablation of ventricular tachycardia in patients without structural heart disease. Circulation 85:1666, 1992.
92. Tchou P, Atassi K, Jazayeri M, McKinnie J, Avitall B, Akhtar M: Etiology of polymorphic ventricular tachycardia in the absence of prolonged QT [abstract]. J Am Coll Cardiol 13:21A, 1989.
93. Zilcher H, Glogar D, Kaindl F: Torsades de pointes: Occurrence in myocardial isch-

aemia as a separate entity: Multiform ventricular tachycardia or not? Eur Heart J *1:* 63, 1980.
94. Nguyen PT, Scheinman MM, Seger J: Polymorphous ventricular tachycardia: Clinical characterization, therapy and the QT interval. Circulation *74:*340, 1986.
95. Olshausen KV, Witt T, Pop T, Treese N, Bethge KP, Meyer J: Sudden cardiac death while wearing a Holter monitor. Am J Cardiol *67:*381, 1991.
96. Eisenberg SJ, Dullet N, Lesh MD, Scheinman MM: Polymorphous ventricular tachycardia in patients with normal cardiac function and QT interval [abstract]. J Am Coll Cardiol *17:*198A, 1991.
97. Eagle KA, Black HR, Cook EF, Goldman L: Evaluation of prognostic classifications for patients with syncope. Am J Med *79:* 455, 1985.
98. Kushner JA, Kou WH, Kadish AH, Morady F: Natural history of patients with unexplained syncope and a nondiagnostic electrophysiologic study. J Am Coll Cardiol *14:*391, 1989.
99. Abi-Samra F, Maloney JD, Fouad-Tarazi FM, Castle LW: The usefulness of head-up tilt testing and hemodynamic investigations in the work-up of syncope of unknown origin. PACE *11:*1202, 1988.
100. Almquist A, Goldenberg IF, Milstein S, et al: Provocation of bradycardia and hypotension by isoproterenol and upright posture in patients with unexplained syncope. N Engl J Med *320:*346, 1989.
101. Sra JS, Anderson AJ, Sheikh SH, et al: Unexplained syncope evaluated by electrophysiologic studies and head-up tilt testing. Ann Intern Med *113:*1013, 1991.
102. Middlekauff HR, Stevenson WG, and Saxon LA: Prognosis after syncope: Impact of left ventricular function. Am Heart J *125:*121, 1993.
103. Luu M, Stevenson WG, Stevenson LW, Baron K, Walden J: Diverse mechanisms of unexpected cardiac arrest in advanced heart failure. Circulation *80:*1675, 1989.
104. Multicenter Postinfarction Research Group: Risk stratification and survival after myocardial infarction. N Engl J Med *309:* 331, 1983.
105. Bigger JT Jr, Fleiss JL, Kleiger R, et al: The relationships among ventricular arrhythmias, left ventricular function, and mortality in the 2 years after myocardial infarction. Circulation *69:*250, 1984.
106. Buxton AE, Marchlinski FE, Flores BT, Miller JM, Doherty JU, Josephson ME: Nonsustained ventricular tachycardia in patients with coronary artery disease: Role of electrophysiologic study. Circulation *75:* 1178, 1987.
107. Wilber DJ, Olshansky B, Moran JF, et al: Electrophysiologic testing and non-sustained ventricular tachycardia: Use and limitations in patients with coronary artery disease and impaired ventricular function. Circulation *82:*350, 1990.
108. Moss AJ: Prospective antiarrhythmic studies assessing prophylactic pharmacologic and device therapy in high risk coronary patients. PACE *15:*694, 1992.
109. DEFIBRILAT Study Group: Actuarial risk of sudden death while awaiting cardiac transplantation in patients with atherosclerotic heart disease. Am J Cardiol *68:*545, 1991.

Index

Note: Page numbers in *italics* indicate figures; page numbers followed by t indicate tables.

Ablation techniques. *See* Catheter ablation; Surgery, for ventricular tachycardia.
Acetabutol, 420
Acidosis
 and bradyarrhythmia, 409
 and ischemia in SCD, 532
 metabolic, in cardiac arrest survivors, 468
 SCD risk, 43
Action potentials
 in acute myocardial ischemia, 53–56, *55*
 during acute-on-chronic ischemia, 322–323
 amphiphile effects, 95
 critical mass for VF, 125
 electrolyte triggers, 328
 of healing infarct, 72–74
 in hypertrophic cardiomyopathy, 164–165, 172
Acyl CoA synthase, 85
Acylcarnitine
 accumulation in early ischemia, 85–87, *86*
 in arrhythmogenesis, 90–92
 and ionic currents, 92–93
Acylcarnitine hydrolase, 87
Adenosine triphosphate (ATP)
 in acute myocardial ischemia, 53, 54
 in acylcarnitine metabolism, 85–87
Adrenergic blocking agents
 alpha and beta, and vagal activity, 116–117
 beta, 419–438
  bradyarrhythmias, 413
  in children, 261, 263
  for hypertension treatment, 427–428, 430t
  in post-myocardial infarction patients, 420–426
   clinical implications, 426–427
   delayed intervention trials, 423–426, 424t
    arrhythmias, 425–426
   early intervention trials, 420–423, 421t
    arrhythmias, 422–423, 422t
  in hypertrophic cardiomyopathy, 171, 172
  for long QT syndrome, 212–213
  mechanisms in SCD prevention, 428–430
  SCD after MI, 306–307, *306*
Advanced cardiac life support (ACLS), out-of-hospital, 451, 455–456
Age factors
 in exercise testing, 353, 356
 risk for sudden death, 6–8, 16
Ajmaline, in Wolff-Parkinson-White syndrome, 222
Alcohol
 and lethal arrhythmias, 333
 SCD risk, 45
 and structural heart disease, 203
Alprenol, 420
Ambulance service, 455–456
American Heart Association
 chain of survival concept, 451
 CPR training, 452
 defibrillation programs, 453–454

American Red Cross, EMS system, 451
Amiodarone
 and ambulatory monitoring, 548, 557, 549t
 and arrhythmogenic right ventricular dysplasia, 227, 234
 in CAST, 443
 for hypertrophic cardiomyopathy, 171, 263
 polymorphic VT caused by, 391
 pretreatment before surgery, 569
 prolonged QT interval, 403
 during resuscitation, 457
 and vagal activity, 116
Amphiphiles
 and calcium, intracellular, 93–94
 and molecular membrane dynamics, 83–85
Amygdala, and ventricular tachycardia, 368
Amyloidosis
 in cardiac arrest survivors, 466
 conduction defects, 286
Aneurysm
 aortic, 14
 intracranial, 15
 thoracic, 14
Aneurysmectomy, 566–567
Angina pectoris
 collateral circulation, 298–299, *298*
 and hypertrophic cardiomyopathy, 166
Angina variants
 coronary artery disease, 23
 in myocardial ischemia, 302–303
  during sleep, 372
 supraventricular tachycardia, 392
Angiography
 acute-on-chronic ischemia, 318–319
 coronary, in cardiac arrest survivors, 470
Angioplasty, percutaneous transluminal coronary (PTCA)
 in asymptomatic ventricular arrhythmias, 522
 in beta-blocker trials, 422
 in coronary artery disease, 533
 in sustained ventricular tachyarrhythmias, 602
Animal models
 acute-on-chronic ischemia, 321–322
 baroreceptive reflexes, 102–107
 critical mass hypothesis for VF, 124–127
 ischemia and infarction. *See* Arrhythmias, lethal.
Anisotropy, critical mass hypothesis, 124
Anorexia, lethal arrhythmias, 333
Anoxia, and bradyarrhythmia, 409
Antiarrhythmic drugs
 in cardiac arrest survivors, 557–559, *558*
 and catecholamine interactions, 358
 and defibrillator interaction, 559
 in exercise testing, 357–362
 in hypertrophic cardiomyopathy, 171
 mechanisms of action, 428–430

619

Antiarrhythmic drugs *(Continued)*
   and noninvasive evaluations. *See* Arrhythmias, noninvasive studies.
   in survivors of acute MI, 524
   triggers of SCD, 394–406, *396–402*
   VT caused by, 389–390
Antidepressants, tricyclic, 267
Antihistamines, polymorphic VT caused by, 391
Anxiety, and bradyarrhythmia, 410–412
Aortic rupture in young athletes, 245, 264, *246*
Aortic stenosis
   and bradyarrhythmia, 412
   congenital, 14, 265, 268
   in young athletes, 247
Apnea
   bradyarrhythmias, 412–413
   and myocardial infarction, 372
   obstructive sleep, 374
   sudden infant death syndrome, 412
Aprindine, in survivors of acute MI, 524
Arrhythmias
   acylcarnitine and lysophosphatidylcholine roles, 90–92
   fatal, in cardiac arrest survivors, 465–466
   in hypertrophic cardiomyopathy, 168–169, 174
   induced, and defibrillator implantation, 595
   lethal, ischemia and infarction role, 51–81
     ventricular
       in acute myocardial ischemia and infarction, 51–59, *53, 54, 55, 58*
       delayed, in subacute myocardial infarction, 59–65, *60, 62–65*
       later phases, 65–74, *66–68, 70, 72, 73*
   malignant, etiology of, 155–159, *156, 158*
   during myocardial ischemia, biochemical mechanisms, 82–101
     acylcarnitine accumulation, 85–87, *86*
     acylcarnitine and lysophosphatidylcholine in arrhythmogenesis, 90–92
     and ionic currents, 92–93
     amphipathic metabolites, and cell coupling, 95–96
     amphiphile accumulation, and calcium changes, 93–94
     lysophosphatidylcholine accumulation, 88–90, *88, 89*
     potassium, extracellular, 94–95
     sarcolemma structure and function, amphiphile effects, 83–85, *84, 85*
   noninvasive studies, 541–553, 550t
     ambulatory electrocardiographic monitoring, 541–542
     and amiodarone therapy, 548, 549t
     in cardiomyopathies, 548–550
     classification types, 542–543, 542t, 543t
     clinical experience, 545–548, 547t
     exercise testing, 545, *546*
     proarrhythmia definition, 544–545, 544t, 545t
     variability of ventricular arrhythmias, 543–544, *544*
   nonischemic, in sudden ischemic death, 28–29
   in post-myocardial infarction beta-blocker trials, 422–423, 425–426, 422t
   reperfusion, 299
   structure/function concept, 34–35, *34*
     structural abnormalities, 35–37
   ventricular
     in arrhythmogenic right ventricular dysplasia, 229–230, *230*
     autonomic innervation. *See* Autonomic nervous system.
     in children, 259–262, 260t
     in congestive heart failure, 430–431
     electrolyte triggers. *See* Electrolytes.
     and exercise testing. *See* Exercise.
     in late phase of myocardial infarction, 147–154
     and left ventricular dysfunction after MI, 193–196, 198
     management and survival post MI, 514–517, 515t
     in myocardial ischemia, 302–304
     and structural heart disease, 203
     in tetralogy of Fallot, 266
     See also Ischemia, acute–on–chronic; Ventricular arrhythmias.
Arrhythmogenic right ventricular dysplasia (ARVD), 226–237
   arrhythmogenic substrate, 230–233, *231, 232*
   atrioventricular conduction disturbances, 227–229, *228, 229*
   in children, 267
   definition, 226–227
   and drug therapy, 234
   hemodynamics, 233
   incidence, 227
   and structural heart disease, 202
   sudden death in, 227
   ventricular arrhythmias, 229–230, *230*
   in young athletes, 233–234, 262
   See also Ventricles, right.
Arteriography, coronary, after resuscitation, 28
Artery(ies)
   coronary. *See* Coronary artery.
   great, transposition of, 266–268, 285
Aspirin therapy, 307
Asthma, and SCD in children, 267
Asystole
   and bradyarrhythmias, 407–408
   in cardiac arrest survivors, 466
   electrical triggers, 392
   during sleep, 374
Atenolol
   arrhythmias in beta-blocker trials, 423
   and bradyarrhythmias, 413
   for hypertension, 428
   mechanisms of action, 429
   in post-MI patients, 420
Atherosclerosis
   in cardiac arrest survivors, 467
   in coronary arteries, 35–36, 35t
   and SCD, 13, 22–23
   in young athletes, 245, *247*
Athletes
   arrhythmogenic right ventricular dysplasia, 233–234
   sudden cardiac death, 238–257
     older athletes, 250–251, *250, 251*
     soldiers, 249–250
     young athletes, 238–250, 262–264
       aortic rupture (Marfan's syndrome), 245, *248*
       aortic valvular stenosis, 247
       cardiac conduction system abnormalities, 247–248, *248*

congenital coronary artery anomalies,
    242–244, *243–245*
coronary heart disease, 245, *247*
definition, 238
demographics and mechanisms, 238–239
hypertrophic cardiomyopathy, 240–242, *241*
idiopathic left ventricular hypertrophy, 242, *242*
mitral valve prolapse, 246
myocarditis, 245–246
normal hearts, 249
preparticipation screening, 251–253, *253*
previous investigations, 239–240, *239, 240*
right ventricular cardiomyopathy (dysplasia), 249, *249*
sarcoidosis, 247
ATPase, Na,K–
    amphiphile effects, 93–94
    in hypertrophic cardiomyopathy, 165
ATRAMI (Autonomic Tone and Reflexes After Myocardial Infarction), 120–121
Atrial fibrillation
    in hypertrophic cardiomyopathy, 169
    multiple wandering wavelets, 137
    and structural heart disease, 203
    in Wolff–Parkinson–White syndrome, 215–223, *216–218*
Atrial flutter, and transposition of great arteries, 266
Atrial premature complexes, in hypertrophic cardiomyopathy, 168–169
Atrial septal defect, 285
Atrioventricular (AV) block
    in arrhythmogenic right ventricular dysplasia, 227–229, *228, 229*
    and bradyarrhythmia, 409
    catheter ablation, 574–577, 576t, *575*
        radio-frequency ablation of re-entry tachycardia, 579–580
    in children, 259–261, 268
    conduction abnormalities, 277–278, *278*
    critical mass for VF, 124
    in hypertrophic cardiomyopathy, 166, 168, 174
    and structural heart disease, 202, 204–206
Atrioventricular bundle (penetrating, branching, and bifurcating portions), 278–282, *279–281*
Atrium
    arrhythmias in exercise testing, 362
    pre-excitation syndrome, 282
Atropine
    and behavioral stress, 368
    and vagal activity, 114–115
Autonomic nervous system
    and bradyarrhythmia, 410–412
    in cardiac arrest survivors, 469–470, 476
    and sudden cardiac death, 43–44, 102–123
        ATRAMI, 120–121
        baroreceptive reflexes
            clinical studies, 107–110, 109t, *108–110*
            experimental studies, 102–107, *103–107*
            heart rate variability, 111–112, *111–112*
            vagal activity, 118–120, *120*
        questions and implications, 112–120
            heart rate variability and BRS, 120, *120*
            myocardial infarction and baroreflex sensitivity, 112–113, *113–114*
            survival with depressed BRS, 113–115, *115*
        vagal activity
            antifibrillatory effect during acute MI, 115–117, *116, 117*
            direct recording, 118–120, *119*
            and ventricular fibrillation, 118, *118*
    and ventricular arrhythmias, 341–349
        afferent denervation, 342
        denervation supersensitivity, arrhythmogenesis, and reinnervation, 343–344
        efferent denervation, 342–343, *345*
        and coronary artery disease, 346–347
        preconditioning ischemia, 343
        scintigraphy, sympathetic, 345–346, *346*
        sympathetic and vagal innervation in ventricle, 341, *342–344*
        sympathetic stimulation and ischemia/infarction, 345

Baroreceptive reflex sensitivity (BRS)
    in cardiac arrest survivors, 469–470
    clinical studies, 107–110, 109t, *108–110*
    depression of, and survival, 113–115
    experimental studies, 102–107, *103–107*
    and heart rate variability, 120, *120*
    after myocardial infarction, 112–113, *113–114*
    during sleep, 375
    and vagal activity, 118–120, *119*
Basketball players
    arrhythmogenic right ventricular dysplasia, 233
    sudden cardiac death, 238
Behavioral stress, and arrhythmias, 368–371
Bendrofluazide, 427, 428
Bendroflumethiazide, 428
Beta-Blocker Heart Attack Trial (BHAT), 423–426
    circadian variations, 9
Beta-Blocker Pooling Project (BBPP) Research Group, 426
Beta-blockers. *See* Adrenergic blocking agents, beta.
BHAT. *See* Beta-Blocker Heart Attack Trial.
Biopsy, myocardial, in structural heart disease, 203
Blacks, SCD statistics, 8, 14
Blood flow, coronary
    and hypertrophic cardiomyopathy, 166
    during sleep, 372
Blood pressure
    and baroreflex response, 103–104
    in cardiac arrest survivors, 476
    during exercise, 350
    in hypertrophic cardiomyopathy, 173–174
    and left ventricular dysfunction, 191
Botulism, and sudden infant death syndrome, 412
Bradyarrhythmia, 407–415
    in cardiac arrest survivors, 466
    in idiopathic dilated cardiomyopathy, 155, 157
    mechanisms of sudden death, 409–413, 409t
        and acute myocardial infarction, 413, 513
        aortic stenosis, 412
        apnea-bradycardia, 412–413
        autonomic neural control, death provoked by fear or anxiety, 410–412, *411*
        after electrical cardioversion, 409–410
        sleep apnea syndromes, 412–413
        sudden infant death syndrome, 412
    mortality, 408–409
    prevalence, 407–408, *408*
Bradyasystolic cardiac arrest, 457

Bradycardia
  electrical triggers, 392
  polymorphic VT, 391
Bretylium, 456–457
British Heart Foundation, 454
Bulimia, lethal arrhythmias, 333
Bundle branch block
  hemodynamically tolerated sustained VT, 505–506
  in idiopathic dilated cardiomyopathy, 157
  radio–frequency ablation, 583–584, *584*

Calcium
  in acute myocardial ischemia, 53–55
  channels, acylcarnitine and
    lysophosphatidylcholine effects, 93–94
  in hypertrophic cardiomyopathy, 164, 166, 172
  intracellular, amphiphile accumulations, 93–94
  in ischemia and reperfusion, 40
  and lethal arrhythmias, 333–336
  proarrhythmic actions, 400–402
  in ventricular hypertrophy, 37
Calcium channel blockers
  for hypertrophic cardiomyopathy, 171, 172
  SCD after MI, 306–307, *306*
Cardiac arrest
  bradyarrhythmia, 407–409
  documented ventricular fibrillation, 465–485
    clinical evaluation, 467–468
    incidence, 465
    laboratory evaluation
      invasive, catheterization and angiography, 470
      noninvasive
        ambulatory Holter monitoring, 468–469
        autonomic nervous influence, 469–470
        exercise stress testing, 469
        left ventricular function, 468
        signal-averaged ECG, 469
    pathophysiology of fatal arrhythmias, 465–466
    programmed electrical stimulation (PES), 470–475
      inducible arrhythmias, 470–474, 471t, *473*
      noninducibility, 474–475
    structural cardiac abnormalities, 466–467
    survivors with no structural heart disease, 478
    survivors with specific conditions, 475–478
      ischemic heart disease, 475–477
      nonischemic heart disease, 477–478
  hemodynamically tolerated sustained VT, and CAD, 502–504
  and idiopathic dilated cardiomyopathy, 159
  out-of-hospital. *See* Out-of-hospital cardiac arrest.
  tachyarrhythmic, without acute MI, 608–610
  See also Electrophysiological-electropharmacological tests in cardiac arrest survivors.
Cardiac Arrhythmia Pilot Study (CAPS), 440–442
Cardiac Arrhythmia Suppression Trial (CAST), 439–449
  arrhythmic end points, 303
  cardiac arrest survivors, 469
  Cardiac Arrhythmia Pilot Study (CAPS), 440–442
  CAST-II, 446–448, *447*
  clinical and scientific rationale, 439–440
  critical mass hypothesis for VF, 124
  design of trial, 442–446, 446t, *445*
  lethal proarrhythmias, 395

proarrhythmias, 545t
PVC reduction, 34, 543, 547
survivors of acute MI, 524
Cardiocardiac sympathovagal reflex, 112
Cardiomegaly, and left ventricular dysfunction, 191
Cardiomyopathy
  in cardiac arrest survivors, 466–467
  hypertrophic, 163–189
    in cardiac arrest survivors, 477–478
    in children, 259, 268
    functional and structural abnormalities, 163–169
      cardiac morphology, 165–166
      cellular function, 164–165
      electrophysiology, 168–169
      hemodynamics, 166–167
      myocardial perfusion, 166
      neurohumoral function, 167–168
    hemodynamically tolerated sustained VT, 504–505
    incidence, 163
    medical and operative treatment, 170–171
    noninvasive studies, 549–550
    nonsustained ventricular tachycardia, 486–489
    predictors and associated factors, 169–170
    prevention of sudden death, 180–181
    process of sudden death, 175–179, *175–178*
    specific factors and sudden death, 171–175
      action potential duration, 172
      atrioventricular conduction, 174
      calcium ion regulation, 172
      diastolic dysfunction, 173
      ischemia, myocardial, 172–173
      left ventricular outflow tract, 173
      miscellaneous factors, 174–175
      myocardial mass, 172
      myocyte disarray and fibrosis, 172
      neurohumoral dysfunction, 174
      peripheral vasodilation, 173–174
      sinus node dysfunction, 174
      supraventricular arrhythmias, 174
      ventricular arrhythmias, 174
    structural heart disease, 202
    theory of sudden death, 179–180
    in young athletes, 240–242, 262–263, 262t, *241*
  idiopathic dilated, 155–162
    ambulatory monitoring, 548–549
    in cardiac arrest survivors, 477
    in children, 267
    etiology of malignant arrhythmias, 155–159, *156, 158*
    hemodynamically tolerated sustained VT, 504
    monomorphic VT, 390
    nonsustained ventricular tachycardia, 487–489
    risk assessment, 159
    therapeutic factors, 159–160
  right ventricular (dysplasia), in young athletes, 249, *249*
  and SCD, 13, 14, 37, *38*
Cardiopulmonary resuscitation, out-of-hospital, 450–452, *453*
Cardioverter-defibrillator, implantable. *See* Defibrillators.
Carnitine-acylcarnitine translocase, 87
Carnitine acyltransferases, 86–87
CAST. *See* Cardiac Arrhythmia Suppression Trial.
Catecholamines
  and antiarrhythmic drugs, 358

and behavioral stress, 368
in beta-blocker mechanisms, 428–429
in exercise, 350–351, 362
in hypertrophic cardiomyopathy, 167–168
pericardial, 341
VT triggered by, 506
Catheter ablation, 574–587, 602
   at atrioventricular junction, 574–577, 576t, *575*
   in atrioventricular nodal re-entry tachycardia, 579–580, *580*
   in children, 261
   direct-current, in ventricular tachycardia, 582, 583t
   in idiopathic dilated cardiomyopathy, 157
   radio-frequency
      accessory pathways, 577–579, *578*, *579*
      ventricular tachycardia, 582–585, *584*, *585*
   and sudden death, 282–284
   supraventricular tachycardia, 574
   ventricular tachycardia and SCD, 580–582, *581*, *582*
   in Wolff–Parkinson–White syndrome, 219, 577
Catheterization, cardiac
   in cardiac arrest survivors, 470
   diagnostic assessment, 533
   in structural heart disease, 203
Cell coupling, and amphipathic metabolites, 95–96
Central nervous system triggers for SCD, 367–384
   behavioral stress and arrhythmias, 368–371, 369t, *369–371*
   sleep states, 371–375
      autonomic tone, 371–372
      heart rhythm pauses and arrhythmias, 374–375, *374*
      myocardial perfusion and arrhythmias, 372, *373*
      power spectrum analysis, 375, *376*
   T-wave alternans, 375–379, *377*
      electrophysiological basis, 379
      parasympathetic nervous system effects, 378–379
      sympathetic nervous system effects, 376–378, *378*
Cerebrovascular accident, and hypertrophic cardiomyopathy, 175
Chagas's disease, in cardiac arrest survivors, 466
Chest pain
   in coronary thrombosis, 26–28
   in SCD, 293
   in young athletes, 238
Children, sudden cardiac death in, 258–273
   apparently healthy children, 258–262, 258–259t
      arrhythmias, primary, 259–261, 260t
      mitral valve prolapse, 261–262
      myocarditis, 259
   athletes, 262–264, 262t
      aortic rupture, 264
      coronary artery abnormalities, 263–264
      hypertrophic cardiomyopathy, 263
   criteria, 258
   incidence, 258
   known heart disease, 264–267, 264t
      aortic stenosis, 265
      arrhythmogenic right ventricular dysplasia, 267
      cardiomyopathy, idiopathic dilated, 267
      Ebstein's malformation, 267
      pulmonary vascular obstructive disease, 265
      tetralogy of Fallot, 265–266
      transposition of great arteries, 266–267

      long QT syndrome, 209–214
      noncardiac sudden death, 267–268, 267t
      prevention, 268–269
Chloroform anesthesia, ventricular fibrillation, 44
2-[5-(4-Chlorophenyl)-pentyl]-oxirane-2-carboxylate (POCA), 87, 91
Cholesterol
   in cardiac arrest survivors, 476
   in sarcolemma, 83
Chromosome 11, in long QT syndrome, 209
Circadian rhythms
   in cardiac arrest survivors, 476
   power spectrum analysis, 375
   and sudden cardiac death, 9–11, 295–296, 307, 367, *10*, *295*, *296*
Classification
   SCD codes, 11
   sudden cardiac death, 198–199
   ventricular arrhythmias, 542–543, 542t, 543t
CoA
   in acylcarnitine metabolism, 85–87
   in lysophosphatidylcholine metabolism, 89
Cocaethylene, 45
Cocaine
   and SCD in children, 267
   SCD risk, 45
   and structural heart disease, 203
Codes for SCD, 11
Collagen, in hypertrophic cardiomyopathy, 165
Conduction system abnormalities, 274–289
   atrioventricular bundle (penetrating, branching, and bifurcating portions), 278–282, *279–281*
   atrioventricular node, 277–278, *278*
   critical mass hypothesis, 124
   in exercise testing, 360
   in lethal arrhythmias, 56
   method of study, 274–275
   during myocardial ischemia, 82
   during onset of fibrillation, 129, 133
   sinoatrial node, 275–277, *276*, *277*
   sudden death
      after ablative procedures, 282–284, *284*
      in known diseases, 286–287
         myocarditis, 287
         QT-interval prolongation, 287
      after operation for congenital heart disease, 284–286, *285*, *286*
      in pre-excitation, 282, *283*
      sudden infant death syndrome, 287
      summit of ventricular septum, 287
   VT vs. VF, 138
   See also Heart, conduction system abnormalities.
Congenital heart disease
   postoperative hemodynamically tolerated sustained VT, 505
   and SCD, 14
   See also specific diseases.
Congestive heart failure. *See* Heart failure, congestive.
Connective tissue, in hypertrophic cardiomyopathy, 165
CONSENSUS. *See* Cooperative North Scandinavian Enalapril Survival Study.
Contraction band necrosis, 27
Cooperative North Scandinavian Enalapril Survival Study (CONSENSUS), 433

Coronary artery
  anomalies
    in cardiac arrest survivors, 466
    and hypertrophic cardiomyopathy, 175
    and structural heart disease, 202
    in young athletes, 242–244, 262–264, *243, 244*
  in hypertrophic cardiomyopathy, 166
  left anterior descending, occlusion of, 67–71
  pathology in SCD, 21–31
    acute ischemia vs. chronic nonischemic
        tachyarrhythmia, 28–29
    coronary heart disease, 22–23
    definitions, 21–22
    morphological studies, 23–27
      coronary thrombosis, 25–27, 26t
      plaque instability, 24–25, *24*
    myocardial infarction, 28
    ventricular fibrillation mechanisms, 27–28
      ambulatory monitoring, 27–28
      myocardial lesions, 27
      resuscitation studies, 28
  See also Coronary artery disease.
Coronary artery bypass surgery (CABG), 531–540
  acute-on-chronic ischemia, 319, 320
  and bradyarrhythmia, 409
  cardiac pathology in SCD, 531–532
  diagnostic assessment, 533
  ischemia as precipitating factor, 532
  after MI, 307–308
  prevalence of SCD after surgery, 533–535,
      534–537
  primary and secondary prevention of SCD,
      532–533
  revascularization in preventing recurrent SCD,
      535–538
Coronary artery disease (CAD)
  acute-on-chronic ischemia, 318–319
  angiography, 296–297
  behavioral stress, 370–371
  in cardiac arrest survivors, 466
  in children, 264
  diagnostic assessment, 533
  and efferent sympathetic denervation, 346–347
  exercise testing. *See* Exercise.
  heart rate variability, 108
  hemodynamically tolerated sustained VT, 498–504
    and cardiac arrest, 502–504
    clinical presentation and electrophysiological
        findings, 498–499
    patient outcome, 499–502, 500t
      antiarrhythmic therapy, 502, 503t
  monomorphic VT, 390
  nonsustained ventricular tachycardia, 487
  prodromal symptoms, 293
  and SCD, 3
    epidemiology, 293–296
    out of hospital, 152
  tachyarrhythmic cardiac arrest without acute MI,
      608–610
  in young athletes, 262
Coronary Artery Surgery Study (CASS)
  acute-on-chronic ischemia, 320
  angiographic studies, 296
  cardiac arrest survivors, 470, 533–535, *534, 535*
  exercise testing, 353, 355
Coronary heart disease
  atherosclerotic, 13

  in athletes, 245, 250–251, *247, 250, 251*
  nonatherosclerotic, 13–14
  risk factors for SCD, 3, 5, 16–17, 16t
  and SCD, 3, 22–23
  structural abnormalities, 35–36, 35t
Cost effectiveness
  of beta-blocker therapy, 427
  of implantable defibrillators, 598–599
CPI Ventak defibrillator, 588–590
Creatine kinase, and left ventricular dysfunction,
      190–191
Critical mass hypothesis for ventricular fibrillation,
      124–127
Cyclic nucleotides, 378
Cytochrome oxidase, 87

Deafness, in long QT syndrome, 209–210
Defibrillation, ventricular
  critical mass for VF, 126
  out-of-hospital programs, 452–456
Defibrillator Implantation as Bridge to Later
      Transplant (DEFIBRILAT) trial, 477
Defibrillators, 588–599
  vs. amiodarone therapy, 557
  and antiarrhythmic drug interaction, 559
  and anti-ischemic therapy, 307–308
  arrhythmias, induced, 595
  background, 588
  and bradyarrhythmia, 409
  in children, 261, 263, 268
  complications, 595, 596t
  current status and technology, 588–591, *589, 590*
  follow-up, 591
  future trends, 596–599
    cost effectiveness, 598–599
    data storage, 597
    generator size, 598
    nonthoracotomy implants, 598
    supraventricular vs. ventricular tachycardias,
        597–598
    tiered therapy, 596–597, *596, 597*
  in high-risk patients, 602–605, 603t, 604t, *605*
  for hypertrophic cardiomyopathy, 181
  implantation after MI, 150
  left ventricular ejection fraction, 595
  New York Heart Association functional class, 595
  vs. other therapeutic strategies, 605–608, 606–608t
  patient selection, 593–595
  predischarge testing and programming, 591
  vs. surgical ablation, 564
  in structural heart disease, 206
  in VT and VF, 591–593, 591t, *592–594*
Definitions
  coronary artery pathology, 21–22
  hemodynamically tolerated sustained VT, 496
  proarrhythmia, 544–545
  of SCD, 3, 11–12
  in VT surgery, 563
Demographics, SCD in athletes, 238–239
Depolarization
  in acute myocardial ischemia, 57–58
  electrolyte triggers, 328
  in long QT syndrome, 211, 212
Derived suppression theory, 32
Diabetes
  in children, 264

plaque instability, 25
risk factor for SCD, 17
Diastolic dysfunction, in hypertrophic cardiomyopathy, 166–167, 173
Dieting, lethal arrhythmias, 333
Digitalis, potassium effects, 330–331
Digoxin, 431, 433
Disopyramide
　in exercise testing, 360
　for hypertrophic cardiomyopathy, 171
　in Wolff–Parkinson–White syndrome, 222
Diuretics
　for congestive heart failure, 431, 433
　for hypertension, 428
　polymorphic VT caused by, 391
　potassium effects, 330–331, 333
Diurnal variations, 296
DNA marker, long QT syndrome, 209
Drug use
　and arrhythmogenic right ventricular dysplasia, 234
　in cardiac arrest survivors, 468
　and SCD in children, 267
　and structural heart disease, 203
Dyspnea, 293

Ebstein's malformation
　in children, 267
　and Wolff–Parkinson–White syndrome, 218
Echocardiography
　in cardiac arrest survivors, 468
　in children, 260
　of hypertrophic cardiomyopathy, 163
　left ventricular dysfunction, 192–193
　screening of athletes, 252–253
　in structural heart disease, 203
Edrophonium, 117
EIS. *See* European Infarction Study.
Eisenmenger syndrome, 14, 265
Ejection fraction, left ventricular. *See* Left ventricular ejection fraction.
Electrical stimulation
　during onset of fibrillation, 131–136
　programmed (PES)
　　in cardiac arrest survivors, 470–475
　　　inducible ventricular arrhythmias, 470–474, 471t, *473*
　　　noninducibility as baseline PES, 474–475
　　　nonsustained ventricular tachycardia, 488–491
Electrical triggers of SCD, 385–393
　asystole, 392
　bradycardia, 392
　supraventricular tachycardia, 392
　ventricular tachycardia
　　monomorphic, 386–390
　　　premature beats, 386, *387, 388*
　　　repetitive concealed re-entry, 386–390, *389, 390*
　　polymorphic, 391–392
　　　and normal QT interval, 391–392
　　　in prolonged QT interval, 391
　　progression to fibrillation, 385–386
Electrocardiography
　ambulatory monitoring, 27–28
　arrhythmic mechanisms, 300–301, *300, 301*
　in children, 260

electrolyte effects, 330
of hemodynamically tolerated sustained VT, 498, 498t
in hypertrophic cardiomyopathy, 170
in idiopathic dilated cardiomyopathy, 155–156
of left ventricular dysfunction, 196
in long QT syndrome, 210–212
screening of athletes, 252
signal-averaged
　asymptomatic ventricular arrhythmias, 518–522, 519t
　in cardiac arrest survivors, 469
　nonsustained ventricular tachycardia, 491–492
　risk stratification of myocardial infarction, 150
　in Wolff–Parkinson–White syndrome, 220–221, *220*
Electroencephalography, during sleep, 374–375, *374*
Electrolytes
　in cardiac arrest survivors, 467–468
　during exercise, 350–351
　in idiopathic dilated cardiomyopathy, 156, 159–160
　and ischemia in SCD, 532
　SCD risk, 43
　triggers for ventricular arrhythmias, 327–340
　　calcium, 333–336
　　diuretic effects, 330–333
　　magnesium, 331, 333–335
　　potassium, 328–336, *328–333*
　　sodium, 335–336
Electromechanical dissociation, 457
Electrophysiological-electropharmacological tests in cardiac arrest survivors, 554–561
　antiarrhythmic drugs, 557–559, *558*
　and cardioverter-defibrillator interactions, 559
　candidates for serial testing, 554–556, 555t
　drug efficacy, 556–557
　amiodarone therapy, 557
Electrophysiological Study vs. Electrocardiographic Monitoring (ESVEM), 548, 557, 601
Electrophysiology
　acute-on-chronic ischemia, 322–323
　asymptomatic ventricular arrhythmias, 523–524
　in hypertrophic cardiomyopathy, 168–169, 175–178
　in ischemia and reperfusion, 38–43, 304, *305*
　in nonsustained ventricular tachycardia, 488–491
　of pharmacological triggers of SCD, 394–406
　in structural heart disease, 37, 204
　of sudden cardiac death, 14, 17
　T-wave alternans analysis, 379
　of Wolff–Parkinson–White syndrome, 219
　See also Arrhythmias; Ventricular arrhythmias in ischemia and infarction.
Embolism
　platelet, in coronary thrombosis, 27
　pulmonary, 15
Emergency medical services (EMS). *See* Out-of-hospital cardiac arrest.
Emergency rooms, SCD incidence, 4–9
Enalapril, 433
Encainide
　in CAPS trial, 441
　in CAST, 443, 469
　lethal proarrhythmias, 44, 395
　in survivors of acute MI, 524
　VT caused by, 389–390

Endocardial catheter mapping
  vs. epicardial mapping, 569
  preoperative, 563–564, *564*
  single point vs. multiple site, 568–569
  techniques, 565
Environmental factors, cardiac arrest survivors, 476–477
Enzymes
  in lysophosphatidylcholine metabolism, 89, *89*
  membrane-bound, 83
Epicardial border zone in ventricular tachyarrhythmias, 67–71, *70, 72*
Epicarditis, in atrioventricular bundle, 278–279
Epidemiology of SCD, 3–20
  cardiac arrest survivors, 476–477
  causes, 13–15, 15t, *14*
    atherosclerotic coronary disease, 13
    nonatherosclerotic coronary disease, 13–14
    noncardiac causes, 14–15, 15t
    noncoronary cardiac causes, 14
  data interpretation, 11–13
    biases, 11–12
    ICD codes, 11
    prodromal symptoms, 12–13
  definitions, 3, 293
  incidence, 3–11
    circadian, daily, and seasonal variation, 8–11, 295–296, *10*
    international data, 6, 6t, *7*
    time trends, 8–9, *10*
    U.S. data, 3–5, 5t, *4*
  risk factors, 8–9, 16–17, *10*
    coronary heart disease causes, 161–17, 16t
    electrocardiographic abnormalities, 17
    psychosocial factors, 17
    sex differences, 17
Epinephrine, 456
Ergonovine, 206
Erythromycin, 44
Esophageal pacing, in Wolff–Parkinson–White syndrome, 222
ESVEM. *See* Electrophysiological Study vs. Electrocardiographic Monitoring.
European Coronary Surgery Study, 533
European Dilated Cardiomyopathy Study, 477
European Infarction Study (EIS), 425–426
European Society of Cardiology, 234
Excitability threshold, 329
Exercise
  and aortic valve stenosis, 265
  arrhythmogenic right ventricular dysplasia, 234
  and hypertrophic cardiomyopathy, 167, 169
  risk factor for SCD, 17
  scintigraphy, acute–on–chronic ischemia, 319
  testing
    in cardiac arrest survivors, 469
    and ventricular arrhythmias, 350–366
      and drug therapy, 545, *546*
      nonsustained VT, 488
      in patient management, 356–362, 359t, *357–360*
      physiological effects, 350–352, *351*
      prevalence, 352–354, 352t
      prognostic significance, 354–356, 355t
      reproducibility, 356
      safety of, 362–363
  trigger for arrhythmias, 296
  and vagal activity, 113–114

Fast Fourier transform analysis, in long QT syndrome, 212
Fatty acids
  free, 64
  oxidation in myocardium, 85, 87
  in sarcolemma, 83
Fatty deposits
  in arrhythmogenic right ventricular dysplasia, 226, 227, 230
  in atrioventricular bundle, 278–279, 285–286
Fear paralysis reflex, and bradyarrhythmia, 410–412
Fibrillation, ventricular. *See* Ventricular fibrillation.
Fibrosis, myocardial
  in arrhythmogenic right ventricular dysplasia, 226, 227
  in children, 259
  in hypertrophic cardiomyopathy, 165, 167, 172
Firefighters, in EMS system, 453
First Intervention Study of Infarct Survival (ISIS–1), 420–422, 430
Flavin adenine dinucleotides, 87
Flecainide
  in CAPS trial, 441
  in CAST, 443, 469
  in exercise testing, 358–361
  lethal proarrhythmias, 44, 395
  in survivors of acute MI, 524
  VT caused by, 389–390
  in Wolff–Parkinson–White syndrome, 222
Football players
  arrhythmogenic right ventricular dysplasia, 233
  sudden cardiac death, 238
Framingham Heart Study
  circadian variations, 9
  SCD and coronary artery disease, 293, 294t

G proteins, in long QT syndrome, 211
Ganglionectomy, for long QT syndrome, 212, 213
Gap junctions, and amphipathic metabolites, 95–96
Generator, of defibrillator, 598
Genetic factors, long QT syndrome, 209–211
Glibenclamide, and sympathetic denervation in ischemia, 345
Glycerol, in sarcolemma, 83
Grading system for ventricular arrhythmias, 439

Haloperidol, 267
HAPPHY trial. *See* Heart Attack Primary Prevention in Hypertension.
Harvey–*ras*1 gene, 209, 211
Heart
  accessory pathways, radio-frequency ablation of, 577–579
  collateral circulation, 298–299, *298*
  conduction system abnormalities in young athletes, 247–248
  congenital disease, and sudden death, 284–286
  critical mass hypothesis for VF, 124–127
  structural abnormalities
    in cardiac arrest survivors, 466–467
    in hypertrophic cardiomyopathy, 165–166, 172
    and sudden death, 202–208
      comparison to other studies, 206–207, 206t
      differential diagnosis, 202–203
      University of Virginia experience, 203–206, 204t, *203, 205*

transplantation, 601–602
vasomotor responses, 296
Heart Attack Primary Prevention in Hypertension (HAPPHY) trial, 428
Heart failure
  congestive
    baroreceptive reflex sensitivity, 109
    in cardiac arrest survivors, 467
    exercise testing, 362
    supraventricular tachycardia, 392
    vasodilator therapy, 430–434
      clinical trials, 431–434, 432t
      prevalence of SCD, 431
      ventricular arrhythmias, 430–431, 431t
  lethal arrhythmias, 333
Heart rate
  in asymptomatic ventricular arrhythmias, 522–523, 523t
  and baroreflex sensitivity, 120, *120*
  in cardiac arrest survivors, 469–470
  and cardiac mortality, 111–112, *111–112*
  during exercise, 350, 360
  and left ventricular dysfunction, 191
  in long QT syndrome, 210–211
  as risk factor for SCD, 17
  during sleep, 372, 375
  and vagal activity, 118–120, *119*
Heberden's angina, 293
Helplessness, and bradyarrhythmia, 410–412
Hematocrit, 17
Hemochromatosis, in cardiac arrest survivors, 466
Hemodynamics
  in arrhythmogenic right ventricular dysplasia, 233
  in hypertrophic cardiomyopathy, 166–167, 170, 173
  left ventricular dysfunction, 192
  sustained VT, 498–504
  in tetralogy of Fallot, 266
  of VT/VF, 43
Hemorrhage, and SCD in children, 267
Heroin, 267
His bundle
  in arrhythmogenic right ventricular dysplasia, 228
  in hypertrophic cardiomyopathy, 166, 168, 174
  Purkinje system, structural electrophysiological abnormalities, 37
Hockey players, arrhythmogenic right ventricular dysplasia, 233
Holter monitoring. *See* Monitoring, ambulatory.
Hydralazine, 431–433
Hypercholesterolemia, 16
Hyperlipidemia, 264
Hypertension
  beta-adrenergic blocking drugs, 427–428, 429t
  plaque instability, 25
  risk factor for SCD, 14, 16
Hypertrophic cardiomyopathy. *See* Cardiomyopathy, hypertrophic.
Hypokalemia, in idiopathic dilated cardiomyopathy, 156
Hypothalamus, and ventricular tachycardia, 368
Hypothermia, and bradyarrhythmia, 409
Hypoxemia, 43
Hypoxia
  and action potential duration, 54–55
  acylcarnitine levels, 87, 91
  and ischemia in SCD, 532

Infarction, myocardial. *See also* Myocardial infarction.
Infections
  in children, 258, 268
  of defibrillators, 595
International Classification of Diseases, 4, 11
International Prospective Primary Prevention Study in Hypertension (IPPPSH), 427–428
International Society and Federation of Cardiology, 234
Iodoacetate, 90
Ion channels
  acylcarnitine and lysophosphatidylcholine effects, 92–93
  lipid accumulations, 64
  in sarcolemma, 83
IPPPSH. *See* International Prospective Primary Prevention Study in Hypertension.
Ischemia
  acute myocardial
    antifibrillatory effects of vagal activity, 115–117, *116, 117*
    critical mass for VF, 125
  acute-on-chronic, 318–326
    animal models, 321–322
    and arrhythmias, 318–319
    clinical studies, 319–321
    electrophysiology, 322–323
    mechanisms of ventricular arrhythmias, 323–324
  autonomic innervation. *See* Autonomic nervous system.
  biochemical membrane mechanisms, 82–101
    acylcarnitine
      accumulation, 85–87, *86*
      and arrhythmogenesis, 90–92
      and ionic currents, 92–93
    amphipathic metabolites, and cell coupling, 95–96
    amphiphiles
      and calcium changes, 93–94
      molecular dynamics, 83–85, *84, 85*
    lysophosphatidylcholine
      accumulation, 88–90, *88, 89*
      and arrhythmogenesis, 90–92
      and ionic currents, 92–93
    potassium, extracellular, 94–95
    sarcolemma structure and function, 83–85, *84, 85*
  electrophysiological effects, 38–43, 42t, *39–42*
  in lethal arrhythmias, 51–81
    ventricular arrhythmias in acute phase, 51–59, 52
      electrophysiological effects, 52–56, *54, 55*
      mechanisms of arrhythmias, 56–59, *58*
      reperfusion arrhythmias, 59
  myocardial activation, 128–131, *130*
    electrolyte triggers, 329
    and hypertrophic cardiomyopathy, 166, 172–173
  precipitating factor for SCD, 532
  silent, stress effects, 370
  in sudden arrhythmic death, 148
  tachyarrhythmic cardiac arrest without acute MI, 608–610
  See also Myocardial infarction.
Ischemic heart disease
  in cardiac arrest survivors, 475–477
    environmental factors, 476–477

Ischemic heart disease *(Continued)*
  epidemiology, 476–477
    myocardial infarction, 475–476
    nonischemic disease, 477–478
    reversible ischemia, 476
  coronary thrombosis, 25–28
  SCD mortality, 4–6, 8, 22
  vs. nonischemic tachyarrhythmia, 28–29
ISIS-1 trial. *See* First Intervention Study of Infarct Survival.
Isopropyl alcohol, 267
Isoproterenol
  denervation supersensitivity, 343
  in Wolff–Parkinson–White syndrome, 222–223
Isosorbide dinitrate, 431

Jervell and Lange–Nielsen syndrome
  in children, 260
  conduction defects, 287
  in exercise testing, 360

Kawasaki disease
  in children, 264
  conduction defects, 286
  and structural heart disease, 202
Keans–Sayre syndrome, conduction defects, 286

Lactate, 320
Lancisi, Giovanni Maria, 3
Left ventricular ejection fraction (LVEF), 190–201
  and baroreceptor reflex sensitivity, 109
  in cardiac arrest survivors, 468
  and defibrillation implantation, 595
    vs. surgical ablation, 564–565
  during exercise, 353, 362
  in hemodynamically tolerated sustained VT, 497
  left ventricular dysfunction, 190–193
    and antiarrhythmic drug assessment, 196–198, 197
    clinical variables, 191
    infarct size, 190–191
    noninvasive evaluation, 191–193
    and ventricular arrhythmias after MI, 193–196, 193t, 195t, *194–195*
    and other noninvasive predictors of arrhythmias, 196, 196t
  risk stratification of myocardial infarction, 150
  sudden cardiac death as end point, 198–199, 199t
  supraventricular tachycardia, 392
  See also Ventricles, left.
Left ventricular outflow tract, in hypertrophic cardiomyopathy, 166–167, 173
Lidocaine
  and bradyarrhythmias, 413
  for premature ventricular complexes, 439
  during resuscitation, 456–457
Life-change score, 17
Lipids, intracellular deposits, 64, 67
Long QT syndrome, 14, 209–214
  in cardiac arrest survivors, 466, 467, 478
  in children, 259–261, 268
  clinical studies, 210–212
    arrhythmogenesis, 211
    patient evaluation, 211–212

conduction defects, 287
critical mass hypothesis, 124
drug-induced, 401, 403
epidemiology, 213
in exercise testing, 360–362
historical background, 209
phenotypic considerations, 209–210, 210t
polymorphic VT, 391
and structural heart disease, 202, 204–206
sudden infant death syndrome, 412
therapy, 212–213
in young athletes, 240
Lopressor Intervention Trial (LIT), 425
Lysophosphatidylcholine
  accumulation in early ischemia, 88–90, *88, 89*
  in arrhythmogenesis, 90–92
  and ionic currents, 92–93
  in resting membrane potential, 53
Lysophosphatidylethanolamine, 53
Lysophosphoglycerides, 53
Lysophospholipase-transacylase, 89

Magnesium
  in idiopathic dilated cardiomyopathy, 156
  trigger of ventricular arrhythmias, 331–335
Magnetic resonance imaging, in cardiac arrest survivors, 468
Mahaim fibers, 282
MAPHY. *See* Metoprolol Atherosclerosis Prevention in Hypertensives.
Mapping, endocardial. *See* Endocardial catheter mapping.
Marfan's syndrome, 14
  in young athletes, 245, 264, 268, *246*
Medical Research Council trials, 427
Medtronic pacemaker defibrillator, 588–591
Membrane potentials in acute myocardial ischemia, 52–56
Meningitis, in children, 267
Metaiodobenzylguanidine, 345–346
Methyl alcohol, 267
Metoprolol
  arrhythmias in beta-blocker trials, 422
  and behavioral stress, 368
  for hypertension, 428
  in post-MI patients, 420
Metoprolol in Acute Myocardial Infarction (MIAMI) trial, 422, 430
Metoprolol Atherosclerosis Prevention in Hypertensives (MAPHY), 428
Mexiletine
  in exercise testing, 361
  for hypertrophic cardiomyopathy, 171
  in survivors of acute MI, 524
MIAMI trial. *See* Metoprolol in Acute Myocardial Infarction.
MILIS. *See* Multicenter Investigation of the Limitation of Infarct Size.
Mitochondria, acylcarnitine metabolism, 85–87
Mitral valve prolapse
  in children, 261–262
  conduction defects, 286
  replacement, 569
  in young athletes, 240, 246
Monitoring, ambulatory
  arrhythmogenic right ventricular dysplasia, 234

asymptomatic ventricular arrhythmias, 439,
    517–518
bradyarrhythmias, 407–408
    in cardiac arrest survivors, 468–469, 556–557
    in children, 260
    in exercise testing, 357
    in hypertrophic cardiomyopathy, 170
    ischemia studies, 301
    long QT syndrome, 211–212
    tetralogy of Fallot, 266
    at time of death, 27–28
    ventricular arrhythmias, 541–542
        and amiodarone therapy, 548, 557, 549t
        cardiomyopathies, 548–550, 550t
Moricizine
    in CAPS trial, 441
    in CAST, 443, 469
    in survivors of acute MI, 524
Mortality rates
    beta-blocker trials, 420, 469
    bradycardic cardiac arrest, 408–409
    in CAST, 443–446
MPIP. See Multicenter Post-Infarction Research
    Group.
Multicenter Diltiazem Postinfarction Trial, 191
Multicenter International Study, 423
Multicenter Investigation of the Limitation of Infarct
    Size (MILIS), 542
Multicenter Post-Infarction Research Group (MPIP),
    444, 542
    left ventricular dysfunction, 191–192, 198
    myocardial ischemia and SCD, 299
Multiple Risk Factor Intervention Trial (MRFIT),
    331
Multiple wandering wavelets
    critical mass for VF, 125
    during ventricular fibrillation, 136–137
Mustard/Senning procedure, 266–267, 284
Myocardial infarction
    acute
        bradyarrhythmias, 413
        critical mass for VF, 124
        potassium effects, 331
    autonomic innervation. See Autonomic nervous
        system.
    and baroreflex sensitivity, 104–107, 112–113, *113*,
        114
    beta-adrenergic blocking drugs, 420–426
        delayed intervention trials, 423–426, 424t
            arrhythmias 425–426
        early intervention trials, 420–423, 431t
            arrhythmias, 422–423, 422t
    coronary artery disease, 23
    late phase, 147–154
        out of hospital deaths, 152–153
        risk stratification, 149–152
            MI with spontaneous sustained VT or VF,
                149–150, *149*
            MI without spontaneous sustained ventricular
                arrhythmias, 150–152, 150t, *151*
        substrate, 147–149, 148t, *149*
    and left ventricular dysfunction
        clinical variables, 191
        infarct size, 190–194, *195*
    lethal arrhythmias, 51–81
        acute phase, 51–59, *52, 54, 55, 58*
        later phases of ventricular arrhythmias, 65–74

subacute phase, delayed ventricular
    arrhythmias, 59–65, *60, 62–65*
monomorphic VT, 390
risk of SCD in survivors, 513–528
    antiarrhythmic drug trials, 524
    asymptomatic high-risk patients, 517–523
        heart rate variability, 522–523, 523t
        signal-averaged ECG, 518–522, *519*, 521t
        ventricular arrhythmias and LV function,
            517–518, 518t
    invasive electrophysiological studies, 523–524,
        523t
    management, 514–517, 515t
    sustained VT/VF
        after 48 hours, 514, 514t
        within 48 hours, 514
in SCD victims, 13, 28, 36
See also Ventricles, left, dysfunction.
Myocardial ischemia, acute, 293–317
    arrhythmias, clinical, 300–306
        clinical observations, 301–304, *302, 303*
        electrocardiographic studies, 300–301, *300, 301*
        electrophysiological studies, 304, *305*
        VF vs. VT, 305–306
    coronary artery disease, 296–299
        acute arterial injury, 297–298, *297*
        angiography, 296–297
        coronary collateralization, 298–299, *298*
        pathology, 297
    and sudden cardiac death, 299–300
    therapeutic strategies, 306–308, *306–308*
Myocarditis
    in cardiac arrest survivors, 466
    in children, 258–259
    conduction defects, 287
    and structural heart disease, 203
    viral, in young athletes, 240, 245–246
Myocardium
    activation during ventricular fibrillation. See
        Ventricular fibrillation.
    contractility during exercise, 350
    electrophysiology of ventricular arrhythmias,
        72–74, *73*
    gap junctions, 95–96
    myocytes, in hypertrophic cardiomyopathy, 165,
        167, 172
    neurotransmitter effects, 367
    perfusion, sleep states, 372
    revascularization, 307–308, *307*
    structural abnormalities, 35–36, 35t
Myopathies
    nonischemic ventricle, and SCD, 37, *38*
    See also Cardiomyopathy.
Myotonia dystrophica, 286

National Center for Health Statistics, 4
National Heart, Lung, and Blood Institute (NHLBI),
    423
    CAPS trial, 440
Neurohumoral function, in hypertrophic
    cardiomyopathy, 167–168, 174
Neuromuscular disorders, conduction defects, 286
Neurotransmitters, direct effect on myocardium, 367
New York Heart Association
    classification of congestive heart failure, 430–431
    functional class, and ICD therapy, 595

Nicotinamide adenine dinucleotides, 87
Norepinephrine, denervation supersensitivity, 343
Norwegian Multicenter Study Group, 423, 426, 427, 430

Obesity, risk factor for SCD, 16
Operative death definition, 563
Out-of-hospital cardiac arrest
  community experience, 450–462
    bradyasystolic cardiac arrest, 457
    chain of survival concept, 450–452, *451*
      cardiopulmonary resuscitation, 451–452
      defibrillation, 452–456, *454, 455*
      EMS system, 451
    drug therapy during resuscitation, 456–457
      amiodarone, 457
      bretylium, 456–457
      epinephrine, 456
      lidocaine, 456–457
    electromechanical dissociation, 457
    outcome studies, 457–458
  electrolyte triggers, 331
  management
    beta-adrenergic blocking drugs, 419–438
    cardiac arrhythmia suppression trial, 439–449
  resuscitation studies, 28
  sudden cardiac death, 4–9, 152–153
Oxotremorine, 116, 117
Oxprenolol, 420, 425, 427
Oxygen
  in hypertrophic cardiomyopathy, 166
  myocardial, during exercise, 350–351

Pacemakers
  and bradyarrhythmia, 409
  in children, 261, 268
Palmitoylcarnitine, 93
Paramedics, in EMS system, 453, 455
Parasympathetic nervous system, T-wave alternans analysis, 378–379
Pentamidine, 44
Perfusion, myocardial, 166
pH changes during exercise, 350–351, 362
Pharmacological triggers of SCD, 394–406, *396–402*
Phenobarbital, 267
Phenytoin, 524
Phosphatidylcholine, 83
Phosphatidylethanolamine, 83
Phosphatidylinositol, 83
Phosphatidylserine, 83
Phospholipase A, 88
Phospholipids, 83
Pinacidil, 345
Plaques in coronary artery disease, 24, *24*
Plasmalogenase, 88
Plasmalogens, 83
Platelet aggregation, 297–298
  in cardiac arrest survivors, 476
  in cardiac pathology, 367, 372
Pokkuri disease, 203
Positron emission tomography, 468
Potassium
  in acute myocardial ischemia, 52–56
  and bradyarrhythmia, 409
  in cardiac arrest survivors, 468
  channels, acylcarnitine and lysophosphatidylcholine effects, 92–93
  equilibrium potential, 64–65
  during exercise, 351, 362
  extracellular, amphiphile effects, 94–95
  SCD risk, 43
  and ventricular arrhythmias, 328–336, *328–333*
Potentials
  action. *See* Action potentials.
  intracellular and extracellular, in acute myocardial ischemia, 53–56, *54, 55*
  membrane, in acute myocardial ischemia, 52–56
Power spectrum analysis, heart rate during sleep, 375
PR interval in exercise testing, 359
Practolol
  mechanisms of action, 429
  in post-MI patients, 420, 423
Prazosin, 431
Pre-excitation syndromes, 14, 282
Premature ventricular complexes (PVC)
  in arrhythmogenic right ventricular dysplasia, 232
  in CAST, 443–444
  after early ischemia, 82
  and fatal VT or VF, 32–34, *33, 34*
  and left ventricular dysfunction, 191
  lidocaine suppression of, 439
  monomorphic VT, 386, *387, 388*
  noninvasive evaluation, 541–542, 547
Prinzmetal's angina, 302
  during sleep, 372
Proarrhythmia definition, 544–545, 544t
Procainamide
  in CAST, 443
  in exercise testing, 360
  for hypertrophic cardiomyopathy, 171
  nonsustained VT conversion to sustained tachycardia, *396*
  in survivors of acute MI, 524
  in Wolff-Parkinson-White syndrome, 222, *221*
Prodromal symptoms
  IHD deaths, 8, 26–27
  of SCD, 12–13
Programmed electrical stimulation (PES). *See* Electrical stimulation.
Propafenone, in Wolff-Parkinson-White syndrome, 222
Propranolol
  and behavioral stress, 368
  denervation supersensitivity, 344
  for hypertension, 427
  in post-MI patients, 420, 422–425
Prostaglandins, pericardial, 341
Protein kinase C, amphiphile effects, 94
Proteins, sarcolemmal, 83
Psychosocial factors, 17
Psychotropic drugs, 44
Pulmonary embolism, 15, 175
Pulmonary vascular obstructive disease, 265
Pulmonary venous congestion, 191
Purkinje fibers
  acylcarnitine and lysophosphatidylcholine in arrhythmias, 90–92
  depolarization, 95
  electrolyte effects, 330
  electrophysiology, 58, 59, 61–65, *62–65*
  ultrastructure, 68

QRS interval, in exercise testing, 359–360, 362
QT interval
  polymorphic VT, 391–392
  prolonged. *See* Long QT syndrome.
Quinidine
  in CAST, 443
  in exercise testing, 360, 361
  for hypertrophic cardiomyopathy, 171
  polymorphic VT caused by, 391
  proarrhythmic response, 44
  trigger of SCD, 394

Racial differences, 6–8
Radio-frequency ablation. *See* Catheter ablation.
Radionuclide ventriculography, 191–192
Rales, and left ventricular dysfunction, 191
Rapid eye movement (REM) sleep, 371–375
Re-entry circuits
  atrioventricular, radio-frequency ablation of, 579–580
  lethal proarrhythmias, 395–398
  myocardial activation, 131–133, *135, 136*
  repetitive concealed, 386–390, *389, 390*
  and ventricular tachyarrhythmias, 66–72, *67, 68, 70, 72*
  VT vs. VF, 138
Refractoriness, 54–56, 299
  during acute-on-chronic ischemia, 322–323
  critical mass hypothesis, 124
  denervation supersensitivity, 343
  nonuniform dispersion of, 131, 133, *132*
  pharmacological triggers, 395–400
Reimbursement, hospital, 9
Renal failure, and bradyarrhythmia, 409
Renin-angiotensin system during sleep, 375
Reperfusion
  arrhythmias, 59, 67, 299
  electrophysiological effects, 40–43, *42*
Repolarization
  in acute myocardial ischemia, 55–56
  electrolyte triggers, 328
Respiratory rate, 191
Resuscitation
  acute-on-chronic ischemia, 318
  cardiopulmonary, out-of-hospital, 28, 450–452, *453*
  and CHD deaths, 9
Revascularization, myocardial. *See* Coronary artery bypass surgery; Myocardium.
Rheumatic heart disease, 466
Risk factors
  CAD and cardiac failure, 293–204
  for idiopathic dilated cardiomyopathy, 159
  invasive electrophysiological studies, 523–524
  See also Myocardial infarction.
Romano-Ward syndrome
  in children, 260
  conduction defects, 287
  in exercise testing, 360–361

Sarcoidosis
  conduction defects, 286
  in young athletes, 247
Sarcolemmal structure and function, 83–85, *84, 85*
Scar tissue, 165

Scintigraphy
  exercise, acute-on-chronic ischemia, 319
  sympathetic, 345–346, *346*
  thallium, in cardiac arrest survivors, 469
Scopolamine, 115
Screening, preparticipation, of athletes, 251–253, *253*
Seasonality of sudden cardiac death, 9–11
Seizure disorders, 267
Seldane, 44
Sex differences
  in exercise testing, 353
  risk factor for sudden death, 6–8, 16–17, 22–23
  SCD in young athletes, 239
Shock, cardiogenic
  in cardiac arrest survivors, 467
  and left ventricular dysfunction, 191
Sick sinus syndrome
  in children, 268
  and transposition of great arteries, 266
Sickle cell trait, 240
Signal transduction, in long QT syndrome, 211
Sinoatrial node, 275–277, *276, 277*
  in hypertrophic cardiomyopathy, 166, 168, 174
Sinus bradycardia
  in long QT syndrome, 211
  sudden infant death syndrome, 412
Sinus of Valsalva, 263–264
Sleep
  and heart rhythms, 371–375
    arrhythmogenesis, 374–375, *374*
    autonomic tone, 371–372
    myocardial perfusion and arrhythmias, 372, *373*
    power spectrum analysis, 375
  and hypertrophic cardiomyopathy, 169, 179
  sleep apnea syndrome, bradyarrhythmias, 412–413
Smoking, and SCD, 14, 16
  in cardiac arrest survivors, 476
  trigger for arrhythmias, 296
Soccer players, 234
Sodium
  and calcium exchange, amphiphile effects, 93–94
  channel blockers
    in CAST, 446
    proarrhythmic actions, 400–403
  and ventricular arrhythmias, 336–337
Sodium/potassium pump
  in acute myocardial ischemia, 53
  in subacute myocardial infarction, 65
Soldiers, 249–250
SOLVD. *See* Studies of Left Ventricular Dysfunction.
Sotalol, 420, 425
Sports
  arrhythmogenic right ventricular dysplasia, 233–234
  See also Athletes.
ST-segment
  in coronary artery disease, 301–303, 307
  in exercise testing, 355
  stress effects, 369–371
Starvation, lethal arrhythmias, 333
Stress
  mental, trigger for arrhythmias, 296
  psychosocial, and bradyarrhythmia, 410–412
Structure/function interactions in SCD, 32–47
  premature ventricular contraction hypothesis, 32–34, *33, 34*

Structure/function interactions in SCD *(Continued)*
  structural abnormalities and fatal arrhythmias, 35–37
    coronary heart disease, 35–36, 35t
    electrophysiological abnormalities, 37
    functional modulation, 38–45
      autonomic nervous system, 43–44
      systemic factors, 43
      toxic and proarrhythmic effects, 44–45
      transient ischemia and reperfusion, 38–43, 42t, *39–42*
    hypertrophy, ventricular, 36–37
    myopathy, ventricular, 37, *38*
  time factors, *33*
Studies of Left Ventricular Dysfunction (SOLVD), 433
Subendocardial resection (SER), for ventricular tachycardia, 563, 567–570
Sudden cardiac death (SCD)
  anatomical features, coronary artery pathology, 21–31
    coronary heart disease, 22–23
    definitions, 21–22
    ischemic vs. chronic nonischemic tachyarrhythmia, 28–29
    morphological studies, 23–27, 26t, *24*
    myocardial infarction, 28
    ventricular fibrillation, induction of mechanisms, 27–28
  arrhythmogenic right ventricular dysplasia, 226–237
    arrhythmogenic substrate, 230–233
    atrioventricular block, 227–229
    definition, 226–227
    and drug therapy, 234
    hemodynamics, 233
    prevalence, 227
    ventricular arrhythmias, 229–230
    in young athletes, 233–234
  in athletes, 238–257
    older athletes, 250–251
    preparticipation screening, 251–253
    young athletes, 238–250
  autonomic nervous system, 102–123
    baroreceptive reflexes
      clinical studies, 107–110, 109t, *108–110*
      experimental studies, 102–107, *103–107*
    heart rate variability, 111–112, *112*
    speculations, 112–120
      ATRAMI, 120–121
      depressed BRS and survival, 113–115
      heart rate variability and BRS, 120
      MI and baroreflex sensitivity, 112–113
      vagal activity
        during acute MI, 115–117
        direct recording, 118–120
        and ventricular fibrillation, 118
  beta-adrenergic blocking drug mechanisms, 428–430
  biochemical membrane mechanisms, 82–101
    acylcarnitine effects, 85–87
    amphiphiles
      and calcium changes, 93–94
      and cell coupling, 95–96
      and molecular membrane dynamics, 83–85
    lysophosphatidylcholine effects, 88–90
    potassium, extracellular, 94–95

cardiomyopathy
  hypertrophic, 163–189
    functional and structural abnormalities, 163–169
    incidence, 163
    medical and operative treatment, 170–171
    predictors and associated factors, 169–170
    prevention of, 180–181
    process of, 175–179, *175–178*
    specific factors, 171–175
    theory of, 179–180
  idiopathic dilated, 155–162
    malignant arrhythmias, 155–159, *156, 158*
    risk assessment, 159
    therapeutic considerations, 159–160
central nervous system triggers, 367–384
  behavioral stress, 368–371, 369t, *369–371*
  sleep states, 371–375, *373–376*
  T-wave alternans, 375–379, *378*
in children, 258–273
  apparently healthy children, 258–262, 258–260t
  athletes, 262–264, 262t
  with known heart disease, 264–267, 264t, 265t
  noncardiac death, 267–268, 267t
  prevention, 268–269
conduction system abnormalities, 274–289
  ablative procedures, 282–284
  atrioventricular bundle, 278–282
  atrioventricular node, 277–278
  congenital heart disease, 284–286
  in known diseases, 286–287
  method of study, 274–275
  pre-excitation, 282
  sinoatrial node, 275–277
coronary artery surgery, 531–540
  cardiac pathology, 531–532
  diagnostic assessment, 533
  ischemia, 532
  primary and secondary prevention of SCD, 532–533
  revascularization role in recurrent SCD, 535–538, *537*
  SCD prevalence after surgery, 533–535, *534, 535*
definitions, 293
electrical triggers, 385–393
  bradycardia and asystole, 392
  supraventricular tachycardia, 392
  ventricular tachycardia
    monomorphic, 386–390, *387–390*
    polymorphic, 391–392
    transition to fibrillation, 385–386
epidemiology, 3–20
  data interpretation, 11–13
  incidence, 3–11
  risk factors, 16–17
  underlying conditions, 13–15
and exercise. *See* Exercise.
in late phase of myocardial infarction, 147–154
  out of hospital death, 152–153
  risk stratification, 149–152
    MI with spontaneous sustained VT or VF, 149–150, *149*
    MI without spontaneous sustained ventricular arrhythmias, 150–152, 150t, *151*
  substrate, 147–149, 149t, *148*
long QT syndrome, 209–214
myocardial infarction, acute, 293–317

anatomical extend of coronary artery disease, 296–299
  angiography, 296–297
  arterial injury, 297–298, *297*
  coronary collateralization, 298–299, *298*
  pathology, 297
cellular mechanisms, 299–300
epidemiology, 293–296, 294t
  circardian variations, 295–296, *295*
myocardial ischemia, acute, 293–317
  clinical arrhythmias, 300–306
    clinical observations, 301–304, *302*, *303*
    electrocardiographic studies, 300–301, *300*, *301*
    electrophysiological studies, 304, *305*
    VT vs. VF, 305–306
  therapeutic strategies, 306–308
    medical, 306–307, *306*
    surgical, 307–308, *307*
pharmacological triggers, 394–406, *396–402*
in structural heart disease, 206–208
structure/function interactions, 32–47
  premature ventricular contraction hypothesis, 32–34
  structural abnormalities, 35–45
  time factors, *33*
therapeutic options. *See* Therapeutic options.
Wolff–Parkinson–White syndrome, 215–225
  mechanism of sudden death, 215, *216*, *217*
  patient profile, 215–218
  risk assessment, 218–223
Sudden infant death syndrome, 287, 412
Sulfinpyrazone, 307
Supraventricular tachycardia
  catheter ablation, 574, 577
  fatal, in cardiac arrest survivors, 466
  vs. VT, 597–598
Surgery
  for ventricular tachycardia, 562–573
    amiodarone pretreatment, 569
    comparison of ablative procedures, 566–568
    definitions, 562–563
    endocardial vs. epicardial mapping, 569
    ideal candidate, 570
    map-guided vs. visually guided resection, 568
    mitral valve modification or replacement, 569
    operative procedures, 565–566, 566t, *567*
    preoperative evaluation, 563–564, *564*
    single point mapping vs. multiple site mapping, 568–569
    surgical ablation vs. ICD implantation, 564, 569–570
  See also Coronary artery bypass surgery.
Sympathetic nervous system
  in beta-blocker mechanisms, 428
  T-wave alternans analysis, 376–378
  See also Autonomic nervous system.
Syncope
  in arrhythmogenic right ventricular dysplasia, 233
  in children, 260, 261
  in idiopathic dilated cardiomyopathy, 159
  in long QT syndrome, 210–212
  neurocardiogenic, and structural heart disease, 203, 206
  in sustained monomorphic VT, 610–611
  of unknown origin, 612
  in young athletes, 238
Syphilis, 14

T-wave alternans, 375–379, *376*, *377*
  electrophysiology, 379
  parasympathetic nervous system, 378–379
  sympathetic nervous system, 376–378, *378*
Tachyarrhythmias
  in idiopathic dilated cardiomyopathy, 155
  and transposition of great arteries, 266
  ventricular
    re-entrant circuits, 66–72, *67*, *68*, *70*, *72*
  See also Ventricular tachyarrhythmias.
Tachycardia
  nonischemic, in sudden ischemic death, 28–29, *38*
  permanent form of junctional reciprocating (PJRT), 230
  sinus, in children, 259
  supraventricular, 203, 392
  ventricular. *See* Ventricular tachycardia (VT).
Tamponade, pericardial, 379
Tetralogy of Fallot, 14, 265–266, 268
  in cardiac arrest survivors, 466
  postoperative hemodynamically tolerated sustained VT, 505
  and sudden death, 284
Thallium scintigraphy, 469
Therapeutic options, 529–617
  cardioverter-defibrillators, 588–599
  catheter ablation, 574–587
  coronary artery surgery, 531–540
  electrophysiological testing, 554–561
  noninvasive techniques, 541–553
  surgery for ventricular tachycardia, 562–573
  in sustained ventricular tachyarrhythmias, 600–617
Thrombolysis, and asymptomatic ventricular arrhythmias, 521–522
Thrombolysis in Myocardial Infarction (TIMI) trial, 422
Thrombosis
  acute-on-chronic ischemia, 319
  coronary artery disease, 23–27, 297–299, *297*
Time factors in SCD, 8–9, *10*, *33*
TIMI trial. *See* Thrombolysis in Myocardial Infarction (TIMI).
Timolol
  mechanisms of action, 429–430
  in post-myocardial infarction trials, 420, 423, 426, 427
Tissue plasminogen activator (tPA), 422, 521
Tocainide, 524
Tolamolol, 368
Torsade de pointes
  and antiarrhythmic agents, 44, 334
  drug-induced, 401, 403
  in hypokalemia, 43
  in idiopathic dilated cardiomyopathy, 156
  in long QT syndrome, 211, 212
  polymorphic VT, 391
Transplantation, cardiac, 601–602
Transposition of great arteries, 266–268
  in cardiac arrest survivors, 466
  and sudden death, 284
Trauma, and bradyarrhythmia, 409
Treadmill testing
  in children, 260
  in Wolff-Parkinson-White syndrome, 221

Triggers of SCD. *See* Autonomic nervous system;
    Bradyarrhythmias; Central nervous system;
    Electrical triggers; Electrolytes; Exercise
    testing; Ischemia; Pharmacological triggers.
Type A personality, 17

Uhl's anomaly
    vs. arrhythmogenic right ventricular dysplasia,
        226, 229, 230, 233
    conduction defects, 286
Urokinase, 521

Vagus nerve activity
    antifibrillatory effect during acute MI, 115–117,
        116, 117
    and CNS stimulation, 368
    direct recording, 118–120, *119*
    during sleep, 375
    and ventricular fibrillation, 118, *118*
    See also Autonomic nervous system.
Valvular heart disease, 13, 14
Vasodilation, peripheral, in hypertrophic
        cardiomyopathy, 167, 173–174
Vasodilatory therapy in congestive heart failure,
        430–434
    large trials, 431–434, 432t
    ventricular arrhythmias, 430–431, 431t
Ventricles
    left
        and baroreceptive reflex sensitivity, 109
        dysfunction
            antiarrhythmic drug assessment, 196–198
                asymptomatic ventricular arrhythmias after
                    MI, 198
                sustained ventricular tachycardia or
                    ventricular fibrillation, 196–197, *197*
                unsustained ventricular tachycardia,
                    197–198
            clinical variables, 191
            infarct size, 190–191
            noninvasive evaluation, 191–193
                echocardiography, 192–193
                radionuclide methods, 191–192, *192*
            and ventricular arrhythmias after MI, 193–196
        dysfunction, in sudden arrhythmic death, 148
        ejection fraction. *See* Left ventricular ejection
            fraction.
        idiopathic hypertrophy, in young athletes, 242,
            242
        systolic dysfunction, and idiopathic dilated
            cardiomyopathy, 159
        wall motion abnormalities, 319
    right, dysplasia
        arrhythmogenic
            hemodynamically tolerated sustained VT, 505
            See also Arrhythmogenic right ventricular
                dysplasia (ARVD).
            in cardiac arrest survivors, 466
            in young athletes, 240, 249, *249*
        septum, conduction defects, 287
Ventricular arrhythmias
    autonomic innervation. *See* Autonomic nervous
        system.
    classification, 542–543, 542t, 543t
    in congestive heart failure, 430–431

electrolyte triggers. *See* Electrolytes.
and exercise testing. *See* Exercise.
in ischemia and infarction, 51–81
    acute phase, 51–59, *52*
        electrophysiological effects, 52–56
            intracellular and extracellular potentials,
                53–56, *54, 55*
            resting membrane potential, 52–53
        mechanisms of arrhythmias, 56–59, *58*
        reperfusion arrhythmias, 59
    later phases, 65–74, *66*
        electrophysiology of myocardial fibers, 72–74,
            73
        re-entrant circuits causing tachyarrhythmias,
            66–72, *67, 68, 70, 72*
    subacute phase, 59–65, *60*
        delayed arrhythmias, 60–61
        infarct development, 61, *62*
        Purkinje fiber electrophysiology, 61–65, *62–65*
management and survival post MI, 514–517, 515t
See also Arrhythmias.
Ventricular fibrillation (VF)
    antiarrhythmic actions, 44–45
    in arrhythmogenic right ventricular dysplasia,
        229–232, *230*
    cardiomyopathies, 32, *38*
    critical mass hypothesis, 124–127
    documented, in cardiac arrest. *See* Cardiac arrest.
    electrophysiological differences from VT,
        3035–306
    in exercise testing, 354–359
    induction of mechanisms, 27–28
    in late phase of myocardial infarction, 147–149
    left ventricular dysfunction, 196–197
    myocardial activation, 128–143
        during, 136–138
            degree of organization, 137–138
            frequency characteristics, 138
            multiple wandering wavelets, 137
        at onset, 128–136
            electrical stimulus, 131–136, *132–136*
            ischemia, 128–131, *130*
        vs. ventricular tachycardia, 138–140, *139*
    potassium effects, 330
    reperfusion arrhythmias, 59
    transition from ventricular tachycardia, 385–386,
        466
    and vagal activity, 102–104, 118, *118*
    in Wolff-Parkinson-White syndrome, 217
Ventricular hypertrophy, 16, 36–37
Ventricular myopathy, 37
Ventricular premature beats. *See* Premature
    ventricular complexes.
Ventricular tachyarrhythmias
    in coronary artery disease, 301–304
    sustained
        therapeutic modalities, 600–617
            absence of coronary artery disease, 610
            cardiac arrest without acute MI, 608–610, *609*
            future directions, 612–613
            ICD therapy, 602–608, 603–608t
            monomorphic VT
                hemodynamically tolerated, 611–612
                with syncope, 610–611
            overview, 600–602, 601t
            polymorphic VT, 612
            syncope of unknown origin, 612
        See also Electrical triggers.

Ventricular tachycardia (VT)
  catheter ablation, 581–582, *581, 582*
    direct-current shocks, 582
    radio-frequency ablation, 582–585
  CNS stimulation, 368
  in exercise testing, 354–359
  in hypertrophic cardiomyopathy, 165
  in idiopathic dilated cardiomyopathy, 155–157
  in late phase of myocardial infarction, 147–149
  and left ventricular dysfunction, 194–196
    sustained, 196–197
    nonsustained, 197–198, 486–495
      definitions, 486
      quantitative risk of SCD, 486–487
        coronary artery disease, 487
        hypertrophic cardiomyopathy, 486–487
        idiopathic dilated cardiomyopathy, 487
      specialized testing, 487–492
        electrophysiological testing, 488–491
        exercise testing, 488
        signal-averaged ECG, 491–492
  polymorphic, absence of QT prolongation, 612
  potassium effects, 330
  structural abnormalities, 32, *38*
  in structural heart disease, 204–205
  surgical treatment. *See* Surgery, for ventricular tachycardia.
  sustained
    definition, 563
    hemodynamically tolerated, 496–512
      absence of CAD, 504–506
        arrhythmogenic right ventricular dysplasia, 505
        cardiomyopathies, 504–505
        postoperative congenital heart disease, 505
      absence of heart disease, 505–506
      in coronary artery disease, 498–504
        clinical presentation and electrophysiology, 498–499
        pathophysiological differences in cardiac arrest, 502–504
        patient outcome, 499–502, 500t
          antiarrhythmic therapy, 502, 503t

electrocardiographic criteria, 498, 498t
grading symptoms, 496, 497t
hemodynamic determinants, 497
monomorphic, with syncope, 610–611
transition to ventricular fibrillation. *See* Ventricular fibrillation.
Ventriculography, radionuclide, 468, 469
Ventritex Cadence defibrillator, 588–591
Verapamil, for hypertrophic cardiomyopathy, 164, 172, 263
Vital capacity, 17

Wenckebach cycle, 168
Wolff-Parkinson-White syndrome, 215–225
  in cardiac arrest survivors, 466, 467
  catheter ablation, 282
  in children, 259, 261, 268
  exercise testing, 362
  incidence, 215
  mechanism of sudden death, 215, *216, 217*
  patient profile, 215–218, *217, 218*
  risk assessment, 218–223
    electrocardiography, 220–221, *220*
    esophageal pacing, 222
    groups of patients, 218–219
    isoproterenol effect, 222–223
    pharmacological challenge, 221–222, *221, 222*
    treadmill stress testing, 221
  structural electrophysiological abnormalities, 37
  and structural heart disease, 203, 203–206
  sudden cardiac death, 577
  supraventricular tachycardia, 392
Worcester Heart Attack Study, 294
World Health Organization, 6

Young patients
  arrhythmogenic dysplasia. *See* Arrhythmogenic right ventricular dysplasia (ARVD).
  conduction system abnormalities, 274–289
  structural heart disease, 202–208
  Wolff-Parkinson-White syndrome, 215–225
  See also Athletes.